CORE CURRICULUM FOR
Neonatal Intensive Care Nursing

CORE CURRICULUM FOR
Neonatal Intensive Care Nursing

Second Edition

Edited by

Jane Deacon, RNC, MS, NNP
Clinical Faculty
University of Colorado Health Sciences Center
School of Nursing
Neonatal Nurse Practitioner
The Children's Hospital and University Hospital
Denver, Colorado

Patricia O'Neill, RN, MS
Adjunct Faculty
Georgetown University School of Nursing
Washington, DC
Professional Education Specialist
Association of periOperative Registered Nurses
Denver, Colorado

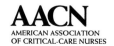

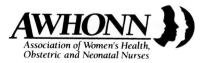

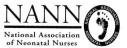

W.B. SAUNDERS COMPANY
A Division of Harcourt Brace & Company

Philadelphia   London   Toronto   Montreal   Sydney   Tokyo

W.B. SAUNDERS COMPANY

A Division of Harcourt Brace & Company

The Curtis Center
Independence Square West
Philadelphia, Pennsylvania 19106

Library of Congress Cataloging-in-Publication Data

Core curriculum for neonatal intensive care nursing / AWHONN
  (Association of Women's Health, Obstetric, and Neonatal Nurses),
  AACN (American Association of Critical-Care Nurses), NANN (National
  Association of Neonatal Nurses) ; [edited by] Jane Deacon, Patricia
  O'Neill. — 2nd ed.
        p.   cm.
  Includes bibliographical references and index.
  ISBN 0-7216-7489-5
    1. Neonatal intensive care Outlines, syllabi, etc.   I. Deacon,
  Jane.   II. O'Neill, Patricia.   III. Association of Women's Health,
  Obstetric, and Neonatal Nurses.   IV. American Association of
  Critical-Care Nurses.   V. National Association of Neonatal Nurses.
    [DNLM: 1. Neonatal Nursing—methods Outlines.   2. Intensive Care,
  Neonatal—methods Outlines.   WY 18.2 C7968 1999]
  RJ253.5.C67 1999
  618.92'01—dc21
  DNLM/DLC
                                                        99-25873

CORE CURRICULUM FOR NEONATAL INTENSIVE CARE NURSING   ISBN 0-7216-7489-5

Printed in the United States of America

Last digit is the print number: 9   8   7   6   5   4   3   2   1

To my husband, Bruce, and children, Jill and Mark,
for their patience and support during the production of this book.
Jane Deacon

To my parents, Larry and Nancy O'Neill, who made all things possible.
Patricia O'Neill

Contributors

Stephanie Amlung, PhD
Manager, Clinical Research, Hill-ROM, Charleston, South Carolina
Families in Crisis

Sharon Anderson, RN, MSN, NNP
Neonatal Nurse Practitioner, St. Peter's University Hospital, New Brunswick, New Jersey
Thermoregulation

Debbie Fraser Askin, RNC, MN
Adjunct Professor, University of Manitoba; Neonatal Nurse Practitioner, St. Boniface General Hospital, Winnipeg, Manitoba, Canada
Ophthalmologic Disorders

Susan Bakewell-Sachs, RN, PhD
Associate Professor and Coordinator, Family Nurse Practitioner Program, The College of New Jersey, School of Nursing, Ewing, New Jersey; Pediatric Nurse Practitioner, The Children's Hospital of Philadelphia, Philadelphia, Pennsylvania
Neonatal Nutrition

Bonnie Barndt-Maglio, MS
Lecturer, Georgetown University, School of Nursing, Washington, D.C.; Principal, Maglio and Associates, McLean, Virginia
Ethical Issues in Neonatal Nursing

Janice Bernhardt, RNC, MS, CNS,C
Perinatal Clinical Nurse Specialist, St. Joseph's Hospital and Medical Center, Paterson, New Jersey
Renal and Genitourinary Disorders

Judy Bildner, RN, MS
Adjunct Clinical Faculty, University of Missouri—Sinclair School of Nursing; Neonatal Advanced Practice Nurse, University of Missouri, Children's Hospital, Columbia, Missouri
Neonatal Pain Management

Sue Botham, BAppSc (Nursing), MHP
Research Nurse, New Children's Hospital, Sydney, New South Wales, Australia
Perinatal Substance Abuse

S. Louise Bowen, RNC, MSN, ARNP
Transport Director, All Children's Hospital, St. Petersburg, Florida
Neonatal Transport

Anne B. Broussard, RNC, DNS, LCCE, FACCE
Associate Professor and Semester Coordinator for Maternal-Child Nursing Course, College of Nursing, University of Southwestern Louisiana, Lafayette, Louisiana
Antepartum-Intrapartum Complications

Deanne Buschbach, MSN, NNP
Clinical Associate, Duke University School of Nursing; Senior Neonatal Nurse Practitioner, Duke University Medical Center, Durham, North Carolina
Physical Assessment of the Newborn Infant

Patricia M. Casey, RNC, MS, NNP
Neonatal Nurse Practitioner Coordinator, New England Medical Center Floating Hospital for Children, Boston, Massachusetts
Respiratory Distress

Wendy Cornell, RN, MS
Nurse Consultant, Boyertown, Pennsylvania
Research

Margaret Crockett, RNC, MS, NNP
Neonatal Clinical Nurse Specialist, Sutter Women's and Children's Services, Sacramento, California
Cardiovascular Disorders

Jane Deacon, RNC, MS, NNP
Clinical Faculty, University of Colorado Health Sciences Center, School of Nursing; Neonatal Nurse Practitioner, The Children's Hospital and University Hospital, Denver, Colorado
Radiologic Evaluation of the Newborn Infant

Paula L. Forsythe, RN, MSN

Clinical Faculty, Frances Payne Bolton School of Nursing, Case Western Reserve University, Cleveland, Ohio, and Kent State School of Nursing, Kent, Ohio; Neonatal Clinical Nurse Specialist, Rainbow Babies and Children's Hospital, University Hospitals Health System, Cleveland, Ohio
Transition of the High-Risk Neonate to Home Care

Sharon M. Glass, RNC, MS, NNP

Neonatal Nurse Practitioner, The Children's Hospital and University Hospital, Denver, Colorado
Hematologic Disorders

Martha Goodwin, RNC, MS, NNP

Neonatal Nurse Practitioner, Children's Mercy Hospital, Kansas City, Missouri
Apnea of the Newborn Infant

Ann M. Gross, RNC, MSN, NNP

Neonatal Nurse Practitioner, The Children's Hospital and University Hospital, Denver, Colorado
Common Invasive Procedures

Harriet A. Harrell, RN, BSN, MPH, CNNP

Adjunct Faculty, College of Nursing, University of Arizona; Director of Neonatal Nurse Practitioners and Outreach Education Coordinator, Section of Neonatology, Department of Pediatrics, Arizona Health Sciences Center, University of Arizona, Tucson, Arizona
Neonatal Delivery Room Resuscitation

Carole Kenner, DNS

Professor and Department Head, Parent Child Health Nursing, University of Cincinnati, Cincinnati, Ohio; Consultant for Education and Programs, National Association of Neonatal Nurses, Petaluma, California
Families in Crisis

Elizabeth Kirby, RN, MS, NNP

Neonatal Nurse Practitioner Coordinator, St. Peter's University Hospital, New Brunswick, New Jersey
Assisted Ventilation

Susan Koch, BSN, MSHA

Program Director of Critical Care Services, The Children's Hospital, Denver, Colorado
Developmental Support in the Neonatal Intensive Care Unit

Nanette Landry, MS, CNM

Volunteer Clinical Faculty, University of Colorado Health Sciences Center, Denver, Colorado; Certified Nurse Midwife, The Medical Center of Aurora, Aurora, Colorado
Uncomplicated Antepartum, Intrapartum, and Postpartum Care

Glenda Louch, RNC, MS, CPNP

Clinical Faculty, University of Colorado School of Nursing; Pediatric Nurse Practitioner, Special Care Clinic, The Children's Hospital, Denver, Colorado
Follow-up of the Preterm Infant and Outcome of Prematurity

Carolyn Houska Lund, RN, MS, FAAN

Assistant Clinical Professor, University of California San Francisco School of Nursing, San Francisco, California; Neonatal Clinical Nurse Specialist, ECMO Coordinator, Children's Hospital Oakland, Oakland, California
Extracorporeal Membrane Oxygenation in the Neonate

Roger G. Martin, RNC, MSN, NNP

Adjunct Clinical Instructor, Department of Pediatrics, University of South Dakota, Vermillion, South Dakota; Neonatal Nurse Practitioner, Sioux Valley Hospital, Sioux Falls, South Dakota
Pharmacology in Neonatal Care

Mary McCulloch, RNC, MS, NNP, CPNP

Adjunct Faculty, University of Utah College of Nursing; Nurse Practitioner Outreach Medical Services, Department of Pediatrics, University of Utah School of Medicine, Salt Lake City, Utah
Neurologic Disorders

Josanne Paxton, RNC, MSN

Adjunct Faculty, University of Arizona; Neonatal Nurse Practitioner, Transport Coordinator, Arizona Health Sciences Center, Tucson, Arizona
Neonatal Infections

Julieanne Schiefelbein, RNC, RM, MAppSc (Nurs), MA(Ed), Grad Dip Clin Teaching, NNP

Neonatal Nurse Practitioner/Clinical Nurse Specialist, Primary Children's Medical Center, Salt Lake City, Utah; formerly at Royal Alexandra Hospital for Children, Sydney, Australia
Genetics and Fetal Anomalies

Carla Shapiro, MN

Lecturer, Faculty of Nursing, University of Manitoba, Winnipeg, Manitoba, Canada
Ophthalmologic Disorders

Leann Sterk, MS, CNP, CNS

Certified Nurse Practitioner, Clinical Nurse Specialist, Rapid City Regional Hospital, Rapid City, South Dakota
Neonatal Orthopedic Conditions

Laura Campbell Stokowski, RN, MS

Staff Nurse, St. John's Hospital, Leavenworth, Kansas
Metabolic Disorders; Endocrine Disorders

M. Terese Verklan, RNC, PhD, CS

Associate Professor, Systems and Technology, and Neonatal Clinical Nurse Specialist, The University of Texas Houston Health Science Center, School of Nursing, Houston, Texas
Legal Issues in the NICU

Robin L. Watson, RNC, MN, CCRN

Neonatal/Pediatric Clinical Nurse Specialist, Harbor–University of California Los Angeles Medical Center, Torrance, California
Gastrointestinal Disorders

Catherine L. Witt, RNC, MS, NNP

Neonatal Nurse Practitioner and Coordinator, Neonatal Nurse Practitioner Services, Presbyterian/St. Luke's Medical Center, Denver, Colorado
Neonatal Dermatology

Christine Zabloudil, BSN, NNP

Staff Nurse in Special Care Nursery, Valley Medical Center, Renton, Washington
Adaptation to Extrauterine Life

Reviewers

Vicky Armstrong, RNC, MSN

Perinatal Outreach Coordinator, Columbus, Ohio

Debbie Fraser Askin, RNC, MN

Adjunct Professor, University of Manitoba; Neonatal Nurse Practitioner, St. Boniface General Hospital, Winnipeg, Manitoba, Canada

Susan Bell, RNC, MS

NICU Charge Nurse, All Children's Hospital, St. Petersburg, Florida

Barbara Carey, RNC, MN, NNP, CPNP

Neonatal Nurse Practitioner, Long Beach, California

Terri Cavaliere, RNC, MS, NNP

Neonatal Nurse Practitioner, North Shore University Hospital; Assistant Clinical Professor, School of Nursing, State University of New York, Stony Brook, New York

Margaret Crockett, RNC, MS, NNP

Neonatal Clinical Nurse Specialist, Sutter Women's and Children's Services, Sacramento, California

Sandra Gardner, RN, MS, CNS, PNP

Director, Professional Outreach Consultation, Aurora, Colorado

Diane Holditch-Davis, RN, PhD, FAAN

Professor and Chair, Department of Children's Health, University of North Carolina, Chapel Hill, North Carolina

Kimberly Horns, PhD, NNP, RNC

Assistant Professor, College of Nursing, Wayne State University, Detroit, Michigan

Kathy Hughes, RNC, MSN, NNP

Neonatal Outreach Coordinator, Children's Hospital Oakland, Oakland, California

Jacqueline Ioli, RN, MSN, CS, CRNP

Advanced Practice Nurse, Hematology, St. Christopher's Hospital, Philadelphia, Pennsylvania

Carole Kenner, DNS

Professor and Department Head, Parent Child Health Nursing, University of Cincinnati, Cincinnati, Ohio; Consultant for Education and Programs, National Association of Neonatal Nurses, Petaluma, California

Cheryl King, RN, MS, CCRN

Neonatal Clinical Nurse Specialist, Presbyterian/St. Luke's Medical Center, Denver, Colorado

Diane Longobucco, RNC, MSN, APRN

Clinical Nurse Specialist, St. Francis Hospital and Medical Center, Hartford, Connecticut

Judy Wright Lott, RNC, DNS, NNP

Associate Professor and Co-Director of NNP Program, College of Nursing, University of Cincinnati, Cincinnati, Ohio

Foreword

Our world and especially health care continues to move faster and faster. This fast and frantic pace often seems to separate us. This is not a good feeling. In these times it is important to build and nourish communities, particularly our nursing community. Being a member of our large nursing community gives us a sense of unity and purpose and ultimately a shared vision. This is especially evident when partnerships like the one created to publish this book are formed. The Association of Women's Health, Obstetric and Neonatal Nurses (AWHONN) joined with the American Association of Critical Care Nurses (AACN) and the National Association of Neonatal Nurses (NANN) to produce this excellent second edition of the *Core Curriculum for Neonatal Intensive Care Nursing*. This combined community has a shared vision of promoting the best outcomes for the health of these sick and fragile newborns and their families. A second shared vision of our community is to bring nurses together so that they may choose to work as a team. This book is a valuable resource in realizing these shared visions. Ths book will be the most utilized nursing care resource at neonatal intensive care nurses' stations everywhere.

The combined energy, talent, and competencies of nurse members from all three associations were tapped by editors Jane Deacon and Patricia O'Neill to contribute their experience and expertise to this revision. It is with gratitude that we thank these editors and all the contributors to the book for this valuable resource created for all who are committed to the care and health of ill or premature infants and their families.

Leith Merrow Mullaly, RNC, MSN, ACCE, IBCLC
1999 AWHONN President

The Association of Women's Health, Obstetric and Neonatal Nurses, an association comprised of 22,000 health care professionals, promotes excellence in nursing practice to improve the health of women and newborns. Through dynamic programs, services, and community outreach, AWHONN strives to enrich not only the health and well-being but also the lives of women and newborns.

Mary G. McKinley, RN, MSN, CCRN
1998–1999 AACN President

The American Association of Critical-Care Nurses is the world's largest specialty nursing organization, with 70,000 members worldwide. Founded in 1969, AACN is dedicated to creating a health care system driven by the needs of patients and families in which critical care nurses make their optimal contribution. AACN is committed to providing the highest quality resources to maximize nurses' contribution to the care of the critically ill.

Frances Strodtbeck, RNC, DNS, NNP
1999–2000 NANN President

The National Association of Neonatal Nurses was founded in 1984 and represents almost 12,000 nurses. The Association's mission is to support and promote neonatal nursing. NANN is a specialty organization that acts as a unified voice to further the work of neonatal nurses in the provision of newborn and family care, facilitates cooperation among nurses in a variety of roles, promotes education for neonatal nursing, fosters advanced nursing practice, enhances the effectiveness of nursing in the promotion of human well-being, promotes ethical and professional conduct, serves as an advocate for the newborn and family, and increases public awareness and understanding of the specialty.

Preface

Providing neonatal intensive care is a multifaceted, constantly evolving area of health care. Those involved in the nursing care of high-risk newborn infants and their families are constantly challenged to integrate the best of themselves, their knowledge of pathophysiology and physical processes, their understanding of family dynamics, and often their very personal struggles with ethics to provide the finest care possible to their tiny patients. The role of the neonatal intensive care nurse is frequently to "bring together" all of the pieces of the puzzle to ensure comprehensive, clinically excellent, and compassionate care to sick newborns and their families.

This second edition of the *Core Curriculum for Neonatal Intensive Care Nursing* is intended to be used as a clinical resource. We have divided it into sections and designed it in outline format so that it can be used as an easy reference for the most current information on problems affecting infants in the NICU. Physiologic problems of the sick newborn are the major focus of this book, but to acknowledge the entire scope of neonatal nursing practice, we have included information on families, ethics, legal issues, research, case management, and the transition to home.

This text is the collaborative effort of three major nursing specialty associations. The Association of Women's Health, Obstetric and Neonatal Nurses (AWHONN), the American Association of Critical-Care Nurses (AACN), and the National Association of Neonatal Nurses (NANN) have all contributed chapter authors and reviewers to this text. Nurses representing various regions in the United States as well as Canada and Australia have also contributed chapters. In fact, this book is the first ever major publication that has brought together so many experts in neonatal nursing, joining them in the common goal of providing a comprehensive resource for the management and care of sick newborns. We are honored to be the editors of such an outstanding collaborative effort.

Our hope is that this book will be brought into your NICU and used as a clinical resource. The format and soft cover were designed specifically to make this a user-friendly manual of neonatal nursing care. We encourage you to mark it up and write notes in the margins so that it becomes an even richer manual of neonatal information to enhance your neonatal nursing practice.

Jane Deacon
Patricia (Beachy) O'Neill

Contents

SECTION III

NEONATAL PATHOPHYSIOLOGY: MANAGEMENT AND TREATMENT OF COMMON DISORDERS ▪ 205

SECTION IV

SOCIAL TRENDS AND FAMILY CARE ▪ 617

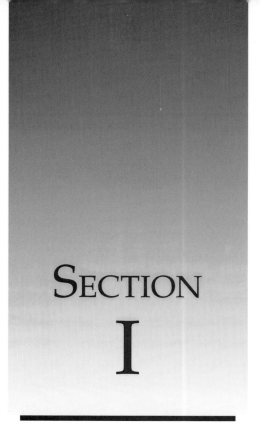

SECTION

I

OBSTETRIC CARE AND THE INFANT IN TRANSITION

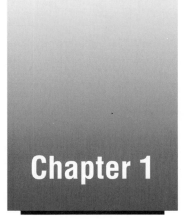

Chapter 1

Uncomplicated Antepartum, Intrapartum, and Postpartum Care

Nanette Landry

Objectives

1. Define term, preterm, and postterm pregnancy.

2. Describe Nägele's rule for estimated date of confinement.

3. Identify normal physiologic changes of each system in pregnancy.

4. Identify three methods of antepartum fetal surveillance.

5. Discuss the normal stages of labor.

6. Contrast low-risk intrapartum fetal monitoring management versus high-risk fetal monitoring management.

7. Identify normal postpartum assessments and management.

Antepartum, intrapartum, and postpartum care is not usually thought of as within the practice parameters of the neonatal nurse. Yet an understanding of the normal processes of pregnancy provides a framework for beginning to understand factors that affect the developing fetus and the high-risk neonate. This chapter discusses uncomplicated antepartum, intrapartum, and immediate postpartum nursing care. In addition, an overview of the normal physiologic changes that can be expected in a healthy mother is included.

Terminology

A. **Duration of gestation:** 280 days—40 postmenstrual weeks, or 10 lunar months.

B. **Trimesters:** division of gestation into three segments of approximately equal duration.
1. First trimester: 0–12 weeks.

2. Second trimester: 13–27 weeks.
3. Third trimester: 28–40 weeks.

C. **Term pregnancy:** 38–42 weeks; preterm: less than 37 weeks; and postterm: longer than 42 weeks.

Normal Physiologic Changes of Systems

Pregnancy affects all body systems. Some of the normal physiologic changes of systems include the following:

A. **Alimentary tract.**

1. There will be an increase in appetite up to 300 kcal/day. The recommended calorie intake for the average woman in pregnancy is 2200 kcal/day. Pregnant teenagers need an additional 100–200 kcal/day.
2. Approximately 70% of pregnancies are affected by morning sickness from weeks 4 through 16.
3. The stomach loses tone and has delayed emptying time.
4. Gastroesophageal junction also relaxes and, in combination with increased intra-abdominal pressure, leads to reflux and resulting heartburn.
5. The small bowel has reduced motility. In the colon, constipation is a problem because of mechanical obstruction from the uterus, reduced motility, and increased water absorption.
6. The gallbladder empties much more slowly in the second and third trimesters, and high residuals increase the chance of gallstone formation from progesterone. High levels of estrogen lead to an increase in bile salts, linking pregnancy to cholestasis and pruritus gravidarum.
7. The liver remains unchanged in pregnancy as far as size and hepatic blood flow are concerned; however, some laboratory values, such as reduced serum albumin, elevated alkaline phosphatase, and elevated serum cholesterol, mimic liver disease. Prothrombin time and serum levels of bilirubin, aspartate aminotransferase, and alanine aminotransferase are unchanged in normal pregnancy.
8. As pregnancy progresses, the stomach and intestines are displaced, causing the physical findings in certain disorders (e.g., appendicitis) to be altered.

B. **Respiratory system.**

1. Hypersecretion of mucus from the nasopharynx leads to nasal stuffiness and epistaxis during pregnancy.
2. The chest wall profile changes, resulting in an expansion of circumference and an increase in the subcostal margin angle. This results in the diaphragm's being elevated by 4 cm in the third trimester.
3. Up to 60–70% of all pregnant women have physiologic dyspnea, with increased tidal volume and reduced $PaCO_2$ levels. Pulmonary function generally is not impaired. Respiratory diseases may be serious during pregnancy.

C. **Skin** (Cunningham et al., 1997).

1. Because of elevated levels of estrogen, spider angiomas (vascular, red elevations with tiny vessels branching out from a central body) are frequently seen on the neck, face, throat, and arms. Palmar erythema—diffuse or blotchy spots on palms—is common in two thirds of white women and one third of black women.
2. Striae gravidarum, or "stretch marks," occur in women with a genetic predisposition to stretching of the skin or connective tissue.
3. Increased pigmentation is due to increased levels of estrogen, progesterone,

and melanocyte-stimulating hormone. This is most marked on the nipples, areolas, perineum, and the midline of the lower portion of the abdomen (commonly called the linea nigra).

4. Sun-sensitive hyperpigmentation of the face, called chloasma or melasma and also referred to as the "mask of pregnancy," results in a dark, blotchy appearance of the face, forehead, and upper lip.

5. During gestation a greater percentage of the hair remains in the anagen (growth) phase, which decreases normal hair loss. Hair loss commonly occurs between 2 and 4 months after delivery and is due to an increase in the telogen (resting) phase of hair growth. The hair will return to a normal growth phase within 6 months to 1 year (Gabbe, Neibyl, and Simpson, 1996).

D. Urinary system.

1. The kidneys enlarge and the ureters dilate. The consequences of these changes include:
   a. An increase in asymptomatic bacteriuria. This can lead to cystitis and pyelonephritis.
   b. Difficulty in diagnosing obstruction on x-ray examination and interference with studies of glomerular filtration, renal blood flow, and tubular function.

2. The glomerular filtration rate increases in pregnancy by 50%, leading to:
   a. An increase in creatinine clearance and a decrease in nitrogen levels.
   b. Increased filtration of sodium, with increased reabsorption of sodium by renal tubules to balance the loss.
   c. A lower threshold at which glucose will be excreted by the kidneys, leading to:
      (1) Inability to use urine glucose measurements in management of pregnant women with diabetes mellitus.
      (2) Increase in susceptibility to urinary tract infections.

E. Cardiovascular system.

1. Cardiac output increases 30–50% in pregnancy and is highest in the second trimester.

2. By the third trimester of pregnancy, the maternal heart rate increases by 15–20 beats above nonpregnant rates.

3. Because the heart is displaced leftward and upward by the enlarging uterus, the cardiac silhouette increases on x-ray films.

4. Altered cardiac sounds in pregnancy include splitting of the first heart sound, systolic flow murmurs (90% of pregnant women), and transient diastolic murmurs (20% of pregnant women).

5. Blood pressure remains normal (at the prepregnancy level) in the first trimester and drops during the second trimester, at approximately 24 weeks' gestation, by 5–10 mm Hg systolic and 10–15 mm Hg diastolic. It returns to normal prepregnancy levels at the end of pregnancy.

6. In late pregnancy, pressure obstruction of the inferior vena cava can occur in the supine position. The resulting 25% fall in cardiac output is called *supine hypotension.*

7. Blood stagnates in the lower extremities because of compression of the pelvic veins and the inferior vena cava. This contributes to dependent edema, varicosities of the legs and vulva, and hemorrhoid formation (Cunningham et al., 1997).

F. Breasts.

1. Early changes in the breasts (beginning by 4 weeks' gestation) include tingling, heaviness, tenderness, and enlargement. These symptoms usually subside at the end of the first trimester.

2. The areolas enlarge and darken.

3. Secretory glands called Montgomery's glands appear on the areolas.
4. Colostrum may be expressed in late pregnancy.

G. Skeletal changes.

1. Compensating for the anteriorly positioned growing uterus, the lower portion of the back curves. This lordosis shifts the center of gravity backward over the lower extremities and causes low back pain, a common complaint in pregnancy.
2. Joints loosen during pregnancy because of the hormone relaxin.
3. These changes and an unsteady gait lead to falls, a common occurrence in pregnancy.
4. Numbness, tingling, weakness, and aching in the upper extremities are a result of marked lordosis. The resulting anterior flexion of the neck produces traction on the ulnar and median nerves.

H. Hematologic changes.

1. Plasma volume is increased by 50% at term.
2. The white blood cell count rises progressively during pregnancy and labor and then returns to normal prepregnancy levels, ranging from 5000 to 12,000 cells/μL and increasing up to 25,000 cells/μL in labor and the early postpartum period.
3. The red blood cell count rises by 18–30% throughout pregnancy, and the plasma volume increases by 50%, reaching its peak at 30–34 weeks. This change in the ratio of red blood cells to plasma causes a drop in hematocrit, resulting in "physiologic anemia of pregnancy." The plasma volume increase levels off as the hematocrit begins to rise, resulting in a more normal ratio of red blood cells to plasma and a rise in hematocrit near term.
4. Platelet count decreases during pregnancy but remains within the normal range.
5. Pregnancy has been called a "hypercoagulable state." Fibrinogen is increased by 50%, and factors VII through X increase. Bleeding and clotting times remain normal. The incidence of thromboembolism increases during pregnancy and is greatest during the postpartum period.
6. Pregnancy is known to result in decreased immunologic function so that the "foreign fetus" is accommodated. This may also account for an abatement of certain autoimmune diseases in pregnancy and an increased susceptibility to certain infections.

Endocrine and Metabolic Changes

A. Thyroid. The thyroid enlarges during pregnancy; however, there is little transplacental transfer of the hormones triiodothyronine (T_3) and thyroxine (T_4). Thyroid-binding globulin total (free and bound) serum T_4 and total T_3 all increase in the first trimester and plateau at approximately 18–20 weeks. There is an inverse relationship between the rise of chorionic gonadotropin concentrations and demonstrating thyrotropin concentrations. High serum chorionic gonadotropin levels are associated with decreased TSH levels. Fetal thyroid function appears to be independent of maternal thyroid function.

B. Carbohydrate metabolism.

1. Carbohydrate metabolism is significantly altered by human placental lactogen, and the effects are in direct proportion to placental mass.
2. The basal metabolic rate is increased by 25%.
3. Peripheral resistance to insulin is referred to as the "diabetogenic effect of

pregnancy." The hormones responsible for this effect are human placental lactogen, progesterone, and estrogen.

4. Glucose is actively transported to the fetus; however, insulin and glycogen do not cross the placenta. Normal pregnancy is characterized by mild fasting hypoglycemia, postprandial hyperglycemia, and hyperinsulinemia. Levels of fatty acids, triglycerides, and cholesterol increase in the fasting pregnant woman. The switch in fuels from glucose to lipids is referred to as accelerated starvation, and ketonuria rapidly appears.

Antepartum Care

A. Initial antepartum visit.

1. A thorough obstetric history should include:
   a. Gravidity—number of pregnancies; parity—number of births.
      (1) A patient's obstetric history is often written as G3, P2, A0, L2, where G is gravity, P is parity, A is the number of abortions, and L is the current number of living children.
      (2) Parity may be subdivided into term and preterm.
      (3) Abortions include all pregnancies terminated before 24 weeks—spontaneous and elective abortions, as well as ectopic pregnancies.
   b. Weeks of gestation achieved with each pregnancy.
   c. Hours of labor.
   d. Type of delivery (i.e., vaginal or operative).
   e. Size of babies at birth.
   f. Any complications.
2. Medical history of the patient and immediate family should include:
   a. Complete medical history.
   b. Infection history.
      (1) Hepatitis.
      (2) Human immunodeficiency virus.
      (3) Herpes.
      (4) Rubella.
      (5) Varicella.
      (6) Sexually transmitted diseases.
   c. Risk assessment.
      (1) Drug or alcohol use.
      (2) Smoking.
      (3) Age.
      (4) Educational level.
      (5) History of emotional problems.
      (6) Support systems.
      (7) Attitude toward pregnancy.
3. Obtain a genetic background to identify factors that may lead to screening for Down syndrome, open neural tube defects (immediate family history), or any other possible genetic defects.
4. Obtain history of current pregnancy.
5. Perform a complete physical examination, including a complete pelvic examination.

B. Initial laboratory work.

1. Blood type and Rh status.
2. Antibody screening test.
3. Hematocrit and hemoglobin; complete blood cell count.
4. Papanicolaou smear.

5. Rubella titer.
6. Serologic tests.
7. Urinalysis for protein, glucose, and evidence of infections.
8. HBsAg (hepatitis B surface antigen).
9. HIV (human immunodeficiency virus), *Chlamydia,* and gonorrhea culture (depending on history and population).
10. Sickle cell screen, Tay-Sachs screen for appropriate population (Gabbe et al., 1996).

C. **Routine and diagnostic laboratory work and procedures (Table 1–1).**

1. At 8–18 weeks: ultrasonography may be indicated to establish accurate dates or to detect genetic abnormalities.
2. Chorionic villus sampling at 9–11 weeks for chromosomal evaluation.
3. At 14–18 weeks: offer maternal serum alpha-fetoprotein (AFP) or maternal serum triple-screen measurements to screen for open neural tube defects, Down syndrome, and other potential problems with the pregnancy. Using the maternal serum triple-screen test enhances the detection rate of Down syndrome.
   a. The maternal serum AFP concentration is low in Down syndrome but elevated in neural tube defects.

Table 1–1
PRENATAL SCREENING TESTS

Test	Reason for Screening Test
Blood type, Rh status, antibody screen	Identifies fetuses at risk of isoimmune disease
Hemoglobin or hematocrit	Baseline laboratory studies: rule out anemia
Rubella antibody screen	Identifies women susceptible to acquiring rubella during pregnancy; susceptible women should be immunized *after* delivery
Tuberculin skin testing	Identifies infected women for treatment
Hepatitis B surface antigen	Identifies women whose offspring can be treated at birth to prevent hepatitis B infection
Serologic test for syphilis (VDRL or rapid plasmin reagin)	Treatment reduces fetal/neonatal morbidity; mandated by law in most states
Human immunodeficiency virus	Identifies women for treatment and perinatal therapy to decrease transmission to the fetus
Urinalysis	
Glucose, ketones, protein	Screen for diabetes, pregnancy-induced hypertension, renal disease
Red blood cells, white blood cells, bacteria	Possible urinary tract infection
Diabetes screen (24–28 wk)	Fasting and glucose tolerance tests to rule out gestational diabetes
Papanicolaou smear	Identifies cervicitis and precancerous and cancerous lesions
Neisseria gonorrhoeae and *Chlamydia** cultures	Identify treatable sexually transmitted diseases, most of which can cause fetal or neonatal morbidity
Triple screen (maternal serum for AFP, human chorionic gonadotropin, estriol)	Tests done at 16–20 weeks at mother's discretion after counseling; AFP screens for neural tube defects, Down syndrome; combination of 3 tests very sensitive in identifying Down syndrome
Other†	

* Some centers also screen for *Mycoplasma hominis* and group B streptococcus colonization.
  † Laboratory tests may vary from one center to another. Certain tests may be ordered if patient is at specific risk (i.e., hemoglobinopathy screen to rule out sickle cell disease in a black patient whose status is unknown or with a family history). Ultrasonography is considered by some to be a screening tool for congenital anomalies.
  Adapted from Clinic Protocol for Department of Obstetrics and Gynecology, University of Colorado Health Sciences Center.
  From O'Neill, P., Thureen, P.J., and Hobbins, J.: Maternal factors affecting the newborn. *In* Thureen, P.J., Deacon, J., O'Neill, P., and Hernandez, J. (Eds.): Assessment and Care of the Well Newborn. Philadelphia, W.B. Saunders, 1999.

  b. Human chorionic gonadotropin level is elevated in Down syndrome.

  c. Unconjugated estriol concentration is low in Down syndrome.

4. At 15–20 weeks: amniocentesis is used for genetic evaluation and measurement of AFP. Other studies, as suggested by the genetic history, may be performed.

5. At 24–28 weeks: a glucose screen for gestational diabetes is performed. A 50 g glucose load is given, and a plasma glucose concentration is determined 1 hour later. A level greater than 140 mg/dL is abnormal.

  a. A glucose tolerance test is performed on all patients with an abnormal screen result. The test includes determination of a fasting plasma glucose concentration, as well as hourly values for 3 hours after a 100 g glucose load. The diagnosis of gestational diabetes is made if two values are elevated (plasma values: fasting, 105 mg/dL; at 1 hour, 190 mg/dL; at 2 hours, 165 mg/dL; and at 3 hours, 145 mg/dL).

6. At 28 weeks: obtain a repeated antibody titer for Rh-negative mothers; administer Rh immunoglobulin, 300 mg, if no anti-D antibody has been detected.

7. Early in the third trimester: obtain repeated hemoglobin and hematocrit determinations to recheck for anemia.

8. At 36–40 weeks: Ultrasonography may be indicated for serial growth evaluation, amniotic fluid volume testing, or placental assessment.

Maternal Infections

A. TORCH infections (Table 1–2).

1. Acronym refers to syndrome of five infectious diseases: toxoplasmosis, other infections (e.g., congenital syphilis), rubella, cytomegalovirus infection, and herpes simplex.

2. All the infectious agents causing TORCH infections cross the placenta and may adversely affect the fetus.

B. Sexually transmitted diseases (Table 1–3).

1. These are transmitted during sexual intercourse.

2. Most cases occur in persons less than 25 years of age. A total of 12 million cases are reported each year.

C. Other communicable diseases (Table 1–4).

1. In all cases, both the fetus and the mother must be examined.

2. Diseases of greatest concern are measles, chickenpox, mumps, mononucleosis, parvovirus infection, and influenza.

D. Chorioamnionitis.

1. An infection of the chorion, amnion, and amniotic fluid that causes perinatal morbidity and death.

2. Usually associated with ruptured membranes but can be found in women with intact membranes.

3. Usually an ascending infection, commonly caused by *Escherichia coli*, group B streptococcus, anaerobic streptococci, and bacteroids.

E. Infection with group B streptococcus.

1. Organism is cultured from the lower portion of the genital tract of 15–20% of all pregnant women between 23 and 26 weeks of gestation (Cunningham et al., 1997).

2. Infection rate is 10 in 1000 infants born to colonized mothers; increases to 40 in 100 infants if there is premature labor and delivery, prolonged rupture of membranes, or intrapartum fever (American College of Obstetricians and Gynecologists [ACOG], 1996).

Table 1–2
TORCH INFECTIONS

Infection/ Incubation	Transmission	Detection	Maternal Effects	Neonatal Effects	Incidence and Prevention
Cytomegalovirus Incubation: unknown	Intimate contact with infected secretions (breast milk, cervical mucus, semen, saliva, and urine) Transplacentally Organ transplantation	IgM titer	Clinically "silent"; only 1–5% acquire symptoms: low-grade fever, malaise, arthralgia, hepatomegaly	Infection is most likely to occur with maternal primary infection 90% of infected infants are free of symptoms at birth, but 5–15% of these may have long-term sequelae, 5% with severe involvement at birth: IUGR, microcephaly, periventricular calcification, deafness, blindness, chorioretinitis, mental retardation, hepatosplenomegaly	Primary occurs in 1–2% of pregnant women 90% of adult population in U.S. are seropositive Rigorous personal hygiene throughout pregnancy to prevent infection if not infected
Herpes simplex virus Incubation: 2–10 days	Intimate mucocutaneous exposure Passage through an infected birth canal Ascending infection, especially with rupture of membranes Transplacentally (rare) if initial infection occurs during pregnancy	Suspect with vesicles on cervix, vagina, or external genital area; painful lesions Presumptive diagnosis by fluorescent antibody or Papanicolaou smear on vesicular fluid Confirm diagnosis by vesicle culture	Painful genital lesions Primary infection commonly associated with fever, malaise, myalgias Numbness, tingling, burning, itching, and pain with lesions Lymphadenopathy Urinary retention	Rare transplacental transmissions have resulted in miscarriages Mortality rate of 5–60% if neonatal exposure is with active primary infection Neurologic or ophthalmic sequelae Disseminated infection in 70% of cases, with jaundice, respiratory distress, and CNS involvement	Estimated 300,000 new cases per year 1:3000–20,000 live births with perinatal transmission Up to 80% of women delivering infected infants have no history of genital herpes; cesarean delivery if known active infection Avoid genital contact when male has penile lesions; use condoms
Rubella Incubation: 14–21 days	Nasopharyngeal secretions Transplacentally	Serologic antibody titer testing (IgG-specific rubella antibody) Virus isolation from throat	Pink maculopapular rash on face, neck, arms, and legs lasting 3 days Lymph node enlargement, fever, malaise, headache History of exposure 3 wk earlier	Fetal infection rate greatest before 11 wk and after 35 wk, but severe sequelae occur with first-trimester infection; includes deafness (60–70%), eye defects (10–30%), CNS anomalies (10–25%), congenital heart disease (10–20%)	Since introduction of vaccine in late 1960s, rubella is rare Occurs more commonly in springtime Vaccine is contraindicated during pregnancy; vaccinate susceptible women postpartum

Table continued on following page

Table 1–2
TORCH INFECTIONS *(Continued)*

Infection/ Incubation	Transmission	Detection	Maternal Effects	Neonatal Effects	Incidence and Prevention
Toxoplasmosis (protozoa, *Toxoplasma gondii*) Incubation: 2–3 wk	Eating raw meat containing *T. gondii* Ingesting *T. gondii* cysts secreted in feces of infected cats Transplacentally Impossible to transmit to others because the infecting organisms are tissue bound and are not secreted	Serologic antibody testing ELISA	90% of infected women have no symptoms Posterior cervical lymphadenopathy Malaise Premature labor and delivery	Severity varies with gestational age (usually, earlier infection results in more severe effects) Neurologic, ophthalmologic, and co-sequelae are variable IUGR Hydrocephalus Microcephaly	Incidence varies throughout world (1–4 infants per 1000 live births) 20–30% of U.S. women have been exposed Incidence of congenital toxoplasmosis infection in U.S. is 1:1000–8000 Reduce contact with cats during pregnancy

TORCH, Toxoplasmosis, other infections (e.g., congenital syphilis), rubella, cytomegalovirus infection, and herpes simplex; *CNS*, central nervous system; *ELISA*, enzyme-linked immunosorbent assay; *IUGR*, intrauterine growth retardation.
From O'Neill, P., Thureen, P.J., and Hobbins, J.: Maternal factors affecting the newborn. *In* Thureen, P.J., Deacon, J., O'Neill, P., and Hernandez, J. (Eds.): Assessment and Care of the Well Newborn. Philadelphia, W.B. Saunders, 1999.

3. All women should be screened at 35–37 weeks' gestation for anogenital group B streptococcus infection. Any woman with positive culture results should be offered chemoprophylaxis even if no risk factors are present (ACOG, 1996).
4. Agreement concerning routine screening and treatment has not been achieved; however, in a consensus developed by the Centers for Disease Control and Prevention (CDC), ACOG, and AAP, the strategy of administering chemoprophylaxis to all women with risk factors is considered to be an acceptable practice. Risk factors include a previous infant with group B streptococcus, known infection with group B streptococcus in this pregnancy, delivery before 37 weeks' gestation, rupture of membranes 18 hours or more before birth, or an intrapartum temperature of 38°C or higher (CDC, 1996).

Assessment of Gestational Age

A. **Last menstrual period (LMP).** Pregnancy may be detected by 5–6 weeks after the LMP. Estimating gestational age by counting from the LMP is a reliable method.
1. A history should include:
   a. Duration of menstrual periods.
   b. Heaviness of menstrual flow.
   c. Menstrual history.
   d. Hormonal contraceptive use.
2. Nägele's rule determines the estimated date of confinement (EDC) or due date by the following formula: EDC = LMP − 3 months + 7 days.

B. **Pelvic examination and fundal height.**

1. Determination of the size of the uterus during an early examination (before 12–14 weeks) is relatively accurate if the mother is of normal height and not grossly obese. Fundal height measurements (in centimeters) are made from 16 to 35 weeks' approximate gestational age and are accurate within 3 weeks. The uterus is generally at the umbilicus at 20 weeks.

Table 1–3
SEXUALLY TRANSMITTED DISEASES

Infection/Agent/ Incubation	Detection	Maternal Effects	Neonatal Effects	Incidence
Acquired immunodeficiency syndrome Human immunodeficiency virus Incubation: variable, months to years	ELISA for screening Western blot or indirect immunofluorescence assay p24 antigen for acute infection before seroconversion		30% chance of transmission from infected mother Syndrome develops in up to 65% of infected infants within a few months after birth	1991: estimated 200,000 cases in U.S.; 0.15% of all women who were delivered were infected
Chlamydiosis Bacterium: *Chlamydia trachomatis* Incubation: variable but >1 wk	Culture of endocervical and urethral specimens ELISA or fluorescent antibody on swab specimen is less sensitive and specific	Most cases asymptomatic Mucopurulent cervicitis Frequently associated with other sexually transmitted diseases Occasionally: premature rupture of membranes, preterm labor, IUGR, infertility, chorioamnionitis	30–40% of exposed infants have conjunctivitis 3–18% have pneumonia	Most common sexually transmitted disease Estimated 4 million cases occur annually in U.S., with prevalence rates in female patients 8–20% 70% of infections may be asymptomatic
Gonorrhea Bacteria: *Neisseria gonorrhoeae*, gramnegative diplococcus Incubation: 10 days	Endocervical, oral, or rectal cultures Genital or blood cultures Gram stain of lesions	60–80% of those infected are free of symptoms Occasionally: pelvic peritonitis, premature rupture of membranes, postpartum endometritis, chorioamnionitis, increased infertility, ectopic pregnancy	Purulent conjunctivitis Sepsis or meningitis	More than 1 million cases are reported in U.S. each year Incidence in pregnancy ranges from 1% to 10%, depending on population
Human papillomavirus Incubation: unknown (3 mo to years)	Single or multiple irregular painless papules in the genital or perianal area Colposcopy used as adjunct in equivocal situations Cervical cytologic testing	Significant number of lesions enlarge during pregnancy Usually multicentric in pregnancy	Potential transmission of laryngeal papillomas Very rare (less than 1 : 1000–1500 pregnancies in which mothers have genital condyloma)	Estimated 40–60 million persons infected worldwide Viral lesions probably more frequent in pregnant women because of increased hormone levels Increasing incidence noted in STD clinics and private offices Peak occurrence at age 15–35 Associated with other STDs
Syphilis Spirochete: *Treponema pallidum* Incubation: 3 wk on average	VDRL test Rapid plasma reagin test Fluorescent treponemal antibody absorption test	Primary chancre: painless ulcerative lesion Secondary syphilis: fever and malaise, red macules on palms or soles of feet Generalized lymphadenopathy Early latent (positive serologic finding <1 year duration) syphilis Latent (cardiovascular) syphilis Neurosyphilis	Vary depending on gestation Stillbirth IUGR Nonimmune hydrops Premature labor	100,000 cases are reported in U.S. each year; 80% of these women are of reproductive age 3850 cases of congenital syphilis in 1992 70–100% fetal transmission rate in primary maternal disease
Trichomoniasis Protozoa: *Trichomonas vaginalis* Incubation: 4–20 days	"Wet prep" saline examination Papanicolaou smear Urinalysis	Malodorous, discolored vaginal discharge Dysuria	Infant contact through infected vagina Usually asymptomatic	Not reported to CDC but estimated in as many as 20% of pregnancies Estimates of 10–15% of all cases of vaginitis

CDC, Centers for Disease Control and Prevention; *ELISA*, enzyme-linked immunosorbent assay; *IUGR*, intrauterine growth retardation.
From O'Neill, P., Thureen, P.J., and Hobbins, J.: Maternal factors affecting the newborn. *In* Thureen, P.J., Deacon, J., O'Neill, P., and Hernandez, J. (Eds.): Assessment and Care of the Well Newborn. Philadelphia, W.B. Saunders, 1999.

Table 1–4
OTHER COMMUNICABLE DISEASES

Infection/Agent/ Incubation	Mode of Transmission	Maternal Effects	Neonatal Effects	Incidence and Prevention
Influenza virus Incubation: 24–72 hr	Respiratory secretions	Usually brief but incapacitating disease Death occurs from secondary bacterial pneumonia	Any risk of malformation has been confined to first trimester Most studies fail to support teratogenicity Teratogenicity is unknown	Killed virus vaccine Vaccine during pregnancy is indicated if mother is at medical risk because of other diseases
Mumps Paramyxovirus Incubation: 16–18 days	Respiratory secretions	Spontaneous abortion rate is increased twofold	Teratogenicity is unknown	Avoid pregnancy for 3 months after vaccination
Parvovirus B19 (fifth disease) DNA virus Incubation: 4–14 days	Respiratory secretions	Erythema Elevated temperature Arthralgia	Spontaneous abortions	Risk for women with primary infection during first 20 wk of pregnancy is 15–17%
Hepatitis B	Sexually Perinatally Transplacentally Blood, stool, and saliva transmission	Fever, jaundice, malaise, hepatosplenomegaly Premature labor	Increased stillbirth rate Infected infants usually symptom free at birth	200,000–300,000 cases in the U.S. each year One third of infants born to HBsAg-positive mother will have HBsAg/HBeAg positivity and anti-HBe negativity
Varicella (chickenpox) Varicella-zoster virus Incubation: 11–21 days	Probably by aerosolized respiratory droplets Portal of entry is respiratory tract Transplacentally	Severe in adults Risk of premature labor as a result of high temperature Risk of varicella pneumonia appears to be increased during pregnancy	2% of infants with maternal infection in first trimester have cutaneous scarring, eye abnormalities, and retardation At risk if maternal rash onset 5 days before to 2 days after delivery; severe disseminated neonatal disease may develop, and one third die	90% of women are immune In U.S. occurs in <0.1% of pregnancies

HBsAg, Hepatitis B surface antigen; *HBeAg,* hepatitis B "e" antigen.
From O'Neill, P., Thureen, P.J., and Hobbins, J.: Maternal factors affecting the newborn. *In* Thureen, P.J., Deacon, J., O'Neill, P., and Hernandez, J. (Eds.): Assessment and Care of the Well Newborn. Philadelphia, W.B. Saunders, 1999.

2. Quickening is the first feelings of fetal movement.
   a. Primigravida: has quickening 18–20 weeks.
   b. Multigravida: has quickening 16–18 weeks.

C. **Fetal heart tones.** Can be detected by an electronic Doppler device as early as 9 weeks and commonly by 12 weeks, and may be auscultated with a fetoscope by 19–20 weeks.

D. **Ultrasonography.**

1. Ultrasonography is most accurate in the first trimester (6–14 weeks), with crown-rump measurement accurately reflecting gestational age plus or minus 3 days.
2. Fetal heart motion can be detected by real-time ultrasonography as early as 6 weeks' gestation by vaginal ultrasonography.
3. Biparietal diameter is the most frequently used method of establishing gestational age; it is most accurate between 12 and 18 weeks (O'Neill, Thureen, and Hobbins, 1999).

4. Abdominal circumference can be used to assess gestational age and intrauterine growth retardation. Combining biparietal diameter and abdominal circumference can give an estimate of fetal weight that is accurate within 10%.
5. Fetal femur length may also be used to determine gestational age. Fetal weight within 7–10% can be determined by combining abdominal circumference and femur length.

E. **Laboratory assessments for documenting fetal lung maturity.**

1. Lecithin/sphingomyelin (L/S) ratio greater than 2:1 occurs when fetal lung surfactant is present in amniotic fluid (at approximately 35 weeks). A level greater than or equal to 2:1 suggests that the baby will not need respiratory support after birth.
2. Phosphatidylglycerol (PG) is also present in amniotic fluid at around 35 weeks and increases rapidly at 37 weeks. Measurement of PG, a component of surfactant, is a more reliable test of lung maturity in mothers with diabetes than is measurement of the L/S ratio. PG is reported as present or not present.
3. Fetal lung maturity assay is another test for lung maturity in the newborn infant that is growing in popularity. It is less expensive, is easier to perform, and has fewer false-negative results than the L/S ratio or PG measurement. Fetal lung maturity measures surfactant/albumin ratio in amniotic fluid. Results are reported as follows: 55 mg/g, mature lungs; >39-55 mg/g, a 20% risk of respiratory distress in the neonate; and <39 mg/g, an 80% risk of respiratory distress in the neonate.

Antepartum Visits

A. **Frequency.**

1. In general, obstetric visits are recommended every 4 weeks until 28 weeks, then every 2 weeks until 36 weeks, and then weekly. Additional visits may be necessary around 18–20 weeks to establish the presence of heart tones with a fetoscope and the presence of quickening or to determine whether the pregnancy shows any signs of complications (Gabbe et al., 1996).

B. **Routine assessments.**

1. Psychosocial assessments.
2. Weight.
3. Blood pressure.
4. Urinary glucose and protein levels.
5. Gestational age in weeks.
6. Fundal height in centimeters.
7. Presence of edema.
8. Fetal heart tones.
9. Fetal movement (after 20 weeks).
10. Fetal presentation.
11. Vaginal bleeding.
12. Prematurity signs and symptoms.
    a. Increased discharge/mucus show.
    b. Contractions, abdominal cramping, intestinal cramping.
    c. Dysuria, frequency of urination, and/or tenderness of costovertebral angle.
    d. Increased pelvic pressure.
13. Signs and symptoms of pregnancy-induced hypertension.
    a. Increased blood pressure, proteinuria, edema.
    b. Epigastric pain.

　c. Nausea and/or vomiting.
　d. Hyperreflexia.
　e. Clonus.
　f. Visual disturbances.
　g. Headaches.
14. Warning signs to report: all of items 12 and 13, above; in addition:
　a. Chills and fever.
　b. Persistent vomiting.
　c. Abdominal pain.
　d. Leakage from vagina.
　e. Change in intensity or frequency of fetal movement.

Antepartum Fetal Surveillance

A. **Nonstress test (NST).** This is the most widely used screening method for fetal well-being.
1. It is indicated for patients at risk of placental insufficiency and may be started as early as 30–32 weeks' gestation. Conditions that are of concern include the following:
　a. Postterm pregnancy.
　b. Diabetes mellitus.
　c. Hypertension.
　d. Previous stillbirths.
　e. Intrauterine growth restriction.
　f. Decreased fetal movements.
　g. Rh disease.
2. Testing is repeated once or twice weekly. With a reactive test result, the perinatal death rate is approximately 5 in 1000.
3. A reactive NST result is two or three fetal heart rate (FHR) accelerations (a FHR acceleration is defined as a 15 beat rise from baseline and return to baseline lasting 15 seconds) during a 20-minute period; a nonreactive test result is either no fetal movements after 40 minutes, in association with FHR accelerations, or no FHR accelerations in association with fetal movements.
4. Whereas a reactive NST result is reassuring, a nonreactive result is an indication for further studies (O'Neill et al., 1999).

B. **Contraction stress test (CST).** CST, the first test of fetal well-being, evaluates the reserve function of the placenta. Indications for use are the same as for use of the NST; the CST is most often used after a nonreactive NST result.
1. CST can be achieved by the following:
　a. Spontaneous contraction test: three spontaneous contractions in a 10-minute period.
　b. Nipple stimulation test: naturally induced oxytocin by stimulation of nipples (endogenous).
　c. Oxytocin challenge test: artificially induced oxytocin by intravenous administration (exogenous).
2. The CST requires three contractions of moderate intensity lasting 40–60 seconds in a 10-minute period. This stimulates a labor pattern and allows the fetus to be stressed as in normal labor. The CST looks for decelerations, or decreases, in the FHR in relation to the onset of uterine contractions.
3. A positive CST result is defined as late decelerations of the FHR that are present with the majority (>50%) of contractions in a 10-minute window. Delivery should be considered with a positive CST result. Findings may also be considered suspect, equivocal, or unsatisfactory, or as showing hyperstimulation. These cases require retesting in the next 24 hours for adequate interpretation of fetal well-being.

4. Frequency of the CST is usually weekly, but the CST can be performed more frequently, as the fetus' condition warrants.

C. **Biophysical profile.**

1. The biophysical profile uses real-time ultrasonography to evaluate five parameters, each receiving either 0 or 2 points; the maximum score is 10 points.
   a. Fetal breathing movements.
   b. Gross body movements.
   c. Fetal tone.
   d. Quantitative amniotic fluid volume.
   e. NST.
2. Management is based on the assigned score:
   a. Score of 8–10 points: normal; weekly tests are indicated.
   b. Score of 6 points: requires repeated test in 4–6 hours or delivery if oligohydramnios is present.
   c. Score of 4 points: suspect chronic asphyxia. Need for delivery will be determined on the basis of gestational age and lung maturity.
   d. Score of 2 points or less: strongly suspect chronic asphyxia; requires delivery regardless of gestational age (O'Neill et al., 1999).

Normal Labor

A. **Phases of labor.** According to Friedman (1955), there are three phases of labor:
1. Latent phase: onset of labor to time when slope of cervical dilation changes.
2. Active phase: approximately 3 cm to complete cervical dilation.
3. Descent phase: coincides with second stage.

B. **Seven cardinal movements of fetal head and body en route to delivery.**

1. Engagement: the head enters the pelvis.
2. Descent: the head descends into the pelvis, past the pelvic brim.
3. Flexion: with flexion of the head, the narrowest diameter of the head is presented to the pelvis.
4. Internal rotation: the head enters the pelvis transversely and then rotates to an anteroposterior position.
5. Extension: the flexed head extends to be delivered.
6. External rotation: the head rotates back to the transverse position.
7. Expulsion: the body is expelled.

Intrapartum Labor Management

A. **Assessments.** Review the prenatal records and determine current status, including the following:
1. Vital signs.
2. Contraction pattern, intensity.
3. Membrane status—intact, ruptured, or leaking.
4. Fetal heart tones.
5. Vaginal findings (if no bleeding or spontaneous rupture of membranes has occurred) to assess:
   a. Dilation of the cervix.
   b. Effacement, or thinning, of the cervix.
   c. Station, or position, of the presenting part in the pelvis. Station 0 represents entrance of the head into the pelvis. As descent occurs, the station is expressed as +1, +2, or +3 and descent is measured in centimeters.

d. Presenting part.

e. Position. The position of the head (i.e., anterior, posterior, or transverse) relative to the pelvis is assessed.

B. **Management of low-risk patient.** The patient should be identified as being at low or high risk on the basis of the available data. A patient determined to be at low risk during labor does not require continuous electronic fetal monitoring. According to ACOG Technical Bulletin No. 207 (1995a), auscultation should be performed at least every 30 minutes after a contraction for 30 seconds. In the second stage of labor, auscultation should be performed every 15 minutes. If electronic monitoring is used, evaluation should continue at the same intervals. Any detectable deceleration of the FHR should alert the nurse to apply the electronic fetal monitor to determine whether the FHR is reassuring.

1. Auscultation. A nonreassuring FHR detected by auscultation for which electronic fetal monitoring should be performed is indicated by the following:

a. A baseline FHR (average rate between contractions) of less than 100 bpm.

b. An FHR of less than 100 bpm 30 seconds after a contraction.

c. Unexplained baseline tachycardia of more than 160 bpm, especially with at-risk patients in whom the tachycardia persists through three or more contractions (10–15 minutes) despite corrective measures.

2. Electronic fetal monitoring. This allows systematic evaluation of the FHR and labor. Contractions should be evaluated for polysystole (more than five contractions in 10 minutes), prolonged contractions lasting more than 90 seconds, and tetanic contractions. These conditions may cause increased stress for the fetus or mother. The baseline FHR should be observed for variability, periodic changes, and trends.

3. FHR patterns reported to be associated with increased incidence of fetal compromise.

a. Severe bradycardia: a rate less than 80 bpm for more than 3 minutes.

b. Repetitive late decelerations: a symmetric fall in the FHR, beginning at or after the peak of the uterine contraction and returning to baseline only after the contraction has ended.

c. Undulating baseline: a pattern of rapid change between tachycardia (rates >160 bpm) and bradycardia (rates <100 bpm).

d. Any nonreassuring pattern associated with explained poor or absent baseline variability: a flat or nearly flat baseline.

e. Absence of accelerations.

Puerperium: "Fourth Trimester"

The period from delivery through the sixth week is known as the "fourth trimester."

A. **Uterine involution.** Involution begins immediately after delivery; the fundus is at the level of the umbilicus.

B. **Placental site regeneration.** Process takes approximately 6 weeks after delivery.

C. **Lochia.** Postdelivery uterine discharge, with changes as follows:

1. Lochia rubra: dark red or reddish brown; 3–4 days.

2. Lochia serosa: pink or brown; 4–10 days.

3. Lochia alba: yellow to white; approximately 10 days after delivery to 4–6 weeks after delivery.

D. **Breasts.** The breasts should be soft until the third or fourth postpartum day, when engorgement occurs. Engorgement resolves spontaneously within 24–36 hours. In non-breast-feeding mothers, lactation ceases within 1 week.

E. Immunizations.

1. Rubella vaccination should be administered in the immediate postpartum period to all women who are not immune (Varney, 1997).
2. Rh(D) immunoglobulin (300 µg given intramuscularly) is administered to the mother within 72 hours of delivery to prevent sensitization from fetal-maternal transfusion of Rh-positive fetal erythrocytes (Varney, 1997).

REFERENCES

American College of Obstetricians and Gynecologists: Fetal Heart Rate Patterns: Monitoring, Interpretation and Management. (Technical Bulletin No. 207.) Washington, D.C., The College, 1995a.

American College of Obstetricians and Gynecologists: Group B Streptococcal Infections in Pregnancy. (Technical Bulletin No. 169.) Washington, D.C., The College, 1995b.

American College of Obstetricians and Gynecologists: Maternal Serum Screening. (Educational Bulletin No. 228.) Washington, D.C., The College, 1996.

American College of Obstetricians and Gynecologists Committee on Obstetrics: Prevention of Early Onset Perinatal Group B Streptococcal Diseases in Newborns. (Committee Opinion No. 173.) Washington, D.C., The College, June 1996.

Centers for Disease Control and Prevention: Prevention of perinatal Group B streptococcal disease: A public health perspective. MMWR Morb. Mortal. Wkly. Rep. 45:1, 1996.

Cunningham, F.R., Macdonald, P.C., Gant, N.F., et al.: Williams' Obstetrics, 20th ed. Stamford, Conn., Appleton & Lange, 1997, pp. 197, 210–211, 333–348.

Friedman, E.A.: Graphic appraisal of labor: A study of 500 primigravidas. Bull. Sloan Hosp. Women, 1:42, 1955.

Gabbe, S.G., Neibyl, J.R., and Simpson, J.L.: Obstetrics: Normal and Problem Pregnancies, 2nd ed. New York, Churchill Livingstone, 1996, pp. 161, 164–170.

O'Neill, P., Thureen, P.J., and Hobbins, J.: Maternal factors affecting the newborn. In Thureen, P.J., Deacon, J., O'Neill, P., and Hernandez, J. (Eds.): Assessment and Care of the Well Newborn. Philadelphia, W.B. Saunders, 1999, p. 7.

Thureen, P.J., Hall, D., Townsend, S., et al.: Fetal assessment, labor and delivery. In Thureen, P.J., Deacon, J., O'Neill, P., and Hernandez, J. (Eds.): Assessment and Care of the Well Newborn. Philadelphia, W.B. Saunders, 1999, p. 7.

Varney, H.: Varney's Midwifery, 3rd ed. Sudbury, Mass., Jones & Bartlett, 1997, pp. 340, 639–649.

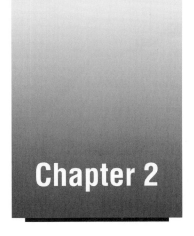

Chapter 2

Antepartum-Intrapartum Complications

Anne B. Broussard

Objectives

1. List maternal risk factors that may exist before pregnancy.

2. Discuss the effects of hypertension and diabetes on the maternal-placental-fetal complex.

3. Categorize intrapartum conditions that may result in complications for the newborn infant.

4. Assess the fetus/neonate for effects of tocolytic drugs.

5. Describe the effect on the fetus/neonate of these intrapartum crises: abruptio placentae, placenta previa, cord prolapse, and shoulder dystocia.

6. List neonatal complications associated with breech delivery.

7. Examine the effect of obstetric analgesia/anesthesia and operative delivery on the newborn infant.

An understanding of maternal complications enhances the ability of the nurse to anticipate and recognize neonatal complications and intervene appropriately. The purpose of this chapter is to provide a comprehensive view of possible neonatal complications resulting from maternal risk factors. These risk factors may exist before the pregnancy or develop during the antepartum and intrapartum periods (see Table 2–1).

Anatomy and Physiology

A. **The fetus.** The fetus is a part of the maternal-placental-fetal complex.

B. **Conditions and substances that affect the pregnant woman.** These have the potential to affect placental functions of respiration, nutrition, excretion, and hormone production. Decreased placental function can in turn adversely affect the fetus.

C. **The placenta.** In addition, the old concept of the placenta as a barrier to noxious substances has long been superseded by the concept of the placenta as a sieve that permits transport of desirable *and* undesirable substances to the fetus. The placental membrane separating maternal and fetal circulations consists of

Table 2–1
PRENATAL HIGH-RISK FACTORS

Factor	Maternal Implications	Fetal/Neonatal Implications
SOCIAL-PERSONAL		
Low income level and/or low educational level	Poor antenatal care Poor nutrition ↑ Risk preeclampsia	Low birth weight IUGR
Poor diet	Inadequate nutrition ↑ Risk anemia ↑ Risk preeclampsia	Fetal malnutrition Prematurity
Living at high altitude	↑ Hemoglobin	Prematurity IUGR
Multiparity > 3	↑ Risk antepartum/postpartum hemorrhage	Anemia Fetal death
Weight < 45.5 kg (100 lb)	Poor nutrition Cephalopelvic disproportion Prolonged labor	IUGR Hypoxia associated with difficult labor and birth
Weight > 91 kg (200 lb)	↑ Risk hypertension ↑ Risk cephalopelvic disproportion	↓ Fetal nutrition
Age < 16 yr	Poor nutrition Poor antenatal care ↑ Risk preeclampsia ↑ Risk cephalopelvic disproportion	Low birth weight ↑ Fetal death
Age > 35 yr	↑ Risk preeclampsia ↑ Risk cesarean birth	↑ Risk congenital anomalies ↑ Chromosomal aberrations
Smoking 1 pack per day or more	↑ Risk hypertension ↑ Risk cancer	↓ Placental perfusion → ↓ O_2 and nutrients available Low birth weight IUGR Preterm birth
Use of addicting drugs	↑ Risk poor nutrition ↑ Risk of infection with IV drugs	↑ Risk congenital anomalies ↑ Risk low birth weight Neonatal withdrawal Lower serum bilirubin level
Excessive alcohol consumption	↑ Risk poor nutrition Possible hepatic effects with long-term consumption	↑ Risk fetal alcohol syndrome
PREEXISTING MEDICAL DISORDERS		
Diabetes mellitus	↑ Risk preeclampsia, hypertension Episodes of hypoglycemia and hyperglycemia ↑ Risk cesarean birth	Low birth weight Macrosomia Neonatal hypoglycemia ↑ Risk congenital anomalies ↑ Risk respiratory distress syndrome
Cardiac disease	Cardiac decompensation Further strain on mother's body ↑ Maternal death rate	↑ Risk fetal death ↑ Perinatal death
Anemia < 9 g/dL hemoglobin (white) < 29% hematocrit (white) < 8.2 g/dL hemoglobin (black) < 26% hematocrit (black)	Iron deficiency anemia Low energy level Decreased oxygen-carrying capacity	Fetal death Prematurity Low birth weight
Hypertension	↑ Vasospasm ↑ Risk irritability of central nervous system → Convulsions ↑ Risk cerebrovascular accident ↑ Risk renal damage	↓ Placental perfusion → Low birth weight Preterm birth
Thyroid disorder Hypothyroidism	↑ Infertility ↓ Basal metabolic rate goiter, myxedema	↑ Spontaneous abortion ↑ Risk congenital goiter Mental retardation → cretinism ↑ Incidence congenital anomalies
Hyperthyroidism	↑ Risk postpartum hemorrhage ↑ Risk preeclampsia Danger of thyroid storm	↑ Incidence preterm birth ↑ Tendency to thyrotoxicosis
Renal disease (moderate to severe)	↑ Risk renal failure	↑ Risk IUGR ↑ Risk preterm birth
Exposure to diethylstilbestrol	↑ Infertility, spontaneous abortion ↑ Cervical incompetence	↑ Spontaneous abortion ↑ Risk preterm birth

Table continued on following page

Table 2–1
PRENATAL HIGH-RISK FACTORS (Continued)

Factor	Maternal Implications	Fetal/Neonatal Implications
OBSTETRIC CONSIDERATIONS		
Previous Pregnancy		
Stillborn	↑ Emotional/psychologic distress	↑ Risk IUGR ↑ Risk preterm birth
Habitual abortion	↑ Emotional/psychologic distress ↑ Possibility diagnostic study	↑ Risk abortion
Cesarean birth	↑ Possibility repeated cesarean birth	↑ Risk preterm birth ↑ Risk respiratory distress
Rh or blood group sensitization	↑ Financial expenditure for testing	Hydrops fetalis Icterus gravis Neonatal anemia Kernicterus Hypoglycemia
Large baby	↑ Risk cesarean birth ↑ Risk gestational diabetes	Birth injury Hypoglycemia
Current Pregnancy		
Rubella (first trimester)		Congenital heart disease Cataracts Nerve deafness Bone lesions Prolonged virus shedding
Rubella (second trimester)		Hepatitis Thrombocytopenia
Cytomegalovirus		IUGR Encephalopathy
Herpesvirus type 2	Severe discomfort Concern about possibility of cesarean birth, fetal infection	Neonatal herpesvirus type 2 Hepatitis with jaundice Neurologic abnormalities
Syphilis	↑ Incidence abortion	↑ Fetal death Congenital syphilis
Abruptio placentae and placenta previa	↑ Risk hemorrhage Bed rest Extended hospitalization	Fetal/neonatal anemia Intrauterine hemorrhage ↑ Fetal death
Preeclampsia/eclampsia (pregnancy-induced hypertension)	See hypertension	↓ Placental perfusion → Low birth weight
Multiple gestation	↑ Risk postpartum hemorrhage	↑ Risk preterm birth ↑ Risk fetal death
Elevated hematocrit > 41% (white) > 38% (black)	Increased viscosity of blood	Fetal death rate 5 times normal rate
Spontaneous premature rupture of membranes	↑ Uterine infection	↑ Risk preterm birth ↑ Fetal death

four tissue layers; it thins to three layers after 20 weeks (Moore and Persaud, 1993).

D. **Placental transport mechanisms.** These mechanisms, including passive and facilitated diffusion, are affected by a number of factors (Martin and Gingerich, 1976; Moore and Persaud, 1993):
1. Placental area.
    a. To supply the increased growth needs of the fetus, the placenta normally increases in size as the pregnancy advances.
    b. A placenta that is not keeping pace with fetal growth or that has decreased

functional area as a result of infarct or separation does not allow optimal transport of materials between fetus and mother.

   c. The outcome of decreased functional placental area can include a decrease in fetal growth, fetal or neonatal distress, and even fetal or neonatal death.

2. Concentration gradient.

   a. Passive and facilitated diffusion of unbound substances dissolved in maternal and fetal plasma occurs in the direction of lesser concentration.

   b. The greater the concentration gradient, the faster the rate of diffusion will be.

   c. Concentration gradients are maintained when dissolved substances are removed from the plasma by metabolism, cellular uptake, or excretion. For example, the excretion of CO_2 from the maternal lungs maintains the concentration gradient for CO_2, permitting fetal plasma CO_2 to cross from fetal plasma to maternal plasma. Inefficient maternal excretion of CO_2 may lead to maternal respiratory acidosis and fetal acidosis.

3. Diffusing distance.

   a. The greater the distance between maternal and fetal blood in the placenta, the slower the diffusion rate of substances will be.

   b. Any edema that develops in the placental villi increases the distance between the fetal capillaries within the villi and the maternal arterial blood in the intervillous spaces, thus slowing the diffusion rate of substances between the maternal and fetal circulations.

   c. Edema of villi may occur in:

     (1) Maternal diabetes.

     (2) Transplacental infections.

     (3) Erythroblastosis fetalis.

     (4) Twin-to-twin transfusion syndrome (donor twin).

     (5) Fetal congestive heart failure.

   d. Thinning of the placental membrane in the second half of pregnancy decreases diffusing distance, thus increasing functional efficiency of the placenta. However, this change also facilitates the passage of drugs in pregnancy and the intrapartum period.

4. Uteroplacental blood flow.

   a. Approximately 73–80% of uterine blood flow reaches the placenta.

   b. Decreased blood flow to the uterus or within the intervillous spaces will decrease the transport of substances to and from the fetus.

   c. Causes of decreased uteroplacental blood flow include:

     (1) Maternal vasoconstriction in hypertension, cocaine abuse, diabetic vasculopathy, and smoking.

     (2) Decreased maternal cardiac output in supine hypotension.

     (3) Decreased maternal blood flow in intervillous spaces resulting from edema of placental villi.

     (4) Hypertonic uterine contractions.

     (5) Severe maternal physical stress.

     (6) Degenerative placental changes near term.

5. Fetal factors.

   a. Fetal tachycardia, often seen with fetal hypoxia, is analogous to an adult's "blowing off CO_2"; the increased heart rate increases the delivery of CO_2 to the placenta for diffusion to the maternal circulation.

   b. Conversely, fetal bradycardia resulting from hypoxia or anoxia causes an increased CO_2 level.

   c. Umbilical cord compression leads to CO_2 accumulation and acidosis.

   d. Fetal pH during labor is usually 0.1–0.15 unit less than the maternal pH; this difference increases the transport of acidophilic substances from the mother to the fetus and reduces albumin binding of drugs, resulting in more free drug in the fetal bloodstream.

Conditions Related to the Antepartum Period

PREECLAMPSIA AND ECLAMPSIA

Hypertension in pregnancy, including preeclampsia, eclampsia, and chronic hypertension, is a major cause of maternal-fetal morbidity and death in the United States (Roberts, 1994). The main pathophysiologic events in preeclampsia are vasospasm, hematologic changes, deposition of fibrin and fibrinogen in vessels, hypovolemia resulting from fluid shifts, and increased CNS irritability.

A. **Incidence.** 5% of all pregnancies (Reeder, Martin, and Koniak-Griffin, 1997).

B. **Etiology/predisposing factors.**

1. The exact cause of preeclampsia and eclampsia has not been determined, although current theories involve an immunologic basis, dietary deficiencies or excesses, and lack of cardiovascular adaptation (Sibai, 1996).
2. Preeclampsia and eclampsia associated with primigravidas, younger and older women, family history of preeclampsia or previous personal history of severe preeclampsia, low socioeconomic class, malnutrition and low weight gain in pregnancy, obesity, diabetes, chronic hypertensive or renal disease, multifetal gestation or large fetus, hydatidiform mole, fetal hydrops, and trisomy 13 (Reeder et al., 1997; Sibai, 1996; Varney, 1997).

C. **Clinical presentation.**

1. Elevated blood pressure (BP) after week 20 of pregnancy: either a BP of 140/90 mm Hg or above, or a rise of 30 mm Hg systolic and/or 15 mm Hg diastolic or more during the early pregnancy baseline.
2. Edema due to salt retention and decreased plasma colloid osmotic pressure, evidenced by sudden and excessive weight gain.
3. Proteinuria due to decreased renal perfusion resulting in development of glomerular capillary endotheliosis.
4. Other signs and symptoms: headache, hyperreflexia with clonus, visual and retinal changes, irritability, nausea and vomiting, epigastric pain, dyspnea, and oliguria.

D. **Potential complications.**

1. Maternal.
   a. Eclampsia (grand mal seizure).
   b. Cardiopulmonary failure.
   c. Hepatic rupture.
   d. Cerebrovascular accident.
   e. Renal cortical necrosis.
   f. Disseminated intravascular coagulation.
   g. HELLP syndrome (*h*emolysis, *e*levated *l*iver function test results, and *l*ow *p*latelet count).
   h. Retinal detachment.
2. Placental/fetal.
   a. Premature placental aging, placental infarction, and decrease in amniotic fluid.
   b. Abruptio placentae in 2–10% of cases (Reeder et al., 1997).
   c. Intrauterine growth retardation (IUGR) resulting from decreased placental blood flow.
   d. Fetal distress.
   e. Preterm delivery.

E. **Assessment and management.**

1. Severe preeclampsia.

a. Hospitalization, with complete bed rest in left lateral recumbent position.

b. Limitation of stimuli such as noise and visitors.

c. Seizure precautions.

d. Frequent assessments of the cardiopulmonary, neurologic, hepatic, renal, and hematopoietic systems for signs and symptoms of progression.

e. High-protein diet (1.5 g/kg per day) with moderate sodium intake (Ladewig, London, and Olds, 1998).

f. Supportive care, including teaching and emotional support of the woman and her family.

g. Laboratory work: complete blood cell count (CBC), liver enzymes, blood urea nitrogen, uric acid, serum creatinine, and 24-hour urinary protein.

h. Placental-fetal function tests: fetal movement; ultrasonography to determine fetal age and detect IUGR; serial nonstress tests, contraction stress tests, biophysical profile, and/or serum estriol levels to detect uteroplacental insufficiency; and amniocentesis to determine fetal lung maturity.

i. Drugs.
   (1) Use of IV magnesium sulfate ($MgSO_4$) as a CNS depressant to prevent convulsions. Monitor fetal heart for changes in short-term cardiac variability.
   (2) Sedation with phenobarbital. Nonstress test may be nonreactive as a result of sedation. Monitor fetal heart for loss of short-term variability.
   (3) Use of hydralazine (Apresoline) for antihypertensive effect. Monitor fetus for signs of hypoxia (tachycardia, bradycardia, late decelerations), which can occur with a sudden decrease in maternal BP.
   (4) Use of labetalol hydrochloride as an antihypertensive agent and to increase uteroplacental perfusion (Clark, Cotton, Hankins, and Phelan, 1994). Monitor fetus for transient bradycardia (Burke and Poole, 1996).
   (5) Low-dose aspirin therapy for women identified as being at risk of having preeclampsia is a more recent pharmacologic therapy. However, it has been shown to increase the incidence of abruptio placentae (Sibai, 1996).

j. Monitoring of fetus for late decelerations caused by decreased uterine perfusion.

k. Delivery by induction or cesarean procedure if fetus is mature or if worsening maternal condition warrants.

2. Eclampsia.
   a. Immediate notification of physician or midwife.
   b. Safety measures for woman during and after convulsion.
   c. Support of respirations with airway, oxygen, and suctioning.
   d. Monitor fetal heart for bradycardia, loss of short-term variability, and late decelerations (Sibai, 1996).
   e. Continuous maternal assessment, including assessment for abruptio placentae.
   f. Laboratory work: CBC, clot observation, serum creatinine, liver function tests, fibrinogen, arterial blood gases, and electrolytes (Sibai, 1996).
   g. Use of IV $MgSO_4$ or diazepam (Valium).
   h. Delivery by induction or cesarean procedure when woman and fetus recover.

3. Assessment of newborn infant for:
   a. IUGR.
   b. Preterm gestational age.
   c. Hypoxia and acidosis.
   d. Specific drug effects on newborn infant:
      (1) Signs of hypermagnesemia when maternal administration of high doses

of $MgSO_4$ occurs near the time of delivery: weakness, lethargy, hypotonia, flaccidity, respiratory depression, poor suck, decrease in gastrointestinal motility, hypotension, urinary retention, and increase in atrioventricular and ventricular conduction.

(2) Hypothermia with maternal administration of diazepam.

(3) Poor suck, decrease in responsiveness, and respiratory depression with maternal administration of phenobarbital.

(4) Thrombocytopenia with maternal administration of hydralazine.

(5) Hypotension, bradycardia, and hypoglycemia with maternal administration of labetalol (Burke and Poole, 1996).

DIABETES MELLITUS

The woman with insulin-dependent diabetes who becomes pregnant and the pregnant woman in whom gestational diabetes develops are at risk during the antepartum period because of altered carbohydrate metabolism. The fetus/neonate is therefore also at risk. Strict control of maternal blood glucose concentration and anticipatory management of the newborn infant are important elements of perinatal care.

A. **Incidence.** 2–3% of all pregnancies. Of these women, 90% have gestational diabetes (Landon, 1996). Another estimate is that gestational diabetes occurs in 1–3% of pregnant women (Barger and Fein, 1997).

B. **Etiology/predisposing factors in gestational diabetes.**

1. In the second half of pregnancy, secretion of estrogen, progesterone, and human placental lactogen increases cellular resistance to insulin. The pancreas of the woman who is predisposed to diabetes cannot meet the increased demand for insulin, and hyperglycemia results.
2. Gestational diabetes is associated with maternal obesity; a family history of diabetes; age more than 40 years; multiparity; and a history of having had an infant who was large for gestational age (LGA), who had a congenital anomaly, whose gestation resulted in hydramnios, or who was stillborn.

C. **Clinical presentation in gestational diabetes.**

1. Polyuria, polydipsia, polyphagia, and excessive weight gain (Barger and Fein, 1997).
2. Abnormally high glucose levels on glucose tolerance tests.

D. **Potential complications.**

1. Maternal.
   a. Hypoglycemic reactions in the first trimester.
   b. Ketoacidosis in the second and third trimesters.
   c. Progression of vasculopathy, nephropathy, and retinopathy with preexisting diabetes.
   d. Hydramnios.
   e. Preeclampsia.
   f. Anemia.
   g. Infections such as monilial vaginitis and urinary tract infections.
2. Fetal/neonatal.
   a. Macrosomia (weight greater than 4000 g) with possible traumatic vaginal delivery. IUGR when the mother has microvascular disease, hypertension, or nephropathy (Enkin, Keirse, Renfrew, and Neilson, 1995).
   b. Fetal death.
   c. Respiratory distress syndrome.
   d. Hypoglycemia, hypocalcemia, and hypomagnesemia.

    e. Polycythemia, hyperviscosity, and hyperbilirubinemia.

    f. Cardiomyopathy with congestive heart failure.

    g. Congenital malformation as a consequence of poorly controlled preexisting diabetes: renal and CNS anomalies, caudal regression syndrome, facial clefts, patent ductus arteriosus, transposition of the great vessels, ventricular septal defect, and small left colon syndrome. The threefold increase in incidence of congenital anomalies can be reduced significantly by preconception control of blood glucose levels (Enkin et al., 1995).

E. **Assessment and management.**

1. In preexisting diabetes:

    a. Preconception counseling is provided, with optimal control of blood glucose levels and use of insulin if necessary (oral hypoglycemic agents are considered teratogenic).

    b. Glycosylated hemoglobin tests may be performed before conception and during the pregnancy to assess glucose control during the previous 1–2 months. Levels beyond the normal range are associated with increased congenital anomalies (Barger and Fein, 1997).

    c. Home blood glucose monitoring, diet, and three or more daily injections of insulin are prescribed to maintain tight control of the blood glucose concentration (98–117 mg/dL), which is associated with decreased risk of macrosomia, perinatal death, and congenital malformations, as well as progressive maternal nephropathy and retinopathy (Enkin et al., 1995).

    d. Renal function tests are performed if hypertension or proteinuria develops. Retinoscopy every trimester in women with long-standing diabetes (Enkin et al., 1995).

    e. Weekly prenatal visits are made after 28 weeks, with fetal assessment by means of nonstress test, contraction stress test, and fetal activity determination.

    f. Early ultrasonography is performed to establish gestational age if necessary, with detailed ultrasonography at 20–24 weeks to detect malformations and late second- and third-trimester sonograms to establish fetal growth. Fetal echocardiography is also recommended (Enkin et al., 1995).

    g. Insulin IV drip is given during labor, with hourly measurement of blood glucose to control blood glucose levels at 60–90 mg/dL.

    h. For women with poorly regulated diabetes, amniocentesis is performed to determine the lecithin/sphingomyelin (L/S) ratio and the presence of phosphatidylglycerol before any decision is made about induction of labor. Delivery is accomplished before term if maternal or fetal complications develop, and immediate delivery by cesarean procedure if fetal distress occurs.

2. In gestational diabetes:

    a. Many authorities recommend that pregnant women with no initial risk factors be screened for gestational diabetes at 28 weeks by determining the fasting blood glucose level and by giving a 1- to 2-hour glucose screening test, followed by a 3-hour 100 g glucose tolerance test if results of the first test are positive (Varney and Reedy, 1997). However, a recent review of randomized, controlled trials does not support this recommendation (Enkin et al., 1995).

    b. Recommend a 2000–2500 calorie diet with no simple carbohydrates.

    c. Assess glucose levels every 2 weeks.

    d. Perform fetal assessment by determining estriol levels and giving a nonstress test twice a week, beginning at 32 weeks. Delivery by induction is delayed until 40–42 weeks if possible (Varney and Reedy, 1997).

3. In neonate:

    a. Assess for gestational age and size (LGA or IUGR).

b. Assess for:
   (1) Respiratory distress.
   (2) Hypoglycemia, hypocalcemia, and hypomagnesemia.
   (3) Polycythemia and hyperviscosity.
   (4) Complications resulting from decreased blood flow, erythrocyte hemolysis, and thrombosis.
   (5) Congenital malformations.
   (6) Birth injuries: fractured clavicles, intracranial bleeding, facial nerve paralysis, brachial palsy, and skull fractures.

Conditions Related to Intrapartum Period

PRETERM LABOR

Preterm labor is defined as labor occurring before week 37 of pregnancy and that results in cervical changes and/or ruptured membranes (Freda and Patterson, 1994). If preterm labor is recognized in time, measures can be taken to stop the contractions. The prognosis for the fetus improves with each week of pregnancy gained.

A. **Incidence.** About 7–9% of all babies in the United States are born before term. Some of these births are necessitated by medical complications, not preterm labor (Freda and Patterson, 1994).

B. **Etiology/predisposing factors.**

1. The exact cause of preterm labor is unknown, although bacterial vaginosis has been implicated in recent studies (Hillier et al., 1995).
2. A number of factors have been associated with an increased incidence of preterm labor: socioeconomic effects (lower socioeconomic status, nonwhite race, poor nutrition, inadequate prenatal care), medical/obstetric history (preterm labor or birth, one or more midtrimester pregnancy losses, short interpregnancy interval, multifetal gestation, uterine anomalies and incompetent cervix, urinary and genital tract infections, polyhydramnios, abruptio placentae, and placenta previa), and lifestyle factors (use of alcohol, cigarettes, and illicit drugs such as cocaine, and stressful work or personal situations) (Varney, 1997).
3. Risk scoring systems, designed to screen women during pregnancy, have only a limited ability to predict preterm labor sensitively. Half of the women who give birth before term do not have any known risk factors (Iams, 1996).

C. **Clinical presentation.**

1. Painless or painful uterine contractions.
2. Low, dull, intermittent or constant backache.
3. Intermittent or constant menstruallike cramping.
4. Intermittent pelvic pressure that may extend along the inner thigh.
5. Abdominal cramps, which may be accompanied by diarrhea.
6. Increased vaginal discharge, which may be mucoid, watery, or slightly bloody.
7. Spontaneous premature rupture of membranes.
8. A generalized feeling that something is wrong.
9. Progressive cervical effacement and dilation unless intervention is performed.

D. **Potential complications.**

1. Maternal.
   a. No particular physical complications other than adverse reactions from tocolytic agents.
   b. Emotional stress and financial problems.

2. Fetal/neonatal.
   a. Preterm birth with an increase in neonatal morbidity and death.
   b. Adverse reactions to tocolytic agents (see below).

E. **Assessment and management.**

1. Screening of pregnant women at the first and subsequent prenatal visits for preterm labor risk factors.
2. Teaching *all* pregnant women the symptoms of preterm labor and the actions to take if they occur (lie down on the left side and drink several glasses of fluid; report to physician or midwife if contractions are still occurring after 1 hour).
3. Helping high-risk women modify their risk factors and take measures to prevent preterm labor (e.g., stop smoking, improve nutrition and hydration, treat infections, decrease work hours and stress, increase bed rest, and avoid nipple preparation that initiates signs of preterm labor).
4. Calcium supplementation may significantly reduce the risk of preterm birth (Enkin et al., 1995).
5. Gentle examination of the cervix of high-risk women at weekly or biweekly prenatal visits to detect changes that are indicative of impending preterm labor. Transvaginal ultrasonography is being used in some centers to detect cervical changes (Iams, 1996).
6. For high-risk women, use of a home contraction monitoring system, with daily telephone counseling from a nurse to increase early diagnosis of preterm labor and provide psychosocial support, is commonly used. However, no definitive proof exists that the monitoring device itself improves neonatal outcome (Enkin et al., 1995).
7. Treatment decisions may be based on the results of a fetal fibronectin test performed on vaginal secretions. The presence of this substance indicates that a woman is at high risk of having a preterm birth within 7–14 days (Escher-Davis, 1996).
8. Episodes of preterm labor may be treated with hospitalization, hydration with IV fluid, bed rest in the left lateral position, sedation, and corticosteroid therapy to reduce the incidence of neonatal morbidity and death from respiratory distress syndrome (Committee on Obstetric Practice, 1994).
9. When appropriate and not contraindicated, use of one of the following drug therapies may prolong pregnancy 24 hours or more, allowing enough time for concurrent corticosteroid therapy to benefit the fetus (Varney, 1997) and/or for transfer of the mother to a hospital with a level III nursery (Enkin et al., 1995):
   a. Ritodrine (Yutopar), given by IV drip, inhibits uterine contractility. Potential fetal/neonatal side effects include tachycardia, hyperglycemia, hypocalcemia, irritability, hypotension, and paralytic ileus (Freda and Patterson, 1994).
   b. $MgSO_4$ can be given by IV drip for uterine relaxation. Monitor the fetus for loss of cardiac variability and the neonate for respiratory depression, hypocalcemia, hypotonia, and drowsiness (Wheeler, 1994).
   c. Terbutaline (Brethine) can be given by IV drip, subcutaneously, or via a subcutaneous pump. For long-term use at home, women can be taught to give themselves terbutaline in programmed continuous and bolus doses via a miniature subcutaneous automatic infusion pump, in conjunction with a home contraction monitoring system. Potential fetal/neonatal side effects are the same as for ritodrine.
   d. Nifedipine, a calcium-channel blocker, is given orally or sublingually. No fetal side effects have been reported as yet (MacMullen, Brucker, and Zwelling, 1997).
10. For women with preterm rupture of the membranes, cultures should be

grown for group B streptococcus and antibiotics administered prophylactically to prevent infection with group B streptococcus in the newborn infant (Iams, 1996).
11. If the measures noted above are not successful, and the cervix continues to efface and dilate, the following measures are important:
    a. To allow the amniotic fluid to cushion the fetal skull, no rupture of the membranes is performed.
    b. The head is delivered in a slow, controlled fashion.
    c. Cesarean delivery is often suggested for the preterm fetus with a breech presentation because of the risk of cord prolapse and the potential risk of difficult delivery of the head.

ABRUPTIO PLACENTAE

In abruptio placentae the placenta separates suddenly and prematurely from the uterine wall during pregnancy or labor. It is a common cause of bleeding in the second half of pregnancy.

A. **Incidence.** 1 in 120 pregnancies, typically before the start of labor (Benedetti, 1996).

B. **Etiology/predisposing factors.**

1. The cause of abruptio placentae has not been definitively established, but there is a high correlation with hypertensive disorders during pregnancy, cocaine and crack use, and trauma.
2. Other factors that are considered predisposing include uterine leiomyomas or anomalies, polyhydramnios and multiple pregnancy, history of previous abruption, and maternal cigarette smoking and poor weight gain.

C. **Clinical presentation.**

1. Types.
    a. Marginal.
    b. Central.
    c. Complete.
2. Maternal signs and symptoms.
    a. Sharp, continuous abdominal pain.
    b. Boardlike and tender abdomen.
    c. Dark or bright red vaginal bleeding (unless the bleeding is concealed behind the placenta), ranging from spotting to frank hemorrhage.
    d. Uterine hyperactivity.
    e. Enlargement of the uterus as blood accumulates.
3. Fetal signs (Varney and Reedy, 1997).
    a. Loss of fetal heart tones or movement.
    b. Tachycardia.
    c. Late or variable decelerations.
    d. Decreased fetal heart rate variability.
    e. Sinusoidal pattern.

D. **Potential complications.**

1. Maternal.
    a. Anemia.
    b. Hypovolemic shock, sometimes resulting in anterior pituitary necrosis (Sheehan's syndrome) (Landon, 1996).
    c. Couvelaire uterus (blood forced between the muscle fibers of the uterus).
    d. Disseminated intravascular coagulation.

     e. Kidney necrosis leading to renal shutdown.
     f. Death.
2. Fetal/neonatal.
     a. Anemia.
     b. Hypoxia and asphyxia.
     c. Hypovolemia.
     d. Neurobehavioral problems such as cerebral palsy (Benedetti, 1996).
     e. 25–30% incidence of death (Benedetti, 1996).

E. **Assessment and management.**

1. Assessment if fetus is stable and maternal hematologic status can be maintained:
     a. Bed rest in left lateral position, close assessment of abdomen for rigidity and pain, and close assessment of vaginal bleeding.
     b. Monitoring of maternal vital signs and continuous monitoring of fetal heart for rate, decelerations, and variability.
     c. Ultrasonography to locate placenta and determine degree of placental separation and location of hematoma (Benedetti, 1996).
     d. Placement of IV line with large-gauge intracatheter for administration of fluids and blood products.
     e. Possible collection of urine for drug screening.
     f. Possible induction of labor and/or vaginal delivery.
2. Preparation for cesarean delivery if fetal distress or severe hemorrhage occurs:
     a. Inform and support parents and ensure that "surgical consent" is obtained.
     b. Order laboratory tests (CBC, type and cross-match blood, coagulation studies).
     c. Prepare abdomen and insert urinary catheter.
     d. Notify NICU and pediatrician.

PLACENTA PREVIA

    Placenta previa is a placenta that is implanted near the cervix (marginal) or, in varying degrees (partial or total), over the cervix. Cervical dilation at or near term is accompanied by bleeding from the placenta. Placenta previa is a common cause of bleeding in the second half of pregnancy.

A. **Incidence.** 1 in 200 pregnancies (Benedetti, 1996).

B. **Etiology/predisposing factors.**

1. The precise cause of placenta previa is unknown, but it occurs most frequently in multiparous and older women.
2. Other associated and predisposing factors include previous placenta previa, history of low-segment cesarean delivery, history of myomectomy or postpartum endometritis, and increased placental size.

C. **Clinical presentation.**

1. Bright red, painless vaginal bleeding. Although the first bleeding episode may be slight in amount, more blood is usually lost in subsequent episodes.
2. Uterine contractions in 20% of cases, but otherwise the uterus is usually soft and nontender (Benedetti, 1996).
3. Finding on ultrasonography at 17 weeks' gestation in 5–15% of pregnant women, with resolution by term 90% of the time (Benedetti, 1996).
4. Failure of presenting part of fetus to become engaged. Fetus may lie transversely or be in breech position.

D. **Potential complications.**

1. Maternal.
   a. Anemia.
   b. Hypovolemic shock.
   c. Endometritis.
   d. Decreased contractile strength of the lower uterine segment, which can lead to postpartum hemorrhage and need for hysterectomy.
2. Fetal/neonatal (White and Poole, 1996).
   a. Hypoxia and asphyxia.
   b. IUGR.
   c. Fetal hemorrhage and death.
   d. Prematurity.
   e. Infection.

E. **Assessment and management.**

1. Marginal or partial placenta previa and low-lying placenta with minimal bleeding are managed conservatively:
   a. Ultrasonography to confirm diagnosis (95% accuracy) and to rule out IUGR.
   b. Bed rest at home or in the hospital with no vaginal examinations.
   c. Avoidance of intercourse and orgasm, which can cause uterine contractions (Varney and Reedy, 1997).
   d. Weekly nonstress test or contraction stress test.
   e. If fetus is mature, possible vaginal examination by physician under double setup (preparation for immediate cesarean delivery). Note that the use of ultrasonography has generally obviated the use of the double setup. Vaginal delivery can be accomplished if bleeding is minimal.
2. Partial or total placenta previa with greater amounts of bleeding are handled as noted above, except that vaginal delivery may not be possible. In addition:
   a. Frequent assessment of vaginal bleeding, with pad counts and/or weighing of pads.
   b. Frequent assessment of maternal vital signs and fetal heart tones, and palpation of abdomen.
   c. Semi-Fowler's position to allow fetus to compress placenta.
   d. Laboratory work: CBC, type and cross-match for possible blood transfusion.
   e. With significant bleeding, placement of IV line with large-gauge intracatheter for blood administration.
   f. Method of delivery:
      (1) Vaginal delivery is performed only if less than 30% of placenta overlies cervix and bleeding remains minimal. Artificial rupture of membranes may be performed to allow presenting part of fetus to compress placental site.
      (2) If a greater degree of placenta previa is present or if bleeding is significant, cesarean delivery is performed.

UMBILICAL CORD PROLAPSE

Umbilical cord prolapse is an event that is life threatening to the fetus and requires immediate and effective management by the nurse. It occurs when the cord falls below the presenting part or is compressed between the presenting part and the pelvis or cervix.

A. **Incidence.** Estimated to occur in 1 of 275 births (about 0.36%) (Dildy and Clark, 1993).

B. **Etiology/predisposing factors.**

1. The fetal presenting part does not fill the pelvic inlet well, and the cord slips past it, often when the membranes rupture.
2. Predisposing factors include malposition (transverse lie and breech presentation), premature or small-for-gestational-age fetus, multifetal pregnancy, polyhydramnios, long cord, cephalopelvic disproportion that prevents fetal engagement, lack of engagement before the onset of labor (as is common with multiparous women) (MacMullen et al., 1997), and compound presentation (Seeds and Walsh, 1996).

C. **Clinical presentation.**

1. Cord is protruding from vagina or is palpable on vaginal examination.
2. In an occult prolapse, cord is not visible or palpable but is located between the presenting part and the pelvis or cervix.
3. Station of presenting part is 0 to −4 cm, and membranes are often ruptured.
4. Fetal heart rate accelerates to 180–200 bpm and then decreases rapidly if adequate treatment is not given. With occult prolapse, variable fetal decelerations may precede these changes.

D. **Potential complications.**

1. Maternal.
   a. Trauma to the birth canal from rapid forceps delivery.
   b. General anesthesia resulting in uterine atony with subsequent postpartum bleeding.
   c. Blood loss from cesarean delivery.
2. Fetal/neonatal.
   a. Perinatal mortality rate increases as increased time elapses between cord prolapse and birth.
   b. Fetal anoxia leading to long-range neurologic complications.
   c. Neonatal infection.

E. **Assessment and management.**

1. Assessments on admission to labor and delivery.
   a. Presenting part and its station.
   b. Dilation of cervix.
   c. Status of membranes.
   d. Estimation of fetal weight and fetal heart rate.
   e. Review of prenatal record for evidence of polyhydramnios.
2. Assessment for presence of polyhydramnios or lack of engagement of presenting part. Ambulation during labor and artificial rupture of membranes may be contraindicated in these and other situations.
3. Assessment after artificial or spontaneous rupture of membranes.
   a. Monitor fetal heart for rate and variable decelerations.
   b. Perform vaginal examination to detect prolapse.
4. If prolapse has occurred:
   a. Keep examining hand in vagina to push presenting part away from cord until delivery of fetus. An alternative measure is to fill the mother's bladder with sterile saline solution to elevate the fetal presenting part so that it is off the cord (Griese and Prickett, 1993).
   b. Have assistant help woman into knee-chest or Trendelenburg's position, with hips elevated and head down.
   c. Have oxygen administered to woman.
   d. Monitor fetal heart rate continuously and palpate cord lightly for continued pulsation.
   e. Tocolytic agents may be used.
   f. For immediate delivery, physician may use internal podalic version to turn fetus to a breech position if woman's cervix is fully dilated; emergency

cesarean delivery may be preferable, especially if cervix is not fully dilated and fetal heart rate is affected.

    g. Provide continuous emotional support of parents.

SHOULDER DYSTOCIA

Shoulder dystocia is defined as a difficult delivery in which the physician or midwife is unable to deliver the shoulders of the infant by the usual maneuvers after delivery of the head.

A. **Incidence.** 0.15–1.7%, with an increased incidence in babies weighing more than 4000–4500 g (Piper and McDonald, 1994).

B. **Etiology/predisposing factors.**

1. The fetal shoulders are too broad to be delivered between the symphysis pubis and the sacrum.
2. Predisposing factors include maternal obesity, excessive weight gain, oversized infant, history of large siblings, maternal diabetes, contracted pelvic outlet, and postdates pregnancy (Varney, 1997).

C. **Clinical presentation.**

1. Slow active phase of labor.
2. Second stage longer than 2 hours, with slow descent of head.
3. After delivery of the head, it recoils against the perineum and restitution does not occur ("turtling"). The usual traction from below, with fundal pressure, is not successful in delivering the baby.

D. **Complications.**

1. Maternal.
   a. Vaginal or perineal lacerations.
   b. Ruptured uterus.
   c. Postpartum hemorrhage or infection.
   d. Bladder trauma.
2. Fetal/neonatal.
   a. Birth injuries such as brachial palsy or fractured clavicle or humerus (White and Poole, 1996).
   b. Anoxia and brain damage.
   c. Intrapartum or neonatal death.

E. **Assessment and management.**

1. Anticipate shoulder dystocia if descent of the head is slow and estimated weight is large. Make sure the woman's bladder is empty before birth occurs (White and Poole, 1996).
2. If shoulder dystocia occurs, physician or midwife will:
   a. Clear infant's airway.
   b. Perform large episiotomy if perineal muscles are tight (Varney, 1997).
   c. Consider anesthesia to relax woman's perineal muscles.
   d. Perform one or several maneuvers to expedite delivery:
      (1) Use the McRoberts maneuver (an exaggerated lithotomy position), turn the woman on all fours to widen the pelvic outlet, or turn the woman on her side to free the sacrum (Varney, 1997).
      (2) Manually rotate shoulders from the anteroposterior to the oblique diameter in the pelvis and have suprapubic pressure exerted to deliver anterior shoulder.
      (3) Use corkscrew maneuver, in which both hands are inserted internally to rotate the posterior shoulder to the anterior position for delivery under

the pubic bone, with the maneuver repeated for the other shoulder (Piper and McDonald, 1994).
  (4) Extract posterior shoulder and arm.
  (5) Fracturing the clavicle to collapse the diameter of the shoulders is necessary on rare occasions (Enkin et al., 1995).
  (6) The Zavanelli maneuver can be used to push the fetal head back into the vagina so that a cesarean delivery can be performed, but it is rarely used (MacMullen et al., 1997).

BREECH DELIVERY

A. **Incidence.** 3–4% of all pregnancies after 37 weeks (Goer, 1995). Incidence increases in multiple gestation and in preterm birth.

B. **Etiology/predisposing factors.**
1. Maternal.
   a. High multiparity with uterine relaxation.
   b. Polyhydramnios with free movement of fetus.
   c. Oligohydramnios with resultant lack of ability of fetus to move from breech position common in second trimester.
   d. Uterine anomalies and leiomyomas.
   e. Contracted pelvis.
2. Placental/fetal.
   a. Placenta previa.
   b. Multiple gestation.
   c. Hydrocephalus or anencephaly or other fetal anomalies.
   d. Fetal death.
   e. Large fetus or preterm fetus.
   f. Cerebral palsy and hip dysplasia (Goer, 1995).

C. **Clinical presentation.**
1. Woman feels fetus kicking in lower abdomen.
2. Fetal heart sounds are heard loudest above umbilicus.
3. Use of Leopold's maneuvers indicates head is in fundal area and breech is in pelvis.
4. On bimanual examination, it is found that the presenting part is soft, no fontanelles are felt, and the genitalia may be identified.

D. **Complications.**
1. Maternal.
   a. Lacerations of the birth canal may occur if the delivery is rapid and forceful.
   b. Usual maternal morbidity is 25–40% if cesarean delivery is performed.
2. Fetal/neonatal complications resulting from vaginal delivery.
   a. Prolapsed cord.
   b. Asphyxia from slow delivery of fetal head or from compression of umbilical cord between pelvis and head during delivery.
   c. Aspiration of amniotic fluid with potential for meconium aspiration syndrome.
   d. Vertebral injury, especially if fetal head is hyperextended (Seeds and Walsh, 1996).
3. Fetal/neonatal complications: incidence is similar in vaginal- and cesarean-born breech babies (Goer, 1995).
   a. Spasticity and cerebral palsy.
   b. Perinatal asphyxia.
   c. Intracranial hemorrhage and skull fractures.

    d. Neonatal seizures.

    e. Developmental delays and mental retardation.

E. **Assessment and management.**

1. A procedure that may help the fetus turn from breech to cephalic presentation is postural exercise in which the woman assumes either the knee-chest or an elevated-hips posture several times a day until the fetus turns (Enkin et al., 1995).

2. The physician may attempt external cephalic version after 37 weeks with or without the use of a uterine relaxant and, if the fetus remains in a cephalic presentation, vaginal delivery (Enkin et al., 1995).

3. Assessments on admission to labor and delivery service.

    a. Perform Leopold's maneuvers and vaginal examination to determine presentation.

    b. Report breech presentation immediately to physician or midwife.

4. Ultrasonography may be ordered to confirm breech presentation, determine degree of flexion of fetal head, evaluate size of fetal head, estimate fetal weight, diagnose fetal anomalies, and locate placenta.

5. A trial of labor for vaginal delivery may be attempted.

    a. The fetus must be between 36 and 42 weeks of gestational age, the fetal position must be a frank or complete breech with the head flexed, and the pelvis must be adequate.

    b. The estimated fetal weight must be less than 3500 g (MacMullen et al., 1997), and no other indications for cesarean delivery must exist.

    c. The nurse should perform, at the time of rupture of the membranes, a vaginal examination to check for prolapsed cord and should monitor the fetal heart tones closely.

    d. Meconium in the amniotic fluid is not necessarily a sign of fetal hypoxia when the fetus is in a breech position. However, meconium aspiration at the time of delivery may be a serious complication.

6. With vaginal delivery, the woman will probably receive a large episiotomy, and Piper's forceps may be used to deliver the baby's head. The nurse may be asked to perform suprapubic pressure to keep the baby's head flexed while the physician or midwife performs certain maneuvers during the delivery.

7. Many physicians will perform cesarean delivery when the fetus is breech in these situations: primigravida, small pelvis, premature rupture of membranes, large fetus, hyperextension of head, footling breech, and preterm fetus.

8. A manual breech extraction with the woman under deep anesthesia may be performed if fetal distress occurs and cesarean delivery cannot be performed immediately.

9. Assessment of the neonate may reveal:

    a. Edema of the external genitalia.

    b. A continuation of the frank breech position for a while after the birth.

    c. Congenital hip dislocation, which is increased in incidence with breech presentation.

Obstetric Analgesia and Anesthesia

Anesthesia complications are the seventh leading cause of maternal deaths in the United States (Dickason, Silverman, and Schult, 1994). Though many of these deaths result from poor technique or overdosage, most anesthesiologists, obstetricians, and midwives would agree that there is no method of pharmacologic pain relief that is completely safe for all laboring women. In addition, side effects or adverse reactions in the woman affect the fetus to some degree. Nonpharmacologic methods of pain management such as labor support, breathing techniques, massage, water immersion, transcutaneous electrical nerve stimulation (TENS) and subcutaneous sterile water injections in the back may provide sufficient pain relief for many women (Simkin, 1995).

OBSTETRIC ANALGESIA

Obstetric analgesia is given by either the intramuscular or the IV route and in as small a dose as possible. Analgesic agents can be given when the woman has reached 4 or 5 cm of dilation, and ideally birth should not occur between 1 and 4 hours after administration (Wakefield, 1994). The most commonly used analgesic is the narcotic meperidine (Demerol); butorphanol (Stadol) and nalbuphine (Nubain) are also commonly used.

A. Potential complications.

1. Maternal.
   a. Respiratory depression.
   b. Nausea and vomiting.
   c. Slowing of labor if given in the latent phase.
   d. Orthostatic hypotension.
   e. Drowsiness and dizziness.
2. Fetal/neonatal.
   a. Decreased fetal activity and short-term variability; late decelerations if mother experiences hypotension.
   b. Neonatal respiratory depression.
   c. Decreased Apgar scores.
   d. Respiratory acidosis.
   e. Neurobehavioral abnormalities.
   f. Hypotonia.
   g. Lethargy.
   h. Thermoregulation problems.

B. Assessment and management.

1. Do not administer analgesics too early or too late in labor.
2. Administer IV analgesics slowly; give during a uterine contraction to minimize amount of drug the fetus receives (Creehan, 1996).
3. Observe woman for side effects and monitor fetus continuously with electronic fetal monitor or periodic auscultation.
4. With maternal hypotension, turn woman on her left side, increase IV infusion of fluids, and closely monitor fetal heart tones as well as woman's BP.
5. Have naloxone (Narcan), oxygen, and ventilatory equipment available for use with the newborn infant if respiratory depression occurs.
6. Document use of analgesic and transmit this information to nursery nurse.
7. In nursery, observe neonate for side effects of maternal analgesia.

OBSTETRIC ANESTHESIA

Several types of anesthesia are used with women in labor and delivery. General anesthesia is used only for emergency cesarean deliveries and complicated vaginal deliveries when it is not possible to have immediate and effective regional anesthesia. Regional anesthesia includes continuous lumbar epidural, spinal, and pudendal block.

A. Potential complications with general anesthesia.

1. Maternal.
   a. Vomiting and aspiration of gastric contents, with chemical pneumonitis as a consequence.

    b. Respiratory depression.

    c. Cardiac irritability and arrest.

    d. Hypotension or hypertension.

    e. Tachycardia.

    f. Laryngospasm.

    g. Postpartum uterine atony.

2. Fetal/neonatal.

    a. Decreased fetal cardiac variability and movements.

    b. Fetal depression in proportion to the amount of anesthesia.

    c. Neonatal respiratory depression.

    d. Hyperbilirubinemia.

    e. Hypotonicity.

B. **Assessment and management with general anesthesia.**

1. The woman must have nothing by mouth while in labor if there is any possibility that she will receive general anesthesia.
2. Note the time of her last meal.
3. Physician may order 30 mL of clear antacid to be administered before general anesthesia to increase the pH of the stomach contents in case of aspiration.
4. Endotracheal tube and cricoid pressure are techniques used by the anesthesiologist to prevent aspiration.
5. Place wedge under right hip to cause displacement of uterus from aorta and vena cava and to prevent supine hypotensive syndrome during surgery.
6. Monitor woman's cardiorespiratory status during and after surgery, and uterine bleeding afterward.
7. Monitor fetus during surgery and newborn infant after surgery for complications.

C. **Potential complications with regional anesthetics.**

1. Maternal.

    a. With spinal and epidural anesthesia:

      (1) 25–75% incidence of hypotension (Hawkins, Chestnut, and Gibbs, 1996).

      (2) Allergic reaction.

      (3) Toxic reaction to overdose or intravascular injection, with convulsions (Hawkins et al., 1996).

      (4) Respiratory paralysis from inadvertent high spinal anesthesia.

      (5) Headaches after spinal anesthesia.

      (6) Failure of anesthetic to be effective.

      (7) Urinary retention during labor and in postpartum period.

      (8) Slowing of labor, with need to use oxytocin and forceps if anesthetic is given too early.

      (9) Formation of a hematoma that compresses the spinal cord, with potential for permanent damage (Hawkins et al., 1996).

    b. With epidural anesthesia:

      (1) Shearing off of epidural catheter.

      (2) Trauma to spinal cord or nerve roots.

      (3) Anterior spinal artery syndrome.

      (4) Transverse arrest or persistent occiput posterior position of the fetal head (Thorp et al., 1993).

      (5) Backache (Enkin et al., 1995).

      (6) "Epidural shakes" and "epidural fever" (involuntary shivering that leads to an elevated temperature) (Lieberman et al., 1997).

    c. With pudendal block.

      (1) Sciatic nerve trauma.

      (2) Perforated rectum.

      (3) Broad-ligament hematoma.

2. Fetal/neonatal.
   a. Toxic reaction from overdose or intravascular injection.
   b. Fetal compromise with prolonged maternal hypotension, as evidenced by late decelerations and decrease in short-term variability.
   c. Hyperthermia with epidural anesthesia (Lieberman et al., 1997).

D. **Assessment and management with regional anesthetics.**

1. Note history of allergies to local anesthetics.
2. Prehydrate with 500–1000 mL IV fluid before spinal or epidural anesthesia to minimize hypotensive effects from sympathetic blockade.
3. Position and reassure woman during administration of anesthetic. To prevent supine hypotension, position woman on alternate side after epidural or spinal anesthetic is given.
4. Monitor woman's BP after administration of spinal or epidural anesthetic; monitor fetal heart after any type of regional anesthesia.
5. Monitor bladder distention, and catheterize if necessary.
6. Monitor for and help to manage complications.
   a. Hypotension.
      (1) Signs and symptoms.
         (a) Drop in BP.
         (b) Dizziness or affected vision.
      (2) Management.
         (a) Increase IV fluids.
         (b) Elevate legs and lower head.
         (c) Displace uterus from aorta and vena cava.
         (d) Administer oxygen and IV ephedrine.
         (e) Monitor fetus for hypoxia and fetus/newborn infant for side effects of ephedrine (tachycardia, jitteriness, and increased muscular activity).
   b. High spinal.
      (1) Signs and symptoms.
         (a) Rising level of anesthesia.
         (b) Difficulty breathing.
      (2) Management.
         (a) Maintain airway and ventilation.
         (b) Reassure woman.
         (c) Monitor fetal heart tones.
   c. Toxic reaction.
      (1) Signs and symptoms.
         (a) Metallic taste.
         (b) Ringing in ears.
         (c) Slurring of speech.
         (d) Numbness of tongue and mouth.
         (e) Convulsions.
         (f) Cardiovascular and respiratory depression.
      (2) Management.
         (a) Cardiorespiratory support.
         (b) Drugs to control convulsions.
         (c) Monitor newborn infant for seizures, bradycardia, apnea, hypotonia.
   d. Allergic reaction.
      (1) Signs and symptoms.
         (a) Bronchospasm.
         (b) Laryngeal edema.
         (c) Urticaria.
      (2) Management: use of IV antihistamine.

Operative Delivery

A. **Incidence.** The cesarean delivery rate in the United States was 20.8% in 1995 but is as high as 40% in some institutions (Curtin and Kozak, 1997).

B. **Indications.**

1. Maternal.
   a. Cephalopelvic disproportion.
   b. Failure to progress in labor.
   c. Previous classic (vertical) uterine cesarean incision.
   d. Pregnancy-induced hypertension.
   e. Cardiac disease.
   f. Diabetes.
   g. Premature rupture of membranes with failed induction.
   h. Active herpes.
2. Placental.
   a. Abruptio placentae.
   b. Placenta previa.
   c. Placental insufficiency.
3. Fetal.
   a. Distress.
   b. Breech or other malpresentation.
   c. Multifetal gestation.
   d. Preterm delivery.

C. **Potential complications.**

1. Maternal.
   a. Infection.
   b. Anemia.
   c. Hemorrhage.
   d. Morbidity and death from anesthesia.
   e. Inadvertent operative injuries.
   f. Pulmonary embolus and atelectasis.
   g. Thrombophlebitis.
2. Fetal/neonatal.
   a. Asphyxia.
   b. Preterm birth.
   c. Respiratory distress caused by retained fluid in the lungs.
   d. Anemia from blood loss caused by incision of placenta and lack of full placental transfusion.

D. **Assessment and management.**

1. Perform usual interventions to prepare woman for operative delivery.
2. Notify infant's physician per policy.
3. Give antacid if ordered.
4. Insert indwelling urinary catheter.
5. Arrange for support person to be with woman for delivery.
6. Remove fetal scalp electrode before surgery.
7. Place wedge under woman's right hip to displace uterus to left to avoid supine hypotension and fetal hypoxia.
8. Suction newborn infant well and observe closely for cardiorespiratory and thermoregulatory status.

REFERENCES

Barger, M., and Fein, E.: High-risk pregnancy. *In* Nichols, F., and Zwelling, E. (Eds.): Maternal-Newborn Nursing: Theory and Practice. Philadelphia, W.B. Saunders, 1997, pp. 622–700.

Benedetti, T.: Obstetric hemorrhage. *In* Gabbe, S., Niebyl, J., and Simpson, J. (Eds.): Obstetrics: Normal and Problem Pregnancies, 3rd ed. New York, Churchill Livingstone, 1996, pp. 499–532.

Burke, M., and Poole, J.: Common perinatal complications. *In* Simpson, K., and Creehan, P. (Eds.): Perinatal Nursing. Philadelphia, J.B. Lippincott, 1996, pp. 109–146.

Clark, S., Cotton, D., Hankins, G., and Phelan, J.: Handbook of Critical Care Obstetrics. Boston, Blackwell Scientific Publications, 1994.

Committee on Obstetric Practice: Antenatal Corticosteroid Therapy for Fetal Maturation. Committee Opinion No. 147. American College of Obstetricians and Gynecologists, 1994.

Creehan, P.: Pain relief and comfort measures during labor. *In* Simpson, K., and Creehan, P. (Eds.): Perinatal Nursing. Philadelphia, J.B. Lippincott, 1996, pp. 227–245.

Curtin, S., and Kozak, L.: Cesarean delivery rates in 1995 continue to decline in the United States. Birth: Issues in Perinatal Care, 24(3), 194–196, 1997.

Dickason, E., Silverman, B., and Schult, M.: Maternal-Infant Nursing Care, 2nd ed. St. Louis, Mosby, 1994.

Dildy, J., and Clark, S.: Umbilical cord prolapse. Contemp. Obstet. Gynecol., 38(11), 23, 1993.

Enkin, M., Keirse, M., Renfrew, M., and Neilson, J.: A Guide to Effective Care in Pregnancy and Childbirth, 2nd ed. New York, Oxford University Press, 1995.

Escher-Davis, L.: Fetal fibronectin: A biochemical marker for preterm labor. AWHONN Voice, 4(3), 1, 6–7, 1996.

Freda, M., and Patterson, E.: Preterm Labor: Prevention and Nursing Management. *In* Damus, K., (Ed.): March of Dimes Nursing Modules. White Plains, N.Y., March of Dimes Birth Defects Foundation, 1994.

Goer, H.: Obstetric Myths Versus Research Realities: A Guide to the Medical Literature. Westport, Conn., Bergin & Garvey, 1995.

Griese, M., and Prickett, S.: Nursing management of umbilical cord prolapse. J. Obstet. Gynecol. Neonatal Nurs., 22(4), 309–311, 1993.

Hawkins, J., Chestnut, D., and Gibbs, C.: Obstetric anesthesia. *In* Gabbe, S., Niebyl, J., and Simpson, J. (Eds.): Obstetrics: Normal and Problem Pregnancies, 3rd ed. New York, Churchill Livingstone, 1996, pp. 425–468.

Hillier, S., Nugent, R., Eschenkach, D., et al.: Association between bacterial vaginosis and preterm delivery of a low-birth-weight infant. The Vaginal Infection and Prematurity Study Group. N. Engl. J. Med. 333(26), 1737–1742, 1995.

Iams, J.: Preterm birth. *In* Gabbe, S., Niebyl, J., and Simpson, J. (Eds.): Obstetrics: Normal and Problem Pregnancies, 3rd ed. New York, Churchill Livingstone, 1996, pp. 743–820.

Ladewig, P., London, M., and Olds, S.: Maternal-Newborn Nursing Care: The Nurse, the Family, and the Community, 4th ed. New York, Addison-Wesley, 1998.

Landon, M.: Diabetes mellitus and other endocrine diseases. *In* Gabbe, S., Niebyl, J., and Simpson, J. (Eds.): Obstetrics: Normal and Problem Pregnancies, 3rd ed. New York, Churchill Livingstone, 1996, pp. 1037–1081.

Lieberman, P., Lang, J., Frigoletto, J., et al.: Epidural analgesia, intrapartum fever, and neonatal sepsis evaluation. Pediatrics, 99(3), 415–419, 1997.

MacMullen, N., Brucker, M., and Zwelling, E. High-risk childbirth. In Nichols, F., and Zwelling, E. (Eds.): Maternal-Newborn Nursing: Theory and Practice. Philadelphia, W.B. Saunders, 1997, pp. 862–931.

Martin, V., and Gingerich, B.: Uteroplacental physiology. J. Obstet. Gynecol. Neonatal Nurs. 5, 16s–25s, 1976.

Moore, K., and Persaud, T.: The Developing Human: Clinically Oriented Embryology, 5th ed. Philadelphia, W.B. Saunders, 1993.

Piper, D., and McDonald, P.: Management of anticipated and actual shoulder dystocia. J. Nurse-Midwifery, 39(2), 91S–105S, 1994.

Reeder, S., Martin, L., and Koniak-Griffin, D.: Maternity Nursing: Family, Newborn, and Women's Health Care, 18th ed. Philadelphia, W.B. Saunders, 1997.

Roberts, J.: Current perspectives on preeclampsia. J. Nurse-Midwifery, 39(2), 70–90, 1994.

Seeds, J., and Walsh, M.: Malpresentations. *In* Gabbe, S., Niebyl, J., and Simpson, J. (Eds.): Obstetrics: Normal and Problem Pregnancies, 3rd ed. New York, Churchill Livingstone, 1996, pp. 469–498.

Sibai, B.: Hypertension in pregnancy. *In* Gabbe, S., Niebyl, J., and Simpson, J. (Eds.): Obstetrics: Normal and Problem Pregnancies, 3rd ed. New York: Churchill Livingstone, 1996, pp. 935–996.

Simkin, P.: Reducing pain and enhancing progress in labor: A guide to nonpharmacologic methods for maternity caregivers. Birth: Issues in Perinatal Care and Education, 22(3), 161–171, 1995.

Thorp, J., Hu, D., Albin, R., et al.: The effect of intrapartum epidural anesthesia on nulliparous labor: A randomized, controlled, prospective trial. Am. J. Obstet. Gynecol., 169(4), 851–858, 1993.

Varney, H.: Varney's Midwifery, 3rd ed. Boston, Jones & Bartlett, 1997.

Varney, H., and Reedy, N.: Screening for and collaborative management of antepartal complications. *In* Varney, H. (Ed.): Varney's Midwifery, 3rd ed. Boston, Jones & Bartlett, 1997, pp. 327–377.

Wakefield, M.: Systemic analgesia: Opioids, ketamine, and inhalational agents. *In* Chestnut, D. (Ed.): Obstetric Anesthesia: Principles and Practice. St Louis, Mosby, 1994, pp. 340–353.

Wheeler, D.: Preterm birth prevention. J. Nurse-Midwifery, 39(2 Supplement), 66S–80S, 1994.

White, D., and Poole, J.: Obstetrical emergencies for the perinatal nurse. *In* Wellman, L. (Ed.): March of Dimes Nursing Modules. White Plains, N.Y., March of Dimes Birth Defects Foundation, 1996.

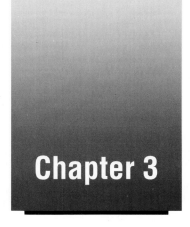

Chapter 3

Adaptation to Extrauterine Life

Christine Zabloudil

Objectives

1. Identify primary features of fetal circulation.
2. Identify physiologic changes that occur during transition to extrauterine life.
3. Identify routine care considerations for a newborn infant during the transition period.
4. Identify signs and symptoms of common problems in the transition period.
5. Define the methods and intervention times for parental teaching.

The transition period is considered to occur from the moment of birth to 6 hours of age, but, more than a period of time, it is a process of physiologic change in the newborn infant that begins in utero as the child prepares for transition from intrauterine placental support to extrauterine self-maintenance. The fetus prepares for transition during the course of gestation in such ways as storing glycogen, producing catecholamines, and depositing brown fat. The neonate's ability to accomplish the transition to extrauterine life will depend on gestational age and on the quality of placental support during gestation.

As the newborn infant adapts during the first hours of life, the level of nursing intervention will vary with the baby's needs. The need for intervention will then determine the level of care required at the end of the transition period.

Anatomy and Physiology

CHARACTERISTICS OF PLACENTAL/FETAL CIRCULATION

A. **Placenta.**

1. Blood oxygenation and elimination of waste products of metabolism. Transfer of O_2 and CO_2 across the placenta is by simple diffusion.
2. High rate of metabolism. Placenta uses one third of all the oxygen and glucose supplied to it by the maternal circulation for its own metabolic needs.

3. Low-resistance circuit. Placenta receives approximately 50% of fetal cardiac output.
4. Uterine venous blood has a PCO_2 of 38 mm Hg, PO_2 of 40–50 mm Hg, and pH of 7.36 as it enters the intervillous space.

B. **Fetal shunts/blood flow (Fig. 3–1) (Moore, 1998).**

1. Umbilical vein (PO_2 32–35 mm Hg) carries oxygenated blood from the placenta to the fetus.
2. Ductus venosus. Forty to sixty percent of the umbilical venous blood bypasses the liver through the ductus venosus to the inferior vena cava (IVC). The venous duct is a low-resistance channel that allows a significant portion of relatively well oxygenated blood to enter the heart directly; the other half passes through the liver and enters the IVC via the hepatic veins. This mixing of blood slightly lowers the PO_2.
3. IVC blood and the blood from the coronary sinuses ($PO_2 = 25–28$ mm Hg). This blood is largely deflected across the right atrium, through the foramen ovale, and into the left atrium. In contrast, most of the blood from the superior vena cava (SVC), also returning to the right atrium, is deflected to the right ventricle (see item 6, below). The crista dividens (lower edge of the septum secundum) separates the flow of blood from the IVC into two streams, with 50–60% of the blood from the IVC being diverted across the foramen ovale into the left atrium (Blackburn and Loper, 1992) and the remainder of blood from the IVC remaining in the right atrium and mixing poorly oxygenated blood from the superior vena cava and coronary sinus.
4. Left atrium. Blood is received from the right atrium via the foramen ovale and mixes with a small amount of blood returning from the lungs via the pulmonary veins.
5. Left ventricular blood ($PO_2 = 25–28$ mm Hg). Virtually all this blood is from the IVC by way of the right atrium–foramen ovale–left atrium pathway. Left ventricular blood is pumped out through the aorta to the brain from the upper part of the aortic arch. Approximately 90% of the blood from the ascending aorta feeds the coronary, carotid, and subclavian arteries and thus the brain and upper extremities.
6. The SVC. Unoxygenated blood returning from the brain and upper extremities is received by the SVC. Ninety-seven percent enters the right atrium and flows to the right ventricle through the tricuspid valve; only 3% flows to the left atrium via the foramen ovale.
7. Right atrium. Some mixing occurs here between the unoxygenated SVC blood and the oxygenated IVC blood not shunted directly into the left atrium via the foramen ovale.
8. Right ventricle. The dominant ventricle ($PO_2 = 19–22$ mm Hg) ejects about 66% of the total cardiac output. Most of the blood is shunted across the ductus arteriosus, away from the lungs, and into the descending aorta to supply the kidneys and intestines. It then divides into two arteries, which subsequently return back to the placenta.
9. Ductus arteriosus. Equal in size to the aorta, it connects the pulmonary artery to the descending aorta. The blood flows right to left (pulmonary artery to aorta) across the ductus arteriosus because of high pulmonary vascular resistance and low placental resistance. Patency is maintained by the low oxygen tension in utero and by the vasodilating effect of prostaglandin E_2.
10. Low pulmonary blood flow (only 8–10% of right ventricular output) results from high pulmonary vascular resistance.
11. Descending aorta supplies kidneys and intestines, divides into two arteries, and returns blood to the placenta for oxygenation.

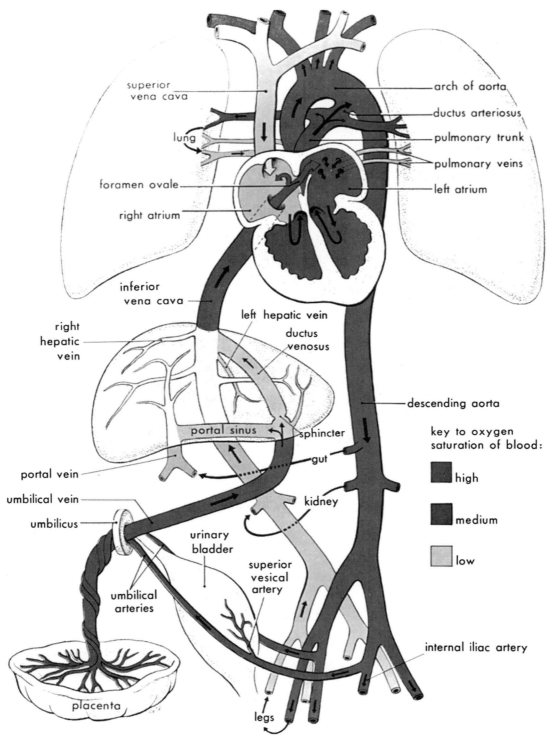

Figure 3–1
Simplified scheme of fetal circulation. Shaded areas indicate oxygen saturation of the blood; arrows show course of fetal circulation. The organs are not drawn to scale. (From Moore, K.L.: The Developing Human: Clinically Oriented Embryology, 6th ed. Philadelphia, W.B. Saunders, 1998.)

FETAL LUNG CHARACTERISTICS

A. **Decreased blood flow.** In part the decrease is caused by compression of the pulmonary capillaries by the fetal lung fluid.

B. **Pulmonary arteries.** The small pulmonary arteries of the fetus have a thick, muscular medial layer; they are very reactive and are actively constricted by low PO_2 normally present during fetal life. Pulmonary vascular resistance increases throughout fetal life.

C. **Lung fluid secretion.** Fetal lungs actively secrete fluid; secretion of fluid is decreased near term. At term the lung contains 30 mL of plasma ultrafiltrate per kilogram of body weight. This is comparable to a postnatal thoracic gas volume of 25 mL/kg. An adequate fluid volume is necessary for lung development. Fluid moves into and out of the lungs through the trachea.

D. **Fetal breathing.** In utero fetal breathing movements have been detected as early as 11 weeks of gestation. They contribute to lung development.

E. **Surfactant.** Surfactant is secreted into the amniotic fluid by the fetal lung before 20 weeks of gestation. The absolute quantity of surfactant increases throughout gestation in both lung and amniotic fluid and can support extrauterine respiration at approximately 34 weeks of gestation.

FETAL METABOLISM AND HEMATOLOGY

A. **Glucose.** Fetal blood glucose concentrations are 70–80% of maternal blood glucose concentrations. Glucose is exchanged via the placenta by facilitated diffusion.

B. **Glycogen.** Large glycogen stores (2–10 times that of an adult) provide large energy reserves to sustain the newborn infant through the transition period.

C. **Hemoglobin.** Fetal hemoglobin has an increased affinity for oxygen. Fetal hemoglobin is progressively replaced by adult hemoglobin from 32–36 weeks of gestation and is approximately 80% of total hemoglobin at term.

LABOR

A. **Placenta.** Maternal placental perfusion ceases with uterine contractions.

B. **Stress hormones.** High concentrations of stress hormones (predominantly norepinephrine) are released as a direct effect of the resultant hypoxia on the adrenal medulla.

CARDIOPULMONARY ADAPTATION AT BIRTH

A. **Cardiovascular adaptation (Fig. 3–2).**

1. Umbilical cord is clamped.
   a. Placenta is separated from the circulation, and the umbilical arteries and veins constrict.
   b. As the low-resistance placental circuit is removed, there is a resultant increase in systemic blood pressure; the systemic vascular resistance then exceeds the pulmonary vascular resistance.
2. The three major fetal shunts (ductus venosus, foramen ovale, and ductus arteriosus) functionally close during transition.
   a. Ductus arteriosus. The lungs now provide more efficient oxygenation of the blood, and the arterial oxygen tension rises. This rise in PO_2 is the most potent stimulus to constriction of the ductus arteriosus (Bloom, 1992).

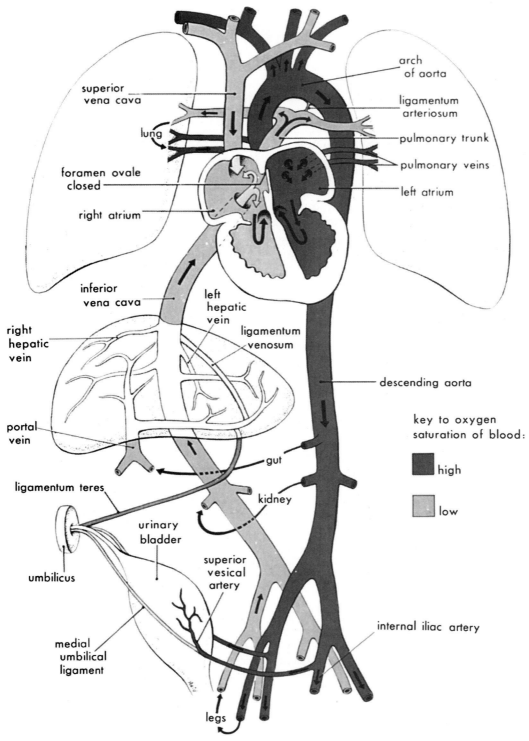

Figure 3–2
Simplified representation of circulation after birth. Adult derivatives of fetal vessels and structures that become nonfunctional at birth are also shown. Arrows indicate course of neonatal circulation. The organs are not drawn to scale. (From Moore, K.L.: The Developing Human—Clinically Oriented Embryology, ed. 6. Philadelphia, W.B. Saunders, 1998.)

Removal of the placenta decreases prostaglandin levels, further influencing closure (Nelson, 1994).
   b. Foramen ovale. The fall in pulmonary vascular resistance results in a drop in right ventricular and right atrial pressure, and the increased systemic vascular resistance results in an increase in left atrial and left ventricular pressures, causing the foramen ovale to close.
      (1) The foramen ovale becomes sealed by the deposit of fibrin and cell products during the first month of life.
      (2) Until the foramen ovale is anatomically sealed, anything that produces a significant increase in right atrial pressure can reopen the foramen ovale and allow a right-to-left shunt.
   c. Ductus venosus. Absent umbilical venous return leads to closure of the ductus venosus. It functionally closes within 2–3 days and becomes the ligamentum venosum.
3. Postnatal circulation (Fig. 3–2) (Moore, 1998).
   a. Systemic venous blood enters the right atrium from the SVC and the IVC.
   b. Poorly oxygenated blood enters the right ventricle and passes through the pulmonary artery into the pulmonary circulation for oxygenation.
   c. The oxygenated blood returns to the left atrium through the pulmonary veins.
   d. This blood passes through the left ventricle and into the aorta to supply the systemic circulation with oxygenated blood.

B. Pulmonary adaptation.

1. The lungs as the organ of gas exchange. Intermittent breathing begins in utero long before delivery and, after birth, is a continuation of movements and reflexes that have been well established.
2. Stimuli for initiating respiration: The mild hypercapnia, hypoxia, and acidosis that result from normal labor is due partially to the intermittent cessation of maternal-placental perfusion with contractions. The decreased pH stimulates the respiratory center directly; the low PO_2 and high PCO_2 stimulate the respiratory center by means of central and peripheral chemoreceptors. Other stimuli include cold, light, noise, and touch.
3. Entry of air into lungs with the first breath.
   a. Aeration of the lungs drives fluid into the interstitium; it is then absorbed through the lymphatic and pulmonary circulation. The rate at which this process occurs is variable, and fine crackling rales may be audible throughout the lungs until this process is completed.
   b. The pulmonary vessels respond to the increase in PO_2 with vasodilation. Pulmonary vascular resistance progressively decreases until adult levels are reached at 2–3 weeks of age.
4. Inspiration of air and expansion of lungs. After the thoracic squeeze (during labor and vaginal delivery this empties the lungs of approximately one third of the fetal lung fluid), the subsequent recoil of the chest wall causes inspiration of air and expansion of the lungs. Negative intrathoracic pressures generated with the first breath may be as high as 40–80 cm H_2O because of the mechanical advantage created by the high resting level of the diaphragm in the nonaerated lung. Subsequent breaths in the normal newborn infant require 15–20 cm H_2O pressure.
5. Respiratory augmentation. Head's paradoxical reflex is a vagally mediated hyperinflation triggered by distention of stretch receptors in the large airways.
6. Work of inspiration. This is mainly (80%) devoted to overcoming the surface tension of the walls of the terminal lung units at the gas-tissue interface. On expiration, the ability to retain air depends on surfactant.
   a. Surfactant is a complete lipoprotein produced by type II alveolar pneu-

mocytes; surfactant release increases in response to increased catecholamine levels at birth.

  b. Surfactant has the ability to lower surface tension at an air-liquid interface.

  c. As surfactant lowers surface tension in the alveolus at end-expiration, it stabilizes the alveoli and prevents collapse.

7. Increase in functional residual capacity with each breath. Less inspiratory pressure is thus required for subsequent breaths.

8. Lung compliance. This improves in the hours after delivery as a result of circulating catecholamines. The increased levels of catecholamines (especially of epinephrine) also clear the lungs by decreasing secretion of lung fluids and increasing their absorption through the lymphatic system.

Routine Care Considerations in the Transition Nursery*

A. **Assessment/observation.**

1. Body measurements. Head circumference, length, and weight are recorded.
2. Vital sign assessment. Vital signs recorded on admission will include heart rate, respiratory rate, and axillary temperature. Universal blood pressure screening in the well newborn infant is not warranted (American Academy of Pediatrics, 1993).
3. Gestational age assessment. Weight, head circumference, and length are graphed against the assessed gestational age and record (refer to Chapter 5).
4. Clinical changes. During the first hours of life, newborn infants follow a sequence of clinical behavior, as summarized in Figure 3–3 (Desmond, Rudolph, and Phitaksphraiwan, 1966). The time sequence of changes is altered in infants with low Apgar scores, immaturity, maternal medications, and intrinsic disease (refer to Chapter 6).
5. Head-to-toe physical examination (refer to Chapter 5). The following findings seen during transition are within normal limits as the infant progresses through the physiologic changes described under cardiopulmonary adaptation, above.
   a. Skin.
      (1) Acrocyanosis. Vasoconstricted peripheral vessels result in a mottled appearance; peripheral pulses are decreased initially. (These findings are sequelae of catecholamine release, mild acidosis, and cold stress.)
      (2) Petechiae of the face and facial bruising. A vertex presentation, a rapid second stage of labor, or a tight nuchal cord may result in these skin changes. (With severe facial bruising, central color may be assessed by looking at the mucous membranes in the mouth.)
   b. Head.
      (1) The newborn infant's head is large relative to the body; during vaginal delivery, considerable molding of the skull bones may take place to facilitate passage through the birth canal. Molding resolves during the first hours and days.
      (2) Caput succedaneum (edema of the presenting part of the scalp, caused by pressure that restricts the return of venous and lymph flow during vaginal delivery), may be present.
   c. Respirations/breath sounds.
      (1) Initially, coarse rales and moist tubular breath sounds. These breath sounds may continue until clearing of lung fluid is complete.

---

*Refer to Chapter 6 for resuscitation of the infant in the delivery room.

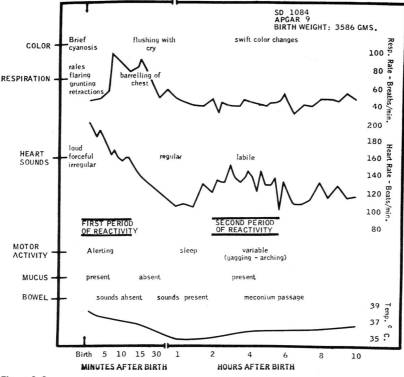

Figure 3–3
Summary of physical findings noted during first 10 hours of extrauterine life in representative high-Apgar-score infant delivered with mother under spinal anesthesia, without premedication. (From Desmond, M.M., Rudolph, A.J., and Phitaksphraiwan, P. Pediatr. Clin. North Am., *13*:651–668, 1966.)

(2) Prolonged expiratory phase.
(3) Respiratory rate, 30–60 breaths per minute.
(4) Grunting and retracting (intercostal and substernal). These findings may be present during the first hours of life as lung fluid is cleared.
d. Heart sounds.
(1) Second heart sound may be loud during first 2 hours; splitting of the second heart sound is usually detectable at 2–4 hours of age and increases during the next 12 hours (pulmonic ahead of aortic component).
(2) Soft grade 2/6 systolic murmur may be present; represents a left-to-right shunt across the ductus arteriosus before its closure.
e. Heart.
(1) Normal heart rate 120–160 bpm; increased initially, with mean peak of 180 bpm, and then decreased or irregular.
(2) Consistently high or low heart rate suggests a pathologic condition.
f. Intestines.
(1) Blood flow is reduced initially.
(2) As the bowel begins to fill with air, normal motility and bowel sounds are present within 15 minutes.
(3) The normal term neonate passes meconium within the first 24 hours after birth. If a term neonate has not passed meconium by 48 hours after birth, the lower gastrointestinal tract may be obstructed (American Academy of Pediatrics [AAP], 1997.)

g. Urinary function.
  (1) Urine is normally passed within the first 24 hours after birth (Gorrie, McKinney, and Murray, 1994).
  (2) Failure to void within the first 24 hours may indicate genitourinary obstruction or abnormality (AAP, 1997).
h. Falling body temperature. Mean low temperature is 35.6° C; lowest temperature is reached at a mean age of 75 minutes after delivery (Desmond et al., 1966).
i. Extremities. Findings may include deformities resulting from intrauterine position.

B. **Thermoregulation considerations in the nursery.** The admission assessment/observation should be done in a controlled environment, such as a radiant warmer or incubator, that both provides warmth and prevents heat loss so that the infant maintains a normal temperature without increasing oxygen consumption, using glucose stores, or exceeding brown fat stores in the process of nonshivering thermogenesis (mediated by norepinephrine released by cold stress) (Philip, 1996). Normal ranges are 36.5–37° C (axillary) and 36.0–36.5° C (skin). Hypothermia and hyperthermia occur when the infant's attempts to maintain a normal temperature fail, which has serious metabolic consequences for the newborn infant (refer to Chapter 4, Thermoregulation).

1. Monitor temperature. Check axillary temperature every 30 minutes to 1 hour during transition while the infant is under a radiant warmer. Avoid hyperthermia (skin temperature greater than 37° C or axillary temperature greater than 37.5° C). NOTE: Monitoring the axillary temperature allows time for successful intervention before a fall in core temperature indicates failure of the body's heat-regulation mechanism.
2. First bath. Delay bath until body temperature has stabilized and is within normal limits. Check temperature 30 minutes after the bath and 1 hour after transfer to open crib.
3. Temperature. Check temperature at least every 4 hours until infant's condition is stable, and then every 8 hours until discharge.
4. Environmental temperature (incubator or warmer). Record environmental temperature with temperature checks of the infant to monitor his or her environmental requirements. NOTE: These requirements can be checked against the normal ranges of neutral thermal environmental temperature needs as a tool in evaluating an infant's condition.

C. **Transition nursery medications.**

1. Eye care. Administered to both eyes before 1 hour of age in infants born by cesarean delivery, as well as those delivered vaginally.
  a. Recommendation. Apply 2 drops of 1% silver nitrate solution or a 1–2 cm ribbon of sterile ophthalmic ointment containing 0.5% erythromycin or 1% tetracycline for prophylaxis of ophthalmia neonatorum due to *Neisseria gonorrhoeae*. Prophylaxis for *Chlamydia trachomatis* requires erythromycin or tetracycline (AAP, 1997).
  b. Procedure. Instill medication into conjunctival sac within 1 hour of birth; medication should not be flushed from the eye after application. A new tube is used for each infant.
  c. Side effects. Sensitivity reaction may be seen. Chemical conjunctivitis can be observed after silver nitrate instillation.
2. Vitamin K_1 (phytonadione). Administer vitamin K within 1 hour of birth.
  a. Recommendation. Every neonate should receive a single parenteral 0.5–1.0 mg dose of natural vitamin K (phytonadione) (AAP, 1997). Administer 0.5 mg if infant weighs less than 1.5 kg or 1 mg if infant weighs more than 1.5 kg. NOTE: Vitamin K may be given orally in 1–2 mg dose; the oral route

was recommended as an alternative by the British Paediatric Association in 1992 but is not recommended by the AAP because oral administration of vitamin K has not been shown to be as efficacious as parenteral administration (AAP, 1997).

b. Risk of deficiency. Maternal dietary inadequacy of vitamin K, hepatic immaturity, reduced liver stores, and absence of intestinal flora predispose the child to deficiency of vitamin K; gut bacteria are a substantial source. Vitamin K is needed to promote the hepatic biosynthesis of vitamin K–dependent clotting factors, including prothrombin (factor II), proconvertin (factor VII), plasma thromboplastin component (factor IX), and Stuart factor (factor X). Deficiency results in hemorrhagic disease of the newborn (HDN).

   (1) Classic HDN. The disease occurs at 1–7 days of life. The infant is healthy at birth but develops cutaneous or gastrointestinal bleeding. Other sites of bleeding include nasal bleeding or bleeding after circumcision. Classic HDN can be prevented with vitamin K prophylaxis.

   (2) Early HDN. Maternal exposure to drugs, including warfarin, anticonvulsants, and antituberculosis drugs, may affect coagulation. Severe or life-threatening hemorrhage may occur during delivery or in the first day of life. Intracranial hemorrhage is a common complication. Early HDN is the only type that cannot be prevented by vitamin K prophylaxis.

   (3) Late HDN. The late form of HDN may occur between 1 and 3 months of life. Acute intracranial hemorrhage is the most common initial finding and is often fatal or neurologically devasting. Other findings include gastrointestinal or mucous membrane bleeding. Late HDN can be prevented by vitamin K prophylaxis.

3. Hepatitis vaccine and hepatitis B immunoglobulin (HBIG) (also see Appendix B).

   a. Rate of infection. Approximately one third of infants born to HBsAg-positive mothers will be HBsAg positive, with rates as high as 70–90% if mothers are HBeAG positive and anti-HBeAG negative (Thureen and Abzug, 1999).

   b. Chronicity. Ninety percent of infected infants will become chronic HBV carriers (Overall, 1992; Burchett, 1998).

   c. Maternal HBsAg positive—treatment recommendations:

      (1) Child is bathed as soon as temperature is stable.

      (2) Hepatitis B vaccine (Engerix-B, 10 µg, or Recombivax-HB, 5 µg) and HBIG, 0.5 mL IM (prepared from plasma to contain a high titer of antibody against HBsAg), should be administered before 12 hours of age (AAP, 1997); may be given concurrently at different sites; 85–95% effective in preventing both HBV infection and the chronic carrier state (Centers for Disease Control, 1991).

      (3) Remaining doses of hepatitis B vaccine are given at 1 and 6 months of age.

   d. Maternal HBsAg negative—treatment recommendations:

      (1) Hepatitis B vaccine should be administered to all infants, including those born to HBsAg-negative mothers.

      (2) Hepatitis B vaccine (Engerix-B, 10 µg, or Recombivax-HB, 5 µg) is administered prior to discharge from the hospital. The second dose is administered at 1–2 months of age and the third dose at 6–18 months of age.

   e. Unknown maternal HBsAg status at delivery. Follow schedule for maternal HBsAg positive. Additional HBIG administration will depend on results of maternal serologic screening done within 12 hours after delivery.

   f. Premature infants with birth weight less than 2 kg born to HBsAg-negative mothers should receive the vaccine just before hospital discharge if the infant weighs more than 2 kg or dose is delayed until 2 months of age when other routine immunizations are given. All premature infants born to HBsAg-positive mothers should receive immunoprophylaxis (HBIG) and vaccine beginning as soon as possible after birth, followed by appropriate postvaccination testing (AAP Committee on Infectious Diseases, 1994).

D. **Glucose needs/first feeding.**

1. The stress of delivery causes increased conversion of fats and glycogen to glucose for the increased energy needs of temperature maintenance, skeletal muscles, and breathing/crying. Breakdown products of this conversion are glucose, free fatty acids, and glycerol.
2. Hepatic glycogen is mobilized immediately after birth in response to the increased catecholamines to provide a continuing source of glucose to the brain in the absence of placental supply; in a healthy term infant, up to 90% of the hepatic glycogen stores may be consumed by 3 hours of life.
3. Blood glucose concentration at birth is about 85% of the maternal level. The last maternal meal, the duration of labor, the mode of delivery, the type and amount of IV fluids administered to the mother, and medications given to the mother all influence the actual concentration of glucose (Cornblath and Schwartz, 1991; Kalhan and Saker, 1997). The glucose level then falls for 1–2 hours, followed by an increase and stabilization at mean levels of 65–71 mg/dL by the age of 3–4 hours in healthy, nonstressed infants (Wilker, 1998).
4. A screening blood glucose test (on capillary whole blood) should be performed in infants with risk factors at 30 minutes to 1 hour of age. A glucose level less than 40 mg/dL at any time in any newborn infant is an indication for evaluation and treatment (Wilker, 1998). The goal is to maintain the glucose value at greater than 40 mg/dL in the first day and greater than 40–50 mg/dL thereafter. NOTE: The whole-blood glucose level on the screening test is usually 10–15% lower than the corresponding serum/plasma level because the erythrocytes will continue to metabolize the glucose in the sample. Risk factors include:
   a. Asphyxia, cold stress, increased work of breathing, and sepsis lead to an increased metabolic response and increased use of glucose.
   b. Reduced stores of glucose in premature and small-for-gestational-age infants.
   c. Hyperinsulinemia in infants of mothers with diabetes or gestational diabetes and in large-for-gestational-age infants, resulting in rapid removal of glucose from the circulation.
   d. Any symptoms of a low blood glucose level. An infant may have jitteriness, irritability, seizures, hypothermia, temperature instability, lethargy, poor feeding, emesis, apnea, pallor, cyanosis, and/or weak or high-pitched cry. (See also Common Problems and Clinical Presentation, item F: Metabolic Problems.) NOTE: Capillary samples from an unwarmed heel may lead to a falsely low glucose value because of stasis of blood and ongoing transfer of glucose to the cells.
5. Early, frequent feedings should be given on demand; frequency is not to exceed 4 hours between feedings (maximum of 3 hours between feedings for infants weighing <2.5 kg). Allow the infant to begin feeding when he or she is demanding nutrition and when evaluation findings are within normal limits; nursing or formula feeding can be used (type of formula is by family's or physician's choice).
   a. Evaluation before feeding.
      (1) Physical examination. Bowel tones are normal, and abdomen is soft and nontender. Sucking reflex is normal, with no excessive mucus. Passage of an orogastric tube is indicated before feeding if questions exist regarding esophageal patency. Anus and nares are patent. Respiratory

rate is less than 70 breaths per minute, and pattern of breathing is normal.
   (2) Contraindications to nippling the feeding or to breast-feeding (consider gavage feeding for these infants).
      (a) Choanal atresia.
      (b) Respiratory rate greater than 70 breaths per minute without other signs of respiratory distress.
      (c) Weak suck.
      (d) Absent coordination of suck and swallow.
   (3) Contraindications to any enteral feedings.
      (a) Cyanosis.
      (b) Severe birth asphyxia.
      (c) Shock.
      (d) Increased work of breathing and oxygen requirement.
      (e) Suspicion of gastrointestinal obstruction.
  b. Sterile-water "test" feeding. It is difficult to evaluate an infant's ability to suck and swallow with sterile water because most infants do not like the taste and on occasion will refuse to suck or swallow; therefore it is advisable to forego "sips of water" in favor of a thorough evaluation before feeding.
  c. Dextrose 5%. Use of dextrose 5% is not indicated as a "test" feeding because studies show that it is as irritating to lungs after aspiration as is formula (Sun, Awnetwant, Collier, et al., 1998). Not indicated after feeding unless:
   (1) Ordered by a physician.
   (2) Requested by mother (e.g., at one night feeding in the nursery or if infant does not settle down after effective nursing).
  d. Guidelines for feeding in transition nursery for transient asymptomatic hypoglycemia:
   (1) May breast-feed or be offered formula (by nipple or gavage) if there are no contraindications to enteral feedings (see Contraindications, item a[3], above), and the infant is active and vigorous.
   (2) Check glucose level 1 hour after feeding is given.
  e. Indications for IV glucose infusion (see Initial Stabilization of the Sick Newborn Infant, below):
   (1) Hypoglycemia is persistent and symptomatic.
   (2) Enteral feedings are contraindicated.
   (3) Oral feedings do not maintain normal glucose levels.
   (4) Initial glucose screening level is less than 20 mg/dL.

E. Ongoing teaching in the transition nursery.

1. Discuss with family the infant's ability to see and hear, with a preference for black-white contrast initially, and the sound of a higher-pitched voice.
2. Demonstrate/point out infant's response to stimuli (tactile, visual, auditory): self-consolability, body movements, gaze, head turning.
3. Discuss physical findings.
  a. Transient: head molding, acrocyanosis, birth trauma, positional deformities.
  b. Permanent: congenital anomalies, birthmarks.
4. A stable infant may stay with the family from birth through recovery to postpartum period with appropriate observation and teaching provided by all staff members in contact with the family unit.

F. Transfer of infant from transition nursery when the following are stable:

1. Temperature, heart rate, respiratory rate.
2. Glucose level.
3. Normal physical assessment findings, or abnormal findings that do not require continuous observation or immediate intervention/treatment.

Recognition of the Sick Newborn Infant

REVIEW OF PERINATAL HISTORY

A. **Ultrasonographic-biophysical profile:** estimated date of confinement, evidence of congenital anomalies, twins, breech, preterm, intrauterine growth retardation.

B. **Medications or history of substance abuse:** alcohol, nicotine, cocaine, opiates, marijuana, amphetamines, tocolytics, anticonvulsants, anticoagulants, and analgesics/anesthetics.

C. **Maternal illnesses:** pregnancy-induced hypertension, diabetes, intrapartum fever/infection (e.g., with group B streptococcus, genital herpes simplex virus, human immunodeficiency virus, varicella), HBsAg positive, thyroid disease, inherited disorders, cardiac disease.

D. **Perinatal fetal distress, delivery complications:** abnormal fetal heart rate pattern, meconium staining of the amniotic fluid, rapid delivery, difficult delivery, rupture of membranes more than 18 hours before delivery.

E. **Cesarean delivery and indications:** breech presentation, fetal distress, placenta previa, abruptio placentae, cephalopelvic disproportion, failure to progress in labor.

PHYSICAL ASSESSMENT

A. **Skin.**

1. Cyanotic.
2. Pale.
3. Mottled.
4. Cool to touch.
5. Poor perfusion.

B. **Respiratory system.**

1. Poor color.
2. Tachypnea.
3. Decreased air entry.
4. Increased work of breathing: grunting, flaring, retracting.
5. Apnea.
6. Unequal breath sounds.
7. Oxygen requirement.

C. **Cardiovascular system.**

1. Abnormal heart sounds such as murmur.
2. Weak, absent, or unequal pulses.
3. Hepatosplenomegaly.

D. **Central nervous system.**

1. Hypertonic or hypotonic.
2. Jitteriness; tremors.
3. Lethargy.
4. Bulging fontanelle (record baseline head circumference).
5. Seizures.
6. Irritability; high-pitched cry.

E. **Morphologic features.**

1. Congenital anomalies (e.g., abdominal wall defects, imperforate anus).

2. Severe birth trauma.
3. Absent or decreased limb movement.
4. Asymmetry.

E. Gastrointestinal tract.

1. Abdominal distention (measure baseline abdominal girth).
2. Increased gastric contents on aspiration.
3. Inability to pass an orogastric tube.
4. Excessive mucus.
5. Emesis soon after birth or after first feeding.

DIAGNOSTIC TOOLS

A. Pulse oximetry (peripheral monitoring of oxygen saturation).

1. Oxygen saturation (SO_2) of blood is that percentage of the total hemoglobin concentration that is chemically combined with oxygen.
2. A baseline PO_2 value should be obtained to confirm the infant's oxygen level.
3. For hyperoxic study, administer 100% oxygen to differentiate between pulmonary and cardiac disease. (In infants with pulmonary disease, saturation will improve, whereas in infants with cyanotic heart disease, little or no change will occur. Use caution to avoid exposing the ductus arteriosus to high oxygen levels in ductal dependent cardiac lesions.)

B. Arterial blood gas determinations. If oxygen requirement persists, pulse oximetry saturations in room air are decreased and cyanosis is present.

C. Chest x-ray examination. Anteroposterior and lateral views are needed if respiratory distress is present or cardiac disease is suspected.

D. Transillumination. Use a high-intensity light placed over the side of the chest in question if pneumothorax or pneumomediastinum is suspected.

E. Whole-blood glucose screening test or serum glucose determination if indicated by history or assessment results (see Routine Care Considerations in the Transition Nursery, item D: Glucose Needs/First Feeding).

F. Hematocrit determination.

1. History of blood loss.
2. Plethoric or pale infant.
3. Twins (to rule out twin-to-twin transfusion).
4. Heel-stick (capillary) samples tend to have higher results of approximately 10%.
5. Hematocrit variations. Highest hematocrit is at 2–4 hours of age and then progressively falls due to the beginning of red blood cell breakdown and the cessation of erythropoiesis in response to a comparatively oxygen-enriched environment.

G. Complete blood cell count with differential examination of the white blood cells.

1. As part of a sepsis diagnostic evaluation.
2. To screen for normal and abnormal hematologic indices.

H. Blood culture as part of a diagnostic evaluation for sepsis.

I. Urine sample collection.

1. Urinalysis.
2. Screening test for drugs of abuse.

J. **Lumbar puncture.** Performed at the discretion of the physician as part of a diagnostic evaluation for sepsis.

K. **Ultrasonography, computed tomography, magnetic resonance imaging.**

1. Cranial evaluation for abnormal CNS findings.
2. Abdominal examination if history of two-vessel cord to rule out renal anomalies.

L. **Echocardiography and electrocardiography.** As part of a diagnostic study for a congenital cardiac defect.

M. **Passage of orogastric tube.**

1. To check patency of esophagus in infants with excessive pooling of mucus in oropharynx.
2. To decompress a distended abdomen.
3. To measure and assess gastric contents (>25 mL and/or significant bile in the stomach indicates obstruction).

COMMON PROBLEMS AND CLINICAL PRESENTATION

A. **Birth trauma (refer to Chapter 20).**

B. **Birth asphyxia.**

1. Birth asphyxia is defined as interference with gas exchange resulting in compromised oxygen delivery, accumulation of CO_2, and a switch to anaerobic metabolism.
2. Fetal distress is indicated by abnormal fetal heart rate pattern, meconium staining of the amniotic fluid, scalp pH less than 7.20, and Apgar scores less than 5 at 1 minute of age and less than 7 at 5 minutes of age.
3. Pathophysiologic sequelae include:
   a. Decreasing PO_2. The tissue hypoxia that ensues leads to anaerobic metabolism with release of lactic acid into the circulation.
   b. Respiratory acidosis from elevated levels of a carbon dioxide.
   c. Metabolic acidosis.
      (1) Results in high pulmonary vascular resistance.
      (2) Leads to decreased surfactant release.
   d. Hypoxic-ischemic damage to less vital organs such as kidney and gut after redistribution of blood to vital organs.
   e. The myocardium depends on its stored reserves of glycogen for energy as its supply of oxygen falls. Eventually this reserve is consumed and the myocardium is simultaneously exposed to progressively lower PO_2 and pH levels. The combined effects lead to reduced myocardial function with decreased blood flow to vital organs (Phibbs, 1994).
4. All newborn infants have some degree of respiratory acidosis and hypoxia during labor and vaginal delivery; a healthy term infant has increased tolerance and reserves. The asphyxiated newborn infant has more prolonged hypoxia and respiratory acidosis and may have additional metabolic acidosis, hypothermia, and hypoglycemia.
5. Clinical findings.
   a. Mild to moderate perinatal asphyxia.
      (1) Extended awake, alert state (45 minutes to 1 hour).
      (2) Dilated pupils.
      (3) Normal muscle tone.
      (4) Active suck.
      (5) Regular or slightly increased respiratory rate.
      (6) Normal or slightly increased heart rate.

b. Moderate to severe perinatal asphyxia.
   (1) Hypothermia.
   (2) Hypoglycemia.
   (3) Pupils constricted.
   (4) Respiratory distress manifested by grunting, flaring, retracting, tachypnea, and oxygen requirement.
   (5) Seizures (subtle and multifocal clonic; 12–24 hours of age).
   (6) Acute tubular necrosis following reduced blood flow to the kidneys.
   (7) Hypotonia initially; lethargy.
   (8) Bradycardia.
c. Severe perinatal asphyxia, which requires constant monitoring in a level II (intermediate care) or level III (intensive care) nursery.
   (1) Pale; poor perfusion.
   (2) Cerebral edema.
   (3) Seizures.
   (4) Apnea.
   (5) Intracranial hemorrhage.

C. Pulmonary problems.

1. Pneumothorax (2% of all births); pneumomediastinum.
   a. Tachypnea, unequal breath sounds, shift of heart tones, distant heart tones.
   b. Transillumination of chest is positive for free air.
2. Retained lung fluid, respiratory distress syndrome (RDS) (because of prematurity or birth asphyxia), pneumonia.
   a. Decreased air entry with RDS and pneumonia.
   b. Increased work of breathing: grunting, flaring, retracting.
   c. Tachypnea, apnea.
   d. Decreased saturations (SO_2), cyanosis, continued oxygen requirement.
3. Aspiration syndromes (meconium, blood).
   a. Coarse rales.
   b. Tachypnea.
   c. Barrel chest.
4. Upper airway obstruction (e.g., choanal atresia or micrognathia).
5. Extrapulmonary (e.g., phrenic nerve injury with resultant diaphragmatic paralysis or eventration of the diaphragm).

D. Cardiovascular problems.

1. Congenital heart disease.
   a. Acyanotic lesions.
      (1) Patent ductus arteriosus with a left-to-right shunt.
      (2) Ventricular septal defect.
      (3) Atrial septal defect.
      (4) Endocardial cushion defect or atrioventricular canal defects.
   b. Obstructive lesions.
      (1) Aortic stenosis.
      (2) Coarctation of the aorta.
      (3) Pulmonary valve stenosis or atresia.
      (4) Hypoplastic left heart syndrome.
   c. Admixture of lesions.
      (1) Normal or increased pulmonary blood flow.
         (a) Complete transposition of the great vessels.
         (b) Truncus arteriosus.
         (c) Anomalous venous connections of the pulmonary veins.
      (2) Decreased pulmonary blood flow.
         (a) Tetralogy of Fallot.
         (b) Tricuspid valve atresia.

2. Persistent fetal shunts.
    a. Patent ductus arteriosus with right-to-left shunt.
    b. Persistent pulmonary hypertension.
3. Clinical findings.
    a. Cyanosis with or without increased work of breathing; decreased oxygen saturations. NOTE: Absence of any signs of abnormal respiratory function in the presence of cyanosis suggests congenital heart disease.
    b. Unequal or absent pulses, bounding pulses, decreased blood pressure in the lower extremities, decreased perfusion.
    c. Increased precordial activity, shift of point of maximal impulse (PMI) of heart tones to right, murmur.
    d. Congestive heart failure, indicated by tachypnea, moist breath sounds, tachycardia, peripheral edema, cardiomegaly, hepatomegaly.

E. Hemodynamics.

1. Acute hypovolemic shock.
    a. Internal hemorrhage resulting from birth trauma; intracranial hemorrhage.
    b. External hemorrhage resulting from placenta previa or abruptio placentae; cord accident; fetal-maternal or twin-to-twin transfusion.
    c. Respiratory distress, pallor, poor perfusion, hypotension, weak or absent pulses, anemia.
2. Polycythemia.
    a. Plethoric, cyanotic, or excessively flushed with crying.
    b. Hypoglycemia.
    c. CNS symptoms including jitteriness, hypotonia, lethargy, seizures.
3. Anemia.
    a. Acute or chronic blood loss.
    b. Hemolysis from sepsis or ABO/Rh blood group incompatibilities.
    c. Reduced red blood cell production, manifested by severe asphyxia, sepsis, aplastic anemia.
    d. Pale skin, murmur, tachypnea, normal arterial blood pressure, signs of congestive heart failure including hepatosplenomegaly and increased vascular markings on x-ray film.

F. Metabolic problems.

1. Hypoglycemia.
    a. Observed in infants who are large or small for gestational age, infants of diabetic mothers, premature infants, and stressed infants such as those with sepsis, cold stress, or respiratory distress.
    b. Clinical findings:
        (1) Jitteriness, irritability.
        (2) Seizures.
        (3) Hypothermia, temperature instability.
        (4) Lethargy.
        (5) Poor feeding, emesis.
        (6) Apnea.
        (7) Cardiorespiratory distress, cyanosis, oxygen requirement.
        (8) Pallor.
        (9) Tachycardia.
        (10) Weak or high-pitched cry.
2. Adverse effects of maternal medications; maternal use of illicit drugs.
    a. Magnesium sulfate. Infants present with respiratory depression, decreased muscle tone, decreased serum calcium concentration.
    b. Tocolytics. Infants may present with hypoglycemia.
    c. Narcotics. Infants present with apnea, respiratory depression, periodic breathing.

    d. Cocaine. Infants may present with apnea, poor muscle tone initially and then irritability and agitation, tremors, feeding difficulties.
    e. Marijuana or methadone. Infants present with hyperthermia, agitation, diarrhea.
    f. Alcohol. Infants have fetal alcohol syndrome with dysmorphic and behavioral abnormalities.

G. **Infection (see also Chapter 17).**

1. Generalized bacterial or viral disease; acquired in utero or nosocomial.
2. Clinical findings. NOTE: Nearly 90% of neonates with early onset group B streptococcus have signs of infection within 12 hours of birth (Mitchell, Steffenson, Hogan, and Brooks, 1997).
    a. Temperature instability.
    b. Tachypnea, apnea.
    c. Respiratory distress, cyanosis.
    d. Tachycardia.
    e. Cool, mottled skin; weak pulses; capillary refill lasting longer than 2 seconds; hypotension.
    f. Disseminated intravascular coagulation.
    g. Hepatosplenomegaly.
    h. Unexplained jaundice.
    i. Purpura, petechiae.
    j. Hypoglycemia or hyperglycemia.
    k. Poor feeding, emesis, abdominal distention.
    l. Lethargy, poor muscle tone.
3. In utero viral infection. Infant may be small for gestational age with microcephaly.

H. **Congenital anomalies.** Frequently obvious on gross examination.
1. Diaphragmatic hernia.
    a. Immediate onset, at birth, of significant respiratory distress.
    b. Shift in heart tones, decreased or unequal breath sounds, bowel tones heard in chest, scaphoid abdomen, cyanosis.
2. Esophageal atresia with or without tracheoesophageal fistula.
    a. Excessive amniotic fluid.
    b. Increased pooling of secretions in oropharynx, respiratory distress; unable to place orogastric tube.
3. Abdominal wall defects: omphalocele, gastroschisis.
4. Limb anomalies: amniotic banding, talipes equinovarus, polydactyly, syndactyly.
5. Neural tube defects.
6. Intestinal obstructions.
7. Chromosomal abnormalities such as trisomy 21 or trisomy 18.
8. Urogenital abnormalities: exstrophy of bladder, hypospadias, epispadias, ambiguous genitalia.

INITIAL STABILIZATION OF THE SICK NEWBORN INFANT

A. **Short-term observation in transition nursery to monitor trends before infant's transfer to NICU.**

1. Infant may be capable of resolving the problem on his or her own if given time (e.g., correction of mild acidosis from asphyxia, clearing of lung fluid, stabilization of blood glucose concentration, stabilization of blood pressure).
2. Monitor and record trends (i.e., improved respiratory rate toward normal, improved perfusion, normal glucose screens).

B. Avoid excessive handling.

1. Organize care and interventions to avoid frequent, unnecessary stimulation of an already stressed infant.
2. Use pulse oximeter and/or cardiorespiratory monitor to reduce hands-on determination of vital signs.
3. Reduce background stimulation such as loud noises or bright lights.
4. Use nonnutritive sucking to lower activity levels and reduce energy needs.
   a. Infant may be more comfortable in a prone position.
   b. Crying can be stressful and is similar to a Valsalva maneuver, with prolonged exhalation, obstructed venous return, quick inspiratory gasp, and right-to-left shunting at the foramen ovale.
   c. Crying depletes energy reserves and increases oxygen consumption.

C. Provide a neutral thermal environment (refer to Chapter 4, Thermoregulation).

1. Observe infant for apnea and hypotension during warming.
2. Avoid hyperthermia.

D. Supply glucose.

1. Oral administration of glucose for a blood glucose level of 20–40 mg/dL; early, frequent feedings by nipple, gavage, or nursing.
   a. Give at least ½ to 1 ounce of formula by nipple or gavage if there are no contraindications to enteral feedings and the infant is free of symptoms (see Routine Care Considerations in the Transition Nursery, above). If condition is stable, infant may be allowed to nurse 5–10 minutes on each breast.
   b. Begin maintenance formula at 50–70 kcal/kg per day or breast-feed on demand every 2–3 hours.
   c. Check blood glucose 1 hour after feeding.
   d. Consider giving a formula designed for premature infants.
      (1) These formulas provide 50% of carbohydrate in the form of glucose polymers that are easily absorbed; salivary amylase retains its activity in the infant's stomach because of increased gastric pH and is effective in digestion of glucose polymers (Blackburn and Loper, 1992).
      (2) Approximately 50% of the fats are provided as medium-chain triglycerides (MCTs). MCTs are absorbed from the stomach; they may also increase the level of plasma ketones, which can be used as an alternative substrate to glucose for brain metabolism (Blackburn and Loper, 1992).
      (3) The process of absorbing fat (fatty acid oxidation and ketogenesis) spares glucose for brain energy needs; free fatty acids and ketones promote glucose production by providing essential gluconeogenic cofactors.
      (4) Healthy newborn infants respond to a protein meal by preferentially increasing glucagon, which elicits a glycemic response.
2. Intravenous administration of glucose for hypoglycemia (see Routine Care Considerations in the Transition Nursery, item D: Glucose Needs/First Feeding) is as follows:
   a. Provide bolus (2 mL/kg) of 10% dextrose in water ($D_{10}W$), followed by an infusion of 6–8 mg/kg per minute; $D_{10}W = 100$ mg/mL.
   b. Monitor therapy with frequent glucose checks and titrate infusion rate and concentration to meet the infant's needs. NOTE: Do not administer an IV bolus of glucose greater than 25% dextrose in water because of reactive hypoglycemia and hypertonicity of the solution. Always follow a glucose bolus with a continuous infusion of glucose.

E. Supply oxygen; assess needs with a pulse oximeter or arterial blood gas determinations and close observation.

1. Extended oxygen use in the transition nurery requires notification of the physician and transfer to a level II or level III setting.
2. Provide warmed, humidified oxygen by oxygen hood, continuous positive airway pressure by nasal prongs, or assisted ventilation by endotracheal tube according to the infant's needs (refer to Chapter 9).
3. Monitor oxygen provided with an oxygen analyzer. Record blow-by oxygen as liters per minute and distance from infant's face.

F. **Supply volume expanders, including blood, normal saline solution, 5% albumin.**

1. For hypotension and blood loss.
2. Requires IV line placement and transfer to level II nursery for continued management and observation, including cardiorespiratory monitoring and blood pressure checks to adjust therapy as necessary.

G. **Naloxone hydrochloride (Narcan).**

1. Administer drug for severe respiratory depression in delivery room and history of maternal narcotic administration within past four hours.
2. Do *not* use naloxone if mother has history of opioid dependency: *may precipitate acute withdrawal symptoms.*

H. **Antibiotics.**

1. As indicated by history, current status of the infant, and initial results of sepis evaluation.
2. Administer via peripheral IV or heparin-lock IV line.

Parent Teaching

BEFORE DELIVERY

A. **History.** Review obstetric history; anticipate needs of infant at delivery.

B. **Complications.** If there are expected complications (preterm delivery, congenital anomalies) and time permits, discuss anticipated plan of care with the family.
1. Discuss plans for managing the infant, including plans for transfer to a level II or III nursery and any special equipment that may be used (oxygen hood, incubator, ventilator, monitors).
2. Allow the parents to tour the NICU if possible.

C. **Parental support.** Encourage parents to express their feelings, fears, misgivings; involve support persons.

AT DELIVERY

A. Place infant on mother's abdomen when possible with uncomplicated deliveries; use family's birth plan as much as possible.

B. After delivery room assessment, return infant to family if infant's condition is stable.

C. Answer questions regarding acrocyanosis, Apgar scores, morphologic findings.

D. Allow parents time to visit, breast-feed, see extended family.

DURING TRANSITION

A. "Introduce" baby to family by noting unique features (dimples, long eyelashes, hair color).

B. Encourage support person to touch and talk to the infant.

C. Discuss physical findings such as caput succedaneum, head molding, positional deformities, birth marks.

D. Discuss infant's sensory capabilities, including seeing, hearing, smell.

E. Listen to the parents. Allow them to express their reactions as they compare their "dream" baby with the real baby they now have (too tiny, not the right sex, deformed, premature).

F. After completion of admission procedures, the infant is returned to the family for feeding and visiting.

G. Allow family to participate in the infant's care, such as giving the first bath or first feeding.

POSTPARTUM PERIOD (EARLY DISCHARGE)

A. Parental involvement. Involve the parents in evaluation of their learning needs; begin teaching as soon as delivery occurs.

B. Short hospital stays and family instruction. With shorter hospital stays, there is less time available for teaching and an increased importance of teaching. This may be the only information many families receive on care of a newborn infant.
1. Classes; videotaped lectures.
    a. Cardiopulmonary resuscitation; safety.
    b. Breast-feeding.
    c. Childbirth preparation.
    d. Developmental milestones.
2. Follow-up visits by nurse to the home and phone calls from postpartum nurses. Encourage families to call the nursery if they have questions about their baby's care.
3. Follow-up visit with primary care provider. Encourage family to select a primary care provider and assist in making an appointment for the first visit.
4. Return visit for newborn screening if needed.

TRANSFER TO LEVEL II OR III SETTING

A. Provide prenatal teaching—if possible, with visits to NICU.

B. Provide information booklets, with location, phone numbers, visiting regulations, parent-to-parent groups, necessary support personnel.

C. Bring mother to infant's bedside if infant is unable to return to mother after delivery. Allow family members to be near infant as much as possible and encourage them to see past the equipment to the infant and his or her special needs (gentle touch, stroking, soft voice, a familiar person).

D. When infant is stable, allow family members to visit in the privacy of their postpartum room or a parent room if condition warrants; for example, an infant with a heparin lock for antibiotics might go to the mother's room to nurse.

E. Provide a picture and footprints of the infant for the family. This is especially important if transfer to a level II or III nursery will be to another facility.

F. Facilitate family in keeping in contact with the transfer facility, and be available to explain information given to the family.

REFERENCES

American Academy of Pediatrics Policy Statement: Routine evaluation of blood pressure, hematocrit, and glucose in newborns (RE9322). Pediatrics, 92(3):474–476, 1993.

American Academy of Pediatrics: Hepatitis B. In Peter, G. (Ed.): 1997 Red Book. Report of the Committee on Infectious Disease, 24th ed. Elk Grove Village, Ill., Author, 1997, pp. 247–260.

American Academy of Pediatrics and American College of Obstetricians and Gynecologists: Guidelines for Perinatal Care, 4th ed. Elk Grove Village, Ill., and Washington, D.C., Authors, 1997, p. 157.

American Academy of Pediatrics Committee on Infectious Diseases: Update on timing of hepatitis B vaccine for premature infants and for children with lapsed immunizations. Pediatrics, 94(3):1994.

Blackburn, S.T., and Loper, D.L. (Eds.): Maternal, Fetal, and Neonatal Physiology. Philadelphia, W.B. Saunders, 1992, pp. 413–414, 420.

Bloom, R.S.: Delivery room resuscitation of the newborn. In Fanaroff, A.A., and Martin R.J. (Eds.): Neonatal-Perinatal Medicine: Diseases of the Fetus and Infant, 5th ed. St. Louis, Mosby–Year Book, 1992, pp. 301–324.

Burchett, S.K.: Viral infections. In Cloherty, J.P., and Stark, A.R. (Eds.): Manual of Neonatal Care, 4th ed. Philadelphia, Lippincott-Raven, 1998, pp. 265–269.

Centers for Disease Control: Hepatitis B virus: A comprehensive strategy for eliminating transmission in the United States through universal childhood vaccination. MMWR. Morb. Mortal. Wkly. Rep., 40:1–19, 1991.

Cornblath, M., and Schwartz, R. (Eds.): Disorders of Carbohydrate Metabolism in Infancy, 3rd ed. Boston, Blackwell Scientific Publications, 1991, p. 55.

Desmond, M.M., Rudolph, A.J., and Phitaksphraiwan, P.: The transitional nursery: A mechanism for preventive medicine in the newborn. Pediatr. Clin. North Am., 13:651–668, 1966.

Gorrie, T.M., McKinney, E.S., and Murray, S.S.: Foundations of Maternal Newborn Nursing. Philadelphia, W.B. Saunders, 1994, p. 497.

Kalhan, C.C., and Saker, F.: Disorders of carbohydrate metabolism. In Fanaroff, A.A., and Martin, R.J. (Eds.): Neonatal-Perinatal Medicine: Diseases of the Fetus and Infant, 6th ed. St. Louis, Mosby, 1997, pp. 1439–1463.

Mitchell, A., Steffenson, N., Hogan, H., and Brooks, S.: Neonatal group B streptococcal disease. MCN; Am. J. Matern. Child Nurs., 22:249–253, September/October 1997.

Moore, K.L.: The Developing Human: Clinically Oriented Embryology, 6th ed. Philadelphia, W.B. Saunders, 1998, pp. 392–393.

Nelson, N.: Physiology of transition. In Avery, G.B., Fletcher, M.A., and MacDonald, M.G. (Eds.): Neonatology: Pathophysiology and Management of the Newborn, 4th ed. Philadelphia, J.B. Lippincott, 1994, pp. 223–247.

Overall, J.C., Jr.: Viral infections in the fetus and neonate. In Feigin, R.D., Cherry, J.D. (Eds.): Textbook of Pediatric Infectious Diseases, 3rd ed. Philadelphia, W.B. Saunders, 1992, pp. 924–959.

Phibbs, R.H.: Delivery room management of the newborn. In Avery, G.B., Fletcher, M.A., and MacDonald, M.G. (Eds.): Neonatology: Pathophysiology and Management of the Newborn, 4th ed. Philadelphia, J.B. Lippincott, 1994, pp. 248–268.

Philip, A.G.S.: Neonatology: A Practical Guide, 4th ed. Philadelphia, W.B. Saunders, 1996, p. 45.

Sun, Y., Awnetwant, E.L., and Collier, S.B., et al.: Nutrition. In Cloherty, J.P., and Stark, A.R. (Eds.): Manual of Neonatal Care, 4th ed. Philadelphia, Lippincott-Raven, 1998, pp. 120–121.

Thureen, P.T., and Abzug, M.J.: Viral infections. In Thureen, P.J., Deacon, J.M., O'Neill, P., and Hernandez, J. (Eds.): Assessment and Care of the Well Newborn. Philadelphia, W.B. Saunders, 1999, p. 324.

Wilker, R.E.: Metabolic problems. In Cloherty, J.P., and Stark, A.R. (Eds.): Manual of Neonatal Care, 4th ed. Philadelphia, Lippincott-Raven, 1998, p. 545.

ADDITIONAL READINGS

American Academy of Pediatrics Committee on Infectious Diseases: Update on timing of hepatitis B vaccination for premature infants and for children with lapsed immunization. Pediatrics, 94:403–404, 1994.

American Academy of Pediatrics Committee on Infectious Diseases and Committee on Fetus and Newborn: Revised guidelines for prevention of early-onset group B streptococcal (GBS) infection. Pediatrics, 99:489–498, 1997.

Avery, G.B., Fletcher, M.A., and MacDonald, M.G. (Eds.): Neonatology: Pathophysiology and Management of the Newborn, 4th ed. Philadelphia, J.B. Lippincott, 1994.

Baker, L., and Stanley, C.A.: Neonatal hypoglycemia. In Bardin, C.W. (Ed.): Curent Therapy in Endocrinology

and Metabolism, 5th ed. St. Louis, Mosby–Year Book, 1994, pp. 376–380.

Blackburn, S.T., and Loper, D.L. (Eds.): Maternal, Fetal, and Neonatal Physiology. Philadelphia, W.B. Saunders, 1992.

Bloom, R.S.: Delivery room resuscitation of the newborn. In Fanaroff, A.A., and Martin, R.J. (Eds.): Neonatal-Perinatal Medicine: Diseases of the Fetus and Infant, 6th ed. St. Louis, Mosby, 1997.

Brooks, C.: Neonatal hypoglycemia, Neonatal Network, 16:15–24, March 1997.

Cornblath, M.: Hypoglycemia in infancy: The need for a rational definition. Pediatrics, 85:834–837, 1990.

Filer, L.J., Jr.: A glimpse into the future of infant nutrition. Pediatr. Ann., 21:633–639, October 1992.

Furdon, S.A.: Recognizing congestive heart failure in the neonatal period. Neonatal Network, *16*:5–11, October 1997.

Gorrie, T.M., McKinney, E.S., and Murray, S.S.: Foundations of Maternal Newborn Nursing. Philadelphia, W.B. Saunders, 1994.

Hammerman, C.: PDA: Clinical relevance of prostaglandins and prostaglandin inhibitors in PDA pathophysiology and treatment. Clin. Perinatol., *22*(2):457–470, 1995.

Hamosh, M.: Digestion in the newborn. Clin. Perinatol. *23*(2):191–209, 1996.

Karp, T.B., Scardino, C., and Butler, L.A.: Glucose metabolism in the neonate: The short and sweet of it. Neonatal Network, *14*(8):17–23, December 1995.

Kays, D.W.: Surgical conditions of the neonatal intestinal tract. Clin. Perinatol., *23*(2):353–373, 1996.

National Association of Neonatal Nurses: Neonatal Hypoglycemia: Guidelines for Practice. This guideline was developed by Elizabeth Estrada Jarosz for NANN. Petaluma, Calif., Author, 1994.

Nichols, F.H., and Zwelling, E.: Maternal-Newborn Nursing: Theory and Practice. Philadelphia, W.B. Saunders, 1997.

Paul, K.E.: Recognition, stabilization, and early management of infants with critical congenital heart disease presenting in the first days of life. Neonatal Network, *14*(5):13–20, August 1995.

Polinski, C.: The value of the white blood cell count and differential in the prediction of neonatal sepsis. Neonatal Network, *15*(7):13–23, October 1996.

Sansoucie, D.A., and Cavaliere, T.A.: Transition from fetal to extrauterine circulation. Neonatal Network, *16*(2):5–12, March 1997.

Serwer, G.A.: Postnatal circulatory adjustments. *In* Polin, R., and Fox, W. (Eds.): Fetal and Neonatal Physiology. Philadelphia, W.B. Saunders, 1998.

Shapiro, C.N.: Epidemiology of hepatitis B. Pediatr. Infect. Dis. J., *12*(5):433–437, 1993.

Simpson, K.R., and Creehan, P.A.: Perinatal Nursing. Philadelphia, J.B. Lippincott, 1996.

Spilman, L.J., and Furdon, S.A.: Recognition, understanding, and current management of cardiac lesions with decreased pulmonary blood flow. Neonatal Network, *17*(4):7–18, June 1998.

Tappero, E.P., and Honeyfield, M.L.: Physical Assessment of the Newborn, 2nd ed. Petaluma, Calif., NICU Ink, 1996.

Tsang, R.C., Lucas, A., Uauy, R., et al.: Nutritional Needs of the Preterm Infant: Scientific Basis and Practical Guidelines. Baltimore, Williams & Wilkins, 1993.

Verklan, M.T.: Diagnostic techniques in cardiac disorders. Pt. 1. Neonatal Network, *16*(4):9–15, June 1997.

Wood, M.K.: Acyanotic cardiac lesions with increased pulmonary blood flow. Neonatal Network, *16*(3):17–25, April 1997.

Wood, M.K.: Acyanotic cardiac lesions with normal pulmonary blood flow. Neonatal Network, *17*(3):5–11, April 1998.

Chapter 4

Thermoregulation

Sharon Anderson

Objectives

1. Identify mechanisms of heat loss and heat production.

2. Describe the effects of cold stress on the neonate.

3. Identify the neonates' limitations in heat production and heat conservation.

4. Define the neutral thermal environment.

5. Discuss effects of hyperthermia.

6. Identify methods used to prevent heat loss.

7. Identify nursing actions to create a physical environment based on thermoregulation principles.

Providing a thermal environment that maintains a core body temperature within a normal narrow range is essential to the survival of the newborn infant. Pierre Budin (1907), the first neonatologist, discovered the need for temperature control after studying the increased survival rates of premature infants whose rectal temperatures were maintained between 36° and 37° C. In his book *The Nursling*, published in 1907, he emphasized the need for temperature control. The work of Budin and many others formed the basis for nursing care of the premature infant. A thorough understanding of thermoregulation is necessary to provide an optimal environment for the neonate to thrive. This chapter will review concepts of thermoregulation and management of the physical environment.

Concepts of Thermoregulation

A. **Homeotherm:** animal (mammal) with the ability to balance heat loss and heat production to maintain a stable deep-body (core) temperature within a very narrow range despite gross variations/changes in the environmental temperature.

B. **Poikilotherm:** animal (reptile) that has little or no ability to produce and regulate heat; takes on the temperature of the environment.

C. **Thermal balance, or equilibrium:** rate of heat generation that is equal to the rate of heat dissipation.

D. **Neutral thermal environment:** narrow range of environmental temperature in which an infant is not required to increase or decrease heat production above natural resting levels and has minimal oxygen consumption.

E. **Thermoneutrality:** optimal thermal condition needed to support internal functions.

F. **Critical temperature:** temperature below thermal neutrality where oxygen consumption increases in an attempt to maintain normal body temperature.

Physiologic Differences Affecting Thermoregulation

Many physiologic differences between the neonate and the adult predispose neonates to the risk of hypothermia.

A. **Adults can produce heat from voluntary muscle activity, involuntary tonic or rhythmic muscle activity (shivering), and nonshivering thermogenesis (cold-induced increase in oxygen consumption and heat production).** Neonates are unable to produce heat through shivering and rely on nonshivering thermogenesis (brown fat metabolism) for heat production.

B. **Heat transfer through the internal gradient is increased in neonates because of their thin layer of subcutaneous fat and large surface-to-volume ratio (three times greater in the term infant and four times greater in the preterm infant than in an adult [LeBlanc, 1991]).** Subcutaneous fat accounts for 16% of body fat in infants, in comparison with 30–35% in adults (Davis, 1980).

C. **Preterm infants have increased evaporative heat loss because of their greater percentage of body water and increased permeability of the skin.**

Control of Body Temperature

A. Heat production.

1. The hypothalamus is the central regulating mechanism (control center) for temperature regulation.
   a. Thermal stimuli providing information to the hypothalamus are derived from the body's skin and deep thermal receptors and from thermal receptors in the preoptic area of the hypothalamus (Thomas, 1994).
   b. The hypothalamus can alter heat production and respond to temperature changes by altering metabolism, motor tone and activity, vasomotor activity, and sweating to produce heat loss or gain.
   c. Asphyxia, central nervous system damage, and drugs such as diazepam can impair heat production mechanisms.
2. The sympathetic nervous system activates heat production in response to cold stress. The process of nonshivering thermogenesis, or brown fat metabolism, is the most important means of heat production in the neonate.
   a. Characteristics of brown fat.
      (1) Situated around the great vessels, kidneys, adrenal glands, axillas, nape of the neck, and between the scapulas.
      (2) Comprises 2–7% of the total body weight in the term newborn infant (Bruck, 1978).
      (3) Present at 26–28 weeks' gestation. Stores increase until 3–5 weeks postnatally unless depleted by cold stress.

(4) Reduced in preterm infants and very low birth weight infants.

(5) Cannot be replenished if used.

(6) Metabolically very active because of cell size, cell number, and the internal mitochondrial structure.

  b. Brown fat metabolism.

    (1) Initiated by stimulation of thermal receptors in skin (primarily the face).

    (2) Controlled by the sympathetic nervous system through release of norepinephrine, which stimulates hydrolysis of brown fat triglycerides into nonesterified free fatty acids and glycerol.

    (3) Produced by the metabolism of fatty acids, which require oxygen and glucose for the thermogenic process.

      (a) The increased oxygen demand may result in hypoxia, metabolic acidosis, pulmonary vasoconstriction, and death.

      (b) Hypoglycemia may occur as a result of rapid consumption of carbohydrate stores for the metabolism of brown fat.

      (c) Heat from this process reaches the skin by direct conduction through body tissues or blood vessels.

B. Heat loss.

1. Fetal thermoregulation is maintained by the dissipation of heat produced by the fetus to the mother across accelerated maternal-environmental temperature and evaporative gradients (placenta, surface to surface, and via the blood). The temperature of the fetus is 0.5° C higher than that of the mother. Fetal hyperthermia induced by maternal infection, dehydration, or increases in environmental temperature may result in seizures or death of the fetus (Baumgart, 1993).

2. Heat is transferred to and from the body surface by four mechanisms: conduction, convection, evaporation, and radiation (NANN, 1997).

  a. Conduction: transfer of heat between two solid objects that are in direct contact.

    (1) Characteristics of transfer of heat by conduction.

      (a) Heat loss may occur when an infant is placed on a cold scale, x-ray cassette, circumcision board, operating room table, or mattress.

      (b) Heat gain may occur when an infant is placed on an object warmer than his own body temperature, such as a chemically activated warming mattress or circulating-water heating pad.

      (c) The rate at which heat is transferred is directly proportional to the size of the temperature gradient.

      (d) The larger the surface area in contact with the object, the greater the heat transfer.

      (e) The greater the ability of a surface to transfer or conduct heat, the greater will be the heat transfer between the two surfaces. Conductive heat loss is greater on highly conductive surfaces such as metal and minimal with insulation such as blankets, clothing, or skin-to-skin contact.

    (2) Mechanisms to decrease conductive heat losses.

      (a) Prewarm surfaces the infant is likely to come in contact with, such as scales, x-ray plates, circumcision boards, operating room tables, and mattresses.

      (b) Preheat incubators, clothing, stethoscopes, heat shields, blankets, and knit caps.

      (c) Use warming blankets or pads. The temperature of these items should not exceed 40° C, and the infant's position should be changed frequently (every 30 minutes) to prevent overexposure of fragile skin to the heat source.

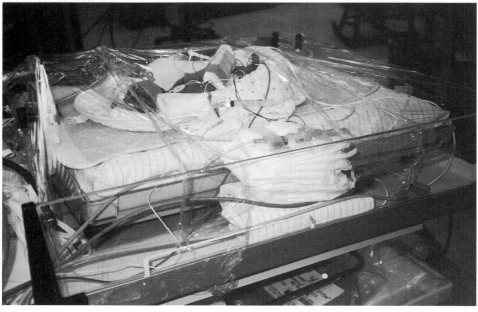

Figure 4–1
Transparent wrap stretched over radiant warmer between side panels to prevent vertical current airflow.

       (d) Use the lowest temperature possible (44° C) if transcutaneous heat probes are used.

   b. Convection: transfer of heat to the air moving across and around the body.

    (1) Characteristics of transfer of heat by convection. The amount of heat loss through convection is dependent on:

       (a) The temperature gradient between the infant and air or liquid. If a large gradient exists between the infant's skin temperature and the environmental temperature, the heat loss or gain is greater.

       (b) The amount of body surface exposed to the air. The infant has a large surface area/body mass ratio, resulting in increased losses by convection.

       (c) The speed of the air movement. Convective losses increase when the infant is exposed to drafts by air vents, cold oxygen, frequent opening of incubator portholes or hoods, or removal of heat-shielding devices.

    (2) Mechanisms to decrease convective heat losses.

       (a) Warm the oxygen used in oxygen hoods.

       (b) Place infants away from drafts or air vents.

       (c) Cluster care activities so that incubator portholes or hoods are opened only when necessary.

       (d) Swaddle infants in cribs with blankets and knit caps.

       (e) Place a light blanket over top of crib if drafts are a concern.

       (f) Clothe and swaddle infants in incubators to reduce exposed surface area and provide external thermal insulation (Perlstein, 1998).

       (g) Maintain raised side panels of radiant warmers to prevent cross-current airflow; use transparent plastic wrap stretched over radiant warmer bed between side panels to prevent vertical-current airflow (Fig. 4–1).

       (h) Provide intrahospital transport (e.g., to x-ray department, operating room) in prewarmed transport incubators.

       (i) Use plastic heat shields in incubator or double-walled incubator to decrease convective losses and diminish airflow (Korones and Bada-Ellzey, 1993).

  c. Evaporation: heat loss by conversion of liquid, usually water, into vapor.

    (1) Characteristics of heat transfer by evaporation. Evaporation:

       (a) Can account for 25% of the infant's total heat loss at delivery.

       (b) Is most pronounced in the delivery room and may result in a decrease of 0.3° C per minute in skin temperature (Sinclair, 1976).

       (c) Includes heat lost through evaporation from the skin or respiratory tract (insensible water loss).

       (d) Is increased in premature infants because of immature keratinization of the epidermal stratum corneum. Keratin formation increases with gestational age and occurs rapidly in the first 1–4 weeks of postnatal life, significantly decreasing evaporative losses.

       (e) Is enhanced in the newborn infant because large surface areas are exposed for evaporative losses from the skin.

       (f) Increases depending on air speed and relative humidity.

       (g) Rises with activity, tachypnea, radiant warmers, and phototherapy.

       (h) Increases with low relative humidity. At a relative humidity of 100%, evaporative heat loss is nonexistent (Sulyok, Jequier, and Ryser, 1982).

       (i) Can be responsible for low birth weight infants losing up to 134 mL/kg per day through insensible water loss when nursed under a radiant warmer (Baumgart et al., 1982).

    (2) Mechanisms to decrease evaporative heat losses.

       (a) Dry the infant immediately after birth or bathing; use prewarmed blankets and towels to dry the infant in the delivery room. Wrap infant with prewarmed blankets and provide a dry, prewarmed stocking cap (D'Apolito, 1994).

       (b) Warm the solutions used on the infant's skin.

       (c) Warm and humidify oxygen.

       (d) Stretch plastic, transparent wrap over the warmer bed between the side panels.

       (e) Bathe under radiant warmer in a draft-free environment.

       (f) Use linens and diapers that direct moisture away from infant's skin.

  d. Radiation: transfer of heat between solid objects that are not in direct contact.

    (1) Characteristics of transfer of heat by radiation. Radiation:

       (a) Is based on temperature gradient. The rate of heat transfer depends on the temperature gradient, surface absorption, and amount of surface area facing the object (LeBlanc, 1987).

       (b) Is the major form of heat loss of infants in incubators.

       (c) Is independent of ambient temperature and other heat loss mechanisms.

    (2) Mechanisms of radiant heat loss or gain.

       (a) When an infant is nursed in a radiant warmer, heat radiates from the radiant heating mechanism toward the baby. Radiant heat loss may occur from the sides of the infant exposed to the cooler room walls (Baumgart, 1990).

       (b) An infant in an incubator transfers heat to the incubator walls; if the walls of the incubator are cold, the infant is cooled even if the ambient temperature of the incubator is warm.

       (c) An incubator or crib placed near a cold wall or window will radiate heat toward the cold object.

       (d) An incubator can act as a "greenhouse" if exposed to sunlight. The acrylic plastic cover will transmit the heat from the sun, and the

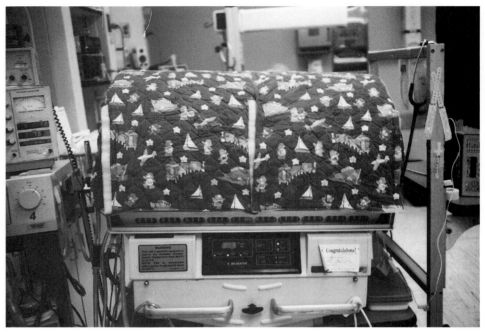

Figure 4–2
Insulating cover placed over an incubator to decrease radiant heat loss.

infant can become overheated. This can also occur with heating lamps or phototherapy lights used with an incubator.
(3) Mechanisms for decreasing radiant heat loss.
  (a) Prewarm incubators, radiant heat warmers, and heat shields.
  (b) Use heat shields and double-walled incubators to prevent heat loss to the cooler room temperature.
  (c) Place incubators away from exterior walls, windows, and direct sunlight.
  (d) Place an insulating cover over an incubator to decrease radiant heat loss (Fig. 4–2).
  (e) Cover external windows with insulating material.

Hypothermia and Cold Stress (Rectal and Axillary Temperature <36.5° C)

A. Consequences of hypothermia and cold stress (Blake and Murray, 1998).

1. Short-term response.
  a. Hypoglycemia, hypoxia, metabolic acidosis caused by metabolism of brown fat, release of fatty acids, and anaerobic metabolism.
  b. Pulmonary vasoconstriction caused by metabolic acidosis.
  c. Increased respiratory distress caused by hypoxia and acidosis.
  d. Feeding intolerance caused by decreased energy to eat and/or digest food.
2. Chronic response.
  a. Impaired weight gain as a result of consumption of calories for heat production.

b. If the degree and duration of cold exposure exceed the infant's ability to compensate, a gradual fall in core temperature will occur, accompanied by respiratory failure, heart failure, depletion of energy resources, and eventually death.

B. **Symptoms of thermal instability.**

1. Apnea.
2. Bradycardia.
3. Tachypnea.
4. Poor perfusion.
5. Acrocyanosis.
6. Oxygen requirement.
7. Seizures.
8. Acidosis.
9. Feeding intolerance.
10. Lethargy.
11. Irritability.
12. Jitteriness.
13. Hypoglycemia.
14. Cyanosis.
15. Abdominal temperature lower than axillary temperature.

C. **Infants at risk of having thermal instability.**

1. Premature infants. Body fat and insulation, ability to maintain a flexed posture, and stores of brown fat are decreased. Surface area/weight ratio and body water content are increased.
2. Small for gestational age infants. Body fat and insulation and stores of brown fat are decreased. Surface area/weight ratio and metabolic rate are increased.
3. Infants stressed because of birth asphyxia, hypoglycemia, respiratory distress, or sepsis.

D. **Treatment of hypothermia.**

1. Warm infant slowly with radiant heat warmer or incubator. Rapid warming has been associated with heat-induced apnea and with hypotension and shock caused by vasodilation.
   a. Recommendations for rewarming infant in an incubator based on the principle of producing heat gain from the environment while eliminating further heat loss from the infant (Perlstein, 1997).
      (1) Warm incubator air over the infant to 36° C and simultaneously increase the humidity to reduce evaporative losses.
      (2) Use a heat shield to decrease radiant losses.
      (3) Monitor with simultaneous axillary, skin, and rectal temperatures.
   b. Considerations while rewarming the infant.
      (1) If the temperature ceases to decrease or begins to rise slowly, maintain the infant's current environment and continue to monitor.
      (2) If the infant's temperature continues to fall, raise the incubator temperature to 37° C, evaluate for missed sources of heat loss, and check that the humidity is greater than 70%.
      (3) If the infant's temperature is still falling 15 minutes later, raise the incubator temperature to 38° C and add a radiant warmer over the incubator to increase the external wall temperature.
      (4) If the infant becomes apneic or exhibits signs of shock, slow the rate of rewarming.
2. Supply heat with the use of chemically activated mattresses or circulating-water heating pads. Avoid hot water bottles, gloves filled with hot water, or heat lamps because they may cause burns.

3. Reduce heat loss by mechanisms discussed under heat loss.
4. Administer oxygen as indicated.
5. Correct abnormalities in acid-base balance.
6. Monitor glucose needs with whole-blood glucose screening tests.

Hyperthermia (Temperature >37.5° C)

Hyperthermia may be iatrogenic or a symptom of a disease process or cold stress. NOTE: An increased axillary temperature with a decreased abdominal temperature may not be hyperthermia; it may be cold stress, which occurs as the infant burns brown fat in that region and causes the axillary temperature to increase.

A. Causes of hyperthermia.

1. Maternal fever, resulting in fever in the neonate during the first minutes of life (fetal temperature is greater than maternal temperature).
2. Overheating from incubators, radiant warmers, or ambient environmental temperature.
3. Phototherapy lights, sunlight.
4. Excessive bundling or swaddling.
5. Infection.
6. CNS disorders such as asphyxia.
7. Dehydration.

B. Effects of hyperthermia.

1. Tachycardia and tachypnea as infant attempts to release excess heat.
2. Sweating in older premature and term infants to increase evaporative loss.
3. Dehydration resulting from increased fluid loss.
4. Increased insensible water loss.
5. Hypoxia and hypoglycemia caused by increased demands for oxygen and glucose.
6. Hypotension and "flushed" skin as a result of peripheral vasodilation to facilitate heat loss.
7. Seizure activity and apnea resulting from effects on the CNS.
8. Poor feeding, decreased activity and tone, weak cry because of CNS depression.
9. Poor weight gain.
10. Shock.

C. Treatment of hyperthermia (Blake and Murray, 1998).

1. Treat cause, such as infection, dehydration, or CNS disorder.
2. Remove external heat sources.
3. Remove anything that blocks heat loss.
4. Move crib or incubator from extra heat sources (e.g., sunlight, phototherapy lights).
5. Remove excess bundling/swaddling materials.
6. Check incubator and radiant warmers for appropriate functioning.
7. Assess thermistor position for appropriate location on the infant.
8. During the cooling process, monitor and record temperatures (skin, axillary, environmental) every 30 minutes.

Managing the Physical Environment

No single environment is appropriate for all sizes and conditions of the neonate. The medical condition of an infant may require some compromise as to the method of providing an optimal thermal-neutral environment.

A. Radiant warmers.

1. Body temperature is maintained and caregivers have easy access for caregiving activities.
2. A servocontrol probe is attached to the infant to maintain skin temperature at a preselected temperature.
3. No feedback or control of the infant's temperature is provided when a radiant warmer is operated in the nonservocontrol mode. This mode can be used to prewarm the bed, but because of the risk of overheating, the warmer should not be operated in this mode when an infant is present (NANN, 1997).
4. Increased convective and evaporative heat losses, which increase insensible water loss.
5. Acrylic plastic heat shields block radiant heat and are not recommended for use in radiant warmers (NANN, 1997). Plastic wrap stretched over the warmer bed will reduce insensible water loss and will not block radiant heat.

B. Incubators.

1. Conductive heat losses are reduced because of the circulation of warm air.
2. Radiant heat is lost to incubator walls of single-walled incubators. Radiant heat loss can be decreased by using double-walled incubators, by using heat shields, and/or by draping a blanket or quilt over the incubator.
3. Humidity can be provided to reduce evaporative losses, but the risk of *Pseudomonas* colonization must be considered.
4. Servocontrol mode can be used, or the desired temperature can be set manually (see Table 4–1 for neutral thermal environmental temperatures).
   a. Servocontrol mode is recommended for the very low birth weight infant or the infant whose temperature fluctuates on manual mode.
   b. With servocontrol mode the body temperature will remain constant, but the environmental temperature may fluctuate and may represent the onset of illness.
5. Ambient and skin temperature fluctuations can occur when the hood or portholes are opened. Plastic sleeves used with the portholes can minimize this loss of heat (NANN, 1997).

C. Temperature probes with servocontrol mode.

1. Temperature probes should be attached to the skin over soft tissue, generally on the abdomen. Do not place probe over bony prominences or extremities (NANN, 1997).
2. The infant must not lie on the probe. This insulates the probe and results in a false high reading of the infant's skin temperature and cooling of air temperature, thus cooling the infant (NANN, 1997).
3. The probe should be covered with a heat reflector if radiant heat or phototherapy is in use.

D. Clothing and other coverings.

1. External insulation is provided.
2. Transfer of heat by radiant, convective, and conductive heat mechanisms is decreased.
3. Evaporative heat loss is reduced because moist air is trapped near the body surface.
4. Use of a hat decreases the metabolic rate and increases body temperature. Hats made of knitted wool, with a gauze or cotton lining, provide the best protection because they allow a higher volume of air to be trapped between the fibers.
5. Use of servocontrol on an incubator with a clothed infant born at 28–31 weeks' gestation can increase weight gain by 50% because evaporative heat losses are diminished and the infants are less active, resulting in more constant skin temperatures (Medoff-Cooper, 1994).

Table 4–1
NEUTRAL THERMAL ENVIRONMENTAL TEMPERATURES

Age and Weight	Range of Temperature (° C)	Age and Weight	Range of Temperature (° C)
0–6 hours		72–96 hours	
< 1200 g	34.0–35.4	< 1200 g	34.0–35.0
1200–1500 g	33.9–34.4	1200–1500 g	33.0–34.0
1501–2500 g	32.8–33.8	1501–2500 g	31.1–33.2
> 2500 g	32.0–33.8	> 2500 g	29.8–32.8
6–12 hours		4–12 days	
< 1200 g	34.0–35.4	< 1500 g	33.0–34.0
1200–1500 g	33.5–34.4	1501–2500 g	31.0–33.2
1501–2500 g	32.2–33.8	> 2500 g	
> 2500 g	31.4–33.8	4–5 days	29.5–32.6
12–24 hours		5–6 days	29.4–32.3
< 1200 g	34.0–35.4	6–8 days	29.0–32.2
1200–1500 g	33.3–34.3	8–10 days	29.0–31.8
1501–2500 g	31.8–33.8	10–12 days	29.0–31.4
> 2500 g	31.0–33.7	12–14 days	
24–36 hours		< 1500 g	32.6–34.0
< 1200 g	34.0–35.0	1501–2500 g	31.0–33.2
1200–1500 g	33.1–34.2	> 2500 g	29.0–30.8
1501–2500 g	31.6–33.6	2–3 weeks	
> 2500 g	30.7–33.5	< 1500 g	32.2–34.0
36–48 hours		1501–2500 g	30.5–33.0
< 1200 g	34.0–35.0	3–4 weeks	
1200–1500 g	33.0–34.1	< 1500 g	31.6–33.6
1501–2500 g	31.4–33.5	1501–2500 g	30.0–32.7
> 2500 g	30.5–33.3	4–5 weeks	
48–72 hours		< 1500 g	31.2–33.0
< 1200 g	34.0–35.0	1501–2500 g	29.5–32.2
1200–1500 g	33.0–34.0	5–6 weeks	
1501–2500 g	31.2–33.4	< 1500 g	30.6–32.3
> 2500 g	30.1–33.2	1501–2500 g	29.0–31.8

Adapted from Scopes, J., and Ahmed, I.: Arch. Dis. Child. *41*:417, 1966. For their table, Scopes and Ahmed had the walls of the incubator 1° to 2° warmer than the ambient air temperatures.
   Generally speaking, the smaller infants in each weight group will require a temperature in the higher portion of the temperature range. Within each time range, the younger the infant, the higher the temperature required. All infants who weighed more than 2500 g were born at more than 36 weeks of gestation.
   From Klaus, M., Fanaroff, A., and Martin, R.: *In* Klaus, M., and Fanaroff, A.: Care of the High-Risk Neonate, 3rd ed. Philadelphia, W.B. Saunders, 1986, pp. 96–112.

E. Kangaroo care (skin-to-skin contact with mother and infant), used to prevent heat loss, especially in the delivery room (Anderson, 1991).

F. Warming of milk to 37° C for infants weighing less than 1500 g will prevent postprandial thermogenesis, increased metabolic rate, cardiovascular effects, and increased oxygen consumption (Gonzales, Duryea, Vasquez, and Geraghty, 1995).

Monitoring Body Temperature

A. Normal rectal and axillary temperatures, 36.5–37.5° C; normal abdominal skin temperature, 36–36.5° C (Gomella et al., 1994).

B. Temperature taking.

1. Core temperature will remain normal until compensatory mechanisms for heat production begin to fail. This is a late indication of hypothermia. Monitoring the core temperature is not recommended because the sigmoid colon turns at a right angle at 3 cm and insertion of the thermometer less then 3 cm will not

accurately reflect core temperature. Insertion to a depth greater than 3 cm risks intestinal perforation (Blake and Murray, 1998).

2. Axillary temperatures are a safe and practical method of monitoring body temperature. The thermometer must be held in the midaxillary space, in compliance with the manufacturer's recommendation, to ensure an accurate reading. In the presence of cold stress and brown fat metabolism, the axillary temperature may remain high. Despite this limitation, the use of axillary temperatures is recommended for monitoring temperature in the neonate.

3. Skin temperature measured by a temperature probe over the abdomen falls first as a result of peripheral vasoconstriction. It is useful to monitor both axillary and skin temperatures simultaneously.

REFERENCES

Anderson, G.C.: Current knowledge about skin-to-skin (kangaroo) care for preterm infants. J. Perinatol., 21(3):216, 1991.

Baumgart, S.: Radiant heat loss versus radiant heat gain in premature neonates under radiant heaters. Biol. Neonate, 57:10–20, 1990.

Baumgart, S.: Incubation of the human newborn infant. In Pomerance, J.J., and Richardson, C.J. (Eds.): Neonatology for the clinician. Stamford, Conn., Appleton & Lange, 1993, p. 140.

Baumgart, S., Langman, C.B., Sosulski, R., et al.: Fluid, electrolyte, and glucose maintenance in the very low birthweight infant. Clin. Pediatr., 21:199–206, 1982.

Blackburn, S.T., and Loper, D.L.: Maternal, Fetal, and Neonatal Physiology: A Clinical Perspective. Philadelphia, W.B. Saunders, 1992, pp. 682–683.

Blake, W.W., and Murray, J.A.: Heat balance. In Merenstein, G.B., and Gardner, S.L. (Eds.): Handbook of Neonatal Intensive Care, 4th ed. St. Louis, Mosby, 1998, pp. 100–115.

Bruck, D.: Heat production and temperature regulation. In Stave, U. (Ed.): Perinatal Physiology. New York, Plenum Press, 1978, pp. 455–492.

Budin, P.: The Nursling. London, Caxton Publishing, 1907.

D'Apolito, K.: Hats used to maintain body temperature. Neonatal Network, 13(5):93–94, 1994.

Davis, V.: The structure and function of brown adipose tissue in the neonate. J. Obstet. Gynecol. Neonatal Nurs., 9:368, 1980.

Gomella, T.L., Cunningham, M.D., and Eyal, F.G.: Neonatology: Management, Procedures, On-Call Problems, Disease and Drugs, 3rd ed. Stamford, Conn., Appleton & Lange, 1994, p. 38.

Gonzales, I., Duryea, E.J., Vasquez, E., and Geraghty, N.: Effect of enteral feeding temperature on feeding tolerance in preterm infants. Neonatal Network, 14(3): 39–43, 1995.

Korones, S.B., and Bada-Ellzey, H.S.: Neonatal Decision Making: Hypothermia. St. Louis, Mosby–Year Book, 1993, pp. 40–41.

LeBlanc, M.H.: The physics of thermal exchange between infants and their environment. Medical Instrumentation, 21:11, 1987.

LeBlanc, M.H.: Thermoregulation: Incubators, radiant warmers, artificial skins, and body hoods. Clin. Perinatol., 18:403, 1991.

Medoff-Cooper, B.: Transition of the preterm infant to an open crib. J. Obstet. Gynecol. Neonatal Nurs., 23(4): 329–335, 1994.

National Association of Neonatal Nurses Guidelines for Practice: Neonatal thermoregulation. Petaluma, CA, 1997, pp. 1–12.

Obstetric-Gynecologic-Neonatal nursing practice resource: Neonatal thermoregulation. Association of Women's Health, Obstetric, and Neonatal Nurses, February 1990.

Perlstein, P.H.: Physical environment. In Fanaroff, A.A., and Martin, R.J. (Eds.): Neonatal-Perinatal Medicine: Diseases of the Fetus and Infant, 6th ed. St. Louis, Mosby, 1997, pp. 450–451.

Perlstein, P.H.: Thermoregulation. Pediatr. Ann., 25:10, 1998.

Sinclair, J.: Metabolic rate and temperature control. In Smith, C.A., and Nelson, N.N. (Eds.): The Physiology of the Newborn Infant, 4th ed. Springfield, Ill., Charles C Thomas, Publisher, 1976, p. 378.

Sulyok, E., Jequier, E., and Ryser, G.: Effect of relative humidity on the thermal balance of the newborn infant. Biol. Neonate, 21:210, 1982.

Thomas, K.: Thermoregulation in neonates. Neonatal Network, 13(2):15–22, March 1994.

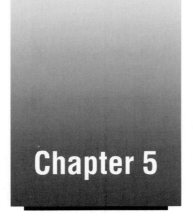

Chapter 5

Physical Assessment of the Newborn Infant

Deanne Buschbach

Objectives

1. Describe methods of determining gestational age prenatally and postnatally.

2. Discuss the classification of newborn infants by birth weight and gestational age, and relate problems that can be anticipated.

3. Review risk factors associated with discordant growth patterns.

4. Describe morbidity and mortality statistics for various classifications and risk groups.

5. Describe the systematic approach to conducting a physical examination of a neonate.

6. Identify and differentiate normal and abnormal findings of a newborn physical examination.

7. Discuss abnormalities that require immediate intervention.

An important objective in neonatology is to decrease morbidity and mortality rates in newborn infants. A thorough physical assessment is essential for early recognition of problems and is important to initiate appropriate timely treatment. This assessment must include a complete perinatal history; evaluation of labor, delivery, and resuscitation; gestational age assessment; and a complete physical examination. This chapter discusses determinants of gestational age, reviews infants identified to be at risk, and describes the systematic approach to conducting a physical examination.

Perinatal History

A complete assessment of the newborn infant begins with a review of the perinatal history. Valuable information may reveal existing pathologic changes and problems that require immediate attention.

A. Prenatal history.

1. Family history.

   a. Inherited diseases such as cystic fibrosis, trisomy, sickle cell anemia, phenylketonuria, and galactosemia.
   b. Familial diseases such as diabetes, mental retardation, cardiac lesions, hyperlipemia, and seizures.
2. Maternal medical history.
   a. Disease processes.
   b. Past hospitalizations.
   c. General health.
   d. Medications before pregnancy.
3. Reproductive history.
   a. Number of pregnancies, gestational age at delivery, delivery mode, and weight and sex of infant(s).
   b. Number of live births and any significant problems at birth or immediately afterward.
   c. Spontaneous and/or elective abortions. Multiple spontaneous abortions would require further testing for future pregnancies.
   d. Neonatal deaths, age of infant(s), and reason for death(s).
4. Pregnancy history.
   a. Prenatal care: when first obtained and how closely followed up.
   b. Blood type and Rh factor.
   c. Prenatal laboratory tests: serologic test for syphilis (VDRL [Venereal Disease Research Laboratory] or rapid plasma reagin [RPR]); screening tests for rubella, blood group incompatibilities (antibodies), hepatitis B, and infection with human immunodeficiency virus; and tests for other sexually transmitted diseases (gonorrhea, chlamydia).
5. Last menstrual period (LMP) and estimated date of confinement (EDC). The estimated date is calculated by using Nägele's rule: Add 7 days to the first day of the LMP and subtract 3 months (regular menstrual cycles are important in the accuracy of this calculation).
6. Results from prenatal testing for fetal well-being:
   a. Ultrasonography. Examination can be performed at any point during the pregnancy. It can provide estimation of gestational age, visualization for anomalies, nonstress testing, and biophysical profile evaluation. Advantages of ultrasonography are that it is relatively inexpensive, is noninvasive, and is readily available (Wapner, Trauffer, and Johnson, 1996a).
   b. Diagnostic amniocentesis. Procedure is performed at 15–18 weeks' gestation. It identifies chromosomal abnormalities, inborn errors of metabolism through enzyme assay, or hemoglobinopathies through DNA analysis. It can help determine the presence of neural tube defects and other anomalies. Disadvantages of amniocentesis are that it is labor intensive, there is a risk of injury to vital fetal structures, results take 1–3 weeks, the procedure is expensive and invasive, there is a risk of infection, and onset of labor is premature in a small percentage (Wapner et al., 1996a).
   c. Chorionic villus sampling (CVS). Procedure is performed at 9–12 weeks after the LMP, is an alternative to genetic amniocentesis, and identifies chromosomal abnormalities, inborn errors of metabolism through enzyme assay, or hemoglobinopathies through DNA analysis. Disadvantages are that accuracy is not as refined as in amniocentesis and that infection and spontaneous abortion are possible (Wapner, Trauffer, and Johnson, 1996b).
   d. Percutaneous umbilical blood sampling (PUBS). Procedure can be performed as early as 16 weeks after the LMP. It involves using real-time ultrasonography to aid in obtaining blood samples from the umbilical cord. It can help in the prenatal diagnosis of inherited blood disorders, karyotyping, and congenital infection and in the evaluation of fetal therapies. Disadvantages are that the procedure is invasive, may result in infection

and/or bleeding, and may cause spontaneous abortion (Blackburn and Loper, 1992b).
   e. Measurement of maternal serum alpha-fetoprotein. The test screens for open neural tube defects.
   f. Triple screen with serum from mother obtained between 15 and 20 weeks' gestation. Results are associated with trisomy 21 and include:
      (1) Decreased alpha-fetoprotein level.
      (2) Increased human chorionic gonadotropin level.
      (3) Decreased level of unconjugated serum estriol (UE$_3$) (Wapner et al., 1996b).
7. Medications and other drugs (over-the-counter, prescription, and "street" drugs) taken during pregnancy.
8. Weight gain, nutrition, and general health during pregnancy.

B. Labor and delivery.

1. Onset of labor.
   a. Spontaneous.
   b. Induced. Note indications for induction.
2. Phases (stages) of labor and duration of labor.
   a. First phase of labor, dilation, begins when regular contractions are 10 minutes apart and ends when dilation of cervix is complete. Average time is 12 hours for primigravidas and 7 hours for multigravidas.
   b. Second phase, expulsion, begins with complete cervical dilation and ends with delivery of the infant. Average time for this phase is 50 minutes for primigravidas and 20 minutes for multigravidas.
   c. Third phase, placental delivery, begins when the baby is born and ends with the delivery of the placenta and membranes. Usual duration of this phase is 15 minutes.
   d. Fourth phase, recovery, begins when the placenta and membranes are delivered and ends approximately 2 hours later as the endometrial arteries constrict and excessive uterine bleeding is prevented.
3. Presence of fetal distress. Terms used in fetal heart rate monitoring (Depp and Kuhlman, 1996):
   a. Normal fetal heart rate: 120–160 bpm.
   b. Fetal bradycardia: sustained fetal heart rate of less than 120 bpm.
   c. Severe fetal bradycardia: sustained fetal heart rate of less than 100 bpm.
   d. Fetal tachycardia: fetal heart rate of more than 160 bpm.
   e. Beat-to-beat variability: reflection of the relationship between the sympathetic and parasympathetic systems. Loss of beat-to-beat variability is worrisome. On fetal heart rate tracing, beat-to-beat variability appears as an irregular, or "jagged," line.
   f. Accelerations: increases in the fetal heart rate for less than 10 minutes in association with fetal movement.
   g. Decelerations: decreases in fetal heart rate for less than 10 minutes in association with fetal stress and hypoxia.
      (1) Early decelerations are related to head compression.
      (2) Late decelerations are related to uteroplacental insufficiency.
      (3) Variable decelerations are related to cord compression.
4. Rupture of membranes.
   a. Artificial or spontaneous.
   b. Time from rupture until delivery.
5. Amniotic fluid volume and appearance.
   a. Volume of amniotic fluid.
      (1) Normal volume at term ranges from 500 to 1500 mL.
      (2) Greater or lesser volumes can be indicators of fetal anomalies.
         (a) Increased fluid (polyhydramnios) can indicate esophageal atresia,

gastrointestinal obstruction, problems with swallowing, hydrops, neural tube anomalies, maternal disease, fetal malformations, genetic disorders, or other problems that impede the elimination of amniotic fluid (Phelan, 1996).

    (b) Decreased fluid (oligohydramnios) can indicate fetal urinary tract anomalies, amnion abnormalities, chronic amniotic fluid leak, fetal illness, maternal illness, or other problems that interfere with amniotic fluid production (Bhutani, 1996).

  b. Appearance of amniotic fluid.
    (1) Clear: normal.
    (2) Green: meconium stained (can be an indication that the fetus has had fetal distress).
    (3) Yellow: Old meconium, old blood, infection.
    (4) Red or pink: blood.
    (5) Cloudy: infection.
6. Type of delivery.
  a. Vaginal.
  b. Cesarean (note indication for operative delivery).
7. Instrumentation.
  a. Forceps assistance.
  b. Vacuum extraction.
8. Type and timing of anesthesia or analgesia.

C. **Resuscitation (refer to Chapter 6).**

1. Apgar scores.
2. Intervention and response.

Assessment of Gestational Age

A. **Purpose of determining gestational age.**

1. Assignment of neonatal classification.
  a. Term infants versus preterm infants (see item F, Classification of the Newborn Infant, below).
  b. Birth weight is plotted on the growth chart in relation to gestational age (see item F, Classification of the Newborn Infant, below).
2. Determination of neonatal mortality risk.
3. Identification of potential morbidity.

B. **Obstetric methods for determining gestational age.**

1. LMP and menstrual history.
2. Pregnancy test.
3. Ultrasonographic evaluation of fetal growth. This test is most accurate when performed before week 12 of pregnancy. Measurement of the crown-rump length and the biparietal diameter of the fetal head are used in estimating fetal age and size.
4. Detection of fetal heart tones (first heard at various weeks of gestation, depending on instrument used for auscultation), fundal height, and quickening (first detected at 17–20 weeks' gestation).
5. Amniotic fluid studies.
  a. Creatinine level increases as pregnancy approaches term.
  b. Bilirubin concentration decreases as pregnancy approaches term.
  c. For the fetal lung maturity profile, the lecithin/sphingomyelin ratio increases, except in infants of diabetic mothers, at 34–36 weeks' gestation. A ratio greater than 2 indicates maturity. These results can be altered by

contamination with meconium and/or blood. Determination of the phosphatidylglycerol level is a qualitative test. A level of 2 µmol/L is considered to indicate lung maturity. These results are not altered by the presence of blood or meconium. A foam stability index (FST or shake test) is grounded in adequate amounts of surfactant, present in the amniotic fluid, to generate a stable foamy layer on the air-liquid interface when the amniotic fluid is mixed with ethanol. Results can be altered by the presence of blood or meconium. Fluorescent polarization (FPOL) determines the microviscosity of the amniotic fluid and lipids compared to albumin. An index of less than 260 indicates maturity. The presence of blood or meconium can alter results (Bhutani, 1996).

C. **Methods of assessing gestational age.**

1. Dubowitz test. Assesses 10 neurologic and 11 physical criteria. These criteria are assigned scores and totaled to give an estimated gestational age (Dubowitz, Dubowitz, and Goldberg, 1970).
2. Ballard Score. A simplified scoring system based on the Dubowitz method. Six neurologic and six physical criteria are used (Fig. 5–1) (Ballard, Khoury, Wedig, et al., 1991).
   a. Unlike the Dubowitz examination, all elements of the Ballard method can be performed on premature, very ill, or fragile babies, therefore giving a more accurate estimate.
   b. Highest reliability when performed within 48 hours of birth.
   c. Accurate within 2 weeks of gestation (Ballard et al., 1991).

D. **Assessment of neurologic signs (Trotter, 1996).**

1. Posture.
   a. Evaluated for increasing flexor and hip adduction with increasing gestational age.
   b. Early in gestation the infant's resting posture is hypotonic.
   c. At 30 weeks there is only slight flexion of the feet and knees.
   d. At 34 weeks the thighs and hips are flexed (frog position), but the arms usually remain extended.
   e. By 35 weeks the beginning of arm flexion can be observed.
   f. By 36–38 weeks the resting posture of the healthy infant is of total flexion with prompt recoil of arms and legs.
2. Square window.
   a. Term describes flexion when the wrist is at a right angle to the forearm.
   b. The angle decreases with increasing gestational age.
3. Arm recoil.
   a. After the arms are flexed for 5 seconds, the arms are fully extended by pulling the hands downward and then releasing them. The degree of arm flexion and the strength of recoil are scored.
   b. A slow response receives a low score, and a vigorous, fully flexed response receives a high score.
4. Popliteal angle.
   a. The angle between the lower leg and thigh, posterior to the knee, is measured.
   b. The angle decreases with increasing gestational age.
5. Scarf sign.
   a. The arm is pulled across the chest and around the neck.
   b. The score is determined by the position of the elbow to the midline of the body.
   c. The infant becomes resistant to this maneuver with increasing gestational age.
6. Heel to ear.

NEUROMUSCULAR MATURITY

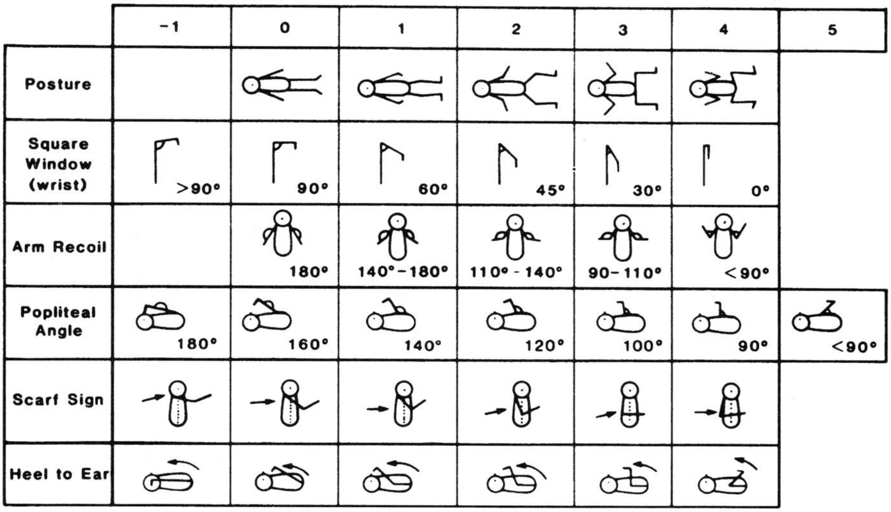

	-1	0	1	2	3	4	5
Posture							
Square Window (wrist)	>90°	90°	60°	45°	30°	0°	
Arm Recoil		180°	140°–180°	110°–140°	90–110°	<90°	
Popliteal Angle	180°	160°	140°	120°	100°	90°	<90°
Scarf Sign							
Heel to Ear							

PHYSICAL MATURITY

Skin	sticky friable transparent	gelatinous red, translucent	smooth pink, visible veins	superficial peeling &/or rash, few veins	cracking pale areas rare veins	parchment deep cracking no vessels	leathery cracked wrinkled
Lanugo	none	sparse	abundant	thinning	bald areas	mostly bald	
Plantar Surface	heel–toe 40–50 mm: –1 <40 mm: –2	>50 mm no crease	faint red marks	anterior transverse crease only	creases ant. 2/3	creases over entire sole	
Breast	imperceptible	barely perceptible	flat areola no bud	stippled areola 1–2 mm bud	raised areola 3–4 mm bud	full areola 5–10 mm bud	
Eye/Ear	lids fused loosely: –1 tightly: –2	lids open pinna flat stays folded	sl. curved pinna; soft; slow recoil	well-curved pinna; soft but ready recoil	formed & firm instant recoil	thick cartilage ear stiff	
Genitals male	scrotum flat, smooth	scrotum empty faint rugae	testes in upper canal rare rugae	testes descending few rugae	testes down good rugae	testes pendulous deep rugae	
Genitals female	clitoris prominent labia flat	prominent clitoris small labia minora	prominent clitoris enlarging minora	majora & minora equally prominent	majora large minora small	majora cover clitoris & minora	

SCORE

Neuro-
  muscular _____
Physical _____
Total _____

MATURITY RATING

score	weeks
-10	20
-5	22
0	24
5	26
10	28
15	30
20	32
25	34
30	36
35	38
40	40
45	42
50	44

Figure 5–1
New Ballard Score, expanded to include extremely premature infants. (From Ballard, J.L., Khoury, J.C., Wedig, K., et al.: J. Pediatr., *119*:417, 1991.)

a. With the hips kept flat on the bed, the foot is drawn toward the head.

b. The distance between the foot and head and the degree of knee extension are noted.

c. The infant demonstrates resistance to this maneuver with increasing gestational age.

E. Assessment of individual physical signs (Trotter, 1996).

1. Skin.
   a. The skin becomes less transparent and develops more texture with increasing gestational age.
   b. By 36–37 weeks the skin has lost its transparency and underlying vessels are no longer visible.
   c. As gestation progresses beyond 38 weeks, subcutaneous tissue begins to decrease, causing wrinkling and desquamation.

2. Lanugo.
   a. Fine, downy hair covers the body of the fetus from 20 to 28 weeks.
   b. At 28 weeks it begins to disappear around the face and anterior aspect of the trunk.
   c. At term a few patches may be present over the shoulders.

3. Plantar creases.
   a. Creases first appear on the anterior portion of the foot, between 28 and 30 weeks gestation, and extend toward the heel as gestation progresses.
   b. An infant with intrauterine growth restriction (IUGR) and early loss of vernix caseosa (a greasy white or yellow material that covers the neonate's skin) may have more plantar creases than expected for size.
   c. After 12 hours, plantar creases are no longer a valid indicator of gestational age because the skin begins to dry.

4. Breast development.
   a. Nipple size and amount of breast tissue are examined.
   b. A 1–2 mm nodule of breast tissue is palpable by about 36 weeks and grows to approximately 10 mm by 40 weeks' gestation (Black, 1978).

5. Eyes and ears.
   a. Eyes are evaluated for fusion of the eyelids.
   b. At 26–30 weeks' gestation, fused eyelids open.
   c. From 27 to 34 weeks' gestation, examination of the anterior vascular capsule of the lens is helpful in determining gestational age by examining the level of remaining embryonic vessels on the lens (Fig. 5–2).
   d. Ears are assessed for formation and amount of cartilage present in the pinna.
   e. Inward curving of the upper pinna usually begins by 34 weeks' gestation and by 40 weeks extends to the lobe.
   f. Before 34 weeks the pinna has little cartilage and will stay folded on itself.
   g. By 36 weeks there is some cartilage, and the pinna will spring back from being folded.

6. Genitalia.
   a. Female infant. Development of the labia minora and majora and prominence of the clitoris are evaluated.
      (1) Early in gestation the clitoris is prominent, with small, widely separated labia.
      (2) By 40 weeks, fat deposits have increased in size in the labia majora, so that the labia majora completely cover the labia minora.
   b. Male infant. Presence of testes, degree of descent into the scrotum, and development of rugae on the scrotum are evaluated.
      (1) The testes begin to descend from the abdomen at 28 weeks.
      (2) At 37 weeks the testes can be palpated high in the scrotum.

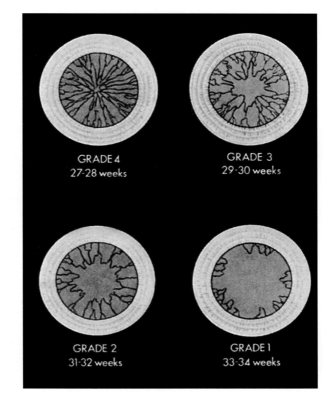

Figure 5–2
Grading system for assessment of gestational age by examination of the anterior vascular capsule of the lens. (From Hittner, H.M., Hirsch, N.J., and Rudolph, A.J.: J. Pediatr. 91:455, 1977.)

GRADE 4
27-28 weeks

GRADE 3
29-30 weeks

GRADE 2
31-32 weeks

GRADE 1
33-34 weeks

(3) At 40 weeks the testes are completely descended and the scrotum is covered with rugae.

(4) As gestation progresses the scrotum becomes more pendulous.

F. Classification of the Newborn Infant.

1. Plot birth weight and gestational age on standard intrauterine growth charts (Fig. 5–3). When comparing the gestational age assessment score and the percentiles of the growth parameters (head, length, and weight), one can identify problems with development, symmetric or asymmetric IUGR, or possible macrosomia related to maternal diabetes.

2. Clinical estimate of gestation is defined by weeks of gestation and is divided into three categories:
   a. Preterm, through 37 weeks.
   b. Term, 38–41 completed weeks.
   c. Postterm, 42 weeks or greater.

3. Plot birth weight and gestational age on standard graphs to determine the neonatal mortality risk by birth weight and gestational age (Fig. 5–4).

4. Infants classified as small for gestational age (SGA) are at less than the 10th percentile for weight. Infants whose size is appropriate for gestational age are between the 10th and 90th percentiles. Large for gestational age (LGA) infants are those above the 90th percentile for weight.
   a. Symmetric IUGR. Weight, length, and head circumference all fall below the 10th percentile.
   b. Asymmetric IUGR. Head circumference and length are normal, with weight below the 10th percentile. The condition is generally associated with

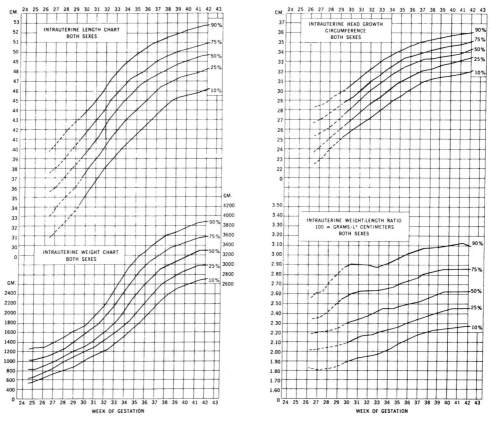

Figure 5–3

Colorado Intrauterine Growth Charts. (From Lubchenco, L.O., et al.: Pediatrics *37*:403, August 1966. Reproduced by permission of *Pediatrics*. Reprinted with permission of Ross Laboratories, Columbus, Ohio, from CO Intrauterine Growth Charts, August 1966, Ross Laboratories.)

impaired placental functioning or poor nutrition with preservation of brain growth.

5. Classification of the newborn infant assists in identification, observation, screening, and treatment of the most commonly occurring problems.

6. A problem list based on morbidity should be formulated for each infant.

G. **Assessment of infants at risk.** Infants determined to be premature, SGA, or LGA require specialized care because they have an increased risk of respiratory disease, metabolic disorders (hypoglycemia, polycythemia), and problems with thermoregulation. Complications associated with LGA and SGA infants are shown in Fig. 5–5.

1. LGA infants.
   a. Birth trauma.
      (1) Head. Trauma may range from a large cephalhematoma to a depressed skull fracture.
      (2) Fractured clavicle.
      (3) Peripheral nerve injuries of the cervical or brachial plexus.
   b. Maternal diabetes. Infant may be large, with an increased weight/length ratio, and has an increased risk of respiratory distress, hypoglycemia, hypocalcemia, polycythemia, hyperbilirubinemia, and congenital anomalies (Goldkrand and Lin, 1987).

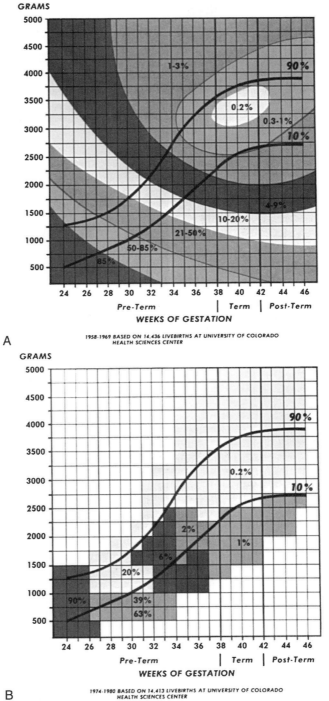

Figure 5–4
Neonatal mortality risk by birth weight and gestational age. (*A* from Lubchenco, L.O., Searls, D.T., and Brazie, J.V.: J. Pediatr. *81*:814, 1972. *B* from Koops, B.L., Morgan, L.J., and Battaglia, F.C.: J. Pediatr., *101*: 969, 1982. *A* and *B* © 1982 Mead Johnson & Co.)

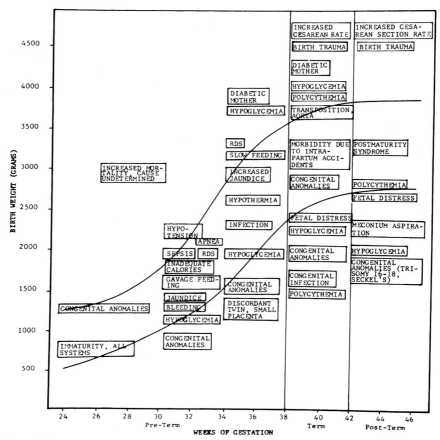

Figure 5–5
Specific neonatal morbidity by birth weight and gestational age. (From Lubchenco, L.O.: The High-Risk Infant. Philadelphia, W.B. Saunders, 1976.)

   c. Beckwith-Wiedemann syndrome. Infant may have macrosomia, macroglossia, umbilical abnormalities (generally omphalocele), and/or hypoglycemia (Jones, 1997b).

   d. Asphyxia caused by CNS trauma during the birth process.

   e. Hypoglycemia.

   f. Thermoregulation problems as a result of CNS trauma or infection.

   g. Increased incidence of cesarean delivery because of size and the complications associated with operative delivery, such as increased respiratory distress, adverse effects of anesthesia, and birth trauma resulting from a difficult extraction.

2. SGA infants.

   a. Hypoglycemia occurs frequently in SGA infants because of the high metabolic rate and low glycogen stores (Spear, 1996).

   b. Infants of mothers with advanced diabetes can have IUGR because of poor placental function.

   c. The incidence of fetal distress and asphyxia is increased. SGA infants are at risk for aspiration of amniotic fluid, which may contain meconium. Complications of meconium aspiration include respiratory distress, pulmonary air leaks, and hypoxia.

   d. Congenital infection can result in SGA/IUGR infants.

   e. Chromosomal defects are commonly seen in SGA/IUGR infants.

f. Thermoregulation problems may be due to a high demand for metabolic fuel. The SGA infant does not have adequate adipose tissue for insulation or stores of brown adipose tissue to maintain body temperature.

g. Polycythemia (venous hematocrit >65% during the first week of life) occurs with placental transfusion; with increased red blood cell production in utero caused by endocrine, metabolic, or chromosomal disorders; or with chronic hypoxia.

Physical Examination

A. Overview.

1. A brief physical examination should be performed in the delivery room to rule out obvious congenital anomalies, birth injuries, and cardiorespiratory distress. A complete examination should be performed within 24 hours of birth.
2. The infant must be kept warm during the examination by using an overhead heat source or by uncovering and examining one body area at a time to avoid hypothermia.
3. The infant will generally be the most cooperative during an examination performed 1–2 hours after a feeding while in a quietly alert or sleepy state.
4. A systematic, organized approach to physical examination will ensure that no part is overlooked.
5. Certain components of a physical examination may need to be modified to match the infant's state.
6. The physical examination should be documented on the patient record.
7. Abnormalities should be noted and the infant's primary care provider notified.

B. Observation of general condition.

1. Size, contour, and general well-being.
2. Posture.
   a. Healthy term infants exhibit flexion of the extremities.
   b. Breech infants exhibit extension of the legs and head, and frank breech infants have abduction and external rotation of the legs.
3. Activity.
   a. Flexion and extension alternate between arms and legs.
   b. Decreased flexion associated with hypotonia should be evaluated further. This may be seen in preterm infants or may be associated with CNS involvement.
   c. Excessive flexion suggests hypertonicity and may be the result of CNS trauma.
   d. Asymmetric movements of arms, legs, or face may suggest a birth injury such as brachial plexus palsy, a bone fracture, or a congenital anomaly.
4. Skin (Witt, 1996).
   a. Observe for dry, peeling skin; rashes; pustules; petechiae; discoloration; and pigmentation.
   b. Describe skin lesions (see Chapter 24).
5. State. The cry should be robust and vigorous in the term infant. The infant should pass through sleep states (deep sleep, light sleep, quiet, active) and awake states (drowsy, quietly alert, actively alert, crying) (Blackburn, 1992a).
6. Respirations (Askin, 1996).
   a. Respiratory rate, rhythm, and effort.
   b. Nasal flaring. The infant attempts to decrease airway resistance by increasing the diameter of the nares.
   c. Expiratory grunting. The infant attempts to increase intrathoracic pressure to prevent volume loss during expiration as a result of alveolar collapse.

   d. Wheeze. High-pitched ronchi are heard on expiration more loudly than on inspiration because of restricted airways.
   e. Stridor. The airway is partially obstructed.
   f. Intercostal and substernal retractions. The intercostal musculature is used to maintain adequate respirations.
7. Morphologic features.
   a. Congenital defects.
   b. Symmetry of like body parts.
   c. Proportional body parts.
8. Nutrition.
   a. Well-nourished appearance. The infant is adequately grown with appropriate amounts of fat and muscle.
   b. Thin and wasted appearance. This is common in infants with IUGR and in postmature infants.
9. Color.
   a. Mucous membranes are the most reliable indicators of central color in all babies. Central cyanosis indicates low oxygen saturation in the blood, usually demonstrating a cardiac or respiratory dysfunction.
   b. Acrocyanosis (cyanosis of hands or feet) suggests instability of the peripheral circulation and may be the result of cold, stress, shock, or polycythemia. May be a normal finding for 24–48 hours after birth.
   c. Pallor at birth reflects poor perfusion and circulatory failure. Pallor with bradycardia usually indicates anoxia or vasoconstriction found in shock, sepsis, or severe respiratory distress. Pallor with tachycardia can indicate anemia.
   d. Plethora. Ruddy or red appearance may indicate polycythemia.
   e. Jaundice. Yellow skin color may appear in the first 12 hours, is abnormal, and should be investigated. All infants who become jaundiced should be evaluated to rule out pathologic jaundice.

C. **Auscultation and palpation.**

1. Auscultation is best accomplished with a quiet infant.
2. Warm hands and warm stethoscope prevent overstimulation, which may cause the infant to cry.
3. Heart.
   a. Heart rate. Beats are counted for a full minute. Normal range is 110–160 bpm.
      (1) A heart rate less than 110 bpm may indicate bradycardia, which may be associated with anoxia, cerebral defects, or increased intracranial pressure. In deep sleep a term infant may have a heart rate as low as 80–90 bpm. If it does not increase quickly to greater than 100 bpm when the infant awakens, it may represent congenital heart block.
      (2) A sustained heart rate greater than 160 bpm indicates tachycardia, which may be associated with respiratory problems, anemia, shock, medication reaction, congestive heart failure, or supraventricular tachycardia (SVT).
   b. Note rhythm and regularity at the apex.
   c. The point of maximal intensity (PMI) of the heart is normally found lateral to the midclavicular line at the third to fourth interspace. Note its location.
   d. Precordial activity is associated with heart disease, fluid overload, and congestive heart failure. An active precordium can often be seen in premature infants with thin skin and little subcutaneous tissue.
   e. Murmurs are heard frequently in the neonatal period. They are created by turbulent blood flow and can be innocent or pathologic. Pathologic murmurs are due to underlying cardiovascular disease. Soft murmurs (grades 1

and 2) noted in the first 48 hours are often not pathologic but should be followed up.

(1) Continuous murmurs extend beyond the second heart sound into diastole.

(2) Note murmurs for loudness, quality, radiation, location, and timing. The grading scale for murmurs follows (Vargo, 1996):

    (a) Grade 1, barely audible.

    (b) Grade 2, soft but easily audible.

    (c) Grade 3, moderately loud, with no thrill.

    (d) Grade 4, loud, with thrill present.

    (e) Grade 5, loud, and audible with stethoscope placed lightly on chest.

    (f) Grade 6, loud, and audible with stethoscope placed near chest.

(3) Transient murmurs, occurring commonly at 4–8 hours of life, are attributed to closing of the ductus arteriosus or to the change in pulmonary vascular resistance that occurs during the change from fetal to adult circulation.

(4) Note muffled or shifted heart sounds, which may indicate pneumothorax, pneumomediastinum, dextrocardia, or diaphragmatic hernia.

(5) Palpate pulses (palmar, brachial, radial, femoral, popliteal, posterior tibial, and dorsalis pedis) while the infant is quiet. Note rate, rhythm, volume, character, and equality—reflections of cardiac output. The volume and character of pulses (normal pulses are +3) are reflected on a grading scale (Vargo, 1996):

    (a) 0, pulses not palpable.

    (b) +1, very difficult to palpate, weak and thready, easily obliterated with pressure.

    (c) +2, difficult to palpate, may be obliterated with pressure.

    (d) +3, easy to palpate, not easy to obliterate with pressure.

    (e) +4, strong and bounding, not obliterated with pressure.

    NOTE: Bounding pulses can be felt with a patent ductus arteriosus. Absent or decreased femoral pulses are associated with coarctation of the aorta. Decreased pulses are associated with shock.

(6) Blood pressures should be recorded at admission and at discharge (Fig. 5–6). Blood pressures in the lower extremities should be slightly higher than in the upper extremities. A differential in blood pressures greater than 20 mm Hg between upper and lower extremities suggests an obstruction (Vargo, 1996).

4. Chest and lungs.

  a. Respirations should be easy and unlabored.

  b. Newborn infants are obligate nose breathers. Obstruction of the nares will lead to respiratory distress and cyanosis.

  c. The chest should be round, with the anteroposterior diameter equal bilaterally. An increased anteroposterior diameter may suggest pneumothorax or cardiomegaly.

  d. Inspect breasts and nipples for symmetry, size, number, and discharge.

    (1) Supernumerary nipples are small, raised pigmented areas found vertical with the main nipple line 5–6 cm below the normal nipple and require no treatment.

    (2) Enlarged breasts result from effects of maternal estrogen and are transient. Rarely a milklike substance can be produced and is considered a normal finding. The enlargement lasts 1–2 weeks.

    (3) Widespread nipples are noted if the distance between the nipples is greater than 25% of the full chest circumference (Hernandez and Hernandez, 1999). May indicate congenital malformations such as Turner's syndrome.

  e. The respiratory rate and pattern should be noted. A normal respiratory rate

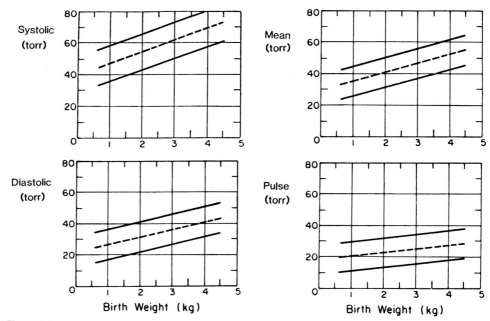

Figure 5–6
Blood pressure by birth weight. (From Versmold, H.T., Kitterman, J.A., Phibbs, R.H., et al.: Pediatrics *67*(5):607, 1981. Copyright © American Academy of Pediatrics, 1981. Reproduced by permission.)

    is approximately 40–60 breaths per minute and can vary somewhat with activity of the infant.

   f. Immediately after birth, fine rales may be audible because of clearing of lung fluid.

   g. Bronchial breath sounds and air entry should be audible bilaterally and should be clear. Rales and rhonchi suggest respiratory disease.

   h. Retractions, nasal flaring, tachypnea, and grunting are all symptoms of respiratory distress.

   i. Asymmetric breath sounds may indicate a tension pneumothorax or diaphragmatic hernia.

   j. Diminished breath sounds may suggest atelectasis, effusion, pneumothorax, or decreased respiratory effort.

5. Abdomen and trunk.

   a. The abdomen is slightly rounded, soft, and symmetric.

   b. A concave abdomen may suggest a diaphragmatic hernia. Decreased abdominal tone may be associated with depressant effects of residual maternal medication, immaturity, or the absence of muscles in the abdominal wall. Prune-belly syndrome is present when there are no muscles in the abdominal wall; it is associated with renal and urinary tract abnormalities.

   c. Abdominal distention may be due to obstruction, infection, masses, or enlargement of an abdominal organ.

   d. Observe infant for abdominal wall defects.

      (1) Omphalocele: protrusion of abdominal contents through a defect in the umbilicus. The thin membrane covering the defect can rupture at birth. The condition is frequently associated with other congenital anomalies (Cooney, 1998).

      (2) Gastroschisis: abdominal wall defect that allows for protrusion of abdominal contents; located lateral (usually to the right) to the umbilical cord and is not covered by a membrane. Abdominal contents usually

show evidence of damage (thick, edematous, matted) caused by extended exposure to amniotic fluid (Cooney, 1998).

    (3) Umbilical hernia: protrusion of part of the intestine, at the umbilicus; covered by skin and subcutaneous tissue.

  e. Palpate the abdomen gently for enlargement of organs or the presence of masses. Auscultate for bowel sounds.

    (1) The liver edge is palpated 1–2 cm below the right costal margin in the midclavicular line. Palpation is begun in the right lower quadrant and progresses upward so that a large liver edge will not be missed. Hepatomegaly may be associated with congenital heart disease, infection, hemolytic disease, or arteriovenous (A-V) malformations.

    (2) A palpable spleen tip more than 1 cm below the left costal margin is abnormal. A normal spleen is rarely palpable.

    (3) Kidneys are palpated by placing one hand under the flank and palpating gently from above with the fingers of the other hand. A normal kidney in a term infant is 4.5–5 cm from pole to pole (Lawrence, 1984). Enlarged kidneys or absence of a palpable kidney suggests further evaluation.

    (4) Abdominal masses are most frequently of urinary tract origin.

    (5) The bladder can be palpated 1–4 cm above the pubic symphysis when urine is present.

  f. Umbilical cord.

    (1) Normally contains two arteries and one vein. A single artery may be associated with an increased incidence of congenital abnormalities, generally of the gastrointestinal, genitourinary, or cardiovascular system.

    (2) The diameter of the cord varies, is related to the quality of Wharton's jelly, and is an indicator of the nutritional status of the infant.

    (3) The cord begins to dry soon after birth and falls off 7–14 days after birth.

    (4) Redness, foul odor, or moisture around the cord may indicate omphalitis and should be investigated immediately.

    (5) Herniation into the umbilical cord, large or small, is a significant finding and should be evaluated to rule out omphalocele.

    (6) Patent urachus is an embryologic communication between the urinary bladder and umbilicus. It is suspected when urine is excreted from the umbilicus (Cilley and Krummel, 1998).

  g. Anus.

    (1) Inspect anal area for presence and patency of an anus. Patency can be determined by passage of meconium or by passing a small rubber catheter 1–2 cm.

    (2) Majority of term neonates pass their first stool within 24 hours. Infants who have not passed their first stool by 24 hours should be examined carefully for signs and symptoms of obstruction. Failure to pass meconium within 48 hours suggests obstruction.

    (3) Passage of stool from the vagina or urethra indicates a rectovaginal or rectourethral fistula.

  h. Back and spine.

    (1) Inspect the infant's back while the child is in a prone position.

    (2) Observe for a flat, straight vertebral column.

    (3) Observe for neural tube defects or signs of underlying abnormalities.

      (a) Sinus tract (can be found anywhere along the spine but is usually noted in the lumbar area).

      (b) Tuft of hair.

      (c) Lipoma.

      (d) Pilonidal dimple.

      (e) Soft, cystic masses or hemangiomas.

(4) Stroke one side of the vertebral column with your finger to check the incurvation reflex. The infant should turn toward the stroked side.

D. Genitalia

1. Male.
   a. The glans should be completely covered with prepuce (foreskin) in the noncircumcised infant.
   b. The normal position of the urinary meatus is at the center of the penile glans.
      (1) Hypospadias is present if the urethral opening is located at the ventral surface of the penis. The three degrees of hypospadias include balanic (glandular), penile, and penoscrotal (perineal). Each describes the location of the meatus (Duckett and Baskin, 1998).
      (2) Epispadias is present if the urethral opening is located on the dorsal surface. This is less common than hypospadias and can vary from an opening on the glans to bladder extrophy (Cavaliere, 1996).
   c. Any abnormality of the genitalia, including micropenis, epispadias, hypospadius, or chordee (bowing of the penis), is a contraindication to circumcision.
   d. Inspect the scrotum for size, rugation, and presence of testes. Testes may be palpable in the inguinal canal in a preterm infant.
      (1) Hydrocele is a collection of fluid in the scrotum that will light up when transilluminated. It is usually transient and can be found either unilateral or bilateral.
      (2) A mass that does not transilluminate may be a tumor or torsion of the testes and is a surgical emergency.
      (3) Swelling and bruising of the scrotum may be evident in a breech delivery.
   e. If external genitalia are ambiguous, further evaluation is necessary.
2. Female.
   a. The labia majora covers the labia minora, clitoris, urethral opening, and external vaginal vault in the term infant.
   b. In a preterm infant the labia majora may not cover the labia minora and the clitoris will be prominent.
   c. An unusually large clitoris may indicate pseudohermaphroditism.
   d. A vaginal skin tag is a common finding and is hypertrophied vaginal tissue. It will regress during the first week of life.
   e. Palpate the labia majora for masses that may indicate hernias or ectopic gonads.
   f. Vaginal discharge is common in the first 48 hours of life.
   g. Ecchymosis and edema of the labia are common in breech deliveries.
   h. Observe for patency of the vaginal opening. There should be a fingertip space between the vagina and the anus in a term female infant.
   i. If external genitalia are ambiguous, further evaluation is necessary.

E. Body part examination.

1. Head.
   a. Note the size, shape, symmetry, and general appearance of the head.
   b. The head is usually 2 cm larger in diameter than the newborn infant's chest.
      (1) Microcephaly: small head size in relation to body size. Usually reflects delayed brain growth.
      (2) Macrocephaly: large head size in relation to body size. May be a result of increased accumulation of cerebrospinal fluid within the ventricles of the brain (hydrocephalus), or may be associated with osteogenesis imperfacta or dwarfism.

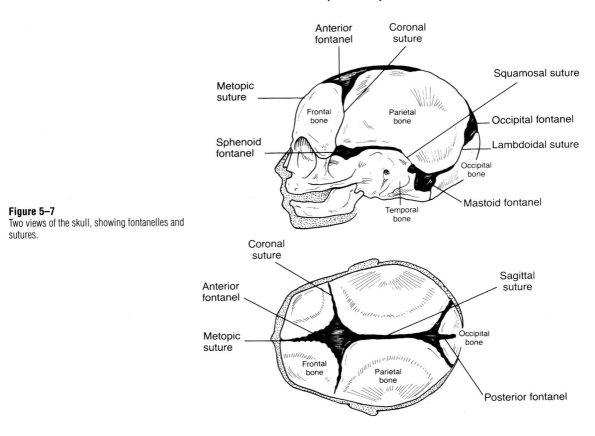

Figure 5–7
Two views of the skull, showing fontanelles and
sutures.

(3) The head of a newborn infant delivered vaginally from a vertex position
will be molded to fit the configuration of the birth canal. The head of an
infant delivered by cesarean birth without labor is usually not molded.
The head of a breech neonate may be flat on top with an increased
anteroposterior measurement.

c. Caput succedaneum: diffuse edema of the scalp resulting from compression
of local blood vessels. The edema crosses suture lines and disappears in a
few days.

d. Cephalhematoma: subperiosteal hemorrhage (bleeding between the periosteum and the skull) resulting from a traumatic delivery. Is limited to the
surface of the bone and does not cross suture lines. Resolution may take up
to several months.

e. Sutures (Fig. 5–7). Placing both thumbs on opposite sides of the suture and
gently pushing alternately, while feeling for motion, check mobility of the
sutures. The mobility of all sutures should be checked.

(1) Craniosynostosis: premature closure of cranial sutures that can lead to
restriction of brain growth.

(2) Craniotabes: soft, demineralized areas of bone in the skull (usually in
the parietal and occipital regions along the lambdoidal suture). When
slight pressure is applied to these areas, the examiner feels a Ping-Pong
effect on the area, as it dents and then returns to normal position. This
condition is time limited and self-resolving.

f. Fontanelles. Check location, number, and size.

(1) The anterior fontanelle is located at the junction of the sagittal and
coronal sutures. It is diamond shaped and measures from 4 to 6 cm at

the largest diameter (measuring bone to bone) and normally closes at 18 months.

(2) The posterior fontanelle is located at the junction of the lambdoidal and sagittal sutures. It is usually triangular and barely admits a fingertip. It closes by 2 months of age.

(3) A third fontanelle may be located between the anterior and posterior fontanelles along the sagittal suture and may vary in size. It may be associated with congenital anomalies.

(4) Large fontanelles may be seen in hypothyroidism.

(5) A bulging, full, or tense fontanelle may be associated with increased intracranial pressure resulting from hydrocephalus, birth injury, bleeding, or infection.

(6) A depressed fontanelle is a late sign of dehydration.

g. Check the scalp.

(1) Observe for abrasions or lacerations that occasionally occur during delivery as a result of forceps, traumatic delivery, or an internal monitor probe.

(2) Cutis aplasia—localized congenital absence of skin. Lesions occur on the scalp and may be solitary or multiple. A number of syndromes exist that are characterized by the pattern of hair distribution.

(3) Hair whorls—spiral hair growth pattern which are a result of brain growth. Their absence, number (>2), or abnormal placement may represent abnormal brain growth/development.

2. Eyes.

a. Eyes may be edematous for several days after birth due to the delivery process or chemical irritation following eye prophylaxis. Infectious conjunctivitis accompanied by purulent discharge is rarely seen on the first day of life.

b. Subconjunctival hemorrhages occur frequently and result from pressure on the fetal head during delivery.

c. The red reflex is normally present and is the reflection of the ophthalmoscope's light on the retina. The red reflex can range from red (in light-skinned infants) to yellow (in dark-skinned infants). If a red reflex is not visualized, further investigation is necessary. Absence can indicate retinoblastoma, glaucoma, or hemorrhage. With congenital cataracts the red reflex appears white. Cataracts may be the result of intrauterine viral infection or can be inherited as a dominant trait from an affected parent.

d. Observe for pupil response to light and for symmetry of eye movements. Pupils should be equal, round, and react to light (PEARL).

e. Mongolian slanting and epicanthal folds may be ethnically normal, indicative of trisomy 21, or a part of the fetal alcohol syndrome.

f. Tears are not normally produced until 2 months of age.

g. The iris is dark blue until 3–6 months of age; eye color may then change.

3. Ears.

a. Inspect for maturity, symmetry, and size.

b. Observe for unusual shape or abnormal position.

c. The helix of the ear normally attaches to the scalp at a point horizontal to the inner canthus of the eyes.

d. Low-set ears may be associated with various syndromes and chromosomal abnormalities.

e. Check for the presence of ear canals. Visualization of eardrums is not necessary unless indicated by the infant's history or other findings.

f. If hearing loss is considered because of a lack of external canals or other indicators, an audiologist should conduct a hearing examination.

g. Preauricular or auricular skin tags or pits are common and may be associated with renal problems or hearing loss or may be a normal variant.

h. Malformed or malpositioned ears may be associated with renal, chromosomal, or congenital abnormalities.

4. Nose.

a. Note the shape and size of the nose.

b. Positional deformities may result from the birth process, and most will resolve without treatment.

c. Abnormal shape may be associated with a congenital syndrome.

d. Patency of the nostrils must be verified because infants are obligate nose breathers. Place a cold, flat metal object under the nose and observe for fogging from the infant's exhalations.

   (1) Drugs, infections, tumors, or mucus may cause obstruction.

   (2) Choanal atresia is a membranous or bony obstruction in the nasal passage. It may be either unilateral or bilateral. Cyanosis, apnea, noisy breathing, or severe respiratory distress may be evident in the infant with choanal atresia.

5. Mouth.

a. The mouth should be symmetric and positioned in the midline.

b. Microstomia, or very small mouth, may be associated with genetic syndromes such as trisomy 18.

c. Macrostomia, or large mouth, may be associated with mucopolysaccharidosis, Beckwith syndrome, or hypothyroidism.

d. The hard and soft palates are examined to rule out cleft palate.

e. Epstein's pearls are small, white epidermal inclusion cysts commonly found on the hard and soft palates and on the gum margins. They usually disappear after a few weeks.

f. The mucous membranes of the mouth and tongue should be pink. Cyanosis of the tongue and mucous membranes is indicative of a pathologic condition.

g. Observe the lips for the presence of a cleft lip, which can vary from a niche in the lip to a complete separation extending upward into the floor of the nose.

h. Natal teeth are not uncommon and are generally located on the lower gum. If they have poor root formation or are mobile, they are generally removed. There is a risk of ulceration of the tongue, pain with breast-feeding, and dislocation. A pediatric dentist should be consulted for evaluation because these may be primary teeth.

i. Thrush, or oral moniliasis, is common in newborn infants. It is usually contracted from mothers with vaginal moniliasis at the time of delivery. The lacy white material is present on the surface of the oral mucous membranes and does not wipe away with a cotton-tipped swab.

j. Assess for root and gag reflexes, which develop at 36 weeks' gestation, and for suck and swallow reflexes, which develop at 32–34 weeks' gestation.

k. A large tongue (macroglossia), a cleft lip and palate, or a high-arched palate may be associated with other congenital anomalies, such as Beckwith-Wiedemann syndrome, Pompe's disease (a type II glycogen storage disease), and hypothyroidism. A protruding tongue is often seen in trisomy 21. A large tongue may be too big to fit in a normal-size mandible and can obstruct the infant's airway.

l. Observe the jaw for size and relationship to the maxilla. Micrognathia (small jaw) may present a serious airway problem. If the normal-size tongue is too large to fit in the small mandible, it can obstruct the infant's airway. Micrognathia is frequently seen in Pierre Robin syndrome, Treacher Collins' syndrome, and de Lange's syndrome (Jones, 1997c).

6. Face.
    a. Observe for symmetry and location of the eyes, nose, and mouth. The face can be divided into thirds, with one third encompassing the forehead, one third the eyes and nose, and one third the mouth and chin.
    b. Observe for symmetry of the face when the infant is crying. A facial palsy may result from a traumatic delivery.
    c. Observe for wide-spaced eyes (hypertelorism); flat, broad nasal bridge; long philtrum; micrognathia; and size of the mouth. Facial characteristics may be familial or may be associated with chromosomal abnormalities or syndromes.
7. Neck.
    a. Palpate the infant's neck to rule out sternocleidomastoid hematoma, thyroid enlargement, cystic hygroma, thyroglossal duct cyst, or a branchial cleft cyst or branchial sinus.
        (1) Thyroid enlargement is rare and is caused by intrauterine deprivation of thyroid hormone.
        (2) The most common neck mass is a cystic hygroma, which is a multiloculated cyst arising from lymphatic channels usually posterior to the sternocleidomastoid muscle and extending into the scapula and axillary and thoracic compartments. Most hygromas (65%) occur in the neck. The cysts invade and distort local anatomy. The airway can be distorted, and respiratory distress can be evident at birth.
        (3) A thyroglossal duct cyst or a branchial cleft cyst can sometimes be found in the neck.
        (4) A branchial sinus can be found along the sternocleidomastoid muscle and can communicate with deeper structures. Surgical removal may be required to prevent infection.
    b. Webbing or redundant skin may be evident because of excessive skin along the posterolateral line. This is associated with the Turner, Noonan, and Down syndromes.
    c. Inspect the clavicles for fractures, which may occur during delivery. A palpable mass, crepitus (caused by bone ends rubbing together), or tenderness is evident at the fracture site. Arm movement may be limited on the affected side.
8. Extremities
    a. Examine extremities, including hands and feet, for malformations and trauma.
    b. Length, contour, and symmetry of the extremities should be evaluated to rule out fractures resulting from a difficult delivery.
    c. Shape and length of digits and fingernails should be noted.
        (1) Syndactyly—webbing between adjacent digits.
        (2) Polydactyly—supernumerary digits.
        (3) Clinodactyly—congenital deviation of digits.
    d. Full range of motion in each extremity should be evident.
    e. Simian crease is a single palmar crease. It is present in 40% of infants with trisomy 21.
    f. Observe for congenital hip dysplasia.
        (1) Ortolani's maneuver and Barlow's test (Fig. 5–8) can rule out developmental dysplasia of the hip (DDH).
        (2) Asymmetric creases in the buttocks raise suspicion of congenital hip dysplasia.
    g. In metatarsus adductus the feet appear clubbed because of intrauterine positioning. A foot that can be put through the full range of motion is clubbed because of intrauterine positioning.
    h. Talipes equinovarus is a malformation of the ankle and forefoot adduction that will not return to midline with passive dorsiflexion.

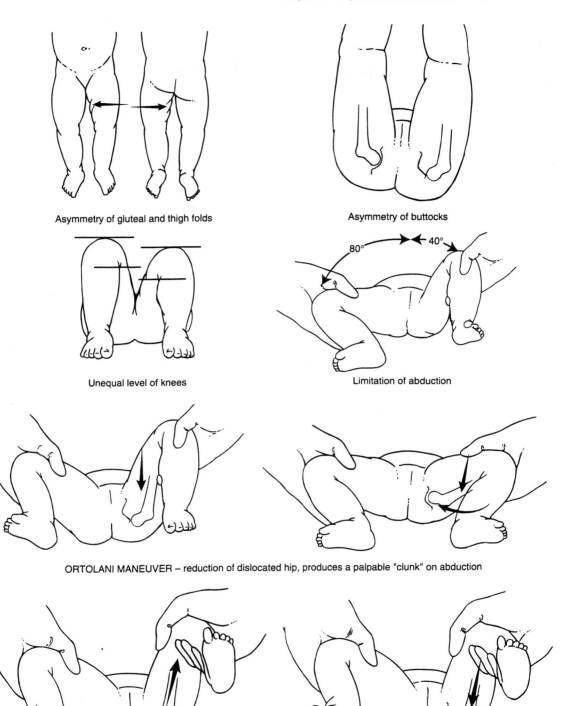

Asymmetry of gluteal and thigh folds

Asymmetry of buttocks

Unequal level of knees

Limitation of abduction

ORTOLANI MANEUVER – reduction of dislocated hip, produces a palpable "clunk" on abduction

BARLOW MANEUVER – dislocation of unstable hip, produces a palpable "clunk" on adduction with gentle downward pressure

Figure 5–8
Assessment of the newborn infant for a dislocated or unstable hip includes gluteal and thigh folds, buttocks, knees, abduction, Ortolani's maneuver, and Barlow's maneuver. (From Nichols, F.H., and Zwelling, E.: Maternal-Newborn Nursing: Theory and Practice. Philadelphia, W.B. Saunders, 1997.)

9. Skin.
   a. The skin is soft, smooth, and opaque. Vernix covers the body of the fetus and decreases with increased gestational age. Discolored vernix occurs with postmaturity, hemolytic disease, and meconium staining.
   b. Skin in a postmature infant may be dry and peeling.
   c. Skin should be warm to the touch. Cold, clammy skin may indicate shock.
   d. Evaluate skin for signs of cyanosis and jaundice.
   e. Capillary refill should be evaluated by depressing the infant's skin over one or more areas. After blanching of the skin, the time required to return to normal skin color is noted. Normal capillary refill time is 2–3 seconds. A capillary filling time greater than 3–5 seconds is prolonged (Vargo, 1996).
   f. Various findings may be evident as a result of the birth process.
      (1) Forceps marks: ecchymoses with rounded contours in the position the forceps were applied.
      (2) Petechiae over the head and neck, typically from a nuchal cord (cord wrapped around the infant's neck).
      (3) Abrasions or lacerations from scalp monitors, vacuum extractions, or scalpels.
   g. Benign lesions (also refer to Chapter 24, Neonatal Dermatology).
      (1) Ecchymosis: large area of subcutaneous hemorrhage usually found over the presenting part in traumatic deliveries.
      (2) Milia: white epidermal cysts or papules found over the forehead, cheeks, and chin. They resolve spontaneously within the first few weeks of life.
      (3) Mongolian spots: macular gray-blue lesions usually located in the lumbosacral area. They are caused by melanocyte infiltration of the dermis and fade with time. They occur in the majority of black, Latin American, Asian, and American Indian infants and in a small number of white infants.
      (4) Vascular nevi: common cutaneous malformations that may occur anywhere on the body. They may be present at birth or may develop in early infancy.
         (a) Nevus simplex or capillary hemangiomas (stork bites): red or pink macular patches with diffuse borders that may be found over the forehead, nape of the neck, glabella, and eyelids. They blanch when pressure is applied and resolve spontaneously.
         (b) Nevus flammeus (port-wine stain): flat, sharply defined lesion, most commonly located on the back of the neck. When present over the face (and possibly involving the upper portion of the trunk), following the branches of the trigeminal nerve (forehead and upper eyelid), it may be associated with Sturge-Weber syndrome (seizures, mental retardation, hemiparesis, and glaucoma). The lesion may fade in time but will not resolve, and will not blanch with pressure.
      (5) Sucking blisters are single blisterlike lesions on the forearm and hands of infants who have sucked on these areas in utero. The lesions will heal and fade in time.
      (6) Erythema toxicum (newborn rash): erythematous macules, each containing a central papule that may be yellow or white. The papules contain eosinophils and are sterile. The eruptions persist for a few days and then resolve spontaneously. They are never located on soles of feet or palms of hands.

F. **Nervous system**

1. Review of the infant's history and gestational age.
   a. A history of familial, genetic, or neurologic diagnosis, birth trauma, difficult

delivery, neonatal depression, abnormal presentation in labor/delivery, prolonged labor, maternal medication/alcohol/drugs, medical problems, difficult transition into extrauterine life, and feeding difficulties may alter a neurologic exam.

   b. Gestational age plays an important role in the neurologic examination because the nervous system is underdeveloped in premature infants. Responses elicited in the premature infant are different from those in the term infant.

2. External examination.
   a. Evaluate for signs of birth trauma: cephalhematoma, forceps marks, intact clavicles, symmetric movement, skin integrity, ecchymosis, petechiae, and edema.
   b. Observe for the presence of skin lesions related to certain neurologic disorders.
     (1) Neurofibromatosis: café au lait spots, greater than 1.5 cm in length or in numbers of 6 or greater (Jones, 1997a).
     (2) Sturge-Weber syndrome: nevus flammeus noted unilaterally, following the trigeminal nerve tract on the face and possibly involving the upper trunk (Jones, 1997a).
     (3) Tuberous sclerosis: areas of hypopigmented (white) macules on the skin (Jones, 1997a)
   c. Assess posture, movement, cry, and muscle tone.
     (1) The resting term infant flexes both upper and lower extremities. The posture of the premature infant becomes more hypotonic with decreasing gestational age.
     (2) The quality of movement in the term infant is smooth. The preterm infant's movements may be jittery and jerky, with tremors. Strength should be equal bilaterally.
     (3) Term infant's cry should be lusty, with normal pitch. A weak cry may indicate a depressed, ill, or premature infant. A high-pitched cry may be present in infants with neurologic or metabolic abnormalities or in drug withdrawal.
     (4) Evaluations for tone can include:
       (a) Checking traction response (pull-to-sit maneuver or head lag).
       (b) Testing the resistance of the upper and lower extremities (scarf sign; leg and arm recoil).
       (c) Checking tendon reflexes.
       (d) Observing for clonus.

3. Assessment of developmental reflexes. The examiner should be able to elicit these reflexes in the normal term infant:
   a. Sucking reflex. When the lips are gently stimulated, the infant will open the mouth and begin to suck. Evaluate the coordination and strength of the suck. This reflex is present at birth even in the premature infant, although it is not as strong as at term.
   b. Rooting reflex. Infant turns head and opens mouth toward the stimulus of stroking of the cheek.
   c. Palmar grasp. When slight pressure is applied in the palm, the infant grasps the finger applying the pressure. Attempts to remove the finger will elicit a tighter grasp. The grasp should be equal bilaterally.
   d. Tonic neck reflex (fencing position). The infant must be laying supine. When the infant's head is turned to one side, the infant will extend the upper extremity on the side where the head is turned and will flex the upper extremity on the opposite side.
   e. Moro reflex—(startle reflex) Support the infant's head and neck a few centimeters off the mattress. Allow the head to drop into a supportive hand. With this rapid movement the infants should extend their arms and open

their hands. They will then flex their arms back toward their chest and close their hands.

   f. Stepping reflex. Hold the infant upright, allowing the soles of the feet to touch a flat surface. The infant will alternate stepping movements.

   g. Truncal incurvation reflex (Galant's reflex). Hold the neonate in ventral suspension. Apply firm pressure along his side parallel to his spine. The infant should then flex the pelvis toward the side where stimulation was applied.

   h. Babinski reflex. Apply stimulation to the sole of the foot. The infant will respond with either flexion or extension of the toes.

4. Evaluation of the cranial nerves.

   a. Olfactory nerve (cranial nerve I). The sense of smell is difficult to evaluate in the infant. It can be done, however, with such strong scents as clove or peppermint. When exposed to these smells, the infant may grimace or exhibit the startle reflex.

   b. Optic nerve (cranial nerve II). Visual acuity and fields can be evaluated by using tracking methods. Watch for wandering or persistent nystagmus. Check pupils for size and constriction in response to light.

   c. Oculomotor, trochlear, and abducens nerves (cranial nerves III, IV, and VI). These cranial nerves supply the pupils and the extraocular muscles. Pupils should be equal (round) and reactive to light (PEARL). In addition, eye size and symmetry are evaluated. A "doll's eyes" (vestibular response) test should be performed. This test consists of gently moving the infant's head from side to side. The eyes should move away from the direction of rotation. When the infant's head moves to the right, the eyes should move to the left.

   d. Trigeminal nerve (cranial nerve V). This nerve supplies the sensory nerves in the face and jaw muscles. Test by touching the cheek and eliciting the rooting reflex. One can also evaluate this nerve by the biting and suck reflexes.

   e. Facial nerve (cranial nerve VII). This nerve controls facial movement. Observe for symmetric movement of the face.

   f. Auditory nerve (cranial nerve VIII). This nerve can be tested only grossly without proper auditory equipment. (See item 5, Sensory Function, below.)

   g. Glossopharyngeal nerve (cranial nerve IX). Evaluate and inspect tongue movements and elicit gag reflex.

   h. Vagus nerve (cranial nerve X). This nerve supplies the back of the mouth (soft palate, pharynx, and larynx). Assess the infant's ability to swallow and determine the presence or absence of stridor, hoarseness, or aphonia.

   i. Accessory nerve (cranial nerve XI). This nerve supplies the neck muscles (sternocleidomastoid and trapezius). When the head is turned from the midline to the side, the infant should attempt to bring it back to the midline.

   j. Hypoglossal nerve (cranial nerve XII). This nerve supplies the muscles of the tongue. Evaluate suck, swallow, and gag reflexes.

5. Sensory function.

   a. Touch. Painful stimulus to a foot elicits a withdrawal reflex. The sole of the foot is touched with a pin to provoke flexion of the limb and extension of the contralateral limb. Absence of flexion in the stimulated leg is abnormal.

   b. Response to light. Shining a penlight into the infant's eye results in eyelid closure.

   c. Response to sound. A bell is rung sharply within a few inches of the infant's ear while the infant is lying supine. Response is based on observable attentiveness to the sound. A brain-stem auditory evoked response (BAER) is recommended in the newborn period for all babies.

REFERENCES

Askin, D.F.: Chest and lungs assessment. *In* Tappero, E., and Honeyfield, M. (Eds.): Physical Assessment of the Newborn, 2nd ed. Petaluma, Calif., NICU Ink, 1996, p. 73.

Ballard, J.L., Khoury, J.C., Wedig, K., et al.: New Ballard Score, expanded to include extremely premature infants. J. Pediatr., *119*(3):418, 1991.

Bhutani, V.K.: Differential diagnosis of neonatal respiratory disorders. *In* Spitzer, A.R. (Ed.): Intensive Care of the Fetus and Neonate. St. Louis, Mosby, 1996, pp. 494–495, 497.

Black, M.: Assessment of weight and gestational age. Nurs. Clin. North Am., *13*:13–22, 1978.

Blackburn, S.T., and Loper, D.L.: The neuromuscular and sensory systems. *In* Blackburn, S.T., and Loper, D.L. (Eds.): Maternal, Fetal, and Neonatal Physiology. Philadelphia, W.B. Saunders, 1992a, p. 562.

Blackburn, S.T., and Loper, D.L.: The prenatal period and placental physiology. *In* Blackburn, S.T., and Loper, D.L. (Eds.): Maternal, Fetal, and Neonatal Physiology. Philadelphia, W.B. Saunders, 1992b, p. 91.

Cavaliere, T.A.: Genitourinary assessment. *In* Tappero, E., and Honeyfield M. (Eds.): Physical Assessment of the Newborn, 2nd ed. Petaluma, Calif., NICU Ink, 1996, p. 111.

Cilley, F.E., and Krummel, T.M.: Disorders of the umbilicus. *In* O'Neill, J.A., Jr., Rowe, M.I., Grosfeld, J.L., et al. (Eds.): Pediatric Surgery, 5th ed. St. Louis, Mosby, 1998, p. 1033.

Cooney, D.R.: Defects of the abdominal wall. In O'Neill, J.A., Jr., Rowe, M.I., Grosfeld, J.L., et al. (Eds.): Pediatric Surgery, 5th ed. St. Louis, Mosby, 1998, p. 1051.

Depp, K., and Kuhlman, K.: Identification and management of the fetus at risk for acidosis. *In* Spitzer, A.R. (Ed.): Intensive Care of the Fetus and Neonate. St. Louis, Mosby, 1996, pp. 109–114.

Dubowitz, L.M.S., Dubowitz, V., and Goldberg, C.: Clinical assessment of gestational age. In the newborn infant. J. Pediatr., *77*:1–10, 1970.

Duckett, J.W., and Baskin, L.S.: Hypospadias. *In* O'Neill, J.A., Rowe, M.I., Grosfeld, J.L., et al. (Eds.): Pediatric Surgery, 5th ed. St. Louis, Mosby, 1998, p. 1761.

Goldkrand, J.W., and Lin, J.Y.: Large for gestational age: Dilemma of the infant of the diabetic mother. J. Perinatol., *7*:282–287, 1987.

Hernandez, P.W., and Hernandez, J.A.: Physical assessment of the newborn. *In* Thureen, P.J., Deacon, J., O'Neill, P., and Hernandez, J. (Eds.): Assessment and Care of the Well Newborn. Philadelphia, W.B. Saunders, 1999, p. 120.

Jones, K.L.: Connective tissue disorders. *In* Jones, K.L.: Smith's Recognizable Patterns of Human Malformation, 5th ed. Philadelphia, W.B. Saunders, 1997a, p. 495.

Jones, K.L.: Early overgrowth with associated defects. *In* Jones, K.L. (Ed.): Smith's Recognizable Patterns of Human Malformation, 5th ed. Philadelphia, W.B. Saunders, 1997b, pp. 164–165.

Jones, K.L.: Facial defects as major feature. *In* Jones, K.L. (Ed.): Smith's Recognizable Patterns of Human Malformation, 5th ed. Philadelphia, W.B. Saunders, 1997c, p. 250.

Jones, K.L.: P. Hamartoses. *In* Jones, K.L. (Ed.): Smith's Recognizable Patterns of Human Malformation, 5th ed. Philadelphia, W.B. Saunders, 1997d, pp. 507–508.

Lawrence, R.A.: Physical examination. *In* Ziai, M., Clarke, T.A., and Merritt, T.A. (Eds.): Assessment of the Newborn. Boston, Little, Brown, 1984, pp. 86–111.

Phelan, J.: Oligohydramnios and polyhydramnios. *In* Spitzer, A.R. (Ed.): Intensive Care of the Fetus and Neonate. St. Louis, Mosby, 1996, p. 252.

Spear, M.: Intravenous alimentation. *In* Spitzer, A.R. (Ed.): Intensive Care of the Fetus and Neonate. St. Louis, Mosby, 1996, p. 836.

Trotter, C.W.: Gestational age assessment. *In* Tappero, E., and Honeyfield M. (Eds.): Physical Assessment of the Newborn, 2nd ed. Petaluma, Calif., NICU Ink, 1996, pp. 25–31.

Vargo, L.: Cardiovascular assessment of the newborn. *In* Tappero, E., and Honeyfield, M. (Eds.): Physical Assessment of the Newborn, 2nd ed., Petaluma, Calif., NICU Ink, 1996, p. 81, 87, 90.

Wapner, R., Trauffer, and Johnson, A.: Amniocentesis. *In* Spitzer, A.R. (Ed.): Intensive Care of the Fetus and Neonate. St. Louis, Mosby, 1996a, pp. 74, 79.

Wapner, R., Trauffer, P., and Johnson, A.: Chorionic villus sampling. *In* Spitzer, A.R. (Ed.): Intensive Care of the Fetus and Neonate. St. Louis, Mosby, 1996b, p. 92.

Witt, C.: Skin assessment. *In* Tappero, E., and Honeyfield, M.E. (Eds.): Physical Assessment of the Newborn, 2nd ed. Petaluma, Calif., NICU Ink, 1996, p. 41.

ADDITIONAL READINGS

Barness, L.A.: Manual of Pediatric Physical Diagnosis, 4th ed. Chicago, Year Book Medical Publishers, 1979.

Battaglia, F.C.: Intrauterine growth retardation. Am. J. Obstet. Gynecol., *106*:1103–1113, 1970.

Battaglia, F.C., and Lubchenco, L.O.: A practical classification of newborn infants by weight and gestational age. J. Pediatr., *71*:159–163, 1967.

Behrman, R.E.: The field of neonatal-perinatal medicine and neonatal risk. *In* Fanaroff, A.A., and Martin, R.J. (Eds.): Neonatal-Perinatal Medicine, 6th ed. St. Louis, Mosby, 1997.

Blackburn, S.T., and Loper, D.L.: Maternal, Fetal, and Neonatal Physiology: A clinical Perspective. Philadelphia, W.B. Saunders, 1992, pp. 83–84, 89–92, 244–245, 551–565.

Driscoll, J.M.: Physical examination. *In* Fanaroff, A.A., and Martin, R.J. (Eds.): Neonatal-Perinatal Medicine, 6th ed. Philadelphia, J.B. Lippincott, 1997.

Hittner, H.M., Hirsch, N.J., and Rudolph, A.J.: Assessment of gestational age by examination of the anterior vascular capsule of the lens. J. Pediatr., *91*:455–458, 1977.

Kenner, C., Brueggemeyer, A., and Gunderson, L.P. (Eds.): Comprehensive Neonatal Nursing: A Physiologic Perspective. Philadelphia, W.B. Saunders, 1993.

Lubchenco, L.O.: Assessment of gestational age and development at birth. Pediatr. Clin. North Am., *17*:125–145, 1970.

Lubchenco, L.O., and Koops, B.L.: Assessment of weight and gestational age. *In* Avery, G.B. (Ed.): Neonatology, 4th ed. Philadelphia, J.B. Lippincott, 1994.

Merenstein, G.B., and Gardner, S.L.: Handbook of Neonatal Intensive Care, 4th ed. St. Louis, Mosby, 1998.

Moore, K.L., Persaud, T.V.N., Shiota, K.: Color Atlas of Clinical Embryology. Philadelphia, W.B. Saunders, 1994, pp. 63, 72–74, 90–91.

Resnick, M.B., Carter, R.L., Ariet, M., et al.: Effect of birth weight, race, and sex on survival of low-birth-weight infants in neonatal intensive care. Am. J. Obstet. Gynecol., *161:* 184–187, 1989.

Sahu, S.: Birthweight, gestational age, and neonatal risks. Perinatol./Neonatol., *8:*28–36, 1984.

Sweet, A.V.: Classification of the low-birth-weight in- fant. *In* Klaus, M.H., and Fanaroff, A.A. (Eds.): Care of the High-Risk Neonate, 6th ed. Philadelphia, W.B. Saunders, 1997.

Walker, E.M., and Patel, N.B.: Mortality and morbidity in infants born between 20 and 28 weeks' gestation. Br. J. Obstet. Gynecol., *94:*670–674, 1987.

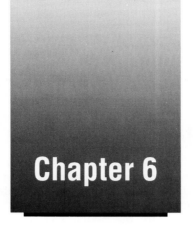

Chapter 6

Neonatal Delivery Room Resuscitation

Harriet A. Harrell

Objectives

1. Describe three anatomically unique features of the neonate that require special consideration during resuscitation.
2. Compare three physiologic characteristics of the neonate that make neonatal resuscitation different from adult resuscitation.
3. List three antepartum, intrapartum, and postpartum factors that indicate the neonate may be at risk of developing asphyxia.
4. Assemble the equipment needed for neonatal resuscitation and discuss maintenance and use.
5. Recite the initial steps of neonatal resuscitation.
6. Discuss the appropriate application of the Apgar scoring system as it relates to neonatal resuscitation.
7. Describe three potential complications of neonatal resuscitation.
8. Construct a plan for postresuscitation care, listing anticipated tests and nursing observations.

Resuscitation involves reestablishing heart and lung function after cardiac arrest or sudden death. Fortunately, neonates rarely have cardiac arrest. The more usual problem is respiratory insufficiency leading to respiratory arrest. If there is no intervention, cardiac arrest will ensue. The goal of resuscitation is to provide quick and efficient interventions, tailored to the neonate's response, that will minimize the effects of hypoxia on the infant. This chapter provides a comprehensive guideline for delivery room resuscitation.

Definitions

Resuscitate: Establish heart and lung function after cardiac arrest or sudden death (adult terminology).
1. Neonates rarely have cardiac arrest.
2. The more usual problem is respiratory insufficiency leading to respiratory arrest; if no intervention is made, insufficiency will lead to cardiac arrest.

Rescue: Save from current or impending danger. This terminology is more appropriate for neonatal delivery room interventions.

Anatomy and Physiology

A. **Physiologic and anatomic characteristics.** These characteristics of the neonate make neonatal resuscitation different from adult resuscitation. In general, the need for cardiopulmonary resuscitation in the neonate begins with respiratory compromise or failure, rather than cardiac arrest. Intervention is often possible before the neonate is compromised to the point of cardiac failure.

1. Large head size/body size ratio. Problems:
   a. Insensible water loss.
   b. Heat loss: no insulating fat layer.
   c. Minimal insulation from hair.
2. Large surface area/body size ratio. Problems:
   a. Insensible water loss.
   b. Heat loss.
3. Decreased muscle mass. Problems:
   a. Decreased ability to flex body to conserve heat.
   b. Decreased ability to generate heat.
4. Decreased subcutaneous fat (premature birth, intrauterine growth restriction). Problems:
   a. Decreased heat production (from brown fat metabolism).
   b. Increased heat loss (from lack of insulation).
5. Immature systems.
   a. CNS. Vasoconstriction is impaired (vasomotor instability).
   b. Neuromuscular system. Neonate is unable to shiver.
   c. Liver. Ability to metabolize drugs is decreased.
   d. Kidneys. Ability to excrete drugs and fluids is decreased; threshold for electrolyte losses is low.
   e. Gastrointestinal tract. Air is swallowed, leading to gastric distention and respiratory compromise.
   f. Metabolism: glucose intolerance.
   g. Lungs: decreased surface area for gas exchange.
   h. Immune system: increased predisposition to infection.
6. Anteriorly situated glottis.
   a. Intubation is difficult.
   b. Neonate is predisposed to airway compromise from positioning.
7. Short neck.
   a. Intubation is difficult.
   b. Neonate is predisposed to airway compromise from positioning.
8. Preferential nasal breathing.
   a. Primary airway is nose, which therefore must be kept clear and patent.
   b. Anatomic patency must be confirmed.
9. Venous access (Fig. 6–1).
   a. Small veins: access is difficult.
   b. Difficulty in restraining infant; thus access is easily lost.
   c. Umbilical access.
      (1) Arterial access.
      (2) Venous access. NOTE: Some medications (e.g., epinephrine, naloxone [Narcan]) can also be given via the endotracheal route while venous access is being established.
10. Veins are small, and skin and tissues are fragile. Care must be taken to avoid undue roughness and trauma.

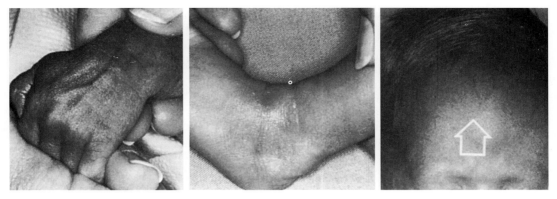

Figure 6–1
Preferred intravenous sites in the neonate for easy and rapid access. (Courtesy of Arizona Health Sciences Center.)

B. Physiology of asphyxia.

1. Perinatal asphyxia may be chronic, ongoing in utero for several days, or acute.
2. Decreased availability of oxygen to tissues as a result of decreased placental blood flow or decreased oxygen content of maternal blood. Tissue hypoxia leads to acidosis and anaerobic metabolism, which lead to increased lactic acid production and further decrease in pH. With placental circulatory compromise, the PCO_2 increases, adding to fetal acidosis. As acidosis worsens, availability of oxygen decreases and the need for glucose increases. Cardiac contractility can be affected by hypoxia, hypoglycemia, and acidosis (Fanaroff and Martin, 1997).
3. Meconium in the amniotic fluid may indicate fetal hypoxia resulting from decreased placental blood flow or maternal hypoxemia.
    a. Fetal tissue hypoxia affects the tone of the anal sphincter, which may relax, allowing passage of meconium into the amniotic sac.
    b. Fetal hypoxia causes gasping respirations in utero; meconium may then be taken into the upper airway. (NOTE: Normal fetal respiratory efforts are minimal, with the net flow of fluid through the lumen of the bronchial tree being outward. However, gasping respirations may allow meconium to enter even the distal airways.)
    c. At delivery, the mouth, nose, and posterior pharynx are suctioned thoroughly before the chest is delivered. Failure to do so may lead to aspiration of meconium into the lower airway when the neonate takes the first breath.
    d. Meconium in the airways may cause airway obstruction by:
        (1) Total blockage of airways, leading to alveolar atelectasis.
        (2) Ball-valve effect. Air enters the alveoli on inspiration, when the partially obstructed airway dilates, allowing air to pass the obstruction. Air becomes trapped in alveoli on expiration, when the airway constricts. This leads to overdistention and alveolar rupture and can precipitate pulmonary air leaks (Avery, 1994). Typical x-ray findings of meconium aspiration reveal areas of atelectasis and air trapping, hyperinflation, and pulmonary air leaks (refer to Chapter 29.).

Risk Factors

Risk factors are warning signs that alert the perinatal team to the possibility of an adverse outcome and the need for anticipatory preparation of neonatal rescue or resuscitation.

A. **Prepartum period (maternal risk factors):** conditions during pregnancy that predispose mother and fetus to stress and can interfere with successful transition of the fetus to extrauterine life.
1. Maternal age more than 35 years or less than 15 years.
2. Diabetes mellitus.
3. Hemorrhage or anemia.
4. Drug abuse.
5. No prenatal care.
6. Polyhydramnios or oligohydramnios.
7. Cardiovascular disease.
8. Prolonged rupture of membranes.
9. Anatomic abnormalities of the uterus.
10. Rh or ABO (blood group) incompatibilities.
11. Hypertension (toxemia, chronic).
12. Multiple gestation.
13. Previous pregnancy complication or fetal loss.
14. Chronic illness (e.g., renal, pulmonary) (Avery, 1994).

B. **Intrapartum period:** conditions that predispose the fetus to difficult transition to extrauterine life or signs that the fetus is not tolerating the stresses of labor. Unsuccessful transition may ensue.
1. Abnormal fetal positioning or presentation (e.g., breech position).
2. Cesarean delivery.
3. Fetal heart rate abnormalities.
4. Intrauterine growth restriction.
5. Intrapartum blood loss, in mother or fetus.
6. Maternal sedation.
7. Maternal fever/infection.
8. Prolonged or difficult labor.
9. Prolonged rupture of membranes.
10. Prolapse of the umbilical cord (Avery, 1994).

C. **Postpartum period:** signs or conditions in the delivery room or during the transitional period that indicate the neonate is having difficulty making all the physiologic changes needed for successful adaptation from intrauterine to extrauterine life.
1. Anomalous airway.
2. Cardiac arrhythmia: tachycardia or bradycardia.
3. Extreme color change.
4. Circulatory compromise.
5. Feeding intolerance.
6. Temperature instability.
7. Meconium staining.
8. Seizures.
9. Prematurity.
10. Postmaturity.
11. Respiratory distress, apnea.
12. Neurologic depression (Avery, 1994).

Anticipation of and Preparation for Resuscitation

Institutional guidelines, protocols, policies, and procedures will dictate the method and frequency of equipment surveillance and staff certification. The Neonatal Resuscitation Program of the American Academy of Pediatrics and the American Heart Association is a national program designed for this purpose

(Bloom and Cropley, 1996). All delivery rooms, emergency departments, birthing centers, nurseries, and postpartum units must be equipped and staffed for neonatal resuscitation at all times. Although many resuscitative events are predictable and can be anticipated, unexpected events must be handled as efficiently as anticipated ones.

A. General preparation.

1. Update staff frequently.
2. Evaluate and update equipment needs frequently.
3. Arrange for periodic evaluation and maintenance of electrical equipment by the biomedical engineering department on a regularly scheduled basis.
4. Schedule periodic evaluation and maintenance of all respiratory equipment.
5. Evaluate and replace supplies every shift (use equipment checklist).
6. Test alerting system for rapid, consistent response of personnel.

B. Delivery room preparation.

1. Identify high-risk situations.
2. Assemble equipment within easy reach and check function.
3. Preheat warmer and blankets.
4. Review resuscitation protocol and familiarize self with drug dosages, concentrations, routes, and side effects.
5. Review size chart for endotracheal tubes.
6. Designate resuscitation team captain and give assignments.
7. Reassure mother, significant others, and obstetrics team that you are present and prepared. Explain that you will notify them of the neonate's well-being as soon as possible.

C. Personnel roles.

1. Personnel designations for neonatal resuscitation are an institutional responsibility. Anyone working with neonates should be able to initiate rescue interventions while additional personnel are responding. In many institutions, a neonatal nurse practitioner is responsible for neonatal resuscitation; in others, an in-house medical staff member is responsible. State law and licensure regulations may dictate who can perform invasive procedures. It is important that each member of the resuscitation team know the scope and level of his or her responsibility, be adequately trained, and have yearly competence assessment.
2. Family support is important and may be the responsibility of the obstetrics nurse if the pediatric personnel are busy. This function (as family supporter) should not be assumed but should be assigned in advance.

D. Non-delivery-room preparation. As with delivery room resuscitation, being prepared for unforeseen events can facilitate success in a time of crisis. Unlike delivery room events, non-delivery-room resuscitation is always unpredictable. The following events may precipitate respiratory or circulatory compromise:

1. Apnea.
2. Choking and/or aspiration.
3. Unwitnessed cardiac arrest.
4. Seizure.
5. Hypoxia or airway obstruction.

Equipment for Neonatal Resuscitation

Not every item on the equipment list (Table 6–1) will be used, but it is important to have sufficient quantities to support a prolonged effort. The

Table 6–1
NEONATAL RESUSCITATION EQUIPMENT LIST

Light source	Extra batteries and bulbs for laryngoscope
Heat source	Noncuffed endotracheal tubes, two of each size: 2.5, 3.0,
Dry, warm, soft blankets	3.5, 4.0
Treatment bed or table with removable or collapsible sides	Endotracheal tube stylets (2)
Clock with second hand or timer	Pectin skin barrier
Wall suction	Adhesive tape, ½ inch and 1 inch wide
Oxygen: wall or cylinder (0–15 L flow)	Alcohol swabs
Air: wall or cylinder (0–15 L flow)	Iodine swabs
Stethoscope: neonatal size	Syringes, 1, 3, 10, and 20 mL
Anesthesia bag, 0.5 L with flow adjustment valve and manometer	Heparinized blood gas syringes
	Needles, 25 and 18 gauge
Self-inflating resuscitation bag, 0.5 L with adapter for 100% oxygen	Intracatheter, 16 gauge (over-the-needle intravascular catheter)
Face masks: premature and newborn sizes	Umbilical catheters, size 3.5F and 5.0F
Oral airways: size 0 and size 1	Three-way stopcock
Laryngoscope with Miller curved and straight blades, size 0 and size 1	Umbilical catheter tray
	Meconium aspiration device
Suction catheters, two of each size: 5F, 8F, and 10F	Epinephrine, 1 : 10,000 concentration
Sterile water for suctioning	Normal saline solution for IV infusion
Sterile normal saline solution ampules for suction or lubrication	Lactated Ringer's solution
	Albumin, 5%
Bulb syringe	Sodium bicarbonate, 4.2%
Cord clamp and sterile scissors	Naloxone hydrochloride (Auvenshine and Enriquez, 1990)
Feeding tube size 8F	

development and improvement of such equipment are ongoing. All new products should be critically evaluated before they are incorporated into existing stock. It is important that staff members be familiar with the equipment they will be using and practice with it frequently.

Decision-making Process

For many years, delivery room resuscitation decisions were based on Apgar scores (Table 6–2). Current recommendations discourage the use of the Apgar score for decision making in resuscitation. Components of the Apgar score are used for assessment and reassessment of resuscitative progress (Covey and

Table 6–2
APGAR SCORE

The Apgar score is a method of evaluating the newborn infant's condition at birth on the basis of five characteristics: heart rate, respiratory effort, muscle tone, reflex irritability, and color. For each parameter the infant receives a score of 0 if it is absent, 1 if it is present but abnormal, and 2 if it is normal. Traditionally scores are assigned at 1 and 5 minutes, but in prolonged resuscitation a score can be assigned at any time to reflect the condition of the infant and the response to resuscitative efforts. With asphyxia, the Apgar characteristics generally disappear in a predictable manner: first the pink coloration is lost, next the respiratory effort, and then tone, followed by reflex irritability and, finally, heart rate.

	Score		
Sign	**0**	**1**	**2**
Heart rate	Absent	Less than 100 bpm	More than 100 bpm
Respiratory effort	Absent	Weak, irregular	Good, crying
Muscle tone	Flaccid	Some flexion of extremities	Well flexed
Reflex irritability (catheter in nose)	No response	Grimace	Cough or sneeze
Color	Blue, pale	Body pink, extremities blue	Completely pink

Table 6–3
PRACTICAL EPIGRAM OF THE APGAR SCORE

> **SIGN**
> A = Appearance (color)
> P = Pulse (heart rate)
> G = Grimace (reflex irritability response to stimulation of sole of foot)
> A = Activity (muscle tone)
> R = Respiration (respiratory effort)
>
> From Covey, M.J., and Butterfield, L.J.: Practical epigram of the Apgar score [letter]. JAMA *181*:353, 1962.
> Copyrighted 1962, American Medical Association.

Butterfield, 1962) (see Table 6–3). Interventions should never be delayed pending the 1-minute Apgar score. The action-evaluation-decision cycle is used (Fig. 6–2).

Neonatal Resuscitation "ABCs"

The steps taken to rescue or resuscitate a neonate are best remembered with the familiar "ABCs" of resuscitation used in all resuscitation programs of the American Heart Association.

A. "ABCs" defined.
1. A = Airway.
   a. Establish and maintain an open airway.
   b. Position infant on back, with neck slightly extended.
   c. Suction mouth, nose, and trachea as needed.
   d. Intubate the trachea if needed to maintain the airway or to remove meconium.
   e. Stabilize and secure endotracheal tube if needed.
2. B = Breathing.
   a. Evaluate respiratory effort and rate.
   b. If infant has apnea, initiate breathing by employing tactile stimulation.
   c. Begin bag-and-mask ventilation if needed.
   d. Initiate bag-to-tube ventilation if trachea is intubated or if use of bag and mask is ineffective.
3. C = Circulation.
   a. Evaluate heart rate.
   b. Evaluate color and perfusion.
   c. Give chest compression by the thumb or two-finger method if needed.

The Action/Evaluation/Decision Cycle

Figure 6–2
Circular process used during neonatal re-suscitation to guide events. (Reproduced with permission. From Bloom, R.S., and Cropley, C.: Textbook of Neonatal Resuscitation. Dallas, Tex., American Heart Association, 1994. [Revised September 1996.] Copyright © American Heart Association.)

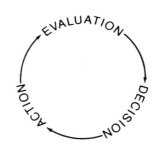

4. D = Drugs/medications.
   a. Epinephrine to stimulate heart by increasing rate and strength of contractions.
   b. Volume expander to increase circulating blood volume when there are signs of hypovolemia, shock, or acute blood loss.
      (1) Whole blood.
      (2) Albumin, 5%.
      (3) Normal saline solution.
      (4) Lactated Ringer's solution.
   c. Sodium bicarbonate, 4.2%, to correct metabolic acidosis.
   d. Naloxone (Narcan) to reverse respiratory depression caused by maternal narcotic administration.
5. E = Environment.
   a. Provide safety for patients and staff.
      (1) Dispose of sharp objects properly.
      (2) Use universal precautions.
   b. Provide humidity, if possible, to prevent metabolic stress.
   c. Provide temperature control to prevent metabolic stress.
   d. Be gentle to prevent unnecessary trauma.

B. **Initial steps.** At most deliveries, the following five steps are the only interventions necessary:
1. Prevent hypothermia, which may increase metabolic requirements.
   a. Place and keep baby in preheated environment (radiant heat source or incubator). Supplement environmental support with:
      (1) Warmed towels.
      (2) Stocking cap.
      (3) Avoidance of drafts.
   b. Maintain dry, warm environment.
      (1) Dry thoroughly.
      (2) Remove wet linen immediately after drying infant and replace with dry linen.
2. Open the airway.
   a. Position infant on the back, with neck slightly extended.
      (1) Do not hyperextend or hyperflex the neck.
      (2) A shoulder pad may help maintain the correct position.
      (3) The infant's head may be turned to the side in this position without airway compromise (Fig. 6–3).
   b. Suction the mouth before the nose is suctioned.
      (1) Use bulb syringe or wall suction. The suction pressure should be 80-100 mm Hg.
      (2) Vigorous or prolonged deep suctioning can result in bradycardia and/or apnea induced by stimulation of the vagus nerve.
      (3) If thick, particulate meconium is present in the amniotic fluid, or if meconium of any consistency is present and the baby's respirations are depressed, intubate the trachea and perform direct tracheal suction until fluid is clear.
         (a) Clinical judgment must be used to decide whether intubation is needed in a vigorous neonate born through meconium-stained fluid.
         (b) If infant is apneic, institute positive-pressure ventilation without delay.
3. Stimulate respirations.
   a. Slap the soles of the infant's feet.
   b. Rub the back.

Positioning

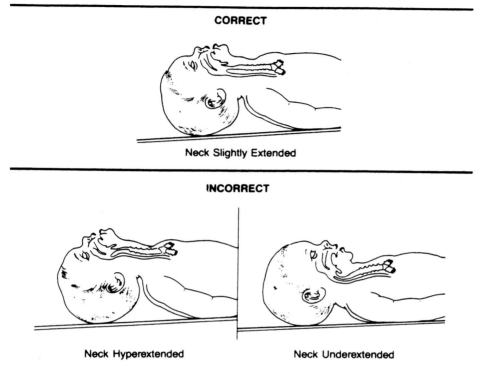

CORRECT

Neck Slightly Extended

INCORRECT

Neck Hyperextended   Neck Underextended

Figure 6–3
Positioning for neonatal resuscitation, appropriate for airway maintenance, bag-and-mask ventilation, and intubation. (Reproduced with permission. From Bloom, R.S., and Cropley, C.: Textbook of Neonatal Resuscitation, 2nd ed. Dallas, Tex., American Heart Association, 1996. Copyright © American Heart Association.)

    c. Make two attempts. If respirations do not begin, proceed on to bag-and-mask ventilation (unless diaphragmatic hernia is suspected, in which case, intubate the trachea and use bag-to-tube ventilation).

4. Evaluate the infant's condition.
    a. Respiratory effort: rate, breath sounds, grunting, flaring, retracting.
    b. Heart rate: count for 6 seconds and multiply by 10. Obtain heart rate by:
       (1) Palpation at the base of the umbilical cord stump.
       (2) Auscultation of the apical heartbeat with a stethoscope.
    c. Color.
       (1) Peripheral cyanosis of hands and feet is usually normal.
       (2) Central cyanosis of tongue and gums is abnormal.

5. Give blow-by oxygen if central cyanosis is present, heart rate is greater than 100 bpm, and respirations are adequate.
    a. Use 100% oxygen.
    b. Withdraw oxygen slowly if baby remains pink.

C. **Positive-pressure ventilation.**

1. Bag-and-mask ventilation.
    a. Initiate for:
       (1) Apnea or gasping respirations.

        (2) Inadequate ventilatory effort.

        (3) Heart rate less than 100 bpm.

   b. Equipment.

        (1) Self-inflating bags must have a reservoir tail to deliver high concentrations of oxygen.

        (2) Anesthesia bags should have a pressure gauge and flow control valve.

        (3) Equipment should always be preset and tested before actual use.

        (4) Mask of proper size should be used to obtain adequate seal.

        (5) Equipment should always be connected to 100% oxygen source at 5–10 L of flow.

   c. Procedure.

        (1) Assemble, set, and test the equipment.

        (2) Position the neonate as in "Initial Steps," item B under Neonatal Resuscitation "ABCs," above.

        (3) Apply mask and ensure proper seal.

        (4) Deliver 15–40 cm H_2O pressure at 40–60 breaths per minute for 15–30 seconds.

           (a) Initial breath: 30–40 cm H_2O pressure.

           (b) Normal lungs: 15–20 cm H_2O pressure.

           (c) Diseased lungs: 20–40 cm H_2O pressure.

        (5) Observe for easy rise and fall of chest.

        (6) Pause to check 6-second heart rate and continue ventilation until neonate begins spontaneous effective breathing and the heart rate is greater than 100 bpm.

        (7) If bag-and-mask ventilation is ineffective or if there is need for prolonged ventilation, endotracheal intubation should be performed.

   d. Exceptions.

        (1) If thick, particulate meconium is present, or if meconium is thin but respirations are depressed, perform intubation and tracheal suctioning before beginning bag-and-mask ventilation.

        (2) If a diaphragmatic hernia is present or is suspected, perform intubation, give bag-to-tube ventilation, and place orogastric tube for gastric decompression.

2. Ventilation by bag to endotracheal tube.

   a. Indications for intervention.

        (1) The neonate does not respond to bag-and-mask ventilation, as evidenced by inadequate chest expansion or continuing low heart rate.

        (2) Diaphragmatic hernia is suspected.

        (3) Prolonged ventilation is required.

        (4) Tracheal suctioning is required.

   b. Equipment.

        (1) Laryngoscope, batteries, bulbs, size 0 and 1 blades (curved or straight).

        (2) Noncuffed, nontapered endotracheal tubes, with vocal cord marks, in a variety of sizes (two each): sizes 2.5, 3.0, 3.5, and 4.0.

        (3) Endotracheal tube stylets.

        (4) Suction equipment with catheters in sizes 5F, 8F, and 10F (two each).

        (5) Neck roll for positioning.

        (6) Adhesive tape; scissors.

        (7) Resuscitation bag (0.5 L), manometer, and masks.

        (8) Oxygen source, flowmeter, and tubing.

   c. Procedure (see Chapter 31).

        (1) Perform intubation.

        (2) Confirm placement.

        (3) Secure tube.

D. Chest compressions.

1. Chest compressions should be initiated when the heart rate is less than 60 bpm or between 60 and 80 bpm and not increasing after 15-30 seconds of ventilation with 100% oxygen.
2. Use one of the following two methods:
   a. Thumb technique.
      (1) Place both thumbs over the lower third of the infant's sternum above the xiphoid process.
      (2) Encircle the infant's chest with your hands to provide support.
   b. Two-finger technique.
      (1) Place the tips of the middle and index fingers of one of your hands over the lower third of the infant's sternum.
      (2) Place your other hand under the infant's back to provide support.
3. Compressions should squeeze the heart between the spinal column and the sternum.
   a. Force of compression should be straight down to avoid rib or lung damage.
   b. Depress the sternum about 1.5–2 cm.
   c. Compress 90 times per minute.
4. Compression/ventilation ratio: 1:3.
   a. Interpose one ventilation for every three compressions. This will equal 30 ventilations and 90 compressions, or 120 events per minute.
   b. Optimally the neonate's trachea should be intubated. If not, place an orogastric tube to vent the stomach.

E. Chemical resuscitation. Most neonatal resuscitations do not require medications or volume expanders. An umbilical catheter or peripheral IV line will need to be placed to administer medications or volume expanders (see Chapter 31). Epinephrine and naloxone hydrochloride (Narcan) can be administered through the endotracheal tube.

1. Indications.
   a. Stimulate the heart.
   b. Increase tissue perfusion.
   c. Correct metabolic acidosis.
   d. Failure of adequate ventilation with 100% oxygen and chest compressions to revive the infant.
2. Drugs and solutions (Table 6–4).
   a. Epinephrine, a cardiac stimulant, increases the heart rate and strength of contractions and causes peripheral vasoconstriction.
      (1) Indications for use:
         (a) Heart rate is less than 80 bpm after ventilation with 100% oxygen, endotracheal tube, and chest compressions.
         (b) Heart rate is undetectable while ventilations and compressions are being started.
      (2) Concentration: 1:10,000.
      (3) Preparation: draw up 1 mL in a 1 mL syringe.
      (4) Dose: 0.1 to 0.3 mL/kg, given rapidly.
      (5) Route: peripheral IV infusion, through endotracheal tube, or through umbilical catheter.
      (6) When given through endotracheal tube, the dose may be diluted in 1–2 mL of normal saline solution or flushed in with 0.5 mL normal saline solution to ensure delivery.
      (7) Response: effect should be evident within 30 seconds of administration. Dosing may be repeated every 3–5 minutes.

Table 6–4
DRUGS AND SOLUTIONS USED IN CHEMICAL RESUSCITATION

Medication	Concentration to Administer	Preparation	Dosage/Route	Rate/Precautions
Epinephrine	1 : 10,000	1 mL	0.01-0.03 mg/kg 0.1-0.3 mL/kg IV or ET	Give rapidly May dilute with normal saline to 1-2 mL if giving ET
Volume expanders	Whole blood 5% Albumin Normal saline Ringer's lactate	40 mL	10 mL/kg IV	Give over 5-10 minutes Give by syringe or IV drip
Sodium bicarbonate	0.5 mEq/mL (4.2% solution)	20 mL or two 10-mL prefilled syringes	2 mEq/kg IV only (4 mL/kg)	Give slowly, over at least 2 minutes Give only if infant is being effectively ventilated
Naloxone hydro-chloride	0.4 mg/mL	1 mL	0.1 mg/kg (0.25 mL/ kg) IV, ET, IM, SQ	Give rapidly IV, ET preferred IM, SQ acceptable
	1.0 mg/mL	1 mL	0.1 mg/kg (0.1 mL/ kg) IV, ET, IM, SQ	

Reproduced with permission. From Bloom, R.S., and Cropley, C.: Textbook of Neonatal Resuscitation, 2nd ed. Dallas, Tex., American Heart Association, 1996. Copyright © American Heart Association.
ET, By endotracheal tube; *IM*, intramuscularly; *SQ*, subcutaneously.

   b. Volume expanders are fluids that increase the neonate's circulating blood volume to correct hypovolemia and facilitate tissue perfusion.
     (1) Indicated when there is suspected or documented blood loss with signs of hypovolemia or shock.
       (a) Weak or absent peripheral pulses.
       (b) Low blood pressure.
       (c) Tachycardia.
       (d) Pale or mottled skin despite good oxygenation.
       (e) Unresponsiveness to resuscitation.
     (2) Solutions.
       (a) Normal saline solution.
       (b) 5% Albumin/plasma substitute.
       (c) Lactated Ringer's solution.
       (d) Whole blood (type O-negative, cross-matched in advance to the mother).
     (3) Preparation: draw up 40 mL.
     (4) Dose: 10 mL/kg in 5–10 minutes.
     (5) Route: peripheral IV line or through umbilical catheter.
     (6) Response: increase in blood pressure, improvement of perfusion of skin, and increase in the intensity of pulses should occur within minutes. Procedure may be repeated if necessary.
   c. Sodium bicarbonate, a base buffer, raises the pH of the blood.
     (1) Indications for use.
       (a) Adequate ventilation has been established.
       (b) Metabolic acidosis has been documented.
       (c) There is evidence of prolonged asphyxia.
     (2) Concentration: 4.2% solution, 0.5 mEq/mL.
     (3) Preparation: open a 10 mL prefilled syringe.
     (4) Dose: 2 mEq/kg, slow IV push (do not exceed 1 mEq/kg per minute).

(5) Route: Peripheral IV infusion or through umbilical catheter.

(6) Response: pH should change and heart rate improve within 30 seconds.

d. Naloxone hydrochloride (Narcan), a short-acting narcotic antagonist, displaces narcotics from receptor sites and reverses the physiologic depressant effects of the narcotic.

(1) Indications for use.

(a) Severe respiratory depression in a neonate born to a mother who has recently been given a narcotic (within 4 hours).

(b) Persistent apnea in a neonate who is being given assisted ventilation and there is a suspicion of maternal narcotics.

(2) Concentration: 1.0 mg/mL or 0.4 mg/mL.

(3) Preparation: draw up 1 mL in a syringe.

(4) Dose: 0.1 mg/kg given rapidly.

(5) Route: may be given by peripheral IV infusion, through umbilical catheter, by intramuscular injection, or through endotracheal tube (may also be given subcutaneously, but onset of effect is slowed).

(6) Response.

(a) Respiratory depression should abate within seconds or minutes (depending on route) after administration. Duration of action is widely variable (1–4 hours). Monitor closely for return of respiratory depression. May be repeated several times if needed.

(b) If given to a neonate of a narcotic-addicted mother, naloxone may precipitate immediate and severe withdrawal, including seizures (Bloom and Cropley, 1996).

Unusual Situations

A. Pulmonary hypoplasia.

1. Definitions and characteristics.

a. Associated with Potter's syndrome, dysplastic renal conditions, chronic amniotic fluid loss, and diaphragmatic hernia.

b. Underdeveloped lungs resulting from insufficient space within the thoracic cavity for normal development.

2. Acute clinical problems.

a. Inability to ventilate lungs adequately.

b. Very high pressures required to expand small, stiff lungs.

c. High risk of pulmonary air leak.

3. Management.

a. Intubate trachea to overcome upper airway resistance.

b. Ventilate with 100% oxygen and as much pressure as necessary to expand the lungs.

c. Transilluminate and auscultate chest frequently, assessing for pulmonary air leaks.

d. Place orogastric tube as soon as possible to prevent gastric and intestinal inflation, which could compromise diaphragmatic excursions.

B. Abdominal wall defects.

1. Definition and characteristics.

a. Gastroschisis: herniation of stomach, liver, and/or intestines through a defect next to the umbilical cord, usually to the right of the cord.

b. Omphalocele: midline herniation of the bowel into the umbilical cord.

c. Exstrophy of the bladder: externalization and aversion of the bladder, urethra, or ureteral orifices through a defect in the lower portion of the abdominal wall.

2. Acute clinical problems.
   a. Fluid and heat loss through exposed viscera (exposure increases surface area).
   b. Potential for visceral damage from drying or trauma.
   c. Increased risk of infection.
3. Management.
   a. Cover defect immediately with sterile 4 × 4's soaked with warm (not hot) normal saline solution and wrap defect with sterile plastic wrap.
   b. Maintain infant in a moist, heated environment.
   c. Place orogastric tube to intermittent suction to prevent gastric and intestinal inflation, which would complicate repair.
   d. Maintain side-lying position to provide support to defect.

C. **Neural tube defects.**

1. Definition and characteristics.
   a. Anencephaly: most severe form, in which neural tube failed to close and brain is exposed.
   b. Encephalocele: defect in closure of the neural tube at proximal end, with outpouching of brain tissue through the skull.
   c. Myelomeningocele: defect in closure at the distal end, with exposure of the neural tube at various levels of the spinal column.
2. Acute clinical problems.
   a. Ethical and legal questions of viability or organ donation from infants with anencephaly.
   b. Heat and fluid losses through open defect.
   c. Increased risk of infection.
   d. Potential for damage of exposed nervous system tissue as a result of trauma.
   e. Difficulty in handling baby because of exposed tissue.
3. Management.
   a. Cover defect with sterile, saline solution–soaked sponges and a plastic barrier to prevent heat and fluid losses.
   b. Maintain baby in a neutral thermal environment.
   c. Keep neonate on side or abdomen.
   d. Assisted ventilation may be given with the neonate on his or her side if necessary.
   e. Manage all defects in the same manner, no matter how severe. Discuss viability issues after resuscitation and stabilization.

D. **Choanal atresia.**

1. Definitions and characteristics.
   a. Bony soft tissue obstruction of the posterior nares; may be bilateral or unilateral.
   b. Respiratory distress immediately after birth because of blockage of the primary airway, the nose.
2. Management.
   a. Stimulate the baby to cry, thereby using the secondary airway (mouth) for ventilation.
   b. Insert an oral airway.
   c. Administer oxygen if needed.
   d. Suction secretions as needed.

E. **Undiagnosed multiple gestation.**

1. Definitions and characteristics.

      a. Unexpected twins, triplets, or quadruplets.
      b. Smaller than average size.
  2. Acute clinical problems.
      a. Inadequate supplies and equipment available to manage multiple prolonged resuscitative efforts.
      b. Immaturity of neonates.
  3. Management.
      a. Always have extra equipment available.
      b. Always stock enough equipment for twins and have backup supplies nearby.
      c. Have a system for calling on secondary resuscitation teams when necessary.

F. **Extremely low birth weight infant.**

  1. Definitions and characteristics.
      a. Immature lungs.
      b. Fragile skin.
      c. Susceptible to trauma from resuscitative intervention.
      d. Susceptible to infection and thermal instability.
      e. Nationwide statistics show that 47–74% of neonates born at less than 26 weeks' gestation survive, and that neonates weighing less than 600 g have a 15–18% survival rate (Hack, Wright, Shankaran, et al., 1995).
  2. Management.
      a. If at all possible, the family and the primary care physician, along with the neonatal team, should explore viability issues and expected outcome before the birth.
      b. Be as gentle as possible with the tiny baby (i.e., drying, ventilating, CPR).

Complications of Resuscitation

A. **Trauma.**

  1. Skin: bruises and abrasions from chest compressions, handling, and tape application and removal.
  2. Mucosa: laryngoscopy can cause trauma to and bleeding of gums, lips, pharynx, and trachea.
  3. Internal organ damage from chest compressions.

B. **Pulmonary air leaks.**

  1. Pneumothorax.
  2. Pneumomediastinum
  3. Pneumopericardium.

C. **Dangers of using umbilical vessel catheters.**

  1. Vessel perforation.
  2. Accidental blood loss.
  3. Clots and emboli.
  4. Organ and vessel endothelial damage from infusion of hypertonic solutions.
  5. Organ ischemia from blockage of major vessels by the catheter tip.
  6. Infection.

D. **Intracranial hemorrhage.**

  1. Subarachnoid.
  2. Periventricular.
  3. Intraventricular.

Postresuscitation Care

The purpose of postresuscitation care is to evaluate the infant's condition for complications and to help diagnose and treat underlying disease.

A. Assess oxygenation, ventilation, and acid-base balance.

1. Check arterial blood gas concentrations.
2. Correlate findings with baby's clinical condition.
3. Correlate findings with transcutaneous monitoring devices.
4. Adjust baby's respiratory support as needed.

B. Monitor glucose concentrations to ensure normoglycemia.

1. Check blood glucose.
2. Treat hypoglycemia and adjust maintenance glucose levels.
3. Perform follow-up glucose checks as ordered.

C. Chest and abdominal x-ray examination for pneumothorax, pneumomediastinum, pneumopericardium, and pneumoperitoneum.

1. Assess endotracheal tube position.
2. Assess umbilical catheter position.
3. Evaluate for lung disease.
4. Rule out fractures and anomalies.

D. Fluids and electrolytes.

1. Calculate fluid volume received during resuscitation.
2. Determine amount needed (in milliliters per kilogram per day).
3. Adjust IV rate as needed.

E. Monitor vital signs.

1. Provide a neutral thermal environment to prevent the sequelae of hypothermia.
2. Assess perfusion and capillary refill in seconds.
3. Monitor blood pressure, preferably arterial.
4. Heart and respiratory rate.

F. Screen for infection.

1. Evaluate maternal history: titers, cultures, pretreatment, and risk factors.
2. Obtain a complete blood cell count, differential cell count, platelet count.
3. Obtain blood and viral cultures and for sensitivity testing as indicated.
4. If index of suspicion is high and neonate's condition is stable, perform lumbar puncture for cerebral spinal fluid analysis.

G. Support family.

1. Report neonate's condition to mother and significant others.
2. Notify social worker of new admission.

REFERENCES

Auvenshine, M.A., and Enriquez, M.G. (Eds.): Comprehensive Maternity Nursing: Perinatal and Women's Health, 2nd ed. Boston, Jones and Bartlett, 1990.

Avery, G.B. (Ed.): Neonatology: Pathophysiology and Management of the Newborn, 4th ed. Philadelphia, J.B. Lippincott, 1994.

Bloom, R.S., and Cropley, C.: Textbook of Neonatal Resuscitation. Dallas, Tex., and Elk Grove Village, Ill., American Heart Association and American Academy of Pediatrics, 1994. [Revised September 1996.]

Covey, M.J., and Butterfield, L.J.: Practical epigram of the Apgar score [letter]. JAMA 181:353, 1962.

Fanaroff, A.A., Martin, R.J. (Eds.): Neonatal-Perinatal Medicine: Diseases of the Fetus and Infant, 6th ed. St. Louis, Mosby, 1997.

Hack, M., Wright, L.L., Shankaran, S. et al.: Very-low-birth-weight outcomes of the National Institute of Child Health and Human Development Neonatal Network, November 1989 to October 1990. Am. J. Obstet. Gynecol., 172:457–464, 1995.

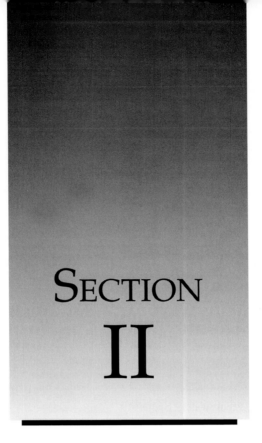

SECTION II

NEONATAL PULMONARY DISORDERS AND MANAGEMENT

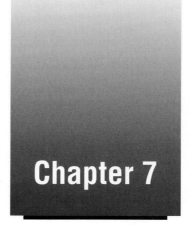

Chapter 7

Respiratory Distress

Patricia M. Casey

Objectives

1. Describe the anatomic and biochemical events associated with lung development.

2. Discuss the physiology of respiration.

3. Describe common respiratory disorders seen in the newborn infant.

4. Discuss common findings in respiratory distress syndrome, meconium aspiration syndrome, pneumonia, pulmonary hypertension, and bronchopulmonary dysplasia.

5. Describe nonpulmonary causes of respiratory distress.

6. Identify treatment strategies for common respiratory problems.

7. Formulate a plan of care for infants with respiratory disorders.

The most common group of life-threatening diseases in newborns are respiratory in origin. This is evidenced by the number of infants admitted to the neonatal intensive care unit (NICU) in respiratory distress. Respiratory distress syndrome, retained lung fluid syndromes, aspiration syndromes, air leaks, and congenital pneumonia account for approximately 90% of all respiratory distress in newborns. Pulmonary disease, however, is not the cause of all respiratory distress in newborn infants. Congenital malformations, metabolic abnormalities, central nervous system disorders, and congenital heart disease may also present with respiratory distress.

This chapter discusses common respiratory problems of the newborn infant, along with pathophysiology, clinical presentation, differential diagnosis, and management. A thorough understanding of respiratory distress is essential for the NICU nurse.

Lung Development

A. **Anatomic events.** Five stages of lung development have been identified and are described as follows (Moore and Persaud, 1993):

1. Embryonic development (weeks 1–5). The endoderm-derived embryonic fore-gut provides a single lung bud that begins to divide; the pulmonary vein

develops and extends to join the lung bud. The trachea develops at the end of the embryonic period. There are three divisions on the right side and two on the left side. These will eventually become the lobes of the lungs.

2. Pseudoglandular period (weeks 5–17). All conducting airways are formed. Cartilage appears; main bronchi are formed; demarcation of major lobes occurs; formation of new bronchi are complete; capillary bed is formed with connecting bronchial blood supply; no connection made with terminal air sacs. The lung resembles an exocrine organ because of surrounding loose mesenchymal tissues, hence the name, pseudoglandular.

3. Canalicular period (weeks 17–24). Formation of gas exchanging acini units (i.e., respiratory units). The appearance of glycogen-rich, cuboidal cells; inclusions for surface-active material storage are seen; capillaries invade terminal airway walls; type II alveolar epithelial cells appear. Airway changes from glandular to tubular and increases in length and diameter. Vascular system proliferates and the capillaries are now closer to the airway epithelium conducting airways. Respiratory bronchioles that will participate in gas exchange can be differentiated. Between weeks 24–26 alveolar sacs are formed; air-blood surface area is limited for gas exchange; type II cells are unable to release surfactant in sufficient quantity to maintain air breathing.

4. Terminal sac period (weeks 24–37). Capillary loops increase; type II cells cluster at alveolar ducts, become numerous and mature; more budding occurs from alveolar ducts, lung size increases rapidly as there is an exponential increase in surface area for gas exchange.

5. Alveolar period (week 37 to 8–10 years). This phase is characterized by continued alveolar proliferation and development.

B. Biochemical events.

1. Surface-active phospholipids line terminal air spaces and maintain alveolar stability by reducing surface tension.
2. Surfactant is a mixture of at least six phospholipids and four apoproteins.
   a. Dipalmitoylphosphatidylcholine is the major surface-active lipid component of surfactant.
   b. Surfactant includes cholesterol and cholesterol esters, proteins, complex carbohydrates, and glycolipids.
   c. Phospholipids are responsible for the surface-active properties of surfactant. Surfactant proteins have recently been found to have important properties.
      (1) Surfactant protein A (SP-A) binds phospholipids, requires calcium ions, and, with surfactant protein B (SP-B), forms the tubular myelin lattice network. SP-A holds the corners of the lattice network together and probably has a role in the recycling of surfactant. SP-A activates alveolar macrophages and thus has a role in host defenses.
      (2) Surfactant protein B (SP-B) is important in the formation of tubular myelin, enhances the uptake of phospholipids by the type II cell, and is also important in the recycling of surfactant.
      (3) Surfactant protein C (SP-C) may have a role in surfactant dispersement and recycling.
      (4) Surfactant protein D (SP-D) is calcium dependent and also may have a role in host defense mechanisms (Whitsett, 1994).
   d. Surfactant reduces surface-tension forces in the alveoli that are capable of producing collapse at expiration (Whitsett, 1994).
      (1) Surfactant is produced in the type II pneumocyte beginning at 24–28 weeks' gestation and continuing to term (Shapiro, 1988). These cells synthesize, store, secrete, and recycle surfactant (Notter, 1988).
      (2) When the lungs are inflated, receptors in type II cells mobilize intracellular calcium, which causes the release of the contents of lamellar bodies

into the air space. After secretion, surfactant can be taken back into type II cells and converted back into lamellar bodies for resecretion, with a turnover time of 10 hours (Moise and Hansen; 1998).

3. The changing pattern of phospholipids in amniotic fluid can be used to assess surfactant production and maturation of pathways.
   a. Material from the fetal lung contributes to amniotic fluid.
   b. Concentrations of various phospholipids can be measured and will assist in determining lung maturity.
4. Sphingomyelin concentration remains stable, with a small peak at 28–30 weeks.
5. Lecithin and phosphatidylinositol concentrations remain low until 26–30 weeks, when an increase begins. A peak occurs at 36 weeks.
6. Phosphatidylglycerol (PG) appears at 30 weeks, peaks at 35–36 weeks, and increases as the phosophatidylinositol level falls.
   a. When PG is present, the risk that RDS will develop in the infant is less than 1%.
   b. PG is measured as absent or present.
   c. Blood and meconium do not affect test results.
7. The lecithin/sphingomyelin ratio (L/S) has been used to assess fetal lung maturity.
   a. An L/S ratio greater than 2:1 is considered to indicate fetal lung maturity.
   b. An infant of a diabetic mother may develop respiratory distress syndrome (RDS) even with a mature L/S ratio (presence of PG ensures lung maturity).
   c. Chronic fetal stress (e.g., maternal hypertension, retroplacental bleeding, maternal drug use, smoking) will tend to accelerate surfactant production, resulting in a mature L/S ratio in premature infants.
8. Fetal lung maturity (FLM).
   a. Measures ratio of surfactant to albumin.
   b. Sample should be free of blood and meconium.
   c. Less than 50 = immaturity; 50–70 = borderline maturity; greater than 70 = mature lungs.

C. **Role of antenatal steroids.**

1. Glucocorticoids (e.g., betamethasone or dexamethasone) affect lung maturation and present a strategy for preventing respiratory distress syndrome (RDS). Betamethasone appears to significantly decrease neonatal death and morbidity (↓ RDS, ↓ incidence of IVH) (NIH Consensus, 1995; Maher, 1994). Steroids accelerate the normal pattern of lung growth by increasing the rate of glycogen depletion and glycerophospholipid biosynthesis. This leads to thinning of the intraalveolar septa and increases the size of the alveoli. The number of surfactant producing type II pneumocytes increases as well as the number of lamellar bodies inside the cells. This leads to increased synthesis of surfactant phospholipids (Blackburn and Loper, 1992). Steroids may also increase the amount of fibroblast pneumocyte factor which affects surfactant production (Blackburn and Loper, 1992).
   a. Treatment with steroids is recommended for:
      (1) Maternal risk of preterm delivery between 24 and 34 weeks.
      (2) Premature rupture of the membranes at less than 30–32 weeks, without chorioamnionitis, because of the risk of IVH.
      (3) Treatment with corticosteroids less than 24 hours prior to delivery is still associated with a decrease in mortality, RDS and IVH. Should be given unless immediate delivery expected.
      (4) Complicated pregnancies where expected delivery is at less than 34 weeks' gestation—unless adverse effect on mother is anticipated (Moise and Hansen, 1998).

   b. Repeated administration of corticosteroids in premature rupture of the membranes is not associated with a higher risk of chorioamnionitis (Ghidini et al., 1997).

   c. When infants receive antenatal steroids and surfactant, an additive effect is observed (Kattwinkel, 1998).

   d. Glucocorticoids are given concurrently with tocolytic agents (e.g., terbutaline, ritodrine, magnesium sulfate) for premature labor.

   e. Betamethsone or dexamethasone is given IV in a 12 mg dose repeated at 12 or 24 hours. The treatment course is repeated weekly until 34 weeks' gestation (Gorrie, McKinney, and Murray, 1994).

2. Thyrotropin-releasing hormone has no additive effect with steroids in reducing RDS or improving outcome for preterm infants. Recent studies recommend antenatal treatment with corticosteroids alone (Ballard et al., 1998; Collaborative Santiago Surfactant Group, 1998).

3. Infants exposed to chronic stress in utero are usually small for gestational age and have more mature lungs (they also have small thymuses and large adrenal glands, suggesting high glucocorticoid levels in utero).

Physiology of Respiration

Refer to Chapters 3 and 9.

Respiratory Disorders

RESPIRATORY DISTRESS SYNDROME/HYALINE MEMBRANE DISEASE

A. Definition.

1. Developmental disorder starting at or soon after birth and occurring most frequently in infants with immature lungs.
2. Increasing respiratory difficulty in first 3–6 hours, leading to hypoxia and hypoventilation.
3. Progressive atelectasis.

B. Incidence (Moise and Hansen, 1998).

1. Approximately 40,000 infants per year affected in the United States.
2. Inversely related to gestational age; 60–80% of infants born at less than 28 weeks are affected.

C. Etiology.

1. Surfactant deficiency.
2. Pulmonary hypoperfusion.
3. Anatomic immaturity.
4. Precipitating factors associated with incidence and/or severity of RDS.
   a. Prematurity.
   b. Cesarean delivery without labor.
   c. Maternal diabetes, especially if infant was born at less than 38 weeks' gestation.
   d. Acute antepartum hemorrhage.
   e. Second twin.
     (1) May be due to greater risk of asphyxia.
     (2) First twin usually smaller, suggesting chronic stress leading to early lung maturation.

      f. Asphyxia at birth.

      g. Male/female ratio of 2:1.

  5. Unlikely factors for RDS development.

      a. Term birth.

      b. Intrauterine growth restriction.

      c. Prolonged rupture of membranes.

      d. Chronic fetal stress.

         (1) Gradual placental insufficiency.

         (2) Pregnancy-induced hypertension.

         (3) Smoking.

         (4) Subacute placental abruption.

         (5) Maternal narcotic addiction.

         (6) Maternal chronic hypertension.

         (7) Prenatal corticosteroids.

D. **Pathophysiology.**

1. Production of surfactant is inadequate, resulting when the utilization of surfactant exceeds the rate of production. This leads to diffuse alveolar atelectasis, edema, and cell injury.
2. Serum proteins, which inhibit surfactant function, leak into the alveoli. The increased water content, immature mechanisms for clearance of lung liquid, lack of alveolar-capillary apposition, and low surface area for gas exchange, typical of the immature lung, also contribute to the disease (Liley and Stark, 1998).

E. **Clinical presentation.**

  1. Almost exclusively in premature infants:

      a. Will appear to be a normally grown, healthy premature infant with good Apgar scores at birth.

      b. Distress begins at or soon after birth.

  2. Increasing respiratory difficulty related to progressive atelectasis. Symptoms are progressive.

      a. Tachypnea (>60 breaths per minute) is usually the first sign; color is maintained.

      b. Audible expiratory grunt.

         (1) Heard during first few hours.

         (2) Caused by forcing of air past a partially closed glottis.

         (3) Used to maintain positive end-expiratory pressure (PEEP) at alveolar level in an attempt to prevent alveolar collapse.

         (4) More pronounced with severe disease.

      c. Intercostal and sternal retractions, seen as ventilatory effort increases. Retractions are a visible sign of chest wall inward collapse during forceful diaphragmatic contractions. A lower portion of fatigue-resistant type I fibers (20% vs 60% in an adult) in the diaphragm and intercostal muscles can quickly lead to fatigue and eventual apnea (Loper, 1997).

      d. Nasal flaring.

      e. Cyanosis due to increasing hypoxemia.

  3. Oxygen requirements increase to maintain arterial PO_2 at 50–70 mm Hg due to decreased lung compliance secondary to decreased surfactant with more physical effort needed to keep terminal airways open resulting in increased work of breathing.

  4. Paradoxical seesaw respirations are seen.

  5. If signs and symptoms are unattended, infant becomes obtunded and flaccid.

      a. Pale gray color obscures severe central cyanosis.

      b. Poor capillary filling time (3–4 seconds).

      c. Progressive edema, usually seen in the face, palms, and soles.

  6. Oliguria is common in the first 48 hours.

7. Breath sounds diminish and lung auscultation is usually described as "poor air entry" despite vigorous effort on the infant's part.
8. Rales occur as the disease progresses.
9. Cardiac murmurs are generally not heard until after 24 hours of age.
10. Tachycardia (heart rate 150–160 bpm) is common and even more prevalent if acidosis and hypoxemia are present.

F. Diagnosis.

1. Signs and symptoms as previously described.
2. Hypoxemia (defined as arterial PO_2 level <50 mm Hg in room air) as a result of right-to-left shunting, responding to supplemental inspired oxygen; respiratory failure secondary to alveolar hypoventilation (PCO_2 >50; pH ≤7.25).
3. Chest x-ray reveals low lung volumes and hazy lung fields with a fine reticulogranular pattern of density with air bronchograms (Wood, 1993).
4. Diagnostic studies.
   a. Chest x-ray examination.
   b. Arterial blood gas (ABG) measurements.
   c. Blood cultures, complete blood cell count. Pneumonia caused by group B streptococcus has similar radiographic features; therefore infection must be considered.
   d. Other blood studies as needed (e.g., electrolytes, calcium and blood glucose levels).

G. Differential diagnosis.

1. Pneumonia. Similar signs, symptoms and radiologic features can be found in neonates with pneumonia and those with RDS.
2. Transient tachypnea of the newborn. TTN can present with the same signs and symptoms but these infants usually require less oxygen, improve quicker and have larger lung volumes on CXR.
3. Pulmonary edema. A primary cardiac disorder with pulmonary edema (caused by patent ductus arteriosus) can mimic RDS.

H. Complications.

1. Pulmonary.
   a. Air leaks.
   b. Pulmonary edema.
   c. Bronchopulmonary dysplasia (BPD).
2. Cardiovascular.
   a. Patent dutus arteriosus.
   b. Systemic hypotension.
3. Renal: oliguria.
   a. Most likely to follow hypoxia, hypotension, or shock ("prerenal" renal failure).
   b. Immature renal function with decreased glomerular filtration in very low birth weight infants.
   c. Natural diuresis will occur at approximately 48–72 hours of age.
4. Metabolic.
   a. Acidosis. Atelectasis with increased work of breathing will lead to hypoxemia and acidemia, which cause vasoconstriction of the pulmonary vasculature. This then limits alveolar capillary blood flow, which further impedes the production of surfactant and compounds the problem (Hagedorn, Gardner, and Abman, 1998).
   b. Hyponatremia or hypernatremia.
   c. Hypocalcemia.
   d. Hypoglycemia.

5. Hematologic.
   a. Anemia—may be iatrogenic due to lab sampling. Hematocrit should be near normal to ensure adequate oxygen carrying capacity.
   b. Disseminated intravascular coagulation. Resulting from infection and/or acidosis. If prolonged bleeding is observed, coagulopathy screen should be obtained.
6. Neurologic
   a. Seizures: may result from an intraventricular hemorrhage (IVH).
   b. Ventilator manipulations, rapid fluid infusions, shock, and acidosis are all factors causing changes in cerebral blood flow and can precipitate a bleed (Minarick and Beachy, 1993).
7. Other.
   a. Secondary nosocomial infections.
   b. Retinopathy of prematurity (ROP).
   c. Displaced endotracheal tubes.
   d. Thrombus formation. Complication of umbilical catheters needed to monitor respiratory status.

I. Management. RDS is a disease that is self-limited and transient. Adequate surfactant can be produced by the premature infant within 48–72 hours.
1. Goal of treatment is supportive until disease resolves and to prevent further lung injury (Moise and Hansen, 1998).
2. Surfactant replacement therapy in multiple controlled trials have shown that treatment with surfactant reduces the morbidity and mortality rates for RDS (Moise and Hansen, 1998; Kattwinkel, 1998). Benefits include:
   a. Improvement in compliance and decreased resistance in surfactant-poor acini, thereby reducing the pressure needed to inflate the lungs and decreased work of breathing.
   b. Improved ventilation in low-volume lung units, which increases the PaO_2, decreases the right-to-left intrapulmonary shunt, and improves overall oxygenation of the infant.
   c. Surfactants approved by U.S. Food and Drug Administration for treatment of RDS:
      (1) Natural surfactants: Survanta, Curosurf, Surfacten, and Alveofact. Composed of minced bovine or porcine lung with added lipids.
      (2) Synthetic surfactants: Exosurf Neonatal and ALEC (artificial lung-expanding compound).
   d. Treatment methods.
      (1) Prophylaxis. Treatment soon after birth: infants born at less than 30 weeks' gestation; dose given via endotracheal tube after initial resuscitation. Additional doses may be given if necessary.
      (2) Rescue. Treatment of infants with established RDS; multiple doses can be given. Studies have shown that surfactant response is improved when it is given early (Kendig et al., 1991; Egberts et al., 1993; Kattwinkel et al., 1993).
3. Provide warm, humidified oxygen to maintain normal PaO_2.
4. Provide continuous positive airway pressure via nasal prongs or endotracheal tube if helpful.
5. Use assisted ventilation for profound hypoxemia (PaO_2 <50 mm Hg) and/or hypercapnia ($PaCO_2$ >60 mm Hg).
6. Provide chest physiotherapy.
7. Perform pulse oximetry and/or transcutaneous monitoring.
8. Verify diagnosis by chest x-ray examination.
9. Other measures.
   a. Stabilize temperature.
   b. Provide adequate fluid and electrolyte intake.

    c. Restore acid-base balance by administration of sodium bicarbonate ($NaHCO_3$) for metabolic acidosis.

    d. Sample and monitor arterial blood gases, electrolytes, calcium, bilirubin, and glucose.

    e. Monitor blood pressure for hypotension. Give volume replacement and pharmacotherapeutic agents (e.g., dopamine or dobutamine) as indicated.

    f. Maintain hematocrit.

    g. Administer antibiotics for associated pneumonia.

    h. Observe infant for complications.

J. **Prevention of RDS.**

1. Maternal glucocorticoid administration prenatally.
2. Use of L/S ratio, fetal lung maturity, and phosphatidylglycerol (PG) determination for timing labor induction or elective cesarean delivery.
3. Obstetric and pediatric management to avoid situations leading to pulmonary circulation compromise in the fetus or newborn infant.
   a. Maternal hypotension.
   b. Oversedation.
   c. Maternal hypoxia.
   d. Fetal distress without prompt delivery.
   e. Delayed resuscitation.
   f. Uncorrected hypoxia or acidosis.
   g. Hypothermia.
   h. Hypovolemia.

K. **Outcome.**

1. Morbidity is related to complications of prematurity.
2. Infants with chronic lung disease improve slowly and progressively if they can be kept infection free. May have episodes of bronchiolitis and pneumonia (especially pneumonia caused by respiratory syncytial virus [RSV]); long-term sequelae are related to specific complications (e.g., BPD, IVH, retinopathy of prematurity [ROP]).
3. Babies who weigh greater than 1500 g who have mild to moderate RDS have the same developmental outcome as babies of the same gestational age without RDS. The infants with the most severe developmental outcomes are those who weigh less than 1500 g and have had an IVH (Hagedorn et al., 1998). Very low birth weight infants have a definite increased risk for school dysfunction (Bennett and Scott, 1997).
4. Cerebral Palsy (CP)—the most prevalent major impairment encountered in premature infants. 40% of all children with CP were born prematurely (Bennett and Scott, 1997). The sickest infants with RDS have a 10–20% chance of major neurologic deficit: CP, hydrocephalus, seizures, and mental retardation diagnosed within the first 2 years of life (Hagedorn et al., 1998).
5. Prognosis for normal development is better in infants with fewer complications.
6. Birth weight relationship exists (lower birth weight is related to greater morbidity).

PNEUMONIA

A. **Definition.** Infection of the fetal or newborn lung; may be intrauterine or neonatal.

1. Intrauterine infection.
   a. Passage of infecting agent by infection of fetal membranes.
   b. Transplacental transmission.
   c. Aspiration of meconium or infected amniotic fluid during delivery.

2. Neonatal infection.
   a. Acquired during nursery stay.
   b. Pathogens are generally different from those acquired in utero.
   c. Results by passage from other infants, equipment, or caretakers.

B. **Incidence.**

1. Varies from center to center and according to causative agent.
2. Bacterial pneumonia incidence is comparable with that of sepsis.
3. The most common neonatal infection; accounts for significant morbidity and mortality.

C. **Etiology.**

1. Risk of infection greatest in premature infants because of immature immune system and lack of protective maternal antibodies (IgG crosses the placenta in the third trimester of pregnancy). Premature infants have decreased levels, absence of secretory IgG, decreased numbers of leukocytes and marrow stem cells, and diminished chemotactic ability.
2. Immature ciliary system in the tracheobronchial tree, leading to suboptimal removal of inflammatory debris, mucus, and pathogens. The number of pulmonary macrophages are insufficient for bacterial clearance (Orlando, 1997).
3. Multiple agents cause neonatal pneumonia (Table 7–1).

D. **Pathophysiology.**

1. Congenital pneumonia.
   a. Infant may be born critically ill or stillborn to mother who has a history of chorioamnionitis. Evidence of pulmonary inflammation is found in 15–38% of stillborn infants at autopsy (Speer and Weisman, 1998). Other factors linked to congenital pneumonia include excessive obstetric manipulation, prolonged labor with intact membranes, and maternal urinary tract infection (Orlando, 1997).

Table 7–1
COMMON ORGANISMS ASSOCIATED WITH NEONATAL PNEUMONIA

TRANSPLACENTAL	AMNIOTIC FLUID
• Rubella	• Cytomegalovirus
• Cytomegalovirus	• Herpes simplex virus
• Herpes simplex virus	• Enteroviruses
• Adenovirus	• Genital mycoplasma
• Mumps virus	• *L. monocytogenes*
• *Toxoplasma gondii*	• *Chlamydia trachomatis*
• *Listeria monocytogenes*	• *M. tuberculosis*
• *Mycobacterium tuberculosis*	• Group B streptococcus (GBS)
• *Treponema pallidum*	• *Escherichia coli*
	• *Haemophilus influenzae* (nontypeable)
AT DELIVERY	**NOSOCOMIAL**
• GBS	• *S. aureus*
• *E. coli*	• *Staphylococcus epidermidis*
• *Staphylococcus aureus*	• GBS
• *Klebsiella* sp.	• *Klebsiella* sp.
• Other streptococci	• *Enterobacter*
• *H. influenzae* (nontypeable)	• *Pseudomonas*
• *Candida* sp.	• Influenza viruses
• *C. trachomatis*	• Respiratory syncytial virus
	• Enteroviruses

From Hansen, T.N., Cooper, T.R., and Weisman, L.E. (Eds.): *Contemporary Diagnosis and Management of Neonatal Respiratory Diseases*, 2nd ed. Newton, Pa., Handbooks in Health Care (division of AMM Co.), 1998, p. 131.

b. Prolonged rupture of membranes (>24 hours); ascending organisms infecting amniotic fluid. If mother is in active labor, contamination occurs more rapidly.

c. Infective organisms may cross the placenta and enter the fetal circulation and cause pneumonia.

d. Infants usually show signs of generalized illness from birth, but signs of illness may be delayed hours to days if the infective fluid is aspirated during delivery.

2. Neonatal pneumonia.

a. Infection occurs days to weeks after birth.

b. Pathogenic organism is acquired from hospital personnel, parents, or other infected infants. Poor hand washing, contaminated blood products, infected human milk, and open skin lesions are common ways of transmitting infection to the neonate (Orlando, 1997).

c. Usual pathogens are coagulase-positive staphylococci, group A streptococci, *Escherichia coli*, and *Staphylococcus epidermidis*.

d. A secondary infection can present as a result of a primary disease, such as infection of the cord stump and circumcision wounds.

E. **Clinical presentation.**

1. Labor >24 hours.

a. Prolonged rupture of membranes (>24 hours).

b. Maternal fever/chorioamnionitis.

c. Foul-smelling or purulent amniotic fluid.

d. Fetal tachycardia.

e. Loss of heart rate pattern variability.

2. Signs and symptoms.

a. Often indistinguishable from those of other forms of respiratory distress and sepsis.

b. Tachypnea, grunting, retractions, cyanosis, hypoxemia, and hypercapnia.

c. With severe involvement, shocklike syndrome, usually in the first 24 hours of life, with recurrent apnea followed by cardiovascular collapse, profound hypoxemia, and persistent pulmonary hypertension. These signs represent a poor prognosis.

3. Physical examination.

a. Physical signs are variable.

b. Diminished breath sounds may be present over one or more areas.

c. In addition, localized dullness, harshness, or rales may be audible.

d. Radiologic findings can mimic those seen with RDS. In addition, pleural effusions can be seen on CXR with GBS pneumonia.

F. **Diagnostic evaluation.**

1. History of any previously mentioned contributing factors is suggestive.

2. Infant may require resuscitation in the delivery room.

3. Chest x-ray findings are variable:

a. Unilateral or bilateral alveolar infiltrates.

b. Diffuse interstitial pattern.

c. Pleural effusions.

4. Samples for blood and viral cultures (including RSV) should be obtained, although results are rarely positive unless there is generalized bacterial sepsis.

5. A complete blood cell count may show neutropenia/leukopenia or may have an abnormal ratio of immature to total neutrophils.

6. Urine collection for latex particle agglutination (LPA) and counterimmuno-electrophoresis (CIE) to detect group B streptococci may be helpful because the results can be obtained faster than culture results.

7. Polymerase chain reaction (PCR) can be used to detect herpesviruses.

8. ABG values should be obtained because metabolic acidosis may be severe.
9. Tracheal aspirate culture should be considered, especially if the infant has an endotracheal tube in place.
10. Cerebrospinal cultures should be grown because meningitis often accompanies pneumonia.

G. Differential diagnosis.

1. RDS.
2. Sepsis.
3. TTN.
4. Meconium aspiration.
5. Lung hypoplasia.
6. Pulmonary hemorrhage.
7. Congenital heart disease.

H. Complications.

1. Meningitis.
2. Gram-negative pneumonia; cardiopulmonary complications similar to those of RDS.
3. Septic shock.
4. Disseminated intravascular coagulation (DIC).
5. Persistent pulmonary hypertension.

I. Management.

1. Antibiotic therapy (see Chapter 17).
2. Maintain normal temperature.
3. Monitor blood pressure and treat hypotension.
4. Oxygen or assisted ventilation to maintain normal ABG concentrations.
5. Correct metabolic acidosis.
6. Provide adequate fluid and electrolyte intake.
7. Monitor for evidence of disseminated intravascular coagulation.
8. Monitor glucose levels.
9. Exchange transfusion, granulocyte transfusion, intravenous immunoglobulin, and granulocyte-monocyte colony-stimulating factors have all been used when conventional treatment has failed.
10. High-frequency oscillatory ventilation and extracorporeal membrane oxygenation have been used for patients who are critically ill with pneumonia, with variable outcomes.
11. Provide support for the family.

RETAINED LUNG FLUID SYNDROMES

A. Definition—delayed clearance of the fetal lung fluid. Referred to as transient tachypnea of the newborn (TTN). Also referred to as Retained Fetal Lung Fluid (RFLF), RDS Type II, "Wet lung."

B. Clinical presentation.

1. Common illness of term and near-term infants.
2. In first few hours, tachypnea results in respiratory rates of 60–120 breaths per minute; grunting and retractions may also be present.
3. Minimal cyanosis may require fractional inspired oxygen of 0.30–0.40; ABGs can show mild respiratory alkalemia, with PCO_2 values often less than 30 mm Hg.
4. Duration may be 1–5 days.

C. **Etiology.**

1. Delay in removal of lung fluid.
2. Excessive amount of lung fluid.

D. **Pathophysiology.**

1. Fetal lung fluid has a higher chloride concentration than plasma, interstitial fluid, or amniotic fluid. During labor, active transport of chloride stops and the fluid is reabsorbed via a protein gradient and removed by the lymphatic system. Two thirds of the lung fluid is removed before birth. Infants born without labor or prematurely do not have the time to reabsorb the fetal lung fluid (Speer and Hansen, 1998). Infants at highest risk for retained fetal lung fluid include:
   a. Birth near or at term.
   b. Cesarean delivery without labor.
   c. Breech delivery.
   d. Second twin.
   e. Small size.
   f. Precipitous delivery.
   g. Delayed cord clamping (results in a transfusion of blood, which may transiently elevate the central venous pressure).
   h. Macrosomia.
   i. Male sex.
   j. Maternal sedation.
   k. Prolonged labor.
2. Delayed clearance of lung fluid by pulmonary lymphatic system. The retained fetal lung fluid accumulates in the peribronchiolar lymphatics and bronchovascular spaces and interferes with forces promoting bronchiolar patency, and results in bronchiolar collapse with air trapping or hyperinflation. Hypoxemia results from continued perfusion of poorly ventilated alveoli and hypercarbia results from mechanical interference with alveolar ventilation. Decreased lung compliance results in tachypnea and increased work of breathing (Lawson, 1998).
3. Aspiration of oropharyngeal secretions may occur.
   a. Amniotic fluid.
   b. Tracheal fluid.
4. Promotion of interstitial fluid results in:
   a. Hypoalbuminemia.
   b. Increased interstitial oncotic pressure.

E. **Diagnosis.**

1. Early signs and symptoms may be difficult to distinguish from those of other respiratory problems; however, they are usually milder.
2. Chest x-ray examination reveals diffuse haziness and streakiness in both lung fields, with clearing at the periphery. Fluid may be present in the interlobar fissures, and mild hyperinflation may be present.
3. Diagnosis is frequently one of exclusion.

F. **Differential diagnosis.**

1. RDS.
2. Pneumonia.
3. Polycythemia (high hematocrit syndrome).
4. Congestive heart failure.
5. Asphyxia.
6. Cold stress (pulmonary vasoconstriction).

G. **Management.**

1. Because diagnosis is not conclusive, other disorders should be ruled out.
2. Supportive management.
   a. Oxygen.
   b. Temperature regulation.
   c. Adequate fluid intake.
   d. Maintain ABGs within normal levels.
   e. Maintain blood glucose at normal levels.
3. If respiratory rate is greater than 60 breaths per minute, delay feedings to avoid possible aspiration.
4. If anything in history indicates risk of infection, broad-spectrum antibiotics (e.g., ampicillin and gentamicin) should be administered until culture results are negative.

H. **Outcome.**

1. These syndromes are self-limited.
2. Oxygen requirement and tachypnea decrease steadily over several days. Infant may remain mildly tachypneic beyond the need for oxygen.
3. Some infants with TTN have high pulmonary artery pressures documented by echocardiography. If hypoxemia and tachypnea persist, a further complication may be persistent pulmonary hypertension of the newborn.

PERSISTENT PULMONARY HYPERTENSION OF THE NEWBORN

A. **Definition.** Persistent pulmonary hypertension of the newborn infant (PPHN) is caused by right-to-left shunting through the fetal shunts at the atrial and ductal levels. It is secondary to persistent elevation of pulmonary vascular resistance (PVR) and pulmonary artery pressure (Harris and Wood, 1996).

B. **Pathophysiology.**

1. After delivery, adequate oxygenation depends on lung inflation, closure of fetal shunts, decreased PVR, and increased pulmonary blood flow.
2. Over the first 12–24 hours of life, PVR falls by 80% of its total decline.
3. When PVR remains high, adaptation from fetal to neonatal circulation is impaired.
4. Neonatal pulmonary vessels have greater vasoactive properties than adult pulmonary vessels and respond to hypoxia and acidosis with vasoconstriction. Numerous factors increase and decrease PVR (Table 7–2).
5. Development of increased vascular smooth muscle contributes to vasospasm. Development of pulmonary artery musculature occurs late in gestation, making PPHN generally a condition of the term and postterm infant.
6. High PVR and pulmonary hypertension impede pulmonary blood flow, which leads to hypoxemia, acidemia, and lactic acidosis.
7. Once vasoconstriction is induced, it can persist even when the precipitating cause is removed (Kinsella and Abman, 1995; Morin and Stenmark, 1995; Steinhorn, Millard, and Morin, 1995).

C. **Etiology (Van Marter, 1998; Weardon and Hansen, 1998).**

1. Maladaptation. The pulmonary vascular bed is structurally normal, but PVR remains high. Maladaptation generally results from active vasoconstriction, which may be transient or persistent.
   a. Hypoxia/asphyxia. This is most commonly associated diagnosis in PPHN. It causes remodeling and abnormal muscularization of small pulmonary arteries. Acute asphyxia may induce persistent pulmonary vasospasm.
   b. Pulmonary parenchymal disease (RDS, meconium aspiration, pneumonia,

Table 7–2
FACTORS THAT MODULATE PULMONARY VASCULAR RESISTANCE IN THE NEAR-TERM AND TERM TRANSITIONAL AND NEONATAL PULMONARY CIRCULATION

Lowers PVR	Increases PVR
Endogenous mediators and mechanisms	Endogenous mediators and mechanisms
Oxygen	Hypoxia
Nitric oxide	Acidosis
PGI_2, E_2, D_2	Endothelin-1
Adenosine, ATP, magnesium	Leukotrienes
Bradykinin	Thromboxanes
Atrial natriuretic factor	Platelet activating factor
Alkalosis	Ca^{2+} channel activation
K^+ channel activation	α-Adrenergic stimulation
Histamine	$PGF_{2\alpha}$
Vagal nerve stimulation	Mechanical factors
Acetylcholine	Overinflation or underinflation
β-Adrenergic stimulation	Excessive muscularization, vascular remodeling
Mechanical factors	Altered mechanical properties of smooth muscle
Lung inflation	Pulmonary hypoplasia
Vascular cell structural changes	Alveolar capillary dysplasia
Interstitial fluid and pressure changes	Pulmonary thromboemboli
Shear stress	Main pulmonary artery distension
	Ventricular dysfunction, venous hypertension

PVR, Pulmonary vascular resistance; *PGI$_2$, E$_2$, D$_2$*, prostaglandins I$_2$, E$_2$, and D$_2$; *ATP*, adenosine triphosphate; *PGF$_{2\alpha}$*, prostaglandin F$_{2\alpha}$.
From Kinsella, J.P., and Abman, S.H.: *J. Pediatr, 126*:853–864, 1995.

other aspiration syndromes) can cause pulmonary vasospasm and may be associated with vascular remodeling.

  c. Bacterial sepsis. The underlying mechanism may be endotoxin-mediated myocardial depression or pulmonary vasospasm associated with high levels of thromboxanes and leukotrienes.

  d. Prenatal pulmonary hypertension.
    (1) Fetal systemic hypertension.
    (2) Premature closure of ductus arteriosus (seen with maternal use of aspirin, prostaglandin inhibitors, phentoyin (Dilantin), lithium, or indomethacin taken in significant amounts).

  e. Any condition preventing normal circulatory transition at delivery (CNS depression, delayed resuscitation, hypothermia).

  f. Hypothermia; hypoglycemia leading to acidosis, which will potentiate vasoconstriction.

  g. Hyperviscosity/polycythemia. This may lead to a functional obstruction of the pulmonary vascular bed.

2. Maldevelopment: abnormal pulmonary vessels. Musculature is hypertrophied and extends into normally nonmuscularized arteries. This excessive muscularization impacts lumen size, which increases vascular resistance. Causes of maldevelopment include:

  a. Intrauterine asphyxia. Increases systemic arterial blood pressure in the fetus and diverts more blood to the lung, resulting in pulmonary vessel development.

  b. Intrauterine aspiration of meconium. Contributes to intrauterine hypoxia.

  c. Fetal ductal closure. Forces cardiac output from the right ventricle through the lungs, resulting in maldevelopment.

  d. Congenital heart disease. Abnormal pulmonary vessels resulting from various defects.

3. Underdevelopment: decreased number of pulmonary vessels. Blood is shunted because there are too few vessels for blood to flow through the lungs, with

decreased cross-sectional area for gas exchange to occur. Severity depends on the timing of the interruption of lung development in utero: reduced numbers of bronchial generations if early (<16 weeks) and decreased number of alveoli if later in gestation. Contributing conditions include:
a. Pulmonary hypoplasia (i.e., Potter's sequence).
b. Space-occupying lesions or lung masses (e.g., diaphragmatic hernia, lung cysts), which prevent normal development of lung tissue and the capillary bed.
c. Congenital heart disease. Pulmonary atresia or tricuspid atresia may lead to decreased blood flow and vascular underdevelopment.

D. Clinical presentation.

1. Near-term, term, or postterm infants.
2. History of hypoxia or asphyxia at birth.
   a. Low Apgar scores.
   b. Infant usually slow to breath or difficult to ventilate.
   c. Meconium-stained fluid, nuchal cord, abruptio placentae or any acute blood loss, and maternal sedation.
3. Respiratory abnormalities.
   a. Symptoms seen before 12 hours of age.
   b. Tachypnea/TTN.
   c. Retractions if airway is obstructed (e.g., because of aspiration).
   d. Cyanosis out of proportion to degree of distress (may not see cyanosis with PaO_2 <50 mm Hg); cyanosis of sudden onset that often is intractable.
   e. Low PaO_2 despite high oxygen concentration administration because of right-to-left shunting.
   f. Chest x-ray can be normal unless aspiration or pneumonia present (will see infiltrates in these cases).
4. Cardiovascular abnormalities.
   a. Blood pressure is usually lower than normal.
   b. Electrocardiogram will show a right axis deviation.
   c. Systolic murmur is heard frequently, usually from a patent ductus arteriosus, foramen ovale, or tricuspid insufficiency. Single loud second heart sound (S_2), resulting from high pulmonary pressures, may be heard.
   d. Echocardiogram shows dilated right side of the heart and evidence of pulmonary hypertension.
   e. Congestive heart failure has been reported occasionally.
5. Metabolic abnormalities.
   a. Hypoglycemia.
   b. Hypocalcemia.
   c. Metabolic acidosis.
   d. Decreased urine output or coagulopathy caused by kidney and liver damage from asphyxia may occur.

E. Diagnosis.

1. It is important to diagnose PPHN but particularly to identify the cause because it may affect treatment.
2. PPHN will be suspected on the basis of history and clinical course.
3. Shunt study. Because of the right-to-left shunting at the level of the ductus arteriosus, there will be a preductal and a postductal PaO_2 difference. Difference in PaO_2 of 10 mm Hg or greater documents ductal shunting.
4. Hyperoxia test. A right-to-left shunt is demonstrated if PO_2 does not increase in 100% oxygen. Cause may be either PPHN or congenital heart disease.
5. Hyperoxia/hyperventilation test. Hyperventilate to pH 7.5–7.55 with $PaCO_2$ less than 25 mm Hg. In PPHN the PaO_2 will increase; in congenital heart disease, the PaO_2 will not increase.

6. An echocardiogram will rule out structural heart disease, evaluate myocardial function, and diagnose right-to-left shunting at the level of the patent ductus arteriosus or foramen ovale.
7. Chest x-ray may or may not be helpful, but should be taken to rule out other lung pathology.
8. Electrolytes, calcium and glucose levels, and complete blood cell count should be checked.

F. **Differential diagnosis.**

1. Congenital heart disease.
2. Pulmonary disease.
   a. Severe disease may mimic PPHN.
   b. Disease may coexist with PPHN.

G. **Complications.**

1. Pulmonary.
   a. Air leaks. Related to high mean airway pressures used in ventilator management.
   b. Bronchopulmonary dysplasia (BPD).
2. Cardiovascular.
   a. Systemic hypotension.
   b. Congestive heart failure.
3. Renal.
   a. Decreased urine output related to asphxia and hypotension.
   b. Kidney damage caused by asphyxia or acute tubular necrosis.
   c. Hematuria.
4. Metabolic.
   a. Hypoglycemia.
   b. Metabolic acidosis.
5. Hematologic.
   a. Thrombocytopenia.
   b. Disseminated intravascular coagulation: depends on precipitating cause of PPHN.
   c. Hemorrhage (e.g., gastrointestinal, pulmonary).
6. Neurologic.
   a. CNS irritability.
   b. Seizures.
7. Iatrogenic.
   a. Thrombus formation or complications of invasive monitoring equipment.
   b. Displaced endotracheal tubes.
8. Other.
   a. Edema.
   b. Abdominal distention.
   c. Side effects of pharmacologic agents used for treatment.

H. **Management.**

1. Main goal is to correct hypoxia and acidosis (major contributing factors) and promote pulmonary vascular dilation, as well as support extrapulmonary systems.
2. Management will depend on the cause of PPHN.
3. Supportive care.
   a. Monitor vital signs.
   b. Temperature stabilization.
   c. Adequate IV fluid infusion.
   d. Monitor electrolytes, glucose, calcium, complete blood cell count, ABGs.
   e. Correction of metabolic abnormalities.

      f. Blood cultures and antibiotics.

      g. Close observation and correction of any complications.

   4. Specialized monitoring.

      a. Umbilical catheters.

        (1) Arterial: blood gas access, arterial pressure monitoring.

        (2) Venous: central pressure monitoring, infusion of vasopressors.

      b. Right radial arterial line.

      c. Transcutaneous monitoring. Preductal and postductal applications can be helpful.

      d. Pulse oximetry. Evaluate oxygen saturation; applications can be preductal and postductal.

   5. Oxygen. Most potent pulmonary vasodilator.

   6. Ventilation.

      a. Conventional mechanical ventilation (CMV).

      b. High-frequency ventilation (HFV); high-frequency oscillatory ventilation (HFOV). Used when CMV fails or when excessive barotrauma is a concern.

      c. Alkalinization for treatment of PPHN (used by many centers). Maintain pH between 7.45 and 7.55; if hyperventilation alone does not accomplish this goal, use of buffers may be needed (e.g., sodium bicarbonate, tromethamine).

        (1) Hyperoxygenation.

          (a) Goal is to keep PaO_2 at greater than 90 mm Hg.

          (b) Danger of retinopathy of prematurity is minimal because most infants are born at or near term.

        (2) Hyperventilation.

          (a) $PaCO_2$ values are at 20–25 mm Hg.

          (b) An aid in reducing acidosis and pulmonary artery pressure caused by the vasodilatory effect of alkalosis.

      d. Inhaled nitric oxide (iNO).

        (1) iNO is a selective pulmonary vasodilator.

          (a) Potent and short acting, with half-life of 3–5 seconds.

          (b) Combines with hemoglobin and becomes inactivated.

          (c) Inactivation results in formation of methemoglobin; levels need to be monitored during treatment.

        (2) Exact dosage has not been determined. Current evidence supports using starting doses of 20 ppm in term newborn infants with PPHN (Kinsella and Abman, 1995 and 1998).

        (3) iNO withdrawal (weaning) needs to be systematic; abrupt discontinuation may be secondary to reported rebound increased PVR. (Kinsella and Abman, 1998).

        (4) Infants with severe parenchymal lung disease/underinflation and PPHN respond better to iNO when it is combined with HFOV.

        (5) iNO treatment of PPHN is still experimental but nearing approval by U.S. Food and Drug Administration.

      e. Surfactant replacement: especially if etiology based on significant parenchymal disease (Kahurinerel, 1998, Kattwinkel, 1998).

      f. Extracorporeal membrane oxygenation (ECMO) may be used when all conventional therapies are unsuccessful.

   7. Minimal stimulation and handling.

      a. Infants will show marked fluctuation (generally decreases) in their PaO_2 if handled or manipulated.

      b. The pulmonary arteries are very reactive to changes in PaO_2; therefore any action that causes a decrease in PaO_2 (e.g., suctioning, blood sampling, vital signs, ventilator changes) will cause further vasoconstriction.

      c. Suction only as needed to maintain a patent airway.

    d. Sedatives and analgesics are used for procedures and treatments.

    e. The bedside nurse must be a strong advocate for these patients and keep noise and environmental stimuli to a minimum.

8. Pharmacologic support.

    a. Muscle relaxants.

      (1) Used when infant's own respirations interfere with assisted ventilation.

      (2) Paralysis prevents resisting the ventilator, reduces pulmonary vascular resistance, and reduces the risk of air leaks and BPD.

      (3) Pancuronium bromide (Pavulon). Dosage: 0.04–0.15 mg/kg every 1–2 hours, or as needed for paralysis (Young and Mangum, 1998).

      (4) Vecuronium. Dosage: 0.1 mg/kg IV every 1–2 hours or as needed (Young and Mangum, 1998).

    b. Vasopressors.

      (1) Goal is to keep the systemic pressure above pulmonary pressure to decrease right-to-left shunting.

      (2) Dopamine is the drug of choice. Dopamine is an endogenous catecholamine, and effect is dependent on dose. Infants must be monitored for effects: blood pressure, urine output, capillary refill, perfusion, and heart rate. Dopamine has a short half-life and must be given by constant infusion. Dosage: 0.5–20 µg/kg per minute of continuous IV infusion. Begin at a low dose and titrate by monitoring effects (Young and Mangum, 1998).

      (3) Dobutamine is a synthetic catecholamine with primary $beta_1$ effects; it is also used for blood pressure support in patients with shock and hypotension related to myocardial ischemia, pulmonary hypertension, and cardiomyopathy (Bell, 1998). Dosage: 2–25 µg/kg per minute by continuous infusion; titrate by monitoring effects (Young and Mangum, 1998).

      (4) Amrinone is a noncatecholamine that stimulates the release of calcium from the sarcoplasmic reticulum in cardiac cells, causing increased contractility. Amrinone also causes decreases in systemic vascular resistance and pulmonary vascular resistance (Bell, 1998). Dosage: a loading dose of 3–4.5 mg/kg is given, followed by a constant infusion of 3–5 µg/kg per minute (Bhatt et al., 1997)

    c. Pulmonary vasodilators.

      (1) iNO (previously described).

      (2) Tolazoline (Priscoline). Alpha-adrenergic antagonist, histamine agonist, and direct vasodilator. Has been used to treat PPHN with mixed results. Seldom used.

      (3) Isoproternol (Isuprel). Dilates the pulmonary arteries and airways, and increases cardiac output. Tachycardia and systemic hypotension may be seen. Dosage: 0.05–0.5 µg/kg per minute continuous IV infusion (Young and Mangum, 1998).

      (4) Other agents. Prostaglandin I_2 (prostacyclin) and nifedipine (calcium-channel blocker) may prove to be more specific and effective. They require further study.

    d. Analgesics and sedatives.

      (1) Fentanyl citrate. In addition to analgesic effect, fentanyl produces a sedative effect. Dosage: 1–4 µg/kg per dose by IV slow push. Repeat as required (usually every 2–4 hours). Frequently used as a constant infusion at 1–5 µg/kg per hour (Young and Mangum, 1998).

      (2) Morphine sulfate. Dosage: 0.05–0.2 mg/kg per dose IV. Repeat as required, usually every 4 hours (Young and Mangum, 1998). Can be used as a constant infusion.

I. Outcome (Wearden and Hansen, 1998).

1. PPHN mortality rate and need for ECMO are 20–40%.
2. Residual chronic lung disease is common.
3. Sensorineural hearing loss is higher among children treated for PPHN.
4. Incidence of abnormal neurologic outcome is 12–25%.

MECONIUM ASPIRATION SYNDROME

A. Definition and etiology of meconium aspiration syndrome (MAS).

1. Meconium is a mixture of epithelial cells and bile salts found in the fetal intestinal tract.
2. With asphyxia in utero, peristalisis is stimulated and relaxation of the anal sphincter occurs, releasing meconium into the amniotic fluid.
3. Aspiration may occur whenever meconium passes into the amniotic fluid, but the risk increases when repeated episodes of severe asphyxia lead to gasping respirations in utero.

B. Incidence. Meconium-stained amniotic fluid (MSAF) is present in approximately 10% of all babies delivered (Blackburn and Loper, 1992).

C. Pathophysiology.

1. Complete or partial airway obstruction can occur.
2. Atelectasis or ball-valve air trapping leading to hyperinflation may be seen.
3. A chemical pneumonitis (probably caused by bile salts) may develop as a result of aspiration of meconium.
4. Asphyxia and the results of chronic hypoxia may predispose these infants to PPHN.

D. Clinical presentation/diagnosis.

1. MAS is a disease of term or postterm infants.
2. MAS is rarely seen in infants born at less than 36 weeks' gestation.
3. Vigorous resuscitation is frequently needed in the delivery room because of central depression.
4. Respiratory distress signs are nonspecific and may include tachypnea, nasal flaring, and retractions.
5. Respiratory distress may range from mild and transient to severe and prolonged.
6. If there has been prolonged placental insufficiency, infants may appear to be wasted, with hanging skinfolds (usually around knees, buttocks, and axillas).
7. Nail beds and skin are usually stained a yellow-green color.
8. The chest may appear to be hyperinflated or barrel shaped.
9. Chest x-ray film shows hyperexpanded, lucent areas mixed with areas of atelectasis throughout lung fields.
10. Expiration phase of respirations may be prolonged.
11. Rales and rhonchi are common on auscultation.
12. No specific laboratory data are useful for diagnosis of MAS.
13. ABGs will show the following:
    a. Respiratory and metabolic acidosis in severe cases.
    b. Low PaO_2 even with 100% oxygen administration.

E. Complications.

1. Pulmonary.
    a. Air leaks (pneumothorax, and pneumomediastinum)—due to ball-valve phenomenon leading to overinflation and air trapping and high ventilator pressures.

b. Pneumonia.
c. PPHN.
d. BPD.
2. Metabolic.
   a. Acidosis.
   b. Hypoglycemia.
   c. Hypocalcemia.
3. Hematologic.
   a. Polycythemia.
   b. Hyperviscosity.
4. Neurologic: will depend on degree of asphyxia.

F. **Management and prevention.**

1. Delivery room management.
   a. Suction nasopharynx, oropharynx, and hypopharynx with delivery of head to remove any meconium before first breath is taken.
   b. Perform tracheal suction by direct laryngoscopy, using direct suction to the endotracheal tube.
   c. Infant may need repeated intubation and tracheal suctioning to remove excessive meconium.
2. Respiratory care.
   a. ABGs to determine degree of respiratory compromise and type of therapy needed.
   b. Oxygen and/or assisted ventilation.
      (1) Use same parameters for therapy as with RDS. May want to use a lower PEEP (to avoid inadvertent PEEP) and a higher respiratory rate to induce alkalosis and prevent PPHN.
      (2) May choose HFV.
      (3) iNO if PPHN develops.
   c. Most recent data suggest the use of multiple doses of surfactant for surfactant inactivation caused by meconium aspiration (Davis and Notter, 1994; Findlay, Taeusch, and Walther, 1996). The use of surfactant in infants with MAS has also decreased the need for ECMO (Lotze et al., 1998).
   d. Use of sedatives and paralysis may be necessary if infant's lungs are ventilated.

G. **Outcome.**

1. The prognosis for infants with mild cases of MAS is generally excellent unless complications such as seizures, PPHN, or severe asphyxia occur during the course of the disease.
2. In more severe cases, neurologic sequelae are common and death may occur despite vigorous, maximal support.

BRONCHOPULMONARY DYSPLASIA

A. **Definition.**

1. In 1967 Northway, Rosan, and Porter originally described the four stages of BPD based on the time that the change occurred (from birth to 30 days of life) and on the type of alveolar and bronchial damage and repair that occurred.
2. Other researchers used various criteria to describe BPD (Bancalari Abdenour, Fellar, and Grannon, 1979; Shennan et al., 1988; Toce et al., 1984).
3. A more clinically useful definition now is: a 36 week post conceptional age infant with an O_2 requirement, an abnormal CXR, and abnormal physical exam findings (Barrington and Finer, 1998; Farrell and Fiascone, 1997).

B. Incidence.

1. Incidence figures vary because of the difference in diagnostic criteria.
2. Overall, BPD seems to be increasing, but the population of infants receiving assisted ventilation has changed since first described (Farrell and Fiascone, 1997).
3. BPD estimates.
   a. Less than 700 g: 85% affected.
   b. Greater than 1500 g: 5% affected.

C. Etiology.

1. Oxygen toxicity can be a cause of BPD.
   a. High inspired oxygen concentrations cause the production of reactive oxygen species and the release of chemotactic factors that attract neutrophils to the lung. Thus begins the inflammatory cycle. Infants with BPD have an ongoing inflammatory process in the lung that causes and continues parenchymal damage (Barrington and Finer, 1998; Farrell and Fiascone, 1997).
   b. Inflammatory mediators and proteolytic enzymes are released. The preterm infant has lower levels of antiproteases such as alpha-1-protease (alpha-1-antitrypsin) and the antioxidant enzymes dismutase and glutathione. Oxidative damage causes the alpha-protease to become inactive. These together make the premature pulmonary system especially vulnerable to oxygen toxicity (Barrington and Finer, 1998).
   c. Oxygen radicals appear in the lung as a result of cellular metabolism and are supplementally provided with treatment for the ongoing pulmonary process (Farrell and Fiascone, 1997).
2. Assisted ventilation with positive pressure and barotrauma contributes to BPD development.
   a. Intubation interrupts normal pulmonary function (mucociliary function is damaged; dead space is increased, leading to increased pressure needs).
   b. Correlation exists between the severity of the initial pulmonary process and BPD (Barrington and Finer, 1998).
   c. Barotrauma is related to the intensity and amount of time exposed to elements of positive-pressure ventilation (peak inspiratory pressure [PIP], inspiratory time, and PEEP). Repeated distention of distal airways during mechanical ventilation of infants with poor alveolar compliance results in ischemia. Because of the immaturity of the pulmonary system, the alveolar capillary unit is further disrupted by mechanical ventilation, leading to pulmonary edema (Farrell and Fiascone, 1997).
3. Increased shunting (left-to-right) via a patent ductus arteriosus (PDA) has been described as a possible cause of BPD.
   a. Improved lung compliance may follow PDA ligation in infants with RDS.
   b. When PDA is a complication of RDS, the risk of BPD development is increased (Bancalari and Gerhardt, 1986; Nickerson, 1985).
4. Excessive fluid intake in the first 4 days of life contributes to the development of BPD (Barrington and Finer, 1998).
5. Colonization by *Ureaplasma urealyticum* has been associated with higher incidence of BPD (Barrington and Finer, 1998).
6. Gestational age plays an important role in the development of BPD.
   a. Damage to the developing lung is more likely in infants weighting less than 1500 g.
   b. Damage may occur with less exposure to the previously noted factors in the low birth weight infant.

D. Pathophysiology. All levels of the tracheobronchial tree are involved.
1. Large airways.

   a. Submucosal glanular hypertrophy.
   b. Increased bronchial smooth muscle.
   c. Bronchial mucosa replaced by metaplastic squamous epithelium.
   d. Submucosal fibrosis.
   e. Inflammatory infiltrates.
   f. Granulation tissue.
   g. Loss of cilia.
   h. Frequent tracheomalacia or bronchiomalacia.
2. Small airways.
   a. Bronchiolar smooth muscle hypertrophy.
   b. Focal mucosal squamous metaplasia.
   c. Chronic inflammation.
   d. Peribronchial edema.
   e. Peribronchiolar fibrosis.
   f. Necrosis with intraluminal debris.
   g. Luminal narrowing.
   h. Excessive production of mucus.
3. Alveoli.
   a. Decreased number of alveoli.
   b. Enlarged alveoli.
   c. Alveolar septal destruction, which leads to emphysematous blebs.
4. Pulmonary vascular bed.
   a. Muscular hypertrophy of the medial layer of pulmonary arterioles.
   b. Fibrosis.
   c. Endothelial cell hyperplasia, which leads to a decreased cross-sectional area.
5. Reactive Airways Disease (Farrell and Fiascone, 1997).

E. **Clinical presentation.**

1. Predisposing risk factors.
   a. Oxygen, intubation, and assisted ventilation.
   b. Gestational age.
   c. Nutritional deficiencies.
   d. Underlying lung disease.
   e. Air leaks.
2. Increase in ventilatory requirements or inability to be weaned from ventilator.
3. Hypoxia, hypercapnia, and respiratory acidosis.
4. Audible rales, rhonchi, and wheezing.
5. Retractions.
6. Increased secretions.
7. Bronchospasm.
8. Electrocardiogram showing right ventricular hypertrophy and right axis deviation.
9. Chest x-ray film showing hyperinflation and cardiomegaly.
10. Fluid intolerance, evidenced by increase in weight, edema, and decrease in urine output, despite no change in fluid intake.

F. **Diagnosis.**

1. Diagnosis of exclusion.
2. Differential diagnosis.
   a. Sepsis.
   b. Pneumonia.
   c. Airway obstruction.
   d. PDA.
3. Chest x-ray findings (see Chapter 29); clinical signs (e.g., tachypnea, hypercapnia, hypoxia, rales) help make diagnosis.

G. **Complications.**

1. Intermittent bronchospasm.
2. Inability to be weaned from ventilator and/or oxygen supplementation.
3. Recurrent infections.
   a. Pneumonia.
   b. Upper respiratory tract infections.
   c. Otitis media.
4. Congestive heart failure from cor pulmonale.
5. BPD "spells."
   a. Infant becomes irritable, agitated, and dusky; has increased respiratory effort, hypoxia, and hypercapnia.
   b. Cause is unknown but may be bronchospasm or increased pulmonary vascular resistance.
6. Gastroesophageal reflux.
7. Developmental delays.
8. Sudden death reported; cause not completely understood (Farrell and Fiascone, 1997).

H. **Prevention.**

1. Administration of antenatal steroids reduces the incidence of RDS and the need for mechanical ventilation.
2. Surfactant rescue therapy decreases mortality rates, and prophylaxis may decrease the incidence of BPD slightly.
3. Some evidence supports the use of early postnatal steroids (e.g., dexamethasone) and warrants further investigation.
4. Gentle ventilation, permissive hypercapnia, and early extubation have all been suggested as ways to decrease BPD but have not yet been confirmed by randomized, controlled trials.
5. Synchronized intermittent mandatory ventilation (SIMV); HFOV. SIMV is associated with less severe BPD because the incidence of pulmonary air leak decreases. A recent trial of HFOV after surfactant therapy demonstrated a decrease in the incidence of BPD (Barrington and Finer, 1998; Farrell and Fiascone, 1997).

I. **Management.**

1. Continued respiratory support.
   a. Continue assisted ventilation.
      (1) Weaning should be *slow,* to allow time for the infant to compensate.
      (2) Decrease the rate because of the need for high peak inspiratory pressure to deliver adequate tidal volume, but always assess each infant individually.
   b. After extubation, oxygen is needed to prevent hypoxia and avoid cor pulmonale.
      (1) Oxygen inhalation alleviates airway constriction seen in infants with BPD.
      (2) Maintain PaO_2 at greater than 55 mm Hg and pH at greater than 7.25.
      (3) Pulmonary vascular resistance is decreased.
      (4) Supplemental oxygen may enhance overall growth of the infant.
   c. Weaning can usually be accomplished by use of pulse oximetry and occasional monitoring of blood gas and/or serum bicarbonate levels (to assess compensation).
2. Use of diuretics to control fluid retention leading to pulmonary edema. Furosemide (Lasix) is used most often. Benefits include decreased airway resistance, increased airway compliance, and a decrease in total body water, extracellular water, and interstitial water (O'Donovan and Bell, 1989).

Complications include renal calcification with long-term use (Hufnagle et al., 1983) and electrolyte disturbances (sodium, potassium, and calcium loss). This can lead to hypochloremic metabolic alkalosis and problems with bone mineralization that can exacerbate osteopenia of prematurity (Hansen and Corbet, 1991). Chlorothiazide (Diuril) has been used with results similar to those seen with furosemide. Follow serum electrolyte values to monitor for hyponatremia, hypokalemia, and metabolic alkalosis.

3. Bronchodilators.
   a. Inhaled bronchodilators which are commonly given to infants with BPD include albuterol, metaproterenol, ipratropium, and cromolyn sodium. The inhaled dose is extremely variable. Long-term outcome data on prolonged treatment with bronchodilators are lacking in this population (Barrington and Finer, 1998).
   b. Systemic bronchodilator: theophylline (aminophylline). Use varies with individual centers; levels must be monitored. Can cause GI irritation.
4. Fluid restriction to help reduce pulmonary edema and right-sided heart failure.
5. Cardiac evaluation for complications.
   a. Cor pulmonale (right ventricular hypertrophy) is a result of pulmonary hypertension and can be seen in infants with BPD.
   b. Electrocardiography and echocardiography should be performed periodically to determine whether right ventricular hypertrophy has developed.
6. Optimal nutrition. Provide increased calories to compensate for increased work of breathing and fluid restriction. Infant may need 150 to 180 kcal/kg per day. Growth failure is common.
7. Monitor for osteopenia beginning at 6 weeks and follow every 2–3 weeks (Rusk, 1998). BPD infants are at high risk due to their gestational age, often protracted respiratory course and medications.
8. Chest physiotherapy and suctioning. These measures are helpful in loosening and removing bronchial secretions. Caregivers must use caution so as not to precipitate a BPD "spell" or cause a rib fracture.
9. Evaluate infant for tracheostomy after 6 to 8 weeks of assisted ventilation and inability to wean off the ventilator. Reduces risk of airway complications (e.g., tracheomalacia, bronchomalacia).
10. Use of steroids.
    a. Use remains controversial.
    b. Steroids inhibit the influx of neutrophils into the lung and decrease the lung inflammation.
    c. Additional benefits include improvement of pulmonary resistance and lung compliance, and the possibility of facilitating extubation.
    d. Complications include impairment of growth, hyperglycemia, systemic hypertension, myocardial hypertrophy, gastrointestinal perforation and gastric ulcerations, and transient adrenal suppression (Parad and Berger, 1998).
    e. Have not been found to have a substantial impact on long term outcomes such as duration of supplemental oxygen requirement, length of hospital stay, or mortality (Parad and Berger, 1998).
    f. Studies investigating the use of inhaled corticosteroids are ongoing (Barrington and Finer, 1998).
    g. Initiation of treatment, selection of candidates, duration of treatment, and dosing regimens remain under investigation. Many institutions have developed their own preferences (Farrell and Fiascone, 1997).
11. Respiratory Syncytial Virus (RSV): BPD infants are at high risk for RSV outbreaks and account for many readmissions with 25% of BPD infants needing assisted ventilation. Treatment modalities include:

   a. Ribavirin. Controversial but is supported by the American Academy of Pediatrics (AAP, 1993). It is administered by inhalation.
   b. RespiGam (RSV IVIG). Decreases the severity of RSV infection, decreases hospitalizations, and reduces the incidence of concurrent otitis media (Welliver, 1998; Impact Study Group, 1998). The AAP recommends prophylaxis to infants who are less than 2 years of age who received supplemental oxygen within the preceding 6 months, infants born at 29–32 weeks' gestation during RSV season, and infants born at less than 29 weeks' gestation (prophylaxis until 12 months of age); prophylaxis is not indicated for infants with cyanotic congenital heart disease (AAP, 1997). Dosage is 750 ml/kg per dose IV, repeated monthly during RSV season (Young, Mangum, 1998). Dosing should resume after recovery if RSV infection develops (Farrell and Fiascone, 1997).
   c. Palivizumab (Synagis). Humanized monoclonal antibody against RSV.
      (1) RSV study group (Impact Study Group, 1998) showed 55% decrease in hospitalizations caused by RSV infection, fewer hospital days, and a lower rate of ICU admissions compared with the control group
      (2) Infants born at less than 35 weeks' gestation and infants with BPD requiring medical management within the preceding 6 months are candidates for treatment
      (3) Dose: 15 mg/kg, intramuscular route, given monthly during RSV season, with the first dose to be given before start of season. (Impact Study Group, 1998).

J. Outcome.

1. Mortality rate is approximately 10–15% by 1 year of age (Davis and Rosenfeld, 1994).
2. After discharge, mortality rate is less than 10%.
   a. Death is usually not caused by respiratory failure.
   b. Complications such as cor pulmonale or infection are the usual causes of death.
3. Some infants will be discharged home with oxygen supplementation.
4. Recurrent pulmonary infections and growth retardation are seen commonly among survivors. The pattern of growth is usually between the 10th and 25th percentiles (Farrell and Fiascone, 1997).
5. Gradual improvement is seen during the first 2 years of life, but pulmonary function and chest x-rays continue to show abnormalities for many years (Dusick, 1997).
6. Neurologic and developmental sequelae.
   a. Cerebral palsy. The most common major neurologic disorder in the first 2 years of life in very low birth weight infants. Disorder related to early neonatal course rather than to BPD (Vohr and Msall, 1997).
   b. Sensorineural hearing loss. Incidence of 0.7–2% in very low birth weight infants. Conductive hearing loss has an incidence of 14–42%. Retinopathy of prematurity is reported at 23–57%, with myopia common (Dusick, 1997).

Chronic Lung Disease in Premature Infants (Pulmonary Insufficiency of Prematurity, Chronic Pulmonary Insufficiency of Prematurity, Wilson-Mikity Syndrome)

A. Definition.

1. Changes in pulmonary structure and function occur without underlying disease.
2. Majority of cases are seen in infants weighing less than 1500 g.

B. **Incidence.** Incidence is unknown. Wide variation in population, clinical practice and definition account for variation in incidence.

C. **Etiology/pathophysiology.**
1. Abnormal distribution of air (overexpansion and atelectasis) due to characteristics of the premature lung.
2. At the end of the first week, the functional residual capacity (FRC) decreases, resulting in hypoxia and hypercapnia, which lead to apnea and atelectasis.
3. Chest x-ray reveals poorly defined, diffuse, hazy lung parenchyma (Cooper, 1998).

D. **Clinical presentation and diagnosis.**
1. Can be seen in premature infants with minimal exposure to increased oxygen.
2. Symptoms appear at 7–10 days of life and include transient cyanosis, hyperpnea, and retractions.
3. Symptoms increase in severity for 2–6 weeks.
4. Increasing oxygen dependency and retention of carbon dioxide.

E. **Management.** Provide supportive care.
1. Oxygen to maintain normal PaO_2.
2. Chest physiotherapy.
3. IV fluids.
4. Caffeine for apnea.
5. Nasal CPAP until about 30 weeks' postconceptional age (Cooper, 1998).

F. **Outcome.**
1. Mortality rates of 10–30% have been reported with these forms of chronic lung disease.
2. Generally there is complete clearing of symptoms by 2–6 months.
3. Condition often resolves with growth.

Pulmonary Air Leaks (Pneumomediastinum, Pneumothorax, Pneumopericardium, Pulmonary Interstitial Emphysema [PIE])

A. **Definition.** Alveolar overdistention and rupture. May occur spontaneously or as a secondary cause, usually when assisted ventilation is used.

B. **Incidence.** In infants receiving assisted ventilation, the incidence ranges from 2% to 8% but among low birth weight infants may be as high as 20% (Whitsett and Pryhuber, 1994; Yu, Wong, Bajuk, and Szymonowicz, 1986).

C. **Pathophysiology.**
1. Generally iatrogenic, resulting from the use of excessive airway pressure during resuscitation or with assisted ventilation.
2. Can occur spontaneously if there is uneven air distribution at birth.
   a. Some areas are expanded, while others remain collapsed.
   b. Infant will generate pressure to expand unopened areas, leading to greater pressure in already expanded areas, which results in the air leak.
3. Frequently, underlying lung disease is present.
   a. Obstructive: such as ball-valve trapping of air, seen with MAS.
   b. Poor lung compliance: such as seen with RDS.
4. Overdistention of alveoli leads to rupture, with gas moving into nonventilated tissues. Air travels via vascular sheaths to the lining of the lung. Interstitial air can dissect around blood vessels or along lymphatics becoming pulmonary

interstitial emphysema (PIE). Air can move from the lining to the mediastinum, resulting in pneumomediastinum, through to the thoracic cavity and visceral pleura, resulting in a pneumothorax. When the air moves along the great vessels to the pericardium, a pneumopericardium results. If air dissects down from the mediastinum through the sheaths of the great vessels, pneumoperitoneum results.

D. Clinical presentation and diagnosis (see Chapter 29 for x-ray findings).

1. Pneumothorax.
   a. Sudden deterioration.
   b. Decreased breath sounds on the affected side, hypotension, skin mottling, and shift of the mediastinum (detected by shift of the point of maximal cardiac impulse on auscultation) to the unaffected side.
   c. Obtain chest x-ray.
   d. Transillumination (translucent glow when fiberoptic light is placed against the skin) of the chest wall may confirm presence of pneumothorax, without having to wait for a chest x-ray.
   e. If the air leak is small, may be asymptomatic.
2. Pneumomediastinum.
   a. Should be anticipated with MAS.
   b. Signs include increased anteroposterior diameter of chest and indistinct heart sounds.
   c. CXR "sail sign," indicating elevation of the thymus surrounded by air.
3. Pneumopericardium.
   a. Immediate presentation with hypotension, muffled heart sound, and bradycardia from cardiac tamponade.
   b. Life threatening.
   c. CXR will show air encircling the heart, halo appearance.
4. Pulmonary interstitial emphysema (PIE).
   a. Difficult to interpret.
   b. Limited to infants with poor lung compliance receiving continuous positive airway pressure or positive-pressure ventilation.
   c. CXR shows microcystic areas throughout one or both lungs; may show hyperinflated lungs and flattened diaphragm.
   d. May progress to pneumomediastinum and/or pneumothorax.
   e. Hypoxia and hypercapnia commonly present.

E. Management.

1. Pneumothorax.
   a. If asymptomatic, will often resolve without treatment.
   b. Symptomatic (tension) pneumothorax requires emergency removal of air. Associated with hypoxia, hypotension, and cardiopulmonary arrest.
      (1) Thoracentesis (needle aspiration to remove air) may be necessary, until a chest tube can be placed, if infant's condition has acutely deteriorated.
      (2) Thoracostomy tube is placed in the anterior chest and connected to underwater-seal drainage system, with continuous negative pressure of 10–15 cm H_2O, and left in place until air ceases to bubble from the chest tube for at least 24 hours and pneumothorax is resolved by chest x-ray examination. The chest tube is then placed to the water seal for 24 hours, and the infant is observed for reaccumulation of air. The chest tube is removed 12–24 hours after the tube has been clamped if the infant remains free of symptoms.
      (3) In asymptomatic infants or non-ventilated infants, administration of 100% oxygen will aid the absorption of the air in the pneumothorax by

the pleural capillaries. Due to the toxic effects of oxygen, this treatment is not recommended for preterm infants.

2. Pneumomediastinum.
   a. Usually not treated.
   b. If associated with pneumothorax (common occurrence), high oxygen concentration to help resolve condition, as described previously.
3. Pneumopericardium. Emergency treatment is required by placement of a long catheter or chest tube into the pericardial sac with constant application of gentle negative pressure.
4. PIE.
   a. If unilateral and persistent, intubation of main-stem bronchus supplying opposite lung may show improvement in condition.
   b. If bilateral, supportive treatment is given (e.g., oxygen, ventilation, fluids).
   c. Minimize positive inspiratory pressure and shorten inspiratory time.
   d. High-frequency ventilation.
   e. Place affected side in dependent position.

F. **Outcome.**

1. Outcome depends on underlying lung pathology.
2. Mortality rate is high with pneumopericardium, bilateral pneumothoraces, and bilateral PIE.
3. In survivors of bilateral PIE, the risk of chronic lung disease is high.

PULMONARY HYPOPLASIA

A. **Definition.** Defective or inhibited growth of the lungs, either unilateral or bilateral. Developmental disorder that results in decreased numbers of alveoli, bronchioles, and arterioles.

B. **Pathophysiology.**

1. Conditions that compress the lungs or limit lung growth (e.g., diaphragmatic hernia) are one cause of pulmonary hypoplasia.
2. Conditions that result in oligohydramnios (e.g., renal disorders, amniotic fluid leakage) are associated with pulmonary hypoplasia caused by thoracic compression.
3. Associated congenital malformations, such as renal dysgenesis (Potter's syndrome), phrenic nerve absence, and vertebral and chromosomal anomalies, should be considered.

C. **Diagnosis.**

1. Often very difficult to diagnose.
2. Any of the above conditions suggestive of pulmonary hypoplasia.
3. Usually present with severe respiratory distress.
4. Higher-than-usual pressures needed for ventilation; pneumothorax common.
5. Hypercapnia difficult or impossible to treat early in disease course.
6. Chest x-ray will usually show decreased volume of the thorax.
7. Symptoms of PPHN possible.

D. **Management.** Treatment is supportive and directed at respiratory failure.
1. Assisted ventilation/HFV: high-frequency ventilation.
2. Treatment of PPHN.
3. iNO (nitric oxide).
4. ECMO.

E. **Outcome.**

1. Degree of hypoplasia determines outcome.

2. Mortality rate is high and may also be affected by the cause of hypoplasia.
3. Management is difficult, but infant can function adequately if treatment and support can be continued until lung growth occurs, although this outcome is rare.

PULMONARY HEMORRHAGE

A. Definition.

1. Localized areas of bleeding into alveoli (generally found at autopsy); also known as hemorrhagic pulmonary edema.
2. Can be a massive generalized bleeding event.

B. Etiology and pathophysiology.

1. Usually occurs as a complication of other disorders such as prematurity, erythroblastosis, intracranial hemorrhage, asphyxia, aspiration, heart disease, sepsis, hypothermia, patent ductus arteriosus, and surfactant replacement.
2. May be due to trauma from improper suctioning technique.
3. Usually results from large increase in capillary hydrostatic pressure; causes capillary rupture and fluid transudation from other capillaries (Welty and Hansen, 1998).

C. Clinical presentation.

1. May present with sudden, severe respiratory distress.
2. Bright red blood can be suctioned from the trachea.

D. Management.

1. Use of assisted ventilation is necessary to maintain gas exchange and PEEP.
2. Transfusion of whole blood.
3. Identify any clotting abnormalities and treat.
4. Treat underlying disease.

E. Outcome.

1. If bleeding is massive, death will occur quickly despite vigorous management.
2. If hemorrhage is small or isolated, infant will recover and outcome will be dependent on underlying disease.

OTHER CAUSES OF RESPIRATORY DISTRESS

A. Upper airway disorders.

1. Choanal atresia: 2–4 in 10,000 births.
   a. Bone or membrane protrudes into nasal passages, causing blockage or narrowing.
   b. Female/male ratio is 2:1.
   c. If condition is bilateral, gasping respirations and cyanosis occur immediately after birth because neonates are obligate nose breathers. Many infants have associated anomalies (Treacher Collins syndrome, tracheoesophageal fistula, palatal abnormalities, CHARGE association [coloboma, heart disease, atresia choanal, retarded growth and development, genital hypoplasia, and ear anomalies]), congenital heart disease.
   d. Signs of distress are intermittent when condition is unilateral.
   e. Failure to pass a catheter through the nasal passages to the posterior oropharynx will make the diagnosis.
   f. Initially treat by placing infant in prone position with a large oral airway taped securely in place (an endotracheal tube can be used if placement of an oral airway is difficult).

    g. Surgical correction of the problem is necessary and consists of perforation of the obstruction and serial dilation by use of obturators.

2. Micrognathia.
    a. Defined as mandibular undergrowth.
    b. Occurs with certain syndromes such as Pierre Robin syndrome, trisomy 18, trisomy 22, and cri-du-chat syndrome (deletion of the short arm of chromosome 5).
    c. Airway distress may be alleviated by prone positioning with the infant's head placed downward.
    d. Use of an oral airway or endotracheal tube will provide an open airway.
    e. If an endotracheal tube is in place, humidification will be needed to prevent the drying of secretions.
    f. Tracheostomy may be necessary.
    g. Generally mandibular growth "catches up" by 6 to 12 months of age.

3. Cystic hygroma.
    a. Form of cystic lymphangioma, with benign water cysts occurring most frequently in the neck (80%); can also be found in the groin, axilla, and mediastinum.
    b. Usually seen at birth.
    c. Mass will occupy the submandibular region and may compromise the airway in 25% of cases.
    d. Symptoms depend on the size and location.
    e. Treatment is related to complications.
       (1) If infant is free of symptoms, surgical excision is performed between 4 and 12 months of age.
       (2) Excision must be performed at an earlier age if the airway is compromised or if infections are recurrent.
       (3) Multiple excisions are usually performed to prevent damage to nerves and vascular structures.

4. Obstruction of larynx or trachea.
    a. Stridor is a major symptom and usually requires no specific treatment, but mechanical causes must be ruled out.
    b. Direct laryngoscopy will reveal structural abnormalities such as polyps, webs, and granulomas.
    c. Hemangiomas of the larynx or trachea may cause obstruction.
    d. Extrinsic compression of the upper airway occurs with thyroglossal duct cyst, cervical neuroblastoma, vascular ring, and double aortic arch.
    e. Laryngotracheomalacia results from collapse of the larynx and cervical trachea, which produces stridor; condition is usually self-limiting and resolves by 6–12 months of age, when the tracheal diameter increases and the cartilage matures.

5. Tracheoesophageal fistula (refer to Chapter 13.)

B. **Thoracic disorders.**

1. Cystic adenomatoid malformation.
    a. Primary pulmonary tissue dysplasia with failure of terminal bronchioles to canalize, which leads to intrapulmonary mass consisting of multiple small cysts.
    b. Two types:
       (1) Lobar cystic adenomatoid malformation, type I. Large cysts in a lobar distribution that replace whole lobe of lung. This type is associated with acites and is more resectable and survivable than type II.
       (2) Diffuse cystic adenomatoid malformation, type II. Entire lung has microscopic cysts, often associated with acites. Resection is not possible; condition usually results in neonatal death (Seeds and Azizkhan, 1990).

    c. Respiratory distress may be seen in newborn infant, or the malformation may cause no symptoms. Sporadic episodes with low rate of recurrence.

    d. May be confused with diaphragmatic hernia or pulmonary sequestration on x-ray.

    e. Treatment of choice is surgical excision of the involved lobe.

2. Bronchogenic cyst.
    a. Mucus-producing cyst.
    b. May cause tracheal, bronchial, or esophageal obstruction.
    c. Distress usually not severe.
    d. Treatment is surgical excision.

3. Congenital lobar emphysema.
    a. Overdistention of one or more lobes of the lung (upper lobes generally affected; 10% in right middle lobe).
    b. Inability of the lung to deflate properly, possibly because of a defect in bronchial cartilage.
    c. Possibility of severe respiratory distress within hours of birth but usually delayed for weeks or months.
    d. Chest x-ray examination: diagnostic (refer to Chapter 29).
    e. Treatment of choice: surgical resection.

4. Chondrodystrophies.
    a. Group of disorders of bone growth, resulting in short stature.
    b. Possible respiratory distress because of small thoracic cavities.
    c. Treatment: based on degree of distress.

5. Neuromuscular disorders.
    a. Conditions resulting in hypotonia, such as spinal muscular atrophy and myotonic dystrophy, result in varying degrees of respiratory distress.
    b. Management will depend on degree of distress.

C. **Central nervous system disorders.**

1. Seizures.
2. Hypoxic-ischemic injury.
3. Intracranial hemorrhages.
4. Drugs.
5. Meningitis.

D. **Cardiovascular and hematologic disorders.**

1. Congenital heart disease.
2. Anemia.
3. Polycythemia.
4. Shock.
5. Sepsis.
6. Respiratory distress, varying from mild to severe.
7. Treatment in relation to underlying cause.

E. **Diaphragmatic disorders (see also Chapter 29).**

1. Diaphragmatic hernia.
2. Diaphragmatic paralysis.
3. Diaphragmatic eventration.

F. **Renal disorders.**

1. Pulmonary hypoplasia results from renal agenesis or renal dysgenesis.
2. Conditions are usually untreatable, and death will occur within hours or days.

REFERENCES

American Academy of Pediatrics Committee on Infectious Diseases: Use of ribavirin in the treatment of respiratory syncytial virus infection. Pediatrics, 92:501–503, 1993.

American Academy of Pediatrics Committee on Infectious Diseases: Respiratory syncytial virus immune globulin intravenous: Indications for use. Pediatrics, 99:645, 1997.

Ballard, R.A., Ballard, P.L., CNAAN, A., et al.: Antenatal thyrotropin-releasing hormone to prevent lung disease in preterm infants. N. Engl. J. Med., 338:493–498, 1998.

Bancalari, E., Abdenour, D.E., Fellar, R., and Gannon, J. BPD: Clinical presentation. J. Pediatr., 95:819–823, 1979.

Bancalari, E., and Gerhardt, T. Bronchopulmonary dysplasia. Pediatr. Clin. North Am., 33:1–20, 1986.

Barrington, K.J., and Finer, N.N. Treatment of bronchopulmonary dysplasia: A review. Clin. Perinatol., 25:177–202, 1998.

Bell, S.G.: Neonatal cardiovascular pharmacology. Neonatal Network, 17(2):7–15, 1998.

Bennett, F.C., and Scott, O.T.: Long-term perspective on premature infant outcome and contemporary intervention issues. Semin. Perinatol. 21:190–201, 1997.

Bhatt, D.R., et al.: Neonatal Drug Formulary, 4th ed. Los Angeles, N.D.F. Publishing, 1997, pp. 36–37.

Blackburn, S.T., and Loper, D.L.: Maternal, Fetal, and Neonatal Physiology: A Clinical Perspective. Philadelphia, W.B. Saunders, 1992, pp. 282–321.

Collaborative Santiago Surfactant Group: Collaborative Trial of Prenatal Thyrotopin-releasing Hormone and Corticosteroids for Prevention of Respiratory Distress Syndrome. Am. J. Obstet. Gynecol., 178:33–39, 1998.

Cooper, T.R.: Chronic pulmonary insufficiency of prematurity. In Hansen, T.N., Cooper, T.R., and Weisman, L.E. (Eds.): Contemporary Diagnosis and Management of Neonatal Respiratory Diseases, 2nd ed. Newton, Pa., Handbooks in Health Care (division of AMM Co.), 1998, p. 149.

Davis, J.M., and Notter, R.H.: Lung surfactant replacement for neonatal abnormalities other than respiratory distress syndrome. In Boynton, B.R., Carlo, W.A., and Jobe, A.H. (Eds.): New therapies for neonatal respiratory failure. New York, Cambridge University Press, 1994, pp. 81–84.

Davis, J.M., and Rosenfeld, W.: Chronic lung disease. In Avery, G.B., Fletcher, M.A., and MacDonald, M.G. (Eds.): Neonatology: Pathophysiology and Management of the Newborn, 4th ed. Philadelphia, J.B. Lippincott, 1994, pp. 453–477.

Dusick, A.M.: Medical outcomes in preterm infants. Semin. in Perinatol., 21(3):164–177, 1997.

Egberts, J., de Winter, J.P., Sedin, G., et al.: Comparison of prophylaxis and rescue treatment with Curosurf in neonates less than 30 weeks' gestation: A randomized trial. Pediatrics, 92:768–774, 1993.

Farrell, P.A., and Fiascone, J.M.: Bronchopulmonary dysplasia in the 1990s: A review for the pediatrician. Pediatrics, 27:129–172, 1997.

Findlay, R.D., Taeusch, H.W., and Walther, F.J.: Surfactant replacement therapy for meconium aspiration syndrome. Pediatrics, 97:48–52, 1996.

Ghidini, A., Salafia, C.M., Miniar, V.K., et al.: Repeated courses of steroids in preterm membrane rupture do not increase the risk of histologic chorioamnionitis. Am. J. Perinatiol., 14:309–313, 1997.

Gorrie, T.M., McKinney, E.S., and Murray, S.S.: Foundations of Maternal Nursing. Philadelphia, W.B. Saunders, 1994, p. 754.

Hagedorn, M.I., Gardner, S.L., and Abman, S.H.: Respiratory diseases. In Merenstein, G.B., and Gardner, S.L. (Eds.): Handbook of Neonatal Intensive Care. 4th ed. St. Louis, Mosby–Year Book, 1998, pp. 437–499.

Hansen, T.N., and Corbet, A.: Disorders of the transition. In Taeusch, H.W., Ballard, R.A., and Avery, M.E. (Eds.): Schaffer and Avery's Diseases of the Newborn, 6th ed. Philadelphia, W.B. Saunders, 1991, pp. 498–514.

Harris, T.R., and Wood, B.R.: Physiologic principles. In Goldsmith, J.P., and Karotkin, E.H. (Eds.): Assisted Ventilation of the Neonate, 3rd ed. Philadelphia, W.B. Saunders, 1996, p. 53.

Hufnagle, K.G., Khan, S.N., Penn, D., et al.: Renal complications of long-term furosemide treatment in preterm infants. Pediatrics 70:360–363, 1983.

Impact Study Group: Palivizuab, a humanized respiratory syncytial virus monoclonal antibody, reduces hospitalization from respiratory syncytial virus infection in high-risk infants. Pediatrics, 102:531–537, 1998.

Jobe, A.H.: The role of surfactant therapy in neonatal respiratory distress. Respiratory Care, 36:695–703, 1991.

Kahurinerel, J.: Multicenter study of surfactant (beractant) use in the treatment of term infants with severe respiratory failure. J. Pediatr., 132:40–47, 1998.

Kattwinkel, J.: Surfactant: Evolving issues. Clin. Perinatol., 25(1):17–32, 1998.

Kattwinkel, J., Bloom, B.T., Delmore, P., et al.: Prophylactic administration of calf lung surfactant is more effective than early treatment of respiratory distress syndrome in neonates 29 through 32 weeks' gestation. Pediatrics, 92:90–98, 1993.

Kendig, J.W., Notter, R.N., Cox, C., et al.: A comparison of surfactant as immediate prophylaxis and as rescue therapy in newborns of less than 30 weeks' gestation. N. Engl. J. Med., 324:865–871, 1991.

Kinsella, J.P., and Abman, S.H.: Recent developments in the pathophysiology and treatment of persistent pulmonary hypertension of the newborn. J. Pediatr., 126:853–864, 1995.

Kinsella, J.P., and Abman S.H.: Controversies in the use of inhaled nitric oxide therapy in the newborn. Clin. Perinatol. 1998 25(2):203–218, 1998.

Lawson, M.E.: Respiratory disorders: Transient tachypnea of the newborn. In Cloherty, J.P., and Stark, A.R. (Eds.): Manual of Neonatal Care, 4th ed. Philadelphia, Lippincott-Raven, 1998, pp. 369–371.

Liley, H.G., and Stark, A.R.: Respiratory disorders. In Cloherty, J.P., and Stark, A.R. (Eds.): Manual of Neonatal Care, 4th ed. Philadelphia, Lippincott-Raven, 1998, p. 329.

Loper, D.L.: Physiologic principles of the respiratory system. In Askin, D.F. (Ed.): Acute Respiratory Care of the Neonate, 2nd ed. Petaluma, Calif., 1997, NICU Ink Books, pp. 1–30.

Lotze, A., Mitchell, B.R., Bulas, D.I., et al.: Mutlicenter study of surfactant (beractant) use in the treatment of term infants with severe respiratory failure. J. Pediatr. 132:40–47, 1998.

Maher, J.E., Cliver, S.P., Goldenberg, R.E., et al.: The effect of corticosteroid therapy in the very premature infant. Am. J. Obstet. Gynecol., 170:869–873, 1994.

Minarick, C.J., and Beachy, P.: Neurologic disorders. *In* Merenstein, G.B., and Gardner, S.L. (Eds.): Handbook of Neonatal Intensive Care, 3rd ed. St. Louis, Mosby–Year Book, 1993.

Moise, A.A., and Hansen, T.N.: Acute, acquired parenchymal lung disease. *In* Hansen, T.N., Cooper, T.R., and Weisman, L.E. (Eds.): Contemporary Diagnosis and Management of Neonatal Respiratory Diseases, 2nd ed. Newton, Pa., Handbooks in Health Care (division of AMM Co.), 1998, pp. 79–95.

Moore, K.L., and Persaud, T.V.N.: The Developing Human. Philadelphia, W.B. Saunders, 1993.

Morin, F.C., III, and Stenmark, K.R.: Persistent pulmonary hypertension of the newborn. Am. J. Respir. Crit. Care Med. *151*:2010–2032, 1995.

National Institutes of Health Consensus Development Panel: Effect of corticosteroids for fetal maturation on perinatal outcomes. NIH Consensus Statement 12(2):1–24, 1994.

Nickerson, B.: BPD: Chronic pulmonary disease following neonatal respiratory failure. Chest, *87*:528–535, 1985.

Nobuhara, K.K., Lund, D.P., Mitchell, J., et al.: Long-term outlook for survivors of congenital diaphragmatic hernia. Clin. Perinatol., 23:873–887, 1985.

Northway, W.H., Rosan, R.C., and Porter, D.Y.: Pulmonary disease following respiratory therapy of hyaline membrane disease. N. Engl. J. Med., *276*:357–368, 1967.

Notter, R.H.: Biophysical behavior of lung surfactant: Implications for respiratory physiology and pathophysiology. Semin. Perinatol., *12*(3):180–212, 1988.

O'Donovan, B.H., and Bell, E.F.: Effects of furosemide on body water compartments in infants with bronchopulmonary dysplasia. Pediatr Res 26:121–124, 1989.

Orlando, S.: Pathophysiology of acute respiratory distress. *In* Askin, D.F. (Ed.): Acute Respiratory Care of the Neonate. Petaluma, Calif., NICU Ink Books, 1997, pp. 37–41.

Parad, R.B., and Berger, T.M.: Chronic lung disease. *In* Cloherty, J.P., and Stark, A.R. (Eds.): Manual of Neonatal Care, 4th ed. Philadelphia, Lippincott-Raven, 1998, p. 384.

Rusk, C.: Rickets screening in the preterm infant. Neonatal Network, 17(1):55–57, 1998.

Seeds, J.W., and Azizkhan, R.G.: Congenital Malformations: Antenatal Diagnosis Perinatal Management, and Counseling. Rockville, Md., Aspen Publishers, 1990.

Shapiro, D.L.: The development of surfactant therapy and the various types of replacement surfactants. Semin. Perinatol., *12*(3):174–179, 1988.

Shennan, A.T., Dunn, M.S., Ohlsson, A., et al.: Abnormal pulmonary outcomes in premature infants: Prediction from oxygen requirement in the neonatal period. Pediatrics, 82:527–532, 1988.

Speer, M.E., and Hansen, T.N.: Transient tachypnea of the newborn. *In* Hansen, T.N., Cooper, T.R., and Weisman, L.E. (Eds.): Contemporary Diagnosis and Management of Neonatal Respiratory Diseases, 2nd ed. Newton, Pa., Handbooks in Health Care (division of AMM Co.), 1998, pp. 95–99.

Speer, M.E., and Weisman, L.E.: Pneumonia. *In* Hansen, T.N., Cooper, T.R., and Weisman, L.E. (Eds.): Contemporary Diagnosis and Management of Neonatal Respiratory Diseases, 2nd ed. Newton, Pa., Handbooks in Health Care (division of AMM Co.), 1998, pp. 130–133.

Steinhorn, R.H., Millard, S.L., and Morin, F.C.: Persistent pulmonary hypertension of the newborn. Clin. Perinatol., 22(2):405–428, 1995.

Toce, S.S., Farrell, P.M., and Leavitt, L.A., et al.: Clinical and roentgenographic scoring systems for assessing bronchopulmonary dysplasia. Am. J. Dis. Child., *138*: 581–585, 1984.

Van Marter, L.J.: Persistent pulmonary hypertension of the newborn. *In* Cloherty, J.P., and Stark, A.R. (Eds.): Manual of Neonatal Care, 4th ed. Philadelphia, Lippincott-Raven, 1998, pp. 364–369.

Vohr, B.R., and Msall, M.E.: Neuropsychological and functional outcomes of low birth weight infants. Semin. Perinatol., *21*(3):202–220, 1997.

Weardon, M.E., and Hansen, T.N.: Persistent pulmonary hypertension of the newborn. *In* Hansen, T.N., Cooper, T.R., and Weisman, L.E. (Eds.): Contemporary Diagnosis and Management of Neonatal Respiratory Diseases, 2nd ed. Newton, Pa., Handbooks in Health Care (division of AMM Co.), 1998, pp. 100–109.

Welliver, R.C.: Respiratory syncytial virus immunoglobulin and monoclonal antibodies in the prevention and treatment of respiratory syncytial virus infection. Semin. Perinatol., 22(1):87–95, 1998.

Welty, S.E., and Hansen, T.N.: Pulmonary hemorrhage. *In* Hansen, T.N., Cooper, T.R., and Weisman, L.E. (Eds.): Contemporary Diagnosis and Management of Neonatal Respiratory Diseases, 2nd ed. Newton, Pa., Handbooks in Health Care (division of AMM Co.), 1998, p. 117.

Whitsett, J.A.: Composition and structure of pulmonary surfactant. *In* Boynton, B.R., Carlo, W.A., and Jobe, A.H. (Eds.): New Therapies for Neonatal Respiratory Failure. New York, Cambridge University Press, 1994 pp. 3–15.

Whitsett, L., and Pryhuber, G.S.: Acute respiratory disorders. *In* Avery, G.B., Fletcher, M.A., and MacDonald, M.G. (Eds.): Neonatology: Pathophysiology and Management of the Newborn, 4th ed. Philadelphia, J.B. Lippincott, 1994, pp. 429–452.

Wood, B.P.: The newborn chest. Radiol. Clin. North Am., *31*:667–676, 1993.

Young, T.E., and Mangum, O.B.: Neofax: A Manual of Drugs Used in Neonatal Care, 11th ed. Raleigh, N.C., Acorn Publishing, 1998.

Yu, V.Y., Wong, P.Y., Bajuk, B., Szymonowicz, W.: Pulmonary air leaks in extremely low birth weith infants. Arch. Dis. Child., *61*:239–241, 1986.

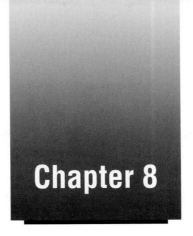

Chapter 8

Apnea of the Newborn Infant

Martha Goodwin

Objectives

1. Define types of apnea seen in the newborn infant.
2. Identify three causes of apnea.
3. Describe the pathogenesis of apnea in the premature infant.
4. Describe the evaluation process for the infant with apnea.
5. Discuss management techniques for controlling apnea.
6. Discuss the current status of home monitoring.

Apnea represents one of the most frequently encountered respiratory problems in the premature infant. It is not known why some infants are affected and others are not, although certain factors have a good predictive value. Apnea that presents in the first 24 hours has historically been perceived as pathologic, while that occurring later has most often been attributed to immaturity. The mechanism of action is not fully understood but can be characterized as an immature respiratory system faced with demands it is ill equipped to handle. This chapter will provide a comprehensive review of apnea of the newborn, including causes, evaluation, treatment and long term home follow up.

Definitions of Apnea

A. **Periodic breathing.**

1. Definition: regular respirations of up to 20 seconds, followed by apneic periods of no longer than 10 seconds, occurring at least three times in succession (Gibson, 1996).
2. Seen in fewer than 2% of well term infants and in 30% to 95% of healthy preterm infants more than 24 hours of age (Barrington and Finer, 1990; Glotzbach et al., 1989).
3. Not accompanied by cyanosis or changes in heart rate.

4. Episodes of periodic breathing in the preterm infant decrease significantly by 39 to 41 weeks' postconception age.
5. Controversy exists as to whether or not periodic breathing is associated with significant apnea or sudden infant death syndrome (SIDS). Recent studies suggest that periodic breathing is not associated with these two entities (Miller and Martin, 1998).

B. Apnea.

1. Definition: cessation of airflow for 20 seconds or longer, or a shorter pause in airflow that is accompanied by bradycardia (heart rate <100 bpm) or cyanosis (Gibson, 1996; Stark, 1991).
2. Most often associated with clinical symptoms such as color change, bradycardia, oxygen desaturation, or change in level of consciousness.
3. Most apnea occurs in the healthy preterm infant without organic disease. Up to 80% of infants weighing less than 1000 g and 25% weighing less than 2500 g at birth will have apnea during their neonatal course (Miller and Martin, 1998).

Types of Apnea

A. Primary apnea.

1. Definition: initial cessation of respiratory movements after a period of rapid respiratory effort as a result of asphyxia during the delivery process.
2. Exposure to stimulation and/or oxygen will usually induce spontaneous respiratory effort.

B. Secondary apnea.

1. Definition: apnea occurring after a period of deep, gasping respirations and fall in blood pressure and heart rate, brought about by prolonged asphyxia during the delivery process. The gasping becomes slower and weaker and then ceases.
2. Infant will not respond to stimulation and will require more vigorous resuscitation.
3. For each minute in secondary apnea before resuscitation, there is a 2-minute delay before gasping is reestablished and another 2 minutes before the onset of regular respirations.
4. It is not usually possible to distinguish primary from secondary apnea at birth (Bloom and Cropley, 1994).

C. Central apnea.

1. Definition: absence of airflow and respiratory effort.
2. Cause of central apnea in the preterm infant is not fully understood.
3. Contributing factors are thought to include (Miller and Martin, 1998):
   a. Chest wall afferent neuromuscular signals and chest wall instability.
   b. Diaphragmatic fatigue.
   c. Immature, paradoxical response of neonate to hypoxia and hypercapnia.
   d. Altered levels of local neurotransmitters in brain-stem region of CNS.
4. Fifteen percent of apnea episodes are central in origin.
5. Closure of upper airway occurs in about half of cases of central apnea (Ruggins and Milner, 1992).

D. Obstructive apnea.

1. Definition: absence of airflow with continued respiratory effort, associated with blockage of airway at level of pharynx (Miller and Martin, 1998) and/or larynx (Ruggins and Milner, 1992).
2. Hyperextension or flexion of the neck may induce obstruction of the airway.

3. May be caused by obstruction of airflow at the mouth or nose as a result of anatomic abnormalities such as macroglossia (Beckwith-Wiedemann syndrome, congenital hypothyroidism) or micrognathia (Pierre Robin sequence).
4. Up to 30% of apnea episodes are obstructive in origin (Ruggins and Milner, 1992).

E. Mixed apnea.

1. Definition: a combination of central and obstructive apnea.
2. Fifty to sixty percent of neonatal apnea episodes are mixed.

F. Idiopathic apnea, or "apnea of prematurity."

1. Diagnosis after exclusion of pathologic processes in the premature infant.
2. Not necessarily associated with the presence of periodic breathing (Barrington and Finer, 1990; Glotzbach et al., 1989; Holditch-Davis, Edwards, and Wigger, 1994).
3. Recurrent apnea seen in preterm infants who show no other abnormalities.
4. Onset within the first week of life, usually at 24–48 hours. If not present within the first week of life, will usually not appear unless later illness develops (Stark, 1991).
5. More likely to be obstructive than central in the first 2 days of life (Barrington and Finer, 1991; Henderson-Smart, 1981; Hertzberg and Lagercrantz, 1987).
6. Episodes of apnea cease by term in 95% of infants: may persist longer in infants born at less than 27 weeks' gestational age.

Pathogenesis of Apnea in the Premature Infant

A. Immature central respiratory center.

1. Decreased afferent traffic occurs as a result of:
   a. Poor CNS myelinization.
   b. Decreased number of synapses.
   c. Decreased dendritic arborization (Gerhardt and Bancalari, 1984; Henderson-Smart, 1981; Miller and Martin, 1998).
2. Decreased amounts of neurotransmitters have been measured in infants with apnea and may play an important role in respiratory control (Kattwinkel, 1977).
3. Fluctuating respiratory center output has been implicated.

B. Chemoreceptors.

1. Located in the medulla (central) and the carotid and aortic bodies (peripheral), chemoreceptors relay information to the respiratory center in the brain about pH, PO_2, and PCO_2 via the vagus and glossopharyngeal nerves.
   a. Hypoxemia is sensed in the carotid and aortic bodies and results in an increase in alveolar ventilation. Premature infants with apnea do not respond to hypoxemia as effectively as infants who do not have apnea (Menendez et al., 1996).
   b. Hypercapnia is sensed centrally. The normal response to an increased arterial PCO_2 is an increase in minute ventilation. Neonates can increase ventilation by only three to four times the baseline values, in comparison with the 10- to 20-fold increase that adults can obtain (Blackburn and Loper, 1992). Premature infants exhibit a blunted response to elevated PCO_2, resulting in ongoing hypoventilation and hypercapnia. This diminished response predisposes them to apnea.
2. Biphasic response of the premature infant to hypoxia.
   a. During the first minute of hypoxia, a brief increase in respiratory effort occurs. It is followed in the next 2–3 minutes by a decrease in respiratory

rate and by periodic breathing, respiratory depression, and apnea. Initial stimulation of the peripheral chemoreceptors is followed by overriding depression of the respiratory centers as a result of hypoxia (Miller and Martin, 1992).

    b. At 7–18 days of postnatal age, an infant can maintain the adult response to hypoxia of sustained hyperventilation.

  3. Depressed response to hypercapnia. The premature infant exhibits decreased sensitivity to increased levels of carbon dioxide, requiring higher levels of carbon dioxide to stimulate respirations (Anderson, Martin, and Fanaroff, 1983; Gerhardt and Bancalari, 1984; Miller and Martin, 1998).

C. Thermal afferents.

1. Apnea is increased in an environment that may be too warm for the infant (Kattwinkel, 1977).
2. Thermal receptors in the trigeminal area of the face produce an apneic response to stimulation by a cold gas mixture (Marchal, Bairan, and Vert, 1987).

D. Mechanoreceptors.

1. Stretch receptors alter the timing of respiration at various lung volumes.
    a. Head's paradoxical reflex: a gasp followed by apnea after abrupt lung inflation.
    b. Hering-Breuer reflex.
        (1) Vagally mediated, it acts to inhibit inspiration and/or prolong expiration.
        (2) Lung inflation initiates inhibitory impulses that terminate inspiration and prolong expiratory time.
        (3) Mechanoreceptors are very active in the neonate but rarely seen in the adult (Blackburn and Loper, 1992; Rigatto, 1992).
2. Pharyngeal collapse and airway obstruction are produced by negative pharyngeal pressure generated during inspiration.
3. Intercostal phrenic inhibitory reflex, an inward movement of the rib cage during inspiration, prematurely ends inspiration (Miller and Martin, 1998).

E. Protective reflexes.

1. Stimulation of the posterior portion of the pharynx with suctioning, endotracheal or gavage tube placement, or gastroesophageal reflux can stimulate apnea (Stark, 1991).
2. Pulmonary irritant receptors can produce an apneic response to direct bronchial stimulation (Martin, Miller, and Waldemar, 1986).
3. Laryngeal taste receptors can produce an apneic response to various chemical stimuli (Kattwinkel, 1977).

F. Sleep state.

1. Eighty percent of the neonate's day is spent in sleep.
2. Respiratory depression occurs predominantly in rapid eye movement (REM) or transitional sleep (Holditch-Davis et al., 1994; Stark, 1991).
    a. May be influenced by central mechanisms at the level of the brain stem (Stark, 1991).
        (1) May be due to a defect in a sleep-related feedback loop or respiratory command (Kriter and Blanchard, 1989).
        (2) Variability of respiratory rhythmicity is seen in active sleep (Miller and Martin, 1992).
    b. May be related to paradoxical respirations in which chest wall movements are out of phase, resulting in rib-cage collapse with abdominal expansion during inspiration. This would lead to a decrease in lung volume and functional residual capacity.

c. May be related to decreased skeletal muscle tone of the tongue and pharynx during sleep, which could lead to increased resistance and obstruction in the upper airway (Miller and Martin, 1998).

Causes of Apnea

A. **Prematurity.**

B. **Hypoxia.**

C. **Respiratory disorders.**

1. Respiratory distress syndrome.
2. Pneumonia.
3. Aspiration.
4. Acidosis.
5. Airway obstruction.
6. Pneumothorax.
7. Atelectasis.
8. Pulmonary hemorrhage.
9. Postextubation status.
10. Congenital anomalies of the upper airway.

D. **Cardiovascular disorders.**

1. Hypotension.
2. Arrhythmias.
3. Congestive heart failure.
4. Patent ductus arteriosus.

E. **Infection.**

1. Sepsis.
2. Pneumonia.
3. Meningitis.
4. Viral infections.
5. Necrotizing enterocolitis.

F. **CNS disorders.**

1. Congenital malformations.
2. Seizures.
3. Asphyxia.
4. Intracranial hemorrhage.
5. Kernicterus.
6. Tumors.

G. **Drugs.**

1. Maternal drugs.
   a. Narcotics.
   b. Analgesics.
   c. Anesthesia.
   d. Beta-blocker antihypertensive agents.
   e. Magnesium sulfate.
2. Neonatal drugs.
   a. Anticonvulsants: phenobarbital, pentobarbital.
   b. Cardiovascular drugs: prostaglandin E_1.
   c. Narcotics/analgesics.
      (1) Fentanyl (Sublimaze).
      (2) Morphine.

(3) Midazolam hydrochloride (Versed).

(4) Lorazepam (Ativan).

H. **Metabolic disorders.**

1. Hypocalcemia.
2. Hypoglycemia.
3. Hypomagnesemia.
4. Hyponatremia.
5. Acidosis.
6. Hyperammonemia.

I. **Hematopoietic disorders.**

1. Polycythemia.
2. Anemia.

J. **Reflex stimulation.**

1. Posterior pharyngeal stimulation.
2. Gastroesophageal reflux.

K. **Environmental factors.**

1. Rapid warming.
2. Hypothermia.
3. Hyperthermia.
4. Elevated environmental temperature.
5. Feeding.
6. Stooling.
7. Painful stimuli.

Evaluation for Apnea

A. **History.**

1. Perinatal risk factors.
   a. Maternal bleeding, drugs, fever, hypertension, prolonged rupture of membranes, polyhydramnios, chorioamnionitis, decreased fetal movements, abnormal fetal presentation.
   b. Fetal hypoxia, trauma.
2. Neonatal risk factors.
   a. Prematurity.
   b. Cardiorespiratory disease.
   c. Metabolic abnormalities.
   d. Temperature instability.
   e. Infection.
   f. Environmental causes.
   g. CNS disorders.

B. **Physical examination.** A complete physical and neurologic examination should be performed. Observe for congenital malformations, especially those involving the airway. Observe for signs of respiratory distress and heart disease. Abnormal behavior, tone, or posturing may be associated with a neurologic focus. An abdominal examination should be performed, which may reveal symptoms related to obstruction, infection, necrotizing enterocolitis, or congestive heart failure.

C. **Documentation of apnea episodes.** A record of apnea episodes should be maintained as part of the infant's record. This allows the caregiver to determine a pattern, if any, to the apnea. It may also provide information about precipitating events or specific events associated with the apnea. Information documented should include the following:

1. Duration of apnea episode.
2. Time of apnea episode and any relation to feeding, activity, stooling, sleep, or procedures.
3. Infant's position: prone or supine, with head of bed elevated or flat.
4. Associated bradycardia.
5. Associated color change and/or oxygen desaturation.
6. Type of stimulation required to resolve the episode:
   a. None, self-resolved.
   b. Gentle tactile stimulation.
   c. Vigorous tactile stimulation.
   d. Oxygen.
   e. Bag-mask ventilation.

D. Laboratory evaluation.

1. Basic evaluation to look for infection, respiratory deterioration, and metabolic problems.
   a. Complete blood cell count, with differential cell and platelet counts.
   b. Blood gas.
   c. Serum glucose, electrolytes, calcium.
   d. Blood culture, lumbar puncture for evaluation of cerebrospinal fluid, urine culture.
2. Extensive laboratory evaluation for less common causes of apnea.
   a. Toxicology screen.
   b. Urine collection for detection of amino acids and organic acids (metabolic screen).
   c. Serum ammonia.

E. Other.

1. Echocardiogram or electrocardiogram: may detect cardiac abnormality or conduction disorders.
2. Electroencephalogram: may confirm suspected seizures.
3. Chest x-ray film: may demonstrate respiratory or cardiac abnormalities.
4. Cranial ultrasound/Computerized tomography: may demonstrate structural abnormalities or hemorrhages.
5. Barium swallow and pH study: to evaluate pharyngeal function or gastro-esophageal reflux.
6. Polysomnogram: examines eye movements, muscle activity, end tidal CO_2, transcutaneous O_2 levels, oral or nasal airway, chest and abdominal wall movements, and cardiorespiratory patterns to detect type of apnea and relate it to sleep state. (Very rarely used.)
7. Pneumogram.
   a. Measures chest wall movement, heart rate, oxygen saturation, and nasal airflow by thermistor or carbon dioxide probe; measures esophageal pH.
   b. No predictive value for sudden infant death syndrome; newer recording monitors are as effective at detecting apnea over a prolonged period (Gibson, Spinner, and Cullen, 1996; National Institutes of Health, 1986; Stark, 1991).

Management Techniques

A. Treat underlying cause if determined.

B. Provide needed medical or surgical intervention.

C. Maintain environmental temperature at the low end of the neutral thermal zone.

D. Avoid triggering reflexes:
1. Vigorous catheter suctioning.
2. Hot or cold to the face.
3. Sudden gastric distention.

E. Maintain infant in the prone position whenever possible. Prone positioning is associated with higher oxygen saturation, shorter gastric emptying time, and decreased incidence of regurgitation and aspiration (Marchal et al., 1987). Supine positioning has been associated with an increase in apnea (Heimler et al., 1992; Kurlak et al., 1994) and severity of apneic episodes (Kurlak et al., 1994). Elevation of the head of the bed by 15 degrees reduces hypoxemic events in preterm infants (Jenni et al., 1997).

F. Maintain the neck in a neutral position, not flexed or hyperextended. Use of a neck roll is recommended.

G. Avoid vigorous manual ventilation to prevent intermittent hyperoxia, hypocapnia, and blunting of the CO_2 response.

H. Provide cutaneous stimulation, which increases the number of external stimuli to compensate for decreased afferent signals to the respiratory center (Marchal et al., 1987). Accomplish by using:
1. Irregularly oscillating water bed.
2. Rocking bed (Groswasser et al., 1995).
3. Touch.

I. Provide other sensory stimulation. Garcia and White-Traut (1993) showed termination of apnea episodes in a limited number of infants treated with oral application of lemon glycerine swabs.

J. Attempt to control apnea by avoiding painful stimuli, loud noises, extremely vigorous tactile stimulation, or potent odors.

K. Consider providing continuous positive airway pressure.
1. Increases end-expiratory lung volumes and splints the upper airway and weak chest wall, thereby improving compliance and oxygenation and decreasing respiratory muscle work so that diaphragmatic movements are less tiring and more effective (Miller and Martin, 1992).
2. Complicates gavage feedings and may increase risk of aspiration. Increases risk of air leak.

L. Pharmacologic therapy.
1. Methylxanthine (aminophylline/theophylline, caffeine), administered orally or intravenously. Used to treat apnea of prematurity after pathologic causes have been eliminated.
   a. Mechanisms of action include:
      (1) Stimulation of central respiratory chemoreceptors.
      (2) Increased ventilatory response to carbon dioxide.
      (3) Increased oxygenation.
      (4) Increased minute ventilation (theophylline).
      (5) Stabilization of oscillations in breathing (theophylline).
      (6) Improved diaphragmatic contractility.
      (7) Relaxation of bronchial smooth muscle (theophylline).
      (8) CNS excitation.
      (9) Increased respiratory drive.

  (10) Increased respiratory muscle activity.

  (11) Increased skeletal muscle activity (Blanchard and Aranda, 1986; Calhoun, 1996; Fanaroff and Martin, 1987).

 b. Pharmacokinetics.

  (1) Half-life of aminophylline/theophylline is approximately 30 hours.

  (2) Half-life of caffeine is approximately 100 hours.

  (3) Both theophylline and caffeine are rapidly absorbed intravenously. Oral absorption of caffeine is rapid, and oral absorption of theophylline is variable.

  (4) Metabolism of caffeine and theophylline takes place in the liver. This is slower in the neonate than in the adult.

  (5) Theophylline is metabolized to caffeine by a metabolic pathway unique to the preterm infant.

  (6) Serum concentrations must be checked to avoid toxic levels (Blanchard and Aranda, 1986; Calhoun, 1996).

 c. Dosage:

  (1) Aminophylline.

   (a) Route: IV.

   (b) Loading dose: 5 mg/kg.

   (c) Maintenance dose: 1–2 mg/kg every 8–12 hours.

   (d) Therapeutic level: 5–15 µg/mL.

  (2) Theophylline.

   (a) Route: by mouth.

   (b) Loading dose: 5 mg/kg.

   (c) Maintenance dose: 1–2 mg/kg every 8–12 hours.

   (d) Therapeutic level: 5–15 µg/mL.

  (3) Caffeine.

   (a) Route: IV or by mouth.

   (b) Loading dose: 10 mg/kg, caffeine base; 20 mg/kg, caffeine citrate.

   (c) Maintenance dose: 2.5 mg/kg, caffeine base; 5 mg/kg, caffeine citrate; every 24 hours.

   (d) Avoid use of caffeine benzoate preparation, which can displace bilirubin from albumin binding sites (Blanchard and Aranda, 1986; Marchal et al., 1987).

   (e) Therapeutic level: 5–20 µg/mL.

   (f) Higher doses and therapeutic levels have been studied, with no reported adverse effects, but not in common use (Lee et al., 1997; Scanlon et al., 1992).

 d. Side effects.

  (1) Caffeine: tachycardia, cardiac dysrhythmias, increased wakefulness, increased active sleep, gastrointestinal distention, gastrointestinal bleeding, and diuresis with sodium loss.

  (2) Theophylline: tachycardia, cardiac dysrhythmias, seizures, jitteriness, feeding intolerance, gastroesophageal reflux, dehydration, hyperglycemia, hypotension, increased cerebrovascular resistance (Calhoun, 1996).

 e. Caffeine versus theophylline.

  (1) Theophylline is a more potent vasodilator (Kriter and Blanchard, 1989).

  (2) Theophylline causes a more rapid and sustained tachycardia (Marchal et al., 1987; Scanlon et al., 1992).

  (3) Caffeine diffuses more rapidly in the CNS (Calhoun, 1996; Marchal et al., 1987).

  (4) Caffeine is given only once a day.

  (5) Caffeine has a wider therapeutic index (Scanlon et al., 1992).

  (6) Caffeine may be effective in apnea not responsive to theophylline and vice versa (Blanchard and Aranda, 1986).

(7) Caffeine has a longer half-life, resulting in smaller changes in its plasma concentration (Calhoun, 1996).

2. Doxapram.

a. Potent respiratory stimulant for apnea refractory to methylxanthine therapy.

b. Mechanism of action thought to be stimulation of the peripheral chemoreceptors at low doses (0.5 mg/kg per hour) and of the CNS at higher doses (Blanchard and Aranda, 1986; Brion et al., 1991).

c. Increases minute ventilation, tidal volume, and mean inspiratory flow and decreases PCO_2 (Brion et al., 1991).

d. Pharmacokinetics.

(1) Half-life is approximately 10 hours in the first few days of life and 8 hours at 10 days of age (Blanchard and Aranda, 1986).

(2) Steady-state levels are reached within 24 hours (Beaudry, Bradley, Gramlich, and LeGatt, 1988).

e. Dosage.

(1) Route: IV.

(2) Dosage range: 0.25–2.5 mg/kg per hour, administered by continuous infusion (Brion et al., 1991; Menendez et al., 1996; Peliowski and Finer, 1990).

(3) Controversy exists over therapeutic and toxic plasma levels. Guidelines include the following:

(a) Therapeutic level: less than 5 mg/L (Hayakawa et al., 1986).

(b) Toxic level: 5 mg/L. Levels greater than 3.5 mg/L may produce side effects (Marchal et al., 1987).

f. Side effects.

(1) Jitteriness, irritability, vomiting, seizures, abdominal distention, increased gastric residuals, hyperglycemia, and glycosuria (Hayakawa et al., 1986; Marchal et al., 1987).

(2) Hypertension, tachycardia, and increased cardiac output.

(3) Increased work of breathing resulting from respiratory stimulation; consequent increased oxygen consumption and carbon dioxide production; increased tidal volume and respiratory rate.

(4) Increased risk of intraventricular hemorrhage if used in first few days of life.

g. Contraindication: Use in newborn infant not recommended because preparation contains benzyl alcohol.

(1) Benzyl alcohol is associated with "gasping syndrome," characterized by metabolic acidosis, renal failure, liver failure, and cardiovascular collapse (Brion et al., 1991).

(2) Cumulative doses might be toxic for the liver, kidney, or brain (Brion et al., 1991; Miller and Martin, 1998).

M. **Assisted ventilation.** Used for apnea resistant to other methods of therapy.

Home Monitoring

A. **Effectiveness of home monitoring.** The Consensus Development Conference Statement on Infant Apnea and Home Monitoring (National Institutes of Health, 1986) states that cardiorespiratory monitoring is effective in preventing death from apnea for certain selected infants but is clearly inappropriate for others, with the primary objective being to serve the best interest of the infant based on the infant's history (Malloy and Hoffman, 1996).

B. **Indications for home monitoring.**

1. Premature infant with symptoms of idiopathic apnea of prematurity who is otherwise ready for hospital discharge.
2. A survivor of an apparent life threatening event (ALTE) defined as apnea, cyanosis, altered muscle tone, choking or gagging. Previously termed a near miss SIDS's.
3. Having two or more siblings with SIDS.
4. Tracheostomy.
5. A sleep apnea syndrome caused by a neurologic disorder, periodic breathing, upper airway abnormality, or idiopathic syndromes.
6. Other conditions of ill or high-risk infants, as determined on an individual basis.

C. **Home monitoring is not indicated in** prevention of SIDS in symptom-free, healthy infants (National Association of Apnea Professionals, 1996; Spinner, Gibson, Wrobel, and Spitzer, 1995; Whitaker, 1995).

D. **Monitoring technology.**

1. Transthoracic impedance combined with electrocardiography is current standard.
   a. Electrodes are placed on infant's chest or inside an adjustable belt worn around the chest.
   b. A small electric current passes between the electrodes. The impedance to this current is measured as the chest wall diameter changes. Monitor senses this change, which is equated with respiration.
   c. Electrocardiograph reads cardiac activity.
   d. High and low limits for respirations and heart rate are set by the clinician.
   e. Monitor is compact and portable, weighing less than 5 pounds. A battery pack is available for use outside the home (Spinner et al., 1995).
2. Technical problems include artifact from signal interference, false alarms caused by shallow breathing, and the monitor's inability to detect obstructive apnea. Incorrect placement of leads can result in false alarms as well (Spinner et al., 1995).
3. Recent advances in technology allow recording of home monitor events for evaluation by the clinician.
   a. Recording of events allows monitoring of compliance.
   b. True events can be distinguished from false alarms.
   c. Fewer rehospitalizations are needed.
   d. Recording is as sensitive as a pneumogram for evaluating whether monitoring can be discontinued.
   e. Fewer monitor days are needed for infants without events (Gibson et al., 1996; Spinner et al., 1995).

E. **Follow-up care.**

1. Multidisciplinary team includes physician, nurse, social worker, and equipment company representatives.
2. Family and other caretakers of the infant are trained in cardiopulmonary resuscitation before hospital discharge. Thorough education in use of the monitor is also provided before discharge.
3. Care includes close telephone contact—within 24 hours after discharge and every week to 2 weeks afterward as needed.
4. Visiting nurse makes home visit within the first week and then as needed.
5. A team member is available 24 hours a day for answering questions and solving problems. Equipment company representative is available as needed for problems and information.
6. Home follow-up does not replace routine clinic follow-up (Gibson et al., 1996; National Association of Apnea Professionals, 1996; Spinner et al., 1995).

REFERENCES

Andersen, J.V., Jr., Martin, R.J., and Fanaroff, M.B.: Neonatal respiratory control and apnea of prematurity. Perinatology-Neonatology, 7(7):65–70, 1983.

Barrington, K., and Finer, N.: Periodic breathing and apnea in preterm infants. Pediatr Res., 27:188–121, 1990.

Barrington, K., and Finer, N.: The natural history of the appearance of apnea of prematurity. Pediatr. Res., 29:372–375, 1991.

Beaudry, M.A., Bradley, J.M., Gramlich, L.M., and LeGatt, D.: Pharmacokinetics of doxapram in idiopathic apnea of prematurity. Dev. Pharmacol. Ther. 11:65–72, 1988.

Blackburn, S.T., and Loper, D.L.: Maternal, Fetal and Neonatal Physiology. Philadelphia, W.B. Saunders, 1992, pp. 262–335.

Blanchard, P.W., and Aranda, J.V.: Drug treatment of neonatal apnea. Perinatology-Neonatology, 10(2):21–28, 1986.

Bloom, R.S., and Cropley, C.: Textbook of Neonatal Resuscitation. Dallas, American Heart Association, 1994.

Brion, L., Vega-Rich, C., Reinersman, G., et al.: Low-dose doxapram for apnea unresponsive to aminophylline in very low birth weight infants. J. Perinatol., 11:359–363, 1991.

Calhoun, L.K.: Pharmacologic management of apnea of prematurity. J. Perinat. Neonat. Nurs., 9(4):56–62, 1996.

Garcia, A.P., and White-Traut, R.: Preterm infants' responses to taste/smell and tactile stimulation during an apneic episode. J. Pediatr. Nurs., 8(4):245–251, 1993.

Gerhardt, T., and Bancalari, E.: Apnea of prematurity. I. Lung function and regulation of breathing. Pediatrics, 74:58–62, 1984.

Gibson, E.: Apnea. In Spitzer, A. (Ed.): Intensive Care of the Fetus and Neonate. St Louis, Mosby–Yearbook, 1996, pp. 470–481.

Gibson, E., Spinner, S., Cullen, J., et al.: Documented home apnea monitoring: Effect of compliance, duration of monitoring, and validation of alarm reporting. Clin. Pediatr., October: 505–513. 1996.

Glotzbach, S.F., Baldwin, R.B., Lederer, B.A., et al.: Periodic breathing in preterm infants: Incidence and characteristics. Pediatrics, 84:785–792, 1989.

Groswasser, J., Sottiaux, M., Rebuffat, E., et al.: Reduction in obstructive breathing events during body rocking: A controlled polygraphic study in preterm and full term infants. Pediatrics, 96(1 Pt1):64–68, July 1995.

Hayakawa, F., Hakamada, S., Juno, K., et al.: Doxapram in the treatment of idiopathic apnea of prematurity: Desirable dosage and serum concentrations. J. Pediatr., 109:138–140, 1986.

Heimler, R., Langlois, J., Hodel, D., et al.: Effect of positioning on the breathing pattern of preterm infants. Arch. Dis. Child., 67:312–314, 1992.

Henderson-Smart, D.: The effect of gestational age on the incidence and duration of recurrent apnoea in newborn babies. Aust. Paediatr. J., 17:273–276, 1981.

Hertzberg, T., and Lagercrantz, H.: Postnatal sensitivity of the peripheral chemoreceptors in newborn infants. Arch. Dis. Child., 62:1238–1241, 1987.

Holditch-Davis, D., Edwards, L.J., and Wigger, M.C.: Pathologic apnea and brief respiratory pauses in preterm infants: Relation to sleep state. Nurs. Res., 43(5): 293–299, 1994.

Jenni, O.G., von Siebenthal, K., Wolf, M., et al.: Effects of nursing in the head-elevated tilt position (15 degrees) on the incidence of bradycardia and hypoxemia episodes in preterm infants. Pediatrics, 100:622–625, 1997.

Kattwinkel, J.: Neonatal apnea: Pathogenesis and therapy. J. Pediatr., 90:342–347, 1977.

Kriter, K.E., and Blanchard, J.: Management of apnea in infants. Clin. Pharm., 8:577–587, 1989.

Kurlak, L.O., Ruggins, N.R., and Stephenson, T.J.: Effect of nursing position on incidence, type, and duration of clinically significant apnoea in preterm infants. Arch. Dis. Child., 71:F16–F19, 1994.

Lee, T.C., Charles, B., Steer, P., et al.: Population pharmacokinetics of intravenous caffeine in neonates with apnea of prematurity. Clin. Pharmacol. Ther., 61:628–640, 1997.

Malloy, M.H., and Hoffman, H.J.: Home apnea monitoring and sudden infant death syndrome. Prev. Med., 25:645–649, 1996.

Marchal, F., Bairan, A., and Vert, P.: Neonatal apnea and apneic syndromes. Clin. Perinatol., 14:509–529, 1987.

Martin, R.J., Miller, M.J., and Waldemar, A.C.: Pathogenesis of apnea in preterm infants. J. Pediatr., 109:733–741, 1986.

Menendez, A., Alea, O.A., Beckerman, R.C., et al.: Control of ventilation and apnea. In Goldsmith, J., and Karotkin, E.: Assisted Ventilation of the Neonate, 3rd ed. Philadelphia, W.B. Saunders, 1996, pp. 69–81.

Miller, M.J., Fanaroff, A.A., and Martin, R.: Respiratory disorders in preterm and term infants. In Fanaroff, A., and Martin, R. (Eds.): Neonatal-Perinatal Medicine, 6th ed. St. Louis, Mosby, 1997, pp. 1055–1059.

Miller, M.J., and Martin, R.J.: Apnea of Prematurity. Clin. Perinatol., 19:789–808, 1992.

Miller, M., and Martin, R.: Pathophysiology of apnea of prematurity. In Polin, R., and Fox, W. (Eds.): Fetal and Neonatal Physiology, 2nd ed. Philadelphia, W.B. Saunders, 1998, pp. 1129–1140.

National Association of Apnea Professionals: Guidelines for the provision of services to families using infant apnea monitors. Neonatal Intensive Care, May/June: 10–15, 1996.

National Institutes of Health: Consensus Development Conference Statement on Infant Apnea and Home Monitoring. NIH Consensus Statement, 6(6):1–10, 1986.

Peliowski, A., and Finer, N.: A blinded, randomized, placebo-controlled trial to compare theophylline and doxapram for the treatment of apnea of prematurity. J. Pediatr., 116:648–653, 1990.

Rigatto, H.: Maturation of breathing. In Hunt, C. (Ed.). Clin. Perinatol., 19:739–756, 1992.

Ruggins, N.R., and Milner, A.D.: Site of upper airway obstruction in preterm infants with problematical apnea. Neonatal Intensive Care, March/April, 1992.

Scanlon, J., Chin, K., Morgan, M., et al.: Caffeine or theophylline for neonatal apnoea? Arch. Dis. Child., 67:425–428, 1992.

Spinner, S., Gibson, E., Wrobel, H., and Spitzer, A.: Recent advances in home infant apnea monitoring. Neonatal Network, 14(8):39–46, 1995.

Stark, A.: Disorders of respiratory control in infants. Respir. Care, 36:673–682, 1991.

Whitaker, S.: The art and science of home infant apnea monitoring in the 1990s. J. Obstet. Gynecol. Neonatal Nurs., 24(1):84–89, 1995.

ADDITIONAL READINGS

Adams, J.A., Zabaleta, I.A., and Slacker, M.A.: Respiratory events during cardiac deceleration in premature newborns. Neonatal Intensive Care, November/December: 18–24, 1995.

Ahmann, E.: Family impact of home apnea monitoring:: An overview of research and its clinical implications. Neonatal Intensive Care, July/August: 26–48, 1993.

Barrington, K.J., Finer, N.N., Torok-Both, G., et al.: Dose-response relationship of doxapram in the therapy of refractory idiopathic apnea of prematurity. Pediatrics, *80:*22–27, 1987.

Devlieger, H., Daniels, H., Marchal, G., et al.: The diaphragm of the newborn infant: Anatomical and ultrasonographic studies. J. Dev. Physiol., *16:*321–329, 1991.

Frank, M.: Theophylline: A closer look. Neonatal Network, *6*(2):7–13, 1987.

Gerhardt, T., and Bancalari, E.: Apnea of prematurity. I. Lung function and regulation of breathing. Pediatrics, *74:*58–62, 1984.

Hayakawa, F., Hakamada, S., Juno, K., et al.: Doxapram in the treatment of idiopathic apnea of prematurity: Desirable dosage and serum concentrations. J. Pediatr., *109:* 138–140, 1986.

Heldt, G.P.: Development of stability of the respiratory system in preterm infants. J. Appl. Physiol., *65*(1):441–444, 1988.

Hodgman, J.E., Hoppenbrouwers, T., and Cabal, L.: Episodes of bradycardia during early infancy in the term-born and preterm infant. Am. J. Dis. Child., *147:*960–964, 1993.

Hodson, W.A., and Troug, W.E.: Critical care of the newborn, 2nd ed. Philadelphia, W.B. Saunders, 1989, p. 73.

Keyes, W.G., Donohue, P.K., Spivak, F.L., et al.: Assessing the need for transfusion of premature infants and role of hematocrit, clinical signs, and erythropoietin level. Pediatrics *84:*412–417, 1989.

Koons, A.H., Mojica, N., Jadeja, N., et al.: Neurodevelopmental outcome of infants with apnea of infancy. Am. J. Perinatol., *10:*208–211, 1993.

Krauss, A.N.: Apnea in infancy: Pathophysiology, diagnosis and treatment. N Y State J. Med., *86*(2):89–96, 1986.

Lott, D.: Home apnea monitoring: An update. Perinatology-Neonatology, July/August: 22–37, 1988.

Meadows, W., Mendez, D., Lantos, J., et al.: What is the legal "standard of medical care" when there is no standard of medical care? Neonatal Intensive Care, May/June: 43, 1992.

Nathanson, I., O'Donnell, J., and Commins, M.: Cardiorespiratory patterns during alarms in infants using apnea/bradycardia monitors. Am. J. Dis. Child., *143:* 476–480, 1989.

Poets, C.F., Stebbens, V.A., and Samuels, M.P.: The relationship between bradycardia, apnea, and hypoxemia in preterm infants. Pediatr. Res., *34*(2):144–147, 1993.

Rowland, T., Donnelly, J., Landis, J., et al.: Infant home apnea monitoring: A five-year assessment. Clin. Pediatr., *26*(8):384–387, 1987.

Ryan, C.A., Finer, N.N., and Peters, K.L.: Nasal intermittent positive-pressure ventilation offers no advantages over nasal continuous positive airway pressure in apnea of prematurity. Am. J. Dis. Child., *143:*1196–1198, 1989.

Strute, H., Greiner, B., and Linderkamp, O.: Effect of blood transfusion on caridorespiratory abnormalities in preterm infants. Arch. Dis. Child., *72:*F194–F196, 1995.

Swanson, J., and Berseth, C.: Continuing care for the preterm infant after dismissal from the neonatal intensive care unit. Mayo Clin. Proc. *62:*613–622, 1987.

Toong, C.L., Charles, B.G., Steer, P.A., and Flenady, V.J.: Saliva as a valid alternative to serum in monitoring intravenous caffeine treatment for apnea of prematurity. Ther. Drug Monit., *18:*288–293, 1996.

Walther, F., Erickson, R., and Sims, M.: Cardiovascular effects of caffeine therapy in preterm infants. Am. J. Dis. Child., *144:*1164–1166, 1990.

Weintraub, Z., Alvaro, R., Kwiatkowski, K., et al.: Effects of inhaled oxygen (up to 40%) on periodic breathing and apnea in preterm infants. J. Appl. Physiol., *72:*116–120, 1992.

Chapter 9

Assisted Ventilation

Elizabeth Kirby

Objectives

1. Identify the concepts of FRC, TV, VC, and TLC and describe their importance in the physiology of ventilation.

2. Describe the concepts of elastic recoil, compliance, resistance, and gas trapping and their importance in ventilating the lungs of the newborn infant.

3. Explain the relationship of fetal hemoglobin, pH, and temperature to the oxyhemoglobin dissociation curve.

4. List potential causes of respiratory and metabolic acid-base disturbance in the newborn infant. Identify ranges of pH, Pao_2, $Paco_2$, HCO_3^-, and base excess/deficit in various respiratory disease states in the newborn infant.

5. Identify treatment modalities for neonates in respiratory distress.

6. Describe various types of mechanical ventilation devices available for the neonate.

7. List nursing interventions required to care for ventilated infants, based on the theories of mechanical ventilation.

8. Differentiate among the three types of high-frequency ventilation: jet, oscillatory, and high-frequency positive-pressure ventilation.

9. Identify the nursing interventions required for high-frequency ventilation that differ from those required for conventional ventilation.

10. Identify changes in patient status that indicate potential complications with assisted ventilation.

11. Describe various medications used to enhance lung status in the ventilated patient.

Caring for an infant requiring assisted ventilation is a challenge. It is necessary for the nurse to understand the normal pulmonary physiology as well as the pathophysiology of pulmonary diseases in the neonate. An understanding of the basic mechanical principles of various ventilators is important to providing optimal care for a neonate. New ventilation techniques are being developed rapidly, and the choices for ventilating the neonate are greater now than ever before. The focus of this chapter is to provide the basic knowledge needed to care for the infant requiring oxygen therapy or mechanical ventilation.

Physiology

A. Definitions (Harris and Wood, 1996).

1. Tidal volume (TV): the amount of air that moves into or out of the lungs with each single breath at rest (6–8 mL/kg).
2. Vital capacity (VC): the volume of air maximally inspired and maximally expired (40 mL/kg).
3. Functional residual capacity (FRC): the volume of gas that remains in the lungs after a normal expiration (30 mL/kg).
4. Total lung capacity (TLC): the amount of air contained in the lung after a maximal inspiration (63 mL/kg).
5. Physiologic dead space: anatomic plus alveolar dead space (Loper, 1997).
   a. Anatomic dead space: the volume of gas within the area of the pulmonary conducting airways that cannot engage in gas exchange.
   b. Alveolar dead space: the volume of inspired gas that reaches the alveoli but does not participate in gas exchange because of inadequate perfusion to those alveoli.
6. Mechanical dead space: gas that fills the ventilator circuit for availability in inspiration, as well as exhaled gas. Minimal dead space is desirable. Excessive dead space can cause increased retention of carbon dioxide.

B. Concepts.

1. Elastic recoil: the natural tendency for a stretched object to return to the original resting volume. With inhalation, alveoli stretch to a certain point, and during exhalation the alveoli return to their original size in an infant with normal lungs.
2. Lung compliance: the change in volume that occurs with a change in pressure (elasticity of the lung). It also refers to the relationship between a given change in volume and the pressure required to produce that change. An infant with severe hyaline membrane disease will have decreased compliance (because of lack of surfactant) requiring increased pressure to overcome the pressure generated by the increased surface tension. The major force contributing to elastic recoil of the lung is surface tension at the air-liquid interface in distal bronchioles and alveoli. The amount of distal airway pressure needed to counteract the tendency of the alveoli and bronchioles to collapse is demonstrated by the Laplace relationship: the relationship between pressure, surface tension, and the radius of a structure. The pressure needed to stabilize an alveolus is directly proportional to twice the surface tension and inversely proportional to the radius of that alveolus.
3. Lung resistance: the result of friction between moving parts. It refers to the relationship between a given change in pressure and a given change in flow. Resistance to gas in a 2.5 mm endotracheal tube (ETT) is higher than in a 3.5 mm ETT because of the narrow lumen of the smaller tube. It takes greater pressure to force air through a small tube. Anatomic sources of resistance in the newborn infant include nasal passages, the glottis, the trachea, and the main bronchi. During intubation the ETT is also a source of resistance.
4. Gas trapping: more gas entering the lung than leaving the lung. A partially occluded ETT can cause gas trapping. Debris from meconium can allow gas into the lung but may occlude the airway during exhalation (known as a ball-valve effect).

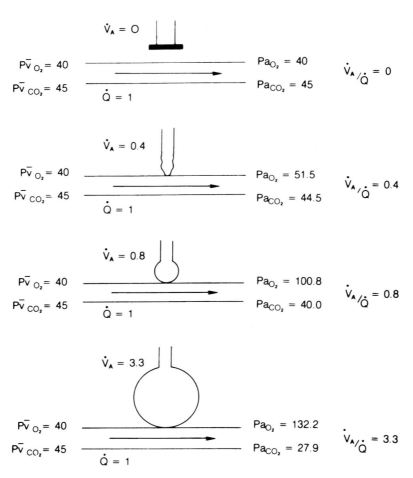

Figure 9–1

Effects of various ventilation-perfusion ratios on blood gas tensions. *A,* Direct venoarterial shunting ($\dot{V}A/\dot{Q} = 0$). Venous gas tensions are unaltered, and arterial blood has the same tension as venous blood. *B,* Alveolus with a low $\dot{V}A/\dot{Q}$ ratio. Only partial oxygenation and CO_2 removal take place in this alveolus because of underventilation in relation to perfusion. *C,* Normal alveolus. *D,* Underperfused alveolus with high $\dot{V}A/\dot{Q}$ ratio. Note that although the oxygen tension is 32 mm greater than alveolus *C,* this results in only a slightly higher saturation and O_2 content. (From Thibeault, D.W., and Gregory, G.A.: Neonatal Pulmonary Care. Norwalk, Conn., Appleton-Century-Crofts, 1986.)

5. Inadvertent positive end-expiratory pressure (PEEP): a result of gas trapping in which volume and pressure increase in the distal airways through end expiration. Providing oxygen by nasal cannula can result in inadvertent PEEP in the small premature infant.

6. Ventilation-perfusion ratio ($\dot{V}A/\dot{Q}C$) (Fig. 9–1). Matching pulmonary ventilation and perfusion is necessary for efficient gas exchange. The relationship between ventilation and perfusion is expressed as a ratio and describes the relationship between alveolar ventilation and capillary perfusion of the lungs. A 1:1 ratio indicates that the alveoli are in perfect contact with the pulmonary capillaries, allowing exchange of O_2 and CO_2. A $\dot{V}A/\dot{Q}C$ ratio of zero indicates

a shunt whereby no ventilation occurs during passage of blood through the lungs. Abnormalities of the $\dot{V}_A/\dot{Q}_C$ ratio may be due to:

    a. Too much or too little ventilation with normal blood flow.

    b. Too much or too little blood flow with normal ventilation.

    c. Combination of the above.

7. Mean airway pressure (MAP): mean or average pressure transmitted to the airways during a series of respiratory cycles (Harris and Wood, 1996). MAP is the sum of the ventilator rate, gas flow through the ventilator circuit, peak inspiratory pressure (PIP), PEEP, and inspiratory time. Increasing MAP can greatly influence the management of respiratory distress in decreasing atelectasis and true intrapulmonary shunting and is a useful tool in determining oxygenation.

C. Oxygen transport.

1. The amount of oxygen that can be delivered to the tissues is dependent on cardiac output and the oxygen content of the blood.

2. Oxygen is transported to tissue cells bound reversibly to hemoglobin and dissolved in plasma O_2. The amount of O_2 that is dissolved in the plasma is small (0.3 mL of O_2 dissolved in 100 mL of plasma per 100 mm Hg of O_2) compared with the amount that is bound to hemoglobin (1.34 mL of O_2 per gram of 100% saturated hemoglobin).

3. The amount of oxygen carried in the blood by hemoglobin depends on the hemoglobin concentration and the percent saturation of the hemoglobin. Adequate saturation is affected by the amount of hemoglobin available. Hemoglobin is almost fully saturated at a P_{O_2} of 80–100 mm Hg.

4. The binding of oxygen to hemoglobin varies with the Pa_{O_2}. The relationship is nonlinear and gives rise to an S-shaped curve—the oxyhemoglobin dissociation curve. The amount of oxygen that combines with hemoglobin at a given P_{O_2} depends on the position of the hemoglobin-oxygen dissociation curve (Fig. 9–2). Factors that determine the position of the dissociation curve are:

    a. Concentration of 2,3-diphosphoglycerate and the proportion of hemoglobin A (adult) to hemoglobin F (fetal).

    b. Temperature.

    c. P_{CO_2}.

    d. pH.

Figure 9–2
Hemoglobin-oxygen dissociation curve. Nonlinear or S-shaped oxyhemoglobin curve and the linear or straight-line dissolved O_2 relationships between the O_2 saturation (Sa_{O_2}) and the P_{O_2}. Total blood O_2 content is shown with division into a portion combined with hemoglobin and a portion physically dissolved at various levels of P_{O_2}. Also shown are the major factors that change the O_2 affinity for hemoglobin and thus shift the oxyhemoglobin dissociation curve either to the left or to the right. *DPG*, 2,3-Diphosphoglycerate. (Modified from West, J.B. Respiratory Physiology: The Essentials, 2nd ed. Baltimore, Williams & Wilkins, 1979, pp. 71, 73.)

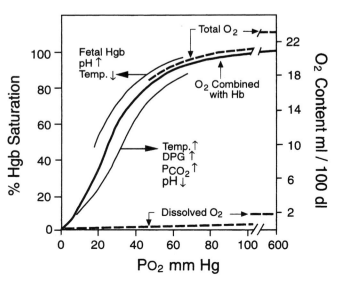

5. With decreased affinity (shift to the right), hemoglobin releases O_2 more easily to the tissues.
6. With increased affinity (shift to the left), oxygen is unloaded less rapidly and efficiently in the peripheral tissues.

D. **Control of breathing.** (Goldsmith and Karotkin, 1996). Control of ventilation (Table 9–1) is affected by both neurologic and chemical factors. The neurologic factors include CNS maturity, sleep state, and reflexes. The chemoreflexes include responses to hypoxemia, hyperoxia, and hypercapnia.

E. **Hypoxia.** Delivery of O_2 to tissues is inadequate. Causes include:
1. Heart failure.
2. Anemia. Hemoglobin available to transport oxygen is reduced although completely saturated. PaO_2 levels are usually normal.

Table 9–1
FACTORS AFFECTING CONTROL OF VENTILATION IN THE SPONTANEOUSLY BREATHING NEONATE

A. Neurologic Factors
1. "Maturity" of the CNS
   a. Degree of *myelination*, which largely determines speed of impulse transmission and response time to stimuli affecting ventilation
   b. Degree of *arborization*, or dendritic interconnections (synapses) between neurons, allowing summation of excitatory potentials coming in from other parts of the CNS, and largely setting the neuronal depolarization threshold and response level of the respiratory center
2. Sleep state (i.e., rapid eye movement, or REM, sleep vs. quiet or non-REM sleep)
   a. *REM sleep* is generally associated with irregular respirations (both in depth and frequency), distortion, and paradoxical motion of the rib cage during inspiration, inhibition of Hering-Breuer and glottic closure reflexes, and blunted response to CO_2 changes
   b. *Quiet sleep* is generally associated with regular respirations, a more stable rib cage, and a directly proportional relationship between Pco_2 and degree of ventilation
3. Reflex responses
   a. *Hering-Breuer reflex*, whereby inspiratory duration is limited in response to lung inflation sensed by stretch receptors located in major airways. Not present in adult humans, this reflex is very active during quiet sleep of newborn babies but absent or very weak during REM sleep
   b. *Head's reflex*, whereby inspiratory effort is further increased in response to rapid lung inflation. Thought to produce the frequently observed "biphasic sighs" of newborn infants that may be crucial for promoting and maintaining lung inflation (and therefore breathing regularity) after birth
   c. *Intercostal-phrenic reflex*, whereby inspiration is inhibited by proprioception (position-sensing) receptors in intercostal muscles responding to distortion of the lower rib cage during REM sleep
   d. *Trigeminal-cutaneous reflex*, whereby tidal volume increases and respiratory rate decreases in response to facial stimulation

   e. *Glottic closure reflex*, whereby the glottis is narrowed through reflex contraction of the laryngeal adductor muscles during respiration, "breaking" exhalation and increasing subglottic pressure (as with expiratory "grunting")

B. Chemical Drive Factors (Chemoreflexes)
1. *Response to hypoxemia (falling Pao_2) or to decrease in O_2 concentration breathed* (mediated by peripheral chemoreceptors in carotid and aortic bodies):
   a. Initially there is increase in depth of breathing (tidal volume), but subsequently (if hypoxia persists or worsens), there is depression of respiratory drive, reduction in depth and rate of respiration, and eventual failure of arousal
   b. For the first week of life, at least, these responses are dependent on environmental temperature (i.e., keeping the baby warm)
   c. Hypoxia is associated with an increase in periodic breathing and apnea
2. *Response to hyperoxia* (increase in Fio_2 breathing causes a transient respiratory depression, stronger in term than in preterm infants
3. *Response to hypercapnia (rising $Paco_2$ or [H^+]) or to increase in CO_2 concentration breathed* (mediated by central chemoreceptors in the medulla):
   a. Increase in ventilation is directly proportional to inspired CO_2 concentration (or, more accurately stated, to alveolar CO_2 tension), as is the case in adults
   b. Response to CO_2 is in large part dependent on sleep state: in quiet sleep, a rising $Paco_2$ causes increase in depth and rate of breathing, whereas during REM sleep the response is irregular and reduced in depth and rate. The degree of reduction closely parallels the amount of rib cage deformity occurring during REM sleep
   c. Ventilatory response to CO_2 in newborn infants is markedly depressed during behavioral activity such as feeding, and easily depressed by sedatives and anesthesia

From Goldsmith, J.P., and Karotkin, E.H.: Assisted Ventilation of the Neonate, 3rd ed. Philadelphia, W.B. Saunders, 1996, p. 26.

3. Abnormal hemoglobin. O_2 is not released to the tissues.
   a. Methemoglobin.
   b. Bart's hemoglobin.
4. Shock.

F. **Hypoxemia.** O_2 content of arterial blood is low because of extrapulmonary or intrapulmonary shunts. The blood has bypassed adequately ventilated alveoli.
1. Intrapulmonary shunt.
   a. Ventilation-perfusion mismatch caused by lung diseases such as atelectasis, hyaline membrane disease, and pneumonia.
   b. Can occur whenever alveoli are inadequately ventilated (hypoventilation).
2. Extrapulmonary shunt.
   a. Cyanotic congenital heart disease. Abnormal heart structure causes blood to bypass the lungs for oxygenation.
   b. Pulmonary artery hypertension. Blood shunts from the right side of the heart to the left side via a patent foramen ovale or ductus arteriosus, or both, causing blood to bypass the lungs.
      (1) Comparison of the PaO_2 or O_2 saturation of preductal and postductal blood can help determine whether a right-to-left shunt is present.
      (2) In the presence of shunting, preductal blood obtained from the right radial artery has a greater than 5% difference in saturation from postductal blood obtained from the umbilical artery or posterior tibial artery.

Treatment Modalities

A. **Blow-by oxygen.** Free flow of O_2 from a bag and mask or flow of O_2 through O_2 tubing near the infant's face may be useful for short-term O_2 delivery to an infant who is breathing but needs an O_2-enriched atmosphere for oxygenation (i.e., in the delivery room, during caregiving activities, during placement of an IV line into the scalp, during weighing). There is no way to determine the exact content of O_2 delivered to the infant. O_2 content depends on O_2 concentration, flow rate, the distance of the O_2 source from the baby, and the ventilatory efforts of the infant.

B. **Oxygen hood.** Warm, humidified oxygen is provided at a measured concentration via a plastic hood placed over the infant's head.
1. Indications are respiratory distress, hypoxemia, and cyanosis.
2. Disadvantages are the necessity of restraining the infant's movements, temperature instability, loss of O_2 when hood is removed, and the possibility that the oxygen tubing will become disconnected from the hood.
3. O_2 concentration must be measured with an appropriately calibrated oxygen analyzer.
4. Pulse oximeter should be used to monitor O_2 saturation.
5. Adequate gas flow is required to avoid CO_2 accumulation within the hood.
6. Hood size should be appropriate to the size of the infant.

C. **Nasal cannula.** Humidified O_2 is delivered at a set flow rate via a cannula, with the flow directed into the nares.
1. Conventional nasal cannula. O_2 is delivered at 100% through the cannula and is regulated by the flow (measured in liters). Low-flow meters are capable of delivering amounts as small as 0.02 L/min.
2. High-flow nasal cannula. Flow is 0.5–2 L/min, with oxygen blended to a known concentration.
3. Indications. A nasal cannula is needed for low oxygen requirement in an oxygen hood (<30%), prolonged oxygen requirement as in chronic lung

disease, transfer or transport, and increased mobility of the infant for feedings or for other developmental activities.

4. Complications. Pressure-related tissue damage may occur because of improper or infrequent changing, O_2 concentration may vary, hypoxemia may result from a displaced cannula, and the cannula may be occluded by nasal secretions (may cause significant respiratory distress).

D. **Continuous positive airway pressure (CPAP).**

1. Mask CPAP: Delivery of positive pressure (2–8 cm H_2O pressure) with variable amounts of O_2 via face mask. Requires appropriate size mask and tight seal around the nose and mouth.
   a. Indications: atelectasis, apnea, respiratory distress, and pulmonary edema.
   b. Advantages: short-term use to assist with alveolar expansion and to inhibit alveolar collapse (atelectasis); intubation not required.
   c. Complications: pulmonary hyperexpansion potentially leading to air leaks (i.e., pneumothorax, pneumomediastinum), aspiration of stomach contents, and ineffective ventilation leading to increasing respiratory difficulty.
2. Nasal CPAP: continuous positive airway pressure (generally 4–8 cm H_2O pressure) delivered by prongs that fit into the nares, in addition to a measured concentration of oxygen.
   a. Indications: atelectasis, apnea, respiratory distress, pulmonary edema, and need for prolonged mask CPAP.
   b. Advantage: intubation not required.
   c. Complications: ineffective ventilation, variable pressure delivery when infant's mouth is open, molding of the head from securing straps, erosion of the septum from poorly fitting prongs, agitation, dislodging of prongs by an active infant, and gastric distention.
3. Nasopharyngeal CPAP: continuous positive airway pressure delivered by ETT, which is passed through one of the nares and positioned with the tip of the tube in the oropharynx.
   a. Indications: atelectasis, apnea, respiratory distress, and pulmonary edema.
   b. Advantage: stable placement of tube, which an infant is less likely to dislodge than with nasal CPAP.
   c. Disadvantages: need for a skilled provider to place the tube, possible damage to the nasal septum and oropharynx, more invasive than other forms of CPAP, variable pressure delivery when infant's mouth is open, and gastric distention.
4. Endotracheal CPAP: continuous positive pressure delivered via an ETT placed orally or nasally into the trachea.
   a. Indications: atelectasis, apnea, respiratory distress, pulmonary edema, improved pulmonary suctioning, upper airway obstruction, and CNS disorders.
   b. Advantage: constant delivery of O_2 and pressure.
   c. Disadvantage: skilled provider required for intubation.
   d. Complications: malpositioned or dislodged tube, trauma resulting from intubation, port of entry for pathogens, hypoventilation, mucous plugging, possible airway injury (subglottic stenosis, laryngomalacia, tracheomalacia) with prolonged use, and increased risk of pulmonary air leaks.
5. Mechanical ventilation: respiratory support of infant using mechanical assistance.
   a. Gas exchange mechanisms in spontaneous and conventional mechanical ventilation:
      (1) Convection (bulk flow) in large airways goes to approximately the eighth bronchial generation. Gas moves along a negative pressure gradient from the upper airways to the alveoli.

(2) Molecular diffusion occurs in terminal airways and alveoli. This is the exchange of gases in adjacent spaces.

(3) The status of alveolar ventilation is determined as follows: Alveolar ventilation = Respiratory rate × (Tidal volume delivered − Anatomic dead-space volume).

b. Indications: respiratory failure (hypoxemia, hypercapnia, and/or acidemia), pulmonary insufficiency, severe apnea and bradycardia episodes, cardiovascular support, CNS disease, and surgery.

c. Advantages: consistent delivery of assisted ventilation and oxygen therapy; decreases the work of breathing.

d. Disadvantages: intubation by skilled provider, x-ray examination to confirm placement, possible intermittent x-ray examinations to verify placement or lung status, continuous monitoring of vital signs and oxygen saturation.

e. Complications: tube malposition or dislodgment, underventilation or overventilation, tracheobronchial injury, pulmonary air leaks, infection, intracranial hemorrhage, bronchopulmonary dysplasia, and retinopathy of prematurity.

TYPES OF ASSISTED VENTILATION

A. **Negative-pressure ventilator (derivative of "iron lung").** Provides ventilation by chest wall movement and eliminates the need for intubation. It requires a sealed chamber to provide negative pressure to the chest, which limits access to the infant for providing routine care. It was used in ventilating newborn infants in the early 1970s. With its limitations and the advent of the pressure-limited time-cycled ventilator, it is seldom used today.

B. **Positive-pressure devices.**

1. Bag-and-mask ventilation. Positive pressure and O_2 are delivered via face mask applied with an adequate seal around the mouth and nose. Maximal pressure can be preset to prevent excessive pressure. A manometer can measure pressure delivered to the patient. Device does not require intubation and can be very effective for short-term use.

2. Volume-limited ventilator. Inspiration ends when a preset volume of gas is delivered, regardless of the pressure reached within the ventilator circuit. A certain amount of gas is trapped in the dead space and compliance of the circuit. A decrease in lung compliance could result in hypoventilation.

3. Pressure-limited ventilator. Inspiratory phase ends when a preset pressure is reached within the ventilator circuit, regardless of the volume of gas delivered during inspiration.

4. Time-cycled, pressure-limited, continuous-flow ventilator. A predetermined pressure of gas is administered, the duration of inspiration and expiration can be adjusted. Ventilator also allows for the infant's spontaneous respiratory efforts, facilitating a gradual reduction of support. This is the most commonly used ventilator in neonatal care.

VENTILATOR MODES

A. **Intermittent mandatory ventilation.** "Breaths" are delivered at a predetermined rate, regardless of where the patient is in the respiratory cycle. The ventilator continues to deliver fresh gas, which allows spontaneous respirations as well. It is possible to stack a ventilator breath on top of a spontaneous breath during either inspiration or expiration. This may lead to air trapping, air leaks, CNS dysfunction, and irregularity of blood pressure and cerebral blood flow.

B. Synchronized ventilation (also referred to as patient-triggered ventilation). Mechanical breaths are delivered in response to a signal derived from the patient and detected as a spontaneous respiratory effort. The goal is to avoid asynchrony of breathing by the patient and breaths given by the ventilator. Asynchrony may lead to air trapping, air leaks, CNS dysfunction, and irregularity of blood pressure and cerebral blood flow.

1. Synchronized intermittent mandatory ventilation.
   a. Preset number of ventilator breaths is synchronized with the onset of spontaneous breaths.
   b. Unassisted breaths occur between ventilator breaths, with continuous flow of gas from the ventilatory circuit.
   c. Initiation of a mechanical breath is in response to the onset of the patient's respiratory effort, resulting in full synchrony.
   d. Partial asynchrony may occur if inspiratory times are different, in that the patient may terminate the inspiratory effort while the ventilator continues to be in the inspiratory phase.
   e. Signal detection is from a chest–abdominal wall movement monitor or from changes in airflow detected in the ventilator circuit.
2. Assist/control mode of ventilation.
   a. A synchronized breath is delivered each time a spontaneous patient breath meeting the threshold criteria is detected, or mechanical breaths are delivered at a preset regular rate if the patient does not exhibit spontaneous respiratory effort (i.e., if the patient has apnea).
   b. A detection system signals the start of inspiratory effort, which allows for synchronous initiation of inspiration.
   c. Asynchronous expiratory-phase breaths may still occur.

Nursing Care of the Patient Requiring Respiratory Support or Conventional Mechanical Ventilation

A. Care of O_2 delivery devices.

1. Oxygen hood. Warm, humidified (to prevent heat loss) O_2, delivered via head hood, is usually blended to select the appropriate amount needed. The percentage of O_2 in the hood must be monitored by a properly calibrated O_2 analyzer placed in the hood near the infant's nose. Ensure a hood of correct size for each infant. To prevent buildup of CO_2, do not block openings in the hood and ensure an adequate flow of 5–7 L/min. Clean and change per unit protocol.
2. Nasal cannula. Remove and clean secretions every 4–6 hours as needed. Inspect surrounding tissue for pressure-related injury. If sudden onset of respiratory distress occurs inspect cannula for secretions and suction nasopharynx for mucus. Change according to unit protocol.
3. Nasopharyngeal or nasal prong CPAP. Ensure that CPAP device is of the correct size to decrease the incidence of pressure necrosis of the nares. Nasal CPAP units come in a variety of sizes and should be short and wide, with thin walls to allow for maximal airflow. They should be soft and flexible and should be easy to secure and maintain. Humidification of 90–100% should be provided in the CPAP system to prevent drying out of the mucous membranes and subsequent formation of thick secretions. Evaluate the need for suctioning every 2–4 hours. Inspect surrounding tissue for pressure-related injury. Secure the device to a stockinette cap or with soft straps provided by some manufacturers. Lightweight tubing is helpful for ease in securing the device and in keeping the unit in the nose. The infant can be positioned supine, on either side, or prone, generally with the head of the bed at approximately a 30-degree

angle. Observe for abdominal distention resulting from excessive air entering the stomach from the CPAP device. Consider aspirating every few hours with an orogastric tube or leaving it in place continuously to vent gas in the stomach. Feeding is not contraindicated during delivery of CPAP. The clinical condition must be evaluated before institution of feedings. During CPAP delivery, feedings must be administered via orogastric tube either intermittently or by continuous drip. Change prongs according to unit protocol, generally every 2–3 days.

4. ETT. After correct placement has been determined, note the depth of the tube at the gum or lip and post at the bedside. This is important for future reference in case the tube slips, reintubation is needed, or to determine suction catheter length. Secure the ETT with tape or other method. Each institution generally develops a method that works well for the staff and patients. Observe for evidence of slipping or tape loosening and secure again when necessary to prevent accidental extubation. Position the infant supine, on either side, or in the prone position, with the head in a neutral position. Be aware that the tube moves with the chin and can move several centimeters with flexion or extension of the head. Signs of extubation include sudden deterioration in clinical status, abdominal distention, crying, decreased chest wall movement, breath sounds in the abdomen, agitation, cyanosis, or bradycardia. Notify the physician or neonatal nurse practitioner if extubation is a concern and prepare for reintubation as soon as possible. Intubation equipment should be readily available. A bag and mask with pressure manometer should also be available at each bedside and should be tested during each shift. Suction the ETT when necessary. Complications of an ETT include palatal grooves (consider a palate protector, which can be made by a pediatric dentist or is commercially available), nasal erosion, subglottic stenosis, tracheoesophageal perforation during insertion of the tube, aspiration, infection, and tracheal granuloma.

5. Tracheostomy tube. Daily changing of the dressing and weekly changing of the tube are usually adequate. Inspect the site for signs of tissue pressure and/or necrosis. Suctioning is necessary to keep the airway clear of secretions. Family members need to be included in this procedure, thus facilitating discharge.

B. **Suctioning the airway.**

1. Nontracheal tubes.
   a. Suctioning of the mouth, nose, and tubes should be performed on an as-needed basis. The presence of a foreign body in the mouth or nose will cause an increase in secretions.
   b. Suctioning can coincide with the cleaning or changing of the tubes or with routine caregiving.
2. Endotracheal tubes.
   a. The amount of secretions will be disease related. Infants with resolving respiratory distress syndrome, patent ductus arteriosus, bronchopulmonary dysplasia, and pneumonia are more likely to require frequent suctioning because of an increased production of mucus. Patients with early-stage respiratory distress syndrome and those with most types of congenital heart disease will not have much mucus and will require less suctioning.
   b. Protocols for suctioning vary from one institution to another and generally include instilling several drops of normal saline solution into the ETT (with thick secretions a dilution of 1:4 sodium bicarbonate may be used in place of normal saline solution), hand ventilating for 30–60 seconds (an increase in fraction of inspired oxygen [FIO_2] may be necessary to maintain oxygenation during the procedure), suctioning, and hand ventilating after suctioning for another 30–60 seconds. In-line suction devices allow suctioning while ventilation continues. Do not advance the suction catheter farther than the distance of the ETT, and do not suction too vigorously.

    c. Vacuum pressure range should be 60–100 mm Hg (Simbruner, Coradello, and Fodor, 1981). A 5F or 6F suction catheter for a 2.5–3.5 ETT, or an 8F suction catheter for a 4.0–4.5 ETT, is usually appropriate.

    d. Hazards of suctioning include hypoxemia, bradycardia, barotrauma, intraventricular hemorrhage, and pneumothorax.

C. **Initiating mechanical ventilation.** The goal of mechanical ventilation is to assist in providing adequate tissue oxygenation and eliminating CO_2.

1. Establish an airway. Endotracheal intubation should be performed by a skilled provider (see Chapter 31, Common Invasive Procedures).

2. Ventilator selection. The ventilator selected for use is based on the patient's condition and disease process, the patient's response to previous ventilatory support, and staff experience and comfort with the device. The most common ventilator used in the NICU is a time-cycled, pressured-limited, continuous-flow device. This type of ventilator allows the operator to adjust peak pressure, PEEP, inspiratory time, flow rate, rate of intermittent mandatory ventilation, inspiratory time, and FIO_2.

3. Parameters to be set and/or monitored during mechanical ventilation.

    a. Rate of intermittent mandatory ventilation. Infants without respiratory failure have a resting respiratory rate of approximately 40/min, whereas infants with respiratory failure may have a respiratory rate of 0 to more than 100/min. A beginning ventilator rate of 30–40/min for an infant with respiratory failure should be adequate. For infants without respiratory failure, a rate of 20–30/min should be adequate. The ventilator rate will affect the ability to blow off CO_2. The rate is adjusted to maintain the arterial tension of CO_2 in the range of 40–50 mm Hg and to avoid excessive respiratory effort, which would exhaust the infant. A rate greater than 40/min may shorten the expiratory phase of ventilation and cause air trapping.

    b. Peak inspiratory pressure (PIP). PIP is the primary factor used for determining tidal volume and affecting PaO_2. Determining the appropriate PIP requires careful and skilled assessment. The complications of excessive PIP include air leaks, decreased venous return, and decreased cardiac output. Factors such as weight, gestational age, disease process, lung compliance, and airway resistance must be considered. Auscultation of breath sounds to assess aeration and compliance is necessary. Experimenting with an anesthesia bag to find the best rate and pressure may be useful and allows the clinician to determine the infant's ventilation needs. Visual inspection of chest wall movement, in conjunction with the use of a pressure gauge connected to the anesthesia bag, may guide your assessment. A beginning PIP of 20 cm H_2O is appropriate for most preterm infants. The lowest PIP that will provide adequate ventilation is ideal, with the goals of preventing barotrauma and decreasing the incidence of air leaks and chronic lung disease (Wung et al., 1985). Certain conditions may warrant use of high PIP, including poor compliance, atelectasis, or pulmonary hypertension. Before connecting the patient to the ventilator, ensure that the inspiratory pressure is correct. Recheck after the connection has been made, and adjust as necessary.

    c. Positive end-expiratory pressure (PEEP). This measure aids in maintaining functional residual capacity, stabilizing and recruiting atelectatic areas for gas exchange, improving compliance, and improving ventilation-perfusion matching in the lung (Spitzer and Stefano, 1993). PEEP is important in assisted ventilation for infants with surfactant deficiency, because of the likelihood of alveolar collapse. Physiologic PEEP is estimated at 2 cm H_2O. Levels lower than 2 cm H_2O are not generally recommended. In most instances, medium levels, about 4–7 cm H_2O, are recommended. Levels greater than 8 cm H_2O are associated with pulmonary air leaks and reduction of cardiac output.

d. Inspiratory/expiratory (I/E) ratio: ratio of time spent in inspiration and time spent in expiration. Determining this time should be based on the underlying reason for ventilation. A physiologic I/E ratio in a nondisease state is equal to 1:2 or 1:3, meaning a short inspiratory time and a long expiratory time. This type of ratio would benefit an infant with distress of unknown cause or with CNS or congenital heart disease. An I/E ratio of 1:1 would be best for infants requiring a high ventilator rate and lower PIP, such as with pulmonary interstitial emphysema. Finally, an inverse I/E ratio of 3:1–2 would be appropriate for treating infants requiring higher mean airway pressure to maintain the PaO_2, such as those with the acute stages of meconium aspiration and resultant persistent pulmonary hypertension (Spitzer and Fox, 1996). Prolonged expiratory time is useful during weaning, when oxygenation is not as problematic. The I/E ratio will affect the PaO_2 and $PaCO_2$. Changes affect mean airway pressure and oxygenation.

e. Flow rate: flow of gas (measured in liters per minute) through the patient's circuit. The flow rate determines the ability of the ventilator to deliver the desired amount of PIP, waveform, I/E ratio, and respiratory rate. A flow rate of at least twice the infant's minute ventilation ensures that the ventilator can reach the desired pressure. Flow rates of 4–8 L/min are common (Spitzer and Fox, 1996). With low flow rates (<3 L/min), inspiratory pressure gradually builds to a peak just before expiration, closely resembling a sine waveform (normal breaths are shaped like a sine waveform). There may be less barotrauma to the airways with a sine waveform. High flows of 4–10 L/min or higher are necessary with square-waveform ventilation or when high rates are used. A square waveform pattern moves the ventilator breath rapidly from the resting or expiratory pressure level to the PIP. Because the PIP is reached sooner than with a sine waveform, the PIP is held for a longer period (Fig. 9–3). This may be advantageous with atelectatic areas of the lung. It may also contribute to barotrauma.

f. Mean airway pressure (MAP): average distending pressure throughout a complete respiratory cycle. It is the major determinant of oxygenation. MAP, which can be manipulated by altering the PEEP, PIP, I/E ratio, flow,

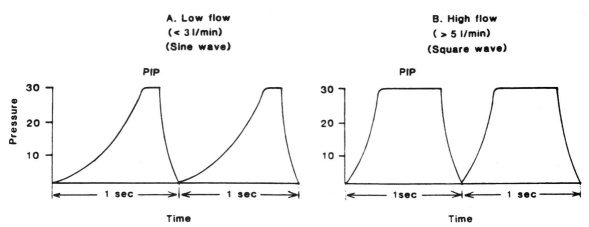

Figure 9–3
Comparison of ventilator waveforms. *A*, Relative sine wave. *B*, Relative square wave. (From Goldsmith, J.P., and Karotkin, E.H. [Eds.]: Assisted Ventilation of the Neonate, 3rd ed. Philadelphia, W.B. Saunders, 1996, p. 169.)

and rate, is digitally displayed on newer ventilators. Separate devices can be attached to older ventilators to display MAP. Increases in oxygenation are directly related to increases in MAP, and increased barotrauma to the lungs can result with high MAP. Close attention to the MAP during ventilation is essential, especially once the underlying disease begins to resolve.

4. For effects of different ventilator changes, see Table 9–2.

High-frequency Ventilation

High-frequency ventilation (HFV) is any of several forms of mechanical ventilation that use small tidal volumes and rapid ventilator rates to ventilate patients with severe respiratory failure. The advantage of HFV over conventional mechanical ventilation is the ability to deliver adequate minute volumes with lower proximal airway pressures.

A. **Gas-exchange mechanisms in HFV.** The tidal volumes used may be less than or equal to anatomic dead-space volume. According to gas-exchange theories for conventional ventilation, alveolar ventilation during HFV should be zero.

B. **Theories of gas exchange during HFV.**

1. Augmented (facilitated) diffusion. Gas molecules diffuse higher in the airways.
2. Coaxial diffusion. Fresh gases travel down the center of the airway, and CO_2 elimination occurs along the periphery of the airway (Fig 9–4).
3. Entrainment. Gas molecules from higher in the airway are pulled into the area of low pressure created behind a high-velocity gas entry point, such as a jet cannula port (Fig. 9–5).
4. Interregional gas mixing ("pendelluft"). Because of the different time constants of the respiratory units, gases in the periphery of the lung may move between alveolar units to provide better matching of ventilation and perfusion.

C. **Effectiveness of gas exchange.** All forms of HFV produce gas exchange with lower PIPs, theoretically reducing the risk of barotrauma.

D. **Types of high-frequency ventilators.**

1. High-frequency positive-pressure ventilation (HFPPV): Infant Star ventilator

Table 9–2
SPECIFIC EFFECTS OF DIFFERENT VENTILATOR CHANGES

INCREASING PIP
1. Increases V_T and $\dot{V}_E$
2. Adds little to MAP unless combined with a reversal of I/E ratio or prolongation of IT
3. Affects maximum dilation of alveoli already open, contributing to barotrauma
4. Opens alveoli with high critical opening pressures

REVERSING I/E RATIO (FOR LENGTHENING IT WHILE RESPIRATORY RATE IS KEPT CONSTANT)
1. Has little effect on V_T or $\dot{V}_E$ beyond the minimum IT needed to deliver V_T or reach desired PIP level (or both)
2. Can contribute on more than one-to-one basis to MAP, depending on original PIP and degree of reversal of I/E ratio
3. Allows expansion of atelectatic alveoli at lower PIP
4. May cause inadvertent PEEP, overinflation of alveoli, and reduction of pulmonary blood flow

INCREASING BACKGROUND CPAP OR PEEP
1. Decreases V_T and $\dot{V}_E$ unless significant atelectasis is overcome
2. Adds to MAP on a one-to-one basis
3. Holds open alveoli and terminal airways on end-expiration, thus raising closing volume and aiding in equal distribution of ventilation
4. Reduces likelihood of inadvertent PEEP

V_T, Tidal volume; $\dot{V}_E$, expired volume per unit time.
From Goldsmith, J.P., and Karotkin, E.H. (Eds.): Assisted Ventilation of the Neonate, 3rd ed. Philadelphia, W.B. Saunders, 1996, p. 62.

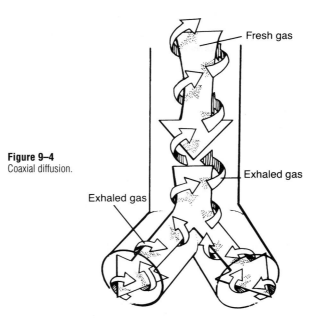

Figure 9–4
Coaxial diffusion.

(Infrasonics, San Diego, Calif.); Volumetric Diffusive respirator (Percussionaire Corp., Sandpoint, Idaho).

a. These conventional mechanical ventilators are adapted to operate at rapid rates.

b. They include ventilators referred to as high-frequency flow interrupters. Flow interrupters are neither oscillators nor jet ventilators. They operate with a microprocessor-controlled pneumatic valve to interrupt the gas flow to achieve a pulsatile flow.

c. Inhalation: active; exhalation: passive. A Venturi system on the Infant Star ventilator facilitates exhalation and prevents inadvertent PEEP. Exhalation is still passive with this feature.

d. Indications for use:
   (1) Severe pulmonary air leaks.
   (2) Lung diseases unresponsive to conventional mechanical ventilation.

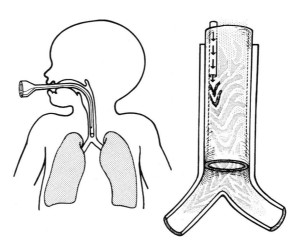

Figure 9–5
Entrainment during high-frequency jet ventilation. Gas molecules near the jet orifice are "entrained," or dragged along with the jet pulse, whereby additional volume is delivered to the patient without substantially increasing static airway pressure. (From Harris, T.R.: *In* Goldsmith, J.P., and Karotkin, E.H. [Eds.]: Assisted Ventilation of the Neonate, 2nd ed. Philadelphia, W.B. Saunders, 1988.)

e. Parameters to be set and/or monitored during HFPPV:
   (1) Amplitude: size of the pressure wave produced by the ventilator. Affects CO_2 elimination.
   (2) MAP: affects optimal lung volume and oxygenation. High MAP can impede venous return, decrease cardiac output, and damage the airways.
   (3) Sighs: conventional breaths given periodically to recruit alveoli and minimize atelectasis. (Sighs are optional with this mode.)
   (4) FIO_2 concentration: set on the ventilator as with conventional ventilation.
f. Complications: inadequate gas delivery during inspiration and incomplete lung emptying during expiration.

2. High-frequency jet ventilation (HFJV): Bunnell Life Pulse Jet Ventilator (Bunnell Inc., Salt Lake City, Utah).
   a. A jet injector or narrow-bore cannula that delivers short, rapid, high-velocity pulses from a pressurized gas source directly into the trachea via a small cannula. Requires the use of a triple-lumen ETT (Hi-Lo Jet Tube), which is specially designed for use during HFJV (requires reintubation) or a triple-lumen ETT adapter ("jet nozzle") that attaches to a standard ETT. The tube has a standard ETT lumen, a pressure-monitoring port located at the distal tip, and a jet injector port located within the tube wall.
   b. Servo-controlled driving pressure: continuously adjusts the pressure of the gas supply to the jet cannula to maintain desired peak airway pressure.
   c. Solenoid valve: opens and closes gas supply to the jet cannula.
   d. Humidification system: built in-line.
   e. Proximal airway pressures: monitored and continuously displayed; used in servo control of pressure delivery.
   f. Conventional ventilator: used in tandem to provide gas for entrainment, PEEP, and background ventilation (sighs).
   g. Exhalation: passive.
   h. Indications for use: effective with disorders in which CO_2 elimination is the major problem. CO_2 elimination is achieved at lower peak and mean airway pressures than with HFPPV or high-frequency oscillatory ventilation.
   i. Parameters to be set and/or monitored:
      (1) PIP: set on both the jet and the conventional ventilator.
         (a) Jet PIP is usually initially set at the same PIP required during conventional ventilation, and the conventional ventilator PIP is lowered by 2–5 cm H_2O.
         (b) A higher conventional PIP may cause interruption of the jet.
      (2) Servo-controlled pressure: internal adjustment of driving pressure by the ventilator as patient compliance and pressure settings change.
         (a) Lower servo-pressure reflects worsening lung disease, airway obstruction, pneumothorax, or kinked ventilator tubing.
         (b) Higher servo-pressure indicates improved lung compliance or a leak in the patient/system.
      (3) PEEP: set on conventional ventilator; displayed on jet ventilator. Value displayed may be lower than value set, because of where and how it is measured. The PEEP provided by the conventional ventilator assists in lung recruitment when atelectasis is a problem.
      (4) Jet valve on time: percentage of time that the jet valve is open; similar to inspiratory time, usually 0.02 second.
      (5) Rate set on jet and conventional ventilators:
         (a) The jet rate is usually 400–500 breaths per minute; Bunnell default setting of 420/min appears to be most effective for that ventilator.

(b) The rate for conventional intermittent mandatory ventilation is usually set between 5 and 20 breaths per minute to provide background ventilation (sigh breaths), which helps to prevent atelectasis.

(6) FIO_2: set on jet and conventional ventilators.

j. Weaning from HFJV is usually accomplished by 7–14 days. Air leaks should be resolved for 1–2 days before switching back to conventional mechanical ventilation. Weaning is accomplished by decreasing the PIP and reducing the HFJV rate to 250–350 breaths per minute. Support from conventional mechanical ventilation is increased using small tidal volume breaths.

k. Patient care assessment.

(1) Patient may undergo reintubation with special ETT that has a jet port and a pressure-monitoring port built in (Fig. 9–6), or an ETT adapter may be attached to the standard ETT.

(2) Suctioning may be performed with HFJV on or off.

(a) Placing jet ventilator on stand-by mode during suctioning may prevent airway damage caused by the shearing force of opposing positive and negative pressures.

(b) Suctioning with the jet ventilator on may help decrease respiratory decompensation during the procedure in some patients.

(c) If suctioning is performed with the jet ventilator running, suction must be applied as the catheter is inserted, as well as when withdrawn, to prevent overpressurization of the circuit and alveolar rupture.

(3) Humidification of gases is important with HFJV in preventing obstruction of the ETT.

(a) Jet port should be irrigated with 0.5 mL normal saline solution or air every 3–4 hours.

(b) Main port of ETT is suctioned as usual.

(4) Tubing to the conventional ventilator must never be kinked, because overpressurization of the circuit and alveolar rupture may occur if expiratory gas cannot escape.

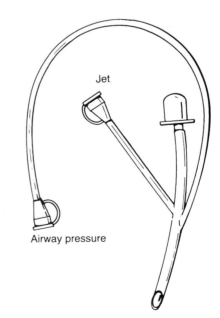

Figure 9–6
Triple-lumen endotracheal tube.

Jet

Airway pressure

(5) Vibration of the chest wall is an indicator of lung compliance, airway patency, and effectiveness of ventilator settings.
  (a) Chest wall vibration must be assessed after head position changes to ensure that the jet port of the ETT has not been occluded by the tracheal wall.
  (b) Sudden decrease in chest wall vibration may indicate a plugged ETT or a pneumothorax.
(6) Vibration may interfere with electrical monitoring of heart rate and respiratory rate.
  (a) Use pulse from arterial line or pulse oximeter to monitor heart rate if necessary.
  (b) Respiratory rate cannot be monitored.
(7) Jet ventilation is more efficient at CO_2 elimination than at oxygenation.
  (a) Increasing the background ventilation rate may improve oxygenation.
  (b) Pressure difference between PIP and PEEP is the major determinant of ventilation.
  (c) MAP is the major determinant of oxygenation.
(8) Patients are generally weaned to a low PIP and then switched back to conventional ventilation before extubation.

l. Complications and problems:
(1) Airway obstruction, which may be indicated by decreased chest wall vibration, increased PCO_2, and decreased servo pressure.
(2) Necrotizing tracheobronchitis (inflammatory injury to tracheal mucosa).
(3) Microatelectasis and poor oxygenation, possible after prolonged HFJV; necessitates return to conventional ventilation.
(4) Air trapping occurs at very high rates or with excessive jet valve on-times.

3. High-frequency oscillatory ventilation (HFOV): SensorMedics model 3100A (SensorMedics Corp., Yorba Linda, Calif.).
a. Piston, or vibrating diaphragm, that moves a small volume of gas toward and then away from patient.
b. Oscillators deliver very little bulk gas. A continuous flow of fresh gas flows past the source that powers the oscillations, producing bias gas flow in a resulting push-pull fashion and thereby eliminating CO_2 buildup and delivering O_2. A low-pass filter allows gas to exit the system while maintaining vibration of gas in the airway (Butler, Bohn, and Bryan, 1980).
c. Proximal airway pressure is monitored by the ventilator, but clinical relevance is questionable because it probably does not reflect alveolar pressure.
d. HFOV allows for the use of higher MAP with less barotrauma, in comparison with conventional-mechanical ventilation and ventilation with small tidal volumes.
e. Exhalation is active, assisted by the oscillating device.
f. Indications for use are:
(1) Severe lung disease that is unresponsive to conventional ventilation.
(2) Pulmonary air leaks, pulmonary interstitial emphysema, pneumothorax, and bronchopleural fistula.
(3) Pulmonary hypoplasia and diaphragmatic hernia: treated with limited success. HFV can be used to stabilize the condition of these patients and as an intermediate step before extracorporeal membrane oxygenation.
(4) Persistent pulmonary hypertension and meconium aspiration syndrome: treated with mixed results. The improved CO_2 exchange may provide a respiratory alkalosis that would result in dilation of the pulmonary vascular bed.
(5) Failure of conventional mechanical ventilation.

g. Parameters to be set or monitored:
  (1) MAP: affects oxygenation.
  (2) Amplitude: size of pressure wave produced by oscillator (another way to describe volume delivered).
  (3) Sighs: conventional breaths given periodically to recruit alveoli and minimize atelectasis.
  (4) FIO_2: set on the ventilator as with conventional ventilation.
  (5) Frequency: 180–900 "breaths" per minute (3–15 Hertz).
h. Patient care and assessment:
  (1) No special ETT is required.
  (2) Suctioning procedure is performed as usual.
  (3) Chest wall vibration is assessed, rather than breath sounds, to determine effectiveness of ventilator settings and lung compliance changes. Breath sounds are not audible during HFOV.
  (4) Vibration may interfere with electrical monitoring of heart rate and respiratory rate.
    (a) Use pulse from arterial line or pulse oximeter for heart rate monitoring if necessary.
    (b) Respiratory rate cannot be monitored.
    (c) Sighs help to reduce microatelectasis and improve oxygenation.
  (5) Complications and problems are:
    (a) Microatelectasis, poor oxygenation.
    (b) Increased incidence of intraventricular hemorrhage in collaborative trial of HFV using oscillators for treatment of respiratory distress syndrome in preterm infants (HIFI Study Group, 1989).
4. Liquid ventilation: currently experimental but thought to be a powerful addition to pulmonary care for the future.
  a. Elimination of the air-liquid interface in the alveolus decreases surface tension, which results in a high degree of solubility for respiratory gases. Perfluorocarbon liquids are being studied as the basis for liquid ventilation.
  b. Indications for use are respiratory distress syndrome and secondary surfactant deficiency.
  c. Monitoring is dependent on the delivery system. The circuit, similar to that used in extracorporeal membrane oxygenation, requires constant monitoring to ensure that there is no loss of tidal volume or any impairment of gas exchange. The circuit allows the fluid to flow into and out of the pulmonary airways, either by gravity or with a pump. Chest wall movement indicates patency and position of the ETT and tidal volume. Change of position is necessary to allow for even distribution of the lung liquid.
  d. Perfluorocarbons provide decreased alveolar surface tension, recruit lung volume, allow ventilation with decreased pressures, improve ventilation-perfusion matching, and clean debris from the lungs.
  e. Research and clinical trials are ongoing.

Nursing Care During Therapy

A. Physical assessment.

1. Observation. One of the most valuable tools in assessing an infant's respiratory status is observation. Does the infant appear to be comfortable while breathing, or does the baby show signs and symptoms of distress by grunting, flaring, and retracting? The Silverman-Anderson score is a screening tool that uses five signs or symptoms to assess respiratory distress in the newborn infant (Fig. 9–7). Assess the skin color of the infant. It should be uniformly pink. Skin color that is blue, dusky, or pale needs to be evaluated further. A dramatic change in

SILVERMAN-ANDERSEN RETRACTION SCORE

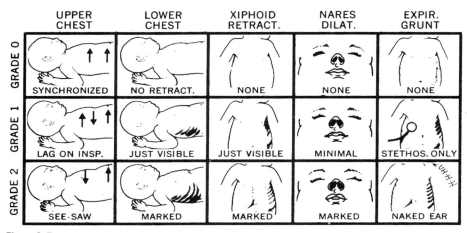

Figure 9–7
Silverman-Andersen scale to assess respiratory distress in the newborn infant. (Adapted from Silverman, W.A., and Andersen, D.H.: Reproduced by permission of Pediatrics, *17*:1–10, copyright 1956.)

skin color needs to be investigated immediately to rule out a pneumothorax versus a mechanical obstruction. Observe the infant's respiratory rate. Is it within the normal range (40–60 breaths per minute)? When observing the respiratory rate, consider variables such as environment, temperature, and the infant's state of activity or inactivity, which can increase or decrease the respiratory rate. Observe whether the chest rises symmetrically; if asymmetrical, suspect a possible pneumothorax, diaphragmatic hernia, or phrenic nerve palsy. With accidental extubation, chest movement may not be observable or may be decreased from previous observations.

2. Auscultation. Listen to the breath sounds carefully to determine differences in the upper and lower lung fields and differences in the left and right lung fields. Is aeration equal bilaterally? Are rales (fine crackles) or rhonchi (coarse crackles) evident? Are other abnormal sounds audible? A finding in a ventilated infant may be louder breath sounds on the right; if so, suspect that the ETT may have slipped into the right bronchus or that a pneumothorax may have occurred, necessitating evaluation. Rule out other noises and their points of origin. Bowel sounds heard in the chest are an indication of a diaphragmatic hernia. In the patient receiving HFV, chest wall vibration is an indicator of lung compliance, airway patency, and effectiveness of ventilator settings. Chest wall vibration must be assessed after repositioning. Sudden decrease in chest wall vibration may indicate a plugged ETT or a pneumothorax.

3. ETT observation. Fogging or condensation in the ETT is a sign that the infant is intubated. The condensation occurs on exhalation and is visible in the ETT. Observation of the tube position more than 1 cm from its desired location may indicate extubation or placement in the right main-stem bronchus.

4. Signs of extubation:
   a. Audible crying.
   b. Absent or decreased breath sounds.
   c. Cyanosis.
   d. Bradycardia.

e. Hypoxemia.
f. Agitation, restlessness.
g. Increased abdominal distention.

B. **Equipment function.** All ventilators used for conventional mechanical ventilation should have been approved by the U.S. Food and Drug Administration and should display rate (intermittent mandatory ventilation), peak inspiratory pressure, PEEP, tidal volume (where applicable), inspiratory time, I/E ratio, mean airway pressure, and O_2 concentration. Ventilators must be plugged into an electrical outlet that provides emergency power in the event of a power failure.
1. All mechanical ventilators should have:
    a. Alarms activated to alert caregivers to ventilator malfunction or disconnection.
    b. Preset pressure relief valves to ensure against administration of excessive PIP and PEEP.
    c. Frequently scheduled inspections by licensed respiratory therapists.
    d. Ventilator tubing changed routinely per unit policy.
    e. O_2 concentration analyzed routinely and documented in the patient record.
    f. Routine cleaning between patient use.
2. The following equipment, to be located in the immediate area of all infants requiring mechanical ventilation, should be checked for proper functioning and replaced as needed:
    a. Laryngoscope with blade.
        (1) Size 0 for infants weighing less than 4 kg.
        (2) Size 1 for infants weighing more than 4 kg.
    b. Sterile ETTs.
        (1) Size 2.5 for infants weighing less than 1000 g.
        (2) Size 3.0 for infants weighing 1000–2000 g.
        (3) Size 3.5 for infants weighing 2000–3000 g.
        (4) Size 4.0 for infants weighing more than 3000 g.
    c. Sterile stylet (plastic coated).
    d. Magill forceps (nasal intubation).
    e. Suction tubing and catheters (suction control gauge set at 80–100 mm Hg).
    f. Sterile orogastric tubes.
        (1) Size 5F for infants weighing less than 1 kg.
        (2) Size 8F for infants weighing more than 1 kg.
    g. Anesthesia bag with manometer and mask: capable of delivering blended O_2, and O_2 source.
    h. Tape, scissors.

C. **Noninvasive monitoring.**

1. All infants receiving O_2 therapy should be considered as potential candidates for mechanical ventilation and should be monitored with the following:
    a. Heart rate monitor: audible beat-to-beat capability and alarm device for bradycardia (<100 bpm) or tachycardia (>180 bpm); should provide visual display of electrocardiogram and actual heart rate.
    b. Respiratory monitor: visual display of respiratory wave pattern and actual respiratory rate; should include alarm device for apnea and tachypnea. Respiratory rate trend mode is preferred.
    c. Blood pressure monitoring: peripheral (cuff) blood pressure or arterial blood pressure monitoring, performed on a scheduled interval and documented on the permanent record.
    d. O_2 analyzer: continuous monitoring of O_2 content of the gas delivered to the patient, with mandatory alarm device for O_2 concentration greater than or less than desired range.

e. Pulse oximetry: continuous monitoring for critically ill infants; intermittent checks with documentation of peripheral O_2 saturations indicated for infants not critically ill.
f. Additional requirements for all infants requiring mechanical ventilation, based on clinical condition:
    (1) Arterial access (usually via umbilical artery catheter) for:
        (a) Blood gas sampling.
        (b) Blood pressure monitoring.
    (2) Transcutaneous PO_2 and PCO_2 monitoring as indicated by clinical status.
2. Pulse oximetry.
    a. Pulse oximetry is a noninvasive and continuous method of measuring hemoglobin O_2 saturation. With the use of red and infrared light, the saturation of hemoglobin bound to O_2 is determined by a digital readout displayed by the monitoring device. The main advantage of pulse oximetry is the short response time in determining O_2 saturation in a neonate. It also reduces the number of invasive blood gas measurements necessary for a particular infant. It can be used in various settings outside the NICU (e.g., in neonatal transport, delivery room care, and surgery). The alarm device will alert attendants if O_2 saturations are at less than or greater than the desired range.
    b. An accurate reading is dependent on several factors, a primary factor being the perfusion status of the infant. The accuracy of pulse oximetry decreases with low-perfusion states. Phototherapy, motion artifact, dyes (ink from footprints), and vasoconstricting drugs (dopamine) can affect saturation readouts. Pulse oximetry does not eliminate the need for blood gas analysis, because clinical signs of ventilation and acid-base balance must still be evaluated. Continuous saturations greater than 96% may indicate that an infant is ready to be weaned from O_2 therapy, depending on the acute or chronic nature of the infant's disease. Wasunna and Whitelow (1987) suggested that saturations greater than 92% may be associated with hyperoxia in the preterm infant. Table 9–3 gives percentage parameters for O_2 saturation monitoring.
3. Transcutaneous monitoring.
    a. Transcutaneous monitoring (TCM) is the measurement of skin O_2 tension rather than arterial O_2 tension. The correlation between skin O_2 tension and arterial O_2 tension is excellent. A heated electrode measures the O_2 flow across the skin (skin PO_2) by making the skin more permeable to O_2, which

Table 9–3
PRACTICAL HINTS FOR O_2 SATURATION MONITORING

Acceptable Limits	Acute	Chronic
	87-95%	90-95%
Oxygen management parameters	Wean from O_2 when infant stable and $StcaO_2$ readings are consistently >95% every 15-30 minutes	Wean from O_2 when infant stable and $StcaO_2$ readings are consistently >95% every 12-24 hours
Blood gas requirements	When $StcaO_2$ <85% or >97% consistently >15-30 minutes Monitoring and electrocardiographic heart rate not correlating and perfusion status poor	When $StcaO_2$ <87% or >95% consistently >1 hour

From Dziedzic, K., and Vidyasagar, P.: Clin. Perinatol., 16(1):179–197, 1989.

occurs when the lipid layer under the skin is altered and the O_2 dissociation curve is shifted to the right. Thus O_2 is not bound as tightly to the hemoglobin molecule and is more readily released to the tissues. The correlation between skin and arterial O_2 tension is best with normal perfusion, body temperature, and blood pressure. The advantage of TCM is the same as for the pulse oximeter. TCM reduces the number of invasive blood gas measurements and also can be used in various settings outside the NICU. The TCM also has several disadvantages. The readout on the TCM is not immediate—a warming period is required (10–20 minutes), and after about 4–6 hours the TCM begins to lose its measurement reliability, requiring change of the probe. The TCM requires frequent calibration during use. The electrode has been reported to cause burns in premature infants, and the probe adhesive may cause skin breakdown in the very low birth weight preterm infant. Further, the readout time of the transcutaneous PO_2 values lags 5–10 seconds behind the PaO_2 value, but the correlation between the PaO_2 value and the transcutaneous PO_2 value is as high as 0.98 (Peabody, 1978). This correlation can change if the infant is in overt shock, with transcutaneous PO_2 values much lower (Rooth, Huch, and Huch, 1987). TCM should be used for trending measurements. The TCM does not replace the need for monitoring arterial blood gases.

    b. Transcutaneous PCO_2 monitoring can be beneficial in caring for infants with respiratory problems characterized by hypercapnia. It is also beneficial in determining complications of pneumothorax or mechanical obstruction before they are clinically evident in the infant. Correlation with transcutaneous PCO_2 is fairly accurate, but transcutaneous PCO_2 values can be overestimated (Herrell et al., 1980).

4. End-tidal CO_2 monitoring.
    a. Measures CO_2 tension through gas analysis during respiration.
    b. Most accurate when infants have normal lung function and a normal ventilation to perfusion ($\dot{V}A/\dot{Q}C$) ratio.
    c. Markedly less accurate in infants with severe lung disease (large alveolar-arterial gradient) and cannot be relied on for accuracy.
    d. May be useful in premature infants with mild to moderate lung disease and in infants with normal lung function.
    e. Transcutaneous CO_2 monitoring is more accurate in the infant with severe lung disease.

D. **Blood gas measurement.** Blood gas measurement is the standard method for monitoring oxygenation, ventilation, and acid-base balance in the ill newborn infant. Different methods are available for obtaining the blood sample, with umbilical arterial catheterization being the most common. Other methods for sampling include the use of indwelling peripheral arterial catheters, intermittent arterial puncture, and capillary sampling. Arterial samples are preferred over capillary samples (heel stick or finger stick) because arterial samples are more reliable in obtaining an accurate PaO_2 value. Capillary samples are useful for measuring PCO_2 and pH in infants with chronic lung disease. All these methods are invasive, with the potential for complications (see Chapter 31, Common Invasive Procedures).

Medications Used During Ventilation Therapy

A. **Bronchodilators.**

1. Aminophylline (theophylline): relaxes smooth muscle, increasing blood flow to the lungs and vital capacity; stimulates cardiac muscle, increasing cardiac output.

     a. Dose: loading dose, 4–6 mg/kg; maintenance dose, 1.5–3.0 mg/kg per dose every 8 to 12 hours; by continuous IV infusion, IV, by mouth (Young and Mangum, 1998).

     b. Monitor: trough level obtained 30 minutes before dose, 48 to 72 hours after therapy is initiated; therapeutic range: apnea: 7 to 12 µg/mL; bronchodilation: 10–20 µg/mL (Young and Mangum, 1998).

     c. Considerations: Holding dose if heart rate exceeds 180 bpm.

     d. Signs of toxicity: gastrointestinal upset, tachycardia, poor weight gain, hyperreflexia, and seizures.

2. Albuterol: achieves bronchodilator effect similar to aminophylline but with less cardiac stimulation; enhances clearance of mucociliary secretions.

     a. Dose: aerosol, 0.1–0.5 mg/kg per dose every 2–6 hours via nebulized solution; oral, 0.1–0.3 mg/kg per dose every 6 to 8 hours (Young and Mangum, 1998).

     b. Monitor: serum concentration not determined; heart rate and respiratory effect monitored.

     c. Considerations: dilution of aerosol preparation with normal saline solution before use; signs of toxicity: tachycardia, arrhythmia, tremors, and irritability.

3. Caffeine: see Chapter 8, Apnea of the Newborn Infant.

4. Isoproterenol (Isuprel): decreases pulmonary artery pressure and resistance with minor cardiac effects, increasing blood flow to lungs.

     a. Dose: 0.05–0.5 µg/kg per minute; maximum dose, 2 µg/kg per minute (Young and Mangum, 1998); continuous IV infusion, IV, or ETT.

     b. Monitor: continuous vital signs; heart rate (may be affected); intra-arterial blood pressure and central venous pressure (preferred); frequent blood/serum glucose evaluation (insulin production may be increased).

     c. Considerations: therapy reserved for severe bronchopulmonary dysplasia and reactive airway disease; signs of toxicity: arrhythmia and tachycardia (can lead to congestive heart failure); hypoglycemia.

B. Diuretics.

1. Furosemide (Lasix): affects chloride transport in the loop of Henle, causes loss of chloride, sodium, potassium, and calcium. Diuresis may decrease pulmonary blood flow, decrease vascular resistance, and increase pulmonary compliance.

     a. Dose: 1–2 mg/kg per dose IV; 1–6 mg/kg per dose by mouth (Young and Mangum, 1998). Interval: premature infant, every 24 hours; term, every 12 hours; full-term >1 month, every 6–8 hours. Long-term therapy: consider a dose every other day.

     b. Monitor: accurate intake and output; specific gravity to evaluate response; frequent electrolyte values to monitor losses and replacement.

     c. Considerations: ototoxic, with transient and permanent hearing losses reported; renal calculi reported with long-term use.

2. Spironolactone (Aldactone): exerts inhibitory effect of aldosterone on the tubules, with resultant increase in sodium losses and sparing of potassium.

     a. Dose: 1–3 mg/kg per dose by mouth every 24 hours (Young and Mangum, 1998).

     b. Monitor: accurate intake and output; specific gravity to evaluate response; electrolyte values after 48 to 72 hours to detect hyperkalemia.

     c. Considerations: may cause rash, vomiting, and diarrhea. Use with caution in infant with impaired renal function.

3. Chlorothiazide (Diuril): inhibits sodium reabsorption in the distal renal tubule; has potentiating effect on furosemide; calcium sparing.

     a. Dose: 10–20 mg/kg per dose by mouth every 12 hours (Young and Mangum, 1998).

    b. Monitor: accurate intake and output; specific gravity to measure response; electrolyte, sodium, potassium, chloride, calcium, phosphorous, magnesium, and bicarbonate concentrations to evaluate losses and replacement.

    c. Considerations: optimal response when used with furosemide or spironolactone; may cause electrolyte disturbances and hyperglycemia; avoid with significant renal or hepatic dysfunction.

4. Hydrochlorothiazide (HydroDiuril): Similar in all respects to chlorothiazide. Dose: 1–2 mg/kg per dose by mouth every 12 hours (Young and Mangum, 1998).

C. **Corticosteroids.**

1. Dexamethasone (Decadron), a long-acting anti-inflammatory medication useful in treatment of chronic lung disease and tracheal edema before and after extubation.

    a. Dose: relative to indication for therapy.

      (1) Bronchopulmonary dysplasia.

        (a) Single 12-day course: 0.25 mg/kg per dose every 12 hours for 3 days. Decrease dose by 50% every 3 days (Young and Mangum, 1998).

        (b) Pulse therapy: 0.25 mg/kg per dose every 12 hours for 3 days. Repeat course at 10-day intervals as needed (Young and Mangum, 1998).

      (2) Tracheal edema: 0.25 mg/kg per dose every 6 to 12 hours for three to six doses. Do not exceed 1 mg/kg per day (Young and Mangum, 1998).

    b. Monitor: serum and urine glucose; blood pressure; gastric aspirates for blood. Echocardiogram is indicated if treatment continues longer than 7 days.

    c. Considerations: adverse effects—hyperglycemia, glycosuria, hypertension, cardiac effects, sodium and water retention, poor weight gain, hypokalemia, hypocalcemia, and increased risk of sepsis.

D. **Paralytic agents.**

1. Pancuronium (Pavulon): pharmacologic relaxation/paralysis of the skeletal muscle to promote improved mechanical ventilation with improved oxygenation/ventilation; decreased barotrauma; decreased fluctuations in cerebral blood flow.

    a. Dose: 0.04–0.15 mg/kg per dose IV push. Interval: every 1 to 2 hours as needed for paralysis (Young and Mangum, 1998).

    b. Monitor: vital signs frequently; blood pressure continuously.

    c. Considerations: mandatory availability of mechanical ventilation before use; adequate pulmonary toilet mandatory because no swallow or gag reflex is present; eye lubricant necessary. Signs of toxicity: tachycardia, hypertension, or hypotension.

2. Vecuronium: similar in all respects to pancuronium. Dose: 0.03–0.15 mg/kg per dose IV push every 1 to 2 hours as needed for paralysis (Young and Mangum, 1998).

E. **Pain control/sedation:** see Chapter 20, Neonatal Pain Management.

Weaning From Conventional Ventilation

A. **Indications.**

1. Clinical status of infant consistent with beginning resolution of pulmonary condition.

2. Ventilation becomes easier with less support and may result in hypocapnia.

B. Techniques.

1. Physical assessment of respiratory status: breath sounds, aeration, chest wall excursion, and spontaneous respiratory rate. Physical assessment of cardiovascular status: color, perfusion, heart rate, pulses, blood pressure, and presence or absence of murmur. Physical assessment of neurologic status: presence of spontaneous respirations, tone, irritability, and reflexes.
2. Radiographic evaluation: useful in documenting improved lung status and absence of pathologic changes.
3. Laboratory analysis: fluid, electrolyte, and hematologic stability.
4. Blood gas analysis: primary information for weaning an infant from conventional mechanical ventilation. If all other assessments indicate improvement, blood gas analysis provides information about the appropriate ventilator settings to adjust. To decrease the PaO_2, alter the MAP: reduce PIP, FIO_2, inspiratory/expiratory time (I/t) ratio, or PEEP. To increase $PaCO_2$, decrease ventilation: decrease rate or tidal volume. During weaning, it is important to try to decrease the most injurious parameters first. O_2 toxic effects from free O_2 radicals damage lung tissue, and O_2 is associated with retinopathy of prematurity. Therefore it is important to keep O_2 use at a minimum. PIP, PEEP, I/t ratio, and rate are all associated with barotrauma, so weaning should be achieved as soon as possible.

C. Extubation from mechanical ventilation. When low ventilator parameters have been achieved (intermittent mandatory ventilation, 10–20/min; PIP, 14–18; FIO_2, 0.21–0.30), the baby should be evaluated for extubation. Is the infant capable of maintaining respiration without ventilator support? Use of CPAP by ETT can be used as a trial to determine whether respirations are adequate. Some infants may need a transition to nasal CPAP, nasal prong, cannula, or O_2 hood.

NURSING CARE DURING WEANING PROCESS

A. Airway management, equipment function, and monitoring of the infant do not change during the weaning process.

B. Frequent assessment of the infant's vital signs, blood pressure, O_2 saturation, and neurologic status is essential. Documentation of this assessment will facilitate appropriate changes in ventilator support.

C. Be alert for decompensation of respiratory or cardiovascular status during this time, and notify the appropriate personnel when necessary.

D. Preparation for extubation:

1. Equipment for reintubation available at the bedside.
2. Suction of ETT and oropharynx.
3. Postextubation equipment ready for use.
4. Blood gas determination after extubation.
5. X-ray examination of chest to rule out atelectasis if decompensation occurs.
6. Frequent physical assessment every 1–2 hours after extubation for 24 hours.
7. Chest physiotherapy and inhalation treatment to help avoid atelectasis if possible.
8. Frequent position changes; suctioning as needed.
9. Explanation of the plan and process to the family before extubation.

Interpretation of Blood Gas Values

The purpose of obtaining blood gas values in the neonate is to determine whether the patient has adequate ventilation and perfusion (Goldsmith and Karotkin, 1996). Blood gas values also facilitate analysis of oxygenation and

Table 9–4
NORMAL ARTERIAL BLOOD GAS VALUES

pH	7.35–7.45
$PaCO_2$	35–45 mm Hg
PaO_2	50–80 mm Hg
HCO_3^-	22–26 mEq/L
Base excess	−2 to +2

acid-base status. Oxygenation is measured by the PaO_2. The PaO_2 is the amount of O_2 dissolved in the serum—3% of the total O_2 content. The remainder of the body's O_2 is bound to hemoglobin. Acceptable arterial blood gas values are illustrated in Table 9–4. Capillary PaO_2 reliability is uncertain. The value is lower than with an arterial specimen. Acid-base balance is indicated by the pH and the base deficit or excess. Ventilation is measured by PCO_2.

A. **Acidosis and alkalosis.** Changes in the pH from the normal range indicate a change in the acid-base status of the infant. An elevated pH, greater than 7.45, is alkalosis, which is caused by excess base or decreased acid in the blood. A decreased pH, less than 7.35, is acidosis, which is caused by decreased base or increased acid in the blood.

1. Respiratory acidosis ($PaCO_2$ >45; pH <7.45), caused by the accumulation of CO_2, the respiratory acid, results from hypoventilation.
2. Respiratory alkalosis ($PaCO_2$ <35; pH >7.35), caused by the decrease of CO_2, results from hyperventilation.
3. Metabolic alkalosis (base excess >+2; increased pH) is caused by a failure to excrete HCO_3^-, which is controlled by kidney function.
4. Metabolic acidosis (base deficit >−2 and <7.45), is caused by failure to retain HCO_3^- or by an increase in blood acid, which is controlled by the kidney.
5. For causes of acidosis and alkalosis, see Table 9–5.

Table 9–5
CAUSES OF ACIDOSIS AND ALKALOSIS

Cause	Mechanism
RESPIRATORY ACIDOSIS (↑ $PaCO_2$, ↓ pH)	
CNS depression	Maternal narcotics during labor, asphyxia, intracranial hemorrhage, neuromuscular disorder, CNS dysmaturity (apnea of prematurity)
Decreased ventilation-perfusion ratio	Obstructed airway, meconium aspiration, choanal atresia
Decreased lung compliance	Hyaline membrane disease, pulmonary insufficiency, diaphragmatic hernia
Injury to the thorax	Phrenic nerve paralysis, pneumothorax
METABOLIC ACIDOSIS (↓ HCO_3^-, pH, AND BASE EXCESS [NEGATIVE VALUE])	
Decreased tissue perfusion	Increased lactic acid production
Sepsis, congestive heart failure	
Renal failure	Increased organic acids
Renal tubular acidosis	Renal loss of base
Diarrhea	Gastrointestinal loss of base
RESPIRATORY ALKALOSIS (↓ $PaCO_2$, ↑ pH)	
Iatrogenic	Excessive mechanical ventilation
Hypoxemia	Increase in alveolar ventilation
CNS irritation (pain)	
METABOLIC ALKALOSIS (↑ HCO_3^-, pH AND BASE EXCESS [POSITIVE VALUE])	
Gastric suction	Loss of acid
Vomiting	Loss of acid
Diuretic therapy	Renal losses of H^+ ion
Iatrogenic	Administration of HCO_3^- (base added)

B. Disorders of acid-base balance (see Chapter 14, Metabolic Disorders).

C. Interpreting a blood gas value.

1. Evaluate the pH. Is there an acidosis or an alkalosis?
2. Evaluate the $PaCO_2$. If it is not normal, does it contribute to the acid-base status? Or is it a compensating factor?
3. Evaluate the HCO_3^- and the base excess or deficit. If they are not normal, do they contribute to the acid-base status? Or are they compensating factors?
4. Evaluate the PaO_2. Is there hypoxia or hyperoxia?
5. From this information, you can attempt to identify the specific cause of the abnormal acid-base status and treat as indicated.

REFERENCES

Butler, W.J., Bohn, D.J., Bryan, A.C., and Froese, A.B.: Ventilation by high-frequency oscillation in humans. Anesth. Analg., 59:577–584, 1980.

Goldsmith, J.P., and Karotkin, E.H. (Eds.): Assisted Ventilation of the Neonate, 3rd ed. Philadelphia, W.B. Saunders, 1996.

Harris, T.R., and Wood, B.R.: Physiologic principles. In Goldsmith, J.P., and Karotkin, E.H. (Eds.): Assisted Ventilation of the Neonate, 3rd ed. Philadelphia, W.B. Saunders, 1996, pp. 22–23.

Herrell, N., Martin, R.J., Pultusker, M., et al: Optimal temperature for the measurement of transcutaneous carbon dioxide tension in the neonate. Pediatrics, 97: 114–117, 1980.

HIFI Study Group: High-frequency oscillatory ventilation compared with conventional mechanical ventilation in the treatment of respiratory failure in preterm infants. N. Engl. J. Med., 320(2):88–93, 1989.

Loper, D.L.: Physiologic principles of the respiratory system. In Askin, D.F. (Ed.): Acute Respiratory Care of the Neonate. Petaluma, Calif., NICU Ink, 1997, pp. 21.

Peabody, J.L.: Clinical limitations and advantages of transcutaneous oxygen electrodes. Acta Anaesthesiol. Scand., 68:76–82, 1978.

Rooth, G., Huch, A., and Huch, R.: Transcutaneous oxygen monitors are reliable indicators of arterial oxygen tension (if used correctly). Pediatrics, 79:283–286, 1987.

Simbruner, G., Coradello, H., Fodor, M., et al.: Effect of tracheal suction on oxygenation, circulation, and lung mechanics in newborn infants. Arch. Dis. Child., 56:326–330, 1981.

Spitzer, A.R., and Fox, W.W.: Positive-pressure ventilation: Pressure-limited and time-cycled ventilators. In Goldsmith, J., and Karotkin, E.H. (Eds.): Assisted Ventilation of the Neonate. Philadelphia, W.B. Saunders, 1996, pp. 175–176.

Spitzer, A.R., and Stefano, J.: Respiratory distress syndrome. In Polin, R., Yoder, M., and Berg, F. (Eds.): Workbook in Neonatology. Philadelphia, W.B. Saunders, 1993, p. 177.

Wasunna, A., and Whitelow, G.L.: Pulse oximetry in preterm infants. Arch. Dis. Child., 62:957–971, 1987.

Wung, J.T., James, L.S., Kilchevsky, E., et al.: Management of infants with severe respiratory failure and persistence of fetal circulation without hyperventilation. Pediatrics, 76:488–494, 1985.

Young, T.E., and Mangum, O.B.: Neofax: A Manual of Drugs Used in Neonatal Care, 11th ed. Raleigh, N.C.: Acorn Publishing, 1998.

ADDITIONAL READINGS

Antunes, M.J., Greenspan, J.S., and Zukowsky, K.: Advanced ventilation in the neonate. Nurs. Clin. North Am., 31:404–422, 1996.

Askin, D.F.: Acute Respiratory Care of the Neonate, 2nd ed. Petaluma, Calif., NICU Ink, 1997.

Askin, D.F.: Interpretation of neonatal blood gases. Part I. Physiology and acid-base homeostasis. Neonatal Network, 16(5):17–21, 1997.

Askin, D.F.: Interpretation of neonatal blood gases. Part II. Disorders of acid-base balance. Neonatal Network, 16(6):23–29, 1997.

Blackburn, S.T., and Loper, D.L.: Maternal, Fetal, and Neonatal Physiology: A Clinical Perspective. Philadelphia, W.B. Saunders, 1992.

Bloom, R.S., and Cropley, C.: Textbook of Neonatal Resuscitation, 3rd ed. Dallas and Elk Grove Village, Ill., American Heart Association–American Academy of Pediatrics, 1994.

Broughton, J.O.: Understanding Blood Gases [reprint 456]. Ohio Medical Products, 1971.

Collins, J.R., and Minton, S. Weaning from HFOV to conventional ventilation. Neonat. Intens. Care, May/June, 39–43, 1996.

Cox, C.A., Wolfson, M.R., and Shaffer, T.H.: Liquid ventilation: A comprehensive overview. Neonatal Network, 15(3):31–43, 1996.

Cvetnic, W.G., Cunningham, M.D., Sills, J.N., et al.: Reintroduction of continuous negative pressure ventilation in neonates: 2-year experience. Pediatr. Pulmonol. 8:245–253, 1990.

Cvetnic, W.G., Waffarn, F., and Martin, J.M.: Continuous negative pressure and intermittent mandatory ventilation in the management of pulmonary interstitial emphysema: A preliminary study. J. Perinatol., 9:26–32, 1989.

Eanes, R.: On the horizon: Liquid ventilation. J. Obstet. Gynecol. Neonatal Nurs., *24*:119–124, 1996.

Hansen, T.N., Cooper, T.R., and Weisman, L.E.: Contemporary Diagnosis and Management of Neonatal Respiratory Diseases, 2nd ed. Newton, Pa., Handbooks in Health Care. 1998.

Lynam, L.E., and Algren, S.: Pulmonary function testing: A tool for managing the mechanically ventilated patient. Neonatal Network, *12*:61–64, 1993.

Myrer, M.L.: New trends in neonatal mechanical ventilation. Crit. Care Nurs. Clin. North Am., *4*:507–513, 1992.

Patel, C.A., and Klein, J.M.: Outcome of infants with birth weights less than 1000 gm with respiratory distress syndrome treated with high-frequency ventilation and surfactant replacement therapy. Neonat. Intens. Care, *November/December*:25–29, 64–65, 1995.

Workman, E., and Donn, S.M.: Synchronized ventilation of the newborn: Impact on care practices. Neonat. Intens. Care, *September/October*:16–18, 1995.

Wung, J.T.: Respiratory management for low birthweight infants. Neonat. Intens. Care, *January/February*:32–33, 1994.

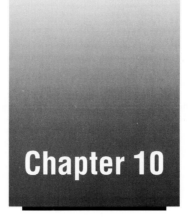

Chapter 10

Extracorporeal Membrane Oxygenation in the Neonate

Carolyn Houska Lund

Objectives

1. Discuss the history of neonatal ECMO and related survival statistics.

2. Discuss indications and contraindications for ECMO.

3. Discuss the criteria used to determine an infant's need for ECMO.

4. Review the technical and mechanical aspects of the ECMO procedure.

5. Review the physiology of extracorporeal circulation.

6. Discuss the general care given to infants undergoing the ECMO procedure and the support provided to their families.

7. Review follow-up and outcome of ECMO survivors.

Extracorporeal membrane oxygenation (ECMO) is the process of prolonged cardiopulmonary bypass (extracorporeal circulation) that provides cardiorespiratory support for infants in reversible, profound respiratory and/or cardiac failure. Despite recent advances in ventilatory management, respiratory failure remains the most frequent cause of neonatal death. ECMO is used as a "rescue" therapy for the 2–5% of critically ill infants who do not respond to maximal conventional ventilatory, medical, and surgical treatments.

ECMO: A Historical Perspective

A. **John Gibbon (1937) invented the first heart-lung machine** and was the first physician to use the technology to perform cardiac surgery successfully. This prototype required direct exposure of the blood to oxygen and a roller pump.

B. **Development of a membrane lung by Clowes (1956)** allowed for separation of the blood and gas phases and dramatically reduced complications (thrombocytopenia, hemolysis, organ failure) of the direct exposure of blood to oxygen.

C. Development of silicone rubber by Kammermeyer (1957) made the membrane lung feasible for long-term support.

D. Kolobow (1969 to 1970) demonstrated the safe use of extracorporeal support for up to 7 days in lambs, using a coiled silicone membrane lung.

E. Prolonged ECMO support for moribund neonates in respiratory failure was attempted from 1965 to 1971. Bartlett began extensive clinical studies and reported improvements in survival and morbidity rates (Bartlett, 1986; Bartlett and Gazzaniga, 1978; Bartlett et al., 1982, 1985).

F. First survivor was successfully treated in 1975.

1. Survival rate of 55% in 1981 (Bartlett et al., 1982).
2. Survival rate of 100% in 1985 (Bartlett et al., 1985).

G. Bartlett's success prompted clinical trials at various centers throughout the United States.

1. These centers reported results similar to those of Bartlett's.
2. O'Rourke et al. (1989), in a prospective clinical trial, demonstrated that the overall survival rate of ECMO-treated infants was 99%, in comparison with 60% of infants treated with conventional mechanical therapy.

H. Neonatal ECMO Registry Report (July 1997) lists a total of 12,692 infants treated since 1975, with an overall survival rate of 80%. A total of 117 ECMO centers reported. Survival by diagnosis was as follows: meconium aspiration syndrome 94%, persistent pulmonary hypertension of the newborn/persistent fetal circulation 82%, respiratory distress syndrome/hyaline membrane disease 84%, pneumonia/sepsis 76%, air-leak syndrome 67%, congenital diaphragmatic hernia (CDH) 59%, and other 76%.

Criteria for Use of ECMO

A. Neonatal ECMO patient criteria (Rosenberg and Seguin, 1995).

1. Gestational age greater than 34 weeks.
2. Birth weight greater than 2000 g.
3. No significant coagulopathy or uncontrollable bleeding.
4. No major intracranial hemorrhage.
5. Mechanical ventilation for less than 10–14 days.
6. Reversible lung injury.
7. No lethal malformations.
8. No major cardiac malformations (except in infants requiring stabilization and life support before or after surgery).

B. Acute and reversible respiratory or cardiac pathology.

1. Respiratory distress syndrome.
2. Meconium aspiration syndrome.
3. Persistent pulmonary hypertension of the newborn.
4. Congenital diaphragmatic hernia.
5. Sepsis.
6. Life support before or after cardiac surgery.
7. Acute respiratory distress syndrome.

C. Cranial and cardiac ultrasonography findings ruling out severe intracranial hemorrhage and cyanotic congenital heart disease.

D. Objective criteria for final selection predictive of greater than 80% mortality rate (Table 10–1). To achieve specificity, each ECMO center must determine its

Table 10–1
NEONATAL ECMO PATIENT QUALIFYING CRITERIA

Alveolar-Arterial Difference in Partial Pressure of Oxygen: 600–624 mm Hg for 4–12 Hours at Sea Level.

$$AaDO_2 = \frac{\text{Atmospheric pressure} - 47 - (PaCO_2 + PaO_2)}{FIO_2}$$

Note: 47 is the partial pressure of water vapor.

Oxygenation Index: 25–60 for 30 Minutes to 6 Hours

$$OI = \frac{MAP \times FIO_2 \times 100}{PaO_2}$$

where MAP is mean airway pressure.

PaO_2: 35–50 mm Hg for 2–12 Hours

Acute Deterioration
PaO_2 ≤30–40 mm Hg
pH ≤7.25 for 2 hours
Intractable hypotension

Reprinted with permission from Rosenberg, E., and Seguin, J.: Selection criteria for use of ECLS in neonates. *In* Zwischenberger, J., and Bartlett, R.H. (Eds.): ECMO: Extracorporeal Cardiopulmonary Support in Critical Care. Ann Arbor, Extracorporeal Life Support Organization, 1995.

own mortality indicators and criteria. Criteria may differ in different disease states, such as septic shock, CDH, or severe air leak caused by barotrauma.

E. **Pre-ECMO stabilization, including optimal ventilatory management and trial of high-frequency ventilation, volume support, vasopressors, vasodilator medications, surfactant, and nitric oxide if indicated.** These should be used at a center where ECMO can be initiated quickly if the infant does not respond adequately.

Venoarterial Perfusion

A. Technique for venoarterial perfusion (VA).

1. Deoxygenated blood is drained from the right side of the heart through a cannula placed in the right atrium via the right internal jugular vein.
2. Venous cannula must be capable of delivering total cardiac output (120–150 ml/kg per minute) to the membrane lung; cannulas of largest possible internal diameter (8–14F) are inserted.
3. Oxygenated blood is returned through a cannula placed into the ascending aorta via the right common carotid artery (Hagedorn, Gardner, and Abman, 1998).

B. Advantages.

1. Technique provides both respiratory and cardiac support by decompressing pulmonary circulation, decreases pulmonary artery and pulmonary capillary filtration pressure, and supports circulation by augmenting the pumping action of the heart (Chapman, Toomasian, and Bartlett, 1988).
2. Positive-pressure ventilation can be reduced to minimal parameters: peak inspiratory pressure, 15–20 cm H_2O; positive end-expiratory pressure, 5–10 cm H_2O; respiratory rate, 10–20/min; and fractional concentration of oxygen in inspired gas (FIO_2), 21%.

C. Disadvantages (Chapman et al., 1988).

1. Emboli (air or particulate) could be infused directly into the arterial circulation.
2. Ligation of carotid artery may affect cerebral perfusion.

Venovenous Perfusion

A. Technique for venovenous (VV) perfusion.

1. Double-lumen cannula is used (size 12F, 14F, or 15F). Deoxygenated blood is drained from the venous limb, positioned in the right atrium.
2. Blood is returned through the arterial limb, also located in the right atrium, with side holes positioned at the tricuspid valve.
3. Blood flow is directed across the valve, into the right ventricle, and through the pulmonary circulation. It returns to the left atrium before entering the systemic circulation via the aorta.

B. Advantages (Cornish et al., 1993).

1. No ligation of the carotid artery is necessary.
2. Oxygenated blood flows through pulmonary circulation, which may help to reverse pulmonary hypertension.
3. Oxygenated blood is provided to the coronary arteries.
4. Emboli (air or particulate) are less likely to result in severe compromise to the infant because blood is not returned directly to the arterial circulation.

C. Disadvantages (Cornish et al., 1993).

1. VV perfusion can be used only with adequate cardiac function because systemic flow is dependent on cardiac output. In the event of cardiac "stun," or decreased function, emergent conversion to VA ECMO may be needed.
2. Recirculation of oxygenated blood can occur. Oxygenated blood returned to the right atrium may be emptied again into the venous side of the double-lumen cannula, rather than across the tricuspid valve.
3. Use of somewhat higher ventilatory support may be required because lower flow rates are achieved with the smaller lumens of the double-lumen cannula.
4. Vasopressor therapy may need to be continued to support blood pressure and ECMO flow.

Circuit Components and Additional Devices

A. Cannulas (Fig. 10–1).

1. Cannulas remove deoxygenated venous blood and return oxygenated blood to the circulation.
2. Before insertion of the cannulas, the infant is paralyzed to prevent respiratory movement and air embolism, and systemic heparin is given to prevent clotting of the cannulas and the circuit (Nugent and Matranga, 1997).
3. In VA ECMO the venous cannula tip is positioned in the right atrium to drain blood flow from the inferior vena cava and the superior vena cava. The arterial cannula tip reaches just to the aortic arch.
4. In VV ECMO the double-lumen cannula is positioned in the right atrium, with the arterial side directed toward the tricuspid valve.

B. Polyvinyl chloride (PVC) tubing.

1. Tubing consists of Luer-Lok connectors, stopcocks, infusion sites, and silicone bladder.
2. Blood circulates through components of circuit; blood is removed from venous side of circuit; and parenteral fluids, medications, and blood products are administered through venous side of circuit.
3. Only platelets are infused on the arterial side of circuit.
4. Precautions and guidelines for placing medications and blood products into

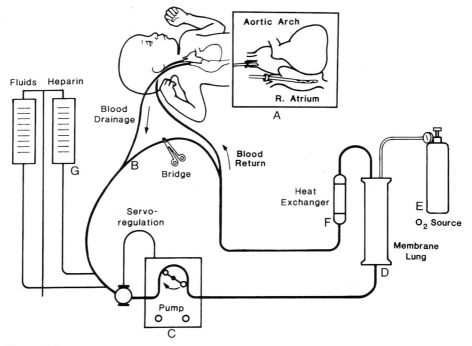

Figure 10–1
Components of ECMO circuit: cannulas, polyvinylchloride tubing, roller head pump, membrane oxygenator (lung), gas source, heat exchanger, and infusion pumps.

the circuit are the same as those for safely administering medications and blood products directly to patients.

C. Silicone bladder for venous pressure monitoring.

1. Collapsible silicone bladder distends with returning venous blood.
2. Inadequate flow (decreased venous return) into the ECMO circuit causes the bladder to collapse, which triggers a microswitch and an audible alarm and stops the roller head pump.
3. When the bladder reexpands, the microswitch reengages the pump and normal pump operation continues.
4. Adequate venous return is critical for maintaining cardiorespiratory support; therefore the cause of decreased return must be recognized and corrected immediately.
5. Servomechanism regulation of ECMO flow can also be achieved by transducers placed in the circuits. Premembrane (venous) pressure and postmembrane (arterial) pressure may be monitored continuously to signal extracorporeal flow problems before collapse of the silicone bladder. This allows for early detection and timely intervention.
   a. Rise in premembrane pressure indicates decreased venous return.
   b. Rise in postmembrane pressure indicates malfunction of membrane oxygenator or heat exchanger.

D. Pumps.

1. Roller head pumps are the most commonly used. They compress and displace the blood in the PVC tubing placed in the pump raceway.

2. Blood is pushed forward, creating gentle suction in the venous cannula and assisting left ventricular function when VA bypass is used.
3. Digital display indicates circuit flow in cubic centimeters per minute.
4. Electrically powered; must be hand cranked or attached to battery pack if power failure occurs.
5. Centrifugal pumps generate flow by means of a spinning motor; commonly used for bypass during cardiovascular surgery and, at some centers, for ECMO bypass.
6. Newly developed "M-pump" is a passively filled, nonocclusive roller pump that does not generate negative pressure.

E. **Membrane oxygenator.**

1. Solid silicone polymer membrane envelope with plastic space screen is wrapped spirally around a spool; encased in a silicone rubber sleeve.
2. Oxygenator of choice because it eliminates the damaging blood-gas interface, ensures constant blood volume, and is relatively easy to operate (Chapman et al., 1988).

F. **Heat exchanger.**

1. Located downstream from the oxygenator.
2. Rewarms blood to 37.2° C (normothermia) before returning it to the infant's circulation.
3. Heat loss occurs from cooling effect of ventilating gases inside the oxygenator and circuit exposure to ambient air temperature.

G. **Bubble detector.**

1. Placed distal (patient side) to heat exchanger to detect air in blood flowing through arterial side of pump as the blood is returned to the patient.
2. In some systems, when air is detected, the roller head pump is shut off and flow to the patient ceases.

H. **Activated clotting time (ACT) monitoring.**

1. Intermittent (every 30–60 minutes) monitor of the infant's ACT (Nugent and Matranga, 1997).
2. Infusion pump for continuous infusion of heparin solution (30–60 U/kg per milliliter) into ECMO circuit (Nugent and Matranga, 1997).
3. Titration of heparin solution to keep ACT within the desired range (180–220 seconds) (Torosian, Statter, and Arensman, 1996).
4. For control of heparin administration, no heparin added to any other medications or fluids (an exception may be the fluids being infused into umbilical or peripheral arterial lines).
5. Factors that influence heparin requirements: thrombocytopenia, abnormal clotting studies, urinary output, and infusions of blood products that contain clotting factors.

I. **Blood gas monitoring.**

1. Mixed venous oxygen saturation ($S\bar{v}O_2$), monitored continuously, is the optimal parameter to assess tissue oxygen delivery. It can be measured through fiberoptic catheters or by using optical reflectance technology. Correlation with co-oximeter values measured by a blood gas machine is required.
2. Arterial blood gas measurements obtained beyond the membrane oxygenator in the ECMO circuit reflect the function of the membrane lung.
3. Patient blood gas values and noninvasive oxygen saturation monitoring are used to assess the recovery of lung function and the infant's acid-base balance.

Physiology of Extracorporeal Circulation

The physiology of extracorporeal circulation has been discussed by Nugent and Matranga (1997) and by Torosian et al. (1996).

A. Blood flow.

1. VA bypass is instituted by draining venous blood into the ECMO circuit; a like amount of oxygenated blood is returned to the arterial circulation.
2. As bypass flow increases, flow through the pulmonary artery decreases faster than bypass flow and reduces total flow in the systemic circulation, causing peripheral and pulmonary hypotension.
3. Blood volume replacement is required for optimal tissue perfusion.
4. ECMO perfusion is nonpulsatile (pulse contour decreases as flow rate increases); kidneys interpret this as inadequate flow and promote the release of renin and aldosterone, which causes sodium retention, extracellular fluid expansion, and a decreased total body potassium concentration.
5. Total patient flow is the sum of ECMO flow and pulmonary blood flow; adequate flow is reached when oxygen delivery and tissue perfusion result in normoxia, normal pH, normal $S\bar{v}O_2$, and normal organ function.
6. Total gas exchange and support are achieved at a flow rate of 120–150 mL/kg per minute.

B. Gas exchange.

1. The membrane lung has two compartments divided by a semipermeable membrane: ventilating gas is on one side, and blood is on the other.
2. Oxygen diffuses into the blood because of a pressure gradient between the elevated oxygen pressure in the gas compartment and the low oxygen pressure in the venous blood.
3. Carbon dioxide diffuses from the blood compartment to the gas compartment as a result of a pressure gradient between venous carbon dioxide pressure and the ventilating gas. The carbon dioxide transfer rate is six times greater than oxygen transfer. The ventilating gas mixture is usually enriched with carbon dioxide to prevent hypocapnia.

C. Blood-surface interface.

1. During ECMO, up to 80% of the cardiac output is exposed to a large artificial surface each minute.
2. Clot formation is prevented by systemic heparinization; platelet destruction is minimized by preexposure of the circuit to albumin.
3. Platelets show the greatest effect of exposure to a foreign surface, as evidenced by decreased platelet count (thrombocytopenia) and function.
4. Hemolysis is monitored regularly by measuring plasma free hemoglobin levels. It is usually not significantly altered by ECMO flow, although increases may indicate problems with red blood cell destruction in the membrane oxygenator or small-lumen cannula.
5. All types of white blood cells decrease in concentration, and phagocytic activity is significantly decreased.
6. After cessation of ECMO, platelets and white blood cell counts return to normal.

Care of the Infant During ECMO

Nugent and Matranga (1997) and Torosian et al., (1996) have discussed the responsibilities of the ECMO specialist and the nurse in the care of the infant during ECMO.

A. Cannulation.

1. Cannulation and initiation of a local anesthetic and systemic analgesia; bypass occur in the NICU after the infant has been given a local anesthetic; the operating room staff is in attendance.
2. See Table 10–2 for nursing responsibilities and interventions.
3. ECMO specialist responsibilities:
   a. Maintain and monitor ECMO circuit.
   b. Assess physiologic stability.
   c. Maintain physiologic parameters such as blood gas values, blood pressure, platelet count, $S\bar{v}O_2$ and arterial oxygen saturation (SaO_2) and ACT.
   d. Assist nurse in general care of infant.
   e. Be prepared for circuit emergencies.

B. During ECMO "run."

1. Bypass is gradually instituted until approximately 80% (120–150 mL/kg per minute) of cardiac output is diverted through the ECMO circuit.
2. At maximal flow, blood gas values should normalize and $S\bar{v}O_2$ is maintained at greater than 70%.

Table 10–2
NURSING RESPONSIBILITIES AND INTERVENTIONS FOR ECMO

Responsibility	Intervention
BEFORE CANNULATION	
Obtain and document base-line physiologic data.	Record weight, length, head circumference.
	Draw blood samples for CBC, electrolytes, calcium, glucose, BUN, creatinine, PT/PTT, platelet count and function, arterial blood gas values.
	Record vital signs: heart rate; respiratory rate; systolic, diastolic, and mean blood pressure; and temperature.
Ensure adequate supply of blood products for replacement.	Draw type and cross-match samples for two units of packed red blood cells and fresh frozen plasma.
	Keep one unit of packed cells and fresh frozen plasma always available in the blood bank.
Maintain prescribed pulmonary support.	Maintain ventilator parameters.
	Administer muscle relaxants if indicated.
Assemble and prepare equipment.	Prepare infusion pumps to maintain arterial lines and infusion of parenteral fluids and medications into the ECMO circuit.
	Place the infant on a radiant warmer with the head positioned at the foot of the bed to provide thermoregulation and access for cannulation.
	Attach infant to physiologic monitoring devices to monitor heart rate, intra-arterial blood pressure, transcutaneous oxygen, and other parameters.
	Insert urinary catheter and nasogastric tube; place to gravity drainage.
	Remove IV lines just prior to heparinization (optional).
	Prepare loading dose of heparin (50-100 units/kg).
	Prepare heparin solution for continuous infusion (100 units/mL 5% dextrose in water).
	Prepare paralyzing drug (pancuronium bromide, 0.1 mg/kg, or succinylcholine, 1-4 mg/kg).
	Assist in insertion of arterial line (umbilical or peripheral).
	Administer prophylactic antibiotics.
DURING CANNULATION	
Monitor cardiopulmonary status during procedure.	Monitor heart rate and intra-arterial blood pressure continuously.
	Obtain blood gas values after paralysis and during cannulation, as indicated by the infant's response to the procedure.
Be prepared to administer cardiopulmonary support.	Have medications and blood products available to correct hypovolemia, bradycardia, acidosis, and cardiac arrest.
Administer medications.	Give loading dose of heparin systemically when vessels are dissected free and are ready to be cannulated.
	Give paralyzing drug systemically just before cannulation of internal jugular vein if infant has not been previously paralyzed. Give analgesia for anesthetic effect.
Reduce ventilator parameters to minimal settings.	Once adequate bypass is achieved, reduce PIP to 16-20 cm H_2O, PEEP to 4 cm H_2O, ventilator rate to 10-20 breaths per minute, and FIO_2 to 21-30%. Patients undergoing VV bypass may require greater respiratory support.

Table continued on following page

Table 10–2
NURSING RESPONSIBILITIES AND INTERVENTIONS FOR ECMO *(Continued)*

Responsibility	Intervention
DURING ECMO RUN Monitor and document physiologic parameters.	Record hourly: heart rate, blood pressure (systolic, diastolic, mean), respirations, temperature, oxygen saturation, ACT, ECMO flow. Measure hourly accurate intake and output of all body fluids (urine, gastric contents, blood); test all stools for occult blood. Assess hourly: color, breath sounds, heart tones, murmurs, cardiac rhythm, arterial pressure waveform, peripheral perfusion. Assess hourly: level of consciousness, reflexes, tone, and movement of extremities; assess neurologic exam including fontanelle tension, pupil size and reaction every 8-12 hours. Record ventilator parameters hourly. Assess weight and head circumference daily.
Monitor and document biochemical parameters.	Draw samples for arterial blood gas values from umbilical or peripheral line as indicated. All other blood specimens are drawn from ECMO circuit by ECMO specialist: electrolytes, calcium, platelets, Chemstrip blood tests, hematocrit every 4-8 hours, CBC, PT/PTT, BUN, creatinine, total and direct bilirubin, plasma hemoglobin, fibrinogen, fibrin split products, and blood culture as indicated.
Administer medications.	Remove air bubbles and double-check dosages before infusion. Administer no medications intramuscularly or by venipuncture. Place all medications and fluids into the venous side of the ECMO circuit. Prepare and administer the arterial line (umbilical or peripheral) infusion. Administer parenteral alimentation.
Provide pulmonary support.	Perform endotracheal suctioning according to individual assessment and need. Maintain patent airway; be alert to extubation or plugging. Obtain daily chest films and tracheal aspirate cultures as indicated. Maintain ventilator parameters.
Prevent bleeding.	Avoid all of the following: rectal probes, injections, venipunctures, heel sticks. Avoid invasive procedures. Do not change nasogastric tube, urinary catheters, or endotracheal tube unless absolutely necessary; use premeasured endotracheal tube suction technique. Observe for blood in urine, stools, and endotracheal or nasogastric tubes.
Maintain excellent infection control.	Change all fluids and tubing daily. Change dressings daily and as needed. Maintain closed system for urinary catheter drainage. Maintain strict aseptic and hand-washing techniques. Use universal barrier precautions.
Provide physical care.	Keep skin dry, clean, and free of pressure points. Give mouth care as needed. Provide range of motion as indicated. Turn side to side every 1-2 hours.
Provide pain management, sedation, stress reduction.	Minimize noise level. Cluster patient care to maximize sleep period. Administer analgesia: fentanyl or morphine as continuous IV drip. Manage iatrogenic physical dependency by following dose reduction regimen.
Be alert to complications and emergencies.	See text.

CBC, Complete blood cell count; *BUN,* blood urea nitrogen; *PT/PTT,* prothrombin time/partial thromboplastin time; *PIP,* peak inspiratory pressure; *PEEP,* positive end-expiratory pressure; *Fio$_2$,* fractional concentration of oxygen in inspired gas.
Adapted from Nugent, J. and Matranga, G.: Extracorporeal membrane oxygenation. In Askin, D. F. (Ed.): Acute Respiratory Care of the Newborn, 2nd ed. Petaluma, Calif., NICU Ink, 1997, pp. 341-368.

3. $S\bar{v}O_2$ is an excellent indicator of adequate flow during VA ECMO because it is a measure of tissue perfusion and efficiency of extracorporeal circulation in meeting metabolic demands.
4. Oxygenation during VV ECMO is assessed by infant's arterial blood gas values and continuous oxygen saturation monitoring via pulse oximetry. $S\bar{v}O_2$ is not an accurate reflection of deoxygenated blood because of recirculation; $S\bar{v}O_2$ is used as a trending parameter during VV ECMO.
5. Ventilator settings are reduced to a minimum; vasopressor therapy and chemical paralysis are usually discontinued; enteral feedings are generally

withheld because of concern about hypoxic injury to the gastrointestinal tract, which has never been exposed to nutrients; and blood loss is quantified and replaced.

6. Emergencies during ECMO:
   a. Circuit emergencies.
      (1) Air embolism.
      (2) Tubing rupture.
      (3) Oxygenator malfunction.
      (4) Accidental decannulation.
      (5) Power failure.
      (6) Gas source failure.
   b. Responsibilities of the nurse during a circuit emergency:
      (1) Notification of physician.
      (2) Ventilation.
      (3) Anticoagulation.
      (4) Chemical resuscitation.
      (5) Blood loss replacement.
   c. Responsibilities of the ECMO specialist during a circuit emergency:
      (1) Clamp catheters.
      (2) Open bridge.
      (3) Remove gas source.
      (4) Repair circuit.

C. **ECMO patient complications (Nugent and Matranga, 1997).**

1. Electrolyte/glucose/fluid imbalance. Sodium requirements decrease; potassium requirements increase because of the action of aldosterone. Calcium replacement may be needed if citrate-phosphate-dextrose anticoagulated blood is used. Hyperglycemia may necessitate a decrease in the glucose concentration of IV fluids.
2. CNS deterioration: cerebral edema, intracranial hemorrhage, and seizures. Deterioration results from initial hypoxia, acidosis, hypercapnia, or vessel ligation.
3. Generalized edema. The extracellular space is enlarged by the distribution of crystalloid solution and the action of aldosterone and antidiuretic hormone. The use of diuretics or hemofiltration may be necessary if edema causes brain or lung dysfunction.
4. Renal failure. Acute tubular necrosis results from pre-ECMO hypotension and hypoxia. Indicators of renal failure are abnormal blood urea nitrogen and creatinine values. Low-dose dopamine therapy and/or hemodialysis may be necessary.
5. Hemorrhage due to thrombocytopenia, coagulopathy.
6. Decreased venous return and/or hypovolemia. These complications are due to inadequate circulating blood volume, pneumothorax, and/or partial venous catheter occlusion or malposition.
7. Hypertension due to overinfusion of blood products, renal ischemia, and excretion of renin-angiotensin.
8. Patent ductus arteriosus. Left-to-right shunting may cause increased blood flow to the lung, necessitating high pump flows without the expected increase in PaO_2. Ligation may be necessary.
9. Cardiac "stun." Transient loss of ventricular contractility (1–3 days) is manifested by hypotension, decrease in aortic pulse pressure, poor peripheral perfusion, and decreased PaO_2. It is possibly due to mismatch between afterload and ventricular contractility during ECMO.
10. Mechanical complications. These include incorrect catheter placement, oxygenator failure, power failure, and accidental decannulation.

D. Weaning/decannulation.

1. Signs of improvement and indicators that the infant is ready to be weaned are as follows:
   a. Improvement of lung fields on chest x-ray examination.
   b. Clinical findings: improved breath sounds, rising PaO_2 on fixed ECMO flow, improvement in lung compliance.
2. Once improvement has been ascertained, flow rate is decreased slowly in 10–20 mL increments until ECMO support is no longer needed to maintain adequate gas exchange at low ventilator settings (Nugent and Matranga, 1997).
3. When flow rate is 50–100 mL/kg per minute, a state of "idling" is achieved; the infant remains at this lowest possible flow rate for 4–8 hours.
4. If improvement in lung function remains stable, cannulas are clamped, heparin is infused directly into the infant, and the circuit is recirculated via a bridge. If blood gas values deteriorate, the cannulas are unclamped and ECMO support is resumed.
5. During VV ECMO the cannulas are not clamped during the "trial off" procedure; gas flow to the membrane oxygenator is discontinued. Low flow rates are maintained, and patient response is assessed by measurement of blood gases.
6. Decannulation proceeds if blood gas values remain satisfactory.
7. Before decannulation, the infant undergoes chemical paralysis and ventilator parameters are increased to compensate for loss of spontaneous respiratory function.
8. After a local anesthetic has been administered, the cannulas are removed. Both the internal jugular vein and the carotid artery are ligated. In some ECMO centers, carotid reconstruction is attempted (Levy and Fackler, 1998). The efficacy of this procedure is still debated because of clot formation at the site of reconstruction.
9. After decannulation, the infant is weaned as tolerated from the ventilator and routine NICU care is resumed.

Post-ECMO Care

A. **Lung recovery is achieved through weaning of the infant from assisted ventilation.** Occasionally the use of steroids and/or diuretics is necessary to improve recovery.

B. **Assessment of neurologic recovery involves clinical evaluation and CT scan.** It may be difficult to assess neurologic status during opiate use or while the infant is recovering from significant illness, so assessment may be deferred until the infant is ready for discharge.

C. **Weaning from opiate analgesics and sedatives involves a gradual reduction of doses and careful monitoring for withdrawal symptoms.** Infants receiving ECMO therapy require opiate infusions or scheduled dosing of opiates and sedatives throughout their course of ECMO to prevent excessive movement, which can dislodge the cannulas (Arnold et al., 1990; Caron and Maguire, 1990; Franck and Vilardi, 1995).

D. **Establishing oral feedings may be difficult.** Prolonged respiratory compromise, the effect of opiates on state control, alterations in swallowing caused by neck dissection during cannula placement, and gastroesophageal reflux, particularly in infants with CDH, are some of the causes of feeding problems in the post-ECMO infant. Feeding difficulties are generally more common in infants with CDH than in those with other diagnoses such as meconium aspiration syndrome or persistent pulmonary hypertension of the newborn.

Parental Support

A. **The ECMO candidate's parents are in crisis.** They are aware that ECMO is a method of last resort with no guarantee of positive result, and the technology is overwhelming.

B. **Parents need concise, accurate information** about their child's condition and the required procedures.

C. **Parent-to-parent support, using parents of "ECMO graduates," is effica-cious and a positive experience.**

D. **Parents should have access to their infant.** The ECMO candidates have an increasingly bright outcome, and every effort should be made to encourage involvement and bonding.

Follow-up and Outcome

The follow-up and outcome of ECMO have been discussed by Bernbaum et al. (1995); Boggs and LaPrade-Wolf (1992); Glass, Miller, and Short (1989); Glass, Wagner, and Coffman (1995); and Kanto (1994).

A. **Critical scrutiny of survivors is essential to assess the value and safety of ECMO.** Survivors should be evaluated at 4–6 months, and then yearly until school age. The following are assessed:
1. Growth and development.
2. Cardiorespiratory development.
3. Cerebrovascular status.
4. Neurologic and psychologic functioning.

B. **Medical morbidity includes poor somatic growth, feeding problems, chronic lung disease, and rehospitalizations.** Predictors include diagnosis of CDH, lower birth weight, and age at initiation of ECMO.

C. **The incidence of sensorineural disabilities among ECMO survivors is 6% (range, 2–18%). The incidence of significant developmental delay is 9% (range, 0–21%) (Glass, Wagner, Papero, et al., 1995; Hofkosh et al., 1991).** Predictors include cardiopulmonary resuscitation before ECMO, neuroimaging abnormalities, and seizures.

D. **School-age ECMO survivors are twice as likely as other children to have neuropsychologic deficits and are at risk of having academic problems.** Predictors include lower birth weight, abnormal findings on neurologic imaging, chronic lung disease, and failure to thrive. However, even children who do not have these risk factors can have neuropsychologic testing to predict the need for special education services.

E. **Psychologic morbidity, including behavioral problems, is also reported and may be due to altered parenting styles and family stress.** Early trauma from severe illness may set the stage for problems in parent-child interactions.

REFERENCES

Arnold, J., Truog, R., Orav, E.J., et al.: Tolerance and dependence in neonates sedated with fentanyl during extracorporeal membrane oxygenation. Anesthesiology, 73:1136–1140, 1990.

Bartlett, R.: Respiratory support: Extracorporeal membrane oxygenation in newborn respiratory failure. *In* Welch, K., et al. (Eds.): Pediatric Surgery. Chicago, Year Book Medical Publishers, 1986, pp. 74–77.

Bartlett, R., and Gazzaniga, A.: Extracorporeal circulation for cardiopulmonary failure. Curr. Probl. Surg., 12(5):1–96, 1978.

Bartlett, R., Andrews, A.F., Toomasian, J.M., et al.: Extracorporeal membrane oxygenation for newborn respiratory failure: Forty-five cases. Surgery, 92:425–433, 1982.

Bartlett, R., Roloff, D.W., Cornell, R.G., et al.: Extracorporeal circulation in neonatal respiratory failure: A prospective randomized study. Pediatrics, 76:479–487, 1985.

Bernbaum, J., Schwartz, I.P., Gerdes, M., et al.: Survivors of extracorporeal membrane oxygenation at 1 year of age: The relationship of primary diagnosis with health and neurodevelopmental sequelae. Pediatrics, 96:907–913, 1995.

Boggs, K., and LaPrade-Wolf, P.: Beyond survival: Strategies for establishing a follow-up program for infants with extracorporeal membrane oxygenation. Neonatal Network, 11:7–13, 1992.

Caron, E., and Maguire, D.: Current management of pain, sedation and narcotic physical dependency of the infant on ECMO. J. Perinatal Neonatal Nurs., 4:63–74, 1990.

Chapman, R., Toomasian, J., and Bartlett, R.: Extracorporeal Membrane Oxygenation Technical Specialist Manual. Ann Arbor, University of Michigan Press, 1988.

Cornish, J.D., Clark, R.H., Ricketts, R.R., et al.: Extracorporeal membrane oxygenation service at Egleston: Two years' experience. J. Med. Assoc. Ga., 82:471–476, 1993.

Franck, L., and Vilardi, J.: Assessment and management of opioid withdrawal in ill neonates. Neonatal Network, 14:39–48, 1995.

Glass, P., Miller, M., and Short, B.: Morbidity for survivors of extracorporeal membrane oxygenation: Neurodevelopmental outcome at 1 year of age. Pediatrics, 83:72–78, 1989.

Glass, P., Wagner, A., and Coffman, C.: Outcome and follow-up of neonates treated with ECMO. In Zwischenberger, J., and Bartlett, R. (Eds.): ECMO: Extracorporeal Cardiopulmonary Support in Critical Care. Ann Arbor, Extracorporeal Life Support Organization, 1995, pp. 327–340.

Glass, P., Wagner, A., Papero, P., et al.: Neurodevelopmental status at age five years of neonates treated with extracorporeal membrane oxygenation. J. Pediatr., 125:104–110, 1995.

Gomez, M.R.: Extracorporeal membrane oxygenation. In Hansen, T.N., Cooper, T.R., and Wiesman, L.E. (Eds.): Comtempory Diagnosis and Management of Neonatal Respiratory Diseases. Newton, Pa., Handbooks in Health Care (AMM Co.), 1995, pp. 258–261.

Hagedorn, M.E., Gardner, S.L., and Abman, S.H.: Respiratory diseases. In Merenstein, G.B., and Gardner, S.L. (Eds.): Handbook of Neonatal Intensive Care, 4th ed. St. Louis, Mosby, 1998, p. 459.

Hofkosh, D., Thompson, A., Nozza, R., et al.: Ten years of extracorporeal membrane oxygenation: Neurodevelopmental outcome. Pediatrics, 87:549–555, 1991.

Kanto, W.P.: A decade of experience with neonatal extracorporeal membrane oxygenation. J. Pediatr., 124:335–347, 1994.

Levy, M., and Fackler, J. Extracorporeal membrane oxygenation. In Cloherty, J.P., and Stark, A.R. (Eds.): Manual of Neonatal Care, 4th ed. Philadelphia, Lippincott-Raven, 1998, pp. 348–353.

Neonatal ECMO Registry Report, July 1, 1997. Ann Arbor, Extracorporeal Life Support Organization, 1997.

Nugent, J., and Matranga, G.: Extracorporeal membrane oxygenation. In Askin, D.F. (Ed.): Acute Respiratory Care of the Newborn, 2nd ed. Petaluma, Calif. NICU Ink, 1997, pp. 341–368.

O'Rourke, P., et al.: Extracorporeal membrane oxygenation and conventional medical therapy in neonates with persistent pulmonary hypertension of the newborn: A prospective randomized study. Pediatrics, 84:957–963, 1989.

Rosenberg, E., and Seguin, J.: Selection criteria for use of ECLS in neonates. pp. 273, In Zwischenberger, J.B., and Bartlett, R.H. (Eds.): ECMO: Extracorporeal Cardiopulmonary Support in Critical Care. Ann Arbor, Extracorporeal Life Support Organization, 1995.

Torosian, M.B., Statter, M.B., and Arensman, R.M.: Extracorporeal membrane oxygenation. In Goldsmith, J.P., and Karotkin, E.H. (Eds.): Assisted Ventilation of the Neonate, 3rd ed. Philadelphia, WB Saunders, 1996, pp. 242–243.

Zwischenberger, J., and Bartlett, R.: ECMO: Extracorporeal Cardiopulmonary Support in Critical Care. Ann Arbor, Extracorporeal Life Support Organization, 1995.

ADDITIONAL READINGS

American Academy of Pediatrics Committee on Fetus and Newborn. Recommendations on extracorporeal membrane oxygenation. Pediatrics, 85:618–619, 1990.

Anderson, H.L., Snedecor, S.M., Otsu, T., and Bartlett, R.H.: Multicenter comparison of conventional venoarterial access versus venovenous double-lumen catheter access in newborn infants undergoing entracorporeal membrane oxygenation. J Pediatr Surg, 28:530–535, 1993.

Faulkner, S.: Mobile extracorporeal membrane oxygenation. Crit. Care Nurs. Clin. North Am., 7:259–266, 1995.

Krause, K., and Youngner, V.: Nursing diagnoses as guidelines in the care of the neonatal ECMO patient. JOGNN, 21:169–176, 1992.

Stolar, C., Crisafi, M., and Driscoll, Y.: Neurocognitive outcome for neonates treated with extracorporeal membrane oxygenation: Are infants with congenital diaphragmatic hernia different? J. Pediatr. Surg., 30:366–371, 1995.

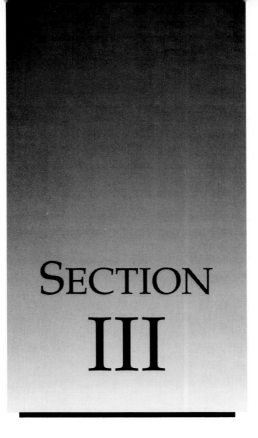

SECTION III

NEONATAL PATHOPHYSIOLOGY: MANAGEMENT AND TREATMENT OF COMMON DISORDERS

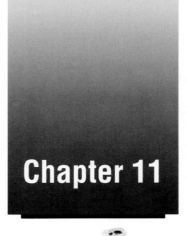

Chapter 11

Cardiovascular Disorders

Margaret Crockett

Objectives

1. Describe how to differentiate between cyanosis that is cardiac in origin and that which is pulmonary in origin.

2. Name the major classifications of congenital heart disease; list two anomalies in each.

3. Define and describe the hemodynamics and resulting clinical signs and the possible treatment of tetralogy of Fallot, coarctation of the aorta, patent ductus arteriosus (PDA), ventricular septal defect (VSD), atrial septal defect (ASD), and hypoplastic left heart syndrome.

4. Describe the basic medical rationale for care of the newborn infant with suspected or identified cardiac defect.

5. Describe basic surgical rationale for treatment of major cardiovascular defects.

6. List signs and symptoms of congenital heart abnormalities of the newborn infant.

7. Describe a cardiac catheterization and list the major postoperative nursing concerns.

8. List the signs and symptoms of PDA and the current medical and surgical interventions.

9. Discuss the treatment modalities employed in congestive heart failure, including the risks and benefits to the neonate.

10. Define the three classifications of shock and list one cause under each category.

Until the twentieth century, there was limited clinical interest in congenital heart disease. In the majority of cases, the anomaly was incompatible with life; in the others, no treatment existed either to remedy the condition or to relieve its symptoms. Today, with advances in medical and surgical therapy, the survival and quality of life of infants with congenital heart disease have markedly improved.

Advances in angiography, echocardiography, and radionuclide imaging, coupled with a more complete understanding of newborn physiology, have led to improvements in diagnostic capabilities without undue risk. Additionally, the advent of deep hypothermia with circulatory arrest permits the total correction of many forms of congenital heart disease in the neonatal period. In some cases, early intervention is essential to prevent long-term morbidity or early death.

In this chapter, topics considered to be of interest to the neonatal nurse are covered. For more detailed coverage, standard pediatric cardiology texts should be consulted.

Cardiovascular Embryology and Anatomy

CARDIAC DEVELOPMENT

The majority of fetal cardiac development (Witt, 1997; Moore and Persaud, 1993) occurs between weeks 3 and 7 of fetal life.

A. Cardiac tube.
1. In the third week of fetal life, a single cardiac tube is formed from two endothelial tubes (endocardial heart tubes). A fusion of the two tubes occurs cranially to caudally.
2. With elongation of the cardiac tube, it expands and loops to the right (Fig. 11–1). A malrotation results in cardiac malposition (i.e., dextrocardia or corrected [L; levocardia] transposition) (Witt, 1997).

B. Cardiac septation: process occurs between weeks 5 and 6.
1. Atrial septum and foramen ovale are formed from two septa and endocardial cushions.
    a. An initial septum (septum primum) grows from the top of the common atrium, extending toward the endocardial cushions (Fig. 11–2, *A*) and leaving an opening (ostium primum) between the rim of the septum primum and the endocardial cushions.
    b. Perforation occurs high in the septum primum to form the ostium secundum; growth of the endocardial cushions eliminates the ostium primum.
    c. A second septum (septum secundum) appears to the right of the septum primum and grows to overlap the ostium secundum. Thus the flapped opening, the foramen ovale, is created (Fig. 11–2, *C*).
2. Ventricular septation results from fusion of the endocardial cushions (forming the membranous portion of the ventricular septum) and dilation and fusion of the ventricles (creating the muscular ventricular septum) (Fig. 11–3).
3. Tissue of endocardial cushion forms the atrioventricular valves.
    a. Tricuspid valve: between right atrium and ventricle.
    b. Mitral valve: between left atrium and ventricle.
4. Abnormal development during cardiac septation can lead to the following:
    a. Ventricular septal defect (VSD), atrial septal defect (ASD), and endocardial cushion defect (atrioventricular canal).
    b. Absence, deformation, stenosis, or atresia of the tricuspid and/or mitral valves.

GREAT VESSEL DEVELOPMENT

A. Single vessel (truncus arteriosus) extends from the ventricles until the fourth week of fetal life.

B. Fifth week: ridges appear within the vessel or trunk. These ridges extend and spiral, separating the truncus arteriosus into the aorta and the pulmonary artery (Fig. 11–4).
1. Swellings at the base of the truncus appear and fuse to form the right and left ventricular outflow tracks.

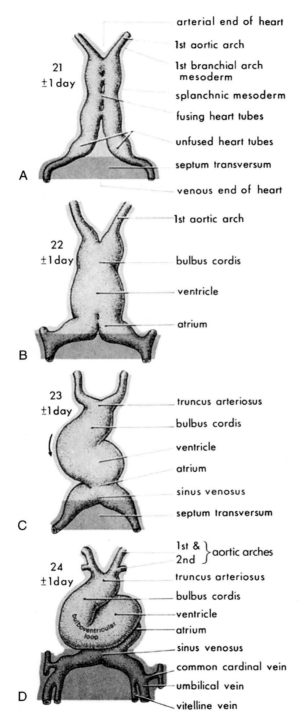

arterial end of heart

1st aortic arch

1st branchial arch mesoderm

splanchnic mesoderm

fusing heart tubes

unfused heart tubes

septum transversum

venous end of heart

1st aortic arch

bulbus cordis

ventricle

atrium

truncus arteriosus

bulbus cordis

ventricle

atrium

sinus venosus

septum transversum

1st & 2nd } aortic arches

truncus arteriosus

bulbus cordis

ventricle

atrium

sinus venosus

common cardinal vein

umbilical vein

vitelline vein

Figure 11–1
Sketches of ventral views of the developing heart (at 20–25 days), showing fusion of the endocardial heart tubes to form a single heart tube. Bending of the heart tube to form a bulboventricular loop is also illustrated. (From Moore, K.: The Developing Human, 4th ed. Philadelphia, W.B. Saunders, 1988, p. 292.)

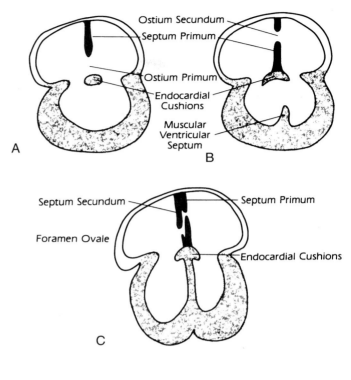

Figure 11–2
Atrial septation. *A,* Septum primum begins to form, extending toward endocardial cushion (note ostium primum). *B,* Ostium primum is closed and perforation (called ostium secundum) forms in septum primum. *C,* Septum secundum forms, creating the foramen ovale. (From Hazinski, M.F.: Congenital heart disease: Part I. Neonatal Network, February 1983, pp. 34–35.)

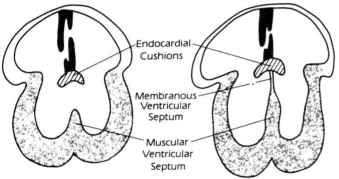

Figure 11–3
Ventricular septation (with muscular and membranous septum). (From Hazinski, M.F.: Congenital heart disease: Part I. Neonatal Network, *4*:34–35, February 1983.)

Figure 11–4
Closing of the truncus arteriosus and division into the pulmonary artery and the aorta. (From Hazinski, M.F.: Congenital heart disease: Part I. Neonatal Network, February 1983, p. 35.)

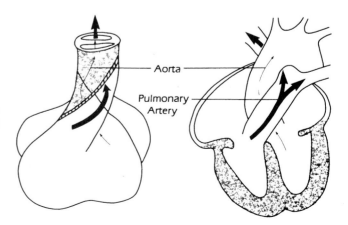

2. The semilunar valves (aortic and pulmonic valves) develop from three ridges of tissue at the opening to the aorta and pulmonary trunk.

C. **Developmental abnormalities of truncal septation include:**

1. Persistent truncus arteriosus.
2. Tetralogy of Fallot.
3. Pulmonary and/or aortic valve atresia or stenosis.
4. Transposition of the great vessels (dextroposition).

CIRCULATORY DEVELOPMENT

A. **Heart contractions begin around 22 days;** the atrium and ventricle muscle layers are continuous. Contractions result in a wavelike peristalsis. The initial circulation is an ebb-and-flow type.

B. **Coordinated contractions** established by the fourth week of gestation provide a unidirectional flow.

C. **Electrical conduction system is functional around 10 weeks, with normal sinus rhythm seen by 16 weeks (Witt, 1997)**

D. **Establishment of fetal circulation.** With completion of atrial and ventricular septation, development of valves between chambers and outflow tracks, and separation of the truncus arteriosus into the great vessels, fetal circulation is established.

E. **Fetal circulation is anatomically and physiologically different from adult circulation.** For a full discussion of fetal circulation and cardiopulmonary adaptation at birth, see Chapter 3, Adaptation to Extrauterine Life.

CARDIOVASCULAR PHYSIOLOGY

A. **Normal circulation (Fig. 11–5).**

1. Oxygen-poor blood enters the right atrium and passes through the tricuspid valve into the right ventricle, where it is pumped through the pulmonary artery to the lungs.
2. As the blood flows through the lungs, it gives up carbon dioxide and gains oxygen.
3. Oxygen-rich blood returns from the lungs through the pulmonary veins. It enters the left atrium and then passes through the mitral valve into the left ventricle, which pumps it through the aortic valve and into the aorta.
4. The aorta then delivers oxygenated blood to all body organs and tissues.

B. **Cardiac depolarization (Guyton and Hall, 1996).**

1. Cardiac depolarization, which results from the electrical discharge across the myocardial cell (total net movement of ions across the cell wall), is measured by the electrocardiograph (ECG).
2. Shortening of muscle fibers (contraction) usually follows cardiac depolarization. Strength of cardiac (ventricular) contraction is measured by blood pressure or arterial pulse palpation.
3. Cardiac electrical activity does not ensure adequate cardiac function.
   a. Congenital defects or surgical injury to the conduction system may result in arrhythmias or heart block.
   b. Electrolyte disturbance (i.e., altered fluid composition surrounding the cells) can affect electrical activity.
      (1) Hypokalemia and hyperkalemia.
      (2) Hypocalcemia and hypercalcemia.
      (3) Hypoxia.
      (4) Acidosis.

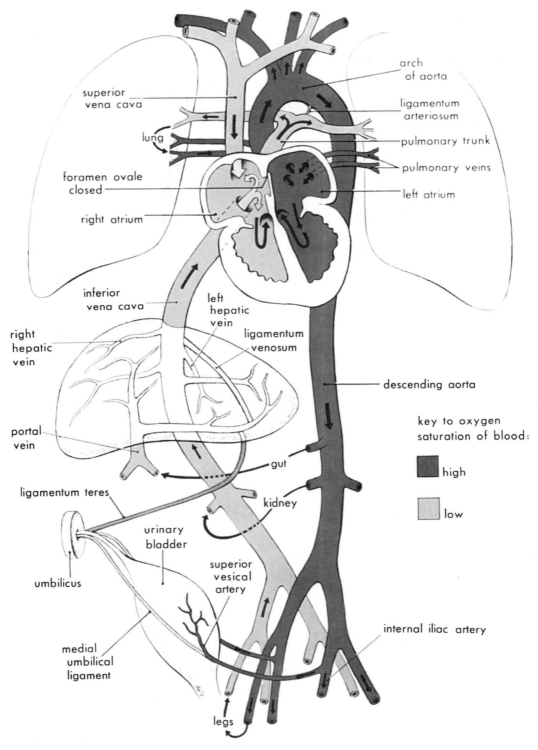

Figure 11–5
Simplified representation of neonatal circulation. Adult derivatives of the fetal vessels and structures that become nonfunctional at birth are also shown. *Arrows* indicate the course of neonatal circulation. (The organs are not drawn to scale.) After birth, the three shunts that short-circuited the blood during fetal life cease to function, and the pulmonary and systemic circulations become separated. (From Moore, K., and Persaud, T.: The Developing Human: Clinically Oriented Embryology, 5th ed. Philadelphia, W.B. Saunders, 1993, p. 345.)

C. Cardiac output.

1. Cardiac output is the volume of blood ejected by the heart in 1 minute. Approximations vary from 120 to 200 mL/kg per minute.
2. Cardiac output = Stroke volume × Heart rate (in liters per minute).
   a. As heart rate fluctuates, so will cardiac output.
      (1) Normal term newborn infants can vary their heart rate range from 59 to 220 bpm in a monitored 24-hour period (Page and Hasking, 1997).
      (2) Significant or persistent bradycardia will result in a drop in the neonate's cardiac output.
   b. Tachycardia seems to be an effective mechanism for improving cardiac output as long as the tachycardia does not compromise diastolic filling time and decrease coronary artery perfusion.
3. Stroke volume is relatively fixed at 1.5 mL/kg and is affected by three factors: preload, contractility, and afterload.
   a. Preload: the volume of blood in the ventricles before contraction.
      (1) Clinically, preload is a measurement of pressure, rather than volume, in the ventricles before contraction.
      (2) Increasing the volume in the ventricles, consequently lengthening the myocardial fibers before contraction, should result in improved stroke volume (Frank-Starling law) (Patterson and Starling, 1914). The newborn infant is capable of increasing stroke volume provided there is no increase in systemic vascular resistance or rapid rise in aortic pressure. Given the neonate's smaller contractile mass, less compliant myocardium, and normal maximization of myocardial fiber length, volume infusions are likely to increase aortic pressure and afterload, resulting in a decline in stroke volume (Bell, 1998).
   b. Contractility: speed of ventricular contraction.
      (1) Cardiac cycle consists of ventricular contraction (systole), followed by ventricular relaxation (diastole). As contraction time decreases, relaxation time (diastole) increases, with an increase in ventricular filling volume (preload) before contraction.
      (2) Ventricular contractility cannot be directly measured. Measurements of cardiac shortening fractions and ejection fraction provide an indirect assessment of contractility.
      (3) Contractility in neonates is influenced by the following:
         (a) Exogenous catecholamine (dopamine/dobutamine) use, which increases blood pressure and cardiac output (Bell, 1998).
         (b) Factors that decrease contractility.
            (i) Acidosis, which impairs myocardial response to catecholamines.
            (ii) Hypoxia.
            (iii) Electrolyte disturbances.
            (iv) Hypoglycemia.
   c. Afterload: the resistance to blood leaving the ventricle.
      (1) Dependent on systemic vascular resistance (SVR) and pulmonary vascular resistance (PVR); if SVR or PVR increases, afterload increases.
      (2) The neonate's myocardium is very sensitive to increased afterload; with small increases in afterload, stroke volume can fall significantly.
      (3) Afterload can be reduced by IV infusion of vasodilators (e.g., nitroglycerin and nitroprusside). Tolazoline and dobutamine can be used to decrease PVR (Bell, 1998).
4. Concepts of blood flow.
   a. Flow ∝ Pressure/Resistance.
   b. Blood flow will always take the path of least resistance.

c. If heart action (pressure) remains unchanged but vasoconstriction or dilation or obstruction to flow (resistance) changes, flow will change (i.e., cardiac output will vary).
d. PVR starts to fall after delivery and declines to levels less than 50% of systemic arterial pressure (Ivy, Neish, and Abman, 1998). This normal decline is influenced by prematurity, low birth weight, and hypoxia episodes.

Congenital Heart Disease

OCCURRENCE

A. **Incidence:** congenital heart disease (CHD) occurs in 8:1000 live births (<1%) (Burton and Cabalke, 1994).

B. **Unknown causes: 85%.** Probably an inherited predisposition combined with an environmental predisposition at a critical period during cardiac development.

C. **Genetic factors.** Chromosomal abnormalities: Overall incidence of CHD in patients with a chromosome aberration is 30%.
1. Incidence of CHD varies with chromosomal abnormality.
   a. Trisomy 21: 50%.
   b. Trisomy 18 and 13: 90%.
   c. Chromosome deletion syndromes 18, 13, 5, and 4: 25–50%.
2. Single-mutant-gene syndromes: 3%. Both autosomal dominant and recessive syndromes have been associated with CHD.

D. **Environmental factors.**
1. Cardiac teratogenesis is associated with maternal ingestion of:
   a. Thalidomide: dramatically illustrates the extraordinarily deleterious effects of prescribed drug on a developing fetus.
   b. Anticonvulsants. All teratogenic syndromes induced by anticonvulsants have associated congenital cardiac defects.
      (1) Phenytoin.
      (2) Carbamazepine (Tegretol).
      (3) Valproate.
      (4) Trimethadione: increased incidence of transposition of the great vessels, tetralogy of Fallot, and hypoplastic left heart syndrome.
      (5) Pentobarbital: no confirmed specific embryopathy but may potentiate the effects of other drugs taken concurrently.
   c. Anticoagulants.
      (1) Warfarin (Coumadin) causes abortion or fetal embryopathic development in weeks 6–9 of gestation. Cardiac malformations have been identified, but no consistent cardiac defect has been noted.
      (2) Heparin, because of its larger molecular weight, does not cross the placenta.
   d. Antineoplastic medications.
      (1) Aminopterin: cardiac manifestations include dextroposition but are not as prominent as other defects resulting from drug ingestion.
      (2) In general, the disorders for which antineoplastic agents are used are serious enough to preclude pregnancy.
   e. Lithium: leads to defects such as Ebstein's anomaly, ASD, and tricuspid atresia.
   f. Retinoic acid.
   g. Isotretinoin.

    h. Alcohol. Fetal alcohol syndrome is accompanied by a variety of cardiac lesions (e.g., VSD with or without subpulmonic and subaortic stenosis, coarctation of the aorta, aortic regurgitation, and ASD).

    i. Amphetamine: induces congenital cardiac conditions.

2. Exposure to environmental hazards such as radiation, heat, and gases may produce teratogenic effects, but there are no specific associated cardiac malformations.

E. Maternal disease and viral infections (Table 11–1).

1. Women with diabetes mellitus have a five times greater risk of their children being born with cardiac anomalies than the general population of pregnant women have. Disorders include VSD, double-outlet right ventricle, transposition of the great vessels, truncus arteriosus, and coarctation of the aorta.

2. Rubella is the only viral illness that produces clinically significant heart disease (Ayers, 1998). Disorders seen are pulmonary stenosis and branch pulmonary artery stenosis, VSD, and ASD.

SEX PREFERENCES ASSOCIATED WITH CARDIAC LESIONS

A. Males.

1. Coarctation of the aorta.
2. Aortic stenosis.
3. Transposition of the great vessels (TGV).

Table 11–1

CLASSIFICATION OF MATERNAL DISEASES AFFECTING THE FETAL CARDIOVASCULAR SYSTEM

CATEGORY I: MATERNAL DISEASES THAT DIRECTLY AFFECT THE FETAL CARDIOVASCULAR SYSTEM (EXCLUDING TERATOGENIC EFFECTS) Pheochromocytoma Hyperthyroidism Diabetes mellitus Collagen vascular disease (e.g., Ro antibody) Smoking Rubella Cytomegalovirus Enterovirus infection Toxoplasmosis Listeriosis Maternal group B streptococcal colonization with fetal invasion Syphilis Inherited metabolic diseases
CATEGORY II: MATERNAL DISEASES THAT MAY INDIRECTLY AFFECT THE FETAL CARDIOVASCULAR SYSTEM AS A RESULT OF ABNORMALITIES OF UTEROPLACENTAL FUNCTION Neoplastic diseases Diabetes mellitus Maternal cardiac disease Anemia (including the hemoglobinopathies) Hypertensive disorders Collagen vascular disease (e.g., lupus anticoagulant and systemic lupus erythematosus) Renal disease (associated with hypertension) Smoking Asthma Cholestatic jaundice of pregnancy Cytomegalovirus Bacterial infections

From Katz, V., and Bowes, W.: Maternal diseases affecting the fetal cardiovascular system. *In* Long, W. (Ed.): Fetal and Neonatal Cardiology. Philadelphia, W.B. Saunders, 1990, p. 135.

B. Females.

1. ASD.
2. Patent ductus arteriosus (PDA).

Approach to Diagnosis of Cardiac Disease

HISTORY

A. Gestational age.

1. Preterm. Babies born prematurely are much more likely to have pulmonary problems resulting in cyanosis than to have CHD, but they do have a higher incidence of:
   a. PDA.
   b. Left-to-right shunts (e.g., VSD or atrioventricular canal).
2. Term. Majority of infants with CHD are term babies.

B. Maternal disease (see Table 11–1).

1. Infants of mothers with uncontrolled diabetes have an increased risk of:
   a. TGV.
   b. VSD.
2. Viral and bacterial illnesses may directly and indirectly affect the fetal cardiovascular system (see Table 11–1).

C. Congenital diseases or syndromes may have associated cardiac anomalies. The following associations have been noted:

1. Trisomy 13: PDA and/or VSD.
2. Trisomy 18: VSD, PDA.
3. Trisomy 21: ASD, VSD, atrioventricular canal, PDA.
4. Turner's syndrome: coarctation of the aorta.
5. DiGeorge syndrome: PDA, peripheral pulmonary stenosis.
6. Rubella syndrome: PDA, peripheral pulmonary stenosis.
7. Fetal alcohol syndrome: VSD, ASD, tetralogy of Fallot.

D. Mode of delivery.

1. Vaginal delivery usual for CHD, with good Apgar scores initially.
2. History of cesarean section and poor Apgar scores more indicative of asphyxia and respiratory distress.

E. Prenatal diagnosis with the use of ultrasonography may identify the infant with CHD before delivery.

CLINICAL PRESENTATION

A. Cyanosis (in the first week may be sole evidence of a heart lesion).

1. With cardiovascular problems, cyanosis is unexpected or gradual in onset.
2. Cyanosis observation.
   a. Dependent on hemoglobin levels; 3.5–5% desaturation of hemoglobin is necessary before cynanosis becomes apparent.
   b. Will be influenced by presence of anemia or polycythemia and the levels of 2,3-diphosphoglycerate.
3. Differentiation between central and peripheral cyanosis.
   a. Peripheral cyanosis results from sluggish movement of blood through the extremities and increased tissue oxygen extraction.
      (1) Persists from birth and can last several days.
      (2) Does not involve mucous membranes.
      (3) May be caused by peripheral vasomotor instability.

    b. Central cyanosis results when blood leaves the heart desaturated.
      (1) Seen as bluish discoloration of tongue and mucous membranes, reflecting arterial desaturation.
      (2) Central cyanosis may present difficulties in differential diagnosis between respiratory and cardiac origin.

B. Respiratory pattern.

1. Useful in the differentiation of cyanosis.
2. Tachypnea (respiratory rate >60) without respiratory distress is associated with congestive heart failure (CHF). In the absence of cyanosis, may indicate a left-to-right shunt lesion.
3. Hyperpnea (increased respiratory depth) is observed in congenital heart lesions resulting in diminished pulmonary blood flow.
4. Crying may exacerbate cyanosis in neonates with CHD because of increased tissue demands for oxygen.

C. Heart sounds.

1. First heart sound (S_1) represents closure of the mitral and tricuspid valves at the end of atrial systole.
    a. Best heard at cardiac apex (fifth intercostal space at sternal border).
    b. S_1 is accentuated with the following:
      (1) Increased cardiac output.
      (2) Increased flow across atrioventricular valves.
      (3) Specific conditions such as:
        (a) PDA.
        (b) VSD with increased mitral flow.
        (c) Total anomalous pulmonary venous connection (TAPVC).
        (d) Arteriovenous malformation.
        (e) Tetralogy of Fallot.
        (f) Anemia.
        (g) Fever.
    c. Conditions decreasing S_1 include the following:
      (1) Decreased atrioventricular conduction.
      (2) CHF.
      (3) Myocarditis.
2. Second heart sound (S_2) occurs at the end of ventricular systole from closure of aortic and pulmonic valves.
    a. Heard best at upper left sternal border.
    b. Split S_2 is a normal occurrence, reflecting closure of aortic valve before the pulmonic valve.
      (1) Increases on inspiration
      (2) Single S_2 is often heard in the first 2 days of life because of increased PVR.
      (3) Splitting of S_2 is influenced by:
        (a) Abnormalities of aortic or pulmonic valves.
        (b) Conditions altering PVR or SVR.
    c. Conditions widening the S_2 are influenced by:
      (1) ASD.
      (2) TAPVC.
      (3) Tetralogy of Fallot.
      (4) Pulmonary stenosis.
      (5) Ebstein's anomaly.
    d. Absent S_2 splits occur in the following:
      (1) Pulmonary atresia and severe pulmonary stenosis.
      (2) Aortic stenosis/atresia.
      (3) Persistent pulmonary hypertension.

(4) L-TGV.

(5) Truncus arteriosus.

3. Third heart sound (S_3).

   a. Follows S_2 and is a low-pitched, broad sound.

   b. Prominent in situations of increased atrioventricular flow and increased ventricular filling (Duff and McNamara, 1998).

     (1) Left-to-right shunts (e.g., ASD, VSD, PDA).

     (2) Anemia.

     (3) Mitral valve insufficiency.

4. Fourth heart sound (S_4).

   a. Occurs just before S_1 and is low pitched.

   b. Rarely heard in the newborn infant.

   c. Always pathologic and indicates altered ventricular compliance.

5. Ejection clicks.

   a. Abnormal (except during first 24 hours of life) and indicate cardiac disease.

   b. Audible for short duration after S_1.

   c. Associated with dilation of the great vessels or deformity of aortic or pulmonic valve.

   d. Other conditions associated with ejection clicks include the following:

     (1) Aortic valve stenosis.

     (2) Truncus arteriosus.

     (3) Tetralogy of Fallot (severe).

     (4) Pulmonary valve stenosis.

     (5) Hypoplastic left heart syndrome.

     (6) Coarctation of the aorta.

6. Murmurs.

   a. Murmurs result from turbulence of blood flow and may be due to:

     (1) Abnormal valves.

     (2) Septal defects.

     (3) Regurgitated flow through incompetent valves.

     (4) High blood flow across normal structures.

   b. Physiologic murmurs have been noted in 60% of neonates in the first 48 hours of life (Braudo and Rowe, 1961). Generally, these murmurs are from:

     (1) Transient left-to-right flow via the ductus arteriosus.

     (2) Increased flow over pulmonary valve associated with fall in PVR.

     (3) Possibly, mild bilateral peripheral pulmonary arterial stenosis because of size and pressure differences between the main pulmonary trunk and the left and right pulmonary arterial branches.

   c. Absence of murmur does not indicate absence of significant cardiac disease.

   d. Evaluation of murmurs includes the following:

     (1) Intensity of sound.

       (a) Murmurs are graded. Those less than grade 3/6 generally present no hemodynamic problems (Duff and McNamara, 1998) (Table 11–2).

Table 11–2
GRADING OF MURMURS

Grade 1	Soft; requires extended listening
Grade 2	Soft; heard immediately
Grade 3	Moderate intensity; no thrill
Grade 4	Loud; often with thrill or palpable vibration at murmur site
Grade 5	Loud; thrill present; audible with stethoscope partially off the chest
Grade 6	Loud; audible with stethoscope off chest

       (b) Presence of a thrill on palpation is associated with a loud murmur of at least grade 4.

  (2) Location within cardiac cycle.

       (a) Systolic: heard during ventricular systole (i.e., between S_1 and S_2).

          (i) Identified as early, mid, or late systolic.

          (ii) Pansystolic (holosystolic): murmurs present for duration of systole. Heard in mitral or tricuspid insufficiency and VSD.

          (iii) Ejection murmurs: turbulence of blood flow leaving the heart; noted in aortic or pulmonic valve stenosis, tetralogy of Fallot, ASD, and TAPVC.

       (b) Diastolic: heard during period of ventricular filling (i.e., between S_2 and S_1).

          (i) Early: results from aortic or pulmonic valve insufficiency.

          (ii) Mid: increased blood flow across normal mitral or tricuspid valve.

          (iii) Late: associated with stenotic mitral or tricuspid valve.

       (c) Continuous: audible throughout cardiac cycle but can be louder in systole or diastole (e.g., PDA).

  (3) Quality of sound.

       (a) Pitch (reflects frequency of vibrations). High-pitched sound generally reflects valve insufficiency on left side of heart, whereas a low-pitched sound reflects right-sided valve insufficiency.

       (b) Other descriptive terms (have less precise meaning):

          (i) Harsh.

          (ii) Blowing.

          (iii) Musical.

  (4) Location on chest of murmur's maximum intensity.

D. Peripheral pulses.

1. Palpate simultaneously on each side and in turn all extremities and carotid.
2. Pulses should be synchronous with equal intensity.
3. Discrepancies (e.g., pulses that are greater in upper than in lower extremities) raise the possibility of an abnormal aortic arch.
4. Weak pulses indicate low systemic output, as seen in the following:
   a. Obstruction of left side of heart (e.g., hypoplastic left heart syndrome or severe aortic stenosis).
   b. Myocardial failure.
   c. Shock.
5. Visible precordial impulse persisting after the first 12 hours of life occurs in defects with volume overload (Verklan, 1997).

E. Blood pressure.

1. Normal values are as follows:
   a. Healthy term infant: mean systolic pressure, 70–75 mm Hg (range, 55–90); mean diastolic pressure, 40–45 mm Hg (range, 30–55).
   b. Premature infant's blood pressure varies with size and gestational age. For infant weighing 1000 g: systolic mean pressure, 50 mm Hg; diastolic mean pressure, 30 mm Hg.
2. Blood pressure values may be affected by body temperature, activity, and posture.
3. Systolic blood pressure of the upper extremities 20 mm Hg above that of lower extremities is suggestive of:
   a. Coarctation of the aorta. PDA may mask these pressure differences.
   b. Aortic arch abnormalities.
     (1) Additionally, blood pressure differences between the upper extremities are seen with aortic arch abnormalities.

Table 11–3
CAUSES OF CONGESTIVE HEART FAILURE IN THE FIRST WEEK OF LIFE

Disease	History	Pulses	ECG	Precordium
Transient myocardial ischemia	+			
Dysrhythmias	±			
Arteriovenous fistula	–	Increased		
Coarctation of the aorta (interrupted aortic arch)	–	Asymmetrical		
Aortic stenosis	–	Decreased	LVH	
Hypoplastic left heart syndrome	–	Decreased	RVH	Hyperactive
Myocarditis	–	Decreased	RVH	Decreased

LVH, Left ventricular hypertrophy; *RVH*, right ventricular hypertrophy.
   From Freed, M.: Congenital cardiac malformations. *In* Taeusch, H.W., Ballard, R.A., and Avery, M.E. (Eds.): Schaffer and Avery's Diseases of the Newborn, 6th ed. Philadelphia, W.B. Saunders, 1991, p. 629.

(2) To evaluate, simultaneously measure blood pressure in both arms and one leg. Either leg can be evaluated, because the blood supply to both legs comes from the descending aorta below the level of the defect.
4. In a term infant, neonatal hypertension is defined as a systolic blood pressure greater than 90 mm Hg and a diastolic pressure greater than 60 mm Hg.
   a. In a premature infant, systolic pressure greater than 80 mm Hg and diastolic pressure greater than 50 mm Hg indicates hypertension.
   b. Renal vein thrombosis resulting from high umbilical artery catheter placement is the most common cause of hypertension.

 Congestive heart failure.

1. CHF is typically associated with congenital heart lesions. The timing of CHF appearance may assist in diagnosis of the lesion (Tables 11–3 and 11–4).
2. See Congestive Heart Failure, below, for other causes and clinical manifestations of CHF.
3. Late-onset CHF may result from bronchopulmonary dysplasia or other pulmonary stressors. (Refer to Chapter 7.)

Table 11–4
CAUSES OF CONGESTIVE HEART FAILURE DURING WEEKS 2 THROUGH 4 OF LIFE

ACYANOTIC (Pao$_2$ >150 mm Hg in 100% O$_2$)
Coarctation of the aorta
Aortic stenosis
Myocarditis
Endocardial fibroelastosis
Patent ductus arteriosus
Aortopulmonary window
Anterievenous fistula
Ventricular septal defect
Atrioventricular canal defects

CYANOTIC (Pao$_2$ <150 mm Hg in 100% O$_2$)
Hypoplastic left heart syndrome
Total anomalous pulmonary venous return
Truncus arteriosus
Transposition and a ventricular septal defect
Tricuspid atresia and a ventricular septal defect
Single ventricle

From Freed, M.: Congenital cardiac malformations. *In* Taeusch, H.W., Ballard, R.A., and Avery, M.E. (Eds.): Schaffer and Avery's Diseases of the Newborn, 6th ed. Philadelphia, W.B. Saunders, 1991, p. 630.

DIAGNOSTIC ADJUNCTS

A. **Arterial blood gas values** are used primarily to help differentiate lung disease versus heart disease as the cause of cyanosis.
1. $PaCO_2$: generally normal in CHD and elevated in pulmonary parenchymal disease.
2. Hyperoxygen test.
   a. Sample arterial PO_2, with infant breathing 100% oxygen versus room air.
      (1) Umbilical artery sample may detect right-to-left shunts via PDA. The lowered PaO_2 is a reflection usually of lung disease and not of primary heart disease.
      (2) Administration of oxygen to infants with cardiac disease resulting in high pulmonary blood flow and CHF will improve oxygen levels (i.e., increased PaO_2) through decreased PVR and increased pulmonary blood flow.
      (3) Most accurate assessment of cardiac versus pulmonary disease can be made if the right radial or temporal (preductal) and umbilical artery samples (postductal) are taken simultaneously.
      (4) Monitoring of preductal and postductal transcutaneous oxygen pressure or pulse oximetry provides a noninvasive evaluation for cardiac versus pulmonary disease.
   b. Preductal PaO_2 increases in 100% oxygen greater than 250 mm Hg indicate lung disease; increases of 100 mm Hg or less are consistent with cardiac disease (Flanagan and Flyer, 1994).

B. **Chest x-ray examination is used to:**
1. Rule out pulmonary parenchymal disease.
2. Identify increased pulmonary markings, as seen in lesions with left-to-right shunting.
3. Evaluate cardiac size and shape.
   a. Cardiomegaly: defined as cardiac/thoracic ratio greater than 0.6.
   b. See Chapter 29 for chest x-ray findings in heart disease.

C. **Electrocardiography (EKG).**
1. Reflects abnormal hemodynamic burdens placed on the heart.
2. Used to determine severity of disease by assessing the degree of atrial or ventricular hypertrophy. Right ventricular predominance is normal shortly after birth. (In utero the right ventricle does most of the cardiac work.)
3. Changes in ST segments or T waves may suggest myocardial ischemia.
   a. Tall, peaked P waves are common in right-sided heart failure.
   b. Wide, notched P waves are seen with left-sided heart failure.
4. EKG is the major diagnostic tool for evaluating arrhythmias and the impact of electrolyte imbalances (e.g., potassium and calcium) on electrical conductivity.
5. Normal EKG values in term neonates:
   a. Heart rate: 125–135 bpm in first week.
   b. Normal sinus rhythm: P wave precedes QRS complex.
   c. P wave: duration 0.04–0.08 second.
   d. PR interval: 0.08–0.14 second. Prolonged interval is seen in first-degree heart block (usually benign).
   e. QRS complex: duration, 0.03–0.07 second. Prolonged complex indicates interventricular conduction delay.
   f. Premature infants have higher resting heart rates with greater variation. Duration of P wave is shorter. PR and QRS intervals are decreased (0.10 and 0.04 second, respectively).

D. Echocardiography.

1. Provides rapid, noninvasive, and painless evaluation of heart anatomy and flow by use of ultrasonic sound waves.
   a. M-mode (single-dimension) echocardiography permits evaluation of anatomic relationships of heart and vessels, including relative sizes of each.
   b. Two-dimensional (real-time) echocardiography has greater versatility, providing more specific information regarding anatomic relationships.
   c. Color-flow Doppler echocardiography shows:
      (1) Patterns of blood flow (i.e., right-to-left versus left-to-right shunting).
      (2) Location of restrictions and/or regurgitation.
   d. Continuous-wave Doppler echocardiography shows the quantity of flow across an obstruction, giving an estimate of pressure gradients.
   e. Contrast echocardiography is accomplished by rapid injection of saline solution in a vein while conducting an ultrasonographic examination. It allows for greater evaluation of flow patterns throughout the heart and identifies the presence of shunts.
2. Although echocardiography allows for rapid bedside diagnosis of cardiac lesions and differentiation from other abnormalities (e.g., sepsis, persistent fetal circulation), it does not replace cardiac catheterization as a diagnostic tool.

E. Cardiac catheterization.

1. An invasive procedure to obtain data (e.g., oxygen saturation and pressure measurements) for definitive diagnosis or in preparation for cardiac surgery.
   a. May be used in palliative treatment (e.g., in the use of balloon atrial septostomy to treat TGV).
   b. Usually reserved for cyanotic heart lesions.
   c. For acyanotic heart lesions, can be delayed until full effect of medical management of CHF is seen.
   d. Treatment modalities during catheterization have included placement of stints, angioplasty, and implanting of devices for closure of an ASD.
2. Procedure: advancement of a catheter through the umbilical, subclavian, femoral, or right internal jugular vessels and into the heart.
   a. If balloon septostomy is anticipated, a large vessel will be needed.
   b. Pressure measurements are made of all chambers and outlet tracts.
3. Concomitant angiography (injection of contrast medium): often performed to achieve maximal cardiac information.
4. Complications.
   a. Mortality risk is approximately 4–6% and is directly related to the underlying cardiopulmonary defect and the patient's condition (Nihill, 1998).
   b. High sodium content of contrast medium contributes to myocardial depression and exerts an osmotic effect, temporarily increasing intravascular volume.
   c. Hemorrhage with catheter insertion or removal may lead to:
      (1) Hypotension.
      (2) Shock.
      (3) Cardiac tamponade if bleeding is in the pericardial sac.
   d. Dysrhythmias are not uncommon (e.g., premature atrial and ventricular beats and tachycardia), because of catheter manipulation.

F. Laboratory data.

1. Complete blood cell count with differential cell count.
   a. Rules out anemia or polycythemia as cause of CHF.
   b. Decreased number of neutrophils and presence of left shift: possible indication of sepsis. Group B beta-hemolytic streptococci can mimic hypoplastic left heart syndrome.

2. Blood glucose concentration. Used to evaluate hypoglycemia as potential cause of cardiomyopathy.
3. Electrolytes (especially potassium and calcium). Both potassium and calcium are major cations in electrical conductivity. Alterations can adversely affect cardiac contractility.

Defects With Increased Pulmonary Blood Flow

PATENT DUCTUS ARTERIOSUS

A. Incidence (fourth most common lesion).
1. Isolated PDA in term gestations: 1:2000 live births.
2. In preterm gestations, 8:1000 live births (Brook and Heyman, 1995).
   a. Incidence is inversely related to gestational age.
   b. Of infants weighing more than 1750 g: 45%.
   c. Of infants weighing less than 1200 g: 80%.
3. Occurs three times more commonly in females than in males.

B. Anatomy: persistent patency of the ductus arteriosus after birth (Fig. 11–6).
1. Fetal patency of this structure is functional, diverting blood away from fluid-filled lungs toward the placenta for oxygen gas exchange.
2. Patency is influenced by several factors.
   a. Increased oxygen tension is a potent stimulant of smooth muscle contraction: decreases patency.
   b. Lack of ductal smooth muscle (e.g., in premature infants) prolongs patency.
   c. Prostaglandins inhibit closure of ductus.

C. Hemodynamics.
1. As PVR falls and SVR rises, a left-to-right shunt via the PDA results in blood flow from the aorta into the pulmonary artery, increasing pulmonary blood flow. The increased pulmonary artery pressure and increased left ventricular pressure and volume lead to bilateral CHF.
2. Because left-to-right flow is dependent on a drop in PVR, infants with pulmonary disease (e.g., hyaline membrane disease) will show symptoms when lung disease improves. Before this time, PVR greater than SVR leads to a right-to-left shunt via the patent ductus (commonly referred to as persistent pulmonary hypertension of the neonate).

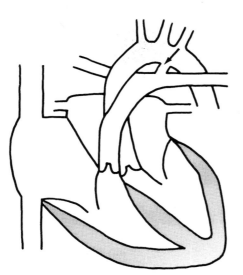

Figure 11–6
Patent ductus arteriosus (PDA). (Redrawn courtesy of G.G. Janos, M.D., 1989.)

D. Clinical features.

1. Characteristically is manifested at 3 to 7 days of life with classic signs of heart failure.
   a. Increased pulmonary vasculature and cardiomegaly.
   b. Bounding peripheral pulses and hyperactive precordium.
   c. Widening pulse pressure (>20 mm Hg).
2. Murmur may be "silent" in 10–20% of the preterm infants despite hemodynamically significant shunt.
3. Radiographic findings consist of cardiomegaly (cardiothoracic ratio >0.60), pulmonary edema, and increased pulmonary vascularity. These "typical" signs may be absent if the infant is receiving positive-pressure ventilation.

E. Management.

1. Dependent on whether shunt is hemodynamically significant. In premature infants the PDA may prolong ventilator use beyond the dictates of the initial lung disease. Early intervention may prevent lung complications of ventilator use (Corbet, 1998).
2. Hemodynamically significant ductus arteriosus includes the following:
   a. Heart rate greater than 170 bpm.
   b. Respiratory rate greater than 70/min.
   c. Hepatomegaly greater than 3 cm below costal margin.
   d. Bounding pulses.
3. Conservative measures are generally employed initially.
   a. Fluid restriction.
   b. Diuretics: if employed with fluid restriction, may lead to electrolyte imbalance, dehydration, and caloric deprivation.
   c. Digitalis.
      (1) In infant weighing less than 1250 g, has little or no benefit and is frequently toxic.
      (2) In combination with indomethacin, increased susceptibility to digoxin toxicity.
   d. Positive end-expiratory pressure: useful in reducing left-to-right shunt via PDA.
4. Indomethacin management includes the following:
   a. As a prostaglandin inhibitor, indomethacin can constrict and close the PDA in some premature infants.
   b. Dosage is 0.2–0.3 mg/kg, given up to three times 8–12 hours apart (Wood, 1998).
   c. Complications are as follows:
      (1) Transient decreased renal function.
      (2) Increased incidence of occult blood loss via gastrointestinal tract.
      (3) Inhibition of platelet function for 7–9 days, with potential for intracerebral hemorrhage.
   d. Ductus recurrence rate is high in infants weighing less than 1000 g who were treated with indomethacin (Corbet, 1998).
   e. Contraindications are as follows (Brook and Heyman, 1995):
      (1) Renal failure (blood urea nitrogen concentration >30 mg/dL, serum creatinine concentration >1.8 mg/dL, urine <6 mL/kg per hour).
      (2) Frank renal or gastrointestinal bleeding.
      (3) Necrotizing enterocolitis: not a contraindication. However, surgical ligation is more rapid, and certain resolution of PDA results in prompt decrease in bowel ischemia from the PDA.
      (4) Platelet count less than 60,000/mm^3.
      (5) Sepsis: proved or strongly suspected.
      (6) Severe pulmonary hypertension with irreversible pulmonary vascular disease.

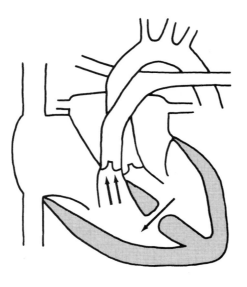

Figure 11–7
Ventricular septal defect *(VSD)*. (Redrawn courtesy of G.G. Janos, M.D., 1989.)

5. Surgical management involves ligation of the PDA.
   a. Surgery carries almost negligible risk.
   b. Surgery carries potential for complications of bleeding with prior indomethacin therapy (risk dependent on time from dose to surgical intervention).
6. Cardiac catheterization and insertion of a vascular occlusion device, consisting of a coil-filled sack that releases from the catheter, has been approved by the U.S. Food and Drug Administration (Allen et al., 1998).

VENTRICULAR SEPTAL DEFECT

A. **Incidence.** At 1:3000 live births, VSDs are the most common of all CHDs.

B. **Anatomy:** abnormal opening in the septum between the right and left ventricle. Sizes range from pinhole to almost complete absence of the ventricular septum (Fig. 11–7).

C. **Hemodynamics.**

1. The degree of hypertrophy of ventricles and the pressure relationships are dependent on the size of the defect. A small defect allows pressure differences between ventricles.
2. PVR less than SVR results in a left-to-right shunt, producing increased pulmonary blood flow and leading to decreased pulmonary compliance and pulmonary edema.
3. Excessive pulmonary artery blood flow eventually results in pulmonary artery hypertrophy and stenosis.
4. High pulmonary artery pressure can delay maturation of pulmonary arterioles.

D. **Clinical features.**

1. Size dependent.
2. Small VSD.
   a. Asymptomatic.
   b. High-pitched pansystolic murmur along left sternal border.
3. Moderate VSD: asymptomatic except for murmur and recurrent respiratory infection.
4. Large VSD.

a. Present at 1–2 months of age with CHF, pulmonary infection, and increased precordial activity.
b. Loud, blowing pansystolic murmur at left lower sternal border.
c. Chest x-ray examination: cardiac enlargement and increased pulmonary vascular markings.

E. Management.

1. Small defects often close spontaneously; 20% of large defects become smaller or close.
2. With mild CHF, management is with digoxin and diuretics.
3. Treatment of significant CHF with poor weight gain despite pharmacologic management is as follows:
   a. Palliative: surgical banding of pulmonary artery to reduce pulmonary blood flow, decrease CHF, and prevent pulmonary vascular resistance.
   b. Surgical: repair by suturing defect or patching defect.
   c. Earlier surgical repair, rather than palliative banding with delayed repair: associated with better results (Graham and Gutgell, 1995).

F. Prognosis: excellent, with spontaneous closure the norm and operative closure required in only a small percentage of the defects. Later course may be complicated by conduction abnormalities or aortic and/or tricuspid insufficiency (Gumbiner and Takao, 1998).

ATRIAL SEPTAL DEFECT

A. Incidence: 1:5000 live births.

B. Anatomy: defect in formation of septum, resulting in a communication between right and left atria. Defect may be an ostium secundum defect, an ostium primum defect, or a partial endocardial cushion defect (Fig. 11–8). By definition, a patent foramen ovale is generally excluded, although symptoms can be the same.

C. Hemodynamics.

1. In early neonatal period, right ventricle pressure is greater than left ventricle pressure, so there is no shunt or only a small right-to-left shunt.
2. As PVR decreases, left-to-right shunt develops with concomitant right ventricular volume overload and hypertrophy.

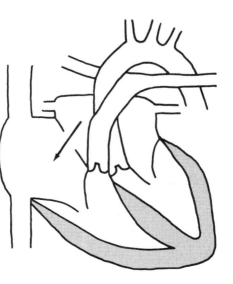

Figure 11–8
Atrial septal defect *(ASD)*. (Redrawn courtesy of G.G. Janos, M.D., 1989.)

D. Clinical features.

1. In isolated defect, generally asymptomatic and unrecognized. If ASD is diagnosed in infancy, 50–100% of the patients have symptoms.
2. CHF from left-to-right shunt and mitral valve insufficiency.
3. Failure to thrive.
4. Recurrent respiratory infections.
5. Systolic murmur at second left intercostal space, persistent split S_2 if shunt is large, diastolic murmur heard at left lower sternal border.
6. Chest x-ray examination: large pulmonary artery blood flow with enlargement of right atrium and ventricle.

E. Management.

1. In asymptomatic ASD, follow-up without early operative repair; spontaneous ASD closure possible.
2. ASD with CHF: medical treatment of CHF and delay of surgical repair.
3. ASD with intractable CHF: early surgical repair (i.e., suturing or patching of defect).
4. Various occluding devices (button, disk, double-umbrella): experimentally placed for closure of ASD. Approval from the U.S. Food and Drug Administration is pending. Complications include residual shunting and embolization of the device (Allen et al., 1998).

F. Prognosis.

1. Spontaneous closure occurs in 14–60% of septum secundum ASDs during the first year (Coburn et al., 1995).
2. Perioperative mortality rate is 3.3%, with good long-term results in survivors. Survival at 5 years of age is 97% and at 10 years, 90% (Coburn et al., 1995).

ENDOCARDIAL CUSHION DEFECT (ATRIOVENTRICULAR CANAL)

A. Incidence: 1:9000 live births. Most common heart defect in Down syndrome.

B. Anatomy.

1. Endocardial cushions form the lower portion of the atrial septum, the upper portion of the ventricular septum, and septal portions of the mitral and tricuspid valves.
2. A wide range of defects are possible, from simple cleft of the mitral and/or tricuspid valves to complete absence of the lower atrial and upper ventricular septa with common atrioventricular valve (i.e., atrioventricular canal) (Fig. 11–9).

C. Hemodynamics.

1. With PVR less than SVR, blood dependently shunts left to right via the ASD and the VSD.
2. Higher pressure of the left ventricle creates obligatory left-to-right shunting via the atrioventricular valve (atrioventricular valve regurgitation). Blood flows from the left ventricle, to the mitral portion of the atrioventricular valve, to the left atrium, to the ASD, and to the right atrium.

D. Clinical features.

1. Isolated ostium primum atrial defect: rarely identified in the neonatal period.
2. Isolated ventricular defect: see clinical features of VSD, above.
3. Complete atrioventricular canal.
   a. Atrioventricular valve regurgitation controls age at presentation.

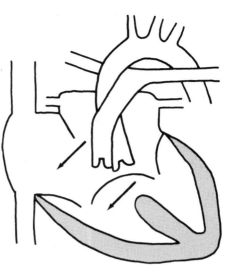

Figure 11–9
Atrioventricular canal *(AVC)*. (Redrawn courtesy of G.G. Janos, M.D., 1989.)

(1) Severe: seen at 1–2 weeks of age with CHF.
(2) Valves competent: seen in first or second month of life.
  b. Active precordium, with a thrill at the left lower sternal border.
  c. Variable murmurs; usually loud pansystolic murmur at the left lower sternal border.
  d. Chest x-ray examination: cardiomegaly, bilateral atrial and ventricular hypertrophy, increased pulmonary markings.

E. Management.

1. Objective: to avoid development of pulmonary vascular obstructive disease.
2. Medical management: to control the CHF.
3. Palliative pulmonary artery banding to decrease pulmonary overload. Does not influence obligatory shunting of the atrioventricular valve.
4. Primary repair with closure of atrial and ventricular septal defects and mitral and tricuspid valve reconstruction (Vick, 1998). Usually undertaken between 2 and 6 months of age.

F. Prognosis.

1. Prognosis is dependent on details of anatomic form and on the presence of significant associated noncardiac anomalies and significant pulmonary obstructive vascular disease.
2. Best results are seen with ostium primum defect or common atrium; long-term prognosis is good.
3. Partial atrioventricular defect has mortality rate of 30% (Feldt et al., 1995).
4. Outlook for complete atrioventricular canal without operation is poor.
5. Mortality rate for surgical repair is around 10% (Gaedeke, 1996; Vick, 1998).

Obstructive Defects With Pulmonary Venous Congestion

COARCTATION OF THE AORTA

A. Incidence: 5–8% of congenital heart lesions.
1. Most common congenital heart defect presenting in week 2 of life.
2. Male dominance: 2:1.

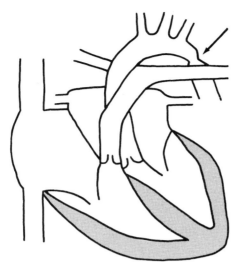

Figure 11–10
Coarctation of the aorta. (Redrawn courtesy of G.G. Janos, M.D., 1989.)

B. **Anatomy:** constriction of aorta distal to left subclavian artery (Fig. 11–10).
1. Usually occurs at insertion site of ductus arteriosus.
2. Preductal coarctation associated with hypoplasia of the aortic arch and intra-cardiac defects.

C. **Hemodynamics.**
1. Isolated coarctation: obstruction to left ventricular outflow, leading to increased left ventricular, left atrial, and pulmonary venous pressures. Pulmonary venous congestion develops.
2. Coarctation with VSD: elevated left ventricular pressure, shunting blood left to right via VSD and causing pulmonary overload.
3. Preductal coarctation: dependent on PDA for distal aorta and lower body blood flow.

D. **Clinical features.**
1. CHF with hepatomegaly.
2. Decreased pulses and blood pressures in the lower extremities.
   a. Decreased blood pressure in left arm, indicative of left subclavian artery as site of coarctation.
   b. Decreased blood pressure in right arm: right subclavian artery arises below coarctation (rare).
   c. Pulses that "wax and wane": related to increase or decrease in PDA blood flow.
3. Heart sounds.
   a. Postductal: no murmur or short systolic ejection click in axilla or back.
   b. Preductal with VSD: harsh pansystolic murmur at left lower sternal border.
   c. Gallop rhythm possible.
4. Chest x-ray examination: enlarged heart with left ventricular hypertrophy and pulmonary vascular congestion.

E. **Management.**
1. Medical management of CHF.
2. Prostaglandin E_1 to dilate ductus arteriosus (preductal lesion).
3. Isolated postductal coarctation: control of CHF first, then delayed surgical correction.
4. Surgical correction: two common repairs.

a. Either resection of abnormal segment and reanastomosis.
b. *Or* subclavian patch across area of obstruction.
c. With associated anomalies, variable approaches according to type of defect.

F. Prognosis.

1. Outcome is dependent on complexity of coarctation, with mortality rates at 1 month ranging from 0% for simple coarctation to 13%; can be higher for complex coarctation associated with VSD or other left-sided obstruction (Chang and Vaughn, 1998).
2. Long-term prognosis after coarctation repair is determined by the presence of residual or recurrent coarctation, persistence of pulmonary hypertension, and residual cardiovascular lesions.
   a. Incidence of recurrence of 25–60% after resection and end-to-end anastomosis has been reported for repair in infancy.
   b. Left subclavian flap operation has reported an incidence of 0–13% for significant recoarctation, with one report of a 25% reoperation rate (Beekman, 1995).
   c. Potential residual complications include persistent hypertension, Horner's syndrome, and mesenteric vasculitis.

AORTIC STENOSIS

A. Incidence: 1:24,000 live births.

B. Anatomy: Presence of stenosis at (with valve cusps thickened or deformed), above (supravalvular), or below (subvalvular) the aortic valve. The myocardium of the left ventricle is hypertrophied (Fig. 11–11).

C. Hemodynamics. Obstruction to left ventricular outflow leads to increased left ventricular pressures and hypertrophy. If aortic stenosis is severe in utero, blood flow through the ventricle is decreased, resulting in left ventricular hypoplasia and left-sided heart syndrome.

D. Clinical features.

1. The infant is free of symptoms at birth.
2. Heart sounds include a systolic murmur along the left sternal border, radiating to the right upper sternal border.

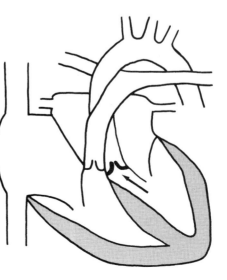

Figure 11–11
Aortic stenosis *(AS)*. (Redrawn courtesy of G.G. Janos, M.D., 1989.)

3. CHF symptoms may be delayed by weeks but progress rapidly after onset.
4. Chest x-ray examination shows cardiomegaly with or without pulmonary venous engorgement.

E. **Management.**

1. Initially, CHF is treated with acidosis management and antibiotic prophylaxis.
2. Percutaneous balloon aortic valvuloplasty is done to delay valvotomy or aortic replacement. Mortality rate is less than 2% (Friedman, 1995).
3. Surgery involves aortic valvotomy.
4. If neonates have CHF initially, they usually remain in failure, and operative relief is necessary.

F. **Prognosis.**

1. Operative risk is high as a result of ventricular hypoplasia and myocardial hypertrophy. Late potential complications include calcification and endocarditis.
2. Aortic stenosis is the most common cause of sudden death in children with heart disease.

Obstructive Defects With Decreased Pulmonary Blood Flow

TETRALOGY OF FALLOT

A. **Incidence:** 1:5000 live births. Most common cyanotic heart lesion.

B. **Anatomy:** classified as a combination of four defects, although Nos. 3 and 4, below, are consequences of Nos. 1 and 2 (Fig. 11–12).
1. Pulmonary stenosis: obstruction of outflow tract.
2. VSD.
3. Aorta overriding VSD.
4. Right ventricular hypertrophy.

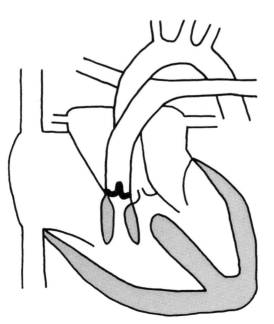

Figure 11–12
Tetralogy of Fallot *(TOF)*. (Redrawn courtesy of G.G. Janos, M.D., 1989.)

C. Hemodynamics.

1. Dependent primarily on degree of pulmonary stenosis and to a lesser extent on VSD size.
2. In severe pulmonary stenosis, blood flow passes from right to left via the VSD, with resulting hypoxia and cyanosis.
3. In mild pulmonary stenosis, blood flows from left to right via the VSD, with CHF resulting.
4. In mild to moderate pulmonary stenosis, blood flow via VSD may be minimal as long as PVR and SVR are balanced. With crying, right-to-left shunting occurs.

D. Clinical features.

1. Presentation is a function of the degree of pulmonary stenosis.
2. Severe obstruction presents in the first days of life with severe cyanosis.
3. Milder pulmonary obstruction presents in the first days of life with mild cyanosis.
4. Chest x-ray examination shows normal heart size with decreased pulmonary markings if hypoxia is present. Classic picture is that of a boot-shaped heart.
5. Traditional "TET spells" (paroxysmal dyspnea and severe cyanosis) are unusual in the first months of life.

E. Management.

1. All palliative treatments involve creation of systemic–pulmonary artery shunts.
   a. Waterston: shunt between ascending aorta and right pulmonary artery (largely abandoned).
   b. Potts: shunt between descending aorta and left pulmonary artery. Largely abandoned because of tendency toward development of pulmonary vascular obstructive disease.
   c. Blalock-Taussig or modified Blalock-Taussig procedure: shunt between right or left subclavian and pulmonary artery.
2. Corrective surgery involves closure of the VSD with a patch and eliminating the pulmonary stenosis by resection. The pulmonary outflow tract may be enlarged by a patch.
   a. Surgical correction is performed after 6 months of age and may be delayed to 2–4 years of age in symptom-free children.
   b. If child has symptoms before 6 months of age, a Blalock-Taussig procedure is generally performed, with full correction at a later time.
   c. Mortality rate in infancy is less than 10% (Daberkow-Carson and Washington, 1998).
   d. Complications/residual effects include decreased or absent pulses in affected arm, inadequate shunt, and CHF resulting from large shunt.

PULMONARY STENOSIS

A. Incidence: 1:14,000 live births.

B. Anatomy: narrowed opening either in pulmonary valve as a consequence of pulmonary valve cusp fusions (Fig. 11–13) or above or below the valve because of tissue hypertrophy.

C. Hemodynamics.

1. In utero, right ventricular hypoplasia can develop, depending on the degree of pulmonary valve stenosis and subsequent decrease in right ventricular blood flow.

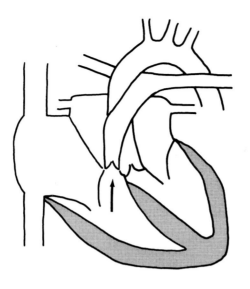

Figure 11–13
Pulmonary stenosis *(PS).* (Redrawn courtesy of G.G. Janos, M.D., 1989.)

2. After birth, the combination of right ventricular hypoplasia and severe pulmonary valve stenosis redirects blood flow from right to left at the atrial level via the foramen ovale. Pulmonary blood becomes dependent on a left-to-right flow via the PDA.
3. In mild stenosis, the pulmonary blood flow is not excessively restricted and is PDA independent. As PVR decreases, atrial right-to-left shunt will decrease and systemic hypoxia improve.

D. Clinical features.

1. Mild pulmonary stenosis: loud systolic murmur at left upper sternal border is the only finding.
2. Moderately severe stenosis.
   a. Murmur is less prominent. Murmur of tricuspid insufficiency may be noted.
   b. Cyanosis is present and increases with PDA closure.
   c. Generally, hepatomegaly is present.
3. Chest x-ray examination: mild cardiomegaly with diminished pulmonary blood flow.

E. Management.

1. Cyanotic neonate.
   a. Initial management: oxygen, bicarbonate, and prostaglandin E_1.
   b. Nonsurgical treatment with balloon valvuloplasty or angioplasty.
      (1) Few complications; effective.
      (2) Treatment of choice for discrete valvular lesion.
   c. Surgical valvotomy or tissue excision if valvuloplasty fails and patient symptomatic.
2. Noncyanotic neonate: conservative management includes catheterization at 6–12 months if stenosis is severe, with subsequent surgery if right ventricular pressure exceeds systemic.

F. Prognosis. Operative mortality rate for surgical repair or angioplasty is less than 5% (Cheatham, 1998; Gaedeke, 1996).

PULMONARY ATRESIA

A. Incidence: 1:14,000 live births.

B. **Anatomy:** complete obstruction of the pulmonic valve, resulting in a hypoplastic right ventricle and tricuspid valve (Fig. 11–14). In the presence of a VSD the right ventricle may be of adequate size.

C. **Hemodynamics.**

1. Venous blood returning to the right atrium goes across the foramen ovale into the left atrium, into the left ventricle, and out the aorta.
2. Blood flow to the lungs is derived entirely from a left-to-right shunt at the ductus arteriosus, which is generally small and tortuous. As the PDA closes, severe hypoxemia ensues.
3. Regurgitant blood flow occurs at the tricuspid valve.

D. **Clinical features.**

1. Mild cyanosis at birth, progressing to intense cyanosis by 24 hours.
2. Heart sounds.
   a. PDA murmur is present.
   b. Systolic harsh murmur is heard at the left and right sternal borders and reflects tricuspid insufficiency.
   c. Chest x-ray examination shows increased heart size with decreased pulmonary markings.

E. **Management.**

1. Initial treatment is use of oxygen and bicarbonate for metabolic acidosis and prostaglandin E_1 to dilate the ductus arteriosus.
2. Mild right ventricle hypertrophy: surgical valvotomy may be effective.
3. With severe hyperplasia of right ventricle and tricuspid valve, initial palliation is variable. Management includes systemic-to-pulmonary shunt, plus the following (see also section E, management, under heading Tetralogy of Fallot, above):
   a. Atrial septectomy.
   b. Pulmonary valvotomy.
   c. Right ventricular outflow tract reconstruction and pericardial patching.
   d. Modified Fontan operation. Attachment of the right atrium to the pulmonary artery may be possible.

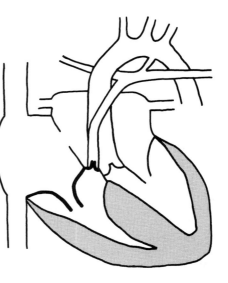

Figure 11–14
Pulmonary atresia. (Redrawn courtesy of G.G. Janos, M.D., 1989.)

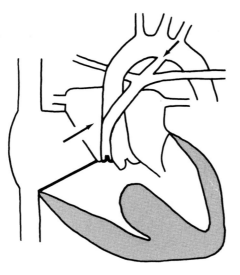

Figure 11–15
Tricuspid atresia. *Arrows* identify shunting through patent foramen ovale and patent ductus arteriosus. (Redrawn courtesy of G.G. Janos, M.D., 1989.)

F. Prognosis.

1. Operative outlook for pulmonary atresia with intact ventricular septum is poor.
2. Reported survival rates range from 20% to 36%, depending on extent of defect, size of right ventricle, and operative procedure (Reddy, Ungerleider, and Hanley, 1998).

TRICUSPID ATRESIA

A. Incidence: 1:18,000 live births.

B. Anatomy: failure of tricuspid valve development with associated patent foramen ovale (Fig. 11–15).
1. VSD is often associated with the hypoplastic right ventricle.
2. Pulmonary atresia or stenosis is possible.
3. Transposition of the great vessels occurs in 30% of the cases.

C. Hemodynamics.

1. Systemic venous blood returns to the right atrium, passing through the foramen ovale into the left atrium and left ventricle. With an isolated defect the pulmonary blood flow is supplied by the left ventricular outflow via the PDA.
2. In the presence of a VSD, some of the blood entering the left ventricle shunts across into the hypoplastic right ventricle and out the pulmonary artery—or out the aorta in the case of coexisting transposition. If severe pulmonary stenosis or atresia is present, blood does not flow through the VSD. (See also item C.1, above.)

D. Clinical features.

1. Cyanosis presents soon after birth with an isolated defect or coexisting VSD and pulmonary outflow tract obstruction. Increasing cyanosis occurs with closure of the ductus.
2. CHF ensues with large VSD and absent pulmonary stenosis (usually in the first month of life).
3. Murmur is absent unless associated with pulmonary stenosis or VSD.
4. Chest x-ray examination shows variable heart size, depending on the degree of pulmonary stenosis; size is generally nondiagnostic.

E. Management.

1. Primary treatment: oxygen, bicarbonate, and prostaglandin E_1 for severe hypoxia.
2. Palliative treatment.
   a. Systemic–pulmonary artery shunt (see section E, Management, under heading Tetralogy of Fallot, above)
   b. Large VSD with no pulmonary stenosis. Pulmonary artery banding is performed to control CHF.
3. Reparative surgery.
   a. Right atrium is connected to either the right ventricular outflow track or the pulmonary artery (Fontan or modified Fontan), so that the right atrium forces blood into the lungs.
   b. Modified Fontan procedure separates oxygenated and unoxygenated blood inside the heart but does not restore normal hemodynamics or anatomy.

F. Prognosis. With the advent of the Fontan procedure, survival rates are 90% and higher (Driscoll 1998).

Mixed Defects

TRANSPOSITION OF THE GREAT VESSELS

A. Incidence: 1:5000 live births; male predominance: 2:1.

B. Anatomy: positions of the great arteries are reversed (i.e., the pulmonary artery arises from the left ventricle and the aorta from the right ventricle). Without other intracardiac defects (e.g., VSD, ASD), an independent, parallel circuit exists (Fig. 11–16). In dextroposition ("D" presentation), aorta is situated to the left of the pulmonary artery.

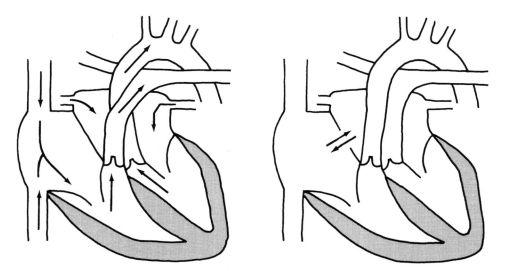

Figure 11–16
Transposition of the great vessels *(TGV). A,* Normal anatomy. *B,* Appearance of the heart with TGV. (Redrawn courtesy of G.G. Janos, M.D., 1989.)

C. Hemodynamics.

1. Oxygenated blood returning from the lungs enters the left atrium and ventricle, exiting via the pulmonary artery and flowing back to the lungs.
2. Desaturated blood returns to the right atrium and ventricle, leaving via the aorta to perfuse the body.
3. Mixing of oxygenated and unoxygenated blood occurs at the ductus arteriosus (as long as patency exists) or through any existing septal defects (ASD, VSD).
   a. Mixing is required for survival.
   b. Shunting occurs from left to right through septal defects or the PDA, ameliorating degree of cyanosis and hypoxia.

D. Clinical features.

1. Cyanosis is present within the first 24 hours of life and becomes progressively more intense.
2. Prominent murmurs are uncommon; VSD (if present) will have a loud murmur.
3. Chest x-ray findings are usually normal; the heart may have an "egg on side" appearance. Pulmonary vasculature may be increased or decreased.

E. Management.

1. Correction of metabolic derangements.
2. Prostaglandin E_1 to maintain patency of the PDA until palliative surgery can be performed.
3. Palliation of choice: balloon septostomy.
   a. Balloon catheter is inserted into the femoral or umbilical vein; it is advanced across the foramen ovale into the left atrium, and the balloon is inflated and pulled across the atrium, creating as ASD.
   b. Procedure rapidly improves systemic and pulmonary circulation admixing, thus increasing PaO_2 (30s) and saturation (70s).
4. Blade septostomy: if atrial septum is too thick to be torn by balloon septostomy or balloon septostomy is unsuccessful. A catheter with a blade is introduced into the left atrium with standard catheterization technique, and a hole is excised in the atrial septum (Neches, Park, and Eltedgin, 1998).
5. Pulmonary artery banding: to prevent pulmonary vascular disease, to decrease CHF, or to exercise the left ventricle before surgery by increasing the ventricular workload.
6. Corrective surgery.
   a. Arterial switch operation (Jatene): detaches aorta, coronary arteries, and pulmonary artery, reattaching to correct ventricles. Procedure is generally performed within first weeks of life and provides both anatomic and physiologic correction.
   b. Mustard or Senning: creates a baffle at the atrium to divert systemic venous blood into the left ventricle and pulmonary artery and pulmonary venous blood into the right ventricle and aorta. These procedures result in physiologic correction only and are generally delayed until the infant is 6 months of age.
7. Rastelli's procedure: intraventricular repair combined with placement of an extracardiac shunt from the right ventricle to the pulmonary artery. Used for TGV with large VSD and extensive left ventricular outflow tract obstruction.

F. Prognosis.

1. Changes in medical operative management make short-term data potentially misleading and long-term data out of date.
2. Survival outcomes are 90–95%, depending on type of repair (Wernosky and Jones, 1998).

3. Complications and other residual effects include dysrhythmias, myocardial ischemia, and aortic and/or pulmonic supravalvular stenosis. The Mustard and Senning procedures have an increased risk of inadequate right ventricular function.

TRUNCUS ARTERIOSUS

A. **Incidence:** 1:33,000 live births.

B. **Anatomy:** a single great vessel arises from both ventricles, overriding a VSD (Fig. 11–17).
1. Type I: From base of the truncus, a single pulmonary trunk arises and divides into the right and left arteries.
2. Type II: Arising from the posterior aspect of the truncus, separate left and right pulmonary arteries.
3. Type III: Pulmonary arteries arise independently from the lateral aspects of the truncus.

C. **Hemodynamics.**
1. Both ventricles pump blood into the common trunk supplying the systemic and pulmonary circulation. As PVR drops, preferential shunting to the pulmonary circulation occurs, increasing blood flow to the lungs and workload of the left ventricle.
2. If pulmonary arteries are stenotic or hypoplastic, blood flow to the lungs is restricted.

D. **Clinical features.**
1. CHF with bounding pulses.
2. Intermittent cyanosis: severe cyanosis with pulmonary artery stenosis.
3. Heart sounds: systolic ejection click with single S_2.
4. Chest x-ray examination: cardiomegaly with increased pulmonary markings. (Exception: If pulmonary artery stenosis exists, decreased pulmonary markings are seen.)

E. **Management.**
1. Early surgical repair is the treatment of choice (Rastelli's procedure).

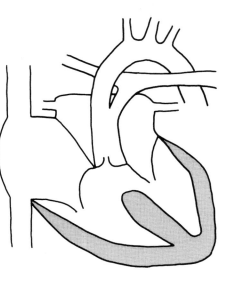

Figure 11–17
Truncus arteriosus. (Redrawn courtesy of G.G. Janos, M.D., 1989.)

a. Homograft between the right ventricle and the pulmonary artery.
b. VSD closure.
c. Connection between aorta and left ventricle alone.
2. Homografts are preferred to synthetic because they are more flexible, easier to use during surgery, and less prone to obstruction.

F. Prognosis.

1. Mortality rate ranges from 10% to 30% if no truncal regurgitation exists (Witt, 1998).
2. Multiple reoperations for conduit or homograft, truncal valve replacement, and potential myocardial problems influence subsequent mortality and morbidity rates.

TOTAL ANOMALOUS PULMONARY VENOUS CONNECTION

A. Incidence: 1:17,000 live births.

B. Anatomy. In TAPVC, pulmonary veins have no connection with the left atrium but drain into the right atrium either directly or indirectly via a systemic venous channel.

1. Presence of a patent foramen ovale or true ASD is required for survival (Fig. 11–18).
2. Varying degrees of pulmonary venous obstruction occur.
3. Three types of TAPVC occur.
   a. Supracardiac. Pulmonary veins attach above the diaphragm, often to the superior vena cava (common form).
   b. Cardiac. Pulmonary veins attach directly to the right atrium or coronary sinus.
   c. Infracardiac. Pulmonary veins attach below the diaphragm (most severe form).

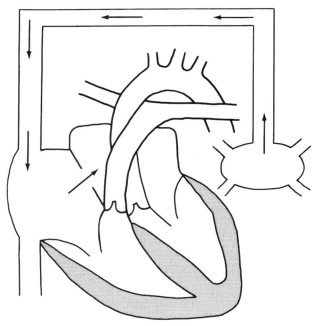

Figure 11–18
Total anomalous pulmonary venous connection *(TAPVC)*. (Redrawn courtesy of G.G. Janos, M.D., 1989.)

C. Hemodynamics.

1. Oxygenated blood from the lungs drains into the right atrium, mixing with the systemic venous return. Part of this flow passes into the left atrium via the patent foramen ovale or ASD, into the left ventricle, and out the aorta. With the normal decrease in PVR, pulmonary blood flow will increase.
2. If obstruction to pulmonary venous return exists, the resulting increase in PVR leads to pulmonary edema and diversion of blood from the pulmonary artery to the aorta via the PDA. Closure of the PDA then increases right-to-left atrial shunting.

D. Clinical features.

1. Nonobstructed.
   a. CHF.
   b. Mild cyanosis.
   c. Heart sounds: systolic ejection click at the lower sternal border and mid-diastolic at the left lower sternal border. Wide split S_2 may be present but is generally nonspecific.
   d. Chest x-ray examination: right ventricle dilation, prominent pulmonary markings; "snowman" appearance.
2. Obstructed.
   a. Cyanosis predominates.
   b. Chest x-ray examination: normal size with pulmonary venous congestion.

E. **Management:** early and occasionally immediate surgical correction.
1. Cardiac catheterization may be omitted to speed time to operation, with surgery based on echocardiography.
2. Anomalous veins are detached and transplanted to the left atrium; the ASD is repaired.

F. Prognosis.

1. Mortality rate for infants with obstructed TAPVC who undergo surgery is 5–50% (Ruth-Sanchez, 1998), with cardiac type less than 5% (Gaedeke, 1996).
2. Long-term prognosis is excellent because TAPVC is closer to a surgically "curable" condition than are most congenital cardiac lesions.

HYPOPLASTIC LEFT HEART SYNDROME

A. **Incidence:** 1:6000 live births.

B. Anatomy.

1. Hypoplastic left ventricle and ascending aorta.
2. Atretic or hypoplastic mitral and aortic valves (Fig. 11–19).

C. Hemodynamics.

1. Obstruction of blood flow through the left side of the heart due to hypoplastic aorta and ventricle leads to pulmonary venous congestion and edema.
2. Blood supply to the descending aorta and to the aortic arch and coronary arteries (retrograde flow) is dependent on the PDA.

D. Clinical features.

1. Asymptomatic at birth.
2. Tachypnea and dyspnea with increasing pulmonary blood flow.
3. CHF: usually presents at 24–48 hours of life.
4. Cyanosis: rarely permanent despite mixing of systemic and pulmonary circulations.

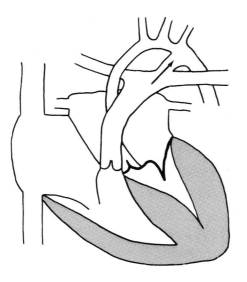

Figure 11–19
Hypoplastic left heart syndrome. (Redrawn courtesy of G.G. Janos, M.D., 1989.)

5. Low output signs as PDA closes.
   a. Severe mottling.
   b. Gray pallor of skin.
   c. Markedly diminished pulses.
6. Chest x-ray examination: cardiomegaly with increased pulmonary blood flow and pulmonary venous congestion.

E. Management.

1. Previously a uniformly fatal lesion; management has been comfort and family support.
2. Initial management.
   a. Prostaglandin E_1 to maintain ductus arteriosus patency and systemic circulation.
   b. Use of inhaled O_2 and nitrogen combination for an inspired O_2 of less than 21%. Nitrogen therapy creates pulmonary hypoxia and vasoconstriction, which may maximize right-to-left shunting and systemic blood flow, with a resulting increase in systemic oxygen saturation.
3. Staged surgical repair.
   a. First stage, or "Norwood" repair.
      (1) Anastomosis of main pulmonary artery to aorta, creating a new aorta.
      (2) Aortopulmonary shunt to provide controlled blood flow to pulmonary arteries.
      (3) Atrial septectomy to ensure pulmonary venous return to the right atrium.
   b. Second stage: bidirectional Glenn's procedure (cavopulmonary anastomosis shunt) or hemi-Fontan procedure done in child between 6 and 9 months of age.
   c. Third stage, or modified Fontan procedure.
      (1) Involves completion of Fontan procedure between 12 and 24 months of age.
      (2) Completion of stages 2 and 3 separates the pulmonary from the systemic circulation.
   d. Disadvantages.
      (1) Two or three open surgeries in first two years of life.
      (2) Single right ventricle supplies the systemic circulation.
   e. Contraindication: significant tricuspid valve or pulmonic valve dysplasia associated with functional disturbances.

4. Heart transplantation.
   a. Provides a structurally and physiologically normal heart in one operation.
   b. Ten to forty percent of infants either undergo staged palliation or die awaiting transplantation (Barber, 1998).
   c. Complications include:
      (1) Increased susceptibility to infections as result of immunosuppression.
      (2) Allograft rejection.
      (3) Systemic hypertension: usually seen only in first year after transplantation.
      (4) Recurrent or residual coarctation: managed with angioplasty or surgical repair.
      (5) Seizures: common neurologic complication.
5. Prognosis.
   a. Comparison of staged repair versus heart transplantation outcomes requires evaluation of numbers of children surviving who completed procedure and numbers of those "lost" through death awaiting procedure or death between stages of procedure.
   b. Heart transplant survival is reported at 68–80% at 5 years (Hsu and Gersony, 1997), with actuarial survival at 61–70% (Freedom and Benson, 1995; Razzouk et al, 1996).
   c. Staged repair survival after completion of the Fontan procedure by the Norwood procedure is reported at 95% (Barber, 1998). Actuarial survival at 4 years is 54% (Freedom and Benson, 1995).

Congestive Heart Failure

ETIOLOGY

A. **CHF is a set of clinical signs and symptoms that indicate a dysfunctional myocardium.**

1. In CHF, cardiac output is unable to meet the body's metabolic requirements.
2. Right and/or left ventricular end-diastolic pressures are elevated, impeding systemic and/or pulmonary venous returns.

B. **Although structural congenital heart defects are the most common cause of CHF, other causes should be considered.**

1. Timing of detection is often helpful in predicting causes, as the diseases causing CHF characteristically show up at certain ages. Tables 11–3 and 11–4 indicate conditions associated with CHF and their time of onset.
2. CHF in utero that is detected at birth may be due to the following:
   a. Profound anemia: erythroblastosis fetalis or twin-to-twin transfusion.
   b. Arrhythmia: superventricular tachycardia or congenital heart block.
   c. Intrauterine infection with myocarditis.
   d. Arteriovenous malformations.
   e. Absent pulmonary valve.
   f. Premature ductus arteriosus closure: maternal use of prostaglandin inhibitor (e.g., aspirin, ibuprofen).
   g. Volume overload: twin-to-twin or mother-to-infant transfusion.

CLINICAL FEATURES

A. **Common signs.**

1. Tachypnea (60–100 respirations per minute at rest).
2. Tachycardia (150–180 bpm at rest).

Table 11–5
MANIFESTATIONS OF AND GUIDELINES FOR ASSESSING THE SEVERITY OF CONGESTIVE HEART FAILURE IN NEONATES AND INFANTS

MANIFESTATIONS OF CHF
Alterations of myocardial performance/initiation of compensatory mechanisms
   Cardiomegaly
   Tachycardia
   Diminished peripheral pulsations and perfusion
   Excessive sweating
   Poor feeding and growth retardation
   Gallop rhythm ± murmur
   Cardiogenic shock: hypotension; tachycardia; poor capillary refill; cool, mottled extremities; decreased output; metabolic
     acidosis
Results of pulmonary venous congestion
   Tachypnea
   Rales
   Dyspnea
   Pulmonary edema
   Hypoxemia
Results of systemic venous congestion
   Hepatomegaly
   Periorbital edema
   Jugular venous distention: difficult to appreciate in the neonate
   Ascites and anasarca: rare, present in hydrops, after cardiac operation or asphyxia

GUIDELINES FOR ASSESSING CHF SEVERITY
1. Mild congestive cardiac failure—presence of any three of the following:
   a. Cardiomegaly (cardiothoracic ratio on chest radiograph of greater than .60), the most reliable sign of the presence of cardiac dysfunction.
   b. Persistent tachycardia (heart rate of greater than 150/minute at rest).
   c. Tachypnea with mild degrees of exertion or at rest (respiratory rate greater than 60/minute).
   d. Scattered rales at base of lungs (retractions will often be present but can be seen in large left-to-right shunts without failure).
2. Moderate congestive cardiac failure—mild congestive cardiac failure criteria are met with the addition of one of the following:
   a. Gallop rhythm.
   b. Hepatomegaly (liver greater than 3 cm below costal margin in the absence of significantly hyperaerated lungs with depressed diaphragm).
   c. Pulmonary edema (with interstitial and alveolar edema radiographically).
3. Severe congestive cardiac failure—presence of cardiogenic shock (hypotension; oliguria; poor capillary refill; cool, mottled extremities; acidosis).

From Monaco, M., and Gay, W.: Congenital cardiac failure. *In* Moller, J., and Neal, W. (Eds.): Fetal, Neonatal and Infant Cardiac Disease. Norwalk, Conn., Appleton & Lange, 1990, pp. 909 and 912.

---

3. Cardiomegaly.
   a. Changes in cardiac contour.
   b. Diminished or engorged pulmonary vasculature.
4. Hepatomegaly (3–5 cm below coastal margin): one of the most useful signs.
5. Pulmonary rales and bronchi.
6. Fatigue or difficulty with feeding.

B. **Less common signs.**

1. Edema: usually not obvious unless CHF is present for some time.
2. Inappropriate sweating.
3. Gallop rhythm.
4. Altered pulses (variable, depending on underlying cause).
5. ECG indicating the following:
   a. Hypertrophy of one or more chambers.
   b. Abnormal mean QRS axis.
   c. Rhythm disturbances.

6. Symptoms of CHF: characterized as those resulting from pulmonary venous or systemic venous congestion or compensatory mechanisms; variable severity (Table 11–5).

MANAGEMENT OF CONGESTIVE HEART FAILURE

A. General measures (appropriate for any heart disease).
1. Use semi-Fowler's or prone position to achieve maximal diaphragmatic excursion and lung expansion.
2. Decrease oxygen consumption.
   a. Maintain neutral thermal environment.
   b. Avoid unnecessary stresses (e.g., heel sticks, radial sticks).
   c. Provide sedation for infant agitation.
   d. Consider assisted ventilation to reduce work of breathing.
3. Provide supplemental oxygen. The amount is dictated by the PaO_2 and the presence of CHD with admixing of arterial and venous blood.
4. Correct acidosis and any metabolic derangements (e.g., hypoglycemia or hypocalcemia).

B. Specific measures.
1. Fluid and nutritional support.
   a. During acute phase, volume intake is reduced, generally to two thirds of maintenance levels.
   b. Use of glucose polymers (Polycose) or medium-chain triglycerides (MCT Oil) enhances caloric content without significant volume increase.
   c. IV infusions of 50% fat emulsions can also be used to increase caloric intake with minimal intake volume.
2. Pharmacologic therapy.
   a. Digoxin therapy (Table 11–6).
      (1) Achieve maximal cardiac output; not as effective in premature babies.
      (2) Digitalize patient (Table 11–6) and observe for bradycardia (discontinue if heart rate <100 bpm).
         (a) Arrhythmias or heart block.
         (b) Hypokalemia.
         (c) Toxic effects: more frequent in premature infants because of a longer serum half-life for digoxin than in term or older infants.

Table 11–6
DIGOXIN DOSAGES AND COMMON SIDE EFFECTS

DIGITALIZING SCHEDULE
Preterm infant
    IV route: 20-30 µg/kg total dose
    PO route: 30-40 µg/kg total dose
Term infant
    IV route: 30-40 µg/kg total dose
    PO route: 40-50 µg/kg total dose
	Total dose is usually divided into three doses, giving one-half, then one-fourth, then one-fourth of the total dose every 8 hours. Check EKG rhythm strip for rate, PR interval, and dysrhythmias before each dose.

MAINTENANCE SCHEDULE
Preterm infant
    IV route: 8-10 µg/kg/day
    PO route: 10-12 µg/kg/day
Term infant
    IV route: 10-12 µg/kg/day
    PO route: 12-14 µg/kg/day
	Total dose should be divided twice a day. Allow 12-24 hours between last digitalizing and first maintenance doses. It takes about 6 days to "digitalize" a patient with maintenance doses alone. The sign of digitalis effect is usually prolongation of the PR interval. The first sign of digitalis toxicity is usually vomiting, dysrhythmias, or bradycardia.

From Daberkow, E., and Washington, R.: Handbook of Neonatal Intensive Care, 2nd ed. St. Louis, C.V. Mosby, 1989, p. 436.

   b. Diuretic therapy.
     (1) Used to eliminate excessive intravascular fluid.
     (2) Furosemide (Lasix), 1–2 mg/kg every 12 hours IV, or 1–3 mg/kg every 12 hours by mouth.
       (a) In severe CHF the IV route is preferable for its rapid onset of action.
       (b) Hypokalemia and hypochloremia are side effects that can result in metabolic alkalosis.
       (c) Urinary losses of calcium occur, placing infant at risk of having nephrocalcinosis.
       (d) Use is contraindicated in renal failure.
     (3) Ethacrynic acid (Edecrin), 1 mg/kg IV.
       (a) Has renal action similar to that of furosemide.
       (b) Complications include gastrointestinal side effects and ototoxic effects.
     (4) Chlorothiazide (Diuril), 20–40 mg/kg per day in two oral doses.
       (a) Administered when less acute oral diuresis is required.
       (b) Does not produce the profound potassium losses seen with furosemide; may reduce urinary calcium losses seen with furosemide.
   c. Inotropic agents.
     (1) May be necessary in severe CHF or cardiogenic shock.
     (2) Most commonly used are isoproterenol, dopamine, and dobutamine.

C. **Cardiology consultation to rule out or establish presence of congenital heart lesion.** Cardiac catheterization, angiocardiography, and surgery may be indicated.

Postoperative Cardiac Management

(McLaughlin, Setzer, and Schleien, 1996)

NONINVASIVE MONITORING

A. **Electrocardiography.**

1. Continuous display should be monitored.
   a. Tachycardia.
   b. Fibrillation.
   c. Asystole.
2. Lead II: assessment of amplitude, axis, and presence and absence of P waves.
3. Lead V_5 changes: septal or lateral wall ischemia.

B. **Blood pressure: manual.**

1. Used to determine accuracy of arterial line (especially radial) reading.
2. Cuff can be used to occlude an arterial catheter leak.
3. Measurement of upper and lower extremities after repair of coarctation of the aorta gives pressure gradient across repair site.
4. Avoid extremity for blood pressure measurement when an artery has been used for surgical repair (e.g., subclavian patch for coarctation of the aorta, Blalock-Taussig shunt).

C. **Pulse oximetry.**

1. Decreasing oxygen saturations may indicate:
   a. Decreased cardiac output.
   b. Increasing intracardiac shunting.
   c. Increased intrapulmonary shunting.
2. Continuous monitoring is useful in pulmonary hypertension. Small decrease

in saturation may be the first sign of increased pulmonary artery pressure with onset of right-to-left shunting.

D. Urinary output.

1. Hourly output rate is a good clinical indicator of renal perfusion.
   a. Invalid in first 2 hours postoperatively after diuretic administration.
   b. Urinary retention can be induced by analgesics.
2. Indwelling catheter is generally not required in those with uncomplicated procedures, stable vital signs, and good peripheral perfusion.

INVASIVE MONITORING

For pressure values from cardiac catheterization, see Table 11–7.

A. Arterial pressure.

1. Mandatory for timely vasoactive medication adjustments.
2. Arterial tracing provides information for analysis of waveform and calculation of pulse pressure.

B. Right-sided cardiac pressures.

1. In patients with normal cardiac anatomy: Right atrial pressure = Right ventricular end-diastole pressure = Central venous pressure.
2. Increasing values seen with:
   a. Right ventricular overload.
   b. Poor ventricular function.
   c. Elevated pulmonary artery pressure, resulting from reactive pulmonary hypertension.
3. Particularly useful for evaluating:
   a. Right-sided cardiac lesions.
      (1) Pulmonic stenosis.
      (2) Tetralogy of Fallot.
   b. Those lesions requiring high right atrial pressures, such as in the Fontan procedure.

C. Pulmonary artery pressure.

1. Catheter is placed through wall of right atrium into pulmonary artery, most commonly during cardiac surgery.
2. Measurements guide the medical management of pulmonary hypertension and are most frequently used in conditions where postoperative pulmonary hypertension is anticipated, as in endocardial cushion repair.
3. Mixed venous oxygen saturation ($S\bar{v}O_2$) monitoring can be obtained from newer pulmonary artery catheters with continuous oximetry capabilities.

Table 11–7
PRESSURE VALUES FROM CARDIAC CATHERIZATION

Pressure	Normal Neonatal Values
Systemic arterial pressure	60-90/20-60 mm Hg (birth to 5 days of age)
Right atrial pressure	3 mm Hg
Right ventricular pressure	30/3 mm Hg
Pulmonary artery occlusion pressure/pulmonary wedge pressure	6-10 mm Hg
Left atrial pressure	8 mm Hg
Left ventricular pressure	100/6 mm Hg

    a. $S\bar{v}O_2$ reflects a balance between oxygen delivery and consumption.

    b. Alterations are seen in:

      (1) Anemia.

      (2) Shock.

      (3) Left-to-right or right-to-left shunts.

    c. Change in $S\bar{v}O_2$ generally precedes detectable hemodynamic changes by several minutes.

D. **Left-sided cardiac pressures.**

1. In patients with normal cardiac anatomy: Left ventricular end-diastolic pressure = Left atrial pressure = Pulmonary artery occlusion pressure = Pulmonary artery wedge pressure.

2. Useful in patients with mitral valve dysfunction, as seen in postendocardial cushion repair.

3. Requires meticulous line care because the risk of air or particulate embolization is high.

E. **Epicardial pacing wires.**

1. Usually attached to right atrium and/or right ventricle.

2. Access to pacing is most important after surgical repairs near the cardiac conduction system. For example:

    a. VSD.

    b. Transposition of the great arteries.

    c. Truncus arteriosis.

    d. Endocardial cushion defects.

HEMODYNAMIC MANAGEMENT

A. **Bradycardia.**

1. Common result of intraoperative cooling; proportional to degree of hypothermia.

2. After extensive atrial surgery, such as arterial switch procedure, TAPVC repair.

3. After injury to sinoatrial node.

4. With conducting problems:

    a. Sinoatrial block.

    b. Sinus asystole.

    c. Atrioventricular junctional block.

5. As a consequence of edema around conduction system (generally resolves in 3–4 days).

B. **Tachycardia.** Observed as a consequence of or in response to:

1. Pain.

2. Agitation.

3. Hypovolemia.

4. Junctional conduction disturbance.

POSTOPERATIVE DISTURBANCES

Heart Failure

Etiology

A. **Most common postoperative event resulting from a neonatal cardiac reserve, limited by:**

1. Decreased myofilament numbers.

2. Decreased ventricle compliance.

3. Greater oxygen consumption, cardiac output, and resting heart rate in the neonate.
4. Nearly maximal neonatal cardiac performance in the absence of stress.

B. **Preload or diastolic filling.**

1. Hypovolemia.
   a. Inadequate volume replacement.
   b. Inadequate mechanical hemostasis.
   c. Impaired clotting.
2. Iatrogenic volume overload.

C. **Inadequate systemic venous return.**

1. Excessive positive end-expiratory pressure.
2. Tension pneumothorax.
3. Atrial baffle obstruction.
4. Postpericardial effusions.

D. **Residual shunting.**

E. **Increased pulmonary vascular resistance.**

F. **Decreased cardiac contractility, resulting from:**

1. Accidental discontinuation of vasoactive drugs.
2. Electrolyte disturbances.
3. Hypoglycemia.
4. Surgical manipulation or damage.

Recognition of Low Cardiac Output

A. **Observation: "just not doing well."**

1. Noninteractive or becoming less interactive with environment.
2. Lack of or decreasing vigor of cries.
3. Awake but "floppy."

B. **Color.**

1. Violet color of mucosa.
2. Gray skin or mottling of skin.

C. **Extremities.**

1. Cool to touch.
2. Lack of or decrease in pedal pulses.
3. Capillary refill time longer than 3 seconds.
4. Edema: often seen postoperatively but also indicative of fluid overload.

D. **Oliguria (urine output <0.5–1 mL/kg per hour).**

E. **Tachycardia.**

1. Gallop rhythm.
2. Distant heart sounds: possible indication of pericardial effusions.

F. **Low arterial blood pressure.**

G. **Respiratory distress.**

1. Retractions, tachypnea, grunting in infant after extubation.
2. Rales: often heard after bypass procedure.

H. **Weight gain disportionate to caloric intake.**

I. X-ray findings.

1. Excessive cardiac size or enlargement of specific chamber.
2. Large cardiac silhouette or "bag of waters" appearance may indicate pericardial effusions.
3. Increased fluffy densities; these are not seen if elevated positive end-expiratory pressure is used in ventilation.

J. Metabolic derangement.

1. Metabolic acidosis, generally resulting from low bicarbonate levels.
2. Low sodium value, in part due to excessive free water.

Management of Low Cardiac Output

A. Use blood for volume replacement.

B. Volume challenge is appropriate in light of cardiopulmonary bypass third spacing.

1. Close monitoring required.
2. Strict intake and output.

C. Provide correction of metabolic disorders (hypocalcemia and hypoglycemia) and acid-base imbalances.

D. Reduce right ventricular afterload.

1. Hyperventilation.
2. Pulmonary vasodilating agents.
   a. Prostaglandin E_1.
   b. Tolazoline.
   c. Nitroglycerin.
   d. Nitroprusside.
   e. Inhaled nitric oxide.

E. Treat rate or rhythm disturbance.

1. Increase heart rate.
   a. Rate of 200–210 bpm is tolerated well, with acceptable myocardial work and oxygen consumption.
   b. Cardioversion can be used for sinus tachycardia.
2. Atrial or atrioventricular pacing is often necessary.

F. Consider pharmaceutical agents.

1. Isoproterenol (Isuprel): acts to decrease pulmonary and systemic vascular resistance (decreases afterload).
2. Nitroprusside or nitroglycerin: reduces afterload.
3. Amrinone or milrinone: increases heart rate and contractility with some vasodilatory properties.
4. Volume replacement: possibly necessary because of vasodilation (maintain preload). Central venous pressure is useful in determining volume needs.
5. Vasopressors (i.e., dopamine, >10 µg/kg per minute, or dobutamine). Potential for increasing PVR. Careful monitoring of effects is necessary.

G. Monitor blood pressure.

Bleeding

A. Provide sedation. Keep infant sedated, avoiding agitation, to prevent hypertension and pressure at active and potential bleeding sites, which may aggravate or disrupt clot formation.

B. **Assess and treat coagulopathy.**

1. Use fresh whole blood for volume and clotting.
2. Use cryoprecipitate for fibrinogen (aids clotting).
3. Evaluate platelets: count is low and function is inadequate because of "bypass" and deep hypothermia.
   a. Give platelet infusion.
   b. Give desmopressin (DDAVP), 0.3 μg/kg, to stimulate platelets to aggregate.

Pulmonary Hypertension/Pulmonary Vasospasm

A. **Avoid hypoxemia and acidosis.**

1. Hypoxia increases PVR.
2. Hyperoxygenate before suctioning; increase fractional inspired oxygen (FIO_2) and hyperventilate; keep suctioning time to minimum.
   a. Pain management or sedation.
   b. Do not disconnect ventilator to suction.

B. **Minimize handling.**

1. Group noxious stimuli when possible; cluster care activities.
2. Give fentanyl or morphine for pain relief.
3. Infant may require sedation for agitation, in addition to analgesia.

Maintenance of Fluid-and-Electrolyte Balance

A. **Hypoglycemia, hypokalemia, and hypocalcemia are potential problems.**

1. All result in decreased myocardial function.
2. Potential for seizures is present.
   a. Poor cardiac output to the brain may cause seizures.
   b. Cardiopulmonary bypass and circulatory arrest also predispose an infant to seizures.
3. Monitor laboratory values and replace electrolytes as needed.

B. **Avoid acidosis.**

1. Metabolic acidosis is common in tissue hypoxia and suboptimal perfusion from lowered cardiac output.
2. Management includes:
   a. Maintenance of slight alkalosis by means of hyperventilation and sodium bicarbonate.
   b. Hyperoxygenation.

C. **Avoid fluid overload.**

1. Maintain meticulous control of infusion rates; carefully label all lines to avoid confusion.
2. Monitor urine output; may require catheter for accuracy, especially if output is minimal.

Shock

Etiology

A. **Shock is a state of inadequate circulating blood volume, resulting in reduced perfusion and oxygenation to the tissues.** Several varieties of shock are recognized.

B. **Hypovolemic shock may be caused by the following:**

1. Blood loss from placental abnormalities (e.g., umbilical cord rupture, abruptio placentae, twin-to-twin transfusion syndrome).
2. Acute blood loss from postnatal hemorrhage.
3. Plasma and fluid losses.
   a. Skin integrity losses (e.g., myelomeningocele, gastroschisis).
   b. Pleural effusions (e.g., erythroblastosis fetalis or nonimmune hydrops).
   c. Body water loss from persistent vomiting, diarrhea, or evaporative skin losses.

C. **Cardiogenic shock may be caused by the following:**

1. Myocardial failure from severe hypoxemia, hypoglycemia, and/or acidemia.
2. Congenital heart lesions.
3. Cardiac arrhythmias.
4. Restriction of cardiac function by:
   a. Tamponade.
   b. Tension pneumothorax.
   c. Excessive levels of ventilatory distending pressures.
5. Myocarditis: often associated with sepsis.

D. **Distributive shock:**

1. Results from impaired peripheral arterial resistance usually caused by sepsis (i.e., release of bacterial toxins).
2. Typically is associated with gram-negative organisms; however, a gram-positive organism may be the causative agent.

Clinical Indicators

A. **Signs of shock are frequently nonspecific.** (Cardiogenic shock may be indistinguishable from CHF.)

B. **Cardiopulmonary status changes.**

1. Tachycardia.
2. Tachypnea and/or apnea.
3. Poor peripheral perfusion.
   a. Pallor (especially with blood loss).
   b. Capillary refill time longer than 3 seconds.
4. Hypotension.

C. **Decreased urinary output.**

D. **Metabolic disturbances.**

1. Metabolic acidosis.
2. Hypoglycemia.
3. Hypothermia.

E. **Evidence of coagulation defects.**

F. **Indicators of blood volume** (or effective blood volume) are as follows:
1. Change in hemoglobin and hematocrit values.
2. Response to fluid challenge of 10 mL of saline solution per kilogram of body weight, while blood pressure and urine output are monitored.
3. Positive Betke-Kleihauer test result indicates fetal-to-maternal transfusion in utero. This test examines the maternal blood for the presence of fetal erythrocytes.

G. **Indicators of cardiac function.**

1. See Cardiopulmonary Status Changes, point B, above.
2. Echocardiogram establishes anatomic defects and/or specific myocardial function abnormalities.
3. Central venous pressure is generally elevated, except during hypovolemic shock.

H. **Indicators of septic shock.**

1. Clinical signs of sepsis or positive culture results.
2. Normal blood pressure in the face of prominent hypoperfusion.
3. Edema or sclerema from capillary protein and fluid leakage.
4. Oliguria, proteinuria.
5. Persistent pulmonary hypertension of the neonate (common).

Management

A. **Shock management: depends largely on prevailing pathogenesis.** A large proportion of the care is supportive.

B. **Supportive care.**

1. Maintain oxygenation and ventilation as dictated by arterial blood gas values.
   a. Give ventilatory support if concurrent pulmonary disease exists.
   b. Tolazoline may be useful in pulmonary hypertension with hypoxemia. Use cautiously in septic shock; systemic hypotension is likely.
   c. Provide neutral thermal environment to decrease oxygen consumption.
   d. Decrease external stress (i.e., handling, peripheral blood sampling).
2. Promptly treat acidosis to avoid adverse effects on myocardial contractility. Sodium bicarbonate is often necessary.
3. Maintain fluid-and-electrolyte balance.

C. **Specific therapies.**

1. Increase blood volume and erythrocyte mass.
   a. Maintain blood pressure and maximize oxygen content.
   b. Treatment of acute blood loss may require large volume transfusion.
   c. Monitoring arterial blood pressure is essential; monitoring of central venous pressure ideally should be included.
   d. *Caution:* In cardiogenic shock, added volume may increase the myocardial workload.
2. Treat the infectious process in septic shock.
   a. Antibiotic therapy should be initiated.
   b. Exchange transfusion with fresh whole blood (controversial) provides neutrophils and removes bacterial toxins.
   c. Give neutrophil transfusion to augment cellular immunity (controversial).
3. Maximize cardiac output.
   a. Inotropic agents: useful in cardiogenic shock to increase cardiac output and support circulation. Start early in septic shock if evidence of oliguria, hypotension, or acidosis exists.
   b. Isoproterenol (Isuprel): increases heart rate and contractility (beta-1-adrenergic effects). Simultaneous effects produce bronchodilation and smooth muscle relaxation (beta-2 effects). Usual dose is 0.05–1.0 mg/kg per minute. Observe for arrhythmias such as premature ventricular contractions.
   c. Dopamine (Intropin): increases cardiac contractility and cardiac output. Effects are dose dependent. At low doses (1–5 µg/kg per minute, IV), selective vasodilation of the renal, mesenteric, cerebral, and coronary vascular beds occurs with little effect on heart rate or blood pressure. With

moderate doses (6–10 µg/kg per minute), increased blood pressure and improved tissue perfusion can be observed. Beneficial effects are dependent largely on adequate blood volume. Correct hypovolemia before the dopamine infusion. At higher doses (>10 µg/kg per minute, IV), vasoconstriction occurs and consists of vasoconstriction of the pulmonary vasculature, increased right ventricular afterload, reduction in pulmonary blood flow, right-to-left shunting through fetal structures, and increased hypoxemia. Tachycardia, dysrhythmias, and ectopic beats can occur as a consequence of dopamine infusion.

    d. Dobutamine (Dobutrex): increases cardiac contractility while exerting limited effects on vasculature. Cardiac output increases, depending on myocardial catecholamine stores. A dose of 2–5 µg/kg per minute, IV, is a reasonable starting dose, with a high dose considered 10 µg/kg per minute or greater (Bell, 1998).

    e. Digitalis should be considered and used selectively, especially in the face of hypoxia or toxic myocardiopathy (see Table 11–6).

4. Correct any tension pneumothorax or cardiac tamponade.

REFERENCES

Allen, H., Beekman, R., Garson, A., et al.: Pediatric therapeutic cardiac catherization. Circulation, *97*:609, 1998.

Ayres, N.: Fetal cardiology. *In* Garson, A., Bricker, J., Fisher, D., and Neish, S. (Eds.): The Science and Practice of Pediatric Cardiology, 2nd ed., vol. 2. Baltimore, Williams & Wilkins, 1998, pp. 2281–2300.

Barber, G.: Hypoplastic left heart. *In* Garson, A., Bricker, J., Fisher, D., and Neish, S. (Eds.): The Science and Practice of Pediatric Cardiology, 2nd ed., vol. 2. Baltimore, Williams & Wilkins, 1998, pp. 1625–1645.

Beekman, R.: Coarctation of the aorta. *In* Emmanouilides, G., Riemenschneider, T., Allen, H., et al. (Eds.): Moss and Adams' Heart Disease in Infants, Children, and Adolescents Including the Fetus and Young Adult, 5th ed., vol 2. Baltimore, Williams & Wilkins, 1995, pp. 1111–1133.

Bell, S.: Neonatal cardiovascular pharmacology. Neonatal Network, *17*(2):7–15, 1998.

Brook, M., and Heyman, M.: Patent ductus arteriosus. *In* Emmanouilides, G., Riemenschneider, T., Allen, H., et al. (Eds.): Moss and Adams' Heart Disease in Infants, Children, and Adolescents Including the Fetus and Young Adult, 5th ed., vol. 1. Baltimore, Williams & Wilkins, 1995, pp. 746–764.

Braudo, M., and Rowe, R.: Auscultation of the heart: Early neonatal period. Am. J. Dis. Child., *101*:575–586, 1961.

Burton, D., and Cabalke, A.: Cardiac evaluation of infants the first year of life. Pediatr. Clin. North Am., *41*:991–1015, 1994.

Chang, A., and Vaughn, A.: Coarctation of the aorta. *In* Chang, A., Hanley, F., Wernovsky, G., and Wessel, D. (Eds.): Pediatric Cardiac Intensive Care. Baltimore, Williams & Wilkins, 1998, pp. 247–256.

Cheatham, J.: Pulmonary stenosis. *In* Garson, A., Bricker, J., Fisher, D., and Neish, S. (Eds.): The Science and Practice of Pediatric Cardiology, 2nd ed., vol. 1. Baltimore, Williams & Wilkins, 1998, pp. 1207–1256.

Coburn, J., Feldt, R., Edwards, W., et al.: Atrial septal defects. *In* Emmanouilides, G., Riemenschneider, T., Allen, H., et al. (Eds.): Moss and Adams' Heart Disease in Infants, Children, and Adolescents Including the Fetus and Young Adult, 5th ed., vol. 1. Baltimore, Williams & Wilkins, 1995, pp. 687–703.

Corbet, A.: Medical manipulation of the ductus arteriosus. *In* Garson, A., Bricker, J., Fisher, D., and Neish, S. (Eds.): The Science and Practice of Pediatric Cardiology, 2nd ed., vol. 2. Baltimore, Williams & Wilkins, 1998, pp. 2489–2513.

Daberkow-Carson, E., and Washington: Cardiovascular diseases and surgical interventions. *In* Merenstein, G., and Gardner, S. (Eds.): Handbook of Neonatal Intensive Care Nursing, 4th ed. St. Louis, Mosby–Year Book, 1998, pp. 500–534.

Driscoll, D.: Tricuspid atresia. *In* Garson, A., Bricker, J., Fisher, D., and Neish, S. (Eds.): The Science and Practice of Pediatric Cardiology, 2nd ed., vol. 2. Baltimore, Williams & Wilkins, 1998, pp. 1579–1587.

Duff, D., and McNamara, D.: History and physical examination of the cardiovascular system. *In* Garson, A., Bricker, J., Fisher, D., and Neish, S. (Eds.): The Science and Practice of Pediatric Cardiology, 2nd ed., vol. 1. Baltimore, Williams & Wilkins, 1998, pp. 693–713.

Feldt, R., Coburn, J., Edwards, W., et al.: Arterioventricular defects. *In* Emmanouilides, G., Riemenschneider, T., Allen, H., et al. (Eds.): Moss and Adams' Heart Disease in Infants, Children, and Adolescents Including the Fetus and Young Adult, 5th ed., vol. 1. Baltimore, Williams & Wilkins, 1995, pp. 704–724.

Flanagan, M., and Flyer, D.: Cardiac disease. *In* Avery, G., Fletcher, M., and Macdonald, M. (Eds.): Neonatology: Pathophysiology and Management of the Newborn, 4th ed. Philadelphia, J.B. Lippincott, 1994, pp. 516–559.

Freedom, R., and Benson, L.: Hypoplastic left heart syndrome. *In* Emmanouilides, G., Riemenschneider, T., Allen, H., et al. (Eds.): Moss and Adams' Heart Disease in Infants, Children, and Adolescents Including the Fetus and Young Adult, 5th ed., vol. 2. Baltimore, Williams & Wilkins, 1995, pp. 1133–1149.

Friedman, W.: Aortic stenosis. *In* Emmanouilides, G., Riemenschneider, T., Allen, H., et al. (Eds.): Moss and Adams' Heart Disease in Infants, Children, and Adolescents Including the Fetus and Young Adult, 5th ed., vol. 2. Baltimore, Williams & Wilkins, 1995, pp. 1087–1110.

Gaedeke, M.: Pediatric and Neonatal Care Certification Review. St. Louis, Mosby–Year Book, 1996, pp. 1–43.

Graham, T., and Gutgell, H.: Ventricular septal defects. *In* Emmanouilides, G., Riemenschneider, T., Allen, H., et al. (Eds.): Moss and Adams' Heart Disease in Infants, Children, and Adolescents Including the Fetus and Young Adult, 5th ed., vol. 1. Baltimore, Williams & Wilkins, 1995, pp. 724–746.

Gumbiner, C., and Takao, A.: Ventricular septal defect. *In* Garson, A., Bricker, J., Fisher, D., and Neish, S. (Eds.): The Science and Practice of Pediatric Cardiology, 2nd ed., vol. 1. Baltimore, Williams & Wilkins, 1998, pp. 1119–1140.

Guyton, A., and Hall, J.: Textbook of Medical Physiology, 9th ed. Philadelphia, W.B. Saunders, 1996, pp. 107–127.

Hsu, D., and Gersony, W.: Medical management of the neonate with congenital heart disease. *In* Spitzer, A. (Ed.): Intensive Care of the Fetus and Neonate. St. Louis, Mosby–Year Book, 1997, pp. 787–796.

Ivy, D., Neish, S., and Abman, S.: Regulation of pulmonary circulation. *In* Garson, A., Bricker, J., Fisher, D., and Neish, S. (Eds.): The Science and Practice of Pediatric Cardiology, 2nd ed., vol. 1. Baltimore, Williams & Wilkins, 1998, pp. 328–347.

McLaughlin, G., Setzer, N., and Schleien, C.: Postoperative management of the cardiac surgical patient. *In* Rogers, M. (Ed.): Textbook of Pediatric Intensive Care, 3rd ed. Baltimore, Williams & Wilkins, 1996, pp. 463–523.

Moore, K., and Persaud, T.: The Developing Human: Clinically Oriented Embryology, 5th ed. Philadelphia, W.B. Saunders, 1993.

Neches, W., Park, S., and Eltedgin, J.: Transposition of the great arteries. *In* Garson, A., Bricker, J., Fisher, D., and Neish, S. (Eds.): The Science and Practice of Pediatric Cardiology, 2nd ed., vol. 2. Baltimore, Williams & Wilkins, 1998, pp. 1463–1503.

Nihill, M.: Catherization and angiography. *In* Garson, A., Bricker, J., Fisher, D., and Neish, S. (Eds.): The Science and Practice of Pediatric Cardiology, 2nd ed., vol. 1. Baltimore, Williams & Wilkins, 1998, pp. 995–1019.

Page, J., and Hasking, M.: An approach to the neonate with sudden dysrhythmia: Diagnosis, mechanisms and management. Neonatal Network, *16*(6):7–18, 1997.

Patterson, S.W., and Starling, J.: On the mechanical factors which determine the output of the ventricles. J. Physiol., *48:* 357, 1914.

Razzouk, A., Chinnock, R., Gundry, S., et al.: Transplantation as a primary treatment for hypoplastic left heart syndrome: Intermediate term results. Ann. Thorac. Surg., 62:1–8, 1996.

Reddy, V., Ungerleider, R., and Hanley, F.: Pulmonary valve atresia with intact ventricular septum. *In* Garson, A., Bricker, J., Fisher, D., and Neish, S. (Eds.): The Science and Practice of Pediatric Cardiology, 2nd ed., vol. 2. Baltimore, Williams & Wilkins, 1998, pp. 1563–1577.

Ruth-Sanchez, V.: Cardiac anomalies restricting blood flow to the left atrium. Neonatal Network, *17*(6):7–17, 1998.

Verklan, M.: Diagnostic Techniques in Cardiac Disorders. Part I. Neonatal Network, *16*(4):9–15, 1997.

Vick, G.: Defects of the atrial septum including atrioventricular septal defects. *In* Garson, A., Bricker, J., Fisher, D., and Neish, S. (Eds.): The Science and Practice of Pediatric Cardiology, 2nd ed., vol. 1. Baltimore, Williams & Wilkins, 1998, pp. 1141–1179.

Wernovsky, G., and Jonas, R.: Transposition of the great arteries. *In* Chang, A., Hanley, F., Wernovsky, G., and Wessel, D. (Eds.): Pediatric Cardiac Intensive Care. Baltimore, Williams & Wilkins, 1998, pp. 289–301.

Witt, C.: Cardiac embryology. Neonatal Network, *16*(1): 43–49, 1997.

Witt, C.: Cyanotic heart lesions with increased pulmonary blood flow. Neonatal Network, *17*(1):7–16, 1998.

Wood, M.: Acyanotic lesion with increased pulmonary blood flow. Neonatal Network, *16*(3):17–24, 1997.

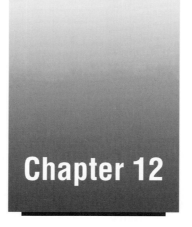

Chapter 12

Gastrointestinal Disorders

Robin L. Watson

Objectives

1. Differentiate between omphalocele and gastroschisis.
2. Describe immediate management for a newborn infant with an abdominal wall defect.
3. Identify four common associations in infants with intestinal obstruction.
4. Identify the clinical presentation of a neonate with tracheoesophageal fistula.
5. Describe x-ray findings in an infant with duodenal atresia.
6. Identify one gastrointestinal disorder that is considered a surgical emergency.
7. Identify the gastrointestinal presentation of infants with cystic fibrosis.
8. Describe the defect in Hirschsprung's disease.
9. Identify the three mechanisms involved in the pathogenesis of necrotizing enterocolitis.
10. Identify the single most important risk factor for the development of necrotizing enterocolitis.
11. Identify the two most important factors in determining prognosis in infants with short bowel syndrome.
12. Describe the clinical presentation of an infant with biliary atresia.
13. Identify the triad of anomalies occurring in prune-belly syndrome.
14. Describe the symptoms of diaphragmatic hernia.
15. Differentiate between unconjugated and conjugated bilirubin.
16. Identify limitations in the normal newborn infant that lead to physiologic jaundice.
17. Compare and contrast physiologic and nonphysiologic jaundice.
18. Describe management of an infant receiving phototherapy.
19. Define "hydrops."
20. Identify four causes of nonimmune hydrops.

Unique embryologic features of the gastrointestinal (GI) tract, such as the obliteration and recanalization of the GI tract, midgut herniation into the umbilical cord, and rotation of the intestines, make the GI tract prone to a variety of congenital anomalies. The majority of neonatal gastrointestinal disorders involve anomalies that may affect any part of the GI tract, from the mouth to the anus. Atresias, stenoses, and functional obstructions account for the vast majority of defects. As for acquired defects, necrotizing enterocolitis is the most common serious GI illness in neonates. This chapter will review the more common GI obstructions, including biliary atresia. In addition, there are a variety of multi-system disorders that have significant GI involvement, such as prune-belly syndrome, congenital diaphragmatic hernia, hyperbilirubinemia, and hydrops fetalis, all of which will be reviewed.

Gastrointestinal Embryonic Development

A. **Week 3.** Liver bud is present; mesentery is forming.

B. **Week 4.** Intestine is present; esophagus and stomach become distinct.

C. **Weeks 5 and 6.** Intestine elongates into a loop and begins to rotate.

D. **Week 7.** Duodenum is temporarily occluded; intestinal loops herniate into umbilical cord, lengthen, and rotate; and urorectal septum fuses with cloacal membrane, separating rectum from developing urinary bladder.

E. **Week 8.** Small intestine recanalizes; villi are present.

F. **Weeks 9 and 10.** Intestines begin to reenter abdominal cavity and continue counterclockwise rotation around the axis of the superior mesenteric artery.

G. **Week 12.** Muscular layers of intestine are present; active transport of amino acids begins; pancreatic islet cells appear; bile appears.

H. **Week 16.** Meconium is present; swallowing is observed.

I. **Week 24.** Ganglion cells are detected in the rectum.

J. **Week 26.** Random peristalsis begins.

K. **Weeks 34–36.** Sucking and swallowing become coordinated.

L. **Weeks 36–38.** Maturity of GI system completed.

M. **Weeks 5–40.** Intestine elongates approximately 100-fold (small intestine is six times the length of the colon).

Functions of the Gastrointestinal Tract

A. Absorption and digestion of nutrients.

B. Maintenance of fluid and electrolyte balance.

C. Protection of host from toxins and pathogens.

Assessment of the Gastrointestinal System

A. History.

1. Presence of GI disease in family.

    2. Presence of genetic syndrome. Major syndromes associated with GI defects include:
      a. Apert's syndrome.
      b. Beckwith-Wiedemann syndrome.
      c. Meckel-Gruber syndrome.
      d. Sirenomelia.
      e. Trisomy 13.
      f. Trisomy 18.
      g. Trisomy 21.
      h. VATER association (*v*ertebral defects, imperforate *a*nus, *t*racheo*e*sophageal fistula, and *r*adial and *r*enal dysplasia); VACTERL association (*v*ertebral abnormalities, *a*nal atresia, *c*ardiac abnormalities, *t*racheo*e*sophageal fistula and/or esophageal atresia, *r*enal agenesis and dysplasia, and *l*imb defects).
    3. Fetal ultrasonography.
      a. Abdomen can be seen by 10 weeks' gestation, stomach by 13 weeks.
      b. Abdomen can be assessed for intactness of abdominal wall, umbilical cord insertion, stomach as fluid-filled chamber, bowel dilation, or indication of obstruction.
      c. Maternal polyhydramnios (>2000 mL) may indicate interference with fetal swallowing or intestinal obstruction.

B. **Abdominal assessment.**

1. Inspection.
    a. Size and shape.
      (1) Should be slightly round, soft, symmetric.
      (2) Distended: intestinal obstruction, infection, enlarged abdominal organ.
      (3) Scaphoid: associated with congenital diaphragmatic hernia.
      (4) Asymmetric: mass, organomegaly, intestinal obstruction.
    b. Muscular development.
      (1) Flat, flabby: prune-belly syndrome.
      (2) Gap between rectus muscles: diastasis recti.
      (3) Externalization of abdominal contents: omphalocele, gastroschisis, bladder exstrophy.
      (4) Hernias: protrusions of peritoneum and intestine through a weakened spot in abdominal wall. Common in three areas:
        (a) Umbilical: common in African American males, Down syndrome, hypothyroidism, Hurler's syndrome, or other mucopolysaccharidosis.
        (b) Inguinal.
          (i) More common in males.
          (ii) Frequently bilateral.
          (iii) May not be evident until second or third month of life.
          (iv) Usually readily reducible.
        (c) Femoral.
          (i) More common in females.
          (ii) Located just below inguinal ligament on anterior aspect of thigh.
    c. Umbilicus.
      (1) Normally is pearly white.
      (2) Green or yellow staining suggests in utero meconium passage.
      (3) Wet, foul smelling, or red: infection.
      (4) Persistent clear drainage: patent urachus.
      (5) Ileal fluid drainage: omphalomesenteric duct.
      (6) Serous or serosanguineous drainage: granuloma.

       (7) Thick, gelatinous: large for gestational age.

       (8) Thin, small: intrauterine growth restriction.

       (9) Normally three vessels: two ventrally situated arteries, one dorsally situated vein.

       (10) Usually falls off after 10–14 days.

  d. Bowel loops.

       (1) Normally not visible.

       (2) Presence: obstruction.

  e. Movements.

       (1) Should move in synchrony with respirations.

       (2) Movements not in synchrony may represent respiratory distress, peritoneal irritation, central nervous system disease.

       (3) Peristalsis: not normally seen.

         (a) May be seen in premature infants with thin abdominal walls.

         (b) Presence: associated with hypertrophic pyloric stenosis.

  f. Veins.

       (1) Superficial veins become more prominent with abdominal distention.

       (2) Dilated veins: venous obstruction.

  g. Perineum: inspected for patency of anus and presence of fistulas.

2. Auscultation.

  a. Done before palpation (to avoid altering sounds).

  b. Bowel sounds.

       (1) Become audible within 15–30 minutes after birth (McCollum and Thigpen, 1998).

       (2) Should have a metallic clicking quality.

       (3) Hyperactive or hypoactive does not necessarily represent pathologic change.

       (4) Increased sounds.

         (a) Malrotation.

         (b) Hirschsprung's disease.

         (c) Diarrhea.

       (5) Decreased or absent sounds.

         (a) Ileus.

         (b) Starvation.

  c. Vascular sounds: bruit, similar to murmur. Caused by turbulent blood flow through the abdominal circulatory system, especially if heard despite position change of infant.

  d. Friction rub: peritoneal inflammation, splenic involvement, hepatic tumor, abscess.

3. Percussion.

  a. Provides information regarding size of organs, presence of masses, fluids, gases. Not significantly useful tool in newborn infant.

  b. Two main sounds to listen for:

       (1) Tympanic: low pitched, heard over gas-filled structures (stomach).

       (2) Dullness: high pitched, short, heard over dense or solid organs (liver, spleen).

4. Palpation.

  a. Performed to assess:

       (1) Abdominal tone.

       (2) Masses.

       (3) Pulsations.

       (4) Fluid.

       (5) Organ enlargement.

       (6) Organ position.

         (a) Liver should be 1–2 cm below right costal margin, midclavicular line.

(b) Spleen rarely palpable. Tip should not be more than 1 cm below left costal margin.

(c) Kidneys are about 4–5 cm in length. Left kidney is easier to palpate.

b. Technique: start in lower quadrants and progress to upper quadrants, using slow, gentle pressure. Place one hand directly behind palpating hand on infant's back. Start with light palpation, progress to deep palpation.

c. Hints to relax infant.

(1) Flex legs.

(2) Use warm hands.

(3) Palpate any known areas of tenderness last.

(4) Use gentle circular motion.

(5) Slowly increase depth of palpation.

C. Diagnostic tests.

1. Gastric aspirate. Measure pH of gastric contents.

2. Apt test.

a. Differentiates maternal from fetal blood.

b. Can be done on gastric fluid or stool.

c. Fluid is centrifuged in 5 mL water; 1 part 0.25 NaOH is added to supernatant. Fluid that remains pink indicates blood is from infant; fluid that turns brown indicates blood is maternal.

3. Stool examination.

a. Usually examined for color, consistency, odor, blood, mucus, pus, tissue fragments, bacteria, parasites.

b. Color may be influenced by diet, dyes, drugs, pathologic change.

(1) Green: indomethacin, meconium.

(2) Greenish black: iron, meconium.

(3) Black: iron.

(4) Pale: biliary atresia.

(5) White: antacids, barium.

c. Odor.

(1) Sweet, yeasty, or acidic in odor suggests carbohydrate malabsorption typical of osmotic diarrhea of viral enteritis.

(2) Stool with purulent odor suggests colitis.

d. pH less than 5.0 in infants suggests carbohydrate malabsorption.

e. Guiaic.

(1) Detects occult blood.

(2) Based on the oxidation of guiaic by hydrogen peroxide in the Hemoccult solution, resulting in an alkaline compound, which turns the test paper blue.

(3) False-positive results: indomethacin, salicylates, steroids.

(4) False-negative results: high doses of vitamin C.

f. Reducing substances. Use of reagent tablets (Clinitest) for evaluation of reducing substances in any fluid other than urine is not supported or approved by the manufacturer.

4. pH probe test: 24-hour pH probe study to diagnose GI reflux.

5. Radiologic studies.

a. X-ray examination (see Chapter 29 for further information).

(1) Bowel gas pattern.

(a) At birth, gut is fluid filled.

(b) Within 30 minutes, gas should be in stomach.

(c) By 3–4 hours, gas should be in small intestine.

(d) By 6–8 hours, gas should be in entire intestine.

(2) Absence of gas below pylorus: possible indication of obstruction.

b. Barium swallow: done to assess structure and function of esophagus, hypertrophic pyloric stenosis, malrotation.

  c. Barium enema: may be used to detect presence of malrotation, Hirsch-sprung's disease, meconium ileus, and meconium plug syndrome. May be therapeutic in meconium ileus and meconium plug syndrome.
6. Ultrasonography: may be used to diagnose suspected cases of pyloric stenosis, duplications, gastroesophageal reflux, or biliary atresia.

Abdominal Wall Defects

A. **Omphalocele.**

1. Definition: herniation of abdominal viscera into umbilical cord, usually covered by a peritoneal sac and with umbilical arteries and veins inserting into apex of defect (Fig. 12–1).
2. Etiology: uncertain, but condition may be caused by incomplete closure of anterior abdominal wall or incomplete return of bowel into abdomen.
3. Incidence: 1:5000 to 1:6000 live births (McCollum and Thigpen, 1998).
4. Associated conditions: 30–50% will have associated anomalies (Rescorla, 1993).
   a. Prematurity (30%); small for gestational age (19%) (McCollum and Thigpen, 1998).
   b. Cardiac defects (19–25%) (Rescorla, 1993).
   c. Intestinal malrotation and/or atresia.
   d. Pentalogy of Cantrell (omphalocele, diaphragmatic hernia, sternal cleft, pericardial defect, intracardiac defect).
   e. Neurologic anomalies.
   f. Genitourinary anomalies.
   g. Skeletal anomalies.
   h. Chromosomal anomalies (45–55%) (Berseth, 1998d).
   i. Beckwith-Wiedemann syndrome.
5. Diagnosis.
   a. Prenatal ultrasonography.
   b. Inspection at birth.

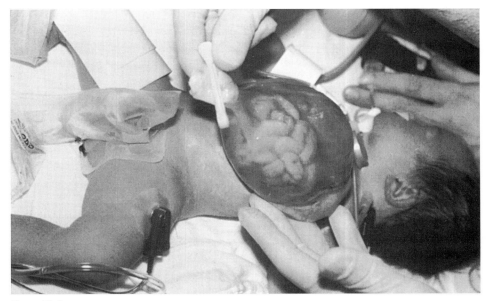

Figure 12–1
Omphalocele.

(1) Omphaloceles differ in size; large defects may include stomach, liver, and spleen, as well as intestines.

(2) Defect can be small; therefore any umbilical cord that is unusually fat should be inspected carefully before clamping to be certain it is not a very small omphalocele.

(3) Sac may rupture before or at time of delivery, exposing the viscera to amniotic fluid.

6. Prognosis.
   a. Mortality rate is related to severity of other defects.
   b. Mortality rate with associated heart disease is 80% but only 30% in absence of heart disease (Berseth, 1998d).

B. **Gastroschisis.**

1. Definition: herniation of abdominal contents through an abdominal wall defect, usually to right of umbilicus. See Table 12–1 for a comparison of omphalocele and gastroschisis.

2. Etiology: unclear; theories include a failure of closure of the lateral fold of the abdominal wall, and an intrauterine vascular accident involving the omphalomesenteric artery, with subsequent disruption of the umbilical ring causing herniation of abdominal contents (Hoyme, Higginbottom and Jones, 1981; Moore and Persaud, 1993).

3. Incidence: occurs two or three times more frequently than omphalocele (Brandt, 1998).

4. Diagnosis.
   a. Prenatal ultrasonography.
   b. Inspection at birth.
      (1) No sac covers the gastroschisis.
      (2) Usually placed to right of umbilicus (Fig. 12–2).
      (3) Gastroschisis usually includes small and large intestines and rarely the liver.
      (4) Intestine is usually thickened, edematous, and inflamed because it has been exposed to amniotic fluid.
      (5) Fascial defect is smaller than the omphalocele.
      (6) Umbilical cord is intact.

5. Associated conditions.
   a. Forty percent of infants are either premature or small for gestational age.
   b. Intestinal malrotation and atresia.
   c. Other anomalies are uncommon.

6. Prognosis. Mortality rate ranges from 10–30% (Berseth, 1998d). Malabsorption is a common prolonged problem postoperatively.

Table 12–1
COMPARISON OF OMPHALOCELE AND GASTROSCHISIS

	Omphalocele	Gastroschisis
Incidence	1:5000 to 1:6000	1:30,000 to 1:50,000
Covering	Present, may be ruptured	None
Site	Umbilical	Paraumbilical, usually to the right
Fascial defect	Small or large	Small
Herniated organs	Intestines; stomach, liver, spleen sometimes	Intestines; rarely liver
Appearance of herniated bowel	Normal, unless sac is ruptured	Often edematous, matted
Associated anomalies	45–55%	10–15%
IUGR	Less common	Common

IUGR, Intrauterine growth restriction.

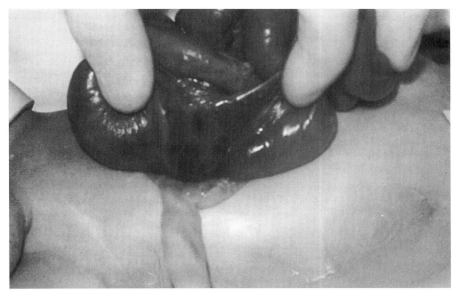

Figure 12–2
Gastroschisis.

C. **Care of the neonate with an abdominal wall defect (omphalocele and gastroschisis)**

1. At the time of delivery, cover the exposed bowel with warm, moist dressings. (Sterile normal saline solution is recommended. In addition, cover the dressing in plastic to prevent evaporated heat loss.) If sterile bowel bag is available, infant is placed in bag from the feet to the axilla. Infants with a ruptured omphalocele or gastroschisis are at higher risk of having fluid, electrolyte, and temperature loss because of exposed bowel.
2. To prevent intestinal vascular compromise from torqued abdominal contents, either position the infant on his or her side or support the defect with a small roll. Handling should be kept to a minimum and done only with sterile gloves.
3. Place infant on a regimen of nothing by mouth (NPO) and insert an orogastric tube. Place orogastric tube on intermittent low suction for gastric decompression. Bowel distended with air can restrict normal blood flow and further compromise the bowel.
4. Begin IV fluid-and-electrolyte therapy and antibiotic therapy as soon as possible. IV fluids are usually increased to approximately 150 mL/kg per day because of increased fluid loss through exposed bowel.
   a. When a sac covers the defect, fluid losses are not as great.
   b. Ideally, IV infusions should not be started in the lower extremities, because postoperative venous stasis results from increased abdominal pressure.
5. Blood studies should be performed: hematocrit, electrolyte values, blood type and cross-match, pH and blood gas values, and clotting times.
6. Assess the infant carefully for associated anomalies, syndromes, or deformations.
7. Most newborn infants with abdominal wall defects require surgical repair. The types of repair include the following:
   a. Primary repair. All intestine is returned to the abdominal cavity, and the fascia and skin are closed. The infant may require prolonged respiratory support because of increased intra-abdominal pressure.

b. **Staged reduction.** Not all the organs are returned to the abdominal cavity during the first surgery; the organs remaining outside the cavity are covered by a pliable plastic (Silastic) sac (silo). The sac is either sutured to the edge of the defect or secured underneath the fascia, allowing gradual reduction of the intestines on a daily basis.

(1) Reduction minimizes the stress on the respiratory and vascular systems by allowing these systems to adjust slowly to the increased pressure of the organs as they are slowly returned to the abdominal cavity.

(2) Reduction can usually be accomplished during a period of 10 days, after which infection becomes a major consideration.

(3) The abdominal wall is closed after the reduction is completed.

c. **Skin flap closure.** Only the skin is pulled over the exposed organs. This method is not a long-term solution and is used when the fascia cannot be initially repaired.

d. **Nonsurgical repair.** The defect is painted with an escharotic agent such as merbromin solution (Mercurochrome) and alcohol and allowed to air dry and epithelialize.

(1) This uncommon procedure is used only if the defect is large, if the infant cannot tolerate surgery, or if the reduction fails.

(2) Systemic side effects are associated with most of the escharotic agents. The health care team should be aware of such effects and assess the infant for them.

8. **Postoperative care.**

a. Pain management is discussed in Chapter 20.

b. Dressing changes are performed with aseptic technique; IV antibiotic therapy is continued postoperatively.

c. Oxygen saturation, urine output, and blood pressure are monitored continuously. Other parameters to watch closely include fluid-and-electrolyte balance, pH, and clotting times.

d. Observe the following for complications: sepsis, intestinal obstruction, respiratory distress, skin necrosis over repaired defect, and venous stasis.

e. When staged reduction is employed, the silo must be suspended from above the infant (usually from the top of incubator or radiant warmer), with a rolled gauze such as Kerlix (manufactured by Kendall) to keep silo contents perpendicular to the infant.

f. Infant will require gastric suction after surgery until gastric output is minimal. Parenteral fluids should be replaced with physiologic IV solutions that account for gastric losses (i.e., suctioned gastric contents should be measured every 4 hours and parenteral fluids increased an equal amount).

g. Feeding is begun very slowly when gastric output is minimal and bowel tones are active.

(1) Low osmolality feeding, such as half-strength formula, breast milk, or mineral-electrolyte solution (Pedialyte) is usually preferred. Feedings are frequently stopped and started for a time.

(2) Most infants will be maintained on hyperalimentation for a while, until feeding is established.

Obstructions of the Gastrointestinal Tract

A. **General considerations.**

1. Obstructions may be either mechanical (in which there is a specific point of obstruction) or functional (usually related to motility) in nature and can be found anywhere from the esophagus to the anus.

2. Obstruction occurs because of an intrinsic or extrinsic blockage (Table 12–2).

Table 12–2
CAUSES OF INTESTINAL OBSTRUCTION IN THE NEWBORN INFANT

Mechanical		Functional
Congenital	*Acquired*	
Intrinsic	Necrotizing enterocolitis	Hirschsprung disease
Atresias	Intussusception	Meconium plug syndrome
Stenoses	Peritoneal adhesions	Ileus
Meconium ileus		Peritonitis
Anorectal malformations		
Enteric duplications		
Extrinsic		Intestinal pseudoobstruction syndrome
Volvulus		
Peritoneal bands		
Annular pancreas		
Cysts and tumors		
Incarcerated hernias		

From Berseth, C.L.: Disorders of the intestines and pancreas. *In* Taeusch, W.H., and Ballard, R.A. (Eds.): Avery's Diseases of the Newborn, 7th ed. Philadelphia, W.B. Saunders Company, 1998c, p. 919.

3. Common associations in infants with intestinal obstruction.
    a. History of polyhydramnios.
        (1) Occurs more often in proximal obstructions.
        (2) Fifteen to twenty percent of polyhydramnios is associated with fetal GI obstructions.
    b. Failure to pass meconium within 24–48 hours. Ninety-four percent of term infants pass meconium by 24 hours, and 99.8% pass meconium by 48 hours (Berseth, 1998a).
    c. Abdominal distention: occurs more often in distal obstructions and tracheoesophageal fistula.
    d. Bilious vomiting: occurs when obstruction is distal to the ampulla of Vater, located in the duodenum.
4. General preoperative management.
    a. Nothing by mouth (NPO).
    b. Gastric decompression.
    c. IV therapy and replacement of fluid losses.
    d. Antibiotics.

B. **Esophageal atresia (EA) and tracheoesophageal fistula (TEF).**

1. Definitions: EA, an interruption in the esophagus; TEF, an abnormal communication between the esophagus and trachea. EA and TEF may occur as separate defects or, more commonly, in association with each other.
2. Incidence: approximately 1:4000 live births (Ross, 1994).
3. Associated anomalies: 50–70% of affected infants. The most common associated anomalies include the following (Rowe et al., 1995):
    a. Cardiac defects (30%): primarily atrial septal defects and ventricular septal defects.
    b. GI anomalies (12%): pyloric stenosis, duodenal obstruction, and imperforate anus.
    c. Esophageal atresia is a frequent component of the VATER or VACTERL association (15%).
4. Etiology: incomplete elongation and separation of esophagus and trachea during fourth week of gestation.
5. Types of TEFs include the following (Fig. 12–3) (Rowe et al., 1995):
    a. Blind proximal pouch with distal tracheoesophageal fistula (most common; 85% of cases).

Esophageal atresia with tracheoesophageal fistula | Isolated esophageal atresia | H-type tracheoesophageal fistula | Esophageal atresia with upper pouch fistula | Esophageal atresia with fistula to proximal pouch

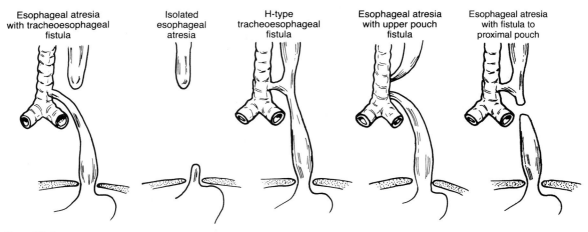

Figure 12–3
Esophageal malformations.

    b. Isolated esophageal atresia without tracheoesophageal fistula (5–7% of cases).

    c. Isolated tracheoesophageal fistula without esophageal atresia (H type of TEF) (2–6% of cases).

    d. Esophageal atresia with fistula between upper pouch and trachea (rare).

    e. Esophageal atresia with fistulas between upper pouch and lower pouches and trachea (rare).

6. Clinical presentation.

    a. Clinical presentation is dependent on the type of tracheoesophageal anomaly.

    b. Accumulation of oral secretions in mouth, drooling.

    c. Inability to pass gastric tube.

    d. Coughing, choking, or cyanosis with feedings.

    e. Abdominal distention.

    f. Recurrent pneumonia (more common in infants with isolated TEF without EA).

7. Diagnosis.

    a. History of polyhydramnios is present.

    b. Gastric tube will stop in the esophageal pouch (will most likely not pass beyond 10 cm).

    c. On x-ray film the gastric tube appears coiled in the upper esophageal pouch. In addition, air in the GI tract indicates the presence of a TEF. A gasless abdomen indicates an isolated EA (refer to Chapter 29).

    d. Use of contrast studies is not recommend because of the risk of aspiration and subsequent chemical pneumonitis.

8. Preoperative care.

    a. See section A, "General Considerations," above.

    b. The head of the bed should be in a 30- to 45-degree upright position to avoid reflux and aspiration of gastric secretions.

    c. A sump catheter on low constant suction should be left in the upper pouch to suction oral secretions.

        (1) The holes in the Replogle tube (Sherwood Medical) are down close to the end of the tube, making this the desired sump tube for use in TEF.

        (2) Assess and maintain patency of the sump tube.

    d. Use comfort measures to prevent crying, which leads to increased swallowed air, abdominal distention, and increased risk of reflux.

9. Surgical repair.

a. Primary repair is ligation of the TEF and anastomosis of the proximal and distal portions of the esophagus.

b. Staged repair is used with infants who are very premature, who have pneumonia or other coexisting life-threatening problems, or in whom the gap between the two esophageal pouches is great.

   (1) Ligation of TEF is performed at initial surgery.

   (2) Gastrostomy tube is placed for feeding after the first surgery.

   (3) Suction to proximal pouch is continued until second surgery.

   (4) Final surgery is usually delayed for 6–12 months in infants with a long gap between pouches. To allow a portal of exit for swallowed saliva, the surgeon creates a spit fistula at the initial procedure, exteriorizing the proximal esophageal pouch to the neck.

c. When end-to-end anastomosis is impossible because the gap between the esophageal pouches is too great, either some other structure must be used to connect the pouches or the upper pouch must undergo an elongation procedure (rarely successful).

10. Postoperative care.

    a. Provide pain management (see Chapter 20).

    b. Maintain elevation of head of bed.

    c. Intubation with low-pressure ventilation protects the tracheal suture line.

    d. Endotracheal tube suctioning should be performed only the length of the endotracheal tube to avoid damage to the tracheal suture line.

    e. Frequent, careful suctioning of the posterior portion of the pharynx with a measured catheter should be performed.

    f. Hyperalimentation and antibiotics are commonly used postoperatively.

    g. There is usually a thoracic drain in place postoperatively; note the color, consistency, and amounts of fluid drainage. Saliva indicates an esophageal leak.

    h. A gastrostomy tube may be placed for gastric decompression and later feedings.

    i. Because of the potential for perforating or damaging the repair, a gastric tube should not be passed.

    j. Gastrostomy feedings may be started 2 days postoperatively. Oral feedings are usually started 7–10 days postoperatively. Contrast esophagram is frequently obtained before oral feedings to confirm that there are no leaks at the esophageal anastomosis.

11. Postoperative complications.

    a. Leaking at site of anastomosis (5–15%), which may lead to sepsis and thoracic empyema (Rowe et al., 1995).

    b. Stricture at site of anastomosis (10–20%). Stricture should be suspected if feeding difficulties exist after the third postoperative week (Berseth, 1998b).

    c. Recurrent fistula, usually resulting from a leak.

    d. Pneumonia.

    e. Sepsis.

    f. Dysmotility of lower esophageal segment.

    g. Unilateral diaphragmatic paralysis.

    h. Tracheomalacia (up to 25%). This complication is occasionally severe enough to require a tracheostomy.

    i. Gastroesophageal reflux is common.

12. Prognosis: survival rate excellent for healthy term infants. Prognosis is dependent on birth weight, presence of other congenital anomalies, especially cardiac, and preoperative condition.

C. Hypertrophic pyloric stenosis.

1. Definition: hypertrophy of the pyloric musculature.

2. Incidence: 1:500 births (Ross, 1994).
   a. Males more likely to be affected than females (4:1 ratio).
   b. More common in white infants.
   c. First born more often affected; at highest risk is the first-born male of an affected mother.
3. Etiology: exact cause unknown. Hereditary component exists because incidence is increased if parent has history of pyloric stenosis.
4. Symptoms usually occur at 3-4 weeks of age but may present up to 5 months after birth. For this reason, pyloric stenosis is not considered a congenital defect.
5. Clinical presentation.
   a. Nonbilious vomiting that becomes projectile with time.
   b. Dehydration.
   c. Hypochloremic and hypokalemic alkalosis.
   d. Visible peristaltic waves in epigastrium.
   e. Palpable pyloric "olive."
   f. Failure to thrive.
6. Diagnosis.
   a. Presence of signs and symptoms.
   b. Confirmation by ultrasonography.
   c. Upper GI tract contrast study.
7. Preoperative care: mainly concerned with correcting the hypokalemia, hypochloremia, and dehydration.
8. Surgical repair is a pyloromyotomy.
9. Postoperative care.
   a. Pain management (see Chapter 20).
   b. Routine wound care.
   c. NPO regimen for 6–8 hours after surgery.
   d. Prevention of perforation of the mucosa at the pyloromyotomy site by avoiding placement of a gastric tube postoperatively.
10. Prognosis: excellent. Generally, complete recovery with no residual effects; some continued vomiting possible in first few days after surgery, followed by quick resolution.

D. Duodenal atresia.

1. Definition: congenital obstruction of the duodenum. The atresia usually occurs distal to the ampulla of Vater.
2. Other types of duodenal obstruction.
   a. Annular pancreas.
   b. Preduodenal portal vein.
   c. Peritoneal (Ladd's) band due to intestinal malrotation.
3. Incidence: approximately 1:10,000 live births (Ross, 1994). Females are more commonly affected than males.
4. Etiology: unknown, but cause may be from a failure of recanalization of the duodenum during weeks 8–10 of fetal life.
5. Associated conditions (other anomalies found in 60–70% of all cases) (McCollum and Thigpen, 1998).
   a. Down syndrome.
   b. Prematurity.
   c. Intestinal malrotation.
   d. Congenital heart disease.
   e. Tracheoesophageal abnormalities.
   f. Anorectal lesions.
6. Clinical presentation.
   a. Bilious vomiting (85%). Nonbilious vomiting does not rule out duodenal atresia or obstruction.

    b. Abdominal distention.

    c. Possible passage of meconium in first 24 hours of life. Bowel movements then cease.

    d. Jaundice.

7. Diagnosis.

    a. History of polyhydramnios.

    b. Prenatal diagnosis by ultrasonography.

    c. X-ray film showing "double bubble" pattern (see Chapter 29).

8. Preoperative care. See section A, "General Considerations," above.

9. Surgery is performed to remove the atretic portions and reanastomose the remaining ends.

10. Postoperative care.

    a. Pain management (see Chapter 20).

    b. Continue total parenteral nutrition (TPN) and antibiotics.

    c. NPO regimen for 3–10 days; delayed gastric emptying is common.

    d. Most infants will have a gastrostomy tube in place postoperatively.

11. Prognosis: excellent. Long-term outcome is primarily dependent on associated anomalies and malformations.

E. **Jejunal or ileal atresia.**

1. Incidence: 1:5000 live births (Rowe et al., 1995). Males and females are equally affected; 55% of intestinal atresias occur in the jejunum or ileum (Berseth, 1998c).

2. Etiology: unknown, but primary cause is believed to result from a mesenteric vascular insult to the small bowel in fetal life.

3. Associated conditions (Rowe, 1995):

    a. Cystic fibrosis (10–12%).

    b. Malrotation (10%).

4. Five types of jejunal or ileal atresia (Fig. 12–4).

    a. Type I: bowel intact, but lumen is obstructed by a septum of tissue (20%).

    b. Type II: blind ends of bowel joined by a fibrous cord; mesentery is intact (30–35%).

    c. Type IIIa: blind ends separated by V-shaped mesenteric defect; most common type (35–40%).

    d. Type IIIb ("apple peel" or "Christmas tree"): blind ends separated by V-shaped mesenteric defect; the proximal intestine coils around a single distal ileal vessel (<1%). This form, although the rarest, is usually familial and carries the highest mortality rate (54%).

    e. Type IV: Bowel has multiple atresias separated by V-shaped mesenteric defects (5–10%).

5. Clinical presentation.

    a. Bilious vomiting.

    b. Abdominal distention that usually presents 12–24 hours after birth. The lower the obstruction, the greater the abdominal distention.

    c. Failure to pass meconium.

    d. Jaundice.

6. Diagnosis.

    a. Presence of symptoms.

    b. History of polyhydramnios.

    c. X-ray films showing dilated loops of bowel and multiple air-fluid levels (refer to Chapter 29).

    d. Barium-enema x-ray film shows a microcolon.

7. Preoperative care: see section A, "General Considerations," above.

8. Surgery.

    a. Primary anastomosis is performed if the proximal and distal ends of bowel are comparable in size.

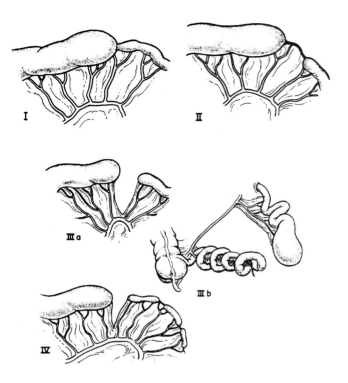

Figure 12–4
Types of jejunal atresia. Type I—mucosal atresia with intact muscularis. Type II—atretic ends are separated by a fibrous band. Type IIIa—atretic ends are separated by a V-shaped gap defect. Type IIIb—apple peel deformity of the distal atretic segment with retrograde blood supply from the ileocolic or right colic artery. Type IV—multiple atresias (string-of-sausage effect). (From Rowe, M.I., O'Neill, J.A., Grosfeld, J.L., et al.: Essentials of Pediatric Surgery. St. Louis, Mosby, 1995, p. 511.)

    b. Stomas are created if there is a large discrepancy in size (proximal is generally larger than distal). After a stoma is healed, irrigation at the small distal stoma will usually help to dilate it so that it can be surgically anastomosed to the proximal bowel.

9. Postoperative care.
    a. Pain management (see Chapter 20).
    b. Continue NPO regimen until normal bowel function is restored (usually 3–7 days).
    c. Continue TPN and antibiotic therapy.
10. Complications.
    a. Ileus.
    b. Peritonitis.
11. Prognosis: excellent, with return to normal bowel function usually within 10 days.

E. Malrotation.

1. Definition: an assortment of intestinal anomalies of rotation and fixation.
2. Etiology: exact cause unknown. Occurs when the intestines do not rotate and/or the mesentery does not fixate appropriately during weeks 6–10 of gestation. Intestines may twist on themselves (midgut volvulus), occluding the intestinal lumen, or around the superior mesenteric artery, occluding intestinal blood supply. Ischemia and bowel necrosis then results.
3. Incidence: unknown; more males affected than females.
4. Associated anomalies.
    a. Intestinal atresia.
    b. Diaphragmatic hernia.
    c. Duodenal obstruction due to peritoneal (Ladd's) bands encircling the duodenum.

   d. Omphalocele.
   e. Gastroschisis.
5. Clinical presentation of acute cases.
   a. Bilious vomiting, suggestive of malrotation with volvulus formation; needs immediate confirmation.
   b. Abdominal distention.
   c. Rectal bleeding.
   d. Abdominal pain.
   e. Signs of shock and sepsis.
6. Clinical presentation of "less acute cases."
   a. Failure to thrive.
   b. Intermittent bilious vomiting.
   c. Abdominal tenderness.
7. Diagnosis.
   a. Presence of symptoms.
   b. X-ray film showing evidence of duodenal obstruction and scanty gas distributed throughout remainder of bowel. An airless abdomen is an ominous sign.
   c. Contrast upper GI tract x-ray film showing distended stomach and a beaklike narrowing at the pylorus; gastric mucosa folds are also seen on the x-ray film.
8. Preoperative care.
   a. See section A, "General Considerations," above.
   b. Malrotation with volvulus is considered a surgical emergency; the primary goal of preoperative care is to get the infant to the operating room as fast as possible to prevent intestinal infarction.
9. Surgical repair. Surgery is aimed at release of strangulation of the bowel.
   a. With midgut volvulus, the intestines usually rotate clockwise, so they are untwisted in a counterclockwise fashion.
   b. If present, peritoneal (Ladd's) bands are divided, relieving duodenal obstruction; the small bowel is placed on right side of abdomen, and colon is placed on left side.
   c. Appendectomy is performed to eliminate appendicitis as a differential diagnosis in the future when the child has abdominal pain.
   d. Necrotic bowel may be resected. If there is no intestinal perforation, some surgeons may wait and perform a second surgery 24–36 hours after the first to resect the bowel (Kays, 1996).
   e. If the length of viable bowel is less than 10–15 cm, most surgeons will close the abdomen without resecting the bowel (Rescorla, 1993).
10. Postoperative care.
    a. Pain management (see Chapter 20).
    b. IV therapy and antibiotics, parenteral nutrition.
    c. Routine wound and stoma care.
    d. The infant should remain on NPO regimen until the return of bowel function (usually in 3–7 days).
11. Prognosis: operative mortality rate is less than 15% (Berseth, 1998c). Morbidity and prognosis depend on the amount of bowel resected. Major postoperative complication is short bowel syndrome.

G. **Meconium ileus.**

1. Definition: mechanical obstruction of the distal ileum due to intraluminal accumulation of thick, inspissated meconium. Although meconium ileus has been reported in a few patients without cystic fibrosis, it is considered a condition unique to cystic fibrosis (Wesson and Haddock, 1996).
2. Incidence. Cystic fibrosis occurs in 1:2000 live births of white infants; 10–15% of children with cystic fibrosis have meconium ileus (Ross, 1994).

3. Etiology: exact cause unknown. Two implicating factors are:
   a. Hyposecretion of pancreatic enzymes, which may play a part in some but not all meconium ileus. As a result, meconium contains an abnormal amount of proteins and glycoproteins, making the meconium thick and viscid.
   b. Abnormal viscid secretions from the mucous glands of the small intestine.
4. Two types of meconium ileus.
   a. Simple meconium ileus.
      (1) Distal segment of small bowel is obstructed with thick, tarlike tenacious meconium, and proximal segment of small bowel is dilated.
      (2) Clinical presentation is usually within 48 hours.
   b. Complicated meconium ileus.
      (1) This type of meconium ileus is complicated because of its association with the following:
         (a) Volvulus.
         (b) Intestinal necrosis and perforation.
         (c) Meconium peritonitis or pseudocyst formation.
      (2) Clinical presentation is usually within 24 hours.
5. Clinical presentation.
   a. Abdominal distention at birth.
   b. Bilious vomiting.
   c. Failure to pass meconium within 12–24 hours.
   d. Palpable, rubbery loops of bowel. Small grapelike pellets of meconium may be palpated distally.
   e. Complicated form has earlier presentation, and these infants appear sicker, with signs of sepsis and respiratory distress.
6. Diagnosis.
   a. Distended bowel loops without air-fluid levels.
   b. X-ray film showing "soap bubble" appearance of distal intestine because of meconium.
   c. Scattered calcifications due to intrauterine intestinal perforations possible in complicated form.
   d. Possible microcolon on contrast radiograph.
   e. Family history of cystic fibrosis: highly suggestive of meconium ileus.
   f. Definitive diagnosis based on diagnosis of cystic fibrosis by a sweat chloride test (sodium and chloride concentrations >60 mEq/L).
7. Nonsurgical management (for simple type only).
   a. A hypertonic contrast enema (Gastrografin or Hypaque) procedure may be successful in dislodging the meconium obstruction and allowing for normal intestinal activity in 25–60% of patients. Usually meconium pellets are passed quickly, followed by liquid meconium for 24 hours after the procedure. A second enema may be required.
   b. Management after enema includes:
      (1) Fluids at one and one-half times maintenance.
      (2) Careful monitoring of urine output, urine specific gravity or osmolality, blood urea nitrogen, creatinine, and serum osmolality.
      (3) Broad-spectrum antibiotics.
      (4) Continued gastric decompression.
   c. Complications of nonsurgical management include the following:
      (1) Hypovolemic shock secondary to rapid fluid shift resulting from hypertonic solution used for enema.
      (2) Intestinal perforation.
8. Preoperative care. See section A, "General Considerations," above.
9. Surgical management.
   a. Used with complicated meconium ileus and when nonsurgical intervention has failed.

(1) In uncomplicated cases, surgeons will evacuate meconium from the bowel either manually or through an enterotomy.

(2) In extreme cases in which bowel necrosis has occurred, all compromised intestine is resected and the proximal and/or distal segment is exteriorized.

(3) A T-tube may be inserted into the distal segment for postoperative irrigation.

b. Postoperative care.

(1) Pain management (see Chapter 20).

(2) Continuation of NPO regimen and gastric decompression until normal bowel function is restored (approximately 3–7 days).

(3) Antibiotics.

(4) Irrigation of distal stoma or T-tube with a radiopaque agent (Gastrografin) or acetylcysteine around postoperative day 3.

10. Postoperative complications.

a. Volvulus.

b. Gangrene.

c. Perforation.

11. Prognosis: operative mortality rate <20%. Morbidity is primarily related to signs and symptoms of cystic fibrosis.

H. **Meconium plug syndrome.**

1. Definition: a mechanical obstruction, usually of the distal segment of the colon and the rectum, that occurs from thick, inspissated meconium in the absence of an abnormality of ganglion cells or enzymatic deficiency.

2. Etiology: unclear; results from diminished colonic motility and meconium clearance.

3. Risk factors.

a. Maternal diabetes, probably due to the increased fetal glycogen production leading to decreased bowel motility.

b. Neonatal hypermagnesemia: usually occurs after mother has been treated with magnesium sulfate for pregnancy-induced hypertension; the decreased bowel motility is secondary to myoneural depression.

c. Prematurity.

d. Hypotonia in infant with CNS disease.

e. Sepsis.

4. Clinical presentation: usually within first 3 days of life.

a. Multiple dilated loops of bowel on physical examination.

b. Bilious vomiting.

c. Abdominal distention.

d. Failure to pass meconium.

5. Diagnosis.

a. Presence of symptoms.

b. X-ray film showing multiple distended loops of bowel (refer to Chapter 29).

c. Water-soluble contrast enema resulting in intraluminal plug. Such an enema will commonly dislodge the plug, and no further interventions will be required.

6. Differential diagnosis. A biopsy for Hirschsprung's disease and a sweat test for cystic fibrosis will rule out these disorders.

I. **Hirschsprung's disease.**

1. Definition: congenital absence of ganglionic cells in the submucosal and myenteric plexuses of the colon.

a. Length of bowel involvement is dependent on the time during which migration of neuroblasts ceased.

   b. Eighty percent of Hirschsprung's disease cases involve only the rectosig-moid region (Ross, 1994).
   c. Three percent of Hirschsprung's disease cases involve the entire colon (Ross, 1994).
2. Incidence: 1:5000 live births. Males are affected four times more often than females (Ross, 1994).
3. Etiology: thought to be related to interrupted migration of ganglionic cell precursors before week 12 of gestation. The lack of intestinal ganglion cells prevents the inhibitory relaxation normally regulated by parasympathetic nerves. The affected segment is unable to relax, and functional obstruction ensues. Familial occurrences may exist, especially in long-segment Hirschsprung's disease.
4. Associated anomalies: not common but may include colonic atresia or imperforate anus; 3–10% of children with Down syndrome have Hirschsprung's disease.
5. Clinical presentation.
   a. Early symptom is failure to pass meconium within 24–48 hours after birth.
   b. Bilious vomiting occurs.
   c. Late symptom is the inability to stool normally. Abnormal stooling since birth is a common symptom of Hirschsprung's disease. As the obstruction continues, enterocolitis may develop, with fever, abdominal distention, and diarrhea. The infant usually has symptoms in the first several weeks and then has diarrhea, abdominal distention, and/or vomiting. In advanced cases, urinary obstruction may occur secondary to mechanical compression of the ureters and bladder.
6. The most common complication is acute enterocolitis caused by:
   a. Bowel wall distention and ischemia.
   b. Bacterial invasion leading to sepsis.
7. Diagnosis.
   a. Suggested by a barium enema that shows a nondistensible rectal ampulla, with a dilated bowel above.
   b. Retained barium in the rectum for more than 24 hours after the procedure is suggestive of Hirschsprung's disease.
   c. Anal manometry is useful in very-short-segment agangliosis or in patients who have normal findings on contrast studies.
   d. Confirmed by rectal biopsy showing the absence of ganglion cells.
   e. Increased acetylcholinesterase content in rectal tissue is identified by histochemical staining.
   f. Only a small percentage of cases (15%) are diagnosed in the neonatal period (Kirschner, 1996).
8. Preoperative care: see section A, "General Considerations," above.
9. Treatment is surgery. Although there is growing experience with a complete pull-through repair in the neonatal period, a staged repair is most common. Initially, a colostomy is created. At 6 months to 1 year of age, a pull-through procedure is performed with an end-to-end anastomosis at the anus.
10. Postoperative care.
   a. Pain management (see Chapter 20).
   b. Routine ostomy care.
   c. NPO regimen and parenteral nutrition until oral feedings can be begun.
   d. Close observation for shock and recurrent enterocolitis.
11. Prognosis: excellent. Mortality rate increases when diagnosis is delayed and enterocolitis occurs. Enterocolitis is the leading cause of death. Approximately 10% of patients will have subsequent elimination problems such as constipation, staining, and delayed toilet training.

J. Imperforate anus.

1. Definition: a broad spectrum of anorectal malformations characterized by a stenotic or atretic anal canal. A fistula between the rectum and the perineum, vagina in females or urethra in males, may also occur.
2. Incidence: 1:5000 live births (Ross, 1994).
3. Etiology: failure of differentiation of the urogenital sinus and cloaca during embryologic development.
4. Common associations: anomalies, including vertebral, genitourinary, cardiovascular, and gastrointestinal malformations, in 20–75% of infants (McCollum and Thigpen, 1998).
5. Classification: high or low, depending on level of defect (i.e., above or below a line drawn from the symphysis pubis to the coccyx [pubococcygeal line]). Level of defect significantly influences outcome regarding fecal continence (Fig. 12–5).
   a. High imperforate anus.
      (1) More common and generally more complex.
      (2) Occurs more frequently in males.
      (3) Rectourinary and rectovaginal fistulas are common associations.
      (4) High imperforate anus with sacral anomaly can be associated with lack of innervation of the bowel and/or bladder, causing incontinence.
      (5) Diagnosis is made by physical inspection, x-ray film, contrast x-ray film, and ultrasonography. An inverted lateral radiograph may be obtained to determine the level of the air-filled rectal pouch in relation to the pubococcygeal line.
      (6) Surgical intervention is always necessary, with the procedure dependent on the level of the anorectal pouch. High and intermediate pouches are treated with a colostomy and a definitive pull-through procedure performed after the infant is approximately 8 months of age and weighs 18 pounds.
   b. Low imperforate anus.
      (1) Male/female ratio closer to 1:1.
      (2) Perineal fistula is a common association.
      (3) Diagnosis is made by physical inspection, x-ray and contrast x-ray examination, and ultrasonography. An infant with anal stenosis or

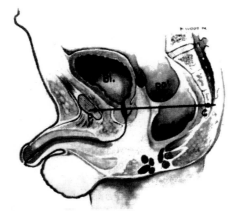

Figure 12–5
Imperforate anus. Rectal pouch 1 *(RP¹)* sits above the pubococcygeal line *(PC)* and would be classified as a "high type" anomaly. Rectal pouch 2 *(RP²)* sits below the PC line and represents a "low type" anomaly. The level of the rectal pouch is crucial in decisions of management. *Bl,* Bladder. (From Ross, A: Intestinal obstruction in the newborn. Reproduced by permission of *Pediatrics in Review,* 15:338–347, 1994, p. 346.)

imperforate anal membrane may have a normal-appearing rectum, with the condition detected only after the absence of stooling is noted.

    (4) Surgical intervention is always necessary, with the procedure dependent on the level of the anorectal pouch. A low pouch can usually be repaired by anoplasty with good results.

6. Infants with a fistula are at risk for hyperchloremic acidosis as a result of colonic absorption of urine.
7. Preoperative care: see section A, "General Considerations," above.
8. Postoperative care.
   a. Pain management (see Chapter 20).
   b. NPO regimen and gastric decompression continued until normal bowel function is restored.
   c. Routine ostomy care if applicable.
9. Postoperative complications: depend on the level of the defect, whether there is innervation of the bowel, and what type of repair is performed.
10. Prognosis: excellent with low imperforate anus; however, with high imperforate anus, 50% or more of these children will have bowel incontinence and may require additional surgery.

K. **Necrotizing enterocolitis (NEC).**

1. Definition: an acquired disease that affects the GI system, particularly that of premature infants. It is characterized by areas of necrotic bowel, most commonly in the terminal ileum but may affect both small and large intestine.
2. Incidence: 1–10% of all admissions to the NICU; approximately 90% of cases occur in preterm infants (Vanderhoof, Zach, and Adrian, 1994). Occurs sporadically and in clusters.
3. Single most important risk factor: prematurity. The following make preterm infants highly susceptible (Neu, 1996):
   a. Decreased immunologic factors in the intestinal tract.
   b. Increased gastric pH.
   c. Immature intestinal barrier.
   d. Decreased intestinal motility.
4. Etiology: unclear and multifactorial. A combination of three mechanisms has been suggested as the pathogenesis of NEC:
   a. Intestinal ischemia. Conditions that may cause mucosal ischemia include the following:
     (1) Asphyxia or hypoxia.
     (2) Hypotension.
     (3) Hypovolemia.
     (4) Hypothermia.
     (5) Umbilical line.
     (6) Polycythemia.
     (7) Exchange transfusion.
     (8) Patent ductus arteriosus.
     (9) Severe stress.
   b. Bacterial colonization of the intestinal tract. Organisms most commonly associated with NEC include *Klebsiella, Escherichia coli, Enterobacter,* and *Pseudomonas* (Neu, 1996).
   c. Enteral feedings.
     (1) Of all infants who have NEC, 90–95% have had enteral feedings. Breast milk may provide some protective ingredients.
     (2) Breast milk provides ingredients that protect against symptomatic infection, including NEC. However, NEC can occur in infants who have received breast milk (Buescher, 1994).

(3) An increase in enteral feedings of greater than 20–30 mL/kg per day has been associated with an increased incidence of NEC (Kliegman, 1993).

(4) Hyperosmolar formula and medications increase the risk of having NEC (McCollum and Thigpen, 1998).

5. Onset is usually between days 3 and 10 of life. Preterm infants are more likely than term infants to have NEC at an older age (Vanderhoof et al., 1994).

6. Clinical presentation varies and includes any or all of the following findings:
   a. Abdominal distention (earliest sign).
   b. Abdominal tenderness.
   c. Bloody stools.
   d. Gastric residuals.
   e. Bilious vomiting.
   f. Lethargy.
   g. Apnea and bradycardia.
   h. Hypoperfusion.
   i. Hypotension due to third-space fluid loss from the intravascular space into the extracellular (third-space) compartment.
   j. Temperature instability.
   k. Visible loops of bowel.
   l. Abdominal erythema (usually indicates peritonitis).

7. Laboratory findings include the following:
   a. Leukocytosis or leukopenia.
   b. Thrombocytopenia.
   c. Electrolyte imbalances.
   d. Acidosis.
   e. Hypoxia.
   f. Hypercapnia.
   g. Presence of blood in stools.
   h. Carbohydrate malabsorption, reflected by reducing substances in stool; may be an early sign of NEC.
   i. Disseminated intravascular coagulation (DIC).

8. X-ray findings.
   a. Pneumatosis intestinalis (air within the wall of the intestine) (see Chapter 29).
   b. Air into the portal venous system (see Chapter 29).
   c. Pneumoperitoneum (free air in the abdomen; represents intestinal perforation) (see Chapter 29).

9. Nonsurgical medical treatment for necrotizing enterocolitis includes the following:
   a. NPO regimen; duration depends on clinical status.
   b. Gastric decompression.
   c. Antibiotics, 3–14 days, depending on clinical status.
   d. Frequent complete blood cell counts and electrolytes to evaluate infant for thrombocytopenia and electrolyte imbalances.
   e. Serial x-rays films (usually every 6 hours).
   f. Respiratory support as needed.
   g. Circulatory support as needed to prevent hypotension. Fresh-frozen plasma, dopamine, and/or dobutamine should be considered.
   h. Platelet transfusions for thrombocytopenia.
   i. Fresh-frozen plasma for DIC; consider use of vitamin K.
   j. Careful monitoring of intake and output. "Third-spacing" of fluids is common.
   k. Frequent abdominal girth measuring.
   l. Close watch of blood glucose.

10. Surgical treatment is used if medical management is not possible or fails. Indications for surgery include the following (Ricketts, 1994):
    a. Absolute indications.
       (1) Pneumoperitoneum.
       (2) Intestinal gangrene (as diagnosed with paracentesis).
    b. Relative indications.
       (1) Progressive acidosis.
       (2) Progressive thrombocytopenia.
       (3) Leukopenia or leukocytosis.
       (4) Progressive pneumatosis.
       (5) Persistent, fixed dilated loop of bowel.
       (6) Abdominal wall edema or erythema.
       (7) Portal vein gas.
11. Surgical procedure consists of the following:
    a. Resection of obvious necrotic bowel and creation of stomas is the most common procedure.
    b. Placement of peritoneal drains without surgery has been successful in very sick infants weighing less than 1000 g with perforation (Ricketts, 1994).
    c. If a large amount of bowel appears to be involved, at the initial exploration the bowel resection is limited to obviously necrotic bowel; a second exploration is performed within 24–48 hours to reevaluate bowel viability (Ricketts, 1994).
12. Postoperative care includes the following:
    a. Pain management (see Chapter 20).
    b. Placement of a central venous line for TPN.
    c. Maintenance of fluid and electrolyte balance.
    d. Antibiotic therapy (both a penicillin derivative and an aminoglycoside).
    e. Gastric decompression.
    f. Observation of stomas for color and drainage.
    g. NPO and TPN regimens until the bowel is functioning, followed by the slow resumption of feedings with a diluted formula.
13. Prognosis.
    a. Overall survival rate for all cases is 70% (Ricketts, 1994).
    b. Strictures occur in 21–39% of infants with resection and creation of stomas. Strictures are less common in infants who have a primary anastomosis (Ricketts, 1994).
    c. Other GI sequelae include enteric fistulas and short bowel syndrome (malabsorption and diarrhea).

Short Bowel Syndrome

A. **Definition:** syndrome of malabsorption and malnutrition as a result of bowel shortening (Ricketts, 1994).

B. **Etiology.**

1. NEC (most common, as high as 50%) (Ricketts, 1994).
2. Multiple intestinal atresias.
3. Midgut volvulus.
4. Extensive Hirschsprung's disease.
5. Omphalocele or gastroschisis.

C. **Clinical presentation:** dependent on length of small bowel and site of intestinal loss (Ricketts, 1994).

1. Loss of stomach is well tolerated if vitamin B_{12} is periodically given parenterally to prevent anemia.

2. Loss of jejunum can result in nutritional deficiencies, steatorrhea, and cholestasis.
3. Loss of ileum has significant metabolic and nutritional consequences.
    a. Vitamin deficiencies (especially fat-soluble vitamins A, D, E, and K).
    b. Watery or fatty diarrhea.
    c. Cholelithiasis, due to depletion of bile acids (normally reabsorbed in ileum).
4. Loss of ileocecal valve results in small bowel colonization with colonic bacteria and less time for digestion and absorption of nutrients in the small intestine.
5. Loss of the colon may result in hypovolemia, dehydration, and electrolyte disturbances.

D. Treatment.

1. TPN regimen; cyclic administration often used.
2. H_2 antagonists for gastric hypersecretion.
3. Slow introduction of feedings, beginning with elemental formulas.
4. Provision of nonnutritive sucking.
5. Cholestyramine for steatorrhea.
6. Antiperistaltic agents for persistent diarrhea.
7. Vitamin B_{12} may be given every 6 months if ileum is lost.
8. Careful monitoring of complications of TPN.
9. Any of a variety of surgical procedures to increase intestinal surface area or decrease intestinal motility.
10. Intestinal transplantation: successful for only a small number of infants; reserved for infants in whom medical and other surgical management has been unsuccessful or who have life-threatening complications of TPN (Ricketts, 1994; Vanderhoof, 1996).

E. Prognosis. Both length of small bowel and site of intestinal loss influence survival of infants receiving enteral nutrition.
1. With an intact ileocecal valve, infants with as little as 11 cm of small bowel can survive (Ricketts, 1994).
2. Without an intact ileocecal valve, infants require at least 25 cm of small bowel for survival (Ricketts, 1994).

Biliary Atresia

A. Definition: obstruction of bile flow in the extrahepatic bile duct system.

B. Incidence: 1:10,000 live births, with a slight preponderance in females (McCollum and Thigpen, 1998).

C. Etiology: exact mechanism unknown. Although once thought to be a congenital defect, biliary atresia is now believed to be caused by an inflammatory process that obliterates the bile duct system (McEvoy and Suchy, 1996). May begin in utero or postnatally.

D. Associated anomalies: occurrence in 10–25% of infants; include cardiovascular disorders, polysplenia, preduodenal or absent portal vein, malrotation, situs inversus, and intestinal atresias (McEvoy and Suchy, 1996).

E. Clinical presentation.

1. Normal appearance at birth, with gradual manifestation during first month of life. Progressive disease leads to cirrhosis of the liver and subsequent portal hypertension.
2. Jaundice.
3. Skin green-bronze color (because of increased direct bilirubin concentration).
4. Acholic stools (meconium is normal in color).

5. Enlarged and hard liver.
6. Splenomegaly.
7. Hemorrhoids.
8. Engorged abdominal veins.
9. Ascites.
10. Bloody stools.
11. Hyperbilirubinemia, with 50% of total bilirubin being direct bilirubin (McEvoy and Suchy, 1996).
12. Elevated serum levels of aminotransferase, alkaline phosphatase, gamma-glutamyltranspeptidase, and 5'-nucleotidase.

F. **Diagnosis.**

1. Liver ultrasonography.
2. Liver biopsy.
3. Operative cholangiography.

G. **Surgical management.**

1. Resection of atretic segments and end-to-end anastomosis: possible in only a few cases.
2. Hepatic portoenterostomy (Kasai procedure). Entails the creation of an intestinal conduit between the liver surface and small intestine. This is most successful when performed by 2 months of age (McEvoy and Suchy, 1996). The conduit is sometimes exteriorized temporarily to allow assessment of bile flow.
3. Liver transplant.

H. **Postoperative management.**

1. Pain management (see Chapter 20).
2. NPO and parenteral nutrition regimens.
3. Gastric decompression.
4. Assessment of bile flow and replacement as appropriate (if exteriorized).
5. Careful monitoring of fluids and electrolytes.

I. **Long-term management.**

1. Administration of fat-soluble vitamins.
2. Administration of prophylactic antibiotics to decrease risk of cholangitis.
3. Use of formulas with medium-chain triglycerides.
4. Choleretic agents such as phenobarbital, Actigall or steroids may be given to increase bile flow.
5. Careful monitoring for hemorrhage secondary to portal hypertension and bleeding tendencies.

J. **Prognosis.**

1. Without treatment, most infants will die by 2 years of age (McEvoy and Suchy, 1996).
2. Survival for infants with surgical intervention is 45–85% (McCollum and Thigpen, 1998).

Multisystem Disorders with Gastrointestinal Involvement

PRUNE-BELLY SYNDROME

A. **Definition:** triad of congenital anomalies consisting of absence of abdominal musculature, genitourinary tract abnormalities, and cryptorchidism (undescended testes). Most common genitourinary defects are:
1. Megaloureter.

2. Cystic renal dysplasia
3. Urethral obstruction.
4. Megacystitis.

B. **Incidence:** 1:35,000 to 1:50,000 live births. Approximately 95% of affected infants are male.

C. **Etiology:** unclear, but may be the result of a generalized developmental defect of abdominal parietes and mesenchyma. The condition is rarely familial, and no cytogenic abnormality has been discovered.

D. **Associated anomalies.**

1. GI tract anomalies (30%) (Berseth, 1998d).
2. Cardiac anomalies (20%) (Berseth, 1998d).
3. Pulmonary hypoplasia.
4. Imperforate anus.
5. Patent uracus.

E. **Diagnosis.**

1. Prenatal ultrasonography. May show bladder distention and dilated ureters, but these are only suggestive.
2. History of oligohydramnios: suggestive of renal pathologic changes.
3. Inspection at birth: shapeless, flat abdomen with wrinkled skin.

F. **Treatment.**

1. Surgery may be required for repair of associated defects in the renal and urinary systems.
2. Measures to improve abdominal musculature include use of abdominal binders and reconstructive surgery, but these are only palliative and cosmetic.
3. Cryptorchidism is surgically repaired by orchiopexy.

G. **Long-term considerations.**

1. Infant may require use of Credé method to empty bladder.
2. Constipation is a common problem.

H. **Prognosis:** Approximately 20% of infants die during the first month of life from renal dysplasia or hypoplasia. Renal failure develops in childhood in approximately 30% of the infants who survive (Berseth, 1998d).

CONGENITAL DIAPHRAGMATIC HERNIA

A. **Definition:** herniation of abdominal organs into the thoracic cavity through a defect in the diaphragm.

B. **Etiology:** failure of the pleuroperitoneal membranes to fuse with the diaphragm (Moore and Persaud, 1993). Congenital diaphragmatic hernia (CDH) can be either a sporadic or a familial disorder (Guzzetta et al., 1994).

C. **Incidence:** 1:1000 to 1:6000 live births (Berseth, 1998d).

D. **Associated findings and anomalies.**

1. Herniation of the intestine into the chest results in hypoplasia of the ipsilateral lung. Displacement of the mediastinum into the chest may also cause hypoplasia of the contralateral lung.
2. Pulmonary vascular bed may be hypoplastic due to lung hypoplasia, resulting in pulmonary hypertension.
3. Ductus arteriosus or foramen ovale usually remains patent because of pulmonary hypertension and right-to-left shunting.
4. Associated anomalies are reported to be greater than 40% (Guzzetta et al., 1994)

and include CNS, cardiovascular, skeletal, GI, and genitourinary defects. Intestinal malrotation is present in all cases.

5. Of diaphragmatic hernias, 85–90% occur on the left (Holland, Price, and Bensard, 1998).

6. The defect can vary from a small slit to the complete absence of the diaphragm on the affected side.

E. Clinical presentation.

1. Respiratory distress and cyanosis at birth or shortly after birth.
2. Decreased breath sounds on ipsilateral side of the chest.
3. Hypoxemia, hypercapnia, and respiratory acidosis.
4. Hypoperfusion and hypoxia due to right-to-left shunting through the ductus arteriosus, foramen ovale, and intrapulmonary shunts.
5. Heart tones may be shifted from their normal point of maximal intensity.
6. Barrel chest.
7. Scaphoid abdomen.

F. Diagnosis.

1. Prenatal ultrasonography.
2. History of polyhydramnios.
3. X-ray films showing air-filled loops of intestine within the chest and a mediastinal shift (see Chapter 29).

G. Immediate treatment and preoperative care.

1. Prophylactic surfactant treatment at birth has had some success in improving oxygenation in infants with CDH (Katz, Wiswell, and Baumgart, 1998).
2. CDH is no longer considered a surgical emergency (Rowe, O'Neill, and Grosfeld, 1995; Guzzetta et al., 1994). Immediate treatment must be prompt and aggressive. Two primary considerations are as follows:
   a. Establishment of adequate perfusion and oxygen status.
   b. Correction of acid-base imbalances.
3. Gastric decompression should be performed as soon as possible to prevent entrance of air into the herniated intestine.
4. Intubation and positive-pressure ventilation. Bag-mask ventilation should be avoided to prevent gastric distention.
5. Mechanical ventilation.
   a. Hyperventilation is controversial. Although hyperventilation induces respiratory alkalosis and pulmonary artery vasodilation, it may result in ventilation-induced lung injury (Bohn, Pearl, Irish, and Glick, 1996).
   b. Permissive hypercapnia has been shown to improve outcomes (Bohn et al., 1996).
   c. The usefulness of high-frequency oscillatory ventilation is uncertain (Bohn et al., 1996).
6. Carefully monitor infant for pneumothorax, which is more common in the contralateral side of the chest.
7. Inotropes are used to increase systemic blood pressure and decrease right-to-left shunting.
8. Inhaled nitric oxide (iNO) may be considered.
   a. iNO has been used in neonates with severe hypoxemia to improve oxygenation. iNO dilates the pulmonary arteries, decreases pulmonary vascular resistance, and decreases a right-to-left shunt across the ductus arteriosus.
   b. Usefulness of iNO in neonates with CDH is still being investigated.
   c. Likely to be beneficial in infants whose hypoxemia is caused by high pulmonary vascular resistance. Unlikely to be beneficial in infants whose hypoxemia is caused by pulmonary hypoplasia (Bohn et al., 1996).

9. Extracorporeal membrane oxygenation (ECMO) is instituted if ventilation does not effectively stabilize infant's pulmonary status.

H. **Surgical repair.**

1. Primary closure of the diaphragmatic defect is usually possible.
2. When primary closure is not possible, a synthetic patch or muscle flap can be used to close the diaphragmatic defect.

I. **Postoperative special considerations.**

1. Appropriate pain management should be initiated (see Chapter 20).
2. Gastric decompression should continue until the bowel is functioning (approximately 7–10 days).
3. A chest tube for drainage should be placed on water seal (without suction) to prevent acute mediastinal shift.
4. Pulmonary management should be carried out very carefully because of hypoplastic lungs and potential for pulmonary hypertension and pneumothorax. If pulmonary management fails, ECMO or iNO may be considered.
5. Blood pressure and perfusion may be especially problematic, and vasopressors such as dopamine and/or dobutamine may be required.

J. **Prognosis:** Survival is approximately 50% and is dependent on degree of pulmonary hypoplasia and preoperative status (Rowe et al., 1995). Onset of symptoms after 1 day of age increases the survival rate (Holland et al., 1998).

Hyperbilirubinemia

A. **Natural history.**

1. Visible jaundice develops in more than 50% of all newborn infants (Gartner, 1994).
2. Most newborn infants will appear jaundiced when their serum bilirubin concentration is greater than 7 mg/dL. Jaundice first appears on the face and progresses caudally as serum bilirubin levels increase.

B. **Bilirubin metabolism (Fig. 12–6).**

1. Synthesis.
   a. Bilirubin is produced from the breakdown of heme-containing proteins.
      (1) Major heme-containing protein is erythrocyte hemoglobin (produces 75% of all bilirubin). Catabolism of 1 g of hemoglobin produces 34 mg of bilirubin.
      (2) A small percentage (approximately 25%) of bilirubin comes from the breakdown of other proteins, such as myoglobin, cytochromes, catalase, and peroxidases.
   b. Normal neonates will produce 6–10 mg of bilirubin per kilogram per day.
   c. Newborn infants produce twice as much bilirubin per day as adults do.
2. Transport.
   a. Newly synthesized bilirubin is referred to as unconjugated, is measured as indirect bilirubin, and is fat soluble. The latter reason explains its propensity for fatty tissues such as subcutaneous and brain tissue.
   b. Bilirubin binds to albumin for transport in the blood to the liver.
   c. Each gram of albumin can bind with approximately 8.5–10 mg of bilirubin (Blackburn, 1995).
   d. The binding of bilirubin to albumin is reversible; factors that can decrease albumin-bilirubin binding include:
      (1) Metabolic derangements: acidosis, hypoxia.
      (2) Hypothermia.

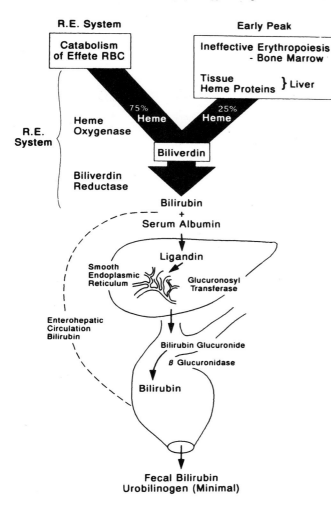

Figure 12–6

Neonatal bile pigment metabolism. *R.E.,* Reticuloendothelial; *RBC,* red blood cells. (From Maisels, M.J.: Jaundice. *In* Avery G.B., Fletcher, M.A., and Macdonald, M.G. (Eds.).: Neonatology: Pathophysiology and Management of the Newborn, 4th ed. Philadelphia, J.B. Lippincott, 1994, pp. 635.)

  (3) Infection.
  (4) Drugs: salicylates, sulfonamides, sodium benzoate, indomethacin, ampicillin (when rapidly injected).
  (5) Free fatty acids: from emulsified fats (Intralipid), starvation, hypothermia, hypoglycemia, and anoxia.
 e. Bound bilirubin does not usually enter the CNS and is nontoxic.
 f. When available albumin binding sites are saturated, unconjugated bilirubin circulates as free bilirubin and can cross the blood-brain barrier, causing kernicterus.
3. Liver uptake, conjugation, and excretion.
 a. Once in the liver, bilirubin detaches from albumin and enters the hepatocyte.
 b. Within the hepatocytes, bilirubin binds to protein Y (ligandin), protein Z, and glutathione *S*-transferase for transport to the smooth endoplastic reticulum for conjugation.
 c. Inside the smooth endoplasmic reticulum of the hepatocyte, bilirubin is converted to glucuronic acid with the aid of glucuronyl transferase.
  (1) This process depends on adequate amounts of glucose and oxygen.
  (2) The converted bilirubin is referred to as conjugated, is measured as direct bilirubin, and is water soluble.

    d. This water-soluble form of bilirubin is then excreted into the bile and eventually into the duodenum to be excreted later in the stool.

    e. In the small intestine, the high concentration of beta-glucuronidase in newborn infants can convert this bilirubin back into the fat-soluble form, which is easily absorbed from the small intestine into the portal circulation. Because the venous blood supply leaving the intestines goes directly to the liver, this process is referred to as the enterohepatic circulation. The enterohepatic circulation may explain why infants with GI obstructions distal to the ampulla of Vater have hyperbilirubinemia.

4. Fetal bilirubin metabolism.
    a. Conjugation is limited in the fetus because there is limited fetal hepatic blood flow.
    b. Unconjugated bilirubin in the fetus is cleared by the placenta.
    c. Conjugated bilirubin in the fetus is not cleared by the placenta and may accumulate in fetal tissue.
    d. Small amounts of bilirubin can normally be found in amniotic fluid between 12 and 37 weeks' gestation. Increased amounts of bilirubin in the amniotic fluid may indicate hemolytic disease or fetal intestinal obstruction below the bile ducts.

C. **Factors influencing bilirubin levels.**

1. Incidence: higher in infants of Chinese, Japanese, Korean, Native American, and Greek descent.
2. Perinatal events.
    a. Delayed cord clamping, which increases erythrocyte volume.
    b. Breech presentation and delivery with the use of vacuum extraction or forceps, which produce bruising and subsequent erythrocyte destruction.
    c. Use of oxytocin. The mechanism is unclear but may involve hemolysis.
    d. Use of epidural bupivacaine. The mechanism is unclear but may involve hemolysis due to changes in erythrocyte deformability.
    e. Asphyxia.
        (1) Inability of liver to process bilirubin.
        (2) Intracranial hemorrhage.
3. Maternal diabetes. Possibly related to hypoxia, polycythemia, or delayed hepatic uptake of bilirubin.
4. Early feeding, which decreases serum bilirubin by decreasing the reabsorption of bile caused by increased gut motility. Feeding introduces bacteria into the gut, which contributes to the conversion of bilirubin to urobilin, a substance that cannot be reabsorbed.

D. **Physiologic jaundice.**

1. Jaundice is the clinical manifestation of hyperbilirubinemia.
2. Physiologic jaundice is the manifestation of the normal hyperbilirubinemia seen in newborn infants and is a diagnosis of exclusion.
3. Chemical hyperbilirubinemia (bilirubin ≥2 mg/dL) is present in essentially all newborn infants during the first week of life because of the limitations and abnormalities of bilirubin metabolism (MacMahon, Stevenson, and Oski, 1998).
4. Physiologic jaundice occurs in 45–60% of term infants and 60% of preterm infants (Blackburn, 1995).
5. Physiologic jaundice is due to a combination of the following:
    a. Increased bilirubin load to liver.
        (1) Newborn infants have a larger red blood cell mass.
        (2) The life span of red blood cells is shorter in neonates (70–90 days, vs 120 days in adults).
        (3) Newborn infants produce a greater amount of bilirubin from sources other than red blood cells.

(4) Neonates have an increased reabsorption of bilirubin from the intestine (enterohepatic circulation) secondary to decreased GI motility, increased beta-glucoronidase activity, and decreased intestinal flora.
   b. Decreased hepatic uptake secondary to decreased ligandin and binding of Y- and Z-proteins by other anions.
   c. Defective conjugation secondary to decreased glucuronyl transferase activity.
   d. Decreased excretion of bilirubin.
6. Bilirubin levels generally peak on day 3 of life in fullterm infants and day 5–6 in preterm infants.
7. Hyperbilirubinemia in preterm infants is an exaggerated form of physiologic jaundice, mainly because of decreased glucuronyl transferase activity in the liver cell (Gartner, 1994).
8. Bilirubin is a potent antioxidant and may have protective properties against oxygen-free radicals during the newborn period (Gartner, 1994).

E. Breast-feeding and jaundice.

1. Breast-fed infants have higher bilirubin levels than bottle-fed infants.
2. Breast-feeding versus breast-milk jaundice.
   a. Breast-feeding jaundice.
      (1) Early onset, starting at 2–4 days of life.
      (2) Related to inadequate frequency of breast-feeding during early days of lactation and subsequent decreased fluid and caloric intake.
      (3) Can be avoided by breast-feeding 10–12 times a day and avoiding glucose water supplementation (Blackburn, 1995).
   b. Breast-milk jaundice.
      (1) Late onset, usually starting at 4–7 days of life.
      (2) Occurs in 10–30% of breast-fed newborn infants in weeks 2–6 of life.
      (3) Recognized as prolonged physiologic jaundice.
      (4) Related to the ingredients in breast milk. Mechanisms may include the following (Blackburn, 1995):
         (a) Decreased conjugation secondary to interference of uridine diphosphoglucuronyl transferase by pregnanediol.
         (b) Decreased conjugation due to increased concentration of free fatty acids because of high levels of lipoprotein lipase in human milk.
         (c) Increased enterohepatic circulation due to increased beta-glucuronidase activity in breast milk.
3. Treatment.
   a. The American Academy of Pediatrics (AAP) does not encourage the interruption of breast-feeding in healthy term infants (AAP, 1994).
   b. Mother's preference and physician's judgment are important considerations.
   c. The following options are acceptable (AAP, 1994):
      (1) Observe.
      (2) Continue breast-feeding; start phototherapy.
      (3) Supplement breast-feeding with bottle feeding, with or without phototherapy.
      (4) Temporarily discontinue breast-feeding; substitute bottle feeding.
      (5) Temporarily discontinue breast-feeding; substitute bottle feeding and start phototherapy.
   d. Bilirubin levels should decrease rapidly after discontinuance of breast-feeding. If levels do not decrease by 72 hours, breast-milk jaundice is not the diagnosis.
   e. When breast-feeding is begun again, bilirubin levels may increase slightly but not to previous high levels.
   f. Provision of water or dextrose supplements to healthy breast-fed infants is not recommended. Supplementation decreases milk intake and maternal

breast stimulation, which may negatively influence milk supply (Blackburn, 1995).

F. **Pathologic unconjugated hyperbilirubinemia.** (For blood incompatibilities, see Chapter 16.)
1. A pathologic reason for unconjugated hyperbilirubinemia is suggested by any of the following criteria (MacMahon et al., 1998):
   a. Jaundice that appears in the first 24 hours of life.
   b. Total serum bilirubin level that increases by more than 5 mg/dL per day.
   c. Total serum bilirubin level that exceeds 12.9 mg/dL in a term infant or 15 mg/dL in a preterm infant.
   d. Direct serum bilirubin level that exceeds 1–2 mg/dL.
   e. Jaundice lasting for more than 1 week in a term infant or 2 weeks in a preterm infant.
2. Etiology.
   a. Hemolysis.
      (1) ABO/Rh incompatibilities.
      (2) Bacterial and viral sepsis (especially *t*oxoplasmoses, *o*ther [congenital syphilis and viruses], *r*ubella, *C*MV, and *h*erpes simplex virus [TORCH] infections).
      (3) Inherited disorders of red blood cell (RBC) metabolism.
         (a) RBC membrane defects (e.g., spherocytosis, elliptocytosis).
         (b) RBC enzyme defects (e.g., glucose-6-phosphate dehydrogenase deficiency).
      (4) Inherited disorders of bilirubin metabolism (e.g., Crigler-Najjar syndrome types I and II, Gilbert's disease).
      (5) Conditions acquired secondary to maternal drug use and microangiopathies.
   b. Extravasation of blood.
      (1) Cephalhematoma.
      (2) Pulmonary, cerebral, or retroperitoneal hemorrhage.
   c. Swallowed blood.
   d. Increased enterohepatic circulation.
      (1) Delayed feeding.
      (2) Intestinal obstructions.
   e. Decreased hepatic function and perfusion.
      (1) Hypoxia.
      (2) Asphyxia.
      (3) Sepsis.
   f. Hypothyroidism.
   g. Hypopituitarism.
   h. Inborn errors of metabolism (with both unconjugated and conjugated hyperbilirubinemia).
      (1) Galactosemia.
      (2) Alpha-1-antitrypsin deficiency.
      (3) Tyrosinosis.
      (4) Hypermethioninemia.
      (5) Cystic fibrosis.

G. **Bilirubin toxic effects.**

1. Definitions.
   a. Kernicterus: neuropathologic findings of yellow staining and neuronal injury in basal ganglia.
   b. Bilirubin encephalopathy: caused by kernicterus; used to describe acute and chronic sequelae of hyperbilirubinemia (Connolly and Volpe, 1990).

2. Etiology.
   a. Unbound (free) bilirubin can cross the blood-brain barrier, where it stains and injures brain cells.
   b. Mechanism by which neuronal injury occurs is unclear.
   c. Factors that decrease albumin-bilirubin binding or alter the integrity of the blood-brain barrier put the infant at risk of having bilirubin toxic effects.
3. Clinical presentation.
   a. Early signs: blunted Moro's reflex, lethargy, weak suck, high-pitched cry, and hypotonia.
   b. Later signs: fever, hypertonia, opisthotonus, and upward gaze.
   c. Neurologic sequelae in survivors: hearing loss, choreoathetoid cerebral palsy, and mental retardation.
4. Treatment. There is no treatment for kernicterus. Prevention of elevated bilirubin levels is the most effective strategy.

H. Management of unconjugated hyperbilirubinemia.

1. The goal of treating hyperbilirubinemia is to prevent bilirubin toxic effects.
2. Although kernicterus is rare, there is evidence that healthy term infants are at risk (Maisels and Newman, 1995).
3. Guidelines for treating hyperbilirubinemia in healthy term infants are listed in Table 12–3.
4. Management of hyperbilirubinemia in low birth weight infants is determined by clinical status, age, weight, and history (Table 12–4).
5. In hemolytic disease, phototherapy is begun immediately.
6. All infants discharged before 48 hours after birth should be followed up by a health care practitioner within 2–3 days of discharge for assessment of jaundice (AAP, 1994).

I. Phototherapy.

1. Most effective in decreasing nonhemolytic hyperbilirubinemia.
2. Mechanism for phototherapy action.

Table 12–3
MANAGEMENT OF HYPERBILIRUBINEMIA IN HEALTHY TERM NEONATE*

Age (hr)	TSB Level, mg/dL (µmol/L)			
	Consider Phototherapy*	*Phototherapy*	*Exchange Transfusion if Intensive Phototherapy Fails†*	*Exchange Transfusion and Intensive Phototherapy*
≤24‡	—	—	—	—
25-48	≥12 (170)	≥15 (260)	≥20 (340)	≥25 (430)
49-72	≥15 (260)	≥18 (310)	≥25 (430)	≥30 (510)
>72	≥17 (290)	≥20 (340)	≥25 (430)	≥30 (510)

TSB, Total serum bilirubin.

*Phototherapy at these TSB levels is a clinical option, meaning that the intervention is available and may be used *on the basis of individual clinical judgment.*

†Intensive phototherapy should produce a decline of TSB of 1 to 2 mg/dL within 4 to 6 hours and the TSB level should continue to fall and remain below the threshold level for exchange transfusion. If this does not occur, it is considered a failure of phototherapy.

‡Term infants who are clinically jaundiced at ≤24 hours old are not considered healthy and require further evaluation.

From American Academy of Pediatrics Provisional Committee for Quality Improvement and Subcommittee on Hyperbilirubinemia: Practice parameter: Management of hyperbilirubinemia in the healthy term newborn. Pediatrics, *94*:558–565, 1994, p. 560. Used with permission. © American Academy of Pediatrics 1994.

Table 12–4
MANAGEMENT OF HYPERBILIRUBINEMIA IN LOW BIRTH WEIGHT INFANTS

Birth Weight	Indirect Bilirubin Concentrations					
	5-6 mg/dL	**7-9 mg/dL**	**10-12 mg/dL**	**12-15 mg/dL**	**15-20 mg/dL**	**>20 mg/dL**
≤1000 gm	Phototherapy	————→*	Exchange transfusion†	——————————————————————————————→		
1001-1500 gm	Observe and repeat BR	Phototherapy	————————→	Exchange transfusion	——————————————————→	
1501-2000 gm	Observe and repeat BR	————————→	Phototherapy	————————→	Exchange transfusion	————————→
>2000 gm	Observe	Observe and repeat BR	Phototherapy (<2500 gm)	Phototherapy (>2500 gm)	————————→	Exchange transfusion

BR, Bilirubin.
*Perform binding tests (titration with bilirubin and Sephadex gel filtration) if an infant under phototherapy approaches the next treatment interval.
†Exchange if albumin binding is saturated, or if serum indirect bilirubin continues to rise.
From Cashore, W.J., and Stern, L.: The management of hyperbilirubinemia. Clin Perinatol., *11*:339–357, 1984 p. 353.

a. Photo-oxidation.
   (1) Accounts for only 15% of photodecomposition of bilirubin (Shaw, 1998).
   (2) Involves oxidation of bilirubin to water-soluble products excreted in urine.
b. Photoisomerization.
   (1) Major mechanism of phototherapy action.
   (2) Involves the conversion of bilirubin to water-soluble structural and configurational isomers that can be excreted by the liver without conjugation.
3. Effectiveness: influenced by energy output of phototherapy unit, spectrum of light, and amount of infant's body surface area exposed to light.
4. Delivery methods.
   a. Bilirubin can absorb light of only certain wavelengths (blue, violet, green). Photodecomposition of bilirubin occurs most effectively with lights having an output close to the maximum absorption peak of bilirubin (450–460 nm). Lights that emit blue wavelengths of approximately 425–475 nm achieve this most effectively.
   b. Not all blue lights are equally effective. Only "special blue" lights (labeled F20 T12/BB) are more effective than white lamps (Halamek and Stevenson, 1997).
   c. Disadvantages of these lights are that they create a difficult environment in which to work, and they distort an infant's color.
   d. White lamps, tungsten-halogen lamps, and fiberoptic "blankets" are effective alternatives and do not make the baby look cyanotic.
   e. Advantages of the fiberoptic "blankets" are that eye patches are not needed and that the infant can be held while phototherapy is maintained.
5. Management of phototherapy and of the infant receiving phototherapy.
   a. Fluorescent lights should be at a distance of 45–50 cm from the infant to provide optimal irradiance.
   b. Manufacturer's instructions should be followed for appropriate distance of spotlights.
   c. When bank lights are used, lamps should be covered with Plexiglas to protect the infant from ultraviolet light.
   d. Fluorescent lights should be placed at least 2 inches from the top of an incubator.
   e. Recommendations for changing lamp bulbs range from 200 to 2000 hours of use because of decreased energy output. Use of a spectroradiometer

is probably a more useful strategy to ensure optimal irradiance. Light irradiance of 4–6 μW/cm² per nanometer, as measured by spectroradiometer, is required for optimal phototherapy efficacy (Shaw, 1998).

   f. Infants receiving phototherapy need to have as much skin exposed as possible.

   g. All infants receiving phototherapy need to have their eyes covered with eye patches to protect them from the strong light. Phototherapy may be temporarily discontinued to remove eye patches, provide visual stimulation, and allow the parents to hold and feed the infant.

   h. Turn the infant frequently to allow all areas of the skin to be exposed.

   i. Temperature control is important to monitor whether the infant is in an open crib, an incubator, or an overhead warmer.

   j. Monitor fluids carefully.
     (1) Phototherapy increases insensible water loss. Up to 25% more fluid may be required (Poland and Ostrea, 1993).
     (2) Phototherapy may cause diarrhea with further fluid loss.

   k. Monitor bilirubin levels after phototherapy is discontinued. A rebound of 1–2 mg/dL can be expected.

6. Side effects.
   a. Loose stools.
   b. Hyperthermia.
   c. Bronze baby syndrome.
   d. Dehydration.
   e. Skin rashes.
   f. Lethargy.
   g. Abdominal distention.
   h. Hypocalcemia.
   i. Lactose intolerance.

7. Home phototherapy: an option that decreases hospitalization time for an otherwise healthy newborn infant. Temperature control and fluid intake need to be monitored carefully.

J. Exchange transfusion.

1. The decision to perform an exchange transfusion should be made while taking into consideration the bilirubin level, how quickly the level is rising, the gestational age of the infant, and the age (in hours and days) of the infant (Tables 12–2 and 12–3).

2. Early exchange transfusion is indicated in babies with significant hemolytic disease such as hydrops fetalis, particularly with cord bilirubin levels greater than 4.5 mg/dL and cord hemoglobin less than 11 g/dL.

3. A double-volume exchange transfusion removes 85–90% of the infant's RBC volume and 25% of the infant's total bilirubin.

4. Administration of albumin, 1 g/kg 1 to 2 hours before the transfusion, may increase albumin-bilirubin binding and facilitate movement of bilirubin from the tissues into the intravascular space, thereby increasing the amount of bilirubin exchanged. This therapy remains controversial, because the albumin equilibrates with extravascular albumin quickly and may facilitate movement of bilirubin from the intravascular space into the extravascular space (Shaw, 1998).

5. Procedure for exchange transfusion.
   a. Sick infants should always be treated for hypoglycemia, acidosis, and temperature control before the start of an exchange transfusion.
   b. The infant is restrained on a radiant warmer and placed on a cardiorespiratory monitor. Oxygen and suction should be available at the bedside.
   c. Ideally, an umbilical artery catheter and umbilical venous catheter are placed (see Chapter 31 for procedure).

d. The initial blood removed should be sent to the laboratory for complete blood cell count (CBC), bilirubin and calcium, and blood cultures.

e. The exchange should be done in aliquots of 3–5 mL/kg every 3–5 minutes (Edwards and Fletcher, 1993; Taeusch, 1996).

f. Accurate recording of blood volumes exchanged is essential during the procedure.

g. Watch carefully for hypocalcemia. The citrates found in the anticoagulants (acid-citrate-dextrose and CPD-adenosine) bind to calcium. Symptoms of hypocalcemia include the following:

(1) Irritability.

(2) Tachycardia.

(3) Prolonged Q-T interval.

h. Calcium gluconate should be administered if the infant has hypocalcemia. Normal dose is 1 mL of 10% solution.

i. Always have a resuscitation cart nearby during an exchange transfusion.

j. Evaluate medications. Medications known to decrease significantly during exchange transfusions should be administered after the transfusion (e.g., ampicillin, gentamicin, digoxin, phenobarbital, vancomycin).

6. Complications of exchange transfusions.

a. Embolization.

b. Thrombosis.

c. NEC.

d. Electrolyte imbalance.

e. Overheparinization.

f. Thrombocytopenia.

g. Infection.

h. Cardiac arrhythmias and arrest.

i. Hyperglycemia or hypoglycemia.

7. Postexchange care. Phototherapy should be continued after exchange transfusion.

a. Recheck bilirubin levels every 4 hours. Rebound usually occurs within 1 hour after the exchange.

b. Check blood glucose levels frequently.

c. Observe closely for signs of complications, such as infection, electrolyte imbalance, NEC, and thrombosis.

K. **Alternative therapies.**

1. Early feeding: decreases the enterohepatic circulation.

2. Binding agents: agar and activated charcoal bind bilirubin in the gut and decrease the enterohepatic circulation.

3. Phenobarbital: increases hepatic ligandin concentration.

4. Metalloporphyrins: decrease enzymatic processes necessary for bilirubin production from heme.

L. **Conjugated hyperbilirubinemia (direct).**

1. Causes of elevated conjugated bilirubin.

a. Liver cell injury.

(1) Cholestatic jaundice related to use of parenteral nutrition.

(2) Infection.

(a) Viral.

(b) Bacterial.

(c) Parasitic.

(3) Hepatitis.

(4) Drugs.

b. Bile flow obstruction.

(1) Biliary atresia.

        (2) Extrahepatic obstruction (choledochal cyst, trisomy 13 or 18, or poly-splenia).

        (3) Intrahepatic obstruction (choledochal cyst, bile duct stenosis, bile duct rupture, tumors, cystic fibrosis).

    c. Excessive bilirubin load.

    d. Maternal-fetal blood group incompatibility (i.e., ABO, Rh; see Chapter 16).

  2. Management of conjugated hyperbilirubinemia.

    a. A thorough examination to evaluate for hepatomegaly, splenomegaly, petechiae, chorioretinitis, and microcephaly should be performed.

    b. Assess liver function (aspartate aminotransferase, activated clotting time), prothrombin time, partial thromboplastin time, and serum albumin levels.

    c. Test for ABO and Rh incompatibility (see Chapter 16).

    d. Management is related to the causative factor(s).

Hydrops Fetalis

A. **Definition:** generalized subcutaneous edema in fetus and neonate. Usually accompanied by ascites and pleural and/or pericardial effusions.

B. **Classification.**

1. Alloimmune hydrops occurs when maternal antibodies cross the placenta and destroy fetal erythrocytes. ABO and Rh incompatibilities are the most common causes of alloimmune hydrops fetalis.

2. Nonimmune hydrops occurs for reasons other than those cited above (see section C, Etiology of Nonimmune Hydrops Fetalis, below).

C. **Etiology of nonimmune hydrops fetalis (NIHF).**

  1. Cardiovascular (most frequent cause).

    a. Heart block.

    b. Paroxysmal atrial tachycardia, atrial flutter.

    c. Cardiac malformation.

  2. Hematologic.

    a. Alpha-thalassemia.

    b. Glucose-6-phosphate dehydrogenase deficiency.

    c. Chronic fetal-maternal or twin-to-twin transfusion.

    d. Hemorrhage.

    e. Bone marrow failure.

  3. Renal.

    a. Nephrosis.

    b. Renal vein thrombosis.

    c. Renal hypoplasia.

    d. Urinary obstruction.

  4. Infection.

    a. Syphilis.

    b. Rubella.

    c. Cytomegalovirus.

    d. Congenital hepatitis.

    e. Toxoplasmosis.

    f. Parvovirus.

  5. Pulmonary.

    a. Pulmonary hypoplasia.

    b. Cystic adenomatoid malformations.

    c. Pulmonary lymphangiectasis.

6. Placenta and cord (uncommon).
   a. Chorioangioma.
   b. Umbilical vein thrombosis.
   c. Arteriovenous malformation.
7. Maternal.
   a. Toxemia.
   b. Diabetes.
8. Gastrointestinal.
   a. In utero volvulus.
   b. Meconium peritonitis.
9. Chromosomal.
   a. Achondroplasia.
   b. Turner's syndrome.
   c. Trisomy 13, 18, 21.
   d. Triploidy.
   e. Aneuploidy.
10. Of all cases of hydrops, 20% are of unknown or rare miscellaneous causes (Hinkes and Cloherty, 1998).

D. Clinical presentation.

1. Prenatal findings in NIHF include uterine size greater than normal for gestational age, sudden increase in abdominal girth or weight gain, abdominal pain.
2. Preterm labor occurs in 87% of NIHF cases (Moore and Tipton, 1997).
3. Massive edema, often restricting joint movement.
4. Ascites.
5. Hepatosplenomegaly.
6. Cardiomegaly.

E. Associated laboratory findings.

1. Anemia.
2. Hypoalbuminemia.
3. Reticulocytosis.
4. Thrombocytopenia.

F. Diagnosis.

1. Vigorous prenatal diagnosis with ultrasonography is essential.
2. Echocardiography.
3. Serologic testing for isoimmunization and infection.
4. Chromosomal testing.

G. Management.

1. Antenatal.
   a. Fetal transfusion (for isoimmune hemolytic anemia).
   b. Maternal digitalis (for heart rhythm abnormalities).
   c. Delivery.
2. Neonatal.
   a. Resuscitation is frequently required.
   b. Paracentesis may be required for difficulties with ventilation.
   c. Thoracentesis or chest tubes may be required for hydrothorax.
   d. Partial exchange transfusion may be necessary if the hematocrit is less than 30%.
   e. Fresh frozen plasma may be given for hypoalbuminemia.
   f. Inotropes may be given to improve cardiac output.

g. A complete head-to-toe neonatal assessment should be performed to determine the etiology of the hydrops if it is unknown (including echocardiogram, ultrasound of GI and renal systems).

h. Provide phototherapy when indicated.

H. **Prognosis.** Prognosis in NIHF is very poor and is related to the underlying cause.

REFERENCES

American Academy of Pediatrics Provisional Committee for Quality Improvement and Subcommittee on Hyperbilirubinemia: Practice parameter: Management of hyperbilirubinemia in the healthy term newborn. Pediatrics, 94:558–565, 1994.

Berseth, C.L.: Developmental anatomy and physiology of the gastrointestinal tract. In Taeusch, W.H., and Ballard, R.A. (Eds.): Avery's Diseases of the Newborn, 7th ed. Philadelphia, W.B. Saunders, 1998a, pp. 893–904.

Berseth, C.L.: Disorders of the esophagus. In Taeusch, W.H., and Ballard, R.A. (Eds.): Avery's Diseases of the Newborn, 7th ed. Philadelphia, W.B. Saunders, 1998b, pp. 908–913.

Berseth, C.L.: Disorders of the intestines and pancreas. In Taeusch, W.H., and Ballard, R.A. (Eds.): Avery's Diseases of the Newborn, 7th ed. Philadelphia, W.B. Saunders, 1998c, pp. 918–927.

Berseth, C.L.: Disorders of the umbilical cord, abdominal wall, uracus, and omphalomesenteric duct. In Taeusch, W.H., and Ballard, R.A. (Eds.): Avery's Diseases of the Newborn, 7th ed. Philadelphia, W.B. Saunders, 1998d, pp. 933–940.

Blackburn, S.: Hyperbilirubinemia and neonatal jaundice. Neonatal Network, 14(7):15–25, 1995.

Bohn, D.J., Pearl, R.P., Irish, M.S., and Glick, P.L.: Postnatal management of congenital diaphragmatic hernia. Clin. Perinat., 23:843–872, 1996.

Brandt, M.L.: Gastrointestinal surgical emergencies of the newborn. In Taeusch, W.H., and Ballard, R.A. (Eds.): Avery's Diseases of the Newborn, 7th ed. Philadelphia, W.B. Saunders, 1998, pp. 979–994.

Buescher, E.S.: Host defense mechanisms of human milk and their relations to enteric infections and necrotizing enterocolitis. Clin. Perinatol., 21:247–262, 1994.

Connolly, A.M., and Volpe, J.J.: Clinical features of bilirubin encephalopathy. Clin. Perinatol., 17:371–380, 1990.

Dennery, P.A., and Stevenson, D.K.: Neonatal hyperbilirubinemia. In Polin, R.A., Yoder, M.C., and Burg, F.D. (Eds.): Workbook in Practical Neonatology, 2nd ed. Philadelphia, W.B. Saunders, 1993, pp. 79–98.

Edwards M.C., and Fletcher, M.A.: Exchange transfusions. In Fletcher, M.A., and MacDonald, M.G. (Eds.): Atlas of Procedures in Neonatology, 2nd ed. Philadelphia, J.B. Lippincott, 1993, pp. 363–374.

Gartner, L.M.: Neonatal jaundice. Pediatr. Rev., 15:422–432, 1994.

Guzzetta, P.C., Anderson, K.D., Newman, K.D., et al.: General surgery. In Avery G.B., Fletcher, M.A., and Macdonald, M.G. (Eds.).: Neonatology: Pathophysiology and Management of the Newborn, 4th ed. Philadelphia, J.B. Lippincott, 1994, pp. 914–951.

Halamek, L.P., and Stevenson, D.K.: Neonatal jaundice and liver disorders. In Fanaroff, A.A., and Martin, R.J. (Eds.): Neonatal-Perinatal Medicine: Diseases of the Fetus and Newborn, 6th ed. St. Louis, Mosby, 1997, pp. 1345–1389.

Hinkes, M.T., and Cloherty, J.P.: Neonatal hyperbilirubinemia. In Cloherty, J.P., and Stark, A. (Eds.): Manual of Neonatal Care, 4th ed. Boston, Little, Brown, 1998, pp. 175–210.

Holland, R.M., Price, F.N., and Bensard, D.D.: Neonatal surgery. In Merenstein, G., and Gardner, S. (Eds.): Handbook of Neonatal Intensive Care, 4th ed. St. Louis, Mosby, 1998, pp. 625–646.

Hoyme, H.E., Higginbottom, M.C., and Jones, K.L.: The vascular pathogenesis of gastroschisis: Intrauterine interruption of the omphalomesenteric artery. J Pediatr., 98:228–231, 1981.

Katz, A.L., Wiswell, T.E., and Baumgart, S.: Comtemporary controversies in the management of congenital diaphragmatic hernia. Clin. Perinatol., 25:219–248, 1998.

Kays, D.W.: Surgical conditions of the neonatal intestinal tract. Clin. Perinatol., 23:353–376, 1996.

Kirschner, B.S.: Hirschprung's disease. In Walker, W.A., Durie, P.R., Hamilton, J.R., et al. (Eds.).: Pediatric Gastrointestinal Disease: Pathophysiology, Diagnosis, Management, vol 1, 2nd ed. St. Louis, Mosby, 1996, pp. 980–983.

Kliegman, R.M.: Necrotizing enterocolitis: Differential diagnosis and management. In Polin, R.A., Yoder, M.C., and Burg, F.D. (Eds.): Workbook in Practical Neonatology, 2nd ed. Philadelphia, W.B. Saunders, 1993, pp. 449–470.

MacMahon, J.R., Stevenson, D.K., and Oski, F.A.: Physiologic jaundice. In Taeusch, W.H., Ballard, R.A. (Eds.): Avery's diseases of the newborn, 7th ed. Philadelphia, W.B. Saunders, 1998, pp. 1003–1007.

Maisels, M.J., and Newman, T.B.: Kernicterus in otherwise healthy, breast-fed term newborns. Pediatrics, 96:730–733, 1995.

McCollum, L.L., and Thigpen, J.L.: Assessment and management of gastrointestinal dysfunction. In Kenner C., Lott, J.W., and Flandermeyer A.A. (Eds.): Comprehensive Neonatal Nursing: A Physiologic Perspective, 2nd ed. Philadelphia, W.B. Saunders, 1998, pp. 371–408.

McEvoy, C.F., and Suchy, F.J.: Biliary tract disease in children. Pediatr. Gastroenterol. I, 43:75–98, 1996.

Moore, K.L., and Persaud, T.V.N.: The Developing Human: Clinically Oriented Embryology, 5th ed. Philadelphia, W.B. Saunders, 1993.

Moore, T.R., and Tipton, E.E.: Amniotic fluid and nonimmune hydrops fetalis. In Fanaroff, A.A., and Martin, R.J. (Eds.): Neonatal-Perinatal Medicine: Diseases of the Fetus and Infant, 2nd ed. St. Louis, Mosby, 1997, pp. 312–326.

Neu, J.: Necrotizing enterocolitis: The search for a unifying pathogenic theory leading to prevention. Pediatr. Clin. North Am., 43:409–432, 1996.

Poland, R.L., and Ostrea, E.M.: Neonatal hyperbilirubinemia. In Klaus, M.H., and Fanaroff, A.A. (Eds.): Care of the High-Risk Neonate, 4th ed. Philadelphia, W.B. Saunders, 1993, pp. 302–322.

Rescorla, F.J.: Surgical emergencies in the newborn. *In* Polin, R.A., Yoder, M.C., and Burg, F.D. (Eds.): Workbook in Practical Neonatology, 2nd ed. Philadelphia, W.B. Saunders, 1993.

Ricketts, R.R.: Surgical treatment of necrotizing enterocolitis and the short bowel syndrome. Clin. Perinatol., 21:365–387, 1994.

Ross, A: Intestinal obstruction in the newborn. Pediatr. Rev., 15:338–347, 1994.

Rowe, M.I., O'Neill, J.A., Grosfeld, J.L., et al.: Essentials of Pediatric Surgery. St. Louis, Mosby, 1995.

Shaw, N.: Assessment and management of hematologic dysfunction. *In* Kenner C., Lott, J.W., and Flandermeyer, A.A. (Eds.): Comprehensive Neonatal Nursing: A Physiologic Perspective, 2nd ed. Philadelphia, W.B. Saunders, 1998, pp. 520–563.

Taeusch, H.W.: Hematologic tests and procedures. *In* Taeusch, H.W., Christianson, R.O., and Buescher, E.S. (Eds.): Pediatric and Neonatal Tests and Procedures. Philadelphia, W.B. Saunders, 1996, pp. 599–621.

Vanderhoof, J.A.: Short bowel syndrome in children and small intestinal transplantation. Pediatr. Clin. North Am., 43:533–550, 1996.

Vanderhoof, J.A., Zach, T.L., and Adrian, T.E.: Gastrointestinal disease. *In* Avery, G.B., Fletcher, M.A., and Macdonald, M.G. (Eds.).: Neonatology: Pathophysiology and Management of the Newborn, 4th ed. Philadelphia, J.B. Lippincott, 1994, pp. 605–629.

Wesson, D.E., and Haddock, G.: Congenital anomalies. *In* Walker, W.A., Durie, P.R., Hamilton, J.R., et al. (Eds.).: Pediatric Gastrointestinal Disease: Pathophysiology, Diagnosis, Management, 2nd ed. St. Louis, Mosby, 1996, pp. 555–563.

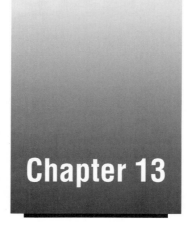

Chapter 13

Neonatal Nutrition

Susan Bakewell-Sachs

Objectives

1. Describe the effects of prematurity on the physiology of digestion and absorption.

2. Identify nutritional deficiencies most common in preterm and term infants.

3. Describe basic nutritional requirements for term and preterm infants and factors that influence these requirements.

4. Describe the standards used to assess growth in preterm infants.

5. Identify nutritional components, uses, methods of delivery, complications, and nursing care issues for parenteral nutrition.

6. Identify the appropriate uses, routes of delivery, components, complications, and nursing care routines for parenteral nutrition.

7. Describe assessment of an infant's readiness for enteral nutrition.

8. Describe minimal enteral feedings and their use in preterm infants.

9. Review the use of human milk feedings for preterm infants and related nursing care issues.

10. Review the use of commercial premature infant formulas for enteral nutrition management.

11. Describe the various methods for enteral feedings and the advantages and disadvantages of each.

12. Describe assessments used to determine infant nutritional status.

13. Describe risks and interventions for feeding intolerances and nutritional deficiency states in preterm infants.

Neonatal nurses face challenges in helping to meet the basic nutritional requirements and supporting the growth needs of high-risk and preterm newborn infants. Tremendous advances in technology and pharmacology permit the survival of even extremely prematurely born infants, who require specialized care and support for immature body systems. Nutritional care is of vital importance for these preterm infants, who have been deprived of transplacentally acquired nutrient stores and who have rapid extrauterine growth rates. Other high-risk infants have special needs related to illness-associated metabolic demands and physiologic instability.

Neonatal nurses with knowledge of the effects of prematurity on gastrointestinal functioning, the special nutritional needs of preterm infants, and methods of delivering nutritional support can better assess infant status and contribute to nutritional management. This chapter reviews the nutritional requirements of preterm and high-risk infants, methods for providing parenteral and enteral nutrition, and nursing interventions for optimal nutritional care.

Anatomy and Physiology of the Preterm Infant's Gastrointestinal Tract

A. **Anatomic and functional development of the gastrointestinal (GI) tract.**

1. Anatomic development. GI tract resembles that of a term newborn infant by 20 weeks' gestation (Blackburn and Loper, 1992; Carver and Barness, 1996).
2. Functional development.
   a. Limited before 26 weeks' gestation and continues after birth (Carver and Barness, 1996).
   b. Sucking movements occur in utero as early as 13–15 weeks' gestation, but functional coordination of suck, swallow, and breathing is not developed until closer to 36–38 weeks (Hill and Rath, 1993).
   c. By 28 weeks the fetus has the biochemical and physiologic capacities for limited digestion and absorption (Carver and Barness, 1996).
   d. Preterm infants have limited lactase levels, which rise postnatally but should be adequate to handle slowly initiated lactose-containing enteral feedings (Neu and Koldovsky, 1996). Lactase reaches mature levels around 36–40 weeks (Hill and Rath, 1993). Other carbohydrate-digesting enzymes, disaccharidases, are functionally active after 27–28 weeks' gestation.
   e. Fat digestion begins in the stomach, where a portion of milk fat is digested and partial hydrolysis occurs as a prerequisite to intestinal fat digestion. Gastric lipase activity is already high at 25 weeks' gestation, remains constant up to 34 weeks, when it peaks, and then decreases slightly before term. Gastric fat digestion is greater in preterm infants fed mother's milk (25%) than in those fed formula (14%), likely because of the bile salt–dependent lipase of human milk (Hamosh, 1996).
   f. Pancreatic lipase has a limited contribution to fat digestion in neonates compared to that in adults. Pancreatic lipase activity is lower in preterm than in term infants and is lower in preterm infants who are small for gestational age (SGA) than in those who are appropriate in size for gestational age (Hamosh, 1996).
   g. Protein enzyme activity increases rapidly after birth in premature and term infants (Hamosh, 1996).
   h. Preterm infants have limited production of gut digestive enzymes and growth factors.
   i. Immature motor function limits the ability to move nutrients through the GI tract and is evidenced by lack of sucking coordination, decreased esophageal sphincter tone, delayed gastric emptying, and slow intestinal transit (Berseth, 1996). Peristalsis and intestinal motility reach mature function during the third trimester (Hill and Rath, 1993).

B. **Postnatal development of the GI tract.**

1. GI motility is the main limiting factor in providing enteral nutrition to preterm infants (Berseth, 1996).

2. Diet is a major factor in the regulation of GI growth and function (Carver and Barness, 1996).
   a. Oral nutrients can have direct or indirect effects through stimulation of hormone secretion.
   b. Vitamins and minerals, such as iron and zinc, are growth factors.
   c. Folic acid and vitamin B_{12} are necessary for DNA synthesis.
   d. Vitamin D hydroxylation influences calcium and phosphorous absorption.
   e. A variety of amino acids are essential for growth.
   f. Diet composition influences enzyme activities and gut flora, which may then affect GI development and function.
   g. Increased oral nutrient intake and increased rate of weight gain lead to earlier maturation of the small-intestine epithelium.
3. Systemically administered growth factors (e.g., by means of parenteral nutrition) can stimulate GI growth and maturation.

C. **Nutrient store deficiencies of preterm infants.**

1. Energy.
   a. Fat provides 9 kcal/g and is therefore the major energy source for neonates (Hamosh, 1996). Significant fat accretion occurs in the fetus between 24 weeks and 40 weeks. At 24 weeks the body composition is less than 2% stored fat, at 32 weeks 5%, and at 40 weeks 15%. Essential fatty acids are important for brain growth and function.
      (1) Sources of fat for the newborn infant include:
         (a) Release of free fatty acids stored in adipose tissue.
         (b) Absorption of fat from human milk or formula (approximately 50% of calories from fat).
         (c) IV lipids.
      (2) Preterm infants have low adipose tissue stores at birth.
   b. Carbohydrate is the second major energy source for neonates. The human neonate's brain is glucose dependent, accounting for 75% of fetal glucose consumption. During the third trimester, glucose is stored as glycogen in the liver.
      (1) Term infants have sufficient energy stores in the form of glycogen and fat for use during the relative starvation state that normally occurs during the first few days of life.
      (2) Preterm infants have limited fat and glycogen stores and will quickly exhaust endogenous energy sources if sufficient exogenous energy is not provided. Nutritional support should ideally begin by 24–72 hours of life to give enough nonprotein calories to prevent existing tissue catabolism. Dextrose alone will result in the use of muscle catabolism for energy (Thureen and Hay, 1993).
2. Vitamins and minerals.
   a. Nutrients such as vitamins A and E, and minerals and trace elements, such as calcium, phosphorus, iron, copper, zinc, selenium, chromium, manganese, molybdenum, cobalt, fluoride, and iodine, normally accumulate at an appreciable rate, predominantly in the third trimester of pregnancy. Levels of these nutrients are therefore low in preterm infants.
   b. These nutrients play an essential role in promoting normal tissue growth and repairing injured tissue. Trace elements also play an important role in numerous metabolic pathways (Zlotkin et al., 1995).
3. Inadequate quantities of many essential nutrients. Prevention of further depletion of reserves and achievement of comparable intrauterine accretion rates are difficult and sometimes not possible.
4. Inadequate nutrition. The growth and development of all organ systems are affected.

Standards for Adequate Growth

A. Intrauterine growth curves.

1. Widely accepted.
2. Standard for adequate growth: normal fetus at postconceptional age similar to that of preterm newborn infant.
3. May be an inappropriate standard for adequate growth for preterm infants for the following reasons:
   a. Because of immature organ systems of the preterm infant, it is impossible, even with total parenteral nutrition and commercially prepared preterm infant formulas, to match the transplacental provision of nutrients.
   b. As gestational age decreases, extrauterine provision of comparable nutrients becomes increasingly difficult and may be undesirable in extremely low birth weight or critically ill infants.
   c. Severe illness affects both nutrient demands and nutrient use (Wahlig and Georgieff, 1995).
   d. Overly aggressive attempts to attain comparable intrauterine growth may result in the following:
      (1) Acidosis.
      (2) Fluid overload.
      (3) Promotion of patent ductus arteriosus (PDA) (Shaffer and Weismann, 1992).
      (4) Increased risk of bronchopulmonary dysplasia (BPD) secondary to PDA.

B. Postnatal growth curves for preterm infants.

1. Weight and head circumference are based on birth gestational age.
2. Growth curves attempt to account for early postnatal water weight loss.
3. Growth curves reflect a slower growth velocity than is seen with intrauterine growth curves.
4. Clinicians must bear in mind that definitive criteria for adequate growth remain controversial.
5. Anthropometric measurements and standardized growth curves are necessary tools for assessing growth and nutrition.
   a. Growth charts for very low birth weight (VLBW) preterm male and female infants were developed from growth percentiles obtained during the Infant Health and Development Program and are now published by Ross Products Division, Abbott Laboratories (Infant Health and Development Program, 1990). (See Chapter 5, p. 82.)
   b. Whether based on intrauterine or postnatal criteria, a standardized growth curve that is reflective of a comparable population with respect to geographic location/climate, ethnic, and socioeconomic variables must be selected or developed by each institution.

Nutritional Requirements and Feeding for Term Infants

A. Caloric and fluid requirements.

1. Healthy newborn infants require approximately 100–120 kcal/kg per day for adequate growth and development.
2. Adequate caloric intake is generally achieved by intake of 150–180 mL/kg per day when formula with 20 kcal per ounce or human milk is used.

B. Protein, fat, and carbohydrate.

1. Total caloric intake should be represented by the following:
   a. Protein: 7–12%.
   b. Fat: 35–55%.
   c. Carbohydrate: 35–55%.
2. Human milk and commercial infant formulas supply these nutrients within acceptable ratios. Infant formulas are designed to approximate the nutrients in human milk.
3. Vitamins, minerals, and trace elements.
   a. Vitamin deficiency in healthy term infants is rare.
   b. Human milk and formulas provide adequate amounts of vitamins to meet the needs of most infants. However, supplements of fluoride and iron are often recommended, especially for breast-fed infants.
   c. Recommended daily requirements and intakes are described elsewhere (Moran and Greene, 1998).
4. Human milk and term-infant formulas.
   a. Human milk is the ideal food for term infants. All healthy mothers should be encouraged to breast-feed their infants.
      (1) Human milk may be deficient in vitamin D, especially for dark-skinned infants who are not exposed to adequate amounts of sunlight. Vitamin B_{12} is often deficient in the milk of strictly vegetarian women who do not take supplements.
      (2) The unique absorption of iron and zinc from human milk results in only rare deficiencies of these minerals, despite their low content in human milk. Supplemental feedings, however, (i.e., formula, cereal, fruit) decrease iron and zinc absorption from human milk.
   b. Commercial formulas for term infants are cow milk or soy based. Although both types support adequate weight gain for term infants, soy-based formulas are not recommended unless the infant exhibits signs and/or symptoms of lactose intolerance or milk-protein allergy.
5. Supplements. Controversy exists regarding supplementation of human milk or formulas with additional vitamins and minerals. Some recommendations for supplementation are as follows:
   a. Iron.
      (1) Iron supplementation may be beneficial for exclusively breast-fed infants beginning at 4 months of age.
      (2) Iron supplements may be given in the form of ferrous sulfate, multivitamins with iron, iron-fortified formula, or iron-fortified cereal.
   b. Vitamin D.
      (1) Adequate amounts are supplied in formula when intake is adequate.
      (2) Vitamin D supplements (200 to 300 IU/day) are recommended for those infants born at term whose exposure to sunlight is less than 30 minutes a week while wearing only a diaper or at least 2 hours a week while fully clothed but with no hat (Slusser and Powers, 1997).
   c. Fluoride.
      (1) Fluoride supplementation is recommended after age 6 months, when the concentration of fluoride in the drinking water is less than 0.3 ppm.
      (2) For ages 6 months to 3 years, the dose is 0.25 mg/day (Orth, 1997).
      (3) In areas where drinking water is adequately treated with fluoride, breast-fed infants may not require supplementation (Slusser and Powers, 1997).
      (4) If fluoride in the local water supply is less than 0.3 ppm, the supplementation recommendation is 0.25 mg/day.
      (5) If the fluoride content in the local water supply is more than 0.3 ppm, no supplementation is recommended.

d. Vitamin B_{12}. Supplementation in the amount of 0.3 to 0.5 µg/day is recommended for infants whose mothers eat no animal products and take no vitamin B_{12} supplements (Slusser and Powers, 1997).

Nutritional Requirements for Preterm Infants

A. General considerations.

1. Recommendations for nutritional requirements and advisable intakes must be used as guidelines for meeting nutritional requirements.
2. Individual infant nutritional needs may be highly variable.
3. Gestational age and birth weight influence nutrient body stores at birth, as well as digestive, absorptive, and metabolic capabilities.
4. Estimated requirements vary for parenteral and enteral routes.
5. Day-to-day clinical status of the infant will determine nutrient requirements.
6. Consensus recommendations for nutritional needs of transitional (<2 weeks of age) preterm infants are presented in Table 13–1. A comparison of enteral intake recommendations for growing preterm infants in stable condition is presented in Table 13–2.

B. Specific recommendations.

1. Water.
   a. Requirement = Amount of water lost from insensible water loss + Fecal and urine water + Amount retained in newly synthesized tissue.
   b. Actual requirements are highly variable and are dependent on the clinical status of the infant.

Table 13–1
CONSENSUS RECOMMENDATIONS FOR NUTRITIONAL NEEDS OF TRANSITIONAL (<2 WEEKS OF AGE) PRETERM INFANTS

	Estimated Requirements (per kilogram per day)		Nutrients (per 100 kcal)
	Parental	*Enteral*	
BIRTH WEIGHT <1000 g			
Energy (kcal/kg)	35–90+	110–120	100
Protein (g)	0–3.8	3.6–3.8	3–3.6
Sodium (mg)	0–23	0–23	0–20
Chloride (mg)	0–35	0–35	0–30
Potassium (mg)	0–39	0–39	0–33
Calcium (mg)*	60–90	120–230	100–192
Phosphorus (mg)*	47–70	60–140	50–117
Magnesium (mg)	4.3–7.2	7.9–15	6.6–12.5
BIRTH WEIGHT >1000 g			
Energy (kcal/kg)	35–90+	110–120	100
Protein (g)	0–3.6	3.0–3.6	2.5–3.0
Sodium (mg)	0–23	0–23	0–20
Chloride (mg)	0–35	0–35	0–30
Potassium (mg)	0–39	0–39	0–33
Calcium (mg)	60–90	120–230	100–192
Phosphorus (mg)	47–70	60–140	50–117
Magnesium (mg)	4.3–7.2	7.9–15	6.6–12.5

*Assuming fluid intake of 120-150 mL/kg per day.
Data from Tsang, R., Lucas, A., Uauy, R., and Zlotkin, S. (Eds.): Nutritional needs of the preterm infant. Baltimore, Williams & Wilkins, 1993, Appendix, Table A.1.

Table 13–2
COMPARISON OF ENTERAL INTAKE RECOMMENDATIONS FOR GROWING PRETERM INFANTS IN STABLE CLINICAL CONDITION

Nutrients per 100 kcal*	Consensus Recommendations		AAP-CON	ESPGAN-CON
	<1000 g	*>1000 g*		
Water, mL	125–167	125–167	—	115–154
Energy, kcal	100	100	100	100
Protein, g	3.0–3.16	2.5–3.0	2.9–3.3	2.25–3.1
Carbohydrate, g			9–13	7–14
Lactose, g	3.16–9.5	3.16–9.8	—	—
Oligomers, g	0–7.0	0–7.0	—	—
Fat, g			4.5–6.0	3.6–7
Linoleic acid, g	0.44–1.7	0.44–1.7	0.4+	0.5–1.4
Linolenic acid, g	0.11–0.44	0.11–0.44		>0.055
$C_{18:2}/C_{18:3}$	>5	>5	—	5–15
Vitamin A, IU	583–1250	583–1250	75–225	270–450
With lung disease,	2250–2333	2250–2333	—	
Vitamin D, IU	125–333	125–333	270	800–1600/day
Vitamin E, IU	5–10	5–10	>1.1	0.6–10
Supplement, HM	2.9	2.9	—	—
Vitamin K, µg	6.66–8.33	6.66–8.33	4	4–15
Ascorbate, mg	15–20	15–20	35	7–40
Thiamine, µg	150–200	150–200	>40	20–250
Riboflavin, µg	200–300	200–300	>60	60–600
Pyridoxine, µg	125–175	125–175	>35	35–250
Niacin, mg	3–4	3–4	>0.25	0.8–5.0
Pantothenate, mg	1–1.5	1–1.5	>0.30	>0.3
Biotin, µg	3–5	3–5	>1.5	>1.5
Folate, µg	21–42	21–42	33	>60
Vitamin B_{12}, µg	0.25	0.25	>0.15	>0.15
Sodium, mg	38–58	38–58	48–67	23–53
Potassium, mg	65–100	65–100	66–98	90–152
Chloride, mg	59–89	59–89	—	57–89
Calcium, mg	100–192	100–192	175	70–140
Phosphorus, mg	50–117	50–117	91.5	50–87
Magnesium, mg	6.6–12.5	6.6–12.5	—	6–12
Iron, mg	1.67	1.67	1.7–2.5	1.5
Zinc, µg	833	833	>500	550–1100
Copper, µg	100–125	100–125	90	90–120
Selenium, µg	1.08–2.5	1.08–2.5	—	—
Chromium, µg	0.083–0.42	0.083–0.42	—	—
Manganese, µg	6.3	6.3	>5	1.5–7.5
Molybdenum, µg	0.25	0.25	—	—
Iodine, µg	25–50	25–50	5	10–45
Taurine, mg	3.75–7.5	3.75–7.5	—	—
Carnitine, mg	2.4	2.4	—	>1.2
Inositol, mg	27–67.5	27–67.5	—	—
Chlorine, mg	12–23.4	12–23.4	—	—

AAP-CON, American Academy of Pediatrics Committee on Nutrition; *ESPGAN-CON*, European Society of Paediatric Gastroenterology and Nutrition Committee on Nutrition of the Preterm Infant; *HM*, human milk.
  *Based on a need for 120 mg/kg per day.
  From American Academy of Pediatrics Committee on Nutrition: Pediatric Nutrition Handbook, 4th ed. Elk Grove Village, Ill., Author, 1998, p. 56. Reproduced with permission. © American Academy of Pediatrics.

   c. Minimum requirement is approximately 120–150 mL/kg per day for a growing preterm infant receiving 110–120 kcal/kg per day with enteral feedings or approximately 120–150 mL/kg per day for an infant receiving parenteral fluids (Tsang, Lucas, Uauy, and Zlotkin, 1993).
   d. Factors that increase fluid requirements include:
     (1) Abnormal fluid losses (ileostomy, colostomy, chest tubes).
     (2) Diarrhea, vomiting.

      (3) Increase in activity level.

      (4) Labile body temperature, fever, cold stress.

      (5) Low environmental humidity.

      (6) Phototherapy.

      (7) Prematurity.

      (8) Radiant warmers.

      (9) Renal dysfunction (glycosuria, acute tubular necrosis).

      (10) Third spacing.

  e. Factors that result in decreased fluid requirements include:

      (1) Birth asphyxia.

      (2) BPD.

      (3) PDA.

      (4) Postoperative status.

      (5) Congestive heart failure.

      (6) Meningitis.

      (7) Renal failure.

2. Calories.

  a. Energy intake = Energy stored + Energy expended + Energy excreted.

  b. Generally, a human milk or formula intake of 120 kcal/kg per day will meet the requirements of stable, growing preterm infants (Table 13–3). Meeting this goal requires that human milk be supplemented at least with protein, and with calories if volume is restricted. Some infants may require as much as 150–165 kcal/kg per day for catch-up growth.

  c. Parenteral requirements are about 20% less than enteral requirements, or about 80–100 kcal/kg per day.

  d. Adequate caloric intake should be assessed on the basis of appropriate daily weight gain, or 18–20 g/kg per day for preterm infants (Putet, 1993).

  e. Factors that increase caloric requirements are as follows:

      (1) Acute or chronic respiratory disease.

      (2) Fluctuations of ambient temperature outside the limits of neutral thermal range.

      (3) Hypothermia, hyperthermia.

      (4) Increased cardiac output; left-to-right shunting.

      (5) Increased muscular activity, agitation, and pain.

      (6) Infection.

      (7) Malabsorption of prematurity.

      (8) Short gut syndrome or other malabsorption syndromes.

      (9) Small for gestational age.

      (10) Periods of rapid growth.

Table 13–3
ESTIMATION OF CALORIC REQUIREMENTS FOR LBW INFANTS

Metabolic or Physical Activity	Calories Needed (kcal/kg per day)
Energy expended	40–60
Resting metabolic rate	40–50
Activity	0–5
Thermoregulation	0–5
Fecal losses	15
Specific dynamic action (energy cost of digestion and metabolism)	15
Growth	20–30
Total	90–120

Adapted from American Academy of Pediatrics Committee on Nutrition: Pediatric Nutrition Handbook, 4th ed. Elk Grove Village, Ill., Author, 1998, p. 57. Reproduced with permission. © American Academy of Pediatrics.

3. Protein.
   a. Necessary for cell growth and synthesis of enzymes and hormones.
   b. Requirement = Growth needs + Losses through skin, urine, and feces.
   c. Precise requirements are not available, and there are several formulas for estimation.
   d. Protein intake of 3–3.8 g, with protein intake being 7–12% of total caloric intake, is generally recommended (Micheli and Schutz, 1993).
   e. For proper protein utilization, 24–32 nonprotein kilocalories must be delivered for each gram of protein administered.
   f. Must consider amino acid constituents.
      (1) In addition to the eight essential amino acids necessary for cell growth, preterm infants require four conditionally essential amino acids: histidine, taurine, cysteine, and tyrosine (Blackburn and Loper, 1992; Pereira, 1995).
      (2) Preterm infants have a limited ability to use excess amino acid and, with unbalanced amino acid intake, are at risk for hyperammonemia, azotemia, metabolic acidosis, and altered plasma amino acid profiles.
      (3) Amino acid requirements for extremely preterm infants range from 2.5 to 3.5 g/kg per day, with higher amounts being used for the smallest preterm infants during active growth (Pereira, 1995).
      (4) The essential and conditionally essential amino acids are present in immature human milk and preterm-infant formulas in adequate amounts. Cysteine has poor solubility in aqueous solutions, so minimal amounts are present in commercial parenteral amino acid preparations.
   g. Whey-predominant formulas are better suited metabolically for preterm infants and are provided in preterm-infant formulas (60:40) to resemble human milk more closely. Human milk has a whey/casein ratio of 70:30, whereas the whey/casein ratio of cow's milk is 18:82 (Schanler, 1995).
   h. Adequate protein intake may not be achievable with unfortified human milk, especially if the infant is fluid restricted or very small (<1200 g).
4. Fat.
   a. Fat is a major source of energy for growing preterm infants and necessary for transport of fat-soluble vitamins.
   b. Guidelines for fat intake are as follows:
      (1) American Academy of Pediatrics Committee on Nutrition (AAP-CON, 1998) recommends 4.5–6.0 g fat per 100 kcal of enteral intake for stable, growing preterm infants. For preterm infants weighing less than 1000 g, enteral fat intake should be 3–4 g/kg per day (Pereira, 1995).
      (2) Preterm infants on fluid-restriction regimens may require higher fat content to meet caloric needs.
      (3) Intake should be approximately 35–55% of total caloric intake.
   c. Good source of energy because of high caloric content and lack of osmolality; however, not all fats are well absorbed by preterm infants.
   d. Human milk provides about 50% of energy from fat; commercial formulas provide 40–50%.
   e. Because of fatty acid composition, organization of the human fat milk globule, and presence of bile salt–stimulated lipase, the fat of human milk is more easily digested and absorbed by low birth weight infants than is fat derived from cow's milk. The lipase in human milk is heat labile and inactivated when pasteurized (63° C) (Innis, 1993). Combining fresh human milk (40%) with formula (60%) has been shown to result in an increase in fat absorption in low birth weight infants, in comparison with use of formula alone (Schanler, 1995).
   f. Medium-chain triglycerides (MCTs) are more easily absorbed than long-chain fatty acids in preterm infants; MCTs are absorbed by passive diffusion and do not require bile salts.

    g. Premature infant formulas use a combination of MCTs and shorter-chain vegetable fatty acids from vegetable oil.

    h. Linoleic acid is an essential fatty acid and should account for at least 3% of total calories (0.4+ g/100 kcal) (AAP-CON, 1998). This amount is achieved with adequate intake of human milk and commercial premature-infant formulas. Linolenic acid is also an essential fatty acid for preterm infants; recommended intake for stable, growing premature infants is 0.11–0.44 (Tsang et al., 1993).

    i. Recent research has emphasized the importance of very long chain fatty acids—arachidonic acid and docosahexaenoic acid—which are derivatives of linoleic and linolenic acids and are found in human milk but not cow's milk. These fatty acids have been associated functionally with cognition, growth, and vision (Schanler, 1995).

5. Carbohydrates.

    a. Glucose is essential for brain function.

    b. Glucose intake must be adequate to maintain serum levels greater than 40 mg/dL. Glucose can be manufactured from other carbohydrates, protein, and fats, so there is not an absolute intake requirement. The usual dose of glucose provided parenterally during the transitional neonatal period is 4–6 mg/kg per minute and can be met by 10% dextrose at infusion rates of 60 to 90 mL/kg per day (Shaffer and Weismann, 1992). Preterm infants rapidly become hypoglycemic with inadequate glucose intake. Hyperglycemia can also be a problem with extremely premature infants. Hyperglycemia contributes to hyperosmolality and may be a risk factor for intracranial hemorrhage in those infants.

    c. Carbohydrate intake should provide 35–55% of total calories. Lactose, or a combination of lactose and other sugars, is the preferred carbohydrate for enteral nutrition.

    d. Lactose is the carbohydrate in human milk and is the predominant carbohydrate in most milk-based formulas for term infants. The lactose content of human colostrum is lower than that of mature milk.

    e. Lactose may promote the growth of nonpathogenic lactobacillus, which may be somewhat protective against pathogens such as *Klebsiella, Escherichia coli,* and *Enterobacter* (Neu and Koldovsky, 1996).

    f. Low intestinal mucosal lactase activity in preterm infants may affect digestion of lactose and may result in the slow advance of feedings, especially in small infants. Concern regarding lactase deficiency should not be used to support the use of elemental formulas rather than human milk.

    g. It is uncertain whether the addition of glucose polymers facilitates better tolerance by preterm infants than 100% lactose.

    h. A combination of lactose and glucose polymers, sucrose, or other partially hydrolyzed starches is used as a carbohydrate source in many preterm infant formulas.

6. Electrolytes.

    a. Sodium, potassium, and chloride are necessary for growth and play a significant role in water and acid-base balance.

    b. Preterm infants have limited renal sodium-conservation mechanisms during the transitional neonatal period. Whether additional sodium chloride should be provided along with additional fluids and whether insensible water losses should be replaced with water and nutrients (not electrolytes), while excretion of excess extracellular fluid is permitted, remain controversial (Arant, 1993).

    c. After reduction of the extracellular fluid, loss of body weight slows and urinary excretion of sodium chloride decreases. The sodium requirement for stable, growing preterm infants is 2–4 mEq/kg per day (Pereira, 1995; Tsang et al., 1993).

     d. Factors that influence electrolyte balance include the following:

        (1) Abnormal or immature renal function.

        (2) Diuretic therapy.

        (3) Increased gastrointestinal losses from diarrhea, vomiting, or gastric suction.

        (4) Gestational age.

        (5) Sepsis.

        (6) Insensible water losses.

     e. Preterm infant formulas provide higher amounts of sodium, potassium, and chloride than term infant formulas and are generally sufficient for growing preterm infants.

     f. Preterm human milk has higher sodium and chloride levels than mature human milk (after 4 weeks), but levels may still be insufficient to meet infant needs; close monitoring of electrolyte levels is therefore warranted.

  7. Vitamins and minerals.

     a. Exact requirements of vitamins and trace minerals by preterm infants have not been established. Preterm-infant formulas provide greater amounts than term-infant formulas to prevent deficiencies, provide stores equivalent to those accumulated by a term infant, and avoid toxic effects of excess amounts (Moran and Greene, 1998; Zlotkin, Atkinson, and Lockitch, 1995).

     b. Preterm infants require more of some vitamins and minerals than term infants because of preterm infants' diminished nutrient stores at birth and the rapid growth that occurs once preterm infants are stable and well.

     c. Tables 13–4 and 13–5 provide advisable enteral intakes of vitamins and minerals, respectively, for growing preterm infants. Vitamin supplements are commonly provided to extremely premature infants because the daily volume of nutrients might not be adequate. Vitamin supplements are usually hyperosmolar and may cause feeding intolerance or diarrhea. To minimize such side effects, one can divide the dose and give it with two or more feedings (Pereira, 1995).

     d. Vitamin A (fat soluble).

        (1) Is a precursor of photosensitive pigments.

        (2) Plays a role in the following:

           (a) Enhancement of light perception.

           (b) Differentiation of epithelial tissues.

Table 13–4
RECOMMENDED MINIMAL ENTERAL INTAKE OF VITAMINS FOR PREMATURE INFANTS

Vitamin	Recommended Intake
A	583 IU/100 kcal
D	≥270 IU/d
E	>1.1 IU/100 kcal and at least 1.0 IU of linoleic acid per gram
K	4 μg/100 kcal (in addition to 1 mg at birth)
Thiamine	>40 μg/100 kcal
Riboflavin	>60 μg/100 kcal
Niacin	>250 μg/100 kcal
C	30 mg/100 kcal
B_6	>35 μg/100 kcal, or a minimum of 15 g per gram of protein
B_{12}	>0.15 μg/100 kcal, or 0.3–0.5 g/d
Folic acid	20–50 μg/d
Pantothenic acid	>300 μg/100 kcal
Biotin	>1.5 μg/100 kcal

Data from Tsang, R., Lucas, A., Uauy, R., and Zlotkin, S. (Eds.): Nutritional Needs of the Preterm Infant. Baltimore, Williams & Wilkins, 1993.

Table 13–5
RECOMMENDED MINIMAL ENTERAL INTAKE OF MINERALS FOR PREMATURE INFANTS

	Recommended Intake (µg/kg per day)	
Mineral	**Transitional Period (0–14 days)**	**Stable/Postdischarge Periods**
Copper	120	120–150
Iodine	11–27	30–60
Manganese	0.75	0.75–7.5
Zinc	500–800	1000*
Iron†		2–3 mg/kg per day
Selenium	1.3	1.3–3.0
Chromium	0.05	0.1–0.5

*Postdischarge supplement of 0.5 mg/kg per day for infants fed human milk.
†When infant is 2 months of age and when full feedings are tolerated, iron supplements are recommended. If iron supplements are started before 2 months of age, vitamin E supplements should also be given. When infant weighs more than 2000 g or when at home, 2-3 mg/kg per day is recommended supplement for breast-fed infants but usually not necessary if iron-fortified formula is used.
Data from Reifen, R.M., and Zlotkin, S.H.: Microminerals. In Tsang, R.C., Lucas, A., Uauy, R., and Zlotkin, S.H. (Eds.): Nutritional Needs of the Preterm Infant. Baltimore, Williams & Wilkins, 1993, pp. 195–207.

    (c) Support of growth.
    (d) Tissue healing.
    (e) Synthesis of protein.
(3) Is stored primarily in the liver. In certain animals, other organs, including the developing lung, are capable of storing vitamin A. It is not known whether the human developing lung is capable of vitamin A uptake and storage. Body content of vitamin A is generally low in preterm infants because of low hepatic stores.
(4) Low vitamin A levels have been found in infants with BPD. It is controversial whether sick preterm infants with BPD should receive supplemental vitamin A in amounts greater than current recommendations (Shenai, 1993).
(5) Absorption is decreased when fat intake is inadequate and when fat absorption is reduced. Absorption is increased in infants fed human milk, possibly because of the presence of a bile salt–stimulated lipase in fresh milk.
(6) Vitamin A levels need to be measured.
    (a) Less than 20 µg/dL constitutes vitamin A deficiency (normal, 40–70 µg/dL).
    (b) Levels should be monitored and supplements given as needed. Intramuscular supplementation of vitamin A at doses of 2000 U on alternate days to preterm infants with respiratory distress syndrome has been shown to reduce the incidence of BPD (Pereira, 1995). Additional research is needed to confirm these beneficial effects.
(7) Deficiency may lead to the following:
    (a) Cellular changes in the epithelial lining of the lung.
    (b) Decreased resistance to infection.
    (c) Night blindness.
    (d) Poor growth.
    (e) Xerophthalmia.
(8) Excess may lead to the following:
    (a) Signs of increased intracranial pressure.
    (b) Bone and joint pain.
    (c) Mucocutaneous lesions.

  (d) Brittle bones.
  (e) Hepatomegaly and hepatic injury.
  e. Vitamin D (fat soluble).
    (1) Facilitates bone mineralization, mainly by stimulating intestinal absorption of calcium and phosphorus.
    (2) Acts directly to mobilize calcium and phosphorus in the bone to the extracellular fluid to maintain circulating calcium levels.
    (3) Role in the development of osteopenia and rickets remains controversial.
    (4) AAP-CON (1998) recommends 270 IU of vitamin D per day for growing preterm infants.
  f. Vitamin E (fat soluble).
    (1) Contributes to stability of cell membranes by inhibiting the naturally occurring oxidation of polyunsaturated fatty acids.
    (2) Absorption is decreased in infants born at less than 32 weeks' gestational age.
    (3) Absorption is greater from human milk than from formulas (Gross, 1993).
    (4) Iron supplementation interferes with vitamin E absorption and activity. High intake of polyunsaturated fatty acids increases vitamin E requirements.
    (5) Supplementation may be used to prevent hemolytic anemia associated with prematurity.
    (6) Supplementation has been associated with an increased incidence of necrotizing enterocolitis (NEC) and intraventricular hemorrhage.
    (7) Preterm infant formulas provide a minimum of 0.7 IU per 100 kcal and at least 1 IU of vitamin E per gram of linoleic acid. How much additional supplementation is needed is unclear because these formulas exceed minimum requirements. The AAP-CON (1998) recommends further that preterm infants receive an additional oral vitamin E supplement of 5 to 25 IU/day because of limited stores at birth, poor fat absorption, and rapid postnatal growth (Gross, 1993). Infants fed human milk may require less supplementation than formula-fed infants.
  g. Vitamin K (fat soluble).
    (1) Necessary for manufacturing several clotting factors (e.g., prothrombin and factor VII).
    (2) All newborn infants, term and preterm, require 0.5–1 mg vitamin K, given intramuscularly, at birth.
    (3) Deficiency may result in hemorrhagic disease of the newborn infant (refer to Chapter 3).
  h. Calcium, phosphorus, and magnesium.
    (1) Necessary for tissue structure and function, particularly bone mineralization.
    (2) Low stores at birth make the preterm infant susceptible to rickets if adequate intakes are not provided during growth.
    (3) Calcium and phosphorus retention and absorption are interdependent.
    (4) Alkaline phosphatase levels at greater than 500 mg/dL or radiologic evidence of rickets indicates a need to increase calcium and phosphorus intake.
    (5) Calcium, phosphorus, and alkaline phosphatase levels should be monitored periodically to assess bone mineralization status. Decreased calcium and phosphorus levels or increased alkaline phosphatase levels indicate bone demineralization (Frentner, 1995).
    (6) Human milk and term-infant formulas provide inadequate amounts of calcium and phosphorus for growing preterm infants.
    (7) Human milk fortifiers (Enfamil Human Milk Fortifier and Similac

Natural Care) can supplement human milk to supply adequate amounts of calcium and phosphorus.

(8) Preterm-infant formulas (Similac Special Care and Enfamil Premature) have increased amounts of calcium, phosphorus, and magnesium and appear to be adequate for most preterm infants. Similac Neosure and Enfamil 22 provide more calories (22 calories per ounce), calcium, phosphorus, and magnesium than term-infant formulas but less than preterm-infant formulas and are designed for use after hospital discharge, until 6 months of age, in infants who need additional calories and minerals.

(9) Hypophosphatemia (serum concentration <4 mg/dL) is common in premature infants fed human milk and should be considered an early warning sign of decreased bone mineralization.

i. Folate.

(1) AAP-CON (1998) recommends a daily folate intake of 33 µg/d for growing preterm infants.

(2) Preterm infant formulas and fortified human milk contain two to three times the amount of folic acid in term infant formulas. It is not clear whether supplementation in addition to these amounts should be provided routinely to all extremely premature infants.

j. Iron.

(1) Important for synthesis of hemoglobin, myoglobin, and iron-containing enzymes.

(2) Difficult to provide extrauterine iron to achieve fetal accretion rates because of poor enteral absorption.

(3) Early physiologic anemia of prematurity is not benefited by iron therapy.

(4) Iron supplementation.

(a) AAP-CON (1998) recommends iron supplementation of 2 mg/kg per day for all preterm infants by the age of 2 months or when birth weight is doubled. Iron supplementation has been shown to reduce the incidence of iron deficiency anemia significantly at 6 and 11 months of age (Pereira, 1995).

(b) Vitamin E supplementation may be needed for premature infants receiving iron supplementation.

(c) Iron supplementation is required for infants being treated for early physiologic anemia of prematurity with erythropoietin.

k. Zinc.

(1) Plays a role in carbohydrate and energy metabolism and in protein catabolism and synthesis and is a cofactor of insulin and at least 40 enzymes. Zinc is necessary for all stages of cell growth and development.

(2) Hepatic stores are limited in the preterm infant.

(3) Absorption is enhanced by the presence of an amino acid such as histidine or cysteine and is inhibited by the presence of phytate (found in soy formula), fiber, and large amounts of dietary calcium. Zinc is better absorbed from human milk than from formula.

(4) Deficiency causes the following (Reifen and Zlotkin, 1993):

(a) Skin lesions.

(b) Anorexia.

(c) Growth failure.

(d) Decreased wound healing.

(e) Hair loss.

(f) Retarded bone age.

(g) Depressed immune function.

(5) Zinc levels should be monitored; levels less than 40 g/dL should be considered low.

Parenteral Nutrition

Parenteral nutrition (PN) is indicated for initiation of nutrition support for preterm neonates and can be used in conjunction with enteral nutrition to provide partial daily requirements for certain infants.

A. Indications for PN in the neonatal period.

1. Surgical gastrointestinal disorders (e.g., gastroschisis, tracheoesophageal fistula, malrotation, intestinal obstruction).
2. Short bowel syndrome.
3. Serious acute alimentary diseases (e.g., NEC).
4. Congenital anomalies.
5. Renal failure.
6. Special circumstances (e.g., cystic fibrosis, cardiac cachexia, hepatic failure, sepsis).
7. Birth weight less than 1500 g and gestational age less than 32 weeks.
8. Insufficient caloric or nitrogen content.
9. Severe respiratory or cardiac disease.

B. PN administration.

1. Peripheral route.
   a. Should be used to provide nutritional support when enteral intake is not possible or does not provide sufficient caloric requirements.
   b. Is less invasive than central administration, but IV access may become problematic if PN is required for several weeks or more.
   c. Requires that dextrose concentrations be limited to less than 12.5% to prevent irritation of small peripheral vessels and that protein concentration be limited to 2 g/dL.
   d. Can provide up to 80–90 kcal/kg per day with combination dextrose and lipid emulsions.
2. Central route.
   a. Dextrose concentrations are not restricted in comparison with peripheral route; therefore more adequate nutritional support may be achieved.
   b. Increased risk of the following:
      (1) Mechanical complications.
      (2) Sepsis.
      (3) Thrombosis of large vessels.
   c. Percutaneous central venous catheters are commonly being used in NICUs. They provide long-term venous access and may be placed at the bedside by advanced practice nurses or medical staff (Chathas and Paton, 1997).
   d. Surgically placed central venous catheters (i.e., Broviac or Hickman) provide long-term venous access but have risks of surgery and anesthesia; they may be more stable than percutaneous central venous catheters because of the sutured cuff.
3. General considerations for PN.
   a. Because of the lack of digestive losses and energy expenditure for food digestion in the GI tract, nutrient intakes for PN are different from those for enteral nutrition.
   b. Assessment of nutritional status and complications related to PN differ from those associated with enteral nutrition. Table 13–6 provides a suggested nutritional assessment monitoring schedule for infants receiving PN.

C. Guidelines for determining appropriate intake, compositions of available preparations, and guidelines for IV administration.

1. Calories. Parenteral requirements are about 20% less than enteral intake, or about 80–90 kcal/kg per day.

a. Caloric values must be adjusted to meet activity levels, body temperature, and degree of stress.

b. Activity and catabolic states can cause a 25–75% increase in metabolic demands.

2. Water.

a. Minimum requirement approximately 100–150 mL/kg per day.

b. Water requirement varies with gestational and postnatal age and environmental conditions, such as incubator versus radiant heat source and phototherapy. Incubators and heat shields can reduce insensible water losses, while radiant warmers and phototherapy increase these losses.

3. Nutrients (Table 13–7).

a. Protein.

   (1) Available preparations:

   (a) Pediatric crystalline amino acid solutions.

   (i) Require no further metabolism before protein utilization.

   (ii) Amount of amino acids provided ranges from 2 to 4 g/kg per day.

   (b) Amino acids (4 kcal/g).

Table 13–6
SUGGESTED MONITORING SCHEDULE FOR INFANTS RECEIVING PN

Parameter	Frequency	Purpose/Comments
Weight	Daily during acute phase to weekly	Indicator of fluid retention and adequacy of caloric intake
Length	Weekly	To assess adequacy of growth
Head circumference	Weekly	To assess adequacy of growth
Serum glucose	Variable*	Glucose tolerance; can use glucometer
Urinary glucose	Daily	To assess glucose tolerance
Serum electrolytes (and carbon dioxide)	Initially 3-4 times a week to weekly	To determine appropriateness of levels in PN
BUN and creatinine	3 times per week†	To assess renal function; to detect deficient or excessive protein intake (blood urea nitrogen and creatinine >17 : 1)
Hematocrit	Weekly	To detect anemia (possibly caused by lack of iron or vitamins)
Iron, total iron-binding capacity, reticulocyte count	As indicated	To determine cause of anemia; to evaluate response to therapy
Differential blood cell count	As indicated	If signs of infection appear
Triglycerides	4 hours after any rate increase	To assess tolerance of lipids (to determine whether they are being cleared from the serum)
Serum calcium, phosphorus, magnesium	3 times a week to weekly	To assess adequacy of intake
Alkaline phosphatase	Weekly	To detect early rickets
Liver function studies	Weekly†	To assess liver function (detect cholestasis)
Serum protein (electrophoresis for albumin/globulin and prealbumin/transferrin)	Weekly†	Indicators of protein nutrition: prealbumin has half-life of 3-4 days, making it a good choice for monitoring nutritional improvement; transferrin is not reliable in iron-deficient patients; albumin has a long half-life (14-18 days), making it slow to respond to nutritional therapy
Vitamin A	Monthly	To assess adequacy of intake
Zinc, copper	Monthly	To assess adequacy of intake

*Monitor closely while initiating PN and during glucosuria and evaluate during any interruption of PN and for 2 to 3 days after cessation of PN to determine degree of hypoglycemia.
†Before starting PN and lipids, obtain baseline values for weight, length, serum glucose, electrolytes, renal and liver function, complete blood cell count, and triglycerides.
Data from American Academy of Pediatrics Committee on Nutrition: Pediatric Nutrition Handbook, 4th ed. Elk Grove Village, Ill., Author, 1998, and Moore, M. C.: Neonatal Network, 6:33, 1987.

Table 13–7
RECOMMENDED CALORIE, CARBOHYDRATE, FAT, FLUID, AND PROTEIN INTAKE FOR PN

Component Weight	% Total Calories	Basis of Equivalent Calculation
Carbohydrates	35–55	
Fat	35–55	0.5–3 g/kg per day
Protein	7–12	3–4 g/kg per day
Kcal		80–100 kcal/kg per day
Fluid		80–150 mL/kg per day

Data from Tsang, R., Lucas, A., Uauy, R., and Zlotkin, S. (Eds.): Nutritional Needs of the Preterm Infant. Baltimore, Williams & Wilkins, 1993.

      (2) Formula for calculating amount of protein an infant is receiving: Protein dose = Weight (in kilograms) × %Amino acid/dL IV fluid × Number of 100 mL increments of IV fluid received (LeFrak-Okikawa, 1988).

  b. Fat.

      (1) Available preparations:

        (a) Supplied by soy and/or safflower oil preparations, which provide essential fatty acids.

        (b) Ten percent lipid preparations: 1.1 kcal/mL.

        (c) Twenty percent lipid preparations: 2.2 kcal/mL.

        (d) Soybean oil–based lipid emulsions: recommended over safflower oils because of potential risk of development of linolenic acid deficiency and hypertriglyceridemia with safflower oils (Pereira, 1995).

        (e) Lipid emulsions, preferably 20% (0.5–1 g/kg per day), for prevention of deficiency of essential fatty acids. For maintenance of energy balance, IV lipid, 0.5–1 g/kg per day, should be introduced as component of PN by 24–48 hours of age. That dose can be increased by 0.5–1 g/kg per day in progressive daily or alternate-day steps, as tolerated, up to 3–4 g/kg per day, based on serum triglyceride clearance (Van Aerde, Feldman, and Clandinin, 1998).

      (2) Guidelines for parenteral fat administration:

        (a) To calculate amount of fat an infant is receiving, use the following formula: Lipid dose = Milliliters of fat per day ÷ 10 or 5 ÷ Weight (in kilograms). (Note: divide by 10 if 10% preparation is used; divide by 5 if 20% preparation is used) (LeFrak-Okikawa, 1988).

        (b) Ten percent preparations may be used when IV fat administration is initiated, especially for VLBW infants. Rates of 0.15–0.2 g/kg per hour are suggested to prevent the complications associated with rapid infusion.

        (c) Lipid tolerance may be enhanced by adding 1 U heparin per milliliter of infusate (0.5 U/mL for VLBW premature infants). Heparin enhances the release of lipoprotein and hepatic lipases into the circulation (Pereira, 1995).

        (d) Twenty percent preparations are commonly used and are generally well tolerated. They are especially useful for infants requiring a great caloric intake but are fluid restricted (e.g., infants with BPD).

        (e) Reduced phospholipid concentration in 20% emulsions enhances triglyceride clearance and reduces the accumulation of cholesterol and phospholipid in low-density lipoproteins (Pereira, 1995).

  c. Carbohydrates.

      (1) Carbohydrate source: glucose monohydrate (dextrose), 3.4 kcal/g.

        (a) Dextrose preparations are made according to the infant's tolerance.

(b) Standard dextrose concentrations are available in 5% or 10% solutions (percentage: grams of dextrose per deciliter of solution). Other concentrations may be tailored to the individual needs of the infant.
  (2) Guidelines for carbohydrate administration:
      (a) Glucose infusion rates of 5–6 g/kg per day are necessary for minimal caloric intake, protein metabolism, and growth.
      (b) Dextrose concentrations may be increased by 1–2 mg/kg per minute each day (until the maximal percentage is obtained for the route being used), as long as serum glucose remains at less than 150 mg/dL and urinary glucose at less than 0.5%. The maximal glucose infusion rate is 12–14 mg/kg per minute—the rate of glucose oxidation by the liver. Higher rates increase the risk of fatty infiltration of the liver.
      (c) Insulin may be added to PN to enhance glucose tolerance in infants exhibiting hyperglycemia. The infant's glucose status must then be monitored closely (as often as every 15 minutes) until the infant's condition is stable and whenever changes in dextrose concentrations or insulin rates are made (LeFrak-Okikawa, 1988).
  d. Calcium and phosphorus.
      (1) PN preparations for infants receiving fluids of at least 120–150 mL/kg per day should contain 60–90 mg of calcium and 47–70 mg of phosphorus per kilogram per day (Tsang et al., 1993).
      (2) Because of the precipitation of minerals in parenteral fluids, it is not possible to supply the extremely premature infant with adequate amounts of parenteral calcium and phosphorus to meet in utero fetal accretion rates.
  e. Vitamins and minerals (Tables 13–8 and 13–9).

D. **Complications associated with PN administration.**

1. Potential complications associated with protein administration.
   a. Excessive protein intake is associated with metabolic disturbances (hyperammonemia, metabolic acidosis, azotemia, and hyperaminoacidemia).

Table 13–8
SUGGESTED VITAMIN DOSAGES FOR INFANTS RECEIVING PN

	Infant Weight	
Vitamin (unit/day)	<1 kg	>1 kg
C (mg)	35–50	52
A (U)	700–1500	700–2500
D (U)	40–160	40–160
B$_1$ (mg)	0.3–0.8	0.2–0.35
B$_2$ (mg)	0.4–0.9	0.15–0.2
B$_6$ (mg)	0.3–0.7	0.15–0.2
Niacin (mg)	5–12	4–6.8
Pantothenic acid (mg)	1.50	1–2
E (mg)	2–4	3.5
Biotin (µg)	6–13	5–8
Folic acid (µg)	40–90	56
B$_{12}$ (µg)	0.3–0.7	0.3
K (µg)	6–10	8–10

Data for <1 kg weight from Pereira, G.: Nutritional care of the extremely premature infant. Clinics in Perinatology, 22(1):61–75, 1995. Data for >1 kg weight from Tsang, R., Lucas, A., Uauy, R., and Zlotkin, S. (Eds.): Nutritional Needs of the Preterm Infant. Baltimore, Williams & Wilkins, 1993.

Table 13–9
SUGGESTED MINERAL INTAKE FOR INFANTS RECEIVING PN

Mineral	Amount (per kg)
Sodium	2–4 mEq
Potassium	2–4 mEq
Calcium	0.45–4 mEq
Phosphorus	0.5–2 mmol
Magnesium	0.25–1 mEq
Zinc	400 μg
Copper	20 μg
Manganese	1 μg
Chromium	0.2 μg
Selenium	3 μg

Data from the American Academy of Pediatrics Committee on Nutrition: Pediatric Nutrition Handbook, 4th ed. Elk Grove Village, Ill., American Academy of Pediatrics, 1998.

    b. Cholestasis and cholestatic jaundice (direct bilirubin >1.5 mg/dL) may occur as a result of excessive protein intake or long-term PN. Factors that may increase the risk of cholestasis and jaundice include:
        (1) Prolonged periods without enteral feeding and conditions that contribute to ineffective utilization and metabolism of protein.
        (2) Hepatitis.
        (3) GI surgery.
        (4) Viral infections (e.g., infection with cytomegalovirus).
  2. Potential complications associated with fat administration.
    a. Inadequate fat intake may lead to deficiency of essential fatty acids and may be evidenced by the following:
        (1) Dry, scaly skin.
        (2) Poor growth.
        (3) Poor platelet aggregation.
        (4) Thrombocytopenia.
        (5) Deficiencies of fat-soluble vitamins.
    b. IV lipids may be contraindicated for infants with severe hyperbilirubinemia because fatty acids compete with bilirubin for binding sites on plasma albumin.
    c. Frequent assessment of triglyceride levels is necessary for all jaundiced infants receiving IV lipids.
  3. Potential complications associated with carbohydrate administration.
    a. Hyperosmolarity.
    b. Hyperglycemia (serum glucose >150 mg/dL) or glucosuria (urinary glucose >0.5%); frequently seen in VLBW infants and infants with sepsis.
    c. Hypoglycemia resulting from insufficient glucose administration or excessive insulin administration.
  4. Additional complications associated with PN.
    a. Dehydration caused by hyperglycemia.
    b. Vitamin imbalance.
        (1) Vitamin A. In parenteral solutions, decreases significantly within 24 hours because of adherence to infusion-pump tubing and photodegradation (Blackburn and Loper, 1992; Moran and Greene, 1998).
        (2) Riboflavin. Destroyed by exposure to light; half may be lost in a 24-hour period, with greater loss during phototherapy.
    c. Inadequate calcium and phosphorus intake, leading to increased risk of rickets.
    d. Trace element deficiency.

    e. Extravasation of IV site.

    f. Infection; contributing factors:

       (1) Indwelling venous catheter.

       (2) Preterm infant's limited immunologic response to infection.

       (3) Excellent medium for bacterial and fungal growth provided by lipid preparation.

5. Measures to prevent or minimize complications associated with PN.

    a. Double-check all PN calculations and solutions before administration to patient.

    b. Use volumetric chamber for 4-hour aliquots of PN to avoid overhydration in the event of infusion-pump malfunction.

    c. Record hourly intake and assess IV site.

    d. Readjust fluid volume, dextrose concentration, protein and/or fat intake, and insulin supplementation as soon as problems are identified.

    e. If possible, PN should be decreased and enteral feedings initiated to stimulate bile production as soon as possible.

    f. Pharmacy preparation of PN under laminar air-flow hood.

    g. Filter central PN with an in-line filter.

    h. Wash hands scrupulously before handling any PN tubing or IV sites.

    i. Use aseptic technique for all dressing and tubing changes.

    j. Use opaque coverings for PN bottles and tubing to reduce vitamin A and riboflavin loss.

    k. If alkaline phosphatase levels exceed 500 mg/dL:

       (1) May need to increase further the doses of calcium and phosphorus in PN.

       (2) If calcium and phosphorus doses are maximal, supplementation with calcium and phosphorus via a separate infusion site may be necessary to supply adequate amounts of these minerals while avoiding the risk of precipitation in the PN solution.

       (3) If possible, begin enteral feedings.

Enteral Feedings: Human Milk and Commercial Formulas

A. Human milk.

1. Term infants.

    a. Human milk is the ideal food for term infants.

    b. Pooled human milk may be suitable for healthy term infants, although pasteurization will denature constituents.

2. Preterm infants.

    a. Nutritionally, unfortified human milk is inadequate to provide certain nutrients for preterm infants.

       (1) Use of pooled human milk is controversial because preterm human milk is better suited to the preterm infant's needs.

       (2) Human milk, both mature and preterm, is generally deficient in calories, protein, sodium, calcium, and phosphorus for the growing preterm infant. Preterm milk has greater protein (total nitrogen content) content for the first several weeks after birth (Schanler, 1995).

       (3) Fat, protein, and sodium content of human milk decreases during lactation.

    b. Fortified mother's milk may be the optimal food for preterm infants.

       (1) Commercially prepared human milk fortifiers (Similac Natural Care or Enfamil Human Milk Fortifier) enhance protein, calories, vitamin, and mineral content of mother's milk (Table 13–10).

Table 13–10
COMMONLY USED COMMERCIAL INFANT FORMULAS

Product/Calories Per Ounce	Manufacturer	Comments
MILK-BASED FORMULAS FOR TERM INFANTS		
Enfamil With Iron, 20	Mead Johnson	Routine feeding for infants weighing >2000 g.
Similac With Iron, 20	Ross	
Similac PM 60/40, 20	Ross	Low levels of calcium, phosphorus, sodium, potassium and chloride. Whey/casein ratio similar to that of human milk protein. Indicated for infants with renal or cardiovascular diseases who benefit from lower renal solute load. Not iron fortified.
MILK-BASED FORMULAS FOR PRETERM INFANTS		
Enfamil Premature Formula, 24	Mead Johnson	Growing LBW infant (<2000 g) feeding. Increased energy, higher concentration of whey-predominant protein, decreased lactose load, blend of medium chain triglycerides, higher concentration vitamins, minerals, and trace elements.
Similac Special Care, 24	Ross	
Similac Neosure, 22	Ross	Growing VLBW (<1500 g) and LBW infant feeding for up to first year of life, after hospital discharge. Increased energy and minerals compared with term but less than preterm infant formulas.
Enfamil, 22	Mead-Johnson	
Enfamil Human Milk Fortifier	Mead Johnson	Powdered human milk fortifier. Increases caloric, protein, and mineral content. Usual dilution: four packages of fortifier per 100 mL expressed human milk.
Similac Natural Care Human Milk Fortifier	Ross	Liquid human milk fortifier. Increases caloric, protein, and mineral content. Designed to be mixed with expressed mother's milk or fed alternatively with human milk.
SOY-BASED FORMULAS		
Isomil, 20	Ross	Recommended for term infants with IgE-mediated reaction to cow's milk protein, for those with lactase deficiency or galactosemia, and for use by vegetarians. Has been demonstrated to be nutritionally equivalent to milk-based formulas in supporting weight gain. Not recommended for preterm infants born weighing less than 1800 g.
ProSobee, 20	Mead Johnson	
Alsoy, 20	Carnation	
I-Soyalac, 20	LomaLinda	
PROTEIN HYDROLYSATE–BASED FORMULAS		
Pregestimil, 20 and 24	Mead Johnson	Indicated for use in infants with allergy to cow's milk and soy protein and for those with malabsorption caused by gastrointestinal or hepatobiliary disease. Protein, fat, and carbohydrate modified. Iron fortified. Available in powder form for easy caloric concentration or as "ready to feed."
Alimentum, 20	Ross	Complete elemental formula for infants. Protein, fat, and carbohydrate modified (See Pregestimil, above).
Nutramigen, 20	Mead Johnson	Protein-modified, lactose-free formula. Indicated for protein allergy or sensitivity and for severe or persistent diarrhea. Iron fortified. Available in powder or as "ready to feed." Generally not used for preterm infants.

Data from American Academy of Pediatrics Committee on Nutrition: Pediatric Nutrition Handbook, 4th ed. Elk Grove Village, Ill., Author, 1998.

    (2) Premature-infant formulas can also be mixed with human milk as a means of nutrient fortification.

    (3) To minimize fat losses from adherence to infusion tubing, use a short length of tubing and position the syringe upright. The fat will rise to the top of the syringe and be infused first.

3. Advantages of human milk (over formula).

    a. Host resistance factors and anti-infective properties.

    b. Enhanced fat, amino acid, and carbohydrate absorption and digestion compared with cow's milk formula.

    c. Improved gastric emptying with human milk, along with many factors that may stimulate GI growth and motility and enhance maturation of the GI tract.

    d. Very long chain fatty acids, which may be important for cognition, growth and vision.

    e. Increased absorption of zinc and iron.

    f. Low renal solute load.

    g. Optimal distribution of calories for term infants: 7% provided as protein, 55% as fat, and 38% as carbohydrate.

    h. Presence of thyroid hormones, which may delay onset of hypothyroidism.

i. Maternal involvement in care of infant.
j. Enteromammary immune system. The mother produces secretory IgA antibody after exposure to foreign antigens and is stimulated to make specific antibodies that are then delivered in her milk, which may improve host defenses in her preterm infant in the NICU (Schanler, 1995). Skin-to-skin contact between mother and infant may enhance this activity.

4. Disadvantages of human milk (compared with formula).
   a. Risk of transmission of infection.
   b. Deficient in protein, calcium, phosphorus, and some vitamins for the growing premature infant.
   c. Higher risk of contamination by pathogenic bacteria during artificial expression, collection, and storage of milk.

5. Establishment and maintenance of adequate milk supply.
   a. Most mothers of preterm or acutely ill infants must establish lactation by expressing milk with a breast pump for several weeks to several months before their infants are able to nurse.
   b. Nurses can play a key role in helping mothers successfully initiate and maintain an adequate supply of milk for their infants.
      (1) A lactation specialist or a breast-feeding support and education group, composed of nurses, physicians, and dietitians, can provide consistent, up-to-date educational and clinical information to staff and families.
      (2) Mothers often need help with obtaining an electric pump for home use, learning how to use the pump, and learning how to collect and store the breast milk. Additionally, mothers need a great deal of ongoing emotional support and follow-up.
      (3) Institutional standards of care for all mothers who wish to breast-feed need to be established.
      (4) The significant benefits of human milk for preterm infants warrants encouraging and actively supporting mothers to pump and provide milk for their infants (Schanler, 1995).

B. Commercially prepared formulas (Table 13–10).

1. Recommendations and standards for commercially prepared formulas were first developed in the 1940s by the U.S. Food and Drug Administration.
2. AAP-CON developed a recommended range of nutrient composition for infant formulas.
3. In 1980 the U.S. Congress passed the Infant Formula Act, which codified the recommendations of AAP-CON and required that all commercially prepared infant formulas meet these standards. The standards were revised in 1986 (AAP-CON, 1998).
4. Formulas can be classified as milk based, soy based, or elemental (i.e., protein, fat, or carbohydrate modified).
   a. Milk-based formulas.
      (1) Appropriate for most infants.
      (2) Term infant formulas, designed to approximate micronutrient content of human milk.
      (3) Have been demonstrated to be equal to human milk in promoting rapid growth during first 6 months of life.
      (4) Preterm infant formulas.
         (a) Provide added calories, protein, vitamins, and minerals to meet the needs of growing low birth weight infants.
         (b) Modifications in fat, protein, and carbohydrate sources enhance the digestibility and absorption of nutrients for infants with immature GI function (Ernst and Gross, 1998).
            (i) Fat: MCTs (25–50%), with vegetable oils.

        (ii) Protein: whey 60%, casein 40%, nonfat cow's milk, and demineralized whey.

        (iii) Carbohydrate: reduced amount of lactose (40–50%) compared with term formulas; glucose polymers (corn syrup solids or hydrolyzed cornstarch) to maintain low osmolality.

  b. Soy-based formulas.

    (1) Lactose free.

    (2) Appropriate for infants with:

      (a) Lactose intolerance.

      (b) Galactosemia.

      (c) IgE-mediated reaction to cow's milk protein.

      (d) Vegetarian diet.

  c. Elemental formulas. Appropriate for infants with:

    (1) Protein (cow's milk and soy) allergy/intolerance.

    (2) Fat malabsorption.

Enteral Feeding Methods

Enteral feedings are achieved via several routes, including oral, nasogastric tube, orogastric tube, and, less commonly, transpyloric tube. The infant's gestational age, clinical condition, and ability to feed orally are factors used to determine the method of enteral feeding (AAP-CON, 1998).

A. **Minimal enteral feedings or trophic feedings** (before 2 weeks of age) have significant long-term advantages for preterm infants (Berseth, 1995). Minimal enteral or trophic feedings are tube feedings given simultaneously with PN. PN supplies the majority of the infant's nutrient intake while the small-volume enteral feedings stimulate growth and maturation of the gastrointestinal tract. As such, minimal enteral feedings are used not to provide nutrition but to encourage functional development of the gut. Minimal enteral feedings varying from 0.1 to 24 mL/kg per day result in a shorter time required to achieve full enteral nutrition and in a lower incidence of feeding intolerance (Berseth, 1995; Pereira, 1995; Premji, 1998).

1. Promotion of gut mucosal development.
2. Stimulation of intestinal motor activity.
3. Increased secretion of GI hormones and peptides.
4. Colonization of the gut with normal flora. Normal flora reduce the possibility of translocation of pathogenic bacteria and resulting infection. Human milk stimulates colonization with lactobacilli and *Bifidobacterium,* which limits colonization by other pathogenic organisms.
5. Improvement in metabolic status.
6. Reduction in the liver enzyme abnormalities associated with PN methods. Decreases the incidence of cholestasis and lowers serum bilirubin and alkaline phosphatase levels.

B. **When to initiate feedings and what method to use are controversial issues.** Several criteria that are applied in making feeding decisions are as follows:

1. Initiation of enteral feedings is generally withheld for 3–5 days after severe perinatal asphyxia, as a precaution against NEC (Pereira, 1995).
2. Episodes of apnea and bradycardia are not necessarily contraindications for enteral feedings, but feedings may need to be postponed or withheld if apnea-bradycardia and/or desaturation episodes become acutely severe or frequent.
3. GI peristalsis must be confirmed and assessed by auscultating bowel sounds, monitoring stooling patterns, and measuring abdominal girth.
4. GI perfusion is decreased with PDA. Feedings may be postponed until PDA is closed.

C. **Oral feedings are initiated after careful assessment.**

1. Indications for oral feedings. Nurses often have input into assessing readiness for oral feedings (Kinneer and Beachy, 1994). How to assess readiness systematically has not been determined, however, and not all nurseries have specific feeding policies (Kinneer and Beachy, 1994; Siddell and Froman, 1994). Additionally, research has demonstrated differences in terms of successful breast-feeding versus bottle feeding, with competency in breast-feeding occurring at a younger postconceptional age than in bottle feeding (Mathew and Bhatia, 1989; Meier, deMonterice, Crichton, and Mangurten, 1993). Consequently there is great variation in oral feeding practices across the United States. Gestational age and weight are traditional criteria used to determine readiness for oral feedings, with behavioral cues more recently included as criteria. One published care map includes evaluation of oral motor readiness at 32–34 weeks' postconceptional age (Tobin, Sabatte, Sandhu, and Penafiel, 1998).

   a. Infant should be free of signs and/or symptoms of respiratory distress (e.g., respiratory rate <60 breaths per minute; blood gas values within normal limits); clinicians may modify these criteria for infants with chronic lung disease.

   b. Infant demonstrates suck-swallow-breathe coordination with an intact gag reflex (Shaker, 1990). Sucking and swallowing appear to be coordinated by approximately 32–34 weeks' gestation, but the ability to suck, swallow, and breathe is not well coordinated until an infant reaches 37 weeks' gestation (Bu'Lock, Woolridge, and Baum, 1990). All infants need to be assessed individually.

   c. Neonatal behavioral profile that is predictive of oral feeding success does not exist; however, assessment of infant behavioral cues and status and provision of individualized developmental care have been demonstrated to facilitate the transition to oral feeding (Als et al., 1994; Anderson et al., 1990; McCain, 1995). Infant sucking behaviors, such as on fingers and pacifiers, are also reportedly used by nurses to assess readiness for oral feeding (Siddell and Froman, 1994).

2. Oral feeding routine.

   a. Oral feedings are the feeding method of choice for most infants born at greater than 34 weeks' gestation.

   b. A healthy infant born at more than 34 weeks' gestation may have feedings initiated as soon after birth as indicated. Factors to be considered include infant behavior, maternal preference for breast-feeding or bottle feeding, and results of hypoglycemia screening of infants who are small or large for gestational age or whose mothers are diabetic.

   c. For infants born at 32–34 weeks' gestation and/or infants who are in transition from gastric gavage (bolus) feeding:

      (1) Feedings should be offered as oral feedings in a progressive fashion; initially, one to three oral feedings per day (the remainder by gavage), with a slow progression as tolerated by the infant.

      (2) Careful monitoring must take place during feedings to ensure safe intake without complications of aspiration, desaturation (or increased requirement for fractional inspired oxygen), apnea, and bradycardia. Such complications have been reported to occur less frequently during breast-feeding than bottle feeding (Meier and Pugh, 1985; Meier et al., 1993).

3. Advantages of oral feeding.

   a. Facilitates the infant's total digestive capacity.

   b. Allows the infant to self-regulate his or her feeding.

   c. Social behavior states of infants are promoted, especially when there is parental involvement.

    d. Complications of indwelling feeding tubes (e.g., bacterial inoculation, perforation) are avoided.

    e. Parents are not forced to adapt to an invasive care routine in the home setting.

4. Disadvantages of oral feeding.

    a. May be associated with an exaggerated vagal response in preterm infants who are in transition from gavage to bottle feedings.

    b. Increased risk of aspiration in infants who do not coordinate sucking, swallowing, and breathing during oral feeding.

5. Disadvantage of bottle feeding: greater decrease in infant oxygenation during and after feeding, in comparison with breast-feeding (Meier, 1988; Meier and Anderson, 1987).

6. Technique for putting preterm infants to breast.

    a. Recent studies have questioned the practice of postponing breast-feeding until bottle feeding is well established (Meier, 1988; Meier, 1990; Meier and Anderson, 1987; Meier and Pugh, 1985).

        (1) Preterm infants have been able to breast-feed successfully as early as 32 weeks' gestation and may establish mature suck-swallow-breathe coordination earlier with breast-feeding than with bottle feeding (Meier, 1991).

        (2) Breast-feeding may be less physiologically stressful to preterm infants than bottle feeding (Meier, 1988; Meier and Anderson, 1987). This may be related to the intermittent nature of breast-feeding, which permits an intermittent sucking pattern and better regulation of breathing in the preterm infant (Shiao, 1997).

    b. Test-weighing of infants (before and after breast-feeding) with an electronic scale has been shown to be a reliable method of determining infant intake of human milk (Meier et al., 1990).

D. Gavage feedings.

1. Enteral feeding of infants born at less than 32 weeks' gestation and/or infants who are unable to feed orally with safety.

2. Orogastric versus nasogastric gavage feedings. Four studies suggest that the use of indwelling nasogastric tubes results in respiratory compromise in VLBW preterm infants (Greenspan et al., 1990; Shiao, 1997; Shiao et al., 1995; Van Someren et al., 1984). Shiao et al. (1995) reported lower minute ventilation and tidal volume with the tube in place, with lower oxygen saturation, pulse rate, and less forceful sucking during attempts at oral feedings with the tube in place. The nasal route is easier to secure, however, which may decrease the risk of tube displacement and the potential for aspiration.

3. PN, if necessary, to supplement enteral intake when feedings are being initiated.

4. Intermittent intragastric gavage feeding routine.

    a. A size 5–8.0F feeding tube is inserted by a standard measuring technique: from the nose to the ear to the lower end of the sternum and adding 1 cm, or from the ear to the nose to a point midway between the xiphoid process and the umbilicus (Weibley et al., 1987). Orogastric tube measurement is from the mouth to the ear to the lower end of the sternum. Size 5F is desirable for nasally placed tubes (Lefrak-Okikawa and Meier, 1993).

    b. The tube should be secured in place with tape.

    c. Proper placement should be assessed after insertion and before each feeding by aspirating stomach contents.

    d. A polyvinylchloride tube may be left in place for 1 day or may be removed after each feeding, depending on clinical preferences. (Because frequent insertion of tubes may cause mucosal trauma and is stressful for infants, the use of an indwelling tube is recommended.) Tubes made of a soft, pliable plastic (Silastic) or polyurethane do not harden with time and may be left in place for several weeks to months, but it is slightly more difficult to secure them with tape because the outer surface is slippery.

e. Most nurses check for residual before each feeding; however, practice regarding refeeding or not refeeding is inconsistent (Hill and Rath, 1993; Hodges and Vincent, 1993). If the residuals are routinely discarded, monitor the infant for signs and symptoms of electrolyte imbalance and metabolic complications (Premji, 1998).

f. Administer feedings by gravity within 15–30 minutes; gravity allows for a natural "burp" through the tube and avoids direct, forceful pressure into the GI tract.

g. During a feeding the infant should be closely observed for intolerance and complications (e.g., oxygen desaturation, emesis, bradycardia, apnea).

h. Nonnutritive sucking on a pacifier should be offered during the feeding (Bernbaum, Pereira, Watkins, and Peckham, 1983; Measel and Anderson, 1979).

i. After a feeding the tube should be cleared with air or sterile water and then capped off to air. A tube that is to be removed after each feeding is removed by pinching it off and withdrawing it quickly.

j. After a feeding the infant should be burped and then placed in a bed with the head elevated at a 30-degree angle.

5. Indications for continuous gavage feedings.

a. VLBW infants whose gastric capacity is limited, infants receiving minimal enteral feedings, and infants who require a steady influx of glucose (e.g., infant with severe hypoglycemia and diabetic mother).

b. Infants with chronic lung disease, minimal oxygen reserve, or apnea.

c. Infants with endotracheal tube in place.

d. Infants with malabsorptive syndromes (e.g., short bowel syndrome, post-NEC, neonatal abstinence syndrome).

e. Intractable gastroesophageal reflux.

6. Continuous nasogastric feeding routine.

a. See previous discussion in section 4, "Intermittent intragastric gavage feeding routine," items a through f.

b. A 4-hour feeding volume should be aseptically prepared and purged through the appropriate infusion-pump tubing. (Syringe infusion pumps are recommended because of their low priming volume and low cost.) Nurses must be vigilant in avoiding inadvertent infusion into an IV site.

c. For human milk feedings, infusion-pump tubing should be changed every 4 hours (i.e., with each 4-hour feeding volume setup) to eliminate exponential bacterial growth in expressed mother's milk (Lefrak-Okikawa and Meier, 1993; Lemons et al., 1983; Meier and Brown, 1996). Placing the pump so that the syringe is vertical, with the tubing coming from the top and below level of the infant, will facilitate improved fat delivery because fat rises to the surface of the milk (Schanler, 1995).

d. After insertion, taping, and assessment for proper placement, the infant's feeding tube is connected to the infusion-pump tubing.

e. The infusion pump is programmed to deliver the appropriate volume to the infant at the appropriate rate.

f. Hourly enteral feeding intake should be recorded.

g. Assess every 2–4 hours (Norris and Steinhorn, 1994):

(1) Gastric residuals. Up to 2–3 hours of infusion volume may be normal if there are no other signs of feeding intolerance.

(2) Abdominal girth.

(3) Bowel sounds. Hyperactive bowel sounds may indicate intolerance.

(4) Infant's behavior. Agitation may indicate abdominal discomfort.

7. Advantages of gavage feedings. Infants who are unable to feed orally with safety are given the benefits of enteral nutrition (e.g., stimulation of bile flow and feeding-induced hormones, improved weight gain).
8. Disadvantages of gavage feedings.
   a. Possible bacterial inoculation of the GI tract via feeding tube and milk.
   b. Potential risks associated with improper placement of feeding tube.
   c. No possibility of self-regulated feeding.
   d. Limited parental involvement in some nursery settings.
9. Advantages of continuous (vs intermittent) gavage feedings.
   a. Better control of fluid and caloric administration.
   b. Possibly more tolerable for VLBW infants or for infants who have had GI injury or surgery.
10. Disadvantages of continuous (vs intermittent) gavage feedings.
    a. Higher risk of aspiration when infant is unattended.
    b. Gastric readiness for bolus feedings not promoted (i.e., stomach capacity remains small).
    c. Alteration of enteric gut hormone secretion because cyclic surges in gut hormones are not accommodated.
11. Disadvantages of intermittent bolus gavage feedings.
    a. Decreased oxygenation during feeding (Herrell, Martin, and Fanaroff, 1980).
    b. Impaired pulmonary function after feeding (Blondheim, Abbasi, Fox, and Bhuthani, 1993).
    c. Decreased mean cerebral blood flow velocity (Nelle, Hoecker, and Linderkamp, 1997).
12. Note of caution: Infants must be observed individually for subtle physiologic changes during feedings.

E. Transpyloric feedings.

1. Not recommended for routine use because feedings bypass the stomach and may result in fat malabsorption (Pereira, 1995).
2. Recommended for infants who are at great risk of aspiration (e.g., infants with gastroesophageal reflux, those receiving nasal continuous positive airway pressure). Risk is minimized because the end of the tube is located beyond the pyloric sphincter.
3. Transpyloric feeding routine.
   a. Nasojejunal tube (Silastic or polyurethane) is inserted by using a standard measuring technique (i.e., from the tip of the infant's nose to the knee).
   b. Placement is assessed by checking pH of aspirated fluid (pH of 5–7 indicates transpyloric placement). X-ray confirmation may also be indicated (Hill and Rath, 1993).
   c. An orogastric feeding tube is inserted before the feeding for assessment of gastric residuals. The presence of gastric residuals indicates decreased or reduced intestinal motility.
   d. Infusion pump and tubing should be prepared and connected to the feeding tube as outlined previously in section D, "Gavage feedings," subsection 4, "Intermittent intragastric gavage feeding routine." Transpyloric feedings are administered only continuously and deliver a small volume to the narrow lumen of the duodenum or jejunum (AAP-CON, 1998).
4. Advantage of transpyloric (vs gastric gavage) feedings: less chance of aspiration because feedings are administered below the pyloric sphincter.
5. Disadvantages of transpyloric (vs gastric) feedings.
   a. Increased risk of intestinal perforation from the tubing, although this risk is reduced with the use of silicone tubes, which are soft (AAP-CON, 1998; Hill and Rath, 1993).

    b. May require tube verification by x-ray examination, as well as increased nursing time to place the tube; both are costly.

    c. May induce symptoms of fat malabsorption (i.e., frequent stooling and increased excretion of fat and potassium) because the stomach enzymes are not able to aid in the digestive process.

E. **Gastrostomy feedings.**

1. Indications for gastrostomy feedings.
   a. Congenital anomalies of the GI tract requiring surgical intervention.
   b. Inability to suck and swallow (e.g., because of severe neurologic insult).
   c. Need for long-term gavage feedings.
2. Gastrostomy feeding routine.
   a. Residuals are assessed before each feeding by unclamping and lowering the gastrostomy tube or by aspirating gastric contents.
   b. Feedings are administered by gravity for 15–30 minutes or may be delivered by continuous drip.
   c. Tube should be cleared with water or air after feeding is finished.
   d. Tube may be left unclamped after feedings at a level of 10–12 cm above the patient for "burping" or clamped after feeding, depending on infant's tolerance and comfort.
   e. Tube migration should be evaluated with any sign of feeding intolerance.
   f. Gastrostomy site should be assessed regularly for leakage around the tube.
3. Advantages of gastrostomy feedings.
   a. Possibility of enteral feedings if oral or gavage routes are not feasible (e.g., esophageal atresia).
   b. More comfortable feeding method than gavage feedings for infants with long-term oral feeding problems.
4. Disadvantages of gastrostomy feedings.
   a. Infant may not be provided with the opportunity to develop suck-swallow-breathe coordination and oral motor development. Nonnutritive sucking and introduction of oral feedings as indicated permits development.
   b. See previous discussion in section D, Gavage feedings, subsection 8, Disadvantages of gavage feedings, items a through d.

Nutritional Assessment

A. **Anthropometric measurements.**

1. Monitor at following intervals:
   a. Weight: daily during acute phase, unless condition is too medically unstable. Infant may be weighed less frequently toward end of hospitalization.
   b. Length and head circumference: weekly.
2. Plot weight, head circumference, and length on growth curves weekly.
3. Monitor intake.
   a. Fluid, protein, and caloric intake should be calculated daily.
   b. Need for vitamin and mineral supplements should be assessed at least weekly.
   c. Laboratory values should be monitored at regular intervals (Merenstein and Gardner, 1998). Growing preterm infants may require weekly measurement of electrolytes, calcium, phosphorus, total protein, albumin, and hemoglobin, and twice-monthly measurement of alkaline phosphatase activity. (See Table 13–6 for suggested laboratory monitoring while the infant is receiving PN.)

B. **Feeding tolerance.**

1. Premature infants are at risk of having a variety of problems related to enteral

feedings as a result of the physiologic limitations of the preterm infant's GI tract (see Anatomy and Physiology of the Preterm Infant's Gastrointestinal Tract at the beginning of this chapter).

2. During the initiation of feedings and until full feedings are maintained and well tolerated, the nurse should assess the following before each feeding or every 2–4 hours during continuous feedings:
   a. Presence of bowel sounds.
   b. Correct placement of gastric or transpyloric tube, if present (see previous sections on gavage and transpyloric feeding methods).
   c. Gastric residuals.
   d. Abdominal girth measurement: compare with previous measurements.
   e. Observation of distended bowel loops on abdominal surface.
3. Frequency, amount, and consistency of stools must be noted with each stool and documented.
   a. Slow GI motility may lead to constipation and result in gastric distention, gastric residual, and possibly vomiting.
   b. Glycerine suppositories may be needed to facilitate stooling.
4. All stools should be checked for occult blood and reducing substance once feedings are started.
   a. If result of test for occult blood is positive, further evaluation is needed. Occult blood may be present if maternal blood was swallowed, if meconium stools are still being passed, after esophageal or gastric irritation from feeding tubes, and if infant has rectal fissures.
   b. Reducing substance in stools may signify carbohydrate malabsorption but may also be a normal finding in infants who are breast fed.
      (1) Results of tests for reducing substance are accurate only when fresh stool is used, because bacteria in stool decrease the sugar content within minutes.
      (2) Carbohydrate malabsorption has been detected in infants with NEC and may represent an early predictor of the infant's risk of NEC.
         (a) In tests for reducing substances with a Clinitest tablet, a finding of 3+ for three consecutive stools is significant (LaGamma and Browne, 1994).
         (b) In the absence of significant indicators of NEC, a reduction in the concentration of carbohydrate or in feeding volumes may alleviate the problem until GI function matures.

Nursing Interventions to Facilitate Tolerance of Enteral Feedings

A. Nonnutritive sucking during gavage feedings (Medoff-Cooper and Ray, 1995).

1. May accelerate maturation of the sucking reflex and facilitate more rapid transition from gavage to oral feedings.
2. May improve weight gain.
3. Lessens behavioral distress caused by stressors (DiPietro, Cusson, Caughy, and Fox, 1994).
4. Results in pleasurable facial and oral stimulation (e.g., firm facial stroking during bathing and after tube changes can help to decrease oral defensiveness) (Cox, 1997).

B. Position of infant during and after feedings (Blackburn and Loper, 1992).

1. Prone or side-lying position lessens gastric emptying time and decreases the chance of regurgitation and aspiration.

2. Position achieved by elevating the head of the bed lessens gastric emptying time.

C. **Flexed, semi-upright position of infant during oral or gavage feedings (Blackburn and Loper, 1992).**

1. Promotes flexed posture.
2. Encourages social interaction.
3. Decreases the chance of regurgitation and aspiration.

D. **Reduction in both stress and stimulation before or during feedings.**

1. Reduces fluctuations in oxygenation, which may interfere with GI perfusion and function.
2. Promotes infant behavior conducive to social interaction.

REFERENCES

Als, H., Lawhon, G., Duffy, F., et al.: Individualized developmental care for the very low-birth-weight preterm infant: Medical and neurofunctional effects. JAMA, 272:853–858, 1994.

American Academy of Pediatrics Committee on Nutrition: Vitamin and mineral supplement needs in normal children in the United States. Pediatrics, 66:1015–1012, 1980.

American Academy of Pediatrics Committee on Nutrition: Nutritional needs of low-birth-weight infants. Pediatrics, 75:976–986, 1985.

American Academy of Pediatrics Committee on Nutrition: Pediatric Nutrition Handbook, 4th ed. Elk Grove Village, Ill.: The Academy, 1998.

Anderson, G.C., Behnke, M., Gill, N.E., et al.: Self-regulatory gavage to bottle feeding for preterm infants: Effect on behavioral state, energy expenditure, and weight gain. In Funk, S.G., Tornquist, E.M., Champagne, M.T., et al. (Eds.): Key Aspects of Recovery: Nutrition, Rest, and Mobility. New York: Springer, 1990, pp. 83–97.

Arant, B.S.: Sodium chloride and potassium. In Tsang, R.C., Lucas, A., Uauy, R., and Zlotkin, S. (Eds.): Nutritional Needs of the Preterm Infant: Scientific Basis and Practical Guidelines. Baltimore, Williams & Wilkins, 1993, pp. 157–175.

Bernbaum, J.C., Pereira, G.R., Watkins, J.B., and Peckham, G.: Nonnutritive sucking during gavage feeding enhances growth and maturation in preterm infants. Pediatrics, 71:41–45, 1983.

Berseth, C. Minimal enteral feedings. Clin. Perinatol., 22:195–205, 1995.

Berseth, C. Gastrointestinal motility in the neonate. Clin. Perinatol., 23:179–190, 1996.

Blackburn, S., and Loper, D.: Maternal, Fetal, and Neonatal Physiology: A Clinical Perspective. Philadelphia, W.B. Saunders, 1992.

Blondheim, O., Abbasi, S., Fox, W., and Bhuthani, V.: Effect of enteral gavage feeding rate on pulmonary functions of very low birth weight infants. J. Pediatr., 122:751–755, 1993.

Bu'Lock, F., Woolridge, M.W., and Baum, J.D.: Development of coordination of sucking, swallowing and breathing: Ultrasound study of term and preterm infants. Dev. Med. Child Neurol., 32:669–678, 1990.

Carver, J.D., and Barness, L.A.: Trophic factors for the gastrointestinal tract. Clin. Perinatol., 23:265–285, 1996.

Chathas, M.K., and Paton, J.B.: Meeting the special nutritional needs of sick infants with a percutaneous central venous catheter quality assurance program. J. Perinatal and Neonatal Nurs., 10(4):72–87, 1997.

Cox, J.H.: Bronchopulmonary dysplasia. In J. Cox (Ed.): Nutrition Manual for At-Risk Infants and Toddlers. Chicago, Ill., Precept Press, 1997, pp. 158–166.

DeBear, K.: Sham feeding: Another kind of nourishment. Am. J. Nurs., 10:1142–1143, 1986.

DiPietro, J., Cusson, R., Caughy, M., and Fox, N.: Behavioral and physiologic effects of nonnutritive sucking during gavage feeding in preterm infants. Pediatr. Res., 36:207–214, 1994.

Ernst, J., and Gross, S.: Types and methods of feeding for infants. In Polin, R., and Fox, W. (Eds.): Fetal and Neonatal Physiology, 2nd ed. Philadelphia, W.B. Saunders, 1998, pp. 363–383.

Frentner, S.: Metabolic bone disease. Central Lines, 11:1, 4, 16, 1995.

Greenspan, J., Wolfson, M., Holt, W., and Shaffer, T.: Neonatal gastric intubation: Differential respiratory effects between nasogastric and orogastric tubes. Pediatr. Pulmonol. 8:254–258, 1990.

Gross, S.: Vitamin E. In Tsang, R.C., Lucas, A., Uauy, R., and Zlotkin, S. (Eds.): Nutritional Needs of the Preterm Infant: Scientific Basis and Practical Guidelines. Baltimore, Williams & Wilkins, 1993, pp. 101–109.

Hamosh, M.: Digestion in the newborn. Clin. Perinatol., 23:191–209, 1996.

Herrell, N., Martin, R.J., and Fanaroff, A.: Arterial oxygen tension during nasogastric feeding in the preterm infant. J. Pediatr., 96:914–916, 1980.

Hill, A., and Rath, L.: The care and feeding of the low-birth-weight infant. J. Perinatal Neonatal Nurs., 6:56–68, 1993.

Hodges, C., and Vincent, P.A.: Why do NICU nurses not refeed gastric residuals prior to feeding by gavage? Neonatal Network, 12(8):37–40, 1993.

Infant Health and Development Program: Enhancing the outcomes of low-birthweight, premature infants. JAMA, 263:3035–3042, 1990.

Innis, S.: Fat. In Tsang, R.C., Lucas, A., Uauy, R., and Zlotkin, S. (Eds.): Nutritional Needs of the Preterm Infant: Scientific Basis and Practical Guidelines. Baltimore, Williams & Wilkins, 1993, pp. 65–86.

Kinneer, M., and Beachy, P.: Nipple feeding premature infants in the neonatal intensive-care unit. J. Obstet. Gynecol. Neonatal Nurs., 23(2):105–112, 1994.

LaGamma, E.F., and Browne, L.E.: Feeding practices for infants weighing less than 1500 g at birth and the pathogenesis of necrotizing enterocolitis. Clin. Perinatol., 21(2):271–306, 1994.

Lefrak-Okikawa, L.: Nutritional management of the very low birth weight infant. J. Perinatal Neonatal Nurs., 2(1):66–77, 1988.

Lefrak-Okikawa, L., and Meier, P.: Nutrition: Physiologic basis of metabolism and management of enteral and parenteral nutrition. In Kenner, C., Brueggemeyer, A., and Gunderson, L. (Eds.): Comprehensive Neonatal Nursing. Philadelphia, W.B. Saunders, 1993, pp. 414–433.

Lemons, P.M., Miller, K., Eitzen, H., et al.: Bacterial growth in human milk during continuous feeding. Am. J. Perinatol., 1:76–80, 1983.

Mathew, O.P., and Bhatia, J.: Sucking and breathing patterns during breast- and bottle-feeding in term neonates. J. Dis. Child., 143:588–592, 1989.

McCain, G.C.: Promotion of preterm infant nipple feeding with nonnutritive sucking. J. Pediatr. Nurs., 10(1):3–8, 1995.

Measel, C.P., and Anderson, G.C.: Nonnutritive sucking during tube feedings: Effect on clinical course in premature infants. J. Obstet. Gynecol. Neonatal Nurs., 8:265–272, 1979.

Medoff-Cooper, B., and Ray, W.: Neonatal sucking behaviors: State of the science. Image, 27(3):195–200, 1995.

Meier, P.: Bottle and breastfeeding: Effects on transcutaneous oxygen pressure and temperature in preterm infants. Nurs. Res., 37:36–41, 1988.

Meier, P.: Nursing management of breastfeeding for preterm infants. In Funk, S.G., Tornquist, E.M., Champagne, M.T., et al.: (Eds.): Key Aspects of Recovery: Nutrition, Rest, and Mobility. New York, Springer, 1990.

Meier, P.: Breast feeding the premature infant. Clinical Update '91: Gastrointestinal Dysfunction. Denver, Conference of the National Association of Neonatal Nurses, 1991.

Meier, P., and Anderson, G.C.: Responses to bottle and breast feeding in small preterm infants: A report of five cases. Am. J. Maternal-Child Nurs., 12:97–105, 1987.

Meier, P., and Brown, L.: State of the science: Breastfeeding for mothers and low birth weight infants. Nurs. Clin. North Am., 31:351–365, 1996.

Meier, P., deMonterice, D., Crichton, C., and Mangurten, H. Suck-breath patterning during breast and bottle feeding for preterm infants. Symposium presentation in Medoff-Cooper, B. (Chair): Toward an objective measure of feeding readiness in preterm infants. Proceedings of ANA Council of Nurse Researchers: 1993 Scientific Session (p. 462). Washington, D.C., American Nurses Association, 1993.

Meier, P.P., Lysakowski, T.Y., Engstrom, J.L., et al.: The accuracy of test-weighing for preterm infants. J. Pediatr. Gastroenterol. Nutr., 10:62–65, 1990.

Meier, P., and Pugh, E.J.: Breastfeeding behavior of small preterm infants. Am. J. Maternal-Child Nurs., 10:396–401, 1985.

Merenstein, G., and Gardner, S.: Neonatal nutrition. In Handbook of Neonatal Intensive Care, 4th ed. St. Louis, Mosby, 1998.

Micheli, J.-L., and Schutz, Y.: Protein. In Tsang, R.C., Lucas, A., Uauy, R., and Zlotkin, S. (Eds.): Nutritional Needs of the Preterm Infant: Scientific Basis and Practical Guidelines. Baltimore, Williams & Wilkins, 1993, pp. 29–46.

Moran, J.R., and Greene, H.L.: Vitamin requirements. In Polin, R., and Fox, W. (Eds.): Fetal and Neonatal Physiology, 2nd ed. Philadelphia, W.B. Saunders, 1998, pp. 344–353.

Nelle, M., Hoecker, C., and Linderkamp, O.: Effects of bolus tube feeding on cerebral blood flow velocity in neonates. Arch. Dis. Child. Fetal Neonatal Ed., 76:F54–56, 1977.

Neu, J., and Koldovsky, O.: Nutrient absorption in the preterm neonate. Clin. Perinatol., 23:229–243, 1996.

Norris, M.K., and Steinhorn, D.M.: Nutritional management during critical illness in infants and children. AACN Clinical Issues, 5(4):485–492, 1994.

Orth, A.M.: Dental health. In Fox, J.A. (ed.): Primary Health Care of Children. St. Louis, Mosby, 1997, pp. 235–243.

Pereira, G. Nutritional care of the extremely premature infant. Clin. Perinatol., 22:61–75, 1995.

Polin, R., and Fox, W. (Eds.): Fetal and Neonatal Physiology. Philadelphia, W.B. Saunders, 1992.

Premji, S.: Ontogeny of the gastrointestinal system and its impact on feeding the preterm infant. Neonatal Network, 17(2):17–24, 1998.

Putet, G.: Energy. In Tsang, R.C., Lucas, A., Uauy, R., and Zlotkin, S. (Eds.): Nutritional Needs of the Preterm Infant: Scientific Basis and Practical Guidelines. Baltimore, Williams & Wilkins, 1993, pp. 15–28.

Reifen, R., and Zlotkin, S. Microminerals. In Tsang, R.C., Lucas, A., Uauy, R., and Zlotkin, S. (Eds.): Nutritional Needs of the Preterm Infant: Scientific Basis and Practical Guidelines. Baltimore, Williams & Wilkins, 1993, pp. 195–207.

Schanler, R.: Suitability of human milk for the low birthweight infant. Clin. Perinatol., 22:207–221, 1995.

Shaffer, S., and Weismann, D.: Fluid requirements in the preterm infant. Clin. Perinatol., 19:233–250, 1992.

Shaker, C.S.: Nipple feeding premature infants: A different perspective. Neonatal Network, 8(5):9–17, 1990.

Shenai, J.: Vitamin A. In Tsang, R.C., Lucas, A., Uauy, R., and Zlotkin, S. (Eds.): Nutritional Needs of the Preterm Infant: Scientific Basis and Practical Guidelines. Baltimore, Williams & Wilkins, 1993, pp. 87–100.

Shiao, S.-Y.: Comparison of continuous versus intermittent sucking in very-low-birth-weight infants. J. Obstet. Gynecol. Neonatal Nurs., 26(3):313–319, 1997.

Shiao, S.-Y., Youngblut, J.M., Anderson, G.C., et al.: Nasogastric tube placement: Effects on breathing and sucking in very-low-birth-weight infants. Nurs. Res., 44:82–87, 1995.

Siddell, E., and Froman, R.: A national survey of neonatal intensive-care units: Criteria used to determine readiness for oral feedings. J. Obstet. Gynecol. Neonatal Nurs., 23(9):783–789, 1994.

Slusser, W., and Powers, N.: Breastfeeding update. Part 1. Immunology, nutrition, and advocacy. Pediatr. Rev. 18:111–119, 1997.

Thureen, P., and Hay, W.: Conditions requiring special nutritional management. In Tsang, R.C., Lucas, A., Uauy, R., and Zlotkin, S. (Eds.): Nutritional Needs of the Preterm Infant: Scientific Basis and Practical Guidelines. Baltimore, Williams & Wilkins, 1993, pp. 243–265.

Tobin, C.R., Sabatte, E., Sandhu, A.S., and Penafiel, E.: A neonatal care map based on gestational age. Neonatal Network, 17(2):41–51, 1998.

Tsang, R., Lucas, A., Uauy, R., and Zlotkin, S.: Nutritional Needs of the Preterm Infant: Scientific Basis and Practical Guidelines. Baltimore, Williams & Wilkins, 1993.

Van Aerde, J.E., Feldman, M., and Clandinin, M.T.: Accretion of lipid in the fetus and newborn. *In* Polin, R., and Fox, W. (Eds.): Fetal and Neonatal Physiology, 2nd ed. Philadelphia: W.B. Saunders, 1998, pp. 458–477.

Van Someren, V., Linnett, S., Stothers, J., et al.: An investigation into the benefits of resisting nasoenteric feeding tubes. Pediatrics, *74:*379–383, 1984.

Wahlig, T., and Georgieff, M.: The effects of illness on neonatal metabolism and nutritional management. Clin. Perinatol., *22:*77–95, 1995.

Weibley, T.T., Adamson, M., Clinkscales, N., et al.: Gavage tube insertion in the premature infant. Am. J. Maternal-Child Nurs., *12:*24–27, 1987.

Zlotkin, S., Atkinson, S., and Lockitch, G.: Trace elements in nutrition for premature infants. Clin. Perinatol., *22:*223–240, 1995.

ADDITIONAL READINGS

Aynsley-Green, A., Adrian, R.E., and Bloom, S.R.: Feeding and the development of enteroinsular hormone secretion in the preterm infant: Effects of continuous gastric infusions of human milk compared with intermittent boluses. Acta Paediatr. Scand., *71:*379–383, 1983.

Churella, H.R., Bachhuber, W.L., and MacLean, W.C.: Survey: Methods of feeding low-birth-weight infants. Pediatrics, *76:*243–249, 1985.

Costarino, A., and Baumgart, S.: Water as nutrition. *In* Tsang, R.C., Lucas, A., Uauy, R., and Zlotkin, S. (Eds.): Nutritional Needs of the Preterm Infant: Scientific Basis and Practical Guidelines. Baltimore, Williams & Wilkins, 1993, pp. 1–14.

Frank, L., and Sosenko, R.S.: Undernutrition as a major contributing factor in the pathogenesis of bronchopulmonary dysplasia. Am. Rev. Respir. Dis., *138:*725–729, 1988.

Georgieff, M.K., and Sasanow, S.R.: Nutritional assessment of the neonate. Clin. Perinatol., *13:*73–89, 1986.

Goldman, A., Sadhana, C., Keeney, S., et al.: Immunologic protection of the premature newborn by human milk. Semin. Perinatol., *18:*495–501, 1994.

Greer, F.R., McCormick, A., and Loker, J.: Changes in fat concentration of human milk during delivery by intermittent bolus and continuous mechanical pump infusion. J. Pediatr., *105:*745–749, 1984.

Kavanaugh, K., Mead, L., Meier, P., and Mangurten, H.: Getting enough: Mothers' concerns about breastfeeding a preterm infant after discharge. J. Obstet. Gynecol. Neonatal Nurs., *24:*23–32, 1995.

Lawrence, P.B.: Breast milk: Best source of nutrition for term and preterm infants. Pediatr. Clin. North Am., *41:*925–941, 1994.

Lemons, P., Stuart, M., and Lemons, J.A.: Breast-feeding the premature infant. Clin. Perinatal Neonatal Nurs., *13*(1):111–122, 1986.

Ostertag, S.G., LaGamma, E.F., Reisen, C.E., et al.: Early enteral feeding does not affect the incidence of necrotizing enterocolitis. Pediatrics, *77:*275–280, 1986.

Pickler, R., Higgins, K., and Crummette, B.: The effect of nonnutritive sucking on bottle-feeding stress in preterm infants. J. Obstet. Gynecol. Neonatal Nurs., *22:* 230–234, 1993.

Pridham, K., Sondel, S., Chang, A., and Green, C.: Nipple feeding for preterm infants with bronchopulmonary dysplasia. J. Obstet. Gynecol. Neonatal Nurs., *22:*147–155, 1993.

Shenai, J.P., Chytil, F., and Stahlman, M.T.: Vitamin A status in neonates with bronchopulmonary dysplasia. Pediatr. Res., *19:*185–189, 1985.

Smith, S., and Kirchhoff, K.: Metabolic bone disease in very-low-birth-weight infants: Assessment, prevention, and treatment by neonatal nurse practitioners. J. Obstet. Gynecol. Neonatal Nurs., *26:*297–302, 1997.

Vanderhoof, J.: Short bowel syndrome. Clin. Perinatol., *23:*377–386, 1996.

Wharton, B.A., Bremer, H.J., Orzalesi, M., et al. (Committee on Nutrition of the Preterm infant, European Society of Paediatric Gastroenterology and Nutrition): Nutrition and Feeding of Preterm Infants. Oxford, Blackwell Scientific Publications, 1987.

Wils, S., and Meier, P.: Helping mothers express milk suitable for preterm and high-risk infant feeding. Am. J. Maternal-Child Nurs., *13:*121–123, 1988.

Ziegler, E.E., O'Donnell, A.M., Nelson, S.E., et al.: Body composition of the reference fetus. Growth, *40:*329–341, 1976.

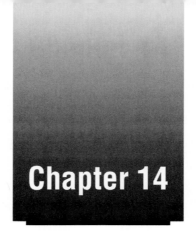

Chapter 14

Metabolic Disorders

Laura Campbell Stokowski

Objectives

1. Describe metabolic control in the mature and the premature newborn infant.

2. Discuss hypoglycemia and hyperglycemia in the neonate.

3. Describe fluid and electrolyte homeostasis in the neonate.

4. Discuss acid-base balance and disorders.

5. Identify specific disorders of metabolism in the neonate.

An essential part of the successful transition to extrauterine life is the achievement of metabolic control. Because mature control of metabolic processes may not occur for many weeks after birth, premature and other stressed neonates can have transient disturbances of glucose, fluid, electrolyte, and acid-base balance. Permanent metabolic disorders, such as those caused by inborn errors of metabolism, may also manifest in the newborn period. Both transient and permanent metabolic derangements can be life-threatening, so caretakers must monitor metabolic functions closely in their neonatal patients.

Glucose Metabolism and Disorders

GLUCOSE HOMEOSTASIS

Glucose is vital for cellular metabolism throughout the body. Blood glucose concentration is determined by the balance between intake/production of glucose and glucose use by the body.

A. **Glucose production.**

1. Glucose intake not required for immediate energy needs is converted to *glycogen* via *glycogenesis* and stored in the liver, heart, and skeletal muscles. During fasting, glycogen is released from the liver in a reverse process known as *glycogenolysis*.

2. The other main source of glucose is *gluconeogenesis:* production of glucose in

the liver by means of nonglucose precursors such as lactate, pyruvate, glycerol, and amino acids.

B. **Glucose metabolism.** Glucose can be metabolized in the body in several ways: production of energy, storage as glycogen, and conversion to gluconeogenic precursors. In the brain, however, because glucose is the primary source of fuel, it is completely oxidized to provide 99% of cerebral energy production (Halamek and Stevenson, 1997). This process is dependent on a number of important enzymes and reactions.

1. Glucose molecules are transported across the blood-brain barrier and into brain cells by glucose transporter (GLUT) proteins.
2. Within the cytoplasm, glucose is metabolized by *glycolysis* to pyruvate. Pyruvate is then oxidized to *acetyl–coenzyme A* (acetyl-CoA), which is transported to the mitochondrion for entry into the citric acid cycle. The end products are carbon dioxide, water, and energy released in the generation of *adenosine triphosphate* (ATP).
3. Of importance to the neonate is that, during hypoglycemia, other substrates (ketone bodies, lactate, glycerol, and amino acids) can also be converted to pyruvate, enter the citric acid cycle, and produce ATP, thus serving as a source of energy for the brain.

C. **Hormonal regulation** of glucose homeostasis.

1. Insulin. Secreted by the pancreatic beta cells in response to an increase in plasma glucose, insulin decreases the blood glucose level by promoting glycogen formation, suppressing hepatic glucose release, and driving peripheral uptake of glucose. Insulin does not control entry of glucose into the brain or liver.
2. Glucagon. Secreted by the pancreatic alpha cells, glucagon promotes glycogenolysis and gluconeogenesis. Glucagon is called a *counterregulatory hormone* because it opposes the effect of insulin by raising the blood glucose level. Other counterregulatory hormones include catecholamines, cortisol, and growth hormone.

D. **Fetal glucose homeostasis.**

1. Glucose reaches the fetus by facilitated diffusion across the placenta at a concentration of about 80% of the mother's.
2. Glycogen storage for postnatal energy needs begins early in gestation, with most glycogen accumulating during the third trimester.
3. Fetal insulin, important for fetal growth, is detectable early in gestation, but the response to a glucose load is not fully developed even at term.
4. The fetus is capable of gluconeogenic activity, using substrates such as lactate if needed to meet metabolic demands in utero.

E. **Neonatal glucose homeostasis.** With the loss of the maternal glucose source, the neonate must assume control of glucose homeostasis and regulate it during intermittent feeding, and yet still must ensure an adequate supply of fuel for the brain and other organs. Early events in this process:

1. After cord clamping, the neonate's blood glucose concentration falls, reaching a nadir at 1–2 hours of age.
2. In the first postnatal hours, the neonatal brain metabolizes lactate, which is abundant, so that even though the glucose concentration is low, the brain is not fuel deficient.
3. The neonate gradually mobilizes glucose to meet energy needs by secreting glucagon and catecholamines and suppressing insulin release. Hepatic glycogen is rapidly depleted if feeding is not established early.
4. Thus, even if a healthy term newborn infant is not fed soon after birth, blood glucose levels rise at 3–4 hours of age.

HYPOGLYCEMIA

A. Pathophysiology.

1. The immediate postnatal drop in the blood glucose concentration is physiologic. Failure to increase glucose concentrations after 4 hours is pathologic. Subsequently, hypoglycemia is usually a result of inadequate hepatic glucose production that cannot meet peripheral demand.
2. During hypoglycemia, the brain increases blood flow to improve glucose delivery and uses alternate fuels such as ketone bodies if they are available.
3. Healthy term infants produce ketones effectively on days 2 and 3 of life, protecting their brains from fuel deficiency if the blood glucose level falls while feeding becomes established. However, the ability of preterm infants and of infants who are small for gestational age to mount a counterregulatory ketogenic response at any time is severely limited, so these babies are heavily dependent on an adequate glucose supply (Hawdon, Ward Platt, and Aynsley-Green, 1992; Hawdon and Ward Platt, 1993).
4. Prolonged hypoglycemia, when not compensated by a supply of alternative fuels, induces biochemical changes at the cell level that may damage the neuronal and glial cells of the brain. It is believed that an accumulation of excitatory amino acids during hypoglycemia leads to prolonged cellular depolarization with entry of water and calcium into the cell, first impairing neuronal growth and eventually causing cell death (Aynsley-Green, 1996). In addition, the hypoglycemic brain may be more vulnerable to the damaging effects of ischemia. Degrees of ischemia and hypoglycemia that alone would not result in brain injury might do so in combination (Volpe, 1995).

B. Etiologies and precipitating factors.

1. Inadequate production or supply of glucose.
   a. Prematurity: immature counterregulatory response to low glucose concentration, insufficient glycogen stores.
   b. Intrauterine growth retardation: low glycogen and fat stores, inadequate metabolic control.
   c. Delayed feedings, insufficient breast-feeding, or fluid restriction.
2. Increased glucose requirement: perinatal asphyxia, respiratory distress, hypothermia, polycythemia/hyperviscosity, infection, adrenal hemorrhage.
3. Increased uptake of glucose related to hyperinsulinism.
   a. *Infant of the diabetic mother* (see following section).
   b. *Persistent neonatal hyperinsulinism and nesidioblastosis:* autosomal recessive disorders thought to be caused by regulatory defects in beta cell function.
   c. *Beckwith-Wiedemann syndrome:* of unknown cause; characterized by macrosomia, hypoglycemia, and dysmorphic features.
   d. High glucose infusion and tocolytics used before delivery. Beta-adrenergic agonists such as terbutaline can stimulate fetal pancreatic beta cells.
4. Other factors.
   a. Inborn errors of carbohydrate, protein, or lipid metabolism.
   b. Endocrine deficiencies (e.g., hypopituitarism).
   c. Iatrogenic: position of tip of umbilical artery catheter near the pancreas.

C. Clinical presentation and assessment.

1. Most neonates are free of symptoms. Signs often linked with hypoglycemia are nonspecific and may occur in conjunction with other clinical conditions, making them unreliable markers for hypoglycemia. These signs are:
   a. Tremors; jitteriness.
   b. Abnormal cry: high pitched or weak.
   c. Respiratory distress: apnea, irregular respirations, tachypnea, cyanosis.

  d. Stupor, hypotonia, refusal to feed.
  e. Seizures.
2. Growth is discordant with gestational age: small or large for gestational age.
3. Some disorders have recognizable features at presentation:
  a. Beckwith-Wiedemann syndrome: macroglossia, abdominal wall defect, ear pit.
  b. Hypopituitarism: microphallus, midline facial defect.

D. **Definition of hypoglycemia.**

1. The lowest level of blood glucose and the longest time it can be tolerated by the neonate without cerebral injury are not presently known. No single value divides "normal" from "abnormal" blood glucose concentrations in all infants. Statistical norms provide a starting point in defining hypoglycemia, but the critical threshold of blood glucose concentration needs to be individualized according to the neonate's clinical status (Volpe, 1995). Even in a relatively healthy population, risk factors for hypoglycemia, feeding status, and the awareness of the possible presence of alternative fuels must all be taken into account when the lowest acceptable glucose level is defined for a given infant. Furthermore, *blood glucose level* can provide only an approximation of *cerebral glucose level;* thus the lowest desirable blood glucose level may be altered by the presence of conditions that impair cerebral blood flow or increase cerebral glucose utilization (Volpe, 1995).
2. A widely used cutoff point for *plasma glucose concentration* is 40 mg/dL; this is the typical threshold for intervention. Contrary to previous suggestions that the preterm infant can withstand lower blood glucose levels than the term infant, some now advocate that the preterm infant's blood glucose level be maintained at greater than 46 mg/dL, because ketones will not be produced (Hawdon et al., 1993a; Koh, 1996).

E. **Diagnostic studies.**

1. Point-of-care blood glucose screening.
  a. Common bedside methods, used for speed and convenience, use whole blood, an enzymatic reagent strip, and a color chart or reflectance meter. Their reliability is questioned because:
    (1) They may underestimate the true glucose level because whole blood gives a reading 10–15% lower than the plasma value.
    (2) They may fail to detect clinically important hypoglycemia because of unpredictable measurement error.
    (3) They are sensitive to error from technical and operator variables such as timing, blotting, and distribution of blood droplets.
  b. Newer devices have been shown to approximate laboratory values more closely, with fewer errors. These include absorption photometry with enzymes to hemolyze erythrocytes before analysis and electrochemical glucose meters (Innanen et al., 1997; Vadasdi and Jacobs, 1993).
2. Laboratory confirmation of point-of-care testing is essential when hypoglycemia is suspected. Blood samples should be placed on ice and analyzed within 30 minutes of drawing to prevent continued metabolism of glucose by blood cells.
3. In suspected hyperinsulinism, testing may include concurrent insulin and glucose levels (insulin level will be inappropriately elevated), ketone and free fatty acid levels (which will be low because release of these fuels is suppressed by hyperinsulinism), and cortisol and growth hormone levels.

F. **Patient care management.**

1. Identify infants at risk with perinatal history, physical examination, body

measurements (weight, length, and head circumference), and gestational age assessment.

2. Prevent hypoglycemia in infants at risk by providing glucose substrate through early enteral feedings (formula or human milk) or IV glucose at 4–6 mg/kg per minute. When tolerated, feedings are preferred over parenteral glucose because milk provides more energy than the equivalent volume of IV fluid and may contribute more essential nonglucose substrate.

3. Assess glucose status with blood glucose screening.
   a. Perform blood glucose screening test on infants at risk 1–2 hours after initiation of feeding or IV administration of glucose. Continue screening at increasingly longer intervals (e.g., every 2–4 hours, before feedings) for 24–48 hours and after changes to the feeding or IV regimen.
   b. Clinically unstable babies and any infant with signs of a possible low blood glucose concentration require regular monitoring.
   c. Routine blood glucose screening of healthy term infants without risk factors is not presently recommended (American Academy of Pediatrics, 1993). In settings where routine blood glucose screening of all newborn infants is conducted, it is not helpful to perform such tests before 2 hours of age because of the physiologic postnatal fall in the blood glucose level, which is of no importance (Hawdon et al., 1993b).

4. If hypoglycemia persists despite feeding, correction is with IV glucose infusion. A minibolus (dextrose 10% in water, 2–3 mL/kg), followed by continuous infusion, rapidly raises the blood glucose level but does not treat the underlying hormonal and metabolic causes of the hypoglycemia.

5. Monitoring of blood glucose levels must then continue, for documentation of the resolution of hypoglycemia with IV therapy and subsequently during the transition to full enteral feedings.

6. Persistent hypoglycemia raises the possibility of hyperinsulinism, although some infants without biochemical hyperinsulinism also have transiently high glucose requirements. Those with true hyperinsulinism may require:
   a. High IV glucose infusion rates (12–16 mg/kg per minute). Delivery of concentrated glucose (>12.5%) requires a central line for safe administration.
   b. Hormonal therapy, which may include glucagon, diazoxide, and somatostatin. Hydrocortisone is mandatory when pituitary failure is suspected.
   c. Subtotal or total pancreatectomy, if severe, persistent hyperinsulinism is unresponsive to medical therapy.

G. Complications.

1. Hypoglycemia will often recur when a bolus of glucose is not followed by a continuous infusion.
2. Necrosis of skin and other tissue caused by extravasation of peripheral glucose infusions. Elevation of the affected area and subcutaneous injections of hyaluronidase may limit the damage.

H. Outcome. Because glucose is essential for cerebral metabolism, a serious potential consequence of hypoglycemia is neurologic impairment, including both intellectual and motor deficits. Even moderate, asymptomatic hypoglycemic episodes were associated with poorer neurodevelopmental outcome at 18 months of age in a large study (Lucas, Morley, and Cole, 1988). In general, outcome studies show that neonates with seizure-associated hypoglycemia have the worst neurologic prognosis (Halamek and Stevenson, 1998).

INFANT OF THE DIABETIC MOTHER

A. Pathophysiology. The hormonal and metabolic changes that complicate diabetic pregnancy can adversely affect the developing fetus and neonate in a number of ways.

1. Early in gestation during organogenesis, the abnormal metabolic milieu is teratogenic, resulting in a higher incidence of congenital malformations.
2. Throughout pregnancy and particularly in the third trimester, the pregnant diabetic woman is increasingly insulin resistant and often has hyperglycemia and hyperaminoacidemia. Excess glucose and amino acids are freely delivered to the fetus, but maternal insulin is not. These nutrients stimulate the fetal pancrease to produce insulin to use the excess fuels resulting in beta-cell hyperplasia and hyperinsulinemia. This, in turn, causes a high rate of fetal growth, increased deposition of fat and visceral enlargement, and subsequent macrosomia.
3. After birth the neonate's pancreas continues to produce insulin, and available glucose is rapidly used. The newborn infant of a diabetic mother (IDM) may exhibit an exaggerated and persistent hypoglycemia.
4. The IDM is at risk of having neural impairment because, even with plentiful adipose tissue, ketogenesis and lipolysis are suppressed by hyperinsulinemia, leaving the brain without a supply of alternative fuels for metabolism during hypoglycemia.

B. Clinical presentation and assessment.

1. Hypoglycemia: may occur immediately after birth without symptoms. In one large retrospective series, hypoglycemia (defined as serum glucose <40 mg/dL) occurred in about one third of IDMs. The majority of those responded rapidly to treatment, but 10% had persistent hypoglycemia despite treatment (Cordero, Treuer, Landon, and Gabbe, 1998).
2. Macrosomia/large size for gestational age (≈35% of IDMs) (Cordero et al., 1998). Some infants are small for gestational age because of placental insufficiency in advanced stages of diabetes.
3. Increase in preterm births in association with diabetic pregnancy. Hyperbilirubinemia in IDMs may be secondary to prematurity.
4. Respiratory distress syndrome and other conditions such as transient tachypnea of the newborn infant. Fetal hyperinsulinemia may inhibit surfactant production, delaying lung maturation.
5. Polycythemia (venous hematocrit >65%). Babies with polycythemia do not always look plethoric, so the hematocrit must be measured.
6. Hypocalcemia, hypomagnesemia.
7. Cardiomyopathy, visceromegaly.
8. Congenital malformations. Cardiac defects (especially transposition), neural tube defects, sacral agenesis, and caudal regression are 3–4 times more frequent than in the general population.

C. Diagnostic studies.

1. Blood glucose screening with laboratory confirmation of plasma glucose.
2. Other laboratory analyses, including calcium and magnesium levels and venous hematocrit.
3. X-ray examination if fractures from traumatic delivery are suspected.
4. Echocardiography.

D. Patient care management.

1. Anticipate problems of IDM before delivery. Tight control of intrapartum glucose levels may reduce the incidence of neonatal hypoglycemia (Curet et al., 1997).
2. Provide early feeding of human milk or formula, orally or via gavage tube if the infant does not feed well. IV administration of glucose is necessary for infants too small or sick to tolerate enteral feeding.

E. **Complications.**

1. Seizures resulting from cerebral fuel deficiency.
2. Shoulder dystocia. Macrosomic infants delivered with forceps or vacuum extraction may have brachial plexus injury (Erb's palsy) or fractures.
3. Renal vein thrombosis (secondary to polycythemia/hyperviscosity).

F. **Outcome.**

1. Increased perinatal mortality rate results from relatively high rates of congenital malformations, stillbirths, and premature delivery.
2. Morbidities associated with IDM include neurologic sequelae, developmental delay, behavioral differences, obesity, and diabetes.
3. Maternal complications, including poor glycemic control, vascular disease, infection, and pregnancy-induced hypertension, are associated with poorer perinatal outcome. Improved outcomes are seen in IDMs when the maternal diabetes is metabolically controlled.

HYPERGLYCEMIA

A. **Pathophysiology.** The glucose intolerance occasionally seen in the extremely low birth weight (ELBW) infant is not fully understood. Normally an infant responds to an exogenous glucose supply with a rise in insulin, suppressing endogenous glucose production and enhancing peripheral uptake of glucose. Though clinically stable ELBW infants are capable of regulating glucose in this manner, a number of them nonetheless become hyperglycemic. Hepatic glucose production in this latter group continues in the presence of hyperglycemia and circulating insulin. This represents a failure of glucose autoregulation involving both the pancreas and liver of infants with hyperglycemia (Hawdon et al., 1992).

B. **Etiologies and precipitating factors.**

1. Extreme prematurity and intrauterine growth restriction (IUGR).
2. Excessive glucose load (>6–8 mg/kg per minute).
3. Stress related to clinical problems such as sepsis or infection.
4. Transient neonatal diabetes mellitus.
5. Dexamethasone therapy for chronic lung disease.

C. **Clinical presentation and assessment.** Onset can be as early as 24 hours of age; usually before 3 days of life. There is no characteristic clinical presentation; diagnosis is by measuring blood glucose concentration.

D. **Diagnostic studies.**

1. Definition of hyperglycemia: plasma glucose concentration greater than 150 mg/dL.
2. Urinary glucose. Very low birth weight (VLBW) infants have a low renal threshold for glucose and may spill sugar at blood glucose levels as low as 80–100 mg/dL.
3. Investigation for possible underlying cause (sepsis workup to rule out infection or insulin level to rule out neonatal diabetes mellitus).

E. **Patient care management.**

1. Monitor blood glucose of infants at risk of developing hyperglycemia, particularly when fluid intake is increased on day 2 or 3 of life.
2. Decrease glucose load to allow the blood glucose level to stabilize in a normal range (<125 mg/dL).
3. Begin feeding, if feasible, to promote tolerance of a higher glucose load.
4. Insulin is sometimes administered to ELBW infants along with parenteral

nutrition in an attempt to normalize blood glucose levels without reducing caloric intake. Insulin is also used to treat transient neonatal diabetes.

E. Complications.

1. Potential complications of severe, prolonged hyperglycemia are osmotic diuresis and neurologic injury from the effects of hyperosmolarity of extracellular fluid (ECF) in the brain. It is thought that this mechanism might also contribute to the development of intraventricular hemorrhage in preterm infants.
2. Insulin management may be difficult in the ELBW infant; blood glucose levels can fluctuate widely. A precisely controlled continuous infusion pump is essential.

Fluid Balance and Disorders

FLUID BALANCE

A. Fluid homeostasis in the fetus and neonate.

1. Body water composition. Water, the most abundant component of the body, is distributed in two main compartments: intracellular fluid (ICF) and ECF; the latter is composed of intravascular and interstitial spaces. As gestation progresses, the fetus undergoes changes in total body water (TBW) and its distribution:
   a. Early in gestation, water makes up 95% of total body weight, with the majority in ECF compartments.
   b. By term, water makes up 75% of body weight and a greater proportion has shifted from ECF to ICF compartments. These changes are largely due to increases in body fat content.
2. Fluid adjustments after birth.
   a. In the immediate postnatal period, the newborn infant must clear residual lung fluid, the reabsorption of which leads to increased ECF after birth. Coupled with the acute increase in intravascular volume that occurs with cord clamping, this results in a higher ECF volume than the neonate requires.
   b. A physiologic contraction of ECF volume with diuresis in the first week of life results in a postnatal weight loss of 5–10% of birth weight in term infants.
3. Because homeostasis of postnatal fluid is more challenging for preterm infants, it has been extensively studied. Three phases have been described (Lorenz et al., 1995):
   a. Prediuretic phase. Urine output is minimal (may be <1 mL/kg per hour); insensible water loss (IWL) is high and variable.
   b. Diuretic phase. Urine output is increased (up to 7 mL/kg per hour); IWL remains high, and body weight decreases 1–3% per day, to as much as 10–15% of birth weight. Urinary sodium loss (natriuresis) accompanies diuresis. In some infants, this phase begins on the first day of life.
   c. Postdiuretic phase. Urine output falls to normal levels (1–3 mL/kg per hour). Weight loss slows and body weight stabilizes.

B. Regulation of fluid balance.

1. Renal mechanisms.
   a. Because water and electrolyte balance is regulated by the placenta, the role of the fetal kidneys is primarily to maintain amniotic fluid volume. Fetal nephrons are functional but immature until 34 weeks. Renal blood flow, renal tubular function, and glomerular filtration rate (GFR) are all immature in the fetus and in the extremely premature infant.

   b. After birth, renal blood flow increases as renal vascular resistance falls. Improved renal function in the days after birth from increased GFR is more pronounced in the term than in the preterm infant.
   c. Both term and preterm infants can dilute urine; however, when faced with a rapid fluid load, the preterm infant may have a delayed response, resulting in fluid retention.
   d. Reabsorption of sodium, bicarbonate, and glucose is limited in the newborn infant.
2. Hormonal mechanisms.
   a. Antidiuretic hormone (ADH) is released by the posterior pituitary in response to a variety of stimuli including hypotension and hypoosmolality. ADH influences water balance by stimulating the kidneys to conserve water. In the absence of ADH, the distal tubules remain impermeable to water, which is excreted as urine.
   b. Because of decreased responsiveness to ADH, neonates cannot efficiently concentrate urine in response to fluid deprivation.

C. **Postnatal influences on fluid balance.** Fluid losses in the neonatal period are from renal and extrarenal sources, including the nonmeasurable IWL of the skin and respiratory tract. Factors that may affect IWL in the neonatal period are listed in Table 14–1. The thermal environment is particularly important to fluid balance.
1. Renal losses. Urine output ranges from 1 to 4 mL/kg per hour. Lower or higher rates correspond with prediuretic and diuretic phases of fluid homeostasis.
2. Transepidermal water loss (TEWL). TEWL occurs as body water diffuses through the immature epidermis and is lost to the atmosphere. Skin features such as poor keratinization, high water content, low subcutaneous fat, large surface area, and high degree of skin vascularity all predispose the infant to high evaporative losses.
   a. TEWL can be as high as 200 mL/kg per day in the ELBW infant, compared with 10–15 mL/kg per day in the term infant. At 24 weeks' gestation, the TEWL rate is similar to the free evaporation of water (Rutter, 1996).
   b. TEWL is highest on the first day of life, decreasing rapidly on subsequent days as the barrier function of the skin improves.
   c. TEWL is closely related to ambient relative humidity. TEWL is much higher when the infant is nursed at a low ambient humidity; under these conditions, TEWL can even exceed the fluid excreted as urine on the first day of life (Sedin, 1996).
   d. If TEWL is not controlled, fluid needs are more difficult to estimate; fluid imbalances can result.

Table 14–1
INFLUENCES ON IWL

Factors That May Increase IWL	Factors That May Decrease IWL
Extreme prematurity	Increasing gestation
Postnatal age <1 wk	Increasing postnatal age
Low relative ambient humidity	High relative ambient humidity
Radiant warmer use	Incubator use
High ambient temperature	Neutral thermal environment
Hyperthermia	Heat shields/plastic blankets
Convection; drafts	Humidification of inspired gases
Ventilation with dry gases	Ointments or transparent dressings on skin
High minute ventilation	Clothing
Phototherapy	
Activity	

IWL, Insensible water loss.

3. Respiratory losses: roughly 0–10 mL/kg per day; related to temperature and humidity of inspired gases and to minute ventilation.
4. Stool losses: estimated to be 5 mL/kg per day in the first week of life, increasing to 10 mL/kg per day thereafter.
5. Other losses: possible gastric drainage, ostomies, surgical wounds.

D. **Fluid therapy.**

1. Goal of fluid therapy. The goal is to permit the physiologic, adaptive fluid and electrolyte changes to occur appropriately, not to replace completely all losses in the early postnatal period. (Lorenz, 1997; Shaffer and Weismann, 1992). A degree of negative water and sodium balance in the first few postnatal days may be obligatory in some infants.
2. Fluid volumes. No fixed fluid administration schedules are appropriate for all infants. General principles:
   a. During the first 3–5 days after birth, fluid intake should be at a level to allow a reasonable weight loss and yet avoid intracellular dehydration. Provision of 60–100 mL/kg per day, depending on the degree of control over IWL, is a typical starting point. Extremely premature infants require more fluid relative to body weight because of larger IWLs. Fluids given to correct shock, hypoglycemia, or acidosis must be taken into account.
   b. Fluid intake is gradually increased on subsequent days to 150–175 mL/kg per day, although fluids may be restricted longer for infants with severe cardiorespiratory disorders, renal failure, and postasphyxial syndrome.
   c. Infants with ongoing fluid losses (chest tube, gastric drainage, diarrhea) need replacement of these volumes with appropriate fluids.
   d. It is generally recommended to use birth weight, rather than current body weight, to calculate fluids on a per-kilogram basis early in life.
3. Fluid constituents.
   a. Dextrose 10% in water is most commonly used for initial fluid therapy. Dextrose 7.5% or 5% in water may be prescribed initially for infants who weighed less than 1 kg at birth, because of the incidence of hyperglycemia in this population.
   b. Electrolytes are not usually added to maintenance IV fluids for the first 24–48 hours after birth. Serum electrolyte levels and urine output are used to determine when to add these electrolytes to IV fluids.

E. **Assessment of fluid balance.** Quantifying fluid requirements can involve guesswork, so close monitoring of hydration status is imperative. Some infants need a fluid balance assessment as often as every 6–8 hours.

1. Body weight. Weight changes with alterations in fluid balance only if there is a net change in TBW; internal shifts of body fluid may not be detected by weight alone. Because the procedure for weighing the ELBW infant is prone to errors and a significant source of stress for the infant, some NICUs have abandoned weighing tiny babies altogether, especially in the first few days. Others use in-bed electronic scales, which are reliable but can be affected by the amount of equipment attached to the infant and how it is handled during weighing (Engstrom et al., 1995).
2. Urine volume. For greatest possible accuracy, urine output must be measured right after it occurs; urine collected onto diapers lying under radiant warmers may evaporate before the diapers are weighed for determination of output. Simulation studies show that evaporation rates are highest when urine volumes are small and when diapers are not closed (Fox, 1992).
3. Specific gravity of urine: an indirect measure of urine osmolality; if normal (1.002–1.012), specific gravity reflects a normal urine osmolality (100–300 mOsm/L). It is unreliable if glucose, blood, or protein is present.

4. Assessment parameters: quality of skin turgor, mucous membranes, presence of edema, appearance of eyes, and level of anterior fontanelle. Hemodynamic assessment includes pulse quality, blood pressure, and perfusion (capillary refill time, temperature, and acid-base balance).
5. Laboratory evaluation of hydration status: serum sodium level, osmolality, blood urea nitrogen, creatinine, and/or hematocrit.

DISORDERS OF FLUID BALANCE

Disorders of fluid balance in the newborn infant do not always fit neatly into categories such as "fluid depletion" or "fluid excess"; some involve elements of both. One such disorder is septic shock, in which low intravascular volume (a fluid deficit) can coexist with interstitial and cellular edema (a fluid surplus). For simplicity, an attempt is made here to group clinical conditions according to the primary effect on total body water (e.g., decreased, as in dehydration, or increased, as in congestive heart failure), even though overlap may exist.

FLUID DEPLETION

A. **Pathophysiology.** Fluid can be lost from the body acutely or gradually. Sudden loss of body fluid can result in signs and symptoms of shock. If lost fluid is not restored, the body will attempt to compensate by retaining sodium and water. Gradual or chronic fluid loss, even though central blood pressure may be maintained, can result in serious metabolic disturbances.

B. **Causes and precipitating factors.**

1. Extreme prematurity (<28 weeks' gestation, <800 g). The large TEWL and rapid contraction of the ECF result in a sodium excess that cannot be excreted efficiently by the kidneys. If fluid intake is inadequate, *hyperosmolar hypernatremic dehydration* ensues.
2. Acute blood loss/hypovolemia: hemorrhagic losses at birth, postnatal internal hemorrhage, surgical blood loss, or the removal of large volumes for laboratory tests.
3. Diarrhea.
4. *Diabetes insipidus* (pure renal water loss from failure to secrete or respond to ADH). This condition is treated with intranasally administered arginine vasopressin (DDAVP).
5. Abdominal or pleural cavity exposure during surgery.
6. Unreplaced losses from gastric suction.
7. Medications that may cause diuresis: caffeine and theophylline.
8. Breast-feeding malnutrition: inadequate intake in a breast-fed infant with a cycle of reduced milk production and decreasing demand, resulting in severe malnutrition, dehydration, and hypernatremia.

C. **Clinical presentation and assessment.**

1. Weight loss if net reduction in TBW.
2. Low urine output (<0.5 ml/kg per hour); possibly high specific gravity. Urine output may be normal or even high in the ELBW infant during postnatal diuresis.
3. Poor skin turgor (gently pinched skin is slow to retract), dry skin and mucous membranes.
4. Hemodynamic changes: tachycardia or decreased pulses with peripheral vasoconstriction (pale, cool, mottled skin with prolonged capillary filling time), increased core-peripheral temperature differential, central blood pressure either normal or low.
5. In breast-feeding malnutrition, possible excessive sleepiness, disinterest in feeding, or irritability.

D. Diagnostic studies.

1. Serum sodium can be low, normal, or high, depending on the cause of dehydration/fluid loss.
2. With dehydration, blood urea nitrogen and creatinine may be elevated.
3. Hematocrit may be increased or decreased with blood loss.
4. Blood gas values may reveal metabolic acidosis in the infant with hypovolemia.

E. Patient care management.

1. Hypovolemic states (shock, hemorrhage) are managed acutely with volume replacement and vasoactive inotropic agents, as described elsewhere in this text.
2. The type of fluid given to replace other fluid deficits depends on the constituents of lost fluid (e.g., free water loss, electrolyte loss) and the infant's electrolyte levels.
3. Management of severe dehydration in the breast-feeding infant involves replacing the free water deficit slowly over several days to avoid a rapid fall in serum osmolality. This is to allow the brain cells, which have already begun to adapt to the hyperosmolar ECF, to return to their normal state without injury (Molteni, 1994).

F. Fluid management of hypernatremic hyperosmolar dehydration in the preterm infant.

1. Prevention of TEWL is more effective than replacing these losses. This is because fluid lost is mostly solute free, whereas replacement fluids contain solutes that can aggravate hyperosmolality (Sedin, 1996).
2. The single method or combination of methods most effective in reducing TEWL has yet to be proved. The following strategies all decrease TEWL to some degree, by raising ambient humidity and/or by preventing TEWL directly at the skin level.
   a. Use of incubators rather than radiant warmers. TEWL is higher under radiant warmers, but this is believed to be due to lower ambient relative humidity and air currents on the radiant warmer, rather than an effect of the radiant energy (Kjartansson et al., 1995).
   b. Supplemental humidity. Devices to saturate the air immediately surrounding the infant (mist tents, "swamping") are used with both incubators and radiant warmers. The humidity level can be raised in most incubators by filling a water reservoir. Newer models are available with servo-controlled humidity, a dynamic system that maintains higher and more stable humidity levels. These incubators allow the nurse to select a desired relative humidity level, and the actual level is continuously monitored and displayed. On radiant warmers the provision of supplemental humidity requires the use of plastic film to contain heated, humidified air directed over the infant. Humidifier temperature, air flow setting, and seasonal ambient relative humidity variations can significantly affect the achievable humidity level with this setup (Seguin, 1997).
   c. Heat shields or plastic film "blankets" increase ambient humidity by using the infant's own trapped evaporative losses.
   d. Semipermeable dressings (adhesive or nonadhesive) reduce TEWL without altering maturation or microflora of treated skin (Knauth et al., 1989; Mancini et al., 1994).
   e. Topical preservative-free ointment (such as Aquaphor) reduces TEWL for 6 hours after application (Nopper et al., 1996).
3. Reduce respiratory water losses by using humidified gas mixtures.
4. If no further reductions in IWL can be made, fluid intake must be increased,

albeit cautiously. Giving too much fluid in response to hypernatremic dehydration can aggravate hyperglycemia and increase the risk of heart failure, pulmonary edema, and CNS injury. It is usually recommended to give just enough fluid to maintain the serum sodium in the high normal range (145–150 mEq/L) during the first 24–72 hours of life (Costarino and Baumgart, 1991).

5. Restrict sodium (unless the baby is hyponatremic), adding gradually when serum sodium level decreases and diuresis begins.
6. Monitor hydration closely. Weight loss up to 20% in ELBW infants is often accepted if other parameters indicate adequate hydration.

G. Complications.

1. High TEWL, which equates with high evaporative heat loss, with risk of hypothermia.
2. Excessive weight loss.
3. Hypotension; tissue damage; metabolic acidosis from hypoperfusion.
4. Impaired excretion of drugs when urine output is minimal.
5. Electrolyte imbalances from slow excretion of daily solute load.
6. Renal failure and vascular thrombosis: possible result of severe dehydration.

FLUID EXCESS

A. Pathophysiology.
The spectrum of disease that can cause body fluid excess in the neonate is broad. Many of the disorders are characterized by *edema*, which is the abnormal accumulation of ECF within the interstitial spaces. Edema can be caused by:

1. Low colloid osmotic pressure (decreased plasma protein concentration).
2. Increased capillary permeability to water and protein (caused by hypoxia).
3. Increased hydrostatic pressure within the capillaries.
4. Impaired lymphatic drainage of interstitial fluids and proteins.

With some of the disorders associated with these pathologic processes, a combination of venous congestion, renal failure, and edema suggests a state of fluid overload even when circulating blood volume is low.

B. Etiologies and precipitating factors.

1. Cardiac dysfunction: congenital heart disease, congestive heart failure, patent ductus arteriosus (PDA).
2. Respiratory distress syndrome and bronchopulmonary dysplasia (BPD). Therapeutic use of oxygen and positive-pressure ventilation causes endothelial injury with subsequent fluid leakage.
3. Perinatal asphyxia.
4. Sepsis; necrotizing enterocolitis.
5. Hydrops fetalis.
6. Renal failure.
7. Miscalculation of fluid needs or provision of too much fluid (possibly from failure to account for all sources of fluid such as flush solutions, medications, colloid).
8. Use of neuromuscular blocking agents.
9. *Syndrome of inappropriate antidiuretic hormone* (SIADH): usually associated with CNS infection or injury. ADH secretion is inappropriate to usual osmotic and volume stimuli. The result is fluid retention with hyponatremia, low serum osmolality, and high urinary sodium loss.

C. Clinical presentation and assessment.

1. Weight gain, if there is a net increase in TBW.
2. Urine output: possible decrease.

3. Edema: peripheral, generalized, pulmonary.
4. Hemodynamic changes: dependent on intravascular volume status. When increased, there may be symptomatic PDA, tachycardia, and increased pulses or blood pressure. With congestive heart failure, venous filling pressure is high.

D. Diagnostic studies.

1. Serum osmolality is low (<280 mOsm/L); urine osmolality is normal.
2. In SIADH, osmolalities and sodium levels of urine and serum are diagnostic (urine output is low with high specific gravity and high sodium levels; serum has low sodium level and low osmolality).

E. Patient care management. In addition to therapy aimed at the underlying disease process:

1. Precise fluid management with fluid restriction is necessary. Daily fluid calculations must take into account renal function and extra fluids given to administer medications and flush intravascular catheters.
2. Diuretics may be used in some situations.
3. Infants with severe edema and low intravascular volume (shock) present a challenge. Circulating blood volume must be maintained with volume expanders and pressor agents, but maintenance fluid must be minimized.
4. Edema may predispose the infant to necrotic injury of the skin. The skin must be protected from pressure with careful repositioning, support, and the use of a nonrigid sleeping surface, such as a gel- or water-filled mattress.

F. Complications.

1. Fluid sequestration in static body fluid compartments ("third spacing") can result in a loss of effective blood volume, compromising delivery of oxygen and nutrients to tissues throughout the body. This can lead not only to serious metabolic imbalances but also to permanent tissue damage.
2. Excessive fluid administration early in life has been associated with worsening of respiratory distress syndrome and development of BPD, symptomatic PDA, and necrotizing enterocolitis.

Electrolyte Balance and Disorders

SODIUM

A. Sodium homeostasis.

1. Functions of sodium (Na). Na, the major extracellular cation, is closely involved in water balance. Na and other electrolytes are found in varying concentrations in all body fluid compartments. They determine the tonicity of the fluid compartment and influence the passage of water through the vascular and cell membranes, thereby controlling the osmotic equilibrium between compartments. With a surfeit of Na, blood becomes hypertonic, causing a shift of fluid from intracellular to extracellular spaces, which results in cellular dehydration. A deficit of Na causes hypotonicity and fluid shifts into the cells (edema).
2. Regulation of Na. Cellular transport of Na is achieved by the sodium-potassium pump, which maintains the electrochemical sodium and potassium gradients across the cell membrane. Renal (GFR, tubular function) and hormonal (aldosterone, ADH) mechanisms influence the body content of Na. Although preterm infants can excrete sodium, low GFR early in life may hamper this ability. In addition, minimal responsiveness to aldosterone and ADH contributes to a baseline salt-wasting tendency.
3. Positive Na balance: Na intake greater than Na losses. This is a prerequisite for the growth of new tissue.

B. Hyponatremia.

1. Pathophysiology. A low serum Na reflects either an excess of body water relative to normal body Na content or a primary Na depletion. When urinary Na wasting occurs, a proportionate loss of water *(isotonic dehydration)* can reduce ECF volume and lead to oliguria.
2. Causes and precipitating factors.
    a. Prematurity (renal and hormonal immaturity, with tendency to excrete Na). Preterm infants are most vulnerable to hyponatremia just after the period of postnatal extracellular volume contraction (Modi, 1998).
    b. Conditions associated with low intravascular volume (e.g., shock). Baroreceptor stimulation of ADH results in reduced renal water excretion and a dilutional hyponatremia.
    c. Dilutional hyponatremia from excessive free water intake.
    d. Renal losses related to medications (furosemide, methylxanthines).
    e. Inadequate Na intake during period of rapid growth, especially in preterm infants fed exclusively human milk. Called "late hyponatremia" because it occurs after the first week of life.
3. Clinical presentation and assessment.
    a. Usually asymptomatic, but apnea, irritability, twitching, or seizures can occur if Na drops acutely or falls to less than 115 mEq/L.
    b. Infants with late hyponatremia may fail to gain weight.
4. Diagnostic studies.
    a. Serum Na low (<130 mEq/L) and osmolality low (<280 mOsm/L). Serum Na can be factitiously low in the presence of hyperlipidemia.
    b. Urine Na excretion rate to rule out excessive Na losses.
5. Patient care management.
    a. Provide Na supplementation after postnatal diuresis begins (usually on day 2). Maintenance Na requirement is 1–4 mEq/kg per day and is usually given as sodium chloride, though Na-acetate or Na-bicarbonate may be used if the infant has metabolic acidosis.
    b. A chronic hyponatremic state is corrected gradually over 48–72 hours to prevent injury to brain cells (Modi, 1998).
    c. Monitor weight, urine output, parameters of hydration, and adequacy of intravascular volume (monitoring of central venous pressure, capillary refill time, and core-peripheral temperature differential).
    d. When hyponatremia is associated with an excess of body water, fluids are restricted. True SIADH is managed with fluid restriction and monitoring of Na, osmolality, and urine output.
    e. Some human milk fortifiers supply additional dietary sodium.
6. Complications.
    a. Acute drops in the serum Na can lead to a shift of fluid into brain cells and cellular edema. This may result in apnea and seizures.
    b. The degree to which the infant's brain may be able to adapt to chronic hyponatremia is not known; however, chronic hyponatremia does impair skeletal and tissue growth.

C. Hypernatremia.

1. Pathophysiology. Hypernatremia usually reflects a deficiency of water relative to total body Na content and thus is actually a disorder of water balance rather than one of Na balance.
2. Causes and precipitating factors.
    a. Excessive IWL with insufficient fluid intake (even without added Na).
    b. High inadvertent Na intake (saline infusions in arterial catheters, sodium bicarbonate [$NaHCO_3$], medications) or early addition of maintenance NaCl.

    c. Breast-feeding malnutrition in term infants. Elevated human milk Na content accompanying insufficient lactation contributes to the hyperosmolar state (Molteni, 1994).

    d. *Diabetes insipidus:* deficiency of pituitary-secreted ADH, causing loss of water in excess of loss of Na.

3. Clinical presentation and assessment.

    a. Signs of dehydration may be present.

    b. In severe hypernatremia, high-pitched cry, lethargy, irritability, and apnea can progress to seizures and coma.

4. Diagnostic studies: serum Na (>150 mEq/L) and osmolality (>300 mOsm/L).

5. Patient care management.

    a. Gradually restrict Na to avoid sudden fall in plasma osmolality. If maintenance Na administration has not been started, it is usually delayed.

    b. Recalculate fluid intake. Fluids may have been restricted too much in light of insensible losses.

    c. Prevent hypernatremia in ELBW infants. Na supplementation may be withheld longer than usual after birth if serum Na level remains normal. This approach has been shown to reduce the need for additional fluids during the first days of life (Costarino et al., 1992). In addition, measures to reduce TEWL will aid in the prevention of hypernatremia.

    d. The need for saline solutions to maintain catheter patency presents a dilemma. Attempts to lower the infused Na concentration too far result in administration of hypotonic solutions, with risk of hemolysis.

6. Complications. As hypernatremia develops, intracellular water can be drawn out, causing cells to shrink. If this process is rapid, this can affect the brain. Sudden increases in plasma osmolality can also contribute to intraventricular hemorrhage.

POTASSIUM

A. Potassium homeostasis.

1. Functions of potassium (K). The major cation in ICF, K contributes to intracellular osmotic activity and in part determines ICF volume. K plays a fundamental role along with Na in regulating cell membrane potential.

2. Regulation of K. K is distributed both intracellularly and extracellularly. The distribution of K between ICF and ECF is regulated by the sodium-potassium pump and is influenced by acid-base balance, insulin, and glucagon. The excretion of K from the body depends on kidney function, GFR, urine flow rate, and aldosterone sensitivity.

B. Hypokalemia.

1. Pathophysiology. Because K is 90% intracellular, it is assessed indirectly by measuring the quantity in the serum. A subnormal serum K implies insufficient K within the cells, which may impede their function. Muscle cells of the gastrointestinal system and the heart can be affected.

2. Causes and precipitating factors.

    a. Loss of K in the urine (kaliuresis) during postnatal diuresis, before K supplementation is begun.

    b. Inadequate K intake.

    c. Increased gastrointestinal losses from an ostomy or nasogastric tube.

    d. Metabolic alkalosis. A high serum pH drives K into cells, resulting in a low serum K.

    e. Medications including bicarbonate, diuretics, and insulin. Insulin increases cellular uptake of K through stimulation of activity of the sodium-potassium pump.

3. Clinical presentation and assessment. Cardiac effects (flattened T waves, prominent U waves, ST depression), hypotonia, abdominal distention, and ileus.
4. Diagnostic studies: serum K (<3.5 mEq/L).
5. Patient care management.
   a. Begin K supplementation when urine output is well established, usually on the second or third day of life. The maintenance K requirement is 2–3 mEq/kg per day.
   b. Correction of hypokalemic states must be done cautiously, with continuous cardiac monitoring.
6. Complications.
   a. Rapid administration of K to correct hypokalemia can lead to fatal arrhythmias.
   b. Hypokalemia potentiates digitalis toxicity.

C. Hyperkalemia.

1. Pathophysiology. In the ELBW infant, the normal postnatal shift of K from the intracellular to the extracellular compartment is intensified. During the prediuretic phase, this excess K is not efficiently excreted secondary to a low GFR and a low Na excretion rate (Lorenz et al., 1997).
2. Causes and precipitating factors.
   a. Extreme prematurity *(nonoliguric hyperkalemia)*.
   b. Endogenous release of K from tissue destruction, hypoperfusion, hemorrhage, and bruising.
   c. Metabolic acidosis. A low serum pH shifts K out of cells.
   d. Renal failure, with decreased K clearance.
   e. Adrenal insufficiency.
   f. Transfusion with blood stored longer than 3 days.
3. Clinical presentation and assessment. Cardiac effects may be seen: ventricular tachycardia, peaked T wave, widened QRS complex.
4. Diagnostic studies.
   a. Serum K (>6.5 mEq/L) from venipuncture or arterial line. Heel-stick samples are often hemolyzed, rendering results unreliable.
   b. Tests of renal function: blood urea nitrogen, creatinine.
   c. Electrocardiography (EKG) to detect cardiac arrhythmias.
   d. Serum ionized calcium, because hypocalcemia may potentiate cardiac toxicity from hyperkalemia.
5. Patient care management.
   a. For prevention of hyperkalemia, K is withheld from early IV fluids. Serum K is monitored as diuresis (and K excretion) begins; K is added when serum K stabilizes in the 4–4.5 mEq/L range.
   b. Acidosis is corrected.
   c. Diuretics and low-dose dopamine therapy may improve renal excretion of K. Dopamine also enhances K uptake by stimulation of activity of the sodium-potassium pump.
   d. Temporary measures may be needed to reduce the effects of circulating K until the total body K level can be reduced.
      (1) Administration of calcium gluconate will lower the cell membrane threshold transiently, antagonizing the effects on the heart muscle.
      (2) Glucose/insulin infusion to enhance cellular uptake of K.
      (3) $NaHCO_3^-$ (shifts K into cells).
   e. When other measures fail to normalize K:
      (1) Cation exchange resin (Kayexalate). Na is exchanged for K in the intestine to increase excretion of K.
      (2) Exchange transfusion.
      (3) Peritoneal dialysis or continuous arteriovenous hemofiltration for severe, intractable hyperkalemia.

6. Complications.
    a. Hyperkalemia is life-threatening because of the risk of cardiac arrest.
    b. Kayexalate can cause hypocalcemia, hypomagnesemia, and hypernatremia.

CALCIUM

A. Calcium homeostasis.

1. Functions of calcium (Ca). Ca plays a central role in many physiologic processes, maintaining cell membrane permeability and activating enzyme reactions for muscle contraction, nerve transmission, and blood clotting. Ca is vital for normal cardiac function and development of the skeleton, where 99% of the body's Ca is stored.
2. Regulation of Ca.
    a. Parathyroid hormone (PTH) increases serum Ca by mobilizing Ca from bone and intestines and reducing renal excretion of Ca. PTH is stimulated by low serum Ca and magnesium (Mg) levels and is suppressed by high Ca and Mg levels.
    b. Vitamin D acts with PTH to restore Ca to normal levels by increasing absorption of Ca and phosphorus from the intestines and bone.
    c. Calcitonin, a Ca counterregulatory hormone secreted from thyroid C cells, lowers Ca levels by antagonizing the Ca, which mobilizes the effects of PTH.
    d. Phosphorus (P) also inhibits the absorption of Ca (the higher the P, the lower the absorption of Ca).
3. Serum Ca is transported in three forms:
    a. Protein-bound calcium, accounting for 40% of total serum Ca.
    b. Inactivated Ca (complexed with anions such as bicarbonate, lactate, and citrate), accounting for 10% of total serum Ca.
    c. Free ionized calcium (iCa), the physiologically active form that can cross the cell membrane, accounting for 50% of the total serum Ca. Blood pH influences the amount of iCa: acidosis increases iCa, and alkalosis decreases iCa.

B. Fetal Ca metabolism.
Fetal Ca needs are met by active transport of Ca across the placenta. Ca accretion increases during the last trimester as Ca is incorporated into newly forming bones. Because maternal PTH and calcitonin do not cross the placenta, the fetus is relatively hypercalcemic, which suppresses fetal PTH and stimulates fetal calcitonin.

C. Neonatal Ca metabolism.
When the supply of Ca ceases at birth, the neonate depends on stored and dietary Ca to avoid hypocalcemia. After birth, the Ca level declines to its nadir by 24 hours of age, but PTH activity remains low. By 48–72 hours, PTH and vitamin D levels rise and the calcitonin level declines, allowing Ca to be mobilized. The serum Ca level returns to normal despite a low Ca intake.

D. Hypocalcemia.

1. Pathophysiology. Failure to achieve Ca homeostasis after birth can result from inadequate Ca stores, immature hormonal control, inability to mobilize Ca, or interference with Ca use. Hypocalcemia increases cellular permeability to Na ions and increases cell membrane excitability.
2. Causes and precipitating factors.
    a. "Early" hypocalcemia.
        (1) Prematurity: reduced Ca stores and relative hypoparathyroidism (blunted PTH response to hypocalcemia).
        (2) Infant of a diabetic mother (IDM): prolonged delay in PTH production by infant after birth.

(3) Placental insufficiency: reduced Ca stores.

(4) Perinatal asphyxia and stress, which precipitate a surge in calcitonin that suppresses Ca. In addition, tissue damage and glycogen breakdown release phosphorus into the circulation, which decreases Ca uptake.

(5) Maternal anticonvulsant therapy, which affects hepatic enzymes involved in vitamin D metabolism.

(6) Low intake of Ca.

(7) Factors that may decrease iCa even when the total serum Ca is normal: exchange transfusion, intravenous administration of lipid emulsion, alkalosis, or alkali therapy for acidosis.

  b. "Late" hypocalcemia.

(1) Hypomagnesemia.

(2) Transient congenital hypoparathyroidism or secondary hypoparathyroidism from maternal hyperparathyroidism. An increased PTH level in the mother raises the fetal Ca level and suppresses the fetal parathyroid gland. After birth, the suppressed gland cannot maintain a normal Ca level.

(3) *DiGeorge syndrome;* absence of thymus and parathyroid glands.

(4) High-phosphate formulas or cereals. The neonate cannot excrete the excess phosphate; the hyperphosphatemia suppresses Ca.

(5) Intestinal malabsorption.

3. Clinical presentation and assessment.

  a. Early hypocalcemia is usually asymptomatic; signs of neuromuscular excitability (jitteriness, twitching) may be present.

  b. Severe hypocalcemia (neonatal tetany) is rare and presents with jitteriness, seizures, high-pitched cry, laryngospasm, stridor, prolonged QT interval.

4. Diagnostic studies.

  a. Serum total calcium (<7 mg/dL) or ionized Ca (<4.4 mg/dL). The proportion of iCa cannot be reliably predicted from total serum Ca levels.

  b. Magnesium and phosphorus levels; acid-base balance.

5. Patient care management.

  a. Monitor serum Ca of infants at risk: premature, IDM, asphyxiated.

  b. Early, mild hypocalcemia often resolves without treatment.

  c. Serious hypocalcemia is treated with boluses and/or continuous infusions of calcium gluconate (can also be given orally).

  d. Treatment of late hypocalcemia depends on the underlying cause.

6. Complications.

  a. Rapid infusion of Ca can cause bradycardia or cardiac arrest. Boluses, if required, should be administered slowly, for 20–30 minutes by syringe pump, while the heart rate is monitored.

  b. Tissue necrosis and calcifications can result from extravasated Ca. Peripheral infiltrations can be treated with subcutaneously administered hyaluronidase.

  c. Intestinal necrosis and liver necrosis have been reported with Ca infusion given via umbilical catheter.

E. **Metabolic bone disease.**

1. Pathophysiology of metabolic bone disease (MBD). Infants born prematurely can miss all or most of the period of greatest intrauterine mineral accretion, which places them at risk of having inadequate postnatal bone mineralization. The primary cause of MBD is inadequate Ca and P intake, rather than vitamin D deficiency.

2. Causes and precipitating factors.

  a. Prematurity: the more immature the infant, the higher the MBD rate.

  b. Parenteral nutrition: low Ca and P intakes.

    c. Unsupplemented human milk feeding (inadequate Ca and P content) or use of formulas not designed for the preterm infant.

    d. BPD secondary to fluid restriction and use of diuretics, with renal Ca wasting.

3. Clinical presentation and assessment.

    a. MBD is asymptomatic; it is often detected initially on routine x-ray examination.

    b. Skeletal fractures may be seen in the thoracic cage or extremities.

    c. Other reported presentation is late-onset respiratory distress from "softening" of the ribs.

    d. Pain occurs with handling.

4. Diagnostic tests.

    a. Serum: normal Ca, low P, high alkaline phosphatase, and high 1,25-dihydroxyvitamin D levels. Ca and P levels alone are not good indicators of metabolic bone disease.

    b. Urine: low or absent P excretion; increased urinary Ca.

    c. Radiologic bone examinations. Wrist x-ray films at age 6–8 weeks are used to monitor for MBD. Early evidence can be difficult to discern because bone mineral content must decrease by 30% to be visible. Photon absorptiometry may be done in centers where the necessary equipment is available.

    d. X-ray examination. Findings may include "washed out" (undermineralized) bones, known as *osteopenia,* or epiphyseal dysplasia and skeletal deformities, known as *rickets* (Huttner, 1998).

5. Patient care management and prevention of MBD.

    a. Maintain Ca/P ratio in parenteral nutrition at 1.3:1 to 1.7:1.

    b. For enteral feeding, use preterm formulas or human milk supplementation.

    c. Direct supplementation of Ca and P may be needed. Ca given without P will be inadequately used, resulting in hypercalciuria and possibly nephrocalcinosis.

    d. Gentle handling of infants at risk and avoidance of chest physiotherapy are warranted to prevent fractures.

E. Hypercalcemia.

1. Pathophysiology. A rise in the serum Ca level can rapidly overwhelm the infant's compensatory mechanisms for Ca equilibrium. An excess supply of Ca has multiple effects and is potentially lethal.

2. Causes and precipitating factors.

    a. Iatrogenic: overtreatment with Ca or vitamin D.

    b. *Hyperparathyroidism:* primary neonatal disorder or secondary to maternal hypoparathyroidism, with chronic stimulation of the fetal parathyroid gland.

    c. Phosphate depletion: caused by low dietary intake; may be associated with low phosphate content in human milk.

    d. *Subcutaneous fat necrosis:* found over the back and limbs; associated with difficult delivery, hypothermia, and maternal diabetes. Pathogenic mechanism is unknown.

    e. *Familial infantile hypercalcemia.*

    f. *Hypervitaminosis D:* excessive maternal intake of vitamin D.

3. Clinical presentation and assessment.

    a. Hypotonia, weakness, irritability, and poor feeding, all from a direct effect of Ca on the CNS.

    b. Bradycardia.

    c. Constipation.

    d. Polyuria, dehydration (associated with severe hypercalcemia).

    4. Diagnostic studies.
        a. Serum Ca (>11 mg/dL); iCa (>5.8 mg/dL).
        b. In hyperparathyroidism the serum Ca level is high, phosphate levels may be low, and urinary Ca and phosphate excretion are high.
    5. Patient care management.
        a. Hydrate infant and promote excretion of Ca (furosemide has calciuretic action).
        b. Restrict Ca and vitamin D intake; increase phosphate intake.
    6. Complications.
        a. Nephrocalcinosis from hypercalciuria.
        b. Metastatic calcification of damaged cells/tissues throughout the body, including the brain.
        c. Cardiac effects: bradycardia and arrhythmias.

MAGNESIUM

A. Magnesium homeostasis.

1. Functions of magnesium (Mg). Mg is a catalyst for many intracellular enzyme reactions, including muscle contraction and carbohydrate metabolism and is critical for normal parathyroid function and bone-serum Ca homeostasis. Mg is regulated primarily by the kidneys.
2. Fetal and neonatal Mg homeostasis. The fetus receives its supply of Mg by active transport across the placenta. Maternal health and diet can influence the amount of Mg accrued by the fetus. After birth, Mg level falls along with Ca level, then rises to normal within 48 hours.
3. Serum total Mg versus the ionized form. Ionized Mg (iMg) is the biologically active fraction of Mg. Total Mg concentration in the serum does not necessarily reflect iMg activity.

B. Hypomagnesemia.

1. Pathophysiology. A low neonatal Mg level is directly related to the maternal level before birth. Although an acute decline in Mg stimulates PTH release, chronic Mg deficiency suppresses PTH and blocks the hormone's actions on the bone and kidneys. Hypocalcemia ensues.
2. Causes and precipitating factors.
    a. Decreased Mg supply: prematurity, placental insufficiency and intrauterine growth restriction (IUGR), low dietary intake.
    b. Increased Mg losses: renal and intestinal disorders, including renal tubular acidosis, diarrhea, short bowel syndrome.
    c. Endocrine causes: neonatal hypoparathyroidism, maternal hyperparathyroidism.
3. Clinical presentation and assessment.
    a. Tremors, irritability, and hyperreflexia, progressing to seizures.
    b. Failure to respond to therapy for hypocalcemia: hypomagnesemia a possibility.
4. Diagnostic studies: serum Mg level (<1.5 mg/dL).
5. Patient care management.
    a. If hypomagnesemia is severe, administration of magnesium sulfate may be necessary to relieve symptoms until Ca balance is restored.
    b. Seizures are usually unresponsive to anticonvulsant agents.
6. Complications. Overtreatment with magnesium sulfate can result in hypotonia and respiratory depression, hypotension, and cardiac arrhythmias.

C. Hypermagnesemia.

1. Pathophysiology. An excess of Mg is slow to be excreted by the neonatal kidneys. Very high Mg levels can cause CNS and neuromuscular depression.

2. Causes and precipitating factors.
    a. Excessive Mg load: magnesium sulfate treatment in labor, excess adminis-
       tration of Mg to neonate.
    b. Reduced excretion of Mg: renal failure, oliguria.
3. Clinical presentation and assessment (may be asymptomatic).
    a. Respiratory depression, apnea.
    b. Neuromuscular depression: lethargy, poor suck, loss of reflexes, flaccidity,
       hypotonia.
    c. Gastrointestinal hypomotility, abdominal distention.
4. Laboratory and diagnostic studies: high serum Mg (>2.5 mg/dL)
5. Patient care management.
    a. Prepare to resuscitate infants born to mothers receiving large doses of
       magnesium sulfate.
    b. Hypermagnesemia usually resolves with adequate hydration and urine
       output. Mg excretion can be increased with furosemide.
    c. If infant is unresponsive to treatment, exchange transfusion may be neces-
       sary.
6. Complications. Cardiac arrest and respiratory failure are possible.

Acid-Base Balance and Disorders

ACID-BASE PHYSIOLOGY

A. **pH.** Acid-base balance is normal when the pH of the blood is between 7.35
and 7.45. The pH is determined by the hydrogen ion (H^+) concentration in the
ECF. An acid is a hydrogen ion donor; a base is an H^+ receptor. A complex system
of buffers, compensation, and excretion regulates the H^+ concentration, thus
keeping the pH in the normal range.

B. **Buffering system:** the first line of defense against excess H^+ concentration.
Buffers, including bicarbonate (HCO_3^-), plasma proteins, and hemoglobin, act
rapidly to pick up excess H^+. The major buffer, HCO_3^-, teams with H^+ to form
carbonic acid, which dissociates into water and CO_2 to be eliminated. The
normal HCO_3^- level in the neonate is 18–21 mEq/L, lower than in the
adult.

C. **Lung regulation.** The lungs act to lower the H^+ level in the blood by removing CO_2, which is produced as a waste product of cellular metabolism. It is
then transported to the lungs, where it is removed from the body by ventilation.
The rate of CO_2 removal can be increased or decreased by altering minute
ventilation.

D. **Kidney regulation.** The kidney acts to maintain equilibrium between acids
and bases in the body by reabsorbing HCO_3^- and other buffers and by excreting
H^+ and other acids. In this way the body eliminates the daily load of nonvolatile
acids produced by normal metabolism.

E. **Compensation.** When one or more of the body's regulatory systems fail,
other systems have a limited ability to maintain the acid-base equilibrium.
When the pH is outside the normal range (<7.35 or >7.45), compensation has
failed.
1. An acid-base deviation is *respiratory* if it is due to an abnormal P_{CO_2} and
   metabolic if it is due to an abnormal level of plasma HCO_3^-.
2. The lungs attempt to compensate for a metabolic aberration, and the kidneys
   for a respiratory aberration. The result is a change in pH toward normal
   despite an abnormal blood P_{CO_2} or HCO_3^-. The lungs compensate much more
   quickly than the kidneys; however, neither can totally normalize the pH unless
   the underlying disorder is corrected.

DISORDERS OF ACID BASE-BALANCE

Only those disorders classified as primary metabolic problems are discussed here.

A. Metabolic acidosis.

1. Pathophysiology. A pH of less than 7.35 can result from the loss of HCO_3^- (buffering capacity) or from excess acid production. The immature kidneys contribute to acidosis by failing both to reabsorb HCO_3^- and to excrete H^+ when faced with an acid load. When cells do not receive enough oxygen (because of low blood oxygen levels or diminished perfusion), they must use anaerobic metabolism to meet energy needs. This results in the accumulation in the body of lactic acid (lactate), the level of which reflects the severity of tissue oxygen deficiency. Blood lactate may be a more sensitive indicator of tissue hypoxia than pH and base-excess values (Deshpande and Ward Platt, 1997).

2. Causes and precipitating factors.
   a. Loss of HCO_3^-: normal anion gap.
      (1) Prematurity: poor renal conservation of HCO_3^-.
      (2) Renal tubular acidosis: decreased proximal reabsorption.
      (3) Severe diarrhea or ileal drainage.
   b. Excess acid load: ingestion or endogenous production of acid, greater than the ability to excrete it; increased anion gap.
      (1) Lactic acidosis from conditions resulting in hypoxia or hypoperfusion: respiratory distress, congenital heart disease, PDA, sepsis, asphyxia, shock/hypovolemia.
      (2) Inborn errors of metabolism: disorders of organic acid and carbohydrate metabolism.
      (3) Caloric deprivation: catabolism of protein or fat for energy.
      (4) Parenteral amino acid solutions.
      (5) "Late metabolic acidosis" of prematurity, caused by intolerance of cow's milk protein.

3. Clinical presentation and assessment.
   a. Metabolic acidosis occurring early in life is primarily related to systemic illness (e.g., respiratory, cardiac); thus the signs and symptoms are those of the underlying condition(s).
   b. Late metabolic acidosis may present at 1–3 weeks of age by poor growth, hyponatremia, and persistent renal acid excretion (urinary pH <5).
   c. Infants with profound acidosis (metabolic defects such as congenital lactic acidosis) may have respiratory compensation (tachypnea, hyperpnea) or neurologic depression (seizures, coma) reflecting CNS acidosis.

4. Diagnostic studies.
   a. Blood pH less than 7.35: acidemia.
   b. Serum HCO_3^- level less than 18 mEq/L.
   c. *Anion gap* to differentiate between excess acid and insufficient HCO_3^- as cause of acidosis: Anion gap = (Serum Na + K) − (serum Cl + HCO_3^-). Usual range is 8–16 mEq. If high (>20 mEq), acidosis is due to excess acid. If normal with elevated chloride level, acidosis is due to loss of HCO_3^-.
   d. Urinary pH greater than 7 with systemic acidosis: suggests renal tubular acidosis. If low (<5), kidneys are excreting acid.
   e. Plasma lactate level greater than 2.5 mmol/L: may be elevated in some conditions, such as early sepsis, even when the pH is normal (Fitzgerald et al., 1992).

5. Patient care management.
   a. Treat underlying cause of acidosis.
   b. Correction of severe acidosis (pH <7.2) is usually with $NaHCO_3$ (concentration of 0.5 mEq/mL), in a 1–2 mL/kg dose. Administer slowly by

syringe pump or continuous drip; rapid increase in osmolality and pH may be dangerous.

   c. Late metabolic acidosis, if not self-correcting, is sometimes treated with oral $NaHCO_3$.

6. Complications.

   a. Severe acidosis: may depress myocardial contractility and cause arteriolar vasodilation, hypotension, and pulmonary edema.

   b. Impaired surfactant production.

   c. Electrolyte imbalance: decreased iCa, hyperkalemia.

   d. Adverse effects of $NaHCO_3$: cerebral hemorrhage or edema related to wide swings in plasma osmolality. $NaHCO_3$ can also worsen acidosis by rapidly increasing CO_2 if lung disease is present and ventilation is inadequate. $NaHCO_3$ can aggravate hypernatremia and cause tissue injury in extravasation.

7. Outcome. In follow-up studies, metabolic acidosis was correlated with poor developmental outcome in VLBW infants (Goldstein et al., 1995).

B. **Metabolic alkalosis.**

1. Pathophysiology. Metabolic alkalosis results from an excess of HCO_3^- or from a loss of acid.

2. Causes and precipitating factors.

   a. Gain of HCO_3^- from overcorrection of acidosis with $NaHCO_3$.

   b. Loss of H^+ during vomiting or nasogastric suction.

   c. Increased renal acid loss from diuretic therapy.

   d. Rapid ECF reduction (contraction alkalosis).

3. Diagnostic studies: blood pH (>7.45: alkalemia); HCO_3^- (>26 mEq/L).

4. Patient care management.

   a. Decrease $NaHCO_3$ intake if alkali therapy is cause of alkalosis.

   b. Restoring fluid and electrolyte balance is critical.

5. Complications. Severe alkalosis causes tissue hypoxia, neurologic damage, and electrolyte disturbances (increased iCa, hypokalemia).

Inborn Errors of Metabolism

COMMON FEATURES

Occasionally a very ill neonate is admitted to the NICU, and no cause can immediately be found for derangements such as acidosis, hypoglycemia, or seizures. Some of these infants have an inborn error of metabolism (IEM), a genetic biochemical disorder that can lead to irreversible brain damage or death if untreated. There are more than 300 known errors of metabolism, about 100 of which may have neonatal onset. New evidence suggests that inborn errors of metabolism are more common than was previously supposed.

A. **Pathophysiology of IEM.** The gene mutations that cause IEMs produce deficiencies in enzymes, cofactors, transport proteins, and other aspects of cell function. A block in a metabolic pathway can cause an excessive accumulation of substances or a deficiency of others. The pathophysiology of metabolic disorders can be divided into three groups, which describe the basic defect leading to a typical clinical presentation (Saudubray et al., 1994):

1. Disorders that disrupt the synthesis or catabolism of complex molecules, leading to permanent, progressive symptoms that are unrelated to food intake or other events. Examples are peroxisomal and lysosomal disorders.

2. Disorders that interfere with intermediary metabolism, leading to an accumulation of toxic compounds proximal to the metabolic block. Symptoms are

related to food intake and nutritional status. Examples are maple syrup urine disease and galactosemia.

3. Disorders that cause a deficiency in energy production or use, with symptoms arising from both deficient energy production and accumulation of toxic compounds. Examples are congenital lactic acidosis and medium-chain acyl-CoA deficiency.

B. Clinical presentation and assessment.

1. The fetus is usually unaffected because the placenta effectively removes toxins; thus neonates with metabolic disease can appear normal at birth. Within hours, days, or weeks, nonspecific signs appear that may initially be attributed to more common neonatal disorders. A metabolic cause should be considered in any sick neonate until proved otherwise.

2. There are clues that point to the possibility of an IEM:
   a. Acute onset and rapid progression of symptoms, onset of symptoms after an interval of apparent normal health after birth, or symptoms that correspond with the introduction of milk feedings.
   b. Unusual severity and intractability of problems such as metabolic acidosis, or failure of usual therapies.
   c. A history of an unexplained neonatal or infant death in the family.

3. Clinical assessment may reveal all or some of the following:
   a. Neurologic deterioration, ranging from lethargy, irritability, and weak suck to tremors, seizures, hypertonicity, rigidity, and coma.
   b. Gastrointestinal symptoms: vomiting, poor feeding, failure to gain weight.
   c. Respiratory distress from neurologic depression; compensatory hyperpnea or tachypnea from severe metabolic acidosis.
   d. Hepatic symptoms: jaundice, hepatomegaly.
   e. Cardiac symptoms: cardiomyopathy, arrhythmias.
   f. Unusual odor or color of the urine.

C. Diagnostic studies.

1. Diagnosis of an IEM involves several levels of investigation:
   a. General tests such as measurement of blood gases, plasma ammonia (NH_3), lactic acid, blood glucose, urinary ketones, and reducing substances help to determine whether a metabolic defect exists. It is extremely important to obtain acute-phase specimens of blood and urine at the time of symptomatic presentation, before any treatment is given. These can be frozen and saved for later analysis.
   b. Metabolic screening tests of blood and urine are used to classify the disorder for purposes of management.
   c. Enzyme analysis and/or molecular DNA testing of blood, urine, and skin or other tissues provides a definitive diagnosis, but this step may take weeks.

2. Newborn screening is used for early identification of some IEMs.
   a. All 50 U.S. states and Canada screen for phenylketonuria. The battery of tests used by each state for other disorders varies but may include tests for galactosemia, maple syrup urine disease, homocystinuria, biotinidase deficiency, tyrosinemia, and cystic fibrosis (Stoddard and Farrell, 1997).
   b. Newborn screening alone cannot be relied on to detect all inborn errors. There are hundreds of disorders not included on screening panels. Furthermore, a small percentage of infants are never screened. Infants discharged before 24 hours and NICU patients (especially those requiring interhospital transfer) are at increased risk for failing to be screened (Gray et al., 1997).
   c. The optimal time for screening the term newborn infant is as close to discharge as possible. Early discharge infants should be rescreened at 1–2 weeks of age.

d. Hospitalized infants should be screened before day 7 of life. If transfusion or dialysis is required, the specimen should be drawn first. For interhospital transfers, policies should clearly delineate responsibility for obtaining the sample.

D. **Patient care management.**

1. General supportive care: respiratory support, antibiotics, fluids, and correction of electrolyte imbalances, hypoglycemia, and acidosis.
2. Nutrition. In the absence of a specific diagnosis, protein intake is stopped and a high-calorie infusion of glucose and insulin is given to induce an anabolic state.
3. Removal of toxic substances from the body by means of hemodialysis, continuous arteriovenous hemofiltration, peritoneal dialysis, or exchange transfusion (least effective).
4. Elimination of metabolites by complexing them with substances excreted in the urine (sodium benzoate, sodium phenylacetate, carnitine).
5. Administration of certain vitamins (B_{12}, biotin, riboflavin, nicotinamide, pyridoxine, and thiamine) may benefit infants with certain disorders. The vitamins function as cofactors for deficient enzymes, increasing residual enzyme activity.
6. Long-term therapy: dietary. The diet varies with the specific disorder.
7. Newer therapies being pursued: direct enzyme replacement, organ transplantation, and gene therapy.

SPECIFIC DISORDERS OF METABOLISM

Disorders that may have a neonatal onset are listed in Table 14–2. Only the more common disorders will be discussed below.

A. **Disorders of amino acid metabolism.**

1. *Phenylketonuria* is a deficiency of the liver enzyme needed for conversion of phenylalanine to tyrosine. Phenylalanine is produced in the breakdown of tissue protein and the digestion of dietary protein. When conversion to tyrosine is blocked, phenylalanine accumulates in body fluids, causing CNS damage and abnormal brain myelination.
   a. Incidence: 1:15,000.
   b. Presentation: after birth or up to 3 months or more before symptoms appear. Early symptoms are vomiting, poor feeding, irritability, overactivity, infantile eczema, hypopigmented skin and hair, and "musty"-smelling urine.
   c. Management: dietary restriction of phenylalanine.
   d. Outcome: mental retardation if untreated.
2. *Maple syrup urine disease* results from the absence of enzymes required for a step in the degradation of three branched-chain amino acids: leucine, isoleucine, and valine. These amino acids are converted to highly toxic ketoacids that cannot be oxidized and therefore accumulate in the blood.
   a. Incidence: 1:150,000 in general U.S. population (1:176 in Mennonites).
   b. Presentation: normal appearance at birth but, by first 48–72 hours, vomiting, rapid shallow respirations, shrill cry, and hypertonicity, followed by seizures and coma. Urine may have characteristic sweet maple-syrup odor.
   c. Management: reduce protein intake; institute peritoneal dialysis to clear ketoacids from the body. Thiamine may benefit some infants.
   d. Outcome: Neonates die very quickly if untreated. Mental retardation is not avoidable if symptoms occur before treatment.

Table 14–2
INBORN ERRORS OF METABOLISM WITH NEONATAL ONSET

AMINO ACID DISORDERS
Phenylketonuria
Maple syrup urine disease
Nonketotic hyperglycinemia
Hereditary tyrosinemia

ORGANIC ACID DISORDERS
Isovaleric acidemia
Propionic acidemia
Methylmalonic acidemia
Biotinidase/multiple carboxylase deficiency
Glutaric acidemia type II

UREA CYCLE DEFECTS/HYPERAMMONEMIA
Ornithine transcarbamylase deficiency
Carbamyl phosphate synthetase deficiency
Citrullinemia
Argininosuccinic aciduria
Arginase deficiency
Transient hyperammonemia of the newborn

DISORDERS OF CARBOHYDRATE METABOLISM
Galactosemia
Hereditary fructose intolerance
Fructose-1,6-diphosphatase deficiency
Primary lactic acidosis (pyruvate dehydrogenase deficiency, pyruvate carboxylase deficiency)
Glycogen storage disease, types 1A and 1B

DISORDERS OF FATTY ACID OXIDATION
Acyl-CoA dehydrogenase deficiencies (very long, long, medium, and short chain forms)
Multiple acyl-CoA dehydrogenase deficiency
3-Hydroxydehydrogenase deficiencies (short or long chain)
Carnitine transport defect/carnitine uptake defect
Carnitine-acylcarnitine translocase deficiency
Carnitine palmitoyl transferase deficiency, types I and II

OTHER
Lysosomal storage disorders
Peroxisomal disorders (Zellweger syndrome, neonatal adrenoleukodystrophy)
Pyridoxine deficiency
α_1-Antitrypsin deficiency
G6PD deficiency
Cystic fibrosis

CoA, Coenzyme A; *G6PD,* glucose-6-phosphate dehydrogenase.

B. **Disorders of organic acid metabolism.**

1. Pathophysiology. Organic acids are intermediate metabolites of amino acid metabolism. When an enzyme defect prevents metabolism, the affected organic acid accumulates, causing CNS damage and placing a sig nificant burden on the immature kidneys. The most common disorder in this class is *methylmalonic acidemia.*

2. Presentation: metabolic acidosis with compensatory hyperpnea, feeding problems, vomiting, CNS depression, seizures, hypoglycemia, leukopenia, thrombocytopenia, and hyperammonemia. A hallmark is an elevated anion-gap metabolic acidosis. *Isovaleric acidemia* produces an odor reminiscent of "sweaty feet."

3. Management: protein restriction, dialysis, and bicarbonate administration. Carnitine and glycine may be used to provide an alternative pathway for excretion of some organic acids.

C. **Disorders of urea cycle/hyperammonemia.**

1. Pathophysiology. The urea cycle is the major pathway for detoxification of ammonia, a by-product of nitrogen degradation. A defect can occur at any of

the five steps in the cycle, resulting in accumulation of ammonia and profound encephalopathy. The most common urea cycle defect is *ornithine transcarbamylase deficiency.* Preterm infants can also exhibit transient hyperammonemia while on a parenteral nutrition regimen.

2. Presentation. Progressive illness begins at 24–72 hours of life with poor feeding, vomiting, and dehydration. Lethargy precedes seizures, coma, cardiovascular collapse, and death.
3. Diagnostic studies. Blood is drawn to measure ammonia (NH_3); levels are often greater than 1000 µg/dL (normal, <40 µg/dL). If no IEM is found, the diagnosis of *transient hyperammonemia of the newborn* is made by exclusion. Blood gas values may indicate respiratory alkalosis.
4. Management. Stop protein intake and begin dialysis to reduce NH_3 levels. Sodium benzoate and phenylacetate promote elimination of nitrogen.
5. Outcome. Neurologic improvement is seen as NH_3 level declines. The degree of permanent damage depends on the duration of coma resulting from hyperammonemia.

D. **Disorders of carbohydrate metabolism.** The most common disorder in this category with onset in the neonatal period is *galactosemia.*
1. Pathophysiology. Lactose is a disaccharide composed of galactose and glucose. In galactosemia the enzyme that converts galactose to glucose is absent; thus infants cannot digest lactose. The partially metabolized galactose is extremely toxic to the brain, liver, and kidneys.
2. Incidence: 1:40,000 to 1:60,000.
3. Presentation. Vomiting and diarrhea correspond with the introduction of lactose feedings. The infant may have lethargy, hypoglycemia, anemia, jaundice, hepatomegaly, and failure to thrive. Cataracts develop early in life. Many infants also have fulminant gram-negative sepsis because of damage to intestinal mucosa by galactose-1-phosphate, allowing invasion by *Escherichia coli.*
4. Diagnostic studies: blood enzyme analysis and urine reducing substances.
5. Management: lactose-free diet. Sepsis must be aggressively treated.
6. Outcome. Mental retardation and cerebral palsy are consequences of untreated galactosemia. Some neurologic problems occur despite adequate therapy. Cataracts and liver damage are reversible. Secondary ovarian failure is reported to be a long-term complication.

E. **Disorders of fatty acid oxidation (FAO).** FAO disorders now represent the most common inborn errors of metabolism. To date, 18 distinct disorders of FAO have been identified (Boles et al., 1998), the most common defect being *medium-chain acyl-CoA deficiency* (MCAD). Cases of sudden unexplained death have been reported, and a recent study found that approximately 5% of all cases of sudden infant death syndrome may actually have been caused by FAO disorders (Boles et al., 1998).
1. Pathophysiology. Fatty acids are oxidized to provide energy during periods of caloric deprivation (or "fasting"), which can occur during the neonatal period. When the metabolism of lipids is disrupted, what might have been at worst a brief episode of hypoglycemia can become a fatal metabolic crisis. Triglycerides accumulate in the liver, heart, skeletal muscle, and kidneys, leading to organ damage and failure.
2. Presentation. Hypoglycemia can occur within 48 hours of birth, possibly in association with fasting intolerance in an infant who is not breast-feeding well or who has an infection. There may be vomiting and lethargy.
3. Diagnostic studies. Findings include hypoglycemia, metabolic acidosis, hyperammonemia, organic aciduria, and abnormal liver function. Serum ketone bodies are usually not elevated, but fatty acids are.
4. Management. Treat hypoglycemia and avoid even brief periods of fasting.

More frequent, smaller feedings are used, supplemented by IV dextrose during times of illness or infection, when nutritional needs are great but intake is poor.

F. **Glucose-6-phosphate dehydrogenase (G6PD) deficiency.**

1. Pathophysiology. The enzyme G6PD mediates the conversion of glucose-6-phosphate to glutathione, which protects the RBC membrane from oxidation. The affected RBC is then vulnerable to oxidation by chemicals, infection, and certain drugs.

2. Incidence. Deficiency of G6PD is the most common enzyme deficiency in the world and is most prevalent in persons of Mediterranean, Asian, and tropical African descent.

3. Presentation. Clinical forms include *spontaneous chronic hemolytic anemia* (neonates may be jaundiced and anemic) and *episodic hemolysis* (induced by exposure to infection or oxidant substances). The latter group may be free of symptoms at birth; the onset of symptoms occurs 48–96 hours after ingestion of the substance.

4. Diagnostic studies: erythrocyte G6PD activity, hemoglobin, hematocrit, reticulocyte count, and serum bilirubin.

5. Patient care management. No cure is available; management is supportive and preventive.
   a. Treat hyperbilirubinemia, anemia, and infection.
   b. Vitamin E has been used for its antioxidant properties.
   c. Parent education: avoidance of oxidant substances and drugs. These should also be avoided by the mother who is breast-feeding.

6. Complication. Kernicterus can result from severe hyperbilirubinemia.

G. **Cystic fibrosis (CF).**

1. Pathophysiology. CF is a multisystem disorder with generalized dysfunction of the exocrine glands. Symptoms are caused by defective transport of Na and chloride across the epithelial cells lining the exocrine organs. Affected organs are those that secrete mucus (lungs, pancreas, intestines, salivary glands, biliary tract, and genitourinary tract). Mucous secretions are viscous and may plug glands and ducts, causing dysfunction, tissue damage, and infection.

2. Incidence: 1:3,300 live births. The carrier rate is 1:20. More than 400 mutations of the CF gene, known as the CF transmembrane conductance regulator, or *CFTR*, have been identified.

3. Presentation. Neonates are usually free of symptoms unless there is a meconium ileus, which occurs in 10–20% of cases.
   a. In meconium ileus, meconium cannot pass through the distal portion of the ileum, which causes distention, bowel loops, vomiting, and failure to pass meconium.
   b. Other signs are failure to thrive, bulky/fatty stools, prolonged jaundice, and early respiratory infection.

4. Diagnostic studies.
   a. Newborn screening for CF is currently performed in four states by means of a three-tiered approach. First, the immunoreactive trypsinogen (IRT) level is measured from a dried-blood spot. If the level is elevated, DNA analysis for CF mutation(s) is done, followed by a confirmatory sweat test for infants found to be homozygous for the CF gene. Early detection by screening improves nutritional status because treatment can be started sooner than when the disease is diagnosed through conventional means (Farrell et al., 1997).
   b. Sweat test consists of analysis of sodium and chloride levels. It may be difficult to collect enough sweat from the newborn infant.
   c. Abdominal x-ray examination and meglumine diatrizoate (Gastrografin) enema are performed to detect possible bowel obstruction. Typical findings

are dilated proximal bowel and microcolon. Gastrografin is hypertonic and irritating, and it often relieves the obstruction by stimulating bowel activity. Surgical resection of dilated bowel may be necessary.

5. Patient care management. Because the neonate is usually free of symptoms, treatment of CF is aimed at prevention of complications.
   a. Optimal nutrition (enriched diet, vitamin and pancreatic enzyme supplementation), with monitoring of growth and development.
   b. Monitor for and prevent respiratory infection. Chest physiotherapy is used to dislodge thick mucus from the lungs.
   c. Prepare family for discharge: assist in the transition to resources for long-term adaptation to chronic illness. Teaching involves home management and recognition of complications and need for medical follow-up. Genetic counseling should be arranged.
6. Complications.
   a. Volvulus, perforation (can occur in utero) with meconium peritonitis.
   b. Recurrent lower respiratory tract infections.
   c. Malabsorption and malnutrition from pancreatic insufficiency.
   d. Severe hyponatremic dehydration from loss of sodium in sweat.
7. Outcome. The median age of survival is presently 31 years. Heart-lung transplantation has been used in recent years for some patients with end-stage disease. Gene therapy is still experimental but holds promise for children with CF.

REFERENCES

American Academy of Pediatrics: Routine evaluation of blood pressure, hematocrit and glucose in newborns. Pediatrics, 92:474–476, 1993.

Aynsley-Green, A.: Glucose, the brain, and the paediatric endocrinologist. Horm. Res., 46:8–25, 1996.

Boles, R.G., Buck, E.A., Blitzer, M.G., et al.: Retrospective biochemical screening of fatty acid oxidation disorders in postmortem livers of 418 cases of sudden death in the first year. J Pediatr., 132:924–933, 1998.

Cordero, L., Treuer, S.H., Landon, M.B., and Gabbe, S.G.: Management of infants of diabetic mothers. Arch. Pediatr. Adolesc. Med., 152:249–254, 1998.

Costarino, A.T., and Baumgart, S.: Neonatal water metabolism. In Cowett, R.M. (Ed.): Principles of Perinatal-Neonatal Metabolism. New York, Springer-Verlag, 1991.

Costarino, A.T., Gruskay, J.A., Corcoran, L., et al.: Sodium restriction versus daily maintenance replacement in very low birth weight premature neonates: A randomized, blind therapeutic trial. J Pediatr., 120:99–106, 1992.

Curet, L.B., Izquierdo, L.A., Gibson, G.J., et al.: Relative effects of antepartum and intrapartum maternal blood glucose levels on incidence of neonatal hypoglycemia. J Perinatol., 17(2):113–115, 1997.

Deshpande, S.A., and Ward Platt, M.P.: Association between blood lactate and acid-base status and mortality in ventilated babies. Arch. Dis. Child. Fetal Neonatal Ed., 76(1):F15–F20, 1997.

Engstrom, J.L., Kavanaugh, K., Meier, P.P., et al.: Reliability of in-bed weighing procedures for critically ill infants. Neonatal Network, 14(5):27–33, 1995.

Farrell, P.M., Kosorok, M.R., Laxova, A., et al.: Nutritional benefits of neonatal screening for cystic fibrosis. N. Engl. J. Med., 337:963–969, 1997.

Fitzgerald, M.J., Goto, M., Myers, T.F., et al.: Early metabolic effects of sepsis in the preterm infant: Lactic acidosis and increased glucose requirement. J. Pediatr., 121:951–955, 1992.

Fox, M.: Measurement of urine output volume: Accuracy of diaper weights in neonatal environments. Neonatal Network, 11(1):11–18, 1992.

Goldstein, R.F., Thompson, R.J., Oehler, J., et al.: Influence of acidosis, hypoxemia, and hypotension on neurodevelopmental outcome in very low birth weight infants. Pediatrics, 95:238–243, 1995.

Gray, J.E., Sorrentino, J.E., Matheson, G.A., et al.: Failure to screen newborns for inborn disorders: A potential consequence of changes in newborn care. Early Hum. Dev., 48:279–285, 1997.

Halamek, L.P., and Stevenson, D.K.: Neonatal hypoglycemia. I. Pathophysiology and therapy. Clin. Pediatr., 37:11–16, 1998.

Hawdon, J.M., Aynsley-Green, A., Bartlett, K., et al.: The role of pancreatic insulin secretion in neonatal glucoregulation. II. Infants with disordered blood glucose homeostasis. Arch. Dis. Child., 68:280–285, 1993a.

Hawdon, J.M., and Ward Platt, M.P.: Metabolic adaptation in small for gestational age infants. Arch. Dis. Child., 68:262–268, 1993.

Hawdon, J.M., Ward Platt, M.P., and Aynsley-Green, A.: Patterns of metabolic adaptation for preterm and term infants in the first neonatal week. Arch. Dis. Child., 67:357–365, 1992.

Hawdon, J.M., Ward Platt, M.P., and Aynsley-Green, A.: Prevention and management of neonatal hypoglycaemia. Arch. Dis. Child. Fetal Neonatal Ed., 70(1):F60–F64, 1993b.

Huttner, K.M.: Metabolic bone disease of prematurity. In Cloherty, J.P., and Stark, A.R. (Eds.): Manual of Neonatal Care. Philadelphia, Lippincott-Raven, 1998.

Innanen, V.T., Deland, M.E., deCampos, F.M., et al.: Point-of-care glucose testing in the neonatal intensive care unit is facilitated by the use of the Ames Glucometer Elite electrochemical glucose meter. Pediatrics, *130:* 151–155, 1997.

Kjartansson, S., Arsan, S., Hammarlund, K., et al.: Water loss from the skin of term and preterm infants nursed under a radiant heater. Pediatr. Res., 37:233–238, 1995.

Knauth, A.K., Gordin, M., McNelis, W., et al.: Semipermeable polyurethane membrane as an artificial skin for the premature neonate. Pediatrics, 83:945–950, 1989.

Koh, T.H.H.G.: Glucose and the newborn baby: Sweet justice? J. Pediatr. Child Health, 32:281–284, 1996.

Lorenz, J.M.: Assessing fluid and electrolyte status in the newborn. Clin. Chem., 43(1):205–210, 1997.

Lorenz, J.M., Kleinman, L.I., Ahmed, G., et al.: Phases of fluid and electrolyte homeostasis in the extremely low birth weight infant. Pediatrics, 96:484–489, 1995.

Lorenz, J.M., Kleinman, L.I., and Markarian, K.: Potassium metabolism in extremely low birth weight infants in the first week of life. J. Pediatr., 131:81–86, 1997.

Lucas, A., Morley, R., and Cole, T.J.: Adverse neurodevelopmental outcome of moderate neonatal hypoglycaemia. B.M.J., 297:1304–1309, 1988.

Mancini, A.J., Sookdeo-Drost, S., Madison, K.C., et al.: Semipermeable dressings improve epidermal barrier function in premature infants. Pediatr. Res., 36:306–314, 1994.

Modi, N.: Hyponatremia in the newborn. Arch. Dis. Child. Fetal Neonatal Ed., 78:F81–F84, 1998.

Molteni, K.H.: Initial management of hypernatremic dehydration in the breast-fed infant. Clin. Pediatr. (Phila.), 33:731–740, 1994.

Nopper, A.J., Horii, K.A., Sookdeo-Drost, S., et al.: Topical ointment therapy benefits premature infants. J Pediatr., 128:660–669, 1996.

Rutter, N.: The immature skin. Eur J Pediatr., 155(Suppl 2):S18–S20, 1996.

Saudubray, J.M., Poggi, F., Spada, M., et al.: A programmed clinical screening for inborn errors of metabolism in neonates. *In* Farriaux, J.P., and Dhondt, J.L. (Eds.): New Horizons in Neonatal Screening. Amsterdam, Excerpta Medica, 1994.

Sedin, G.: Fluid management in the extremely preterm infant. *In* Hansen, T.N., and McIntosh, N. (Eds.): Current Topics in Neonatology. No. 1. London, W.B. Saunders, 1996.

Seguin, J.: Relative humidity under radiant warmers: Influence of humidifier and ambient relative humidity. Am. J. Perinatol., 14:515–518, 1997.

Shaffer, S.G., and Weismann, D.N.: Fluid requirements in the preterm infant. Clin. Perinatol., 19(1):233–248, 1992.

Stoddard, J.J., and Farrell, P.M.: State-to-state variations in newborn screening policies. Arch. Pediatr. Adolesc. Med., 151:561–564, 1997.

Vadasdi, E., and Jacobs E.: HemoCue B-glucose photometer evaluated for use in a neonatal intensive care unit. Clin. Chem. 39:2329–2332, 1993.

Volpe, J.: Hypoglycemia and brain injury. *In* Volpe, J. (Ed.): Neurology of the Newborn. Philadelphia, W.B. Saunders, 1995.

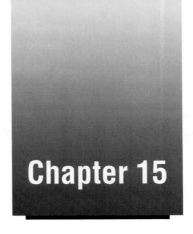

Chapter 15

Endocrine Disorders

Laura Campbell Stokowski

Objectives

1. Describe the components of the endocrine system.

2. Discuss current thinking regarding the definition of hormones.

3. Describe endocrine system regulation.

4. Discuss ways in which endocrine disorders affect the premature infant.

5. Discuss thyroid gland disorders.

6. Discuss adrenal gland disorders.

7. List effective ways to help parents cope with an infant with ambiguous genitalia.

The Endocrine System

The traditional endocrine system is a group of glands (hypothalamus, pituitary, thyroid, parathyroids, thymus, pancreas, adrenals, gonads) and the hormones they produce (Table 15–1). The definition of the endocrine system has evolved recently to encompass not only these classic endocrine glands but every organ and cell in the body that produces and responds to hormones (Chrousos, 1996). Furthermore, hormones are now thought of as being any intracellular messenger—that is, any substance that communicates with a cell distally, locally, or even internally.

A. **Hormones.**

1. Hormones are biologically active substances that exert regulatory functions in cells throughout the body. In composition, hormones are steroids, proteins, glycoproteins, peptides, or amines.
2. To act physiologically, hormones must bind to target cells that have specific receptors for those hormones' molecules. Sensitivity of a target cell to its hormones is critical to normal function.

Table 15–1
MAJOR GLANDS AND HORMONES OF THE ENDOCRINE SYSTEM

Endocrine Gland	Hormones Produced
Hypothalamus	Corticotropin-releasing hormone (CRH) Thyrotropin-releasing hormone (TRH) Gonadotropin-releasing hormone (GnRH) Somatostatin Growth hormone–releasing hormone (GHRH) Prolactin-releasing factor (PRF) Prolactin release–inhibiting hormone (PIH; dopamine)
Anterior pituitary	Adrenocorticotropic hormone (ACTH) Thyroid-stimulating hormone (TSH; thyrotropin) Follicle-stimulating hormone (FSH) Growth hormone (GH) Luteinizing hormone (LH) Prolactin (PRL)
Posterior pituitary	Antidiuretic hormone (ADH; arginine vasopressin) Oxytocin (OCT)
Thyroid gland	Thyroxine (T_4) Triiodothyronine (T_3) Calcitonin
Parathyroid gland	Parathyroid hormone (PTH)
Adrenal medulla	Epinephrine (adrenaline) Norepinephrine (noradrenaline)
Adrenal cortex	Cortisol (hydrocortisone) Aldosterone
Pancreas	Insulin Glucagon Somatostatin

3. Hormones are secreted not only by the major endocrine glands but by non-glandular tissues throughout the body. Many hormones are secreted into the circulation and transported throughout the body to various target tissues. Hormones can also act on cells in the immediate vicinity of their release (*paracrine*) or on the cell that produced the hormone (*autocrine* or *intracrine*).

4. Hormones that circulate in the blood do so both in free form and bound to plasma proteins. It is the free form that is available for receptor binding and that dictates the regulatory influences on hormone release. Furthermore, clinical states of hormone excess and deficiency correlate best with free hormone levels.

B. **Endocrine system regulation (Fig. 15–1).**

1. Many hormones are linked to the hypothalamic–anterior pituitary axis, typified by the classic "negative-feedback loop" regulation of thyroid hormones and cortisol. This type of control begins with hormonal or neural input to the hypothalamus, which produces two substances: *releasing hormones* and *inhibiting hormones.* These are transported via the pituitary portal system to the anterior pituitary. Tropic hormones secreted by the anterior pituitary then regulate the secretions of target organs. As blood concentrations of target hormones reach required levels, a negative message sent to the anterior pituitary inhibits further release of tropic hormones.

2. Other endocrine glands, such as the parathyroids and the pancreatic islets, have a "freestanding" control mechanism. In other words, they are not part of the hypothalamic-pituitary axis. These glands release hormones that stimulate a target tissue to produce an effect, which in turn directly modifies the output of the gland.

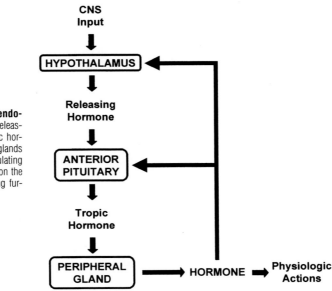

Figure 15–1
Negative feedback loop control of endocrine gland function. Hypothalamic releasing hormones stimulate pituitary tropic hormones, which in turn act on peripheral glands to release hormones. Levels of circulating hormones then exert feedback control on the pituitary and hypothalamus, modulating further output by these glands.

3. In the neuroendocrine relationship, the endocrine and autonomic nervous systems are closely linked in the control of body homeostasis. Hormones act as neurotransmitters, and neurotransmitters are involved in regulating endocrine function. Endocrine glands such as the hypothalamus, the pituitary, and the adrenal cortex respond to neural stimulation. The neuroendocrine system is important in the smooth adaptation of the neonate to the stresses of extrauterine life (Polk and Fisher, 1995).

C. **Endocrine disorders in the neonate.** In addition to well-described neonatal endocrine disorders (hypothyroidism, congenital adrenal hyperplasia), endocrine dysfunction can affect the preterm infant in a variety of ways as a function of maturation. Some of the more common endocrine alterations seen in term and preterm infants will be addressed here. Others, including those involving the parathyroid glands, the posterior pituitary, and the pancreas, are addressed in Chapter 14, Metabolic Disorders.

Thyroid Gland Disorders

THE THYROID GLAND

A. **Normal physiology.**

1. Functions of the thyroid gland.
   a. Concentrates and stores iodide, a trace element required for thyroid hormone synthesis.
   b. Synthesizes *thyroglobulin* (Tg), a thyroid hormone precursor.
   c. Synthesizes and releases the thyroid hormones *thyroxine* (T_4) and *triiodothyronine* (T_3).
2. Thyroid hormone synthesis.
   a. Inorganic iodide is transported from the plasma into thyroid cells.
   b. Iodide is oxidized by thyroid peroxidase and incorporated into tyrosine residues in Tg. This step is known as *organification*.
   c. Iodotyrosines couple within Tg to form T_4 and T_3. Iodinated Tg is then stored outside the thyroid cell.

    d. Tg is resorbed into the cell and proteolyzed to release T_4 and T_3, which diffuse into the circulation.

  3. Thyroid hormone metabolism.

    a. The normal thyroid gland produces mostly T_4 and a small amount of T_3. Most of plasma T_3 (the more potent hormone) is derived from peripheral metabolism *(deiodination)* of T_4.

    b. T_4 enters the cell and is converted to T_3 by enzymes (deiodinases).

    c. Deiodination of the outer ring of T_4 produces T_3. Deiodination of the inner ring of T_4 produces *reverse T_3* (rT_3), a biologically inactive product.

  4. Thyroid hormone transport.

    a. Thyroid hormones circulate in the blood bound to *thyroid-binding globulin* (TBG) and other albumins. Only tiny fractions are in equilibrium as free hormones, but it is this free fraction that is responsible for hormonal activity.

    b. TBG, which is synthesized in the liver, has a high affinity for T_3 and T_4, carrying 70% of circulating hormone. When TBG is deficient, total thyroid hormone concentrations may be lower but free hormone levels are normal.

  5. Mechanisms of thyroid gland regulation.

    a. Hypothalamic-pituitary-thyroid (HPT) axis.

      (1) Hypothalamic thyrotropin-releasing hormone (TRH) is secreted in response to neural input, such as cooling of the skin. TRH stimulates synthesis and release of thyroid-stimulating hormone (TSH; thyrotropin) by the anterior pituitary.

      (2) TSH binds to TSH receptors on thyroid cell membranes and stimulates production of thyroid hormones.

      (3) As thyroid hormone levels rise, further secretion of TSH and TRH is inhibited.

    b. Deiodinase enzymes in the anterior pituitary, brain, heart, liver, and other tissues regulate intracellular T_3 availability.

    c. Autoregulation of hormone synthesis by the thyroid gland itself in relationship to its iodine supply.

    d. Stimulation or inhibition of thyroid function by TSH receptor antibodies.

  6. Physiologic effects of thyroid hormones.

    a. Metabolic processes, such as those involved in oxygen consumption, thermogenesis, cardiac output, erythropoiesis, respiratory drive, gut motility, and carbohydrate, protein, and lipid metabolism.

    b. Growth and differentiation of organs and tissues, including the bones, lungs, and central nervous system. Sufficient thyroid hormones are mandatory for normal brain development.

    c. Thyroid hormones also potentiate the actions of catecholamines by means of increased beta-adrenergic receptor binding.

B. Fetal thyroid development.

1. Fetal thyroid activity begins with synthesis of Tg (week 8), followed by trapping of iodide and limited synthesis of T_4 and T_3 (weeks 10–12).

2. The HPT axis begins to function at mid gestation (weeks 18–20), when iodide uptake increases and the fetal thyroid gland begins to release T_4. Total and free T_4, TSH, and TBG increase progressively until term. The T_3 level remains low until 30 weeks' gestation, rising only in the last 10 weeks as mechanisms for deiodination of T_4 in fetal tissues mature (Fisher, 1997a).

3. The placenta is permeable to TRH, iodide, thyroid autoantibodies, and antithyroid drugs but impermeable to TSH. Maternal thyroid hormones cross the placenta in limited but significant quantities (Vulsma et al., 1989); they may have a role in normal fetal maturation of the central nervous system (Fisher, 1997b). The fetus is dependent on the maternal-placental system for adequate supply of iodide, a critical substrate for fetal thyroid hormone synthesis.

Autoregulation of iodide uptake is not yet mature, so the fetal thyroid is susceptible to inhibitory effects of both iodide deficiency and iodide excess.

C. Neonatal thyroid physiology.

1. At birth, the cooling of the skin and a surge of circulating catecholamines stimulate a sharp rise in the serum TSH level. TSH peaks in the 70–100 mU/L range at 30 minutes of age and then falls to a normal (<20 mU/L) level during the first 3 days of life.
2. The TSH surge stimulates a prolonged rise in thyroid hormone levels. T_4 and T_3 both increase briskly in response to TSH, peaking at 24–36 hours after birth. These changes occur in preterm infants as well but are quantitatively lower. It is speculated that this physiologic hyperthyroid state is important in stimulating thermogenesis of brown adipose tissue (Delange and Fisher, 1995) and in the cardiovascular and pulmonary adaptation to extrauterine life (Rooman et al., 1996).

HYPOTHYROIDISM

Thyroid disorders resulting in low (hypothyroid) states are classified in several ways. First they are considered either permanent (lifelong therapy required) or transient (spontaneously resolving in weeks or months; treatment is temporary or not required at all). Hypothyroidism can also be termed *congenital* (existing from birth) or *acquired*. A third classification relates to the origin of the hypothyroidism:
1. *Primary*. A disorder involving the thyroid gland or some aspect of thyroid hormone synthesis, metabolism, or transport.
2. *Central* (also called secondary/tertiary). Deficient thyroid hormone secretion due to a disorder affecting pituitary control (TSH production) or hypothalamic control (TRH production).

A. Etiology of permanent congenital hypothyroidism (CH).

1. Thyroid abnormalities.
    a. *Thyroid dysgenesis:* absent *(thyroid agenesis)*, hypoplastic, or ectopic gland.
    b. *Familial dyshormonogenesis:* inborn errors of thyroid hormone biosynthesis or metabolism, of which the most common is an organification defect.
2. Extrathyroid abnormalities.
    a. Defects of the pituitary gland (e.g., hypopituitarism) or the hypothalamus.
    b. *TBG deficiency:* X-linked disorder; more common than CH in males.

B. Etiology of transient hypothyroid states.

1. Prenatally acquired:
    a. Maternal autoimmune thyroid disorders characterized by transplacental passage of TSH-receptor blocking antibodies, which inhibit the binding of TSH to the thyroid cell.
    b. Drugs given to the mother that cross the placenta and affect fetal thyroid production. These include propylthiouracil, methimazole, lithium, phenytoin, amiodarone, and radioiodine.
    c. Ingestion of excess iodide or severe deficiency of dietary iodide.
2. Postnatally acquired: transiently impaired thyroid hormone production from exposure to iodine-containing topical disinfectants, ointments, or intravenously administered contrast media. Some studies show an effect of these agents on thyroid function (AvRuskin et al., 1994; Parravicini et al., 1995); others do not (Brown, Bloomfield, and Bednarek, 1997). Preterm infants can absorb and excrete massive amounts of iodine during exposure to these products. Until it is clear that this exposure does not affect thyroid function, minimal use of iodinated substances in the preterm population is usually recommended.

C. **The premature infant.** Several transient hypothyroid states have been described in preterm infants. These states are not universally seen as distinct clinical entities, and there is no agreement as to causes. In many infants, multiple mechanisms may be contributing to the hypothyroid state.

1. *Hypothyroxinemia of prematurity.* Up to 85% of premature infants have low thyroxine levels in the first weeks after birth (Paul et al., 1998). T_4 levels decline to a nadir at 7–14 days of age and then climb to normal within 4–6 weeks. T_4, T_3, and TBG levels in very low birth weight (VLBW) infants are about 60% of those in term infants (Klein et al., 1997). In infants born at less than 30 weeks' gestation, free T_4 levels are low also (Rooman et al., 1996). Low thyroid hormone levels in preterm infants are not surprising because, in the fetus, T_4, free T_4, and TBG all increase only gradually from 20 to 40 weeks' gestation, and T_3 does not rise until after 30 weeks. Thus the infant born between 20 weeks and term has the same underdeveloped thyroid system as the fetus of comparable gestational age. Superimposed on this state of immaturity are the loss of the maternal contributions to the thyroid hormone pool and an increase in T_4 use to meet the stresses of extrauterine life (van Wassenaer et al., 1997a). TSH levels in most preterm infants are normal (e.g., not elevated, as one might expect) because of the relative lack of hypothalamic response to the declining T_4 levels (Rooman et al., 1996).

2. Transient primary hypothyroidism in VLBW infants. Infants weighing less than 1500 g have eight times the incidence of a low T_4/high TSH profile (consistent with hypothyroidism) compared with those weighing more than 2500 g. This differs from the transient hypothyroxinemia described above because of the elevated TSH level. The cause is unknown and may be multifactorial. A few VLBW infants demonstrate a transient hypothyroidism of late onset, with the TSH level rising after 2 weeks of life (Frank et al., 1996).

3. *Nonthyroidal illness* (NTI) syndrome. As in adults, it seems that some nonthyroidal illnesses (e.g., respiratory distress syndrome) can affect thyroid function in the neonate. One effect of NTI is reduced binding of T_4 to TBG (Klein et al., 1997); in addition, hypoxia, hypoglycemia, hypocalcemia, infection, and malnutrition all tend to inhibit conversion of T_4 to T_3 (Fisher and Polk, 1995). Thus the small, sick infant who already has a low T_4 related to prematurity may suffer a further fall in T_4 levels as a result of concurrent illness. Unlike hypothyroxinemia of prematurity, in which free T_4 is often depressed, the free T_4 remains normal or even elevated in many infants with apparent NTI syndrome (Klein et al., 1997). This condition is also known as "low T_3 syndrome" because T_4 is preferentially converted to rT_3 instead of T_3, lowering the serum T_3 level. This may be an adaptive mechanism, reducing the metabolic rate during illness. Alternatively, NTI syndrome could be partially explained by exposure of sicker infants to agents known to affect thyroid function, such as dopamine, which can induce a reversible suppression of TSH and the thyroid axis (Van den Berghe, de Zegher, and Lauwers, 1994). Other agents that may play a role are glucocorticoids (which suppress TSH) and intravenously infused lipid (emulsions) (which inhibit binding of T_4 to TBG).

D. **Clinical presentation and assessment.**

1. Clinical signs and symptoms of CH, which are generally seen only in the most severely affected neonates, reflect the wide-ranging actions of thyroid hormones on metabolism, intestinal motility, cardiac function, temperature regulation, neurologic function, and bone maturation. The earliest signs and symptoms are (Foley, 1996):
   a. Large, open posterior fontanelle (>5 mm)
   b. Birth weight greater than 4 kg; gestation longer than 42 weeks.
   c. Hypothermia.
   d. Abdominal distention.

    e. Poor feeding.

    f. Jaundice lasting more than 3 days.

2. Many of the features commonly associated with hypothyroidism (e.g., macroglossia, dry skin, coarse hair, constipation) are not seen for several weeks after birth.

3. Most transient hypothyroid states in preterm/VLBW infants will not have clinical signs and symptoms readily associated with hypothyroidism.

4. Infants with hypopituitary hypothyroidism may present with midline facial defects (cleft lip and palate), micropenis, and hypoglycemia.

5. Palpation of the neck may identify thyroid enlargement (goiter). A goiter indicates functional thyroid tissue with regard to iodine uptake and is associated with thyroid dyshormonogenesis. Small goiters can be difficult to detect in the short neck of the neonate; extending the neck is helpful.

E. **Diagnostic studies in hypothyroidism** (Table 15–2). Unless the infant is born to a mother with a history of thyroid dysfunction or has obvious clinical signs of hypothyroidism at birth, the diagnosis is usually made after the infant is identified by neonatal screening.

Table 15–2
SUMMARY OF LOW THYROID STATES IN THE NEWBORN INFANT

Screening Results	Possible Conditions	Further Diagnostic Tests	Treatment
T_4 low,* TSH elevated†	**Congenital hypothyroidism** (thyroid agenesis, ectopia, dyshormonogenesis)	Serum TFTs‡; Tg§ level; thyroid scan; ultrasonography; bone age radiography	Thyroid replacement
	Transient hypothyroidism Maternal (drugs, autoimmune) Iodine exposure Some VLBW infants	TSabs, TBabs Urinary iodine level Serum TFTs	Monitoring
T_4 low or low-normal, TSH slightly elevated (borderline)	**Congenital hypothyroidism**	Repeat screen, then test as for congenital hypothyroidism (above)	Thyroid replacement
	Early specimen collection (<24 hours) or false positive	Repeat screen	
T_4 low, TSH normal	**Congenital hypothyroidism** (some functional thyroid: ectopic or hypoplastic)	Repeat screen to detect delayed TSH rise	Thyroid replacement
	Early specimen collection (<24 hours) or false-positive	Repeat screen	
	Prematurity (transient hypothyroxinemia and/or nonthyroidal illness)	Serum TFTs or follow-up screen	Monitoring
	TBG deficiency	Serum TFTs; TBG level; T_3 resin uptake level‖	None
T_4 low, TSH low	**Central hypothyroidism** (hypothalamic-pituitary)	Serum TFTs; TRH stimulation test¶; other tests of pituitary function (cortisol, growth hormone); MRI	Thyroid replacement; other hormonal therapy

TFTs, Thyroid function tests; *TSH,* thyroid-stimulating hormone; *TBG,* thyroid-binding globulin; *MRI,* magnetic resonance imaging; *TSabs,* thyroid-stimulating antibodies; *TBabs,* thyroid-blocking antibodies; *VLBW,* very low birth weight.

    *T_4 low: <6 µg/dL.

    †TSH elevated: >40 mU/L; TSH normal: <10 mU/L; TSH borderline: 20-40 mU/L. Note that a slightly elevated TSH level may be normal in the first 2 days of life.

    ‡May include assays of total and free T_4 and T_3 along with TSH.

    §Tg: thyroglobulin, a thyroid hormone precursor produced by the thyroid gland. A low level suggests thyroid agenesis.

    ‖An indirect measure of protein binding. A high level suggests low binding capacity, as in TBG deficiency.

    ¶TRH stimulation is a test of hypothalmic or pituitary control of thyroid function. A dose of TRH is administered and TSH is measured serially. A subnormal TSH response suggests a deficient pituitary gland, and a delayed response suggests hypothalamic congenital hypothyroidism.

1. Newborn screening for hypothyroidism presently involves a two-tiered approach, although advances in automated screening may soon allow simultaneous testing of various thyroid parameters (American Academy of Pediatrics [AAP], 1993).
   a. T_4 is measured first. If T_4 is low, TSH is measured. A low T_4 concentration with an elevated TSH level is considered to be CH until further testing proves otherwise.
   b. Incidence of CH by screening: 1:4000, with a 2:1 female/male ratio.
   c. Screening recommendations (AAP, 1993).
      (1) Initial heel-stick filter-paper specimen should be drawn on day 2–6 (no later than day 7) of life. If the infant is to be discharged or transferred, the specimen should be drawn first, regardless of age.
      (2) A good-quality blood specimen is needed to minimize measurement errors. Filter-paper circles should be fully saturated on one side of the paper and dried at room temperature without handling or contamination.
   d. A high false-positive rate occurs when samples are drawn during the first 24 hours, when the TSH level may still be physiologically elevated.
   e. Approximately 10% of infants with CH are missed on initial screening; they are detected only through routine second screening in states where this is required (LaFranchi et al., 1985) or on clinical grounds. Some of these infants have compensated hypothyroidism or delayed rise in the TSH level; most seem to have milder forms of hypothyroidism but still require treatment.
   f. Infants at risk of having a missed or delayed diagnosis are those born at home, those who are extremely ill in the neonatal period, and those who are transferred to another hospital at an early age.
2. Thyroid function tests.
   a. When CH is suspected clinically or suggested by initial screening results, confirmatory serum T_4 and TSH measurements are obtained. Free T_4 and T_3 may also be measured, along with other tests, as needed, to determine the cause of abnormal screening results (Table 15–2).
   b. It is important to rule out TBG deficiency in term infants with low T_4 and normal TSH profiles and no clinical signs of hypothyroidism, so that unnecessary treatment is avoided (Fort and Brown, 1996).
   c. If there is a maternal history of a thyroid disorder, serum may be analyzed for the presence of TSH receptor–blocking antibodies.
3. Further evaluation for the cause of a CH blood profile includes ultrasonography of the neck, thyroid radionuclide imaging (to identify normal or ectopic thyroid tissue), and bone age radiography of the knee or foot (delayed bone ossification suggests long-standing thyroid deprivation).

E. **Patient care management.**

1. Congenital hypothyroidism.
   a. Thyroid replacement with synthetic T_4 (L-thyroxine), initially 10–15 µg/kg per day (AAP, 1993). The goal of treatment is to maintain the serum T_4 concentration in the upper half of the normal range, or 10–16 µg/dL (Fisher and Polk, 1995).
   b. Close monitoring of serum T_4 levels and clinical response is needed to prevent overtreatment or undertreatment.
      (1) Overtreatment may lead to advanced bone age, craniosynostosis, and thyrotoxicosis. Early signs are tachycardia, irritability, hyperactivity, poor weight gain, and loose stools.
      (2) Undertreatment leads to clinical hypothyroidism, delayed bone maturation, and neurologic damage.
2. Transient hypothyroidism.

a. Hypothyroxinemia of prematurity, without elevation of the TSH level, is not routinely treated with T_4 supplementation. Despite increasing evidence of associations between low T_4 levels and morbidity and death in premature infants, research to date has not demonstrated clinical or developmental benefits of T_4 supplementation (van Wassenaer et al., 1997b).

b. Because transient hypothyroidism is not always recognized as such in the neonate, replacement therapy for a low T_4–high TSH profile is begun just as it is for established permanent hypothyroidism (AAP, 1993). Evaluation of the permanence of the disease is conducted after the child is 2–3 years of age.

c. Infants who are not treated are usually rechecked at 2-week intervals by repeated filter-paper-specimen or thyroid function tests, to ensure that thyroid function becomes normal. Because of the late-onset TSH rise that can occur in extremely premature infants, it has been recommended that thyroid function tests be repeated at 2 weeks and again at 4–6 weeks of age for these infants (Klein and Mitchell, 1996).

G. Outcome.

1. Congenital hypothyroidism.
   a. CH is one of the most preventable causes of mental retardation. Infants with early diagnosis and early and adequate treatment will have normal IQs (Klein and Mitchell, 1996).
   b. Lifelong thyroid replacement therapy is necessary for normal growth and development.
2. Transient hypothyroidism.
   a. Low T_4 levels in preterm infants are associated with increased severity of neonatal illness, duration of hospitalization, mortality (Reuss et al., 1997), and intraventricular hemorrhage (Paul et al., 1998).
   b. Recent studies indicate an association between low T_4 concentrations in preterm infants and both lower scores on neurodevelopmental outcome measures (Meijer et al., 1992; Reuss et al. 1996; den Ouden et al., 1996) and the incidence of disabling cerebral palsy (Reuss et al., 1996). More research is needed to determine whether transient hypothyroxinemia of prematurity is a harmless physiologic phenomenon or a cause of psychomotor and neurodevelopmental sequelae in this population.

HYPERTHYROIDISM

A. Etiologies.

1. Maternal *Graves' disease* (either active disease during pregnancy or history of disease) is the most common cause of neonatal hyperthyroidism (often referred to as *neonatal Graves' disease*).
2. Rare conditions such as TBG excess and generalized resistance to thyroid hormones can also produce hyperthyroidism in the neonate.

B. Pathophysiology of Graves' disease.

1. Graves' disease is an autoimmune disorder that results in the production of antibodies directed against thyroid antigens such as TSH receptors, thyroglobulin, and thyroid peroxidase (Zimmerman and Lteif, 1998). Most commonly, the mother produces *thyroid-stimulating antibodies* (TSabs), which mimic the action of TSH in stimulating fetal and neonatal thyroid growth and function. However, some mothers will simultaneously produce *thyroid-blocking antibodies* (TBabs), which inhibit the binding of TSH to the thyroid receptor. The effects on the fetus and neonate can therefore be highly variable, depending on the concentration and potency of the two opposing types of antibodies. The clinical

picture also differs between untreated and treated maternal Graves' disease.

2. Effects of active maternal Graves' disease. The fetus may show the effects of hyperthyroidism with tachycardia and, in some cases, development of a fetal goiter detectable by ultrasonography (Polk, 1994). The neonate can exhibit either early or delayed signs of hyperthyroidism. Neonatal effects are usually self-limiting; improvement occurs as the TSabs are degraded in the first 3–12 weeks of life.

3. Effects of treated maternal Graves' disease. Treatment of Graves' disease in the mother is aimed at correcting thyroid hormone levels, usually with antithyroid drugs. Such treatment does not necessarily alter the production of thyroid antibodies, although some drugs may have a partial immunosuppressive effect, reducing the concentration of circulating antibodies (Cooper, 1996). Antithyroid drugs taken by the mother cross to the fetus and block fetal thyroid production. Thus the neonate may actually be hypothyroid at birth, with a delayed onset (up to 10 days) of hyperthyroidism. As maternal antithyroid drugs leave the neonate's circulation, residual TSabs stimulate the neonate's thyroid, and thyrotoxicosis may result. If there are coexisting TBabs, even longer delays (up to 4–6 weeks) are possible before the onset of hyperthyroidism in the infant.

C. Clinical presentation and assessment.

1. Many affected infants are born prematurely and/or exhibit intrauterine growth retardation.

2. Signs and symptoms include irritability, tremor, hyperactivity, flushing of the skin, hyperthermia, sweating, gastrointestinal dysfunction (vomiting, diarrhea), and signs of cardiac stimulation (tachycardia, arrhythmias, congestive heart failure). Eye signs include exophthalmos, eye stare, and lid retraction.

3. Thyromegaly, if present, can worsen during the neonatal period.

4. In severely affected infants, evidence of advanced skeletal maturation (craniosynostosis, frontal bossing) is seen.

D. Diagnostic studies.

1. Total and free T_4 and T_3 are elevated (may initially be normal or low in neonates born to mothers with treated Graves' disease).

2. The TSH is low because of hypothalamic-pituitary feedback-loop suppression.

3. Levels of TSabs and TBabs in the mother and infant may be measured.

E. Patient care management. Clinical and biochemical hyperthyroidism is a medical emergency; the use of some or all of the following can be anticipated:

1. Beta-adrenergic blockers, such as propranolol, to treat cardiovascular overstimulation. Digitalization may also be necessary.

2. Agents to suppress hypersecretion of thyroid hormone:
   a. Propylthiouricil may be administered but will not be effective for several days.
   b. Ten percent potassium iodide or Lugol's iodine solution has been used for acute inhibition of thyroid hormone release.
   c. Radiographic contrast agents (ipodate sodium and iopanoic acid) block peripheral conversion of T_4 to T_3 and inhibit thyroidal secretion of T_4 and T_3 (LaFranchi and Mandel, 1996).

3. A hypothyroid state may be induced by use of the agents mentioned above, making replacement with T_4 necessary.

4. Sedatives may be given for neurologic symptoms.

5. If an enlarged thyroid gland is compressing the trachea, as evidenced by respiratory distress, elevation and extension of the infant's head may help

maintain a patent airway (Dallas and Foley, 1996). In very rare cases, surgery may be necessary to relieve the obstruction.

F. **Complications:** more severe manifestations of thyrotoxicosis, such as congestive heart failure, hepatosplenomegaly, thromobocytopenia, and hyperviscosity syndrome.

G. Outcome.
1. The mortality rate is 16% (Zimmerman and Lteif, 1998).
2. Survivors of severe, prolonged thyrotoxicosis often have permanent neurologic impairment from premature craniosynostosis and the direct effects of excess thyroid hormones on the brain (Fort and Brown, 1996).
3. In a few patients the course of disease lasts months to years, suggesting the onset of true Graves' disease, rather than an effect of maternal antibodies (Dallas and Foley, 1996).

Adrenal Gland Disorders

THE ADRENAL GLAND

A. Anatomy and physiology.
1. The adrenal glands are located at the superior poles of the kidneys. Each highly vascular gland is composed of two distinct endocrine organs: the inner *adrenal medulla* and the outer *adrenal cortex*, which are functionally independent although enclosed within a common capsule.
2. The adrenal medulla produces and stores catecholamines (epinephrine, norepinephrine, dopamine) and is linked to the sympathetic nervous system.
3. The adrenal cortex produces steroid hormones derived from cholesterol (*glucocorticoids, mineralocorticoids,* and *androgens*), known as *adrenocortical hormones.*

B. Adrenocortical hormones.
1. Cortisol, the most important glucocorticoid, has a major role in glucose homeostasis and key regulatory roles in many physiologic processes, including development, growth, inflammatory responses, cardiovascular function, and response to stress.
2. Cortisol is closely regulated by adrenocorticotropic hormone (ACTH) and the hypothalamic-pituitary-adrenal (HPA) axis via a negative-feedback loop. Increased plasma cortisol inhibits secretion of corticotropin-releasing hormone and ACTH, whereas decreased plasma cortisol permits their release. Cortisol is also released in response to stress, such as that caused by hypoglycemia, surgery, extreme heat or cold, decreased oxygen concentration, infection, or injury. During such episodes, glucocorticoids sustain life by activating homeostatic defense mechanisms and, at the same time, by preventing some of these same mechanisms from overresponding.
3. *Aldosterone,* the most important mineralocorticoid, regulates renal sodium and water retention and potassium excretion, thus affecting not only electrolyte balance but blood pressure and intravascular volume as well. Aldosterone is regulated by the plasma renin-angiotensin system and by plasma potassium concentrations. A drop in intravascular volume or the sodium concentration or a rise in the potassium level stimulates the renin-angiotensin system, which in turn stimulates production of aldosterone. Sodium and water are then conserved by the kidneys, and potassium is excreted.
4. Adrenal androgens include dehydroepiandrosterone (DHEA), DHEA sulfate, and androstenedione and are regulated by ACTH. These steroids have minimal androgenic activity but are converted in the peripheral tissues to two more potent androgens: testosterone and dihydrotestosterone.

C. Fetal adrenocortical development.

1. The fetal adrenal gland differs both morphologically and functionally from the mature gland. Beginning at about 8 weeks' gestation, the fetal adrenal cortex differentiates into distinct zones: a large, unique *fetal zone* and a smaller *definitive zone*. The fetal zone is responsible for most of the steroids produced during fetal life. After 25 weeks the definitive zone grows in readiness to assume the principal role in steroid synthesis. Fetal adrenal growth is rapid; at term the gland weighs 8–9 g, twice the size of the adult's. After birth the fetal zone involutes during the first 1–2 months and the adrenal gland shrinks.

2. The fetal adrenal gland and the placenta are an integrated endocrine organ known as the fetoplacental unit. The fetal zone, deficient in a critical enzyme for cortisol synthesis, produces mostly DHEA and DHEA sulfate. These are the precursors for placental estrogen, which is vital to maintenance of the pregnancy and fetal well-being. In turn, the placenta provides pregnenolone, a substrate for fetal cortisol production.

3. Fetal cortisol comes both from the definitive zone of the fetal adrenal cortex and from transplacental transfer. Its rapid metabolism to inactive cortisone protects the fetus from very high cortisol levels. As the fetus nears term, maturation of enzyme systems allows greater conversion of cortisone back to cortisol and synthesis of cortisol from cholesterol. Increases in circulating and local cortisol during the last 10 weeks of gestation (the prenatal cortisol surge) induce the following physiologic changes, which prepare the fetus for extra-uterine life:
   a. Maturation of gut enzymes and islet cells.
   b. Increased metabolism of T_4 to T_3 in the liver.
   c. Maturation of pulmonary surfactant.
   d. Increased conversion of norepinephrine to epinephrine.
   e. Stimulation of hepatic enzymes involved in glucose regulation.
   f. Increased beta-adrenergic receptors in lungs, heart, and brown adipose tissue.

4. Aldosterone production increases throughout pregnancy, preparing the fetus to assume control of salt and water balance after birth.

D. Neonatal adrenocortical function.

1. Plasma cortisol levels are high at the time of birth but begin to fall in the first few days of life. In term infants a nadir is seen on day 4. Likewise, levels of a cortisol precursor, *17-hydroxyprogesterone* (17-OHP), are high at birth but decrease to normal neonatal levels by 12–24 hours of age.

2. Plasma cortisol levels are generally lower in preterm infants, but there is a wide range of variability. Levels of 17-OHP in preterm infants can remain elevated for many weeks even in the presence of low plasma cortisol concentrations, falling only when the activity of 11-beta-hydroxylase (and thus cortisol synthesis) increases (Arnold et al., 1997).

3. In the neonatal period, aldosterone concentration and plasma renin activity are elevated compared with values for older infants. This increase may be necessary for positive sodium balance until the kidneys fully mature. The hyponatremia and urinary sodium loss often seen in preterm infants during the early postnatal weeks are due to a relative mineralocorticoid deficiency as a consequence of immaturity of both the kidneys and the adrenal glands (Dillon, 1995).

E. Adrenal disorders in the neonate.

1. *Congenital adrenal hyperplasia* (see following section).
2. Adrenal hemorrhage (from hemorrhagic diathesis, shock, anoxia, birth trauma).

3. *Hypopituitarism.* The pituitary fails to produce ACTH, and the consequent lack of cortical stimulation results in hypoplasia of the adrenal cortex and adrenal insufficiency.
4. Adrenocortical insufficiency in ill VLBW infants.
   a. Transiently low cortisol levels, seen in some infants, are most likely related to hypothalamic-pituitary-adrenal immaturity (Hanna et al., 1997). This may be a developmental phenomenon, because the fetal cortisol would still be low at the equivalent gestational age. Nevertheless, these low levels are believed to be physiologically inadequate for the stressed infant, leading to clinical adrenal insufficiency and long-term morbidity (Korte et al. 1996).
   b. A low basal cortisol level in the presence of significant stress (severe illness or respiratory distress) suggests an inability of the extremely immature brain to recognize stress in the form of illness (Hanna et al., 1993). More knowledge is needed about development of the stress response and how to recognize periods of hyporesponsivity, which may make the small, sick infant more vulnerable to the effects of stress (Peters, 1998).
5. Adrenal suppression related to postnatal glucocorticoid therapy.
   a. Dexamethasone given to improve pulmonary status, prevent chronic lung disease, and facilitate weaning from the ventilator is associated with temporary suppression of the HPA axis. After prolonged dexamethasone therapy (standard 6-week course with tapering dosages), infants have lower basal cortisol levels and blunted responses to tests of HPA axis functioning. Though most infants recover normal HPA axis function within 1–2 months after therapy, a few exhibit prolonged adrenocortical suppression (Ford et al., 1998).
   b. Other neonatal effects of glucocorticoid therapy include growth failure, hyperglycemia, hypertension, infection, left ventricular hypertrophy, and a diminished ability to respond to subsequent stressful events.

CONGENITAL ADRENAL HYPERPLASIA

A. **Definition:** autosomal recessive conditions resulting from deficient activity of one of the five major enzymes needed for cortisol biosynthesis. A deficiency of the enzyme cytochrome P-450 (P-450$_{c21}$) is the most common type of congenital adrenal hyperplasia (CAH) and is known as *21-hydroxylase deficiency* (21-OHD). Deficiencies of 11-beta-hydroxylase and 3-beta-hydroxysteroid dehydrogenase are less common; the remainder are very rare. CAH has a worldwide incidence of 1:15,000.

B. **Pathophysiology** (Fig. 15–2). Because 21-OHD represents 95% of cases, the remainder of the discussion will pertain to this form of CAH.
1. Lack of fetal P-450$_{c21}$ (21-hydroxylase) prevents conversion of progesterone to its two end-products: cortisol and aldosterone.
2. By reduced negative-feedback regulation, the absence of cortisol causes over-secretion of ACTH, which chronically stimulates the adrenal cortex, resulting in hyperplasia.
3. The cortisol precursor 17-OHP accumulates in the blood because its conversion to cortisol is blocked.
4. The excess 17-OHP enters the unblocked androgen metabolic pathway, and the result is an overproduction of androgens. At a critical stage in fetal development, these androgens cause virilization of the external genitalia in female fetuses. Equally important may be the effects of this androgen exposure on the developing central nervous system.

C. **Clinical presentation.** Three subtypes of CAH related to 21-OHD are traditionally recognized, each of which can give rise to a different clinical picture. Two are known as "classic" CAH: a simple virilizing form and a salt-wasting

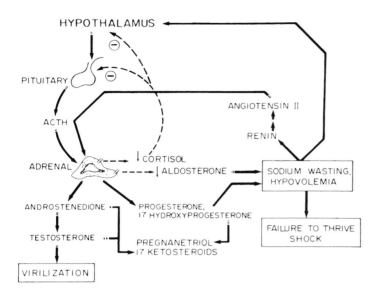

Figure 15–2
Pathophysiology of CAH caused by 21-hydroxylase deficiency. In the absence of cortisol, ACTH stimulates the adrenal cortex to produce virilizing androgens. Diminished production of aldosterone leads to salt wasting and hypovolemia. (From Danish, R.: Abnormalities of sexual differentiation. In Fanaroff, A., and Martin, R. (Eds.): Neonatal-Perinatal Medicine, 4th ed. St. Louis, Mosby, 1987.)

form. A third, "nonclassic" CAH, a milder subtype, presents later in life. Of late it has been suggested that, rather than dividing CAH into types, this complex disorder is best viewed as a disease continuum that reflects the severity of enzyme deficiency (Therrell et al., 1998).

1. *Simple virilizing* (25% of patients).
   a. An incomplete enzymatic block can result in enough aldosterone production to maintain fluid and electrolyte homeostasis. In these infants, clinical signs are few or absent, depending on the degree of enzyme deficiency.
   b. The disease may not be detected until a metabolic emergency occurs, particularly in boys, because genitalia appear normal at birth.
2. *Salt-wasting disease* (75% of patients).
   a. The enzymatic block is more severe, with deficient production of both cortisol and aldosterone. The high sodium excretion that occurs in the absence of aldosterone is called a "salt losing" or "salt wasting" state and can result in profound hyponatremia. Other effects are dehydration and hyperkalemia related to failure of both water conservation and potassium excretion. In addition, effects of glucocorticoid deficiency are impaired carbohydrate metabolism (causing hypoglycemia) and eventual hypotension, shock, and cardiovascular collapse.
   b. Onset of the salt-losing state is delayed for 1–2 weeks after birth. The newborn infant normally has a high aldosterone level in the first week because of slow hepatic clearance, but as aldosterone is used up, the deficient adrenal cortex cannot restore it.

D. Assessment.

1. The earliest signs and symptoms are lethargy, poor feeding, vomiting, diarrhea, dehydration, failure to thrive, apnea, and seizures.
2. Appearance of the genitalia.
   a. In girls with 21-OHD (female karyotype, 46,XX) the external genitalia are masculinized. The phenotype is mild to moderate clitoral hypertrophy, varying degrees of labiosacral fusion, and a urogenital sinus.
   b. In boys with 21-OHD (male karyotype, 46,XY), external genitalia are male, but there can be slight phallic enlargement and hyperpigmentation.

E. Diagnosis of CAH related to 21-OHD. In the past, CAH was not always diagnosed in the neonatal period unless atypical genitalia were noted at birth or the infant had an early salt-wasting adrenal crisis. With the advent of neonatal mass screening, however, CAH is diagnosed in more infants before clinical recognition of the disorder (Therrell et al., 1998).

1. Common diagnostic tests and findings in 21-OHD CAH are as follows:
   a. Serum levels of steroids and precursors are increased: the 17-OHP level is markedly elevated and is hyperresponsive to ACTH stimulation; levels of testosterone and its precursors are increased.
   b. Serum aldosterone and plasma renin activity are measured to detect salt-losing states. The aldosterone level is low in relation to plasma renin activity, which is elevated.
   c. Serum and urine electrolytes reveal hyponatremia, hyperkalemia, and high urine sodium excretion. Other metabolic disturbances include hypoglycemia and metabolic acidosis.
   d. A blood karyotype is obtained to establish genetic sex.
   e. Ultrasonography and/or magnetic resonance imaging are done to visualize the internal structures, including the uterus and adrenal glands.

2. Neonatal screening for CAH is currently performed in 17 states (Therrell et al., 1998). The basis of the test is measurement of 17-OHP, which is elevated in CAH. Some preterm infants and other sick infants have false-positive results because 17-OHP levels are typically higher in these infants. Additionally, blood samples drawn early in life (before 24 hours of age) can give a false-positive screening result because the 17-OHP level may still be physiologically elevated.

F. Patient care management.

1. Goals. Restore physiologic levels of cortisol, suppress ACTH and androgen overproduction, and maintain fluid and electrolyte homeostasis.
2. Hormonal therapy. Administer *hydrocortisone* (glucocorticoid) and *9-alpha-fludrocortisone* (mineralocorticoid).
3. Dietary sodium supplementation to prevent hyponatremia.
4. Additional measures. In a salt-losing state/adrenal crisis, additional measures may include intravenous administration of fluids (glucose and sodium to correct dehydration and metabolic imbalances), treatment of shock, and correction of acidosis.
5. Management of ambiguous genitalia (see later section, Disorders of Sexual Development).
6. Genetic counseling (multiple sibling involvement is common).
   a. Prenatal diagnosis is possible because of molecular genetic techniques, which use samples from chorionic villus sampling or amniocentesis.
   b. Intrauterine treatment can prevent some or all of the virilization of female fetuses. Dexamethasone given to the mother crosses the placenta and suppresses fetal ACTH. Treatment must begin before 8 weeks' gestation and continue to term in affected female fetuses (New, 1998).
7. Parent education. Discuss immediate and long-term management of the disorder, the importance of compliance with therapy, and the need for follow-up of growth and development.

G. Complications.

1. Adrenal crisis can occur with sudden signs of cortisol insufficiency (shock, hypotension, acidosis, hypoglycemia, seizures) plus sodium depletion. This can be triggered by episodes of illness or stress (such as systemic infection or surgery) in the neonatal period. Stress therapy to prevent this complication requires two or three times the usual dosage of hydrocortisone.
2. Consequences of poorly controlled CAH are as follows:
   a. Failure to suppress ACTH and androgen production can result in signs of virilization and accelerated growth or bone maturation.

b. Overtreatment can result in hypertension, pulmonary edema, congestive heart failure, growth failure, adrenal atrophy, and lowered resistance to infection.

H. Outcome.

1. Lifelong hormonal replacement is usually necessary to improve chances for normal growth, pubertal development, and fertility.
2. Missed or delayed diagnosis can result in:
   a. Sudden deterioration or death in infants with undiagnosed CAH.
   b. Progressive virilization in both sexes, with phallic enlargement and growth of facial and pubic hair.
   c. Acceleration of growth and bone maturation. Short stature results from early epiphysial closure.
   d. Sex misassignment, possibly resulting in a later and more traumatic gender change. In some cases, male gender assignments have been retained when late diagnoses were made in genetic females thought to be male from birth (Sripathi et al., 1997).
3. Psychosocial adjustment and psychosexual development in girls with CAH may be altered. Kuhnle and Bullinger (1997) found that, although the overall quality of life did not differ, patients with CAH differed from control subjects in marriage and childbearing rates, body image, and attitudes toward sexuality. Gender change from female to male in adulthood has also been reported (Meyer-Bahlburg et al., 1996).

Disorders of Sexual Development

SEXUAL DIFFERENTIATION

At every stage of fetal sexual differentiation, there is an inherent tendency for the internal and external sexual structures to develop along female lines. Development along male lines requires specific genetic and hormonal influences. Appreciation of the "bipotentiality" of development is fundamental to understanding disorders of sexual development.

A. Fertilization: determination of genetic sex based on X or Y chromosome, contained in the spermatozoon.

B. Primitive gonad development: occurrence in first 5 weeks of gestation.
1. Embryonic gonads form on the genital ridge near the kidneys and are seeded by germ cells that migrate from the yolk sac.
2. At this stage, gonads of male and female embryos are indistinguishable.

C. Gonadal differentiation: beginning at week 6 of gestation.
1. Tendency of the primitive gonad is to become an ovary. Two intact X chromosomes are required for differentiation to a normal ovary.
2. Differentiation to a testis is thought to be activated principally by the testis-determining gene (*SRY*, or sex determining region Y) on the Y chromosome, known as the "switch" because it brings on the first event in differentiation of the male embryo.
3. Primitive Sertoli cells of the testes differentiate first (week 7), followed by the Leydig cells (week 8). The testes begin secreting hormones necessary for further male differentiation. Ovaries differentiate more slowly and do not play an active role in controlling subsequent sexual development.

D. Genital duct differentiation: begins at week 7 or 8 of gestation.
1. Before differentiation, two pairs of primordial ducts form in all embryos: the müllerian ducts and the wolffian ducts.

2. In the absence of furthur hormonal influence, the müllerian ducts become the female urogenital structures (fallopian tubes, uterus, cervix, and upper portion of the vagina) and the wolffian ducts regress.
3. Differentiation of the wolffian ducts into male urogenital structures depends on secretion of antimüllerian hormone by the Sertoli cells and of testosterone, produced by the Leydig cells. These hormones act in a paracrine fashion, causing the adjacent müllerian ducts to regress and the wolffian ducts to persist, forming the excretory ducts to the testes, seminal vesicles, and prostatic glands.
4. The fetal testes begin to descend in the first trimester but do not appear in the scrotum until the last 12 weeks of gestation.

E. **External genital differentiation** (Fig. 15–3): begins at weeks 10–12.
1. Early undifferentiated structures are identical in both sexes: a small genital tubercle, central urogenital slit surrounded by genital folds, and lateral genital swellings.
2. Tendency is for external genitalia to feminize: the genital tubercle forms the clitoris, genital folds become the labia minora, genital swellings form the labia majora, and the genital slit remains open to the vagina.
3. In the presence of testosterone and its metabolite, dihydrotestosterone, genital structures are masculinized: the genital tubercle becomes the glans penis, genital folds form the ventral surface of the urethra and penile shaft, genital swellings become the scrotum, and the genital slit fuses. The enzyme 5-alpha-reductase is required for conversion of testosterone to dihydrotestosterone. The

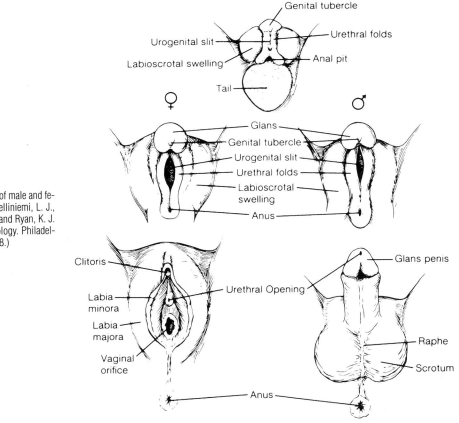

Figure 15–3
Development and differentiation of male and female external genitalia. (From Pelliniemi, L. J., and Dym, M.: *In* Tulchinsky, D., and Ryan, K. J. (Eds.): Maternal-Fetal Endocrinology. Philadelphia. W.B. Saunders, 1980, p. 268.)

presence of testosterone at this time in a female fetus will induce virilization of the external genitalia.
4. Penile growth continues to term under the influence of the pituitary gland. Pituitary luteinizing hormone stimulates the Leydig cells to produce testosterone, which promotes growth of the differentiated penis.

SEXUAL DIFFERENTIATION (INTERSEX) DISORDERS

A. Definitions.

1. *Chromosomal* (or "genetic") sex: the presence or absence of the Y chromosome; also known as the *karyotype* or *genotype.*
2. *Gonadal sex:* the presence of testes or ovaries.
3. *Phenotypic sex:* type of internal and external genitalia. Puberty influences the final phenotype. Another term is *genital sex,* meaning the appearance of the external genitalia.

B. Disorders of gonadal differentiation.

1. *Turner's syndrome* (45,X or variation), a type of gonadal dysgenesis. Affected infants have the female phenotype, with classic somatic features and bilateral streak gonads.
2. *Klinefelter's syndrome* (usually 47,XXY), involving dysgenesis of the seminiferous tubules. This common disorder affects 1 in 1000 newborn male infants but is not generally diagnosed in the neonatal period.
3. *Testicular dysgenesis* (46,XY), with complete or partial failure of testicular differentiation. Partial testicular dysgenesis may present with genital ambiguity because of incomplete masculinization.
4. *Mixed gonadal dysgenesis* (45,X/46,XY). These infants have ambiguous genitalia that are often asymmetric.
5. *True hermaphroditism.* Karyotype can be 46,XX, 46,XY, mosaicism, or 46,XX/46,XY chimerism. Both ovarian and testicular tissues are present, either separately or in combination, in an ovotestis.

C. Disorders of differentiation of the genital duct/external genitalia.

1. Genetic female sex, with masculinized external genitalia (also known as *female pseudohermaphroditism*). Internal organs (gonads, genital ducts) are normal female structures. The degree of masculinization depends on the point during gestation when development was influenced by androgens. Etiologies include:
   a. CAH (21-OHD form).
   b. *Placental aromatase deficiency.* The enzyme aromatase normally catalyzes the conversion of androgens to estrogens. In its absence, excess androgens can virilize both mother and fetus.
   c. Excessive androgen production by the mother (maternal CAH, androgen-producing tumors) or ingestion of certain drugs, such as danazol.
2. Genetic male sex, with incomplete masculinization of external genitalia (also known as *male pseudohermaphroditism*), as a result of defects in the synthesis, metabolism, or receptor sensitivity of androgens. Gonads are normal, but genital ducts fail to develop and external genitalia are ambiguous. Etiologies include:
   a. *Androgen insensitivity syndrome* (AIS). This X-linked recessive disorder is characterized by defects in androgen receptors, preventing binding of testosterone and dihydrotestosterone to genital tissues. Dihydrotestosterone is present but is unable to effect its masculinizing action. There are complete and partial forms, with variable expression.
      (1) Partial AIS is the most common cause of male pseudohermaphroditism. Depending on the severity of the receptor defect, this may result in only

mild undervirilization (small phallus, hypospadias) or genital ambiguity. Infants with genital ambiguity are identified at birth; in others, partial AIS may remain undiagnosed.

(2) AIS is not recognized at birth because the infant's genitalia are female, although a few infants may present with an inguinal or labial mass. Infants with complete AIS have bilateral testes but absent or hypoplastic wolffian duct structures.

b. Defect of androgen biosynthesis. A defect in one of the enzymes required for testosterone synthesis can result in incomplete male sexual differentiation. Three of the enzymes are common to the cortisol pathway, and deficiencies will also result in adrenal insufficiency: cholesterol side-chain cleavage, 3-beta-hydroxysteroid dehydrogenase, and 17-alpha-hydroxylase. Two others, 17,20-desmolase and 17-ketosteroid reductase, are involved only in testosterone synthesis; their absence causes genital ambiguity but not CAH.

c. *Deficiency of 5-alpha-reductase.* This enzyme is required for conversion of testosterone to dihydrotestosterone, the metabolite responsible for masculinization of the external genitalia. Internal structures are normal male, but because of variable degrees of enzyme activity, the external phenotype ranges from ambiguous to female.

d. *Persistent müllerian duct.* The uterus and fallopian tubes fail to regress in an otherwise normal male fetus because of a defect in synthesis, secretion, or response to antimüllerian hormone.

3. Other conditions associated with disorders of sexual development:

a. *Cryptorchidism:* unilateral or bilateral absence of testes in the scrotum, caused by failure of testicular descent. Occurring in 5% of term infants, it is one of the most common urogenital abnormalities of childhood.

b. *Hypospadias:* incomplete fusion of the penile urethra. The urethral meatus is found proximal to the glans penis, somewhere along the ventral surface of the penis or, in severe cases, on the perineum. Hypospadias occurs in approximately 8 of 1000 newborn male infants. Perineoscrotal hypospadias is frequently a feature of abnormal sexual differentiation. First-degree (coronal or glandular) hypospadias does not usually have an endocrine cause.

c. *Micropenis:* an otherwise normally formed penis that measures less than 2.5 cm in stretched length from the pubic bone to the tip of the penis (Zaontz and Packer, 1997). Micropenis results from reduced androgen and/or growth hormone effects during the second or third trimester. Major causes of isolated micropenis include *primary hypogonadism* and *hypopituitarism.* With congenital hypopituitarism, neonates may have persistent hypoglycemia, hypothyroidism, hyperbilirubinemia, and midline craniofacial defects (cleft lip and palate) or septo-optic dysplasia. Birth weight and length are usually unaffected.

D. Clinical presentation.

1. Often, but not always, neonates with disorders of sexual development present with ambiguous genitalia, a term that refers to the fact that a virilized female infant and an undervirilized male infant can have very similar genitalia. In some disorders, there may be only a single atypical genital feature; in still others, genitalia appear "normal" at birth.

2. Other presenting signs and symptoms may relate to a primary endocrine disorder (adrenal insufficiency, hypopituitarism, growth hormone deficiency).

3. Dysmorphic features, such as those of Turner's syndrome, may be associated with cases of gonadal dysgenesis. Many malformation syndromes and other nonendocrine conditions can be associated with genital ambiguity; among

these are trisomy 13, fetal alcohol syndrome, cloacal extrophy, and Smith-Lemli-Opitz syndrome.

E. **Assessment and physical examination.**

1. Examination of the genitalia: close scrutiny not only of babies with clearly atypical genitalia but also of apparent "girls" with inguinal masses, hernias, or clitoromegaly and of apparent "boys" with nonpalpable testes, hypospadias, or unusually small genitalia (Winter and Couch, 1995).

   a. Phallus: size (length and width), presence of *chordee* (downward curvature of the penis, found in some forms of hypospadias), and location of the urethral meatus relative to normal position.

   b. Perineal openings (separate vaginal and urethral openings or a single urogenital sinus): presence of a vagina or a blind vaginal pouch. Observation of voiding may be necessary to locate the urethral opening.

   c. Gonads: presence, location (scrotal sac, inguinal canal, groin), size, and symmetry.

   d. Labiosacral folds: location (posterior or anterior) and degree of fusion (partial or complete).

   e. Pigmentation of external genitalia.

2. Assessment findings.

   a. Genetically female infant. Virilization (Fig. 15–4) can be expressed by degrees of clitoral hypertrophy, nonpalpable gonads in the labiosacral folds or "scrotum," partial or complete fusion of the posterior labia, a single urogenital orifice, and hyperpigmentation of the labia, which may also be rugated. Because complete virilization can be mistaken for bilateral cryptorchidism, any term infant with bilateral undescended testes should receive further evaluation.

   b. Genetically male infant. Hypovirilization (Fig. 15–5) may be expressed by a micropenis (with or without chordee), absence of testes in the scrotum, or incomplete fusion of the genital folds (bifid scrotum, resembling labia majora). A urogenital orifice on the perineum may have a small vaginal pouch. A presumed female infant with unilateral or bilateral inguinal hernia(s) should be examined for complete AIS, because in 75% of these cases, such hernias are present (Viner et al., 1997).

   c. True hermaphrodites and infants with mixed gonadal dysgenesis may present with marked ambiguity that is asymmetric.

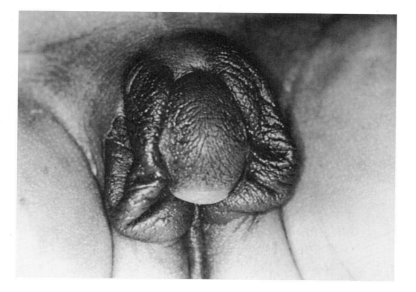

Figure 15–4
Virilization in a 46,XX infant with 21-hydroxylase deficiency. Note clitoral hypertrophy and hyperpigmented and rugated labiosacral folds, resembling an empty scrotum. (Courtesy of Michael S. Kappy, M.D., Ph.D.)

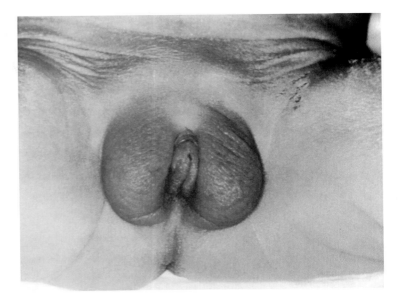

Figure 15–5
Infant with karyotype 46,XY and ambiguous genitalia caused by 5-alpha-reductase deficiency. Note absence of a penis and lack of fusion of labiosacral folds, indicating incomplete virilization. (Courtesy of Michael S. Kappy, MD, PhD.)

F. Diagnosis: a combination of genetic evaluation, clinical and biochemical findings, and examination of internal structures.
1. Family history: a similarly affected infant or family member, ingestion of androgens during pregnancy, maternal virilization, or uncontrolled CAH.
2. Karyotype to determine chromosomal sex.
3. Tests for a possible underlying endocrine disorder.
4. Evaluation of internal structures with ultrasonography, magnetic resonance imaging, radiographic studies (genitography), and/or laparoscopy.
5. More extensive tests and biopsies (molecular biologic studies, enzyme assays of genital skin) for a definitive diagnosis.

G. Care of the parents. Though most people have heard of birth defects and may even know someone whose child was born with one, many will have no prior understanding of the condition of ambiguous genitalia. Indeed, parents in the delivery room may find it incomprehensible that doctors and nurses cannot immediately tell them the sex of their newborn infant. With very little time to consider their reply, staff members (who themselves may never have encountered this situation) must respond to the "simple" question "Is it a boy or a girl?"
1. Communication and education.
    a. When faced with an infant with ambiguous genitalia, staff in the delivery room should not announce a gender, no matter how much pressure they feel to do so, because reversing this gender assignment at a later time may be even more difficult for the parents to accept (Zaontz and Packer, 1997). An option is to tell the parents that a difference in their infant's development prevents determination of the sex in the usual way (i.e., by examining the external genitalia).
    b. Parents should be shown the baby while the differences from more typical features are explained. Open communication regarding planned tests to determine the baby's sex, and when they may expect to hear results, is advocated (Warne and Hughes, 1995).
    c. Later, explanations of fetal sexual development and of the bipotential nature of developing sexual organs are used to help parents understand the influences on the development of their baby's genitalia.

   d. In our technologically advanced society, information about medical disorders, including disorders of sexual development, is literally a few "mouse clicks" away. Both parents and helpful friends or relatives may obtain information from the Internet as fast as, or faster than, they can obtain it from medical professionals. There are websites that cover everything from sexual differentiation of the fetus to personal stories of people who were born with intersex conditions. To prevent confusion on the part of the parents, which may ensue from "information overload" and sometimes conflicting information and opinions, professionals should be aware of the wealth of information available on the Internet, be ready to assist parents in finding what is applicable to their circumstances, and be ready to help them understand what they will discover.

2. Emotional support.
   a. Anticipate parents' reactions, which may include shock, grief, anger, confusion, and disbelief. Frustration with long waits for test results may be expressed.
   b. Provide guidance in dealing with friends and relatives, a significant source of distress for most parents (Warne and Hughes, 1995).
   c. It is suggested that parents delay naming the baby and registering the birth (Witchel and Lee, 1996).
   d. Every effort must be made to encourage parent-infant bonding from the moment of birth.

3. Designation of single spokesperson. Gender assignment decisions are extremely difficult for parents. When a team of professionals is involved in discussions regarding sex-of-rearing assignment, treatment, and prognosis, a single spokesperson should be designated to communicate with the parents (Reiner, 1997a).

4. Counseling for the parents, to begin immediately (Slijper et al., 1998).

H. **Care of the infant.** Most authors outline essentially similar approaches to management of ambiguous genitalia in the newborn infant (Danon and Friedman, 1996; Malasanos, 1997; Warne and Hughes, 1995; Witchel and Lee, 1997). It must be borne in mind that, although current literature reflects the following principles related to gender assignment and surgical repair, even experts do not necessarily agree on these issues (Money and Danon, 1996).

1. Gender assignment.
   a. The birth of an infant with ambiguous genitalia is considered a psychosocial emergency; diagnostic testing must begin immediately. A multidisciplinary team (pediatric endocrinologist, geneticist, pediatric urologic surgeon, radiologist, psychiatrist) may be called on to evaluate the infant or consult on the case.
   b. In the best of circumstances, it can take a minimum of 48–72 hours to get the information needed for some sex-of-rearing decisions. In the interim, sex assignment should not be made or guessed at on the basis of external features alone.
   c. Sex assignment is not determined by any one factor in isolation, such as the chromosomes, gonads, or external anatomy. These and many other factors (e.g., underlying pathophysiology, prognosis for pubertal development, future sexual function, fertility, chances for a satisfactory surgical repair, social factors such as cultural background, and desires of the parents) are considered when sex-of-rearing recommendations are made.
   d. Recommendations for gender assignment.
     (1) Most genetically female infants with CAH are raised as girls, regardless of the degree of virilization, because internal structures are normal and capable of fertility.

    (2) Genetically male infants with defects of androgen synthesis or gonado-tropin deficiencies are usually raised as boys because they may respond to hormonal treatment with phallic growth and testicular descent. A test of stimulation with human chorionic gonadotropin or a trial of testoster-one therapy may be given to some infants to determine whether the genital tissues will respond to androgen at puberty; this process may de-lay gender assignment. Similarly, genetically male infants with 5-alpha-reductase deficiency are raised as boys because they will virilize at puberty and are fertile.

    (3) In most instances, reassignment of a genetically male infant to the female sex is appropriate:

        (a) Micropenis (partial AIS, gonadal dysgenesis, and other causes) if a trial of testosterone therapy fails to result in adequate penile growth.

        (b) Complete or almost complete androgen insensitivity because no further virilization is possible.

        (c) Severe hypospadias that cannot be repaired.

  2. Surgical management.

    a. Surgical repair for the virilized girl involves clitoroplasty, vaginoplasty, and labioscrotal reduction. Some surgeons perform these procedures early in the first year of life in a single operation, with additional procedures at maturity. Minor clitoromegaly does not necessarily need to be repaired (Huma, Crawford, and New, 1995).

    b. Surgery for the genetically male infant being raised as a boy may involve repair of hypospadias and undescended testes in the first year of life. Multistage procedures are often needed for severe hypospadias.

    c. For the genetically male infant raised as a girl, in addition to feminizing genitoplasty, removal of dysgenetic gonads is performed at some point because the risk of later malignancy is high.

I. Complications.

1. Inappropriate sex assignment when the ambiguity was not detected in the neonatal period.
2. Gonadal or genital duct malignancy can occur with gonadal dysgenesis.

J. Outcome.

1. Outcome studies are limited. Information suggests that the affected child and the family can face difficulties that extend well beyond the initial crisis in the neonatal period (Slijper et al., 1998). With patients sometimes "lost to follow-up," professionals may not always be fully aware of the lifelong impli-cations of decisions that were made in the first days of life.
2. Some children undergoing genital surgery will require staged reconstructive procedures and, at puberty, hormonal therapy to induce development of gender-appropriate secondary sexual characteristics.
3. Reproductive capacity varies according to the condition. Fertility is possible in some circumstances (e.g., in a woman with CAH) but is rare or impossible in others (complete AIS, some forms of gonadal dysgenesis).

RECENT CONTROVERSIES IN MANAGEMENT OF AMBIGUOUS GENITALIA

    It is widely believed that, with early sex assignment, early surgical correction, and an environment that accepts the "sex of rearing" with conviction, the psychosocial adjustment, gender identity and role behavior, and sexual orienta-tion of children with disorders of sexual development will not differ from the norm, even when the assigned gender is discordant with the chromosomal sex

(Conte and Grumbach, 1997). However, this belief is being questioned because it is apparent that some sex "reassignments" have not been as successful as hoped. For example, data show that some genetically male individuals reassigned as girls continue to have strong male tendencies, and a few even reverse their gender in adolescence (Reiner, 1997b). Insufficient emphasis may have been given to the lasting effects of androgen exposure on the developing fetal and neonatal brain; in other words, some childrens' brains may be "masculinized" to the point where attempts to impose a female gender identity are doomed to failure. The relative roles of prenatal androgenization (or lack thereof) and sex-of-rearing environment in psychosexual differentiation are a source of debate that is not likely to be resolved soon.

A. **Sex-of-rearing assignment.** Modifications to traditional approaches have been outlined by Diamond and Sigmundson (1997), Reiner (1997a), and Slijper et al. (1998). A number of boys who might in the past have been reassigned as girls (e.g., those with micropenis, traumatic loss of the genitals, and some forms of hypospadias) would be raised in accordance with their genetic sex, as would 46,XY infants with some partial defects in the synthesis of androgens, because these latter boys can virilize at puberty with hormonal therapy (Slijper et al., 1998). Partially virilized girls with CAH are best raised as girls. It is still not known whether genetically female infants with CAH and complete external virilization (extensively fused labia and a penile clitoris) are more likely to develop into the female or male gender role, despite potential fertility as females. Diamond and Sigmundson (1997) recommend that these infants be raised as boys. Data are at present insufficient to predict every intersex child's eventual psychosexual development; for now, many sex-of-rearing decisions remain complex and difficult. In contrast to typical paradigms that stress the emergency nature of the decision making, the time necessary to educate the parents thoroughly, obtain expert opinions, and reach a consensus should be taken (Reiner, 1997a).

B. **Surgical intervention.** Present management of ambiguous genitalia usually involves reconstructive surgery early in life so that the genitalia appear normal and conform to the sex of rearing. Reiner (1997a) found that older children and young adolescents want cosmetically "appropriate" genitalia, and parents may want treatment of their newborn infant's condition. On the other hand, children may suffer as much psychologic trauma from multiple genital reconstructive surgeries as they would by being "different" from typically developed children. It is argued that because such procedures can have an impact on postpubertal sexual function, surgery for cosmetic purposes should be deferred (Diamond and Sigmundson, 1997). This view is shared by some intersex individuals (and former patients) who ask that doctors perform no early genital surgery on affected newborn infants except where medically necessary, such as in severe hypospadias. Because gender reconstruction of any other type is irreversible and in and of itself places the child at unnecessary risk, it would be delayed until the child is old enough to participate in the decision (Intersex Society of North America, 1994).

REFERENCES

American Academy of Pediatrics: Newborn screening for congenital hypothyroidism. Pediatrics, 91:1203–1209, 1993.

Arnold, J., Leslie, G., Bowen, J., et al.: Longitudinal study of plasma cortisol and 17-hydroxyprogesterone in very-low-birth-weight infants during the first 16 weeks of life. Biol. Neonate, 72:148–155, 1997.

AvRuskin, T.W., Greenfield, E., Prasad, V., et al.: De-creased T_3 and T_4 levels following topical application of povidone-iodine in premature neonates. J. Pediatr. Endocrinol., 7(3):205–209, 1994.

Brown, R.S., Bloomfield, S., and Bednarek, F.J.: Routine skin cleansing with povidone-iodine is not a common cause of transient neonatal hypothyroidism in North America: A prospective, controlled study. Thyroid, 7:395–400, 1997.

Chrousos, G.P.: Organization and integration of the endocrine system. *In* Sperling, M. (Ed.): Pediatric Endocrinology. Philadelphia, W.B. Saunders, 1996.

Conte, F.A., and Grumbach, M.M.: Abnormalities of sexual determination and differentiation. *In* Greenspan, F.S., and Strewler, G.J. (Eds.): Basic and Clinical Endocrinology, 5th ed. Stamford, Conn., Appleton & Lange, 1997.

Cooper, D.S.: Treatment of thyrotoxicosis. *In* Braverman, L.E., and Utiger, R.D. (Eds.): Werner and Ingbar's The Thyroid. Philadelphia, Lippincott-Raven, 1996.

Dallas, J.S., and Foley, T.P.: Hyperthyroidism. *In* Lifschitz, F. (Ed.): Pediatric Endocrinology, 3rd ed. New York, Marcel Dekker, 1996.

Danon, M., and Friedman, S.C.: Ambiguous genitalia, micropenis, hypospadias and cryptorchidism. *In* Lifschitz, F. (Ed.): Pediatric Endocrinology, 3rd ed. New York, Marcel Dekker, 1996.

Delange, F., and Fisher, D.A.: The thyroid gland. *In* Brook, C.G.D. (Ed.): Clinical Paediatric Endocrinology, 3rd ed. Oxford, Blackwell Science, 1995.

den Ouden, A.L., Kok, J.H., Verkerk, P.H., et al.: The relation between neonatal thyroxine levels and neurodevelopmental outcome at age 5 and 9 years in a national cohort of very preterm and/or very low birth weight infants. Pediatr. Res., 39:142–145, 1996.

Diamond, M., and Sigmundson, H.K.: Management of intersexuality: Guidelines for dealing with persons with ambiguous genitalia. Arch. Pediatr. Adolesc. Med., 151:1046–1050, 1997.

Dillon, M.J.: Salt and water balance: Sodium-losing states and endocrine hypertension. *In* Brook, C.G.D. (Ed.): Clinical Paediatric Endocrinology, 3rd ed. Oxford, Blackwell Science, 1995.

Fisher, D.A.: Thyroid function in very low birth weight infants. Clin. Endocrinol., 47:419–421, 1997a.

Fisher, D.A.: Fetal thyroid function: Diagnosis and management of fetal thyroid disorders. Clin. Obstet. Gynecol., 40(1):16–31, 1997b.

Fisher, D.A., and Polk, D.H.: Thyroid disease in the fetus, neonate and child. *In* DeGroot, L.J. (Ed.): Endocrinology, 3rd ed. Philadelphia, W.B. Saunders, 1995.

Foley, T.P.: Congenital hypothyroidism. *In* Braverman, L.E., and Utiger, R.D. (Eds.): Werner and Ingbar's The Thyroid. Philadelphia, Lippincott-Raven, 1996.

Ford, L.R., Willi, S.M., Hollis, B.W., et al.: Suppression and recovery of the neonatal hypothalamic-pituitary-adrenal axis after prolonged dexamethasone therapy. J. Pediatr., 131:722–726, 1998.

Fort, P.F., and Brown, R.S.: Thyroid disorders in infancy. *In* Lifschitz, F. (Ed.): Pediatric Endocrinology, 3rd ed. New York, Marcel Dekker, 1996.

Frank, J.E., Faix, J.D., Hermos, R.J., et al.: Thyroid function in very low birth weight infants: Effects on neonatal hypothyroidism screening. J. Pediatr., 128:548–554, 1996.

Hanna, C.E., Jett, P.L., Laird, M.R., et al.: Corticosteroid binding globulin, total serum cortisol and stress in extremely-low-birth-weight infants. Am. J. Perinatol., 14(4):201–204, 1997.

Hanna, C.E., Keith, L.D., Colasurdo, M.A., et al.: Hypothalamic pituitary adrenal function in the extremely low birth weight infant. J. Clin. Endocrinol. Metab., 76:384–387, 1993.

Huma, Z., Crawford, C., and New, M.I.: Congenital adrenal hyperplasia. *In* Brook, C.G.D. (Ed.): Clinical Paediatric Endocrinology, 3rd ed. Oxford, Blackwell Science, 1995.

Intersex Society of North America: Recommendations for Treatment. San Francisco, Calif., 1994 (http://www.isna.org).

Klein, R.Z., Carlton, E.L., Faix, J.D., et al.: Thyroid function in very low birth weight infants. Clin. Endocrinol., 47:411–417, 1997.

Klein, R.Z., and Mitchell, M.M.: Hypothyroidism in infants and children. *In* Braverman, L.E., and Utiger, R.D. (Eds.): Werner and Ingbar's The Thyroid. Philadelphia, Lippincott-Raven, 1996.

Korte, C., Styne, D., Merritt, T.A., et al.: Adrenocortical function in the very low birth weight infant: Improved testing sensitivity and association with neonatal outcome. J. Pediatr., 128:257–263, 1996.

Kuhnle, U., and Bullinger, M.: Outcome of congenital adrenal hyperplasia. Pediatr. Surg. Int., 12:511–515, 1997.

LaFranchi, S.H., Hanna, C.E., Krainz, P.L., et al.: Screening for congenital hypothyroidism with specimen collection at two time periods: Results of the Northwest Regional Screening Program. Pediatrics, 76:734–740, 1985.

LaFranchi, S.H., and Mandel, S.H.: Graves' disease in the neonatal period and childhood. *In* Braverman, L.E., and Utiger, R.D. (Eds.): Werner and Ingbar's The Thyroid. Philadelphia, Lippincott-Raven, 1996.

Malasanos, T.H.: Sexual development of the fetus and pubertal child. Clin. Obstet. Gynecol. 40(1):153–167, 1997.

Meijer, W.J., Verloove-Vanhorick, S.P., Brand, R., et al.: Transient hypothyroxinemia associated with developmental delay in very preterm infants. Arch. Dis. Child., 67:944–947, 1992.

Meyer-Bahlburg, H.F., Gruen, R.S., New, M.I., et al.: Gender change from female to male in classical congenital adrenal hyperplasia. Horm. Behav. 30:319–332, 1996.

Money, J., and Danon, M.: Sexological considerations in patients with a history of ambisexual birth defect. *In* Lifschitz, F. (Ed.): Pediatric Endocrinology, 3rd ed. New York, Marcel Dekker, 1996.

New, M.I.: Diagnosis and management of congenital adrenal hyperplasia. Annu. Rev. Med., 49:311–328, 1998.

Parravicini, E., Fontana, C., Paterlini, G.L., et al.: Iodine, thyroid function and very low birth weight infants. Pediatrics, 98:730–734, 1996.

Paul, D.A., Leef, K.H., Stefano, J.L., et al.: Low serum thyroxine on initial newborn screening is associated with intraventricular hemorrhage and death in very low birth weight infants. Pediatrics, 101:903–907, 1998.

Peters, K.L.: Neonatal stress reactivity and cortisol. J. Perinatal Neonatal Nurs., 11(4):45–59, 1998.

Polk, D.H.: Diagnosis and management of altered fetal thyroid states. Clin. Perinatol., 21:647–661, 1994.

Polk, D.H., and Fisher, D.A.: Fetal and neonatal endocrinology. *In* DeGroot, L.J. (Ed.): Endocrinology, 3rd ed. Philadelphia, W.B. Saunders, 1995.

Reiner, W.: Sex assignment in the neonate with intersex or inadequate genitalia. Arch. Pediatr. Adolesc. Med., 151:1044–1045, 1997a.

Reiner, W. To be male or female—that is the question. Arch. Pediatr. Adolesc. Med., 151:224–225, 1997b.

Reuss, M.L., Paneth, N., Lorenz, J.M., et al.: Correlates of low thyroxine values of newborn screening among infants born before 32 weeks' gestation. Early Hum. Dev., 47:223–233, 1997.

Reuss, M.L., Paneth, N., Pinto-Martin, J.A., et al.: The relation of transient hypothyroxinemia in preterm infants to neurologic development at two years of age. N. Engl. J. Med. 334:821–827, 1996.

Rooman, R.P., Du Caju, M.V.L., Op De Beeck, L., et al.: Low thyroxinaemia occurs in the majority of very preterm newborns. Eur. J. Pediatr., 155:211–215, 1996.

Slijper, F.M.E., Drop, S.L.S., Molenaar, J.C., et al.: Long-term psychological evaluation of intersex children. Arch. Sex. Behav. 27(2):125–145, 1998.

Sripathi, V., Ahmed, S., Sakati, N., et al.: Gender reversal in 46,XX congenital virilizing adrenal hyperplasia. Br. J. Urol., 79:785–789, 1997.

Therrell, B.L., Berenbaum, S.A., Manter-Kapanke, V., et al.: Results of screening 1.9 million Texas newborns for 21-hydroxylase deficient congenital adrenal hyperplasia. Pediatrics, 101:583–590, 1998.

Van den Berghe, G., de Zegher, F., and Lauwers, P.: Dopamine suppresses pituitary function in infants and children. Crit. Care Med., 22:1747–1753, 1994.

van Wassenaer, A.G., Kok, J.H., Briet, J.M., et al.: Thyroid function in preterm newborns: Is T$_4$ treatment required in infants <27 weeks' gestational age? Exp. Clin. Endocrinol. Diabetes, 105(suppl. 4):12–18, 1997a.

van Wassenaer, A.G., Kok, J.H., de Vijlder, J.J., et al.: Effects of thyroxine supplementation on neurologic development in infants born at less than 30 weeks' gestation. N. Engl. J. Med., 336:21–26, 1997b.

Viner, R.M., Teoh, Y., Wiliams, D.M., et al.: Androgen insensitivity syndrome: A survey of diagnostic procedures and management in the UK. Arch. Dis. Child., 77:305–309, 1997.

Warne, G.L., and Hughes, I.A.: The clinical management of ambiguous genitalia. In Brook, C.G.D. (Ed.): Clinical Paediatric Endocrinology, 3rd ed. Oxford, Blackwell Science, 1995.

Winter, J.S.D., and Couch, R.M.: Sexual differentiation. In Felig, P., Baxter, J.D., and Frohman, L.A. (Eds.): Endocrinology and Metabolism, 3rd ed. New York, McGraw-Hill, 1995.

Witchel, S.S., and Lee, P.A.: Ambiguous genitalia. In Sperling, M. (Ed.): Pediatric Endocrinology. Philadelphia, W.B. Saunders, 1996.

Zaontz, M.R., and Packer, M.G.: Abnormalities of the external genitalia. Pediatr. Clin. North Am. 44:1267–1297, 1997.

Zimmerman, D., and Lteif, A.N.: Thyrotoxicosis in children. Endocrinol. Metab. Clin. North Am., 27(1):109–126, 1998.

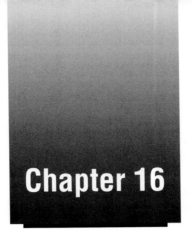

Chapter 16

Hematologic Disorders

Sharon M. Glass

Objectives

1. Differentiate the processes of hematopoiesis and erythropoiesis.

2. Recall erythrocyte and leukocyte development from pluripotent stem cells.

3. Relate the consequences of anemia to the management of the infant.

4. Evaluate the clinical presentation of disseminated intravascular coagulation in relation to the coagulation consumption and fibrinolysis.

5. Describe the etiologic factors of hemorrhagic disease of the newborn.

6. Describe key indicators for nursing assessment of the thrombocytopenic infant.

7. Evaluate the neonatal consequences of maternal immune thrombocytopenic purpura.

8. Discuss the role of partial exchange transfusion in the treatment of neonatal polycythemia.

9. Describe current recommendations for use of blood components.

10. Analyze the components of the complete blood cell count and describe the usefulness of each in the determination of neonatal sepsis.

To meet the objectives, this chapter presents an overview of development of blood cells and coagulation factors and includes normal birth values and common diagnostic tests. Blood products and transfusion therapies are discussed with current recommendations for use. Common hematologic problems and therapies affecting the newborn infant are outlined. An evaluation of the components of a complete blood cell count, useful for identification of sepsis, is included.

Development of Blood Cells

A. **Hematopoiesis:** formation, production, and maintenance of blood cells (Beardsley and Nathan, 1998; Christensen, 1998).
1. Pluripotent stems cells, from which all blood cells derive, are present in the yolk sac at 16 days' gestation.

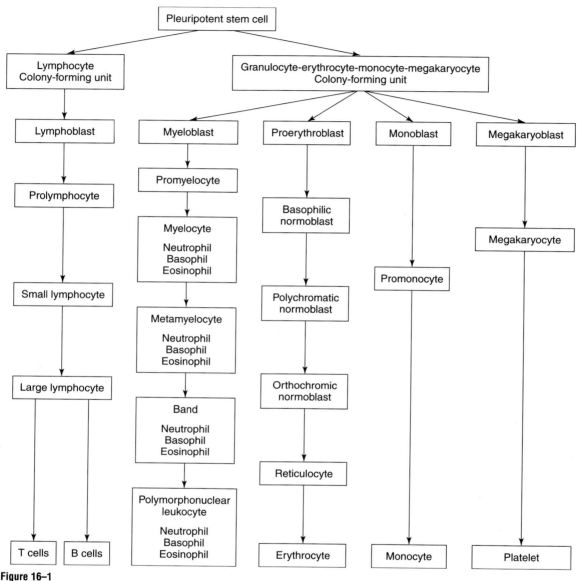

Figure 16–1
Maturation of blood cell components.

2. Circulation begins by day 22, with primitive cells arising intravascularly from vessel walls.
3. Extravascular liver hematopoiesis begins with migration of pluripotent stem cells from the yolk sac, well established by 9 weeks' gestation.
4. Liver hematopoiesis peaks at 4–5 months' gestation and then slowly regresses as medullary (bone marrow) hematopoiesis predominates from 22 weeks' gestation.
5. Sites of extramedullary hematopoiesis (spleen, lymph nodes, thymus, kidneys) aid production of cells during fetal life when long bones are small.
6. Pluripotent cells develop into committed unipotent stem cells (colony-forming units), which evolve into specific cell lines (Fig. 16–1).

7. Stress can influence the rate of differentiation of pluripotent cells yielding different concentrations of committed precursor cells.

B. **Erythropoiesis:** production of erythrocytes (red blood cells [RBCs]).
1. Erythroid precursors develop from a committed unipotent cell, which also differentiates to produce granulocytes, monocytes, and platelets.
2. Erythropoiesis and synthesis of hemoglobin are regulated by a hormone, erythropoietin.
3. Erythropoietin is produced postnatally in the kidneys, but during fetal life extrarenal sites (liver, submandibular glands) predominate.
4. Erythropoietin production is increased in response to anemia and low oxygen availability to tissues and is decreased in response to hypertransfusion.

C. **Hemoglobin:** major iron-containing component of the RBCs.
1. Hemoglobin delivers oxygen from the lungs to the tissue cells through the circulation.
2. By 10 weeks' gestation, fetal hemoglobin (HbF) is the major component of the red cells.
3. Transition from predominant production of HbF to production of adult hemoglobin (HbA) begins at the end of fetal life. RBCs contain 70–90% HbF at birth.
4. HbF has a greater affinity for oxygen than does HbA, resulting in decreased oxygen release to the tissues.
   a. Hemoglobin binds with 2,3-diphosphoglycerate (2,3-DPG) to release an oxygen molecule.
   b. HbF has far less affinity for 2,3-DPG than does HbA.
   c. Levels of 2,3-DPG are directly proportional to gestational age.
5. Normal birth values (Table 16–1).
   a. Values depend on gestational age and volume of placental transfusion (timing of cord clamping, infant position).
   b. Peripheral vasoconstriction and stasis yield higher values from capillary samples.

D. **Hematocrit:** percentage of RBCs in a unit volume of blood.
1. Values rise immediately after birth and then decline to cord levels in the first week.
2. Normal birth values (Table 16–1).
   a. Values depend on gestational age and volume of placental transfusion (timing of cord clamping, infant position).

Table 16–1
NORMAL BLOOD VALUES IN PREMATURE AND TERM INFANTS

Value	Gestational Age (wk)		Term Cord Blood	Day 1	Day 3	Day 7	Day 14
	28	34					
Hb (g/dL)	14.5	15.0	16.8	18.4	17.8	17.0	16.8
Hematocrit (%)	45	47	53	58	55	54	52
Red cells (mm³)	4.0	4.4	5.25	5.8	5.6	5.2	5.1
MCV (μ³)	120	118	107	108	99	98	96
MCH (pg)	40	38	34	35	33	32.5	31.5
MCHC (%)	31	32	31.7	32.5	33	33	33
Reticulocytes (%)	5–10	3–10	3–7	3–7	1–3	0–1	0–1
Platelets (1000 s/mm³)			290	192	213	248	252

Hb, Hemoglobin; *MCV*, Mean corpuscular volume; *MCH*, mean corpuscular hemoglobin; *MCHC*, mean corpuscular hemoglobin concentration.
From Klaus, M.H., and Fanaroff, A.A.: Care of the High-Risk Neonate, 4th ed. Philadelphia, W.B. Saunders, 1993.

    b. Peripheral vasoconstriction and stasis yield higher values from capillary samples.

E. RBCs.

1. Erythroid precursors mature in the bone marrow through the normoblast and reticulocyte stages (Fig. 16–1).
2. Reticulocytes, in the absence of stress, mature 1–2 days in the bone marrow and then another day in the circulation before maturing to erythrocytes.
    a. Reticulocyte count is inversely proportional to gestational age at birth (Table 16–1) but falls rapidly to less than 2% by 7 days.
    b. Persistent reticulocytosis may indicate chronic blood loss or hemolysis.
3. RBC function.
    a. Tissue oxygenation by hemoglobin transport.
    b. Carbon dioxide removal through reaction with carbonic anhydrase.
    c. Hemoglobin can serve as a buffer to maintain acid-base balance.
4. RBC count.
    a. Number of circulating mature RBCs per cubic millimeter (Table 16–1).
    b. Count equals production versus destruction or loss.
    c. RBC life span proportional to gestational age.
        (1) Adult: 100–120 days.
        (2) Term infant: 60–70 days.
        (3) Premature infant: 35–50 days.
    d. Nucleated RBCs are circulating immature (prereticulocyte) red cells.
        (1) Number is inversely proportional to gestational age and declines rapidly in the first week.
        (2) Increase may indicate hemolysis, acute blood loss, hypoxemia, congenital heart disease, or infection.
5. RBC indices: measure of RBC size and hemoglobin content used for designation of anemias (Table 16–1).
    a. Mean corpuscular volume (MCV): average size and volume of a single RBC.
        (1) MCV decreases as gestation progresses and continues to decrease after birth to adult size by 4–5 years.
        (2) Increased MCV: macrocytes.
        (3) Decreased MCV: microcytes.
    b. Mean corpuscular hemoglobin (MCH): average amount (weight) of hemoglobin per single RBC.
        (1) MCH parallels the MCV decrease.
        (2) Increased MCH: hyperchromic cells.
        (3) Decreased MCH: hypochromic cells.
    c. Mean corpuscular hemoglobin concentration (MCHC): average concentration of hemoglobin per single RBC, calculated from the amount of hemoglobin per deciliter of cells.
        (1) MCHC remains constant, with adult values reached by 6 months.
        (2) Increased MCHC: hyperchromic cells.
        (3) Decreased MCHC: hypochromic cells.

F. White blood cells (WBCs).

1. Leukocyte precursors mature in the bone marrow and lymphatic tissues, in the absence of stress, through the promyelocyte, myelocyte, and metamyelocyte stages and enter the circulation at the polymorphonuclear stage (Fig. 16–1).
2. WBCs are carried in the circulation to the extravascular tissues, where they function as an important part of the immunologic system in reaction to foreign protein.
3. Granulocytes, lymphocytes, and monocytes are types of WBCs.
    a. Granulocytes: cell lines include basophils, eosinophils, and neutrophils.

(1) Basophils.
    (a) Important in inflammatory responses.
    (b) Least numerous of the granulocytes: 0.5–1% of total WBC count.
(2) Eosinophils.
    (a) Perform the same functions as neutrophils but are more sluggish in response.
    (b) Important in allergic and anaphylactic responses and most effective granulocyte for parasitic destruction.
    (c) Benign eosinophilia of prematurity, inversely proportional to gestational age, may be seen in infants who receive total parenteral nutrition, multiple blood transfusions, and endotracheal intubation; may be physiologic response to foreign antigens (Bhat and Scanlon, 1981).
    (d) Normally compose 1–3% of total WBC count.
(3) Neutrophils.
    (a) Neutrophils function as phagocytes to ingest and destroy small particles such as bacteria, protozoa, cells and cellular debris, dust, and colloids.
    (b) Stress can increase production and bone marrow release of immature forms.
    (c) Neutrophils are increased at birth but decrease during the first week to reach percentages approximately equal to those of lymphocytes.
b. Lymphocytes.
    (1) Thymus-derived (T) lymphocytes; important in graft-versus-host disease and delayed hypersensitivity reactions.
    (2) Bone marrow–derived (B) lymphocytes; important in the production and secretion of immunoglobulins and antibodies.
c. Monocytes.
    (1) Circulating immature macrophages.
    (2) Transformed into macrophages in tissues (i.e., lung, alveolar macrophage; liver, Kupffer cell macrophages).
    (3) Responsible for clearance of old blood cells, cellular debris, opsinized bacteria, antigen-antibody complexes, and activated clotting factors from the circulation.
4. WBC count.
    a. WBC count is the number of circulating WBCs per cubic millimeter (Table 16–2).

Table 16–2
NORMAL LEUKOCYTE VALUES IN PREMATURE AND TERM INFANTS

Age (h)	Total White Cell Count	Neutrophils	Bands/Metas	Lymphocytes	Monocytes	Eosinophils
TERM INFANTS						
0	10.0–26.0	5.0–13.0	0.4–1.8	3.5–8.5	0.7–1.5	0.2–2.0
12	13.5–31.0	9.0–18.0	0.4–2.0	3.0–7.0	1.0–2.0	0.2–2.0
72	5.0–14.5	2.0–7.0	0.2–0.4	2.0–5.0	0.5–1.0	0.2–1.0
144	6.0–14.5	2.0–6.0	0.2–0.5	3.0–6.0	0.7–1.2	0.2–0.8
PREMATURE INFANTS						
0	5.0–19.0	2.0–9.0	0.2–2.4	2.5–6.0	0.3–1.0	0.1–0.7
12	5.0–21.0	3.0–11.0	0.2–2.4	1.5–5.0	0.3–1.3	0.1–1.1
72	5.0–14.0	3.0–7.0	0.2–0.6	1.5–4.0	0.3–1.2	0.2–1.1
144	5.5–17.5	2.0–7.0	0.2–0.5	2.5–7.5	0.5–1.5	0.3–1.2

Data modified from Xanthou (1970) by Glader (1977).
    From Oski, F.A., and Naiman, J.L.: Hematologic Problems in the Newborn, 3rd ed. Philadelphia, W.B. Saunders, 1982.

b. WBC count is proportional to gestational age, with the total counts of premature infants approximately 30–50% lower than those of term infants.

G. **Platelets.**

1. Small, nonnucleated, disk-shaped cells aid in hemostasis, coagulation, and thrombus formation.
   a. Platelets are derived from megakaryocytes in the bone marrow.
   b. Disrupted endothelium stimulates platelet plug formation and initiates hemostasis.
2. After release into the bloodstream, platelets will circulate 7–10 days before removal by the spleen. In the absence of injury, they circulate freely, without wall adhesion or aggregation with other platelets.
3. Normal range is 150,000 to 400,000/mm^3 in the term and the premature infant. Counts are 20–25% lower in infants who are small for gestational age.

H. **Blood volume.**

1. Volume of blood is measured in milliliters per kilogram of body weight.
2. Factors affecting blood volume are:
   a. Gestational age.
      (1) Term infant: approximately 80–100 mL/kg.
      (2) Preterm infant: approximately 90–105 mL/kg.
   b. Placental transfusion.
      (1) Timing of cord clamping.
      (2) Position of infant relative to placenta (above or below) before cord clamping.
      (3) Timing and strength of uterine contractions.
      (4) Onset of respiration and decrease in pulmonary vascular resistance.
      (5) Cord compression.
   c. Maternal-fetal or fetal-maternal transfusion.
   d. Twin-twin transfusion.
   e. Placenta previa or placental abruption.
   f. Nuchal cord.

Coagulation

Hemostasis is accomplished by biochemical and physiologic events initiated to stop the flow of blood when vessel injury occurs (Esmon, 1998; Kisker, 1998a).

A. **Deficiencies in newborn clotting mechanisms.**

1. Transient diminished platelet function.
2. Transient deficiency of clotting factors II, VII, IX, X, XI, and XII.
   a. Immaturity of hepatic enzymes responsible for production.
   b. Transient deficiency of vitamin K, needed for synthesis of factors II, VII, IX, and X.
   c. Factor concentrations: proportional to gestational age.

B. **Hemostatic mechanisms.**

1. Vascular: damaged vessel contracts, minimizing blood loss.
2. Intravascular: platelet plug formation. Platelet function is stimulated by exposure to damaged endothelial lining. Platelets:
   a. Bloat and develop thornlike projections.
   b. Become sticky and adhere to subendothelial fibers.
   c. Secrete adenosine diphosphate to trigger swelling and adhesiveness in nearby platelets.
   d. Aggregate and form platelet plug.

3. Extravascular.
   a. Pressure effect of surrounding tissue.
   b. Release of tissue thromboplastin by injured tissue.

C. Coagulation process.

1. Cascade of events, each dependent on one another (Fig. 16–2).
2. Formation of thromboplastin by activation of the intrinsic or extrinsic systems in conjunction with calcium, iron, and phospholipids.
   a. Intrinsic system triggered by vascular endothelial injury.
   b. Extrinsic system triggered by tissue injury and release of tissue thromboplastin.
   c. Both systems trigger separate mechanisms (Fig. 16–2) until factor X is activated, beginning the process of prothrombin-to-thrombin conversion. Conversion hydrolyzes fibrinogen (soluble protein in plasma) to fibrin (insoluble, thready polymer) and activates factor XIII, stabilizing fibrin threads into a meshwork to trap platelets and other cells to form the clot.

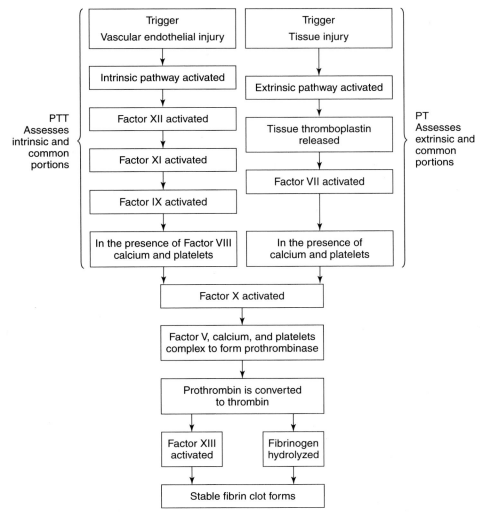

Figure 16–2
Fibrin clot formation through activation of the intrinsic or extrinsic pathways of the coagulation process.

Table 16–3
NORMAL VALUES FOR TESTS OF HEMOSTASIS

Parameter	Fetuses (Weeks' Gestation)			Newborns (n = 60)	Adults (n = 40)
	19–23 (n = 20)	24–29 (n = 22)	30–38 (n = 22)		
PT (s)	32.5 (19–45)	32.2 (19–44)†	22.6 (16–30)†	16.7 (12.0–23.5)*	13.5 (11.4–14.0)
PT (INR)	6.4 (1.7–11.1)	6.2 (2.1–10.6)†	3.0 (1.5–5.0)*	1.7 (0.9–2.7)*	1.1 (0.8–1.2)
APTT (s)	168.8 (83–250)	154.0 (87–210)†	104.8 (76–128)†	44.3 (35–52)*	33.0 (25–39)
TCT (s)	34.2 (24–44)*	26.2 (24–28)*	21.4 (17.0–23.3)	20.4 (15.2–25.0)†	14.0 (12–16)
Factor					
I (g/L Von Clauss)	0.85 (0.57–1.50)	1.12 (0.65–1.65)	1.35 (1.25–1.65)	1.68 (0.95–2.45)†	3.0 (1.78–4.50)
I Ag (g/L)	1.08 (0.75–1.50)	1.93 (1.56–2.40)	1.94 (1.30–2.40)	2.65 (1.68–3.60)†	3.5 (2.50–5.20)
IIc (%)	16.9 (10–24)	19.9 (11–30)*	27.9 (15–50)†	43.5 (27–64)†	98.7 (70–125)
VIIc (%)	27.4 (17–37)	33.8 (18–48)*	45.9 (31–62)	52.5 (28–78)†	101.3 (68–130)
IXc (%)	10.1 (6–14)	9.9 (5–15)	12.3 (5–24)†	31.8 (15–50)†	104.8 (70–142)
Xc (%)m	20.5 (14–29)	24.9 (16–35)	28.0 (16–36)†	39.6 (21–65)†	99.2 (75–125)
Vc (%)	32.1 (21–44)	36.8 (25–50)	48.9 (23–70)†	89.9 (50–140)	99.8 (65–140)
VIIIc (%)	34.5 (18–50)	35.5 (20–52)	50.1 (27–78)†	94.3 (38–150)	101.8 (55–170)
XIc (%)	13.2 (8–19)	12.1 (6–22)	14.8 (6–26)†	37.2 (13–62)†	100.2 (70–135)
XIIc (%)	14.9 (6–25)	22.7 (6–40)	25.8 (11–50)†	69.8 (25–105)†	101.4 (65–144)
PK (%)	12.8 (8–19)	15.4 (8–26)	18.1 (8–28)†	35.4 (21–53)†	99.8 (65–135)
HMWK (%)	15.4 (10–22)	19.3 (10–26)	23.6 (12–34)†	38.9 (28–53)†	98.8 (68–135)

Values are the mean, followed in parentheses by the lower and upper boundaries including 95% of the population.

Abbreviations: *INR*, international normalized ratio; *APTT*, activated partial thromboplastin time; *TCT*, thrombin clotting time; *Ag*, antigenic value; *c*, coagulant activity; *PK*, protein kinase; *HMWK*, high-molecular-weight kininogen.

*$p < .05$.

†$p < .01$.

From Nathan, D.G., and Orkin, S.H. (Eds.): Nathan and Oski's Hematology of Infancy and Childhood, 5th ed. Philadelphia, W.B. Saunders, 1998.

3. Massive intravascular clotting, controlled by concurrent fibrinolysis.
   a. Inactive plasminogen synthesized by the liver is converted to plasmin, an active enzyme, when a fibrin clot is present.
   b. Plasmin begins fibrin clot dissolution, releasing fibrin degradation products (FDPs), also called fibrin split products (FSPs), into the circulation.
   c. FDPs produce an anticoagulant effect by interfering with clot formation and the function of platelets, thrombin, and fibrinogen.

D. **Coagulation tests (Table 16–3).**

1. Platelet count assesses platelet number.
2. Prothrombin time (PT) assesses extrinsic and common portions of the coagulation cascade.
3. Partial thromboplastin time (PTT) assesses intrinsic and common portions of the coagulation cascade.
4. Fibrinogen assesses the circulating level of this protein substrate, required for clot formation.
5. FDP/FSP assesses fibrinolytic activity.
6. Individual clotting factors may be assayed, depending on results of the tests cited above.

Anemia

Low hemoglobin concentration and/or decreased number of RBCs diminishes the oxygen-carrying capacity of the blood and the level of oxygen available to the tissues (Blanchette and Zipursky, 1994; Hume, 1997; Miller, 1995; Oski, Brugnara, and Nathan, 1998).

A. Etiologic factors.

1. Hemorrhage.
   a. Fetal-maternal.
      (1) Spontaneous.
      (2) Traumatic amniocentesis.
      (3) External cephalic version.
   b. Twin-to-twin.
      (1) Monozygotic, monochorial (single) placenta.
      (2) Hemoglobin difference between twins greater than 5 g/dL.
   c. Placental/cord.
      (1) Umbilical cord rupture.
      (2) Cord or placental hematoma.
      (3) Anomalous cord insertion.
      (4) Rupture of anomalous vessels of cord or placenta.
      (5) Accidental incision of cord or placenta.
      (6) Placenta previa or placental abruption.
   d. Internal.
      (1) Intracranial (subdural, subarachnoid, intraventricular), subgaleal.
      (2) Organ rupture (liver, spleen, adrenal, kidney).
      (3) Pulmonary.
   e. External.
      (1) Phlebotomy.
      (2) Iatrogenic (e.g., catheter losses).
2. Hemolysis.
   a. Blood group incompatibilities.
      (1) Rh incompatibility: erythroblastosis fetalis (Miller, 1995; Reid and Toy, 1998).
         (a) Sequence of events. Fetal blood cells containing Rh antigen (Rh positive) enter the maternal circulation; maternal red cells have no antigen (Rh negative); maternal immune system produces antibodies against the foreign fetal antigens; maternal antibodies enter fetal circulation and destroy fetal red cells.
         (b) Predisposing factors.
            (i) Previous pregnancy or abortion.
            (ii) Fetal-maternal hemorrhage during pregnancy.
            (iii) Delivery (vaginal, breech, cesarean).
            (iv) Amniocentesis, chorionic villus sampling.
            (v) External version.
            (vi) Manual removal of placenta.
         (c) Infant presentation.
            (i) Anemia (caused by hemolysis, resulting in increased production of very immature red cells).
            (ii) Tissue hypoxia, acidosis (decreased RBC count and decreased oxygen-carrying capacity of immature cells).
            (iii) Congestive heart failure and hydrops fetalis (fetus attempts to expand blood volume and cardiac output, resulting in generalized edema).
            (iv) Ascites, pleural effusion (fluid collecting in large cavities).
            (v) Hepatosplenomegaly (increased extramedullary hematopoiesis).
            (vi) Petechiae (thrombocytopenia accompanying severe anemia).
            (vii) Hypoglycemia (increased red cell destruction stimulates insulin secretion, resulting in hyperplasia of pancreatic islets and hyperinsulinemia).
            (viii) Positive direct Coombs' test result.

(d) Prophylactic therapy: anti-D immune globulin (RhoGAM).
  (i) Anti-D antibodies injected into maternal circulation (one dose accommodates approximately 15 mL of fetal whole blood or approximately 30 mL of RBCs).
  (ii) Destruction of fetal red cells in maternal circulation, blocking maternal antibody production.
  (iii) Ninety percent effective in prevention of sensitization.
  (iv) Recommended administration at 28 weeks' gestation, within 72 hours after delivery, and after amniocentesis, chorionic villus sampling, percutaneous umbilical blood sampling, or evidence or possibility of fetal-maternal hemorrhage.
(2) ABO incompatibility (Miller, 1995; Wong, 1995).
  (a) More frequently occurring but less severe hemolytic disease than with Rh incompatibility.
  (b) Most often seen in mothers with O blood type (absence of antigen) carrying fetus with A or B blood type (see Table 16–4 for other potential incompatibilities).
  (c) Maternal exposure to naturally occurring A and B antigens in food, bacteria, and pollen initiates maternal production of anti-A, anti-B antibodies and accounts for severity of disease with first pregnancy.
  (d) ABO incompatibility protects against fetal Rh disease because of rapid destruction of fetal A/B cells, preventing Rh antigen exposure and maternal antibody production.
  (e) Infant presentation includes:
    (i) Mild hemolysis, anemia, reticulocytosis.
    (ii) Hyperbilirubinemia (occasionally requiring exchange).
b. Enzymatic defect: glucose-6-phosphate dehydrogenase (G6PD) deficiency (see also Chapter 14, Metabolic Disorders).
  (1) Most common inherited disorder of red cells (sex-linked disease affecting mainly male offspring, occasionally female carriers).
  (2) Interaction of intracellular abnormality (deficiency of red cell enzyme) and extracellular factor (exposure to oxidant stress: drugs, infection), causing hemolysis and shortened erythrocyte life.
  (3) Most common occurrence in American black infants (10–15%) and in infants of Mediterranean, African, and Asian descent.
c. Infection. Intrauterine (viral, protozoan, spirochetal) and postnatal (bacterial) infection may cause neonatal hemolysis, anemia, thrombocytopenia, and disseminated intravascular coagulation.
3. Anemia of prematurity.
  a. Hemoglobin concentration at birth varies only slightly in relation to gestational age.
  b. During the first 2–3 months, hemoglobin concentration falls to the lowest value that occurs at any developmental period.
  c. Anemia of prematurity is considered physiologic because it is characteristic of healthy infants.

Table 16–4
POTENTIAL MATERNAL-FETAL ABO INCOMPATIBILITIES

Material Blood Group	Incompatible Fetal Blood Group
O	A or B
B	A or AB
A	B or AB

 d. Associated factors.
  (1) Rate of decline and nadir are inversely proportional to gestational age.
  (2) Iron concentration is low because of decreased blood volume and decreased concentration of circulating hemoglobin iron.
  (3) Improved extrauterine oxygen delivery causes a temporarily inactive stage of erythropoiesis.
  (4) Erythropoietin production in response to anemia is diminished.
  (5) Shortened red cell life span decreases red cell mass.
  (6) Growth causes dilutional anemia as a result of decreased hemoglobin concentration with expanding blood volume.
  (7) Despite rapid hemoglobin fall, tissue oxygenation is maintained by events responsible for right shift of the hemoglobin-oxygen dissociation curve.
 e. Some infants do manifest symptoms of hypoxemia (poor feeding and weight gain, dyspnea, tachypnea, tachycardia, diminished activity, pallor) in the absence of other problems and require transfusion.
 f. No direct correlation has been established between low hemoglobin levels and the occurrence of apnea (Hume, 1997).
4. Iatrogenic postnatal phlebotomy. Critically ill infants who require frequent monitoring may have excessive amounts of blood removed for diagnostic studies. Removal of greater than 20% of the blood volume over 24–48 hours can produce anemia (Blanchette and Zipursky, 1994).

B. **Clinical presentation:** varies with the volume of hemorrhage and the time period over which the blood is lost.
1. Acute blood loss.
 a. Pallor initially, and then cyanosis and desaturation.
 b. Shallow, rapid, irregular respirations.
 c. Tachycardia.
 d. Weak or absent peripheral pulses.
 e. Low or absent blood pressure, low venous pressure.
 f. Hemoglobin concentration may be normal initially, with rapid decline over 4–12 hours with hemodilution.
2. Chronic blood loss.
 a. Pallor without signs of acute distress.
 b. Possible signs of congestive heart failure with hepatomegaly.
 c. Normal blood pressure, normal or elevated venous pressure.
 d. Low hemoglobin concentration.

C. **Clinical assessment.**

1. Family history.
 a. Bleeding, anemia, splenectomy.
 b. Consanguinity.
 c. Ethnic and geographic origins.
 d. Blood group incompatibilities.
2. Maternal history.
 a. Blood type.
 b. Late third-trimester bleeding.

D. **Physical examination.**

1. Signs of acute or chronic blood loss, as above.
2. Jaundice.
3. Cephalohematoma.
4. Abdominal distention or mass: liver, spleen, adrenal, kidney rupture.
5. Petechiae, purpura.

6. Cardiovascular abnormalities: tachycardia, murmur, gallop rhythm.
7. Hydropic changes.

E. Diagnostic studies.

1. Hemoglobin concentration. Venous hemoglobin values less than 13 g/dL in infants born at 34–35 weeks' gestation or more and in the first week of life are considered abnormal (Blanchette and Zipursky, 1994; Oski et al., 1998). Values vary according to birth weight and postnatal age (Table 16–5).
2. Reticulocyte count. This reflects new erythroid activity and is persistently elevated with ongoing red cell destruction.
3. Peripheral blood smear.
   a. Test evaluates alterations in size, shape, and structure of RBCs that might enhance destruction because of decreased deformability.
   b. Fragmentation of RBCs can be identified.
4. Blood type to identify common blood group antigens: A, B, O, and Rh.
5. Coombs' test.
   a. Positive result on direct Coombs' test indicates presence of maternal IgG antibodies on surface of infant's red cells.
   b. Positive result on indirect Coombs' test means that antibodies against the infant RBCs are present in the maternal serum.
6. Kleihauer-Betke test.
   a. Test identifies fetal hemoglobin in maternal blood.
   b. Calculations indicate volume of fetal-maternal hemorrhage and dose of immune globulin (RhoGAM) required to prevent sensitization.

F. Differential diagnosis: diseases that diminish oxygen delivery to the tissues (pulmonary, cardiac).

G. Complications.

1. Inadequate tissue oxygenation, poor growth.
2. Transfusion.
   a. Transfusion reaction (see Transfusion Therapies, p. 405).
   b. Overhydration with pulmonary congestion.

H. Patient care management (see Transfusion Therapies, p. 405).

1. Emergency treatment for acute blood loss resulting in hypovolemia.
   a. Whole blood or combination of packed RBCs (PRBCs) with crystalloid or colloid.
      (1) Type: group O, Rh-negative.
      (2) Amount: 10–20 mL/kg.
   b. Fresh frozen plasma (FFP), albumin, or saline solution if blood is unavailable.

Table 16–5
SERIAL HEMOGLOBIN VALUES IN LOW BIRTH WEIGHT INFANTS

Birth Weight (g)	Hemoglobin Concentration (g/dL) by Age (in Weeks)				
	2 wk	*4 wk*	*6 wk*	*8 wk*	*10 wk*
800–1000	16.0 ± 0.6	10.2 ± 3.2	8.7 ± 1.5	8.0 ± 0.9	8.0 ± 1.1
1001–1200	16.4 ± 2.3	12.8 ± 2.5	10.5 ± 1.8	9.1 ± 1.3	8.5 ± 1.5
1201–1400	16.2 ± 1.3	13.4 ± 2.8	10.9 ± 1.2	9.9 ± 1.9	—
1401–1500	15.6 ± 2.2	11.7 ± 1.0	10.5 ± 0.7	9.8 ± 1.4	—

Hemoglobin values are presented as grams per deciliter.
   From Oski, F.A.: Hematologic problems. *In* Avery, G.B. (Ed.): Neonatology: Pathophysiology and Management of the Newborn, 4th ed. Philadelphia, J.B. Lippincott, 1994.

2. Nonemergency replacement transfusion: clinical decision based on adequacy of tissue oxygenation in the individual infant.
   a. Oxygen-carrying capacity adequate to maintain cardiopulmonary function can be met by a hemoglobin level of 7 g/dL when intravascular volume is adequate for perfusion (Silberstein et al., 1989).
   b. Consider gestational and postnatal age, intravascular volume, and coexisting cardiac, pulmonary, or vascular conditions.
3. Exchange transfusion.
   a. Treatment of jaundice caused by blood group incompatibility.
   b. Partial exchange if necessary to treat severe anemia of hydrops without increasing intravascular volume.

I. Outcome.

1. Improved tissue oxygenation and resolution of symptoms with replacement transfusion.
2. Long-term outcome varies with degree of anemia and underlying cause.

Hemorrhagic Disease of the Newborn

Hemorrhagic disease of the newborn (HDN) is a hemorrhagic tendency caused by vitamin K deficiency and decreased activity of factors II, VII, IX, and X. A new term, vitamin K–dependent bleeding, is thought to describe more accurately the link between vitamin K deficiency and spontaneous hemorrhage and to exclude newborn infants with bleeding from other causes (Andrew and Montgomery, 1998; Bowman, 1997; Henderson-Smart, 1996; Hilgartner and Corrigan, 1995; Snapp, 1996; Stoeckel, Joubert, and Gruter, 1996).

A. Etiologic factors: primary vitamin K deficiency.
1. Required for activation of clotting factors II, VII, IX, and X and of proteins C and S after liver synthesis.
   a. Vitamin K is important in the formation of calcium-binding sites, which are necessary for functional activation of clotting factors.
   b. In the absence of vitamin K, circulating proteins are decarboxylated; levels of protein induced by vitamin K absence (PIVKA) can be used as an indirect measure of bleeding risk.
2. Suppression of bacterial synthesis.
   a. Intestinal flora is required for vitamin K synthesis.
   b. Newborn intestinal tract is virtually free of bacteria until feedings begin.
   c. Antibiotic therapy can alter normal intestinal bacterial colonization.

B. Clinical presentation: bleeding.
1. Begins at 24–72 hours of age.
2. May be localized or diffuse.
3. Rarely life threatening.
4. Late-onset bleeding possible at approximately 2–3 weeks of age.

C. Clinical assessment: oozing.
1. Localized: frequently gastrointestinal (hematemesis, melena).
2. Diffuse: umbilical cord, circumcision, puncture sites.

D. Physical examination.

1. Diffuse ecchymosis, petechiae.
2. Oozing puncture sites.
3. Abdominal distention.
4. Jaundice.

E. Diagnostic studies.

1. Response to vitamin K administration establishes the diagnosis.
2. PT and PTT are prolonged.
3. Levels of vitamin K–dependent clotting factors are low.
4. PIVKA levels are elevated.

F. Differential diagnosis.

1. Decreased absorption of vitamin K.
   a. Biliary atresia.
   b. Cystic fibrosis.
2. Pharmacologic antagonism of vitamin K (Astedt, 1995).
   a. Anticonvulsants (Dilantin, phenobarbital), anticoagulants (coumarin, warfarin).
      (1) Induce hepatic enzymes and increase vitamin K degradation.
      (2) Inhibit vitamin K transport across the placenta.
      (3) Depress vitamin K–dependent coagulation factors.
   b. Coumarol derivatives: replace with heparin during pregnancy.
   c. Maternal supplementation with oral vitamin K_1 from 36 weeks' gestation to delivery might prevent neonatal hemorrhage associated with anticonvulsant therapy; extra vitamin K given to the mother to increase vitamin K available to the fetus.

G. Complications.

1. Anemia.
2. Intraventricular/intracranial hemorrhage.

H. Patient care management.

1. Prophylactic vitamin K at the time of delivery.
   a. Phytonadione (naturally occurring vitamin K), 0.5–1 mg, intramuscular (IM) administration: premature infants may be given the lower dose.
   b. The American Academy of Pediatrics (AAP) recommends the use of only IM vitamin K at birth (AAP, 1961; AAP, 1993) because of the history of prevention of life-threatening HDN with the parenteral preparation, the unproved risks of cancer, and the need for further research on the efficacy, safety, and bioavailability of oral preparations.
   c. Adequate serum concentrations of vitamin K to prevent classic HDN have been observed after oral administration of 2 mg phylloquinone (vitamin K_1); however, late HDN occurs primarily in breast-fed infants who have not received adequate vitamin K prophylaxis.
      (1) If the oral form is not available, the IV form has been given orally without noted adverse side effects.
      (2) Parental concern with IM administration of vitamin K might stem from:
         (a) Need for injection.
         (b) Early reports (Golding et al., 1992) of an increased incidence of childhood cancer associated with IM vitamin K. Multiple repeated studies have been unable to demonstrate any correlation.
         (c) Readministration of oral dose (2 mg) required at 1–2 weeks and again at 4 weeks in breast-fed infants.
             (i) Commercial formulas contain vitamin K supplement.
             (ii) Intestinal flora of breast-fed infant may produce less vitamin K than that of formula-fed infant.
             (iii) Risk of developing HDN after oral dosing is 13:1, compared with IM dosing.
2. Significant bleeding (hemoglobin concentration <12 g/dL). PRBC infusion may be indicated.

3. Persistent bleeding in premature infant.
  a. FFP infusion may be indicated to replace clotting factors.
  b. Repeated doses of vitamin K are needed.

I. **Outcome.** Prophylactic treatment has virtually eliminated the disease.

Disseminated Intravascular Coagulation

Disseminated intravascular coagulation (DIC) is an acquired hemorrhagic disorder associated with an underlying disease manifested as uncontrolled activation of coagulation and fibrinolysis. Consumption of clotting factors is thought to be initiated by release of thromboplastic material from damaged or diseased tissue into the circulation. In DIC, fibrinogen converts to fibrin to form microthrombi (Andrew, 1997; Beardsley and Nathan, 1998; Fuse et al., 1996; Hilgartner and Corrigan, 1995; Kuehl, 1997; Pugh, 1997).

A. **Common precipitating factors.**

1. Maternal.
  a. Preeclampsia, eclampsia, placental abruption.
  b. Placental abnormalities.
2. Intrapartal.
  a. Fetal distress with hypoxia and acidosis.
  b. Dead twin fetus.
  c. Traumatic delivery.
3. Neonatal.
  a. Infection (bacterial, viral, fungal).
  b. Conditions causing hypoxia, acidosis, and shock.
  c. Severe Rh incompatibility.
  d. Thrombocytopenia.
  e. Tissue injury (birth trauma, breech crush injury).

B. **Clinical presentation (Fig. 16–3).**

1. Hemorrhage: predominant symptom.
  a. Clotting factors and platelets are depleted.
  b. Fibrinolysis is stimulated.
  c. Endogenous thrombin and plasmin are formed.

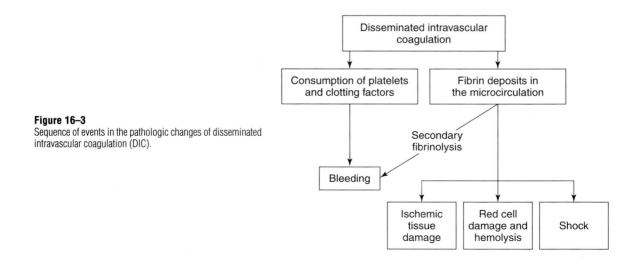

Figure 16–3
Sequence of events in the pathologic changes of disseminated intravascular coagulation (DIC).

2. Organ and tissue ischemia. Microvascular thrombosis (occlusion) by fibrin thrombi causes potential ischemia and necrosis of any organ, particularly the kidneys.
3. Anemia.
   a. Blood loss.
   b. Red cell fragmentation by fibrin strands.

C. Clinical assessment.

1. Review the history for precipitating factors.
2. Concurrent evidence of coagulation and fibrinolysis.

D. Physical examination.

1. Variable signs, depending on underlying disease process.
2. Prolonged oozing from puncture sites or umbilicus.
3. Petechiae, purpura, ecchymosis.
4. Hemorrhage (pulmonary, gastrointestinal, cerebral).
5. Localized necrosis and gangrene resulting from microvascular thrombosis of peripheral vessels.

E. Diagnostic studies.

1. Variable diagnostic studies are performed for delineation of the underlying disease process.
2. Platelet count is low.
3. PT and PTT are both significantly prolonged.
4. Peripheral blood smear identifies microangiopathic hemolytic anemia, abnormalities of red cell shape, cell fragmentation, and decreased number of platelets.
5. Fibrinogen level is low.
6. Fibrinogen-degradation products are significantly increased.
7. D-dimer, sometimes assayed in DIC, is a sensitive marker for endogenous thrombin/plasmin production and can detect much milder forms of DIC.
8. Additional factors and levels might be evaluated: factor VIII and factor II are decreased, as well as protein C, protein S, and antithrombin III.

F. Differential diagnosis.

1. Parenchymal liver disease.
2. Vitamin K deficiency.
3. Microangiopathic disease.
4. Primary fibrinogenolysis.

G. Complications.

1. Microvascular thrombosis.
2. Organ failure resulting from ischemia and necrosis, especially renal.
3. Intraventricular and parenchymal hemorrhage.

H. Patient care management.

1. Aggressive treatment of the underlying disease.
2. Supportive care.
   a. Replacement transfusion with significant bleeding.
      (1) Whole blood for hypovolemia and shock.
      (2) PRBCs for isovolemic anemia.
      (3) Platelets for consumption.
   b. Maintenance of blood pressure.
3. Measures to control DIC.
   a. Replacement of clotting factors.

(1) FFP (replaces all factors, coagulation proteins, and coagulation inhibitors; small amount of fibrinogen).
(2) Platelet concentrates.
(3) Cryoprecipitate (replaces fibrinogen, factor VIII).
(4) Antithrombin III (inhibits coagulation, controls fibrinolysis). High doses (120–250 U/kg per day) might attenuate organ failure and reverse coagulopathy in DIC without heparin therapy.
b. Heparin therapy remains controversial; use if treatment of underlying disease and replacement of clotting factors fail to reverse the process or with evidence of significant large-vessel thrombosis.
(1) Goals are to interrupt fibrin deposition and to achieve normal fibrinogen levels and platelet counts.
(2) Continuous infusion is more physiologic and is safer because intermittent doses may aggravate existing hemorrhage.
(3) Dosage is adjusted to maintain PTT within 60–70 seconds (once achieved, lower-dose heparin therapy may control ongoing consumption).
c. Exchange transfusion.
(1) Rarely tolerated and associated with additional complications (intraventricular hemorrhage, sepsis, thrombocytopenia).
(2) Replaces clotting factors and removes FDP from circulation.
(3) Use fresh heparinized blood or blood stored for less than 72 hours and which has been preserved with citrate-phosphate-dextrose.

I. **Outcome:** related to the prognosis of the underlying disease and the severity of the DIC.

Thrombocytopenia

Thrombocytopenia is an acquired disease in which there is a significant decrease in the platelet count ($<100,000/mm^3$) of the term or premature infant (Beardsley and Nathan, 1998; Blanchette and Rand, 1997; Homans, 1996; Marzich, Strohm, Ayas, and Cochran, 1996).

A. **Etiologic factors.**

1. Platelet destruction.
a. Maternal autoantibodies (autoimmune): idiopathic thrombocytopenic purpura, systemic lupus erythematosus.
(1) Maternal autoantibodies bind to platelet surface antigens, making them susceptible to premature destruction.
(2) IgG antibodies cross the placenta and destroy fetal platelets.
(a) Approximately 10–15% have cord platelet counts of less than $100,000/mm^3$ (half of these have counts $<50,000/mm^3$).
(b) Nadir usually occurs on the second day.
(c) Counts can be depressed for 2–4 months (as long as maternal IgG antibodies remain in circulation).
(d) Recent studies show no evidence of severe intracranial hemorrhage.
(3) Maternal platelet count is low.
b. Neonatal conditions.
(1) Neonatal alloimmune thrombocytopenia.
(a) Analogous to Rh incompatibility.
(i) Fetal platelets contain an antigen lacking in the mother.
(ii) Fetal platelets enter the maternal circulation, resulting in maternal production of antibodies against foreign platelets.

(iii) Maternal antibodies cross into the fetal circulation and coat fetal platelets, which are then destroyed.
(b) Fetal thrombocytopenia can occur as early as 20 weeks' gestation.
(c) Nadir occurs in the first few days; counts normalize by the end of the first month.
(d) About 15–25% have intracranial hemorrhage (approximately 10% in utero).
(e) Maternal platelet count remains normal.
(2) Infection: bacterial or TORCH (*t*oxoplasmosis, *o*ther [congenital syphilis, viruses], *r*ubella, *c*ytomegalovirus, *h*erpes simplex virus).
(a) Megakaryocyte degeneration in bone marrow.
(b) Can cause DIC (platelet consumption).
(c) Activates reticuloendothelial system (increased platelet sequestration).
(d) Platelets may form antigen/antibody complexes with infectious agent.
(3) Thrombotic disorders.
(a) Large-vessel disease (renal vein thrombosis).
(b) Microvascular disease (necrotizing entercolitis, respiratory distress syndrome, persistent pulmonary hypertension of the newborn).
(c) DIC (platelet consumption).
(4) Birth asphyxia. Fetal megakaryocytes may have increased sensitivity to hypoxic injury.
(5) Giant hemangiomas.
(a) Kasabach-Merritt syndrome. Vascular malformation results in platelet and fibrinogen consumption.
(b) Mechanical destruction and sequestration.
(6) Exchange transfusion: shortened survival of transfused platelets.
2. Impaired platelet production (rare, <5%) associated with congenital malformations.
a. Trisomy syndromes (13, 18). Bone marrow hypoplasia affects megakaryocyte production.
b. Thrombocytopenia with absent radii (TAR) syndrome.
(1) Defective megakaryocyte progenitor cell.
(2) Presentation at birth, improvement thereafter.
(3) Anomalies of the radius but not the thumb.
c. Fanconi anemia.
(1) Thumb, skeletal, renal, and CNS anomalies; café-au-lait spots.
(2) Thrombocytopenia: presentation rare in neonatal period; worsens with time.
d. Other, rare syndromes associated with unusually small or giant platelets.
3. Platelet interference: maternal drug ingestion.
a. Interference with platelet aggregation.
b. Meperidine (Demerol), promethazine (Phenergan), acetylsalicylic acid, sulfonamides, quinidine, quinine, thiazides.

B. **Clinical presentation (platelet-type bleeding).**

1. Petechiae, purpura, epistaxis.
2. Ecchymosis over presenting part.
3. Cephalhematoma.
4. Bleeding (mucous membranes, gastrointestinal tract, genitourinary system, umbilical cord, puncture sites, superficial cuts, or abrasions).

C. **Clinical assessment.**

1. Family history: bleeding complications in previous children, other family members.

2. Maternal history.
  a. History of bruising or bleeding, infections, collagen-vascular disease, splenectomy.
  b. Platelet count (low or normal).
  c. Peripheral blood smear (may show low platelet count, increased immature forms).
  d. Medication history.
3. Birth history.
  a. Hypoxia.
  b. Infection risk.

D. Physical examination.

1. Signs of clinical presentation.
2. Jaundice.
3. Intrauterine growth restriction, microcephaly, hepatosplenomegaly with infectious cause (absent with immune etiology).
4. Congenital anomalies consistent with syndromes.

E. Diagnostic studies.

1. Platelet count is low.
2. Peripheral blood smear shows low platelet count and increased immature forms; may show abnormal size.
3. PT and PTT are normal.
4. Bleeding time is prolonged.
5. Maternal blood can be tested for human platelet antigen (HPA) type and for the presence of platelet-specific antibody (up to 2 weeks post partum).
6. In severe cases, platelet typing of mother, father, and infant might be indicated.

F. Differential diagnosis: DIC, vitamin K deficiency.

G. Complications.

1. Cranial hemorrhage with neurologic sequelae in alloimmune disease.
  a. Associated with approximately 12% mortality rate.
  b. Increased incidence in infants weighing less than 1500 g.
2. Entrapped hemorrhage.
3. Anemia.
4. Hyperbilirubinemia.

H. Infant management (see Table 16–5).

1. Supportive care and treatment of underlying disease. Majority of neonatal thrombocytopenias are secondary to other disease processes.
2. Cesarean delivery.
  a. Autoimmune.
    (1) Rarely of benefit for infant.
    (2) Consider if:
      (a) Maternal disease is severe with high antibody levels.
      (b) Prior infant was severely affected.
  b. Alloimmune: maternal HPA typing not routinely done; infants identified postnatally.
3. Platelet transfusion.
  a. Recommended goal: keep platelet count greater than 30,000 in the first 48 hours, and greater than 50,000 if surgery is necessary or infant is premature and at risk for intraventricular hemorrhage.
  b. Autoimmune.
    (1) Rarely needed; platelet counts greater than 20,000/mm^3 usually benign course.

(2) Consider cranial ultrasonography if platelet counts less than 50,000/mm^3.

(3) Consider transfusion if platelet counts less than 20,000/mm^3.

  c. Alloimmune.

(1) Serial transfusions may be necessary.

(2) Obtain HPA type for infant before transfusion.

(3) Transfusion of random donor platelets rarely results in sustained increase because of antibody destruction.

(4) Transfuse maternal platelets (in absence of HPA) that have been washed and resuspended in AB-negative plasma.

  d. Production defects: repeated transfusions usually necessary.

4. Intravenous immune globulin (IVIG).

  a. Eighty percent effective in increasing platelet count.

  b. Effect delayed 12–24 hours.

  c. IgG pooled blood product from multiple donors.

5. Exchange transfusion.

  a. Consider only in infants with life-threatening hemorrhage.

  b. Limited success because IgG has a long half-life and distribution in extravascular tissues.

  c. May be required for hyperbilirubinemia.

6. Steroids.

  a. May be used in infants with platelet counts less than 25,000/mm^3 and clinical bleeding.

  b. May be used for initial treatment of thrombocytopenia resulting from hemangioma.

I. Outcome.

1. Varies with underlying disease, presence of congenital malformations.

2. Autoimmune etiology: usually causes only mild, transient problems, with full recovery of platelet count in 8–12 weeks.

3. Isoimmune etiology: causes mild to moderate problems with full recovery of platelet count in 6–8 weeks.

Polycythemia

Polycythemia is a condition in which infants demonstrate an excess in circulating RBC mass. The venous hemoglobin concentration is greater than 22 g/dL or the venous hematocrit is greater than 65% in the first week of life. Blood viscosity increases with hematocrits greater than 60% and leads to a reduction of blood flow to the organs (Blanchette and Zipursky, 1994; Miller, 1995).

A. Etiologic factors.

1. Intrauterine hypoxia, placental insufficiency. Hypoxia stimulates erythropoiesis, increasing the fetal red cell mass.

  a. Maternal preeclampsia/eclampsia, placenta previa.

  b. Postmaturity syndrome, intrauterine growth restriction.

2. Maternal-fetal and twin-to-twin transfusion.

3. Placental hypertransfusion.

4. Maternal diabetes: possibly resulting from abnormal fetal erythrocyte deformability.

B. Clinical presentation.

1. Many infants are asymptomatic.

2. Plethora.

3. Cyanosis.

4. CNS abnormalities (lethargy, jitteriness, seizures).
5. Respiratory distress (tachypnea, pulmonary edema, pulmonary hemorrhage).
6. Tachycardia, congestive heart failure.
7. Hypoglycemia.
8. Poor feeding behaviors (poor nippling, regurgitation).

C. **Clinical assessment:** History and physical examination usually identify cause.

D. **Physical examination.**

1. Findings may be normal except for plethora and occasionally cyanosis.
2. Symptoms of clinical presentation cannot be attributed to other disease.

E. **Diagnostic studies.** Venous hemoglobin concentration and hematocrit are elevated. Hematocrit values should be determined by microcentrifugation rather than automated Coulter counter to avoid falsely low levels (Villalta, Pramanik, Diaz-Blanco, and Herbst, 1989).

F. **Complications.**

1. Hyperbilirubinemia.
2. Hyperviscosity syndrome: elevated whole blood viscosity associated with reduced blood flow, vascular thrombosis (renal, cerebral, mesenteric), neurologic sequelae, fine motor abnormalities, speech delays up to 2 years of age (Black et al., 1985).

G. **Patient care management.**

1. Partial exchange transfusion.
    a. Controversial in asymptomatic infants.
    b. Desired reduction of hematocrit to less than 60% (blood viscosity is thought to be relatively normal at this level).
    c. Gastrointestinal symptoms: possibility of bleeding, poor feeding tolerance, necrotizing enterocolitis after partial exchange transfusion (Black et al., 1985).
2. Supportive treatment of persistent symptoms.

H. **Outcome.**

1. Gross motor delays, neurologic sequelae, fine motor abnormalities, speech delays seen at 2 years (Black et al., 1985).
2. Lower scores on spelling and arithmetic achievement tests and on gross motor skill tests at 7 years (Delaney-Black et al., 1989).

Inherited Bleeding Disorders

Although inherited bleeding disorders were recognized as early as 600 AD, the specific clotting abnormalities have been delineated only in this century, with the last (deficiency of factor XIII) documented in 1963. These gene disorders are rare, phenotypic expression is extremely variable, and only the most severely affected will be identified in the newborn period (Dragone and Karp, 1996; Edwards, 1998; Kisker, 1998b; Smith, 1990).

A. **Etiologic factors.**

1. Hemophilia.
    a. Ninety percent of infants with hemophilia will have either classic hemophilia (hemophilia A, factor VIII deficiency) or Christmas disease (hemophilia B, factor IX deficiency).

    b. X-linked recessive inheritance.
      (1) Gene is located on the X chromosome.
      (2) Females are carriers; disease is present in male infants because they have only one X chromosome, which carries the abnormal gene (no normal X chromosome as counterbalance).
      (3) Each pregnancy carries a 25% chance of occurrence (50% of the male offspring will be affected).
      (4) Seventy-five percent have a family history of a male with a bleeding disorder.
  2. Von Willebrand's disease.
    a. Autosomal dominant inheritance.
      (1) Males and females are equally affected.
      (2) Each pregnancy carries a 50% chance of occurrence.
      (3) Transmission is vertical (disease is seen in successive generations).
    b. Gene expression markedly variable (family history may be absent despite dominant inheritance).
  3. Factor XIII deficiency: autosomal recessive inheritance.
    a. Both parents are phenotypically normal carriers.
    b. Males and females are equally affected.
    c. In each pregnancy, 25% of the offspring will be affected, 50% will be carriers, 25% will be normal.
    d. Expression is horizontal (deficiency is seen in siblings; skips a generation).

B. Clinical presentation.

1. Rare newborn presentation except for factor XIII deficiency.
2. Usually well infant with delayed bleeding.
3. Clotting screening results usually normal.

C. Clinical assessment.

1. Late bleeding.
    a. Delayed umbilical cord bleeding (>80% with factor XIII).
    b. Circumcision oozing (significant hemorrhage is rare).
    c. Rare intracranial hemorrhage.
2. Family history.

D. Diagnostic studies.

1. PT, PTT, platelet count, fibrinogen level (usually normal).
2. Specific factor assays (identification by factor levels and DNA analysis).
    a. Factor VIII levels should be comparable to normal adult levels in the newborn period.
    b. Factor IX levels are normally low in the neonatal period; however, infants with bleeding presentation will be severely affected, with less than 2% activity (clearly abnormal level).

E. Patient care management.

1. Initial correction is with FFP (contains adequate amounts of all clotting factors except factor VIII).
2. Cryoprecipitate can be used if bleeding persists after use of FFP (enriched with approximately 20 units of factor VIII per milliliter).
3. Diagnosis allows replacement of specific factor.
    a. Recombinant factor VIII is available for classic hemophilia.
    b. Purified (monoclonal antibody) factor IX is available for Christmas disease.
    c. Prothrombin concentrates are not recommended for neonatal use because of thrombogenicity.

F. Outcome: episodic bleeding requiring lifelong replacement.

Transfusion Therapies

A. Recommendations for use of blood components (Blanchette and Rand, 1997; Hume, 1997; Luban, 1995; Manno, 1996; Nugent, 1998; Reid and Toy, 1998):

1. Develop and document criteria indicating need.
2. Use only the blood components required for therapy.
3. Use crystalloid or nonblood colloid whenever possible.
4. Use universal precautions when handling blood products.

B. Written, informed consent has been recommended since 1986 to ensure that families understand risks and explore alternatives:

1. Ethical or religious basis: autonomy—the right of choice.
2. Legal basis: failure to inform adequately and to obtain consent constitutes negligence.
3. Time-consuming: start a few days in advance of need (i.e., include in discussion on the first day of life of sick preterm infants).

C. Informed consent includes discussion of the following:

1. Risks.
   a. Infection.
      (1) Blood is screened for human immunodeficiency virus (HIV), hepatitis B virus (HBV), hepatitis C virus (HCV), human T-cell leukemia/lymphoma virus (HTLV), and *Treponema pallidum* (syphilis).
      (2) Cytomegalovirus transmission can be prevented by using leukocyte-depleted, irradiated products.
      (3) Major risks for transmission via transfusion.
         (a) HIV infection incidence is 1:420,000 (p24 antigen testing soon to be added to routine testing).
         (b) HBV (hepatitis B surface antigen [HBsAg]) infection incidence is 1:200,000; hepatitis B core antigen (HBcAg) is a marker for non-A, non-B hepatitis.
         (c) HCV infection incidence is 1:80,000.
      (4) Predonation questions foster self-elimination of prospective donors with high-risk behaviors.
      (5) Confidential unit exclusion allows donors to designate the elimination of their donation if they recognize risk but want to avoid the embarrassment of refusing to donate.
   b. Transfusion reactions.
      (1) Febrile reactions (most common).
         (a) Probably caused by transfused (passenger) WBCs and/or their cytokine products (RBC and platelet transfusions).
         (b) Leukocyte reduction might prevent reaction.
            (i) Expensive and time-consuming.
            (ii) One unit of PRBCs can contain 1 billion WBCs.
            (iii) WBCs can be removed by centrifugation, or by filtering at donation (prestorage leukocyte depletion), or at transfusion (bedside filtration).
      (2) Allergic reactions.
         (a) Urticaria, angioedema, asthma.
         (b) Higher incidence with multiple transfusions.
         (c) Premedication (antihistamine, antipyretic, steroid) might diminish effect.
      (3) Hemolytic reactions.
         (a) Usually ABO incompatibilities.
         (b) Possible acute or delayed hemolysis.

        (c) Most reactions can be eliminated by typing, screening, and cross-matching.

    c. Graft-versus-host disease.

       (1) Disease may occur in fetus or premature neonate after transfusion.

       (2) Immature immune system may not reject foreign lymphocytes (present in erythrocyte and platelet products); donor lymphocytes proliferate and damage the host (infection and neutropenia).

       (3) Clinical symptoms (within 100 days of transfusion) include rash, diarrhea, hepatic dysfunction, and bone marrow suppression with generalized reduction in all cell lines (pancytopenia).

       (4) Gamma irradiation of blood products will prevent lymphocyte proliferation.

         (a) Mature erythrocytes and platelets are resistant to radiation damage.

         (b) Enhances efflux of potassium ion from red cells (store <28 days, wash to remove excess potassium before transfusion).

2. Expected benefits.

    a. Whole blood (hematocrit approximately 35%).

       (1) Replacement of blood volume.

       (2) Treatment (massive hemorrhage, exchange transfusion).

    b. PRBC (hematocrit approximately 60–90%).

       (1) Improved oxygen-carrying capacity and tissue oxygenation.

       (2) Relief of symptoms of anemia (tachypnea, apnea, periodic breathing, tachycardia, poor weight gain).

       (3) Treatment (active bleeding, hemolytic disease, extracorporeal membrane oxygenation).

       (4) Minimal fluid administration (approximate red cell mass of a whole unit of blood in one-half fluid volume).

    c. Platelets.

       (1) Improved coagulation.

       (2) Treatment (hemorrhage caused by thrombocytopenia or platelet dysfunction).

    d. FFP: replacement of clotting factor deficiency.

    e. Albumin.

       (1) Volume expansion, improved oncotic pressure.

       (2) Treatment (for hypovolemia, third-space losses).

    f. Granulocytes.

       (1) Replacement in life-threatening granulocytopenias.

       (2) Improved survival rates in limited studies using granulocyte transfusions in newborn infants who become neutropenic as a result of consumption during infection.

3. Alternatives.

    a. Directed donation.

       (1) Family and friends with compatible blood type can donate for infant.

       (2) Blood must be irradiated to prevent graft-versus-host disease.

       (3) There is no evidence of overall increased safety in comparison with anonymous volunteer donations.

         (a) Donors might be more truthful (i.e., regarding acceptability for donation) because they know the recipient.

         (b) Donors might be less truthful because they feel pressure to donate.

       (4) Parental donation.

         (a) Maternal plasma is unacceptable for transfusion to neonates because of the possible presence of antibodies directed against inherited paternal antigens on infant's cells.

         (b) Maternal platelets and RBCs can be used if washed before transfusion.

         (c) Paternal donation might be problematic if infant has circulating maternal antibodies produced by stimulation of inherited paternal antigens.

  (5) All blood products from directed donors should be irradiated. Potential antigen similarities between close family members may impede recognition and destruction of foreign lymphocytes.

 b. Erythropoietin (EPO) (Bechensteen et al., 1996; Doyle, 1997; Ohls, Harcum, Schibler, and Christensen, 1997; Strauss, 1997; Widness et al., 1996).

  (1) Recombinant human EPO (r-HuEPO) might be used to treat symptomatic anemia caused by physiologic decline in hematocrit or by blood loss from phlebotomy, or it might be used as a prophylactic therapy to minimize blood product exposure in preterm or sick neonates.

  (2) Plasma EPO levels are lower in anemic preterm infants, suggesting responsibility for hematocrit decline.

   (a) The liver, the initial site of EPO production at early gestation, is less responsive than the kidney to tissue hypoxia caused by anemia.

   (b) EPO pharmacokinetics differ in preterm infants: faster rate of clearance, larger volume of distribution, shorter elimination and mean residence times.

   (c) Clearance increases with duration of r-HuEPO therapy, suggesting the need for progressively higher doses.

  (3) Variable results and small sample sizes hamper clinical trials testing different doses and treatment schedules.

   (a) Therapy with r-HuEPO and iron stimulates erythropoiesis and increases reticulocyte counts.

   (b) Increase in reticulocyte count is dose dependent.

   (c) Oral iron supplement, adequate to support enhanced erythropoiesis, may not be tolerated; intravenous iron therapy has not yet been adequately studied to ensure absence of oxidant injury and toxic metabolites.

   (d) Consistent efficacy of therapy to significantly diminish transfusion need has not yet been demonstrated.

 c. Thrombopoietin. Recombinant human thrombopoietin is currently under development and testing for use as a megakaryocyte enhancer.

 d. Granulocyte colony-stimulating factor (G-CSF): currently under investigation; stimulates growth of neutrophil colonies and induces maturation of promyelocytes to mature neutrophils.

D. Transfusion volumes.

1. Transfusions with PRBCs. For prevention of overhydration, replacement is usually given in increments of 10–15 mL/kg.
2. Partial exchange transfusions.
 a. With normal saline solution: treatment of polycythemia (to reduce hematocrit without reducing blood volume).
 b. With PRBCs: treatment of hydrops fetalis (to correct anemia without increasing blood volume).
 c. Calculations for total exchange volume:

  (1) Volume of normal saline solution to exchange =

$$\frac{\text{Blood volume} \times (\text{Measured hematocrit} - \text{Desired hematocrit})}{\text{Measured hematocrit}}$$

  (2) PRBC volume to exchange =

$$\frac{\text{Blood volume} \times (\text{Desired hematocrit} - \text{Measured hematocrit})}{\text{PRBC hematocrit} - \text{Measured hematocrit}}$$

3. Exchange transfusions.
   a. Single unit of blood (approximately 500 mL) will usually exchange twice the blood volume and remove 70–85% of the infant's blood.
   b. For treatment of hyperbilirubinemia, DIC, and autoimmune thrombocytopenia.
   c. Because preservatives provide a significant glucose load, rebound hypoglycemia may occur.
   d. Preservatives contain citrate, which binds calcium and magnesium; hypocalcemia and hypomagnesemia may occur.
   e. Potassium level rises as blood ages; blood should be less than 5 days old.
4. Platelets.
   a. One unit (approximately 40 mL) provides approximately 5×10^{10} platelets; transfusion of 0.2 platelet unit per kilogram should increase the platelet count by 75,000 to $100,000/mm^3$ (Kisker, 1998b).
   b. Routine volume reduction (platelet concentration) before transfusion is not indicated in infants.
   c. Platelets are separated from single units of whole blood within 6 hours of collection and suspended in small amounts of plasma, or they are obtained by apheresis (single-donor platelets).
5. FFP.
   a. FFP is usually transfused in increments of 10 mL/kg to minimize overhydration.
   b. Transfusion of 15–20 mL/kg replaces all coagulation proteins present in adult concentrations (Kisker, 1998b).
   c. Plasma is obtained from a unit of whole blood and frozen within 6 hours of collection.
6. Cryoprecipitate.
   a. Transfusion volume is usually 1 unit/kg (approximate volume, 15 mL).
   b. One unit contains approximately 100–250 mg of factor I (fibrinogen), approximately 80–100 units of factor VIII (von Willebrand), and 50–75 units of factor XIII (Manno, 1996).
7. Albumin.
   a. For volume expansion, 5% albumin is usually administered in increments of 10 mL/kg; for improvement of oncotic pressure, 25% albumin might be used in increments of 1 gm/kg (4 mL/kg).
   b. Albumin is a major contributor to oncotic pressure because of molecular size and weight.
8. Granulocytes.
   a. Collected by leukapheresis and transfused at a dose of approximately $1–2 \times 10^9$ WBCs/kg (Manno, 1996).
   b. Selectively harvested from whole blood.

Evaluation by Complete Blood Cell Count

An evaluation of certain components of the complete blood cell count might be helpful as an adjunct in the diagnosis of sepsis (Manroe, Weinberg, Rosenfeld, and Brown, 1979; Polinski, 1996).

A. Corroboration of clinical impression by supplemental/screening information.

B. Serial determinations provide more complete information on trends.

C. Automated Coulter counter evaluation. Factors that can alter results:
1. Interreader differences in interpretation of the peripheral smear.

    a. Segmented and band neutrophils exist on a continuum of cellular maturation.

    b. Discrete boundaries are artificial and subject to interobserver bias.

2. Crying for more than 4 minutes: increased WBC count (leukocytosis).
3. Stress: increased WBC count, left shift.
4. Birth asphyxia, maternal hypertension and use of tocolytics: neutropenia (first 72 hours).
5. Hemolytic disease, maternal steroids: neutrophilia (first 72 hours).
6. Central counts lower than peripheral.

D. Response to infection.

1. Evaluation of the total WBC count is insensitive as a predictor of the infection response.
2. Neutrophil count: most sensitive indicator of infant sepsis.

    a. Neutrophil release from the bone marrow is increased.

    b. Number of immature neutrophil forms released into the circulating pool is increased.

    c. Neutropenia, rather than neutrophilia, is more common because of depletion of neutrophil storage pool.

        (1) Neutrophil storage pool consists of neutrophils stored outside the circulation in the bone marrow or layered along vessel walls (margination or marginating pool).

        (2) Infant's neutrophil storage pool is diminished in size compared with that of adults.

        (3) Regulation of marrow neutrophil release is disturbed in the neonate.

3. Absolute neutrophil count (ANC).

    a. Multiply the percentage of total neutrophils by the WBC count.

    b. Normal ranges are:

        (1) Term infants: 1750–5400/mm^3.

        (2) Preterm infants: 1200–5400/mm^3.

    c. Absolute neutrophil count is slightly more sensitive than the total WBC count but, as a single indicator of sepsis, is only approximately 15% predictive.

4. Absolute band form count (ABC).

    a. Multiply the percentage of band forms by the WBC count.

    b. Normally peaks at 1400/mm^3 by 12 hours of age.

    c. May be elevated early in response to infection but is rarely elevated in fatal infection because of rapid exhaustion of marrow reserves and is therefore insensitive as a single indicator of sepsis.

5. Immature/total neutrophil (I/T) ratio.

    a. Total number of immature neutrophil forms (bands, myelocytes, metamyelocytes, promyelocytes) divided by the total number of neutrophils (immature forms plus mature segmented or polymorphonuclear leukocytes; Fig. 16–4).

    b. More sensitive indicator of sepsis because it considers the number of metamyelocytes, which indicates accelerated release from the neutrophil storage pool.

    c. I/T ratio greater than 0.2: probable sepsis.

    d. Neutrophil storage pool depletion: I/T ratio greater than 0.8. Immature forms are all released in response to overwhelming infection.

    e. Factors associated with increased I/T ratio in the absence of sepsis.

        (1) Maternal fever.

        (2) Maternal oxytocin administration.

        (3) Stressful labor.

        (4) Asphyxia.

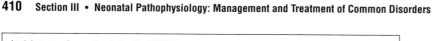

At 6 hours of age the infant's CBC is:

WBC	Polys	Bands	Metamyelocytes	Myelocytes	Lymphocytes
6.0	16	9	3	1	71

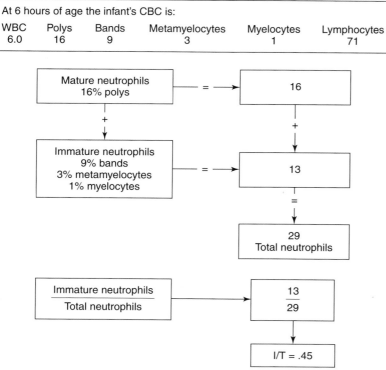

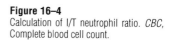

Figure 16–4
Calculation of I/T neutrophil ratio. *CBC,* Complete blood cell count.

    (5) Pneumothorax.
    (6) Intraventricular hemorrhage.
    (7) Seizures.
    (8) Prolonged crying (≥4 minutes).
    (9) Hypoglycemia (blood glucose level <30 mg/dL).
   (10) Surgical intervention.

E. **Evaluation of RBC indices.**
1. Identification of diseases affecting synthesis of hemoglobin.
2. RBC morphology.
    a. Anisocytosis: abnormal variation in size of erythrocytes (severe anemia).
    b. Macrocytosis: diameter greater than 9 μm (micrometer) (increased cell volume: vitamin B_{12} and folic acid deficiencies).
    c. Microcytosis: diameter less than 9 μm (decreased cell volume: iron deficiency, spherocytic and hemolytic anemias).
    d. Poikilocytosis: variation in shape (severe anemia).
    e. Spherocytosis: increased thickness and rounding (decreased deformability and greater susceptibility to destruction; seen in congenital spherocytosis, hemolytic anemias, after transfusion of stored blood).
    f. Target cells: thin, with large diameter, dark center and periphery, with clear ring between periphery and center (hemoglobinopathies, sickle cell/thalassemia, liver disease).
    g. Burr cells: crenations; long spinous processes (hemolytic anemias, DIC, liver disease).
    h. Howell-Jolly bodies: spherical blue bodies in or on erythrocytes; nuclear debris (in asplenia, pernicious anemia).
    i. Nucleated red blood cells: immature red cells with nuclei still present (in chronic blood loss, significant hemolysis, chronic hypoxia, infection).

REFERENCES

American Academy of Pediatrics Committee on Nutrition: Vitamin K compounds and water-soluble analogs: use in therapy and prophylaxis in pediatrics. Pediatrics, 28:501–507, 1961.

American Academy of Pediatrics Vitamin K Ad Hoc Task Force: Controversies concerning vitamin K and the newborn. Pediatrics, 91:1001–1003, 1993.

Andrew, M.: The relevance of developmental hemostasis to hemorrhagic disorders of newborns. Semin. Perinatol. 21:70–85, 1997.

Andrew, M., Montgomery, R.R.: Acquired disorders of hemostasis. In Nathan, D.G., and Orkin, S.H. (Eds.): Nathan and Oski's Hematology of Infancy and Childhood, 5th ed. Philadelphia, W.B. Saunders, 1998, pp. 1677–1718.

Astedt, B.: Antenatal drugs affecting vitamin K status of the fetus and the newborn. Semin. Thromb. Hemost. 21:364–370, 1995.

Beardsley, D.S., and Nathan, D.G.: Platelet abnormalities in infancy and childhood. In Nathan, D.G., and Orkin, S.H. (Eds.): Nathan and Oski's Hematology of Infancy and Childhood, 5th ed. Philadelphia, W.B. Saunders, 1998, pp. 1585–1630.

Bechensteen, A.G., Halvorsen, S., Haga, P., et al.: Erythropoietin (EPO), protein and iron supplementation and the prevention of anemia of prematurity: Effect on serum immunoreactive EPO, growth and protein and iron metabolism. Acta Paediatr., 85:490–495, 1996.

Bhat, A.M., and Scanlon, J.W.: The pattern of eosinophilia in premature infants. J. Pediatr., 98:612–616, 1981.

Black, V.D., Lubchenco, L.O., Koops, B.L., et al.: Neonatal hyperviscosity: Randomized study of effect of partial plasma exchange transfusion on long-term outcome. Pediatrics, 75:1048–1053, 1985.

Blanchette, V.S., and Rand, M.L.: Platelet disorders in newborn infants: Diagnosis and management. Semin. Perinatol., 21(1):53–62, 1997.

Blanchette, V., and Zipursky, A.: Neonatal hematology. In Avery, G.B. (Ed.): Neonatology: Pathophysiology and Management of the Newborn, 4th ed. Philadelphia, J.B. Lippincott, 1994, pp. 638–690.

Bowman, J.: The management of hemolytic disease in the fetus and newborn. Semin. Perinatol., 21:39–44, 1997.

Christensen, R.D.: Developmental hematopoiesis. In Polin, R.A., and Fox, W.W. (Eds.): Fetal and Neonatal Physiology, 2nd ed. Philadelphia, W.B. Saunders, 1998, pp. 1737–1802.

Delaney-Black, V., Camp, B.W., Lubchenco, L.O., et al.: Neonatal hyperviscosity in association with lower achievement and IQ scores at school age. Pediatrics, 83:662–667, 1989.

Doyle, J.J.: The role of erythropoietin in the anemia of prematurity. Semin. Perinatol., 21:20–27, 1997.

Dragone, M.A., and Karp, S.: Bleeding disorders. In Jackson P.L., and Vessey, J.A. (Eds.): Primary Care of the Child With a Chronic Condition. St. Louis, Mosby, 1996, pp. 145–171.

Edwards, T.J.: Hemophilia in the newborn: A case presentation. Neonatal Network, 17(2):67–71, 1998.

Esmon, C.T.: Blood coagulation. In Nathan D.G., and Orkin, S.H. (Eds.): Nathan and Oski's Hematology of Infancy and Childhood, 5th ed. Philadelphia, W.B. Saunders, 1998, pp. 1531–1556.

Fuse, S., Tomita, H., Yoshida, M., et al.: High dose of intravenous antithrombin III without heparin in the treatment of disseminated intravascular coagulation and organ failure in four children. Am. J. Hematol., 53(1):18–21, 1996.

Golding, J., Greenwood, R., Birmingham, K., and Mott, M.: Childhood cancer, intramuscular vitamin K, and pethidine given during labor. Br. Med. J., 305:341–346, 1992.

Henderson-Smart, D.J.: Giving vitamin K to newborn infant: A therapeutic dilemma. Med. J. Australia, 165:414–415, 1996.

Hilgartner, M.W., and Corrigan, J.J.: Coagulation disorders. In Miller, D.R., and Baehner, R.L. (Eds.): Blood diseases of infancy and childhood, 7th ed. St. Louis, Mosby, 1995, pp. 924–986.

Homans, A.: Thrombocytopenia in the neonate. Pediatr. Clin. North Am., 43(3):737–756, 1996.

Hume, H.: Red blood cell transfusions for pretern infants: The role of evidence-based medicine. Semin. Perinatol., 21(1):8–19, 1997.

Kisker, C.T.: Hemostasis. In Polin, R.A. and Fox, W.W. (Eds.): Fetal and Neonatal Physiology, 2nd ed. Philadelphia, W.B. Saunders, 1998a, pp. 1803–1868.

Kisker, C.T.: Pathophysiology of bleeding disorders in the newborn. In Polin, R.A., and Fox, W.W. (Eds.): Fetal and Neonatal Physiology, 2nd ed. Philadelphia, W.B. Saunders, 1998b, pp. 1848–1861.

Kuehl, J.: Neonatal disseminated intravascular coagulation. J. Perinatal Neonatal Nurs., 11(3):69–77, 1997.

Luban, N.L.C.: Blood groups and blood component transfusion. In Miller, D.R., and Baehner, R.L. (Eds.): Blood Diseases of Infancy and Childhood, 7th ed. St. Louis, Mosby, 1995, pp. 54–108.

Manno, C.S.: What's new in transfusion medicine? Pediatr. Clin. North Am., 43(3):793–808, 1996.

Manroe, B.L., Weinberg, A.G., Rosenfeld, C.R., and Brown, R.: The neonatal blood count in health and disease. I. Reference values for neutrophilic cells. J. Pediatr., 95:89–98, 1979.

Marzich, C., Strohm, P.L., Ayas, M., and Cochran, R.K.: Neonatal thrombocytopenia caused by passive transfer of anti-PLA1 antibody by blood transfusion. J. Pediatr., 128:137–139, 1996.

Miller, D.R.: Anemias: General considerations. In Miller, D.R., and Baehner, R.L. (Eds.): Blood Diseases of Infancy and Childhood, 7th ed. St. Louis, Mosby, 1995, pp. 111–139.

Nugent, D.J.: Platelet transfusion. In Nathan, D.G., and Orkin, S.H. (Eds.): Nathan and Oski's Hematology of Infancy and Childhood, 5th ed. Philadelphia, W.B. Saunders, 1998, pp. 1802–1817.

Ohls, R.K., Harcum, J., Schibler, K.R., and Christensen, R.D.: The effect of erythropoietin on the transfusion requirements of preterm infants weighing 750 grams or less: A randomized double-blind, placebo-controlled study. J. Pediatr., 131:661–665, 1997.

Oski, F.A., Brugnara, C., and Nathan, D.G.: A diagnostic approach to the anemic patient. In Nathan, D.G., and Orkin, S.H. (Eds.): Nathan and Oski's Hematology of Infancy and Childhood, 5th ed. Philadelphia, W.B. Saunders, 1998, pp. 375–384.

Polinski, C.: The value of the white blood cell count and differential in the prediction of neonatal sepsis. Neonatal Network, 15(7):13–23, 1996.

Pugh, M.: Lab values and diagnostics of DIC screening in the newborn. Neonatal Network, 16(7):57–64, 1997.

Reid, M.E., and Toy, P.: Erythrocyte blood groups in transfusion. *In* Nathan, D.G., and Orkin, S.H. (Eds.): Nathan and Oski's Hematology of Infancy and Childhood, 5th ed. Philadelphia, W.B. Saunders, pp. 1760–1783.

Silberstein, L.E., Kruskall, M.S., Stehling, L.C., et al.: Strategies for the review of transfusion practices. J.A.M.A., *262*:1993–1997, 1989.

Smith, P.S.: Congenital coagulation protein deficiencies in the perinatal period. Semin. Perinatol., *14*(5):384–392, 1990.

Snapp, B.: Hemorrhagic disease of the newborn and vitamin K. Mother-Baby Journal, *1*(4):17–20, 1996.

Stoeckel, K., Joubert, P.H., and Gruter, J.: Elimination half-life of vitamin K_1 in neonates is longer than generally assumed: Implications for the prophylaxis of haemorrhaghic disease of the newborn. Eur. J. Clin. Pharmacol., *49*:421–423, 1996.

Strauss, R.G.: Recombinant erythropoietin for the anemia of prematurity: Still a promise, not a panacea. J. Pediatr., *131*:653–655, 1997.

Villalta, I.A., Pramanik, A.K., Diaz-Blanco, J., and Herbst, J.J.: Diagnostic errors in neonatal polycythemia based on method of hematocrit determination. J. Pediatr., *115*:460–462, 1989.

Widness, J.A., Veng-Pedersen, P., Peters, C., et al.: Erythropoietin pharmacokinetics in premature infants: Developmental, nonlinearity, and treatment effects. J. Appl. Physiol., *80*:140–148, 1996.

Wong, D.L.: Whaley and Wong's Nursing Care of Infants and Children. St. Louis, Mosby, 1995.

Chapter 17

Neonatal Infections

Josanne Paxton

Objectives

1. Differentiate between humoral and cellular immunologic response in the neonate.

2. List risk factors that predispose a neonate to infection.

3. Describe clinical signs and symptoms of infection.

4. Calculate the absolute neutrophil count and immature/total cell ratio from a complete blood cell count and differential cell count.

5. Identify the common gram-positive and gram-negative organisms responsible for bacterial infections in the neonatal period.

6. Name six antimicrobial agents used to treat neonatal sepsis and discuss indications for and risks of their use.

7. Differentiate between mucocutaneous, systemic, and cutaneous candidiasis.

8. List several clinical manifestations associated with congenital viral infection.

9. Describe the transmission of human immunodeficiency virus and its effect on the immune system.

Infection is a major cause of death during the first month of life, contributing to 13–15% of all neonatal deaths. A review of immunology assists the nurse in understanding neonatal host defense limitations. Interpretations of hematologic studies and identification of risk factors and clinical manifestations can aid in the early detection of neonatal infection.

Group B streptococci and *Escherichia coli* are currently responsible for the majority of early-onset sepsis. Low birth weight infants are at risk of having nosocomial infections caused by coagulase-negative staphylococci. Antibiotic therapy for bacterial infections must be based on the susceptibility of the organism and the achievement of bactericidal concentrations. Congenital viral infections may be asymptomatic at birth or may involve multiple systems. Finally, the human immunodeficiency virus has become a leading cause of immunodeficiency in the neonate, with maternal-infant transmission accountable for the majority of neonatal acquisitions.

This chapter provides the nurse with a comprehensive review of neonatal infections.

Immunology

A. Humoral immunity (Blackburn and Loper, 1992).

1. Immunoglobulin (Polak, Lott, and Kenner, 1994).
   a. Humoral immunity is a specific antibody-mediated response that functions most effectively if there has been previous exposure.
   b. Antibodies are derived from B cells, which have been activated by T cells and antigens (Fig. 17–1).
      (1) B cells mature and are stored in lymph tissue and bone marrow.
      (2) B cells also produce memory cells that recognize antigens on subsequent exposures and initiate an antibody response.
      (3) Antibody functions include:
         (a) Recognition of bacterial antigens.
         (b) Neutralization or opsonization of foreign substances, rendering them susceptible to phagocytosis.
2. Types of immunoglobulin.
   a. Immunoglobulin G (IgG).
      (1) Major immunoglobulin of serum and interstitial fluid.
      (2) Provides immunity against bacterial and viral pathogens.
      (3) Placental transfer to fetus either an active or a passive process.
      (4) Increases gradually until 40 weeks' gestation
      (5) Decreased levels in preterm infants, proportional to their gestational age.
      (6) Decreased levels in postmature and small-for-gestational-age infants, suggesting inhibition of transfer with placental damage.
   b. Immunoglobulin M (IgM).
      (1) IgM does not cross the placenta.
      (2) Synthesis begins early in fetal life, with detectable levels at approximately 30 weeks' gestation.
      (3) Levels may increase (>20 mg/mL) with intrauterine infection.
      (4) Serum levels rapidly increase after birth.

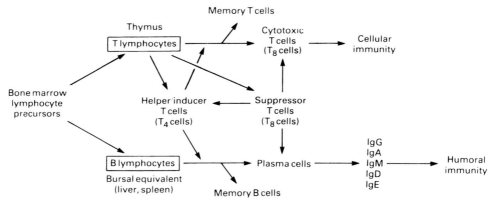

Figure 17–1
Development of cellular and humoral immunity. (From Ganong, W.F.: Review of Medical Physiology, 14th ed. East Norwalk, Conn., Appleton & Lange, 1989.)

   c. Immunoglobulin A (IgA).
     (1) IgA is the most common immunoglobulin in the gastrointestinal tract, respiratory tract, human colostrum, and human milk.
     (2) IgA does not cross the placental barrier.
     (3) Intrauterine synthesis is minimal in an uninfected fetus, and IgA does not become detectable in the newborn infant until 2–3 weeks of life.
     (4) Levels may increase with certain congenital viral infections.
   d. Immunoglobulin E (IgE).
     (1) Present in very small amounts in serum and secretions.
     (2) Major role in allergic reactions.

B. **Cellular immunity.**

1. Specific cellular immunity is mediated by T lymphocytes, which enhance the efficiency of the phagocytic responses.
   a. T lymphocytes migrate to the thymus, where they begin differentiation (see Fig. 17–1).
   b. They are activated by antigens to which they have become sensitized and subsequently become memory or activated T cells.
     (1) Memory cells respond at a later time to the same antigen.
     (2) There are three types of activated T cells.
       (a) Cytotoxic: kill foreign or virus-infected cells.
       (b) Helper: enable B or T cells to respond to antigens and activate macrophages.
       (c) Suppressor: repress responses of specific T and B lymphocytes to antigens.
     (3) T lymphocytes modify the behavior of phagocytic cells and increase their antimicrobial activity.
     (4) Depressed T-cell function may occur as a consequence of neonatal viral infection, hyperbilirubinemia, corticosteroid therapy, or maternal medications taken late in pregnancy.
2. Nonspecific cellular immunity is an inflammatory response involving phagocytosis and includes neutrophils, monocytes, and complement.
   a. Neutrophils are the most numerous of the lymphocytes.
     (1) Neutrophils mature from the bone marrow–committed phagocyte stem cell.
     (2) They are the first line of defense against bacterial infection.
     (3) In a well neonate, a neutrophil reserve is present and exceeds the circulating pool; however, in a septic neonate, the neutrophil reserve pool quickly becomes depleted because of the following:
       (a) Decrease in proliferation or reproduction.
       (b) Decrease in the neutrophil storage pool.
       (c) Decrease in the number of neutrophils that reach the site of infection.
   b. Monocytes are important in the defense against fungal and bacterial infections and are found mainly in the connective tissue.
   c. Complement is the mediator of antigen-antibody reactions.
     (1) Activation by an antibody-dependent mechanism (classic pathway) or antibody-independent mechanism (alternative pathway).
     (2) Purpose.
       (a) Increase neutrophil mobilization from the bone marrow.
       (b) Draw neutrophils to the site of infection.
       (c) Opsonize bacteria for improved phagocytosis.

C. **Summary of neonatal host defense limitations.**

1. Humoral immunity.
   a. Decreased antibody levels.

(1) Poor response to antigenic stimuli.
(2) No production of type-specific antibodies.
   b. Decreased opsonic activity.
     (1) Impaired circulating antibody.
     (2) Depressed complement pathways.
2. Neutrophil response.
   a. Decrease in neutrophil storage pool.
   b. Failure to increase stem cell proliferation during infection.
   c. Altered neutrophil function with respect to chemotaxis, phagocytosis, and bacterial killing.

Transmission of Infectious Organisms in the Neonate

A. **Vertical transmission:** mother to infant.
1. Transplacental acquisition.
   a. Crosses from the placenta to the fetus.
   b. With the exception of *Treponema pallidum* and *Listeria monocytogenes,* an uncommon event because the environment is usually sterile.
2. Ascending acquisition: near time of delivery, when the cervical mucus plug, chorion, and amnion are less than optimal barriers.
3. Intrapartum acquisition: at delivery, during passage of the fetus through a birth canal that is host to a variety of bacteria and to chlamydiae, fungi, yeast, and viruses.

B. **Horizontal transmission:** from nursery personnel and the hospital equipment to the infant; referred to as a nosocomial infection.

Diagnosis and Therapy

CLINICAL ASSESSMENT

Identification of Predisposing Risk Factors

A. **Maternal.**

1. Antepartum.
   a. Poor prenatal care.
   b. Poor nutrition.
   c. Low socioeconomic status.
   d. Recurrent abortion.
   e. Substance abuse.
2. Intrapartum.
   a. Prolonged rupture of membranes (>18 hours).
   b. Maternal group B streptococcal colonization.
   c. Chorioamnionitis: sustained fetal tachycardia, uterine tenderness, purulent amniotic fluid, or unexplained maternal temperature higher than 38° C.
   d. Prolonged or difficult labor.
   e. Premature labor.
   f. Urinary tract infection.
   g. Invasive antenatal procedures.
   h. Maternal infection.

B. **Neonatal.**

1. Low birth weight.
2. Prematurity.
3. Difficult delivery.

4. Birth asphyxia.
5. Meconium staining.
6. Resuscitation.
7. Congenital anomalies (i.e., abdominal wall and spinal defects).

C. **Environmental.**

1. Hospital admission.
2. Length of stay.
3. Invasive procedures.
4. Frequent use of antibiotics.

Clinical Manifestations

A. **Variable nonspecific presentation of sepsis:** appearance of infant "just not right" to nurse or mother, accompanied by subtle changes in feeding and activity. Culture-proven sepsis is relatively rare in the newborn infant; many more infants have signs suggestive of infection at presentation.

B. **Thermoregulation problems.**

1. Fever.
2. Hypothermia.

C. **Neurologic manifestations.**

1. Lethargy.
2. Jitteriness.
3. Irritability.
4. Seizures.
5. Hypotonia or hypertonia.
6. Bulging fontanelles.
7. High-pitched cry.

D. **Respiratory abnormalities:** most common symptom occurring in 90% of infants with sepsis (Guerina, 1998).
1. Grunting.
2. Retractions.
3. Cyanosis.
4. Apnea.
5. Tachypnea.

E. **Cardiovascular manifestations.**

1. Tachycardia.
2. Arrhythmias.
3. Hypotension or hypertension.
4. Cold, clammy skin.
5. Decreased peripheral perfusion.

F. **Gastrointestinal signs.**

1. Poor feeding.
2. Vomiting, diarrhea.
3. Abdominal distention.
4. Increasing feeding residuals.

G. **Skin.**

1. Rash.
2. Pustules.
3. Jaundice.
4. Pallor.

5. Vasomotor instability.
6. Petechiae.

H. Internal organ response.

1. Hepatomegaly.
2. Splenomegaly.

I. Metabolic manifestations.

1. Glucose instability.
2. Metabolic acidosis.

HEMATOLOGIC EVALUATION

A. Complete blood cell count.

1. White blood cell (WBC) count: interpretation is difficult due to the wide range of normal values in the neonate (5000 to 30,000/mm^3) (Oski and Naiman, 1966; Thureen, Deacon, O'Neill, and Hernandez, 1998).
   a. Leukocytosis: an elevated WBC count; may be a normal finding in the newborn infant.
   b. Leukopenia: a depressed WBC count; generally an abnormal finding in the newborn infant.
2. Differential cell count (Fig. 17–2).
   a. Neutrophil count.
      (1) Absolute neutrophil count (ANC).
         (a) ANC is calculated as:

$$\frac{(\% \text{ Segmented forms} + \% \text{ Bands} + \% \text{ Immature cells}) \times \text{Total WBC count}}{100}$$

         (b) Manroe et al. (1979) developed a reference range for the absolute neutrophil count (Fig. 17–3).
      (2) Neutropenia: less than 1500/mm^3.
         (a) Most accurate predictor of infection.
         (b) May be associated with maternal hypertension, confirmed periventricular hemorrhage, severe asphyxia, and reticulocytosis (after 14 days' postnatal age).

Neutrophil: Stages of Maturation

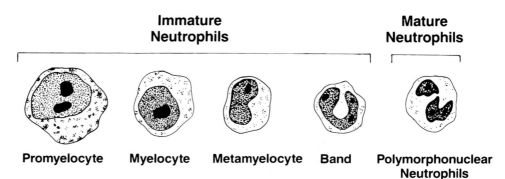

Immature Neutrophils   **Mature Neutrophils**

Promyelocyte   Myelocyte   Metamyelocyte   Band   Polymorphonuclear Neutrophils

Figure 17–2
Neutrophils represent a percentage of the total white blood cell count and are reported as the differential on a complete blood cell count.

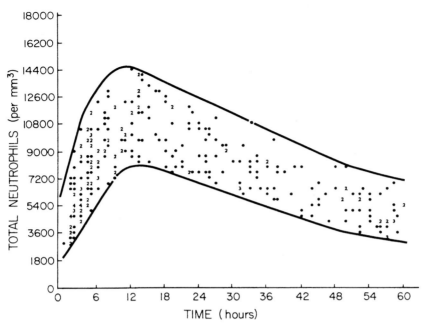

Figure 17–3
Total neutrophil count reference range in the first 60 hours of life. (From Manroe, B.L., Weinberg, A.G., Rosenfeld, C.R., and Browne, R.: The neonatal blood count in health and disease. J. Pediatr., *95*:91, 1979.)

     (3) Neutrophilia.
        (a) Although less predictive, may also suggest presence of infection.
        (b) May be elevated at birth because of neonate's increased neutrophil production and rates of release and demargination from the circulating neutrophil pool.
        (c) Other clinical conditions associated with neutrophilia: hemolytic disease, asymptomatic hypoglycemia, use of oxytocin during labor, maternal fever, stressful labor, pneumothorax, and meconium aspiration.
   b. Immature/total neutrophil (I/T) ratio.
     (1) Less specific than ANC.
     (2) Increase in the I/T ratio also known as a left shift; reflects an increase in immature neutrophils.
     (3) I/T ratio greater than 0.16–0.20 suggestive of infection (Fig. 17–4).
     (4) Calculation of I/T ratio:

$$\frac{\% \text{ Bands} + \% \text{ Immature forms}}{\% \text{ Mature} + \% \text{ Bands} + \% \text{ Immature forms}}$$

   c. Platelet count.
     (1) Normal count: 150,000 to 400,000/mm^3.
     (2) Thrombocytopenia: possible association with bacterial sepsis or viral infection.
     (3) Severe thrombocytopenia: possible association with disseminated intravascular coagulation (DIC).

B. **Additional diagnostic aids.**

1. Detection of bacterial antigens.
   a. Provides a rapid method of diagnosis, although a negative result does not exclude an infectious process.

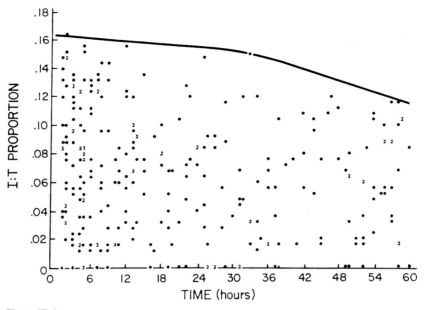

Figure 17–4
Reference range for the proportion of immature to total neutrophils in the first 60 hours of life. (From Manroe, B.L., Weinberg, A.G., Rosenfeld, C.R., and Browne, R.: The neonatal blood count in health and disease. J. Pediatr., *95*:95, 1979.)

    b. Identifies antigens in the blood, urine, and cerebral spinal fluid for *Neisseria meningitidis, Haemophilus influenzae, Streptococcus pneumoniae*, and group B streptococci (GBS).
    c. Does not rely on viable organism; therefore it is possible to obtain positive results even after initiation of appropriate antimicrobial therapy and until suppression of antigen activity has occurred.
    d. Urine latex agglutination for GBS formerly used but, because of high false-positive rate, now replaced by serum testing, which may be useful if the mother is infected with GBS and was treated in labor or in the presence of pneumonia with negative blood culture results. Complicating factors (Harris et al. 1989):
      (1) Detects only GBS, and only 45–55% of neonatal sepsis is due to GBS.
      (2) False-positive rate is 10–15% in asymptomatic infants.
      (3) May have positive result on latex agglutination and negative culture result with low-titer bacteremia or partial treatment.
      (4) Not recommended as a routine screening test for neonatal sepsis.
  2. Hematologic evidence of infection.
    a. Erythrocyte sedimentation rate. Although false-positive results can occur and rates vary widely, levels may rise above the 95th percentile during an infectious process.
    b. C-reactive protein (Mathers and Polhandt, 1987).
      (1) Nonspecific acute-phase reactant is synthesized by the liver in response to interleukin-6, which appears in the blood during an inflammatory process.
      (2) Because of a latency period of 6–8 hours and a stabilization time of 1–2 days after the start of therapy, this test is best performed after the first day infection is suspected.

(3) C-reactive protein is most useful in determining effectiveness of treatment, resolution of disease, and duration of antibiotic therapy.
  c. IgM levels: may rise in the presence of bacterial and/or viral infections.

DIAGNOSTIC EVALUATION

A. **Culture:** isolation of a pathogen in a blood culture obtained by using aseptic technique is diagnostic for infection (Lott and Kilb, 1992).
1. Blood.
  a. Culture specimen obtained from peripheral vein or umbilical vessel.
  b. Procedure.
    (1) Carefully clean infant's skin with an antiseptic such as povidone-iodine solution 10%.
    (2) For maximal bactericidal effect, allow skin to dry for 30 seconds before inserting needle and obtaining culture specimen.
    (3) A minimum of 1–2 mL of blood should be obtained to improve chances for detection of bacteremia. Twenty-three percent of culture results will be falsely negative if less than 1 mL is drawn (Todd, 1991).
  c. May be falsely negative if mother received antibiotics in labor.
  d. Blood culture results to be read at specified intervals, usually 24, 48, and 72 hours, and a final report at 5–14 days.
  e. Ninety-six percent of blood culture results are reliably negative at 48 hours in the absence of maternal antibiotic treatment, and the antibiotics can be discontinued (Philip and Hweitt, 1980). If maternal antibiotics were administered, the clinical course, laboratory tests, and blood culture results should dictate whether to use antibiotic therapy.
2. Cerebrospinal fluid (CSF).
  a. Lumbar puncture. Routine use of lumbar puncture is controversial in early sepsis evaluation. It is frequently unsuccessful or bloody (Schwersenski, McIntyre, and Bauer, 1991) and may also compromise an unstable infant. Meningitis in the absence of bacteremia is uncommon, especially in the neonate with respiratory disease (Weiss, Ionides, and Anderson, 1991). Lumbar puncture may be reserved for infants with central nervous system signs or proven bacteremia.
  b. Abnormal CSF findings.
    (1) A leukocyte count of $100/mm^3$, especially if greater than 60% are polymorphonucleocytes.
    (2) Protein count greater than 100 mg/dL.
    (3) CSF glucose concentration less than 50% of serum level. Obtain serum level before spinal tap to allow for equilibrium to occur between CSF and blood.
    (4) Presence of microorganisms on Gram stain.
  c. Culture.
    (1) Repeat the CSF tap every 24–36 hours until culture is sterile.
    (2) There is a direct correlation between adverse neonatal outcome and persistence of bacteria in the CSF.
3. Urine.
  a. Incidence of contamination with urine obtained by an external collection bag is high. If urine is to be collected, the sample should be obtained by sterile catheterization or suprapubic needle aspiration to avoid contamination and falsely positive results.
  b. If urine is obtained by urethral catheterization, a count greater than 50,000 to 100,000 organisms per milliliter suggests infection.
  c. When culture result is positive, a percutaneous bladder tap should be performed because the urine obtained via bladder tap is presumed to be sterile.

4. Superficial cultures: not recommended because:
   a. Culture result may indicate colonization but does not show bacteremia or sepsis.
   b. Infant may have sepsis in the absence of a positive surface culture result.

B. Follow-up.

1. If a positive culture result has been obtained from blood, CSF, or urine specimen, a follow-up culture specimen should be obtained to document sterilization.
2. Persistent bacteremia may be caused by:
   a. Resistance to antibiotics.
   b. Incorrect administration of antibiotics.
   c. An occult site of infection that may require surgical intervention (e.g., abscess).
   d. Deep IV lines left in place during sepsis.

THERAPY

A. Antibiotic therapy (Table 17–1).

1. Appropriate antibiotic choice depends on the likely organisms, pharmacokinetics, efficacy, and potential toxicity of the antimicrobial agents used.
2. Ampicillin is commonly used in combination with an aminoglycoside for initial treatment of suspected or confirmed bacterial infection.
3. If meningitis is suspected, ampicillin and cefotaxime are the antibiotics of choice until a specific organism has been identified.
4. Third-generation cephalosporins, including cefotaxime and ceftazidime, have increased antimicrobial activity against gram-negative bacilli and enhanced penetration across the blood-brain barrier over gentamicin.
5. Dosage and frequency of administration of antimicrobial agents vary with gestational age and birth weight.
6. Duration of antibiotic therapy is 10–14 days for proven sepsis or 14–21 days for meningitis.
7. If culture results are negative, antimicrobial agents can be discontinued after 48–72 hours.
8. If the mother was treated before delivery, the antimicrobial course may be extended in the face of negative culture results (Gerdes, 1991).

B. Immunotherapy.
The neonate is considered immunocompromised, and defense mechanisms to overcome infections are not yet mature. The administration of blood and tissue factors to enhance the neonatal immune system is under investigation.

1. Intravenous immune globulin (IVIG).
   a. Administration of IVIG may be effective in preventing nosocomial infections, although studies have not been conclusive.
   b. To be useful, IVIG transfusions must contain antibodies specific to the type of infection-causing organism.
   c. IVIG preparations contain protein and varying amounts of IgG, IgA, and IgM (Haque, Zaidi, and Bahakim, 1988).
   d. IVIG acts to neutralize viruses, promote phagocytosis, increase opsonization, and enhance polymorphonucleocyte migration. It prevents neutrophil storage pool depletion by enhancing the neonate's IgG levels for protection against invading bacteria until the immune system is more mature.
   e. Studies continue to determine efficacy of treatment in neonatal infections.
2. Granulocyte transfusion.
   a. Results in an increased number of polymorphonuclear neutrophils, which are responsible for phagocytic action in infection.

Table 17–1
ANTIMICROBIAL CHART FOR NEWBORN INFANTS LESS THAN 7 DAYS OF AGE

Agent	Dose (kg/dose)	Frequency (h)	Indication	Risks
Ampicillin	25-100 mg; slow IV push or IM	q 12	Therapy for sepsis or meningitis gram-positive organisms (e.g., GBS, *L. monocytogenes*)	Seizures in high doses; rash, fever
Cefotaxime	50 mg IM or IV for 30 min	q 12	Sepsis or meningitis caused by gram-negative organisms (e.g., *E. coli, H. influenzae*)	Nephrotoxicity, neutropenia, eosinophilia
Ceftazidime	30 mg IM or IV for 30 min	q 12	Sepsis or meningitis caused by gram-negative organisms (e.g., *E. coli, H. influenzae,* and *Klebsiella*)	Rash, diarrhea, eosinophilia
Ceftriaxone	50 mg IM or IV for 30 min Meningitis: load with 100 mg, then 80 mg	q 12 q 24	Sepsis or meningitis caused by gram-negative organisms (e.g., *E. coli, Klebsiella, H. influenzae,* gonococcal infections)	Displaces bilirubin; eosinophilia, thrombocytosis, pain with IM injections
Clindamycin	5-7.5 mg	≤36 wk: q 12 ≥37 wk: q 8	Bacteremia caused by anaerobic bacteria and some gram-positive cocci: indication for use	Bloody diarrhea, fever, abdominal pain; poor CSF penetration
Erythromycin	10 mg—*by mouth only*	q 6-8	*Chlamydia, Mycoplasma, Ureaplasma*	Contraindicated in patients receiving cisapride and in intrahepatic cholestasis
Gentamicin	2.5 mg 3 mg 2.5 mg IV for 30 min, IM	≤29 wk: q 24 30-36 wk: q 24 ≥37 wk: q 12	Aminoglycoside, initial choice of therapy for sepsis or meningitis, gram-negative organisms	Ototoxicity, nephrotoxicity; monitor serum levels
Methicillin	25-50 mg Slow IV push	q 12	Use if penicillin-resistant *S. aureus* organism, poor CSF penetration	Nephrotoxicity, bone marrow depression, poor CSF penetration
Nafcillin	25-50 mg Slow IV push	q 12	Penicillin-resistant *S. aureus* organisms	Bone marrow depression, irritating to veins
Oxacillin	25-50 mg Slow IV push	q 12	Penicillin-resistant *S. aureus*	Bone marrow depression, rash, nephrotoxicity, poor CSF penetration
Penicillin G	25,000-100,000 units Aqueous penicillin G *IV only* Procaine penicillin G *IM only*	q 12	Gram-positive anaerobes Congenital syphilis	Rare neuromuscular side effects and nephrotoxicity
Tobramycin	2.5 mg 3 mg 2.5 mg IV for 30 minutes, IM	≤29 wk: q 24 30-36 wk: q 24 ≥37 wk: q 12	Aminoglycoside with broad gram-negative coverage	Possible nephrotoxicity and ototoxicity
Vancomycin	20 mg 20 mg 20 mg 15 mg	≤29 wk: q 24 30-33 wk: q 18 34-37 wk: q 12 38-44 wk: q 8	Most gram-positive cocci and rods, methicillin-resistant *S. aureus* and *S. epidermidis*	Nephrotoxicity, ototoxicity, rash, neutropenia, eosinophilia; monitor serum levels

Data from Young, T.E., and Mangum O.B.: Neotax, 11th ed. Raleigh, N.C., Acorn Publishing, 1998; Bhatt, D.R.: Neonatal Drug Formulary, 4th ed. Los Angeles, NDF, 1997; Merenstein, G.B., Gardner, S.L.: Handbook of Neonatal Intensive Care. St. Louis, Mosby, 1998; Lott, J.W.: Neonatal Infection: Assessment, Diagnosis, and Management. Petaluma, Calif., NICU Ink, 1994.

b. May improve survival in infants with sepsis and a decreased neutrophil storage pool (Christensen et al., 1982).

c. Process is both time-consuming and expensive.

d. Risks include fluid overload, graft-versus-host disease, infections, and blood group sensitization.

e. Studies continue to determine the potential for reducing morbidity and mortality rates for infection.

3. Exchange transfusion with fresh whole blood.
   a. Used in severe sepsis to remove bacterial toxins and decrease the bacterial burden, improve peripheral and pulmonary perfusion, and enhance the immune system.
   b. Used widely before 1980; however, prospective studies have not been done to support effectiveness (Vain, Naziumian, and Swarner, 1980).
   c. Adverse reactions include hypoglycemia, acid-base imbalance, thrombocytopenia, and infection.
4. Granulocyte colony-stimulating factor (G-CSF).
   a. Acts to stimulate proliferation of neutrophils; primes neutrophils, thus enhancing their bactericidal and phagocytic activity.
   b. Early trials have demonstrated neutrophil enhancement in neonates without adverse hematologic, immunologic, or developmental defects.
   c. Currently, multicenter trials are evaluating G-CSF for preventing and/or treating late-onset sepsis in low birth weight infants.

History, Sites, and Types of Neonatal Infection

A. **Epidemiologic history.**

1. In 1930s and 1940s: high incidence of group A streptococcus.
2. In 1940s and 1950s: *E. coli* responsible for majority of infections.
3. In 1950s and 1960s: emergence of *Staphylococcus aureus*.
4. From 1970s to 1980s: GBS, *E. coli, L. monocytogenes,* and *H. influenzae* responsible for majority of sepsis during first week of life.
5. In 1990s: *Staphylococcus epidermidis* and methicillin-resistant *S. aureus* have emerged as nosocomial pathogens in the nursery.

B. **Common sites of neonatal infection:** blood, CSF, lungs, and urinary tract.

C. **Types of neonatal infections.**

1. Sepsis.
   a. Incidence of neonatal sepsis varies between 1–8 in 1000 live term births and 1 in 250 live preterm births.
   b. Approximately one third of neonates with bacterial sepsis will have meningitis subsequently (Guerina, 1998).
   c. Six organisms are the most common ones responsible for septicemia:
      (1) Early onset: *E. coli,* GBS, *L. monocytogenes,* and *H. influenzae* (Stoll et al., 1996a).
      (2) Nosocomial: *S. aureus* and *S. epidermidis* (Stoll et al., 1996b).
   d. Presentation is often nonspecific, with subtle signs of temperature instability, lethargy, poor feeding, and glucose instability.
2. Meningitis.
   a. More frequent occurrence during neonatal period than at any other time.
   b. GBS and *E. coli:* majority of pathogens identified in neonatal meningitis.
   c. Acquisition: direct invasion, contamination between CSF space and integumental surfaces, and bacterial dissemination from infected structures.
   d. Clinical manifestations.
      (1) General signs and symptoms of infection at presentation.
      (2) Specific CNS symptoms: increased irritability, alteration in consciousness, poor tone, tremors, seizures, and bulging fontanelle.
   e. CSF culture.
      (1) CSF culture result may be positive even though blood culture result is negative.
      (2) If the CSF culture result is positive, culture must be repeated 24–36 hours after initiation of treatment to ensure adequate therapy.

  f. Antibiotic therapy.
   (1) Prompt initiation is crucial for optimal outcome, and antibiotic may be administered before CSF specimen is obtained.
   (2) Choose antimicrobial agents with good CSF penetration.
   (3) Duration of therapy is dependent on recovered pathogens and clinical response, generally 14–21 days.
  g. Significant sequelae in 20–50% of infants who survive: motor and mental disabilities, convulsions, hydrocephalus, and hearing loss.
 3. Pneumonia.
  a. Transmission.
   (1) Vertical.
    (a) Onset usually from birth to 7 days.
    (b) Most common bacterial pathogen responsible for pneumonia: GBS; however, any organism present in maternal genital tract can cause pneumonia in neonate.
   (2) Horizontal.
    (a) Onset beyond 1 week of life.
    (b) Through human contact or contaminated equipment.
  b. Clinical manifestations: possibly general but usually specific symptoms of respiratory distress.
  c. Diagnosis.
   (1) May be difficult.
   (2) Chest x-ray examination.
    (a) Possible asymmetric densities and pleural effusion.
    (b) Pulmonary granularity present in GBS-related pneumonia; possibly indistinguishable from respiratory distress syndrome in premature infant.
 4. Urinary tract infections.
  a. *E. coli:* most common organism responsible for urinary tract infections; *Klebsiella* and *Pseudomonas aeruginosa:* less common; gram-positive bacteria: rare.
  b. Clinical manifestations.
   (1) General signs are often nonspecific and may include temperature instability, poor weight gain, poor feeding, cyanosis, abdominal distention, hematuria, and proteinuria.
   (2) Localized signs consist of a weak urinary stream and/or bladder distention.
  c. Antimicrobial agents: administer parenterally.
   (1) Oral absorption is erratic.
   (2) There is a 30% association between urinary tract infection and septicemia.
  d. Follow-up.
   (1) Repeat urine culture should be sterile within 36–48 hours after initiation of antimicrobial therapy.
   (2) If a urinary tract infection has been documented in an infant, voiding cystourethrogram should be performed to evaluate the possibility of any congenital abnormalities of the urinary tract.
 5. Neonatal conjunctivitis.
  a. May be caused by a variety of organisms, including *S. aureus, P. aeruginosa, Neisseria gonorrhoeae,* and *Chlamydia trachomatis.*
  b. Manifestations usually include discharge from the eye and conjunctivitis.
  c. Diagnosis is made by a culture and Gram stain, which reveals leukocytes and the causative organism.
  d. Chemical conjunctivitis is usually due to instillation of prophylactic silver nitrate but may occur with topical antibiotics.
  e. Of the ophthalmic antibiotics, methicillin is the antibiotic of choice for

S. aureus, and a combination of carbenicillin and gentamicin are used when *P. aeruginosa* has been identified (also refer to *N. gonorrhoeae,* and *C. trachomatis*).

6. Gastrointestinal disease.
   a. Breast-feeding with the transmission of secretory IgA is important in the prevention of illness (Welsh and May, 1979).
   b. Specific gastrointestinal pathogens.
      (1) Rotavirus.
         (a) Virus is acquired by nosocomial transmission in the NICU.
         (b) Infection may be asymptomatic; infant may exhibit signs and symptoms of severe gastrointestinal distress.
         (c) Symptoms include fever, vomiting, and watery yellow or green diarrhea.
         (d) Detection of the virus is by radioimmunoassay, immunofluorescence, and/or latex agglutination, enzyme-linked immunosorbent assay (ELISA).
         (e) Management includes:
             (i) Replacement of fluids and electrolytes.
             (ii) Elemental diet: may be needed for improved absorption if mucosal damage has occurred.
             (iii) Parenteral nutrition until feedings are well established.
             (iv) Hand washing after contact with infant is essential. Virus is shed in stool 2–3 days before illness is recognized.
             (v) Isolation: may decrease spread of virus.
         (f) Prevention. A rotavirus vaccine (Rv) is now available for the prevention of rotavirus. It is administered at 2, 4, and 6 months of age (AAP, 1999) (see also Appendix B).
      (2) *Clostridium difficile.*
         (a) Gram-positive anaerobic bacillus.
         (b) Causative agent for pseudomembranous colitis.
         (c) Manifested by watery diarrhea, abdominal pain and tenderness, nausea and vomiting, fever, and blood in stool.
         (d) Complications: toxic megacolon, dehydration, and electrolyte disturbances.
         (e) Protective effect: possibly from human milk; neutralizing antibody against *C. difficile* in colostrum.
         (f) Associated with long-term administration of antibiotic therapy.
         (g) May be associated with necrotizing enterocolitis (Lott and Kilb, 1992).
         (h) Intestinal colonization as high as 50% in neonates who generally remain well.
         (i) Treatment: fluid and electrolyte management, antibiotics (generally susceptible to penicillin) (Lott and Kilb, 1992).

Infection With Specific Pathogens

BACTERIAL INFECTIONS

A. Gram-positive organisms.

1. Group B streptococci (CDC, 1996).
   a. Gram-positive spherical bacteria that form pairs or chains during growth.
   b. Twenty identified strains. Groups A, B, and D and *Streptococcus pneumoniae* are responsible for most neonatal infections.
   c. Organism in maternal cervix, vagina, anus, and urethra.
   d. Colonization with GBS in 15–35% of women (Vinal and Huffman, 1997).

   e. Recommendations for intrapartum penicillin therapy:
      (1) History of previous infant with invasive GBS disease.
      (2) Maternal GBS bacteremia with current pregnancy.
      (3) Intrapartum fever.
      (4) Birth at less than 37 weeks' gestation.
      (5) Rupture of membranes more than 18 hours before delivery.
   f. Colonization/disease ratio: approximately 100–200:1.
   g. Most common organism responsible for early-onset bacterial infection in the neonate.
   h. Manifestation of infection: asymptomatic bacteremia, septicemia, pneumonia, or meningitis.
   i. Early-onset infection with GBS.
      (1) Fulminant presentation, typically within first 24 hours of life.
      (2) Most common presentation is with pneumonia and/or meningitis.
      (3) Acquired by vertical transmission.
      (4) Clinical manifestations: respiratory distress, hypotonia, lethargy, poor feeding, abdominal distention, pallor, tachycardia, temperature instability, shock, and seizures.
   j. Late-onset infection with GBS.
      (1) Insidious presentation, usually after 7–10 days.
      (2) Common complication: meningitis.
         (a) In one study, 26% of infants with meningitis died (Wald et al., 1986).
         (b) In 25–50% of neonates, there may be permanent neurologic damage such as mental retardation, spastic quadriplegia, cortical blindness, deafness, uncontrolled seizures, hydrocephalus, and diabetes insipidus.
      (3) Acquired by horizontal transmission.
      (4) Symptoms: fever, lethargy, and bulging fontanelle.
   k. Treatment.
      (1) Antibiotic therapy.
      (2) Fluid management.
      (3) Volume expansion.
      (4) Seizure control.
      (5) Monitoring of electrolytes, fluid balance status, weight, and intake and output.
2. *Staphylococcus.* Gram-positive spherical cells which appear as irregular clusters on Gram's stain. Some species are considered normal flora, and others are pathogenic. Staphylococcal infection can cause mild disease such as local infection from a scalp electrode, or may have widespread manifestations, including osteomyelitis, mastitis, and overwhelming sepsis.
   a. *S. aureus.* A coagulase-positive organism. It is a nosocomial pathogen with the major source of infection being hospital personnel, although also associated with umbilical catheters, endotracheal tubes, and central lines. Colonization occurs in 40–90% of neonates by the fifth day of life. May have widespread manifestations, including osteomyelitis, mastitis, and overwhelming sepsis. Treatment is with methicillin or nafcillin. If methicillin resistant, vancomycin is antibiotic of choice.
   b. *S. epidermidis.* A coagulase-negative organism that is part of the normal skin flora. In recent years it has emerged as a serious pathogen in the preterm infant due to invasive procedures such as endotracheal tubes, umbilical catheters, chest tubes, and central lines which contain a slime-producing agent that can erode the surface of polyethylene catheters and cause colony growth. Many strains are methicillin resistant. Vancomycin is the antibiotic of choice.
3. *Listeria monocytogenes.*
   a. Short gram-positive rod.

    b. Acquired transplacentally or from the vaginal canal of a colonized mother.

    c. Should be suspected in preterm infant who has had passage of meconium or if the maternal history includes prior stillbirth or repeated spontaneous abortions (infection before 28 weeks' gestation frequently results in fetal death) (Lott and Kilb, 1992).

    d. May result in fulminant, disseminated disease with multiorgan involvement.

    e. Symptoms: hypothermia, lethargy, and poor feeding. The infant may have a characteristic salmon-colored rash.

    f. Sensitive to ampicillin.

B. **Gram-negative organisms.**

1. *Escherichia coli.*

    a. Most common gram-negative organism in neonatal period.

    b. Found in female genital tract, with high incidence of colonization in the neonate.

    c. Colonization of human gastrointestinal tract soon after birth; predominant fecal flora throughout life.

    d. Many serotypes of *E. coli.* One form of *E. coli* antigen, K1, is associated with neonatal meningitis.

    e. Possible cause of severe, fulminant infection, leading to respiratory distress, cardiovascular collapse, meningitis, and multiorgan failure and death.

    f. In addition to septicemia, possible cause of localized infection, including cellulitis, pneumonia, septic arthritis, urinary tract infection, and otitis media.

    g. Sensitivity to aminoglycosides such as gentamicin and third-generation cephalosporins.

2. *Pseudomonas aeruginosa.*

    a. Gram-negative, motile, aerobic rod.

    b. Known as "waterbug"; inhabitant of respirators and moist oxygen circuits or environments.

    c. Particular susceptibility to colonization and subsequent development of pneumonia in infant requiring ventilator and receiving antibiotics.

    d. Pathogenic organism in immunocompromised host or where normal defense mechanisms of the skin and mucous membranes are insufficient.

    e. Generally a cause of late-onset disease with respiratory distress.

    f. Treatment: combination of aminoglycoside and anti-*Pseudomonas* penicillin such as carbenicillin, imipenem, piperacillin, or ticarcillin or by ceftazidime, a third-generation cephalosporin.

    g. Also a cause of conjunctivitis in newborn infant. Generally between 5 and 18 days after birth, mild conjunctivitis begins with edema and erythema of the lid, with purulent discharge. May progress quickly, causing corneal perforation, and may also result in virulent necrotizing endophthalmitis and blindness. Parenteral therapy is necessary—typically a parenteral aminoglycoside plus antipseudomonal penicillin or cephalosporin—plus topical aminoglycoside therapy for 7–10 days (Thureen et al., 1999).

3. *Haemophilus influenzae.*

    a. Gram-negative bacillus.

    b. Low rate of maternal genital colonization, although passage to fetus is via the ascending transcervical route.

    c. Chorioamnionitis occurs in all placentas but appears more severe among survivors.

    d. Fifty percent chance of symptomatic infection in colonized infant.

    e. Early-onset fulminant presentation, with pneumonia, respiratory distress, hypotension, and leukopenia.

    f. Mortality rate may be as high as 50%, especially in the very low birth weight infant.

    g. Treatment includes ampicillin and a third-generation cephalosporin. Some strains are resistant to ampicillin (Lott, 1994).

4. *Neisseria gonorrhoeae*

    a. Gram-negative diplococcal bacteria.

    b. Most frequently reported sexually transmitted disease in the United States: approximately 1 million cases annually. Concurrent infections with *C. trachomatis* or *T. pallidum* are common.

    c. Presents in the first week of life with bilateral copious, mucopurulent discharge. Lid and conjunctival edema and erythema are common.

    d. Diagnosis made by Gram stain and confirmed with positive identification on chocolate agar culture. Evaluation for sepsis and meningitis also necessary.

    e. Sequelae: rare, but permanent visual impairment and/or systemic infection possible.

    f. Treatment: third-generation cephalosporin, such as ceftriaxone, until susceptibility testing can be completed. Penicillin G is a secondary choice if the organism is not penicillin resistant. Eye irrigation with saline solution until eye discharge clears is also recommended (Thureen et al., 1999).

    g. Recommended: silver nitrate (1%) aqueous solution or erythromycin (0.5%) ophthalmic ointment in the eyes of all vaginally delivered infants. (NOTE: Eye prophylaxis only minimizes the risk of infection; it does not guarantee prevention.)

C. **Bacterial parasite:** *Chlamydia trachomatis.*

1. Parasite is commonly found in the adult female genital tract. It accounts for approximately 4 million genitourinary tract infections per year—the most common sexually transmitted disease in the United States (Lott, 1994).

2. Delivery through an infected vaginal canal may result in neonatal infection.

3. Conjunctivitis usually is manifested at 5–14 days of age but may be delayed with eye prophylaxis. Symptoms may be minimal. Findings include copious mucopurulent exudate with frequent pseudomembrane formation. Pneumonia, otitis media, and gastroenteritis may also develop.

    a. Diagnosis is by tissue culture isolation from conjunctival, oropharyngeal, genital, or rectal swabs of cells (Lott, 1994).

    b. Treatment for conjunctivitis includes ophthalmic and systemic erythromycin for 14 days. Topical therapy is insufficient to eradicate nasopharyngeal colonization (Thureen et al. 1999).

4. Chlamydial pneumonia is manifested between 4 and 11 weeks postnatally.

    a. Symptoms include a persistent cough, rales, and wheezing.

    b. Chest radiograph may reveal hyperinflation.

    c. Chronic disease may persist even after the acute phase of disease is over.

    d. Treatment is with erythromycin for 14 days.

FUNGAL INFECTION: CANDIDIASIS

Candidiasis is caused by *Candida,* a significant neonatal pathogen. The most common species is *Candida albicans.*

A. Mucotaneous candidiasis.

1. Most common form of candidiasis in the newborn infant.

2. Acquired during passage through the birth canal or from mother during breast-feeding.

3. Appears as pearly white material on the buccal mucosa, dorsum and lateral areas of the tongue, gingivae, and pharynx.

4. Treatment is with oral nystatin oral suspension (100,000 units/mL), 1 mL to each side of mouth every 6 hours for 3 days after symptoms have subsided (Young and Mangum, 1998).
5. May need to treat mother if origin of infection is mother's breast.

B. Cutaneous candidiasis.

1. Presence of oral *Candida* is strongly associated with development of cutaneous candidiasis in the perineal region.
2. May appear initially as erythematous and vesiculopapular lesions, and then develop into fine white, scaly collarettes.
3. Therapy.
   a. Use of topical agents such as nystatin four times a day and continued 2–3 days after the rash has cleared.
   b. Simultaneous treatment with oral nystatin to minimize the risk of recurrence.
   c. Maintenance of area free from moisture and stool.

C. Acute disseminated (systemic) candidiasis.

1. Has emerged as a serious nosocomial infection occurring in very low birth weight infants, with systemic candidiasis developing in as many as 3% (Guerina, 1998).
2. Most frequent sites of infection include the lungs, kidneys, liver, spleen, and brain; several sites may be involved simultaneously.
3. Risk factors include prematurity (immunocompromised state), use of total parenteral nutrition and intravenous fat emulsions, and prolonged use of broad-spectrum antibiotics.
4. Presentation includes respiratory deterioration, abdominal distention, apnea, acidosis, carbohydrate intolerance, hypotension, skin abscesses, temperature instability, and/or erythematous rash.
5. Formation of fungus in urine may lead to urinary tract infection.
6. Diagnosis is made by blood cultures, CSF cultures, microscopic examination of urine and the buffy coat of blood, determination of serum *Candida* antigen, ophthalmologic examination, and renal ultrasonography.
7. Treatment.
   a. Amphotericin B: initial dose of 0.25–0.5 mg/kg IV over 2–6 hours, followed by maintenance doses of 0.5–1 mg/kg per day every 24–48 hours as a daily infusion over 2–6 hours, for 4–6 weeks. Requires close monitoring of hematologic and renal function (Young and Mangum, 1998).
   b. 5-Fluorocytosine: 50–100 mg/kg per day in four divided doses for 3–4 weeks; used in combination with amphotericin B, especially if severe infection or CNS involvement occurs (Merenstein, Adams, and Weisman, 1998).

VIRAL INFECTIONS

A. Mode of transmission.

1. Congenital: acquired in utero during maternal viral infection with exposure to the fetus. Infant presents with disease at birth or shortly thereafter.
2. Intrapartum: acquired at birth from organisms present in the maternal genital tract; onset of neonatal symptoms occurs within 5–7 days or later, depending on incubation period.
3. Postnatal: acquired during neonatal period from breast-feeding (HIV, hepatitis B virus, cytomegalovirus), through blood transmission (cytomegalovirus, hepatitis B virus), or from hospital personnel or family members (enterovirus, respiratory syncytial virus).

B. Viral organisms.

1. Rubella virus.
   a. Generally causes a mild and often asymptomatic infection in children and adults. If acquired during pregnancy, can result in any of a wide range of fetal and neonatal outcomes: spontaneous abortion, congenital malformation, stillbirth, and neonatal disease (e.g., hepatitis, hepatosplenomegaly, jaundice, thrombocytopenia, "blueberry muffin" purpura), asymptomatic fetal infection, or no transmission of virus to the fetus (Cooper, Preblud, and Alford, 1995).
   b. Severity of neonatal disease is increased if infection occurs during the first trimester.
   c. There may be no initial symptoms, although most infected infants will have long-term sequelae such as endocrinopathies, deafness, eye damage, vascular disease, panencephalitis, and developmental delays (Overall, 1992; Sever, South, and Shaver, 1985).
   d. Early manifestations include intrauterine growth restriction, thrombocytopenia, hepatomegaly, jaundice, congenital heart disease (patent ductus arteriosus, peripheral pulmonary artery stenosis, atrial or ventricular septal defects), interstitial pneumonia, cataracts, bone lesions, microphthalmia, lethargy, irritability, bulging fontanelle, and late-onset seizures.
   e. Diagnosis is made by detection of specific rubella IgM; by demonstration of stable or rising rubella IgG titers in serial sera obtained for several months; and/or by cultivation of virus from nasal secretions, throat swab, urine, blood, or CSF. Special cell cultures are required for cultivation of rubella virus.
   f. Prevention measures are as follows:
      (1) Pregnant women should be screened for immunity whether or not they have received prior rubella immunization. Susceptible pregnant women should avoid exposure to infected persons. Pregnant women are not given the vaccine because of the small risk of transmission of virus to the fetus (1.2–1.8%) (Centers for Disease Control [CDC], 1987).
      (2) Seronegative women should be vaccinated post partum, before discharge from the hospital. Vaccine virus is excreted in breast milk, but breast-feeding is not a contraindication to vaccination.
      (3) Routine rubella vaccination should be administered to all infants (American Academy of Pediatrics [AAP], 1998).
   g. Isolation procedures are carried out because respiratory and urinary secretion of virus may occur for several months or more after birth. Transmission-based precautions, in addition to standard precautions, should be used with all infants with suspected congenital rubella during hospitalization.
   h. There is no specific antiviral therapy for congenital rubella or for amelioration of progressive disease after birth.
2. Cytomegalovirus (CMV).
   a. CMV causes the most common congenital viral infection that is spread horizontally by salivary or urinary contamination or by sexual transmission. Infection is more common in crowded conditions, in lower socioeconomic groups, and in breast-fed infants (Stagno, 1995). Up to 90% of the adult population and 70% of children in day care are seropositive. Approximately 2% of women will have a primary CMV infection during pregnancy (Stagno and Whitley, 1985).
   b. Infection may be acquired from cervical secretions at the time of delivery. After birth, the virus may be transmitted in infected maternal secretions or breast milk or through blood transfusions. Overall, with primary maternal infection, 40% of infants are infected, with symptoms manifested at birth

in 10% and with late sequelae occurring in another 5–10% (Stagno and Whitley, 1985).

  c. Clinical manifestations are as follows:

    (1) Congenital infection.

      (a) Symptomatic at birth: growth restriction, hepatosplenomegaly, microcephaly, jaundice, petechiae and purpura, pneumonia, chorioretinitis, and periventricular intracranial calcification. Prognosis is poor, with one third dying in infancy and up to 90% of survivors having severe neurologic sequelae.

      (b) Asymptomatic at birth: 5–15% may have long-term sequelae, the majority having hearing loss and decreased IQ, microcephaly, visual difficulties, and school problems (Stagno, 1995).

    (2) Perinatal or postpartum infection. The majority of infections remain asymptomatic and do not appear to result in any long-term sequelae (Stagno, 1995). Severe disease has occurred in premature infants infected with CMV by means of blood transfusion.

  d. Diagnosis is made by viral isolation from the infant's urine or saliva or by a high anti-CMV IgM titer in the first 2–3 weeks of life or persistant or rising IgG titers in the first 6 months of life. Infants with both congenital and perinatal/postnatal CMV infection excrete virus in their urine for years (Stagno et al., 1983).

  e. There is no proven treatment.

  f. For prevention, pregnant women should be advised to use good handwashing technique. Blood products given to neonates should be treated to reduce the potential for CMV transmission or should be obtained from CMV seronegative donors.

  g. Neither infants with symptomatic CMV infection nor those with diagnosed but asymptomatic CMV infection require isolation, but "standard precautions," particularly for pregnant caretakers, should be enforced.

3. Respiratory syncytial virus (RSV).

  a. Most common respiratory pathogen in infants. It is the major cause of bronchiolitis and pneumonia in infants during the first 3 years of life.

  b. Prevalence. Infection is most prevalent during winter and through early spring (November through April) and is highly contagious. It is transmitted through contact with infected secretions (droplet contamination) resulting from coughing and sneezing. Infection proceeds from the nasal mucosa and spreads from the upper to the lower respiratory tract.

  c. Susceptibility. Initial infection and most serious illness generally occur during the first year of life, especially in infants who were premature or have either chronic lung disease or congenital heart disease.

  d. Presentation.

    (1) Nonspecific: poor feeding, lethargy, apnea, irritability.

    (2) Respiratory symptoms: cough, wheezing, rales, rhonchi, dyspnea, pneumonia, cyanosis, pulmonary infiltrates.

    (3) Increasing respiratory distress, which may result in respiratory failure.

  e. Diagnosis.

    (1) Clinical and epidemiologic findings.

    (2) Rapid viral antigen detection isolated from nasopharyngeal aspirate.

  f. Treatment. Supportive care includes oxygen, hydration, and isolation. High-risk infants may progress to assisted ventilation because of hypoxemia and hypercapnia.

  g. RSV immune globulin (RSVIG). Intravenously administered RSVIG has been approved by the U.S. Food and Drug Administration for use in infants for the prevention of RSV-induced lower respiratory tract disease. RSVIG is ineffective in treating established RSV infection. The AAP (1997d) recommends its use in infants and children younger than 24 months of age with a history of bronchopulmonary dysplasia and in infants born at less than 32 weeks' gestation without this disease. Administration begins before onset of the RSV season.

  (1) RSVIG is an IV preparation administered monthly over 4 hours during the RSV season.

  (2) Palivizumab (Synagis), a new preparation, is a monoclonal antibody that can be administered intramuscularly once monthly (Subramanian, 1998).

  h. Isolation procedures. Transmission-based precautions are used, in addition to standard precautions. May designate cohort of infected infants to prevent widespread infection.

4. Herpes simplex virus (HSV).

  a. Cause of serious disease in fetus and neonate, with incidence estimated at 1 in 3000 to 1 in 20,000 births (AAP, 1997a).

  b. Types of HSV infection.

  (1) HSV-1: nongenital type, although it can infect the genital area.

  (2) HSV-2: genital type; more often associated with neonatal disease.

  c. Transmission. Eighty-five to ninety percent of infections are acquired at the time of delivery. Infections can also occur in utero or postnatally (Whitley and Arvin, 1995). Postnatal infections can be acquired from breast lesions during breast-feeding, from oral lesions through direct contact, and from other infants with HSV infection. The greatest risk to the neonate is in mothers with a primary infection at birth. Transmission occurs in 40–50% of these infants. With reactivation of the disease, transmission occurs in 4–5% of deliveries or fewer (Overall, 1992).

  d. Presentation.

  (1) Intrapartum or postnatal transmission: vesicular lesions, thermal instability, lethargy, respiratory distress, vomiting, poor feeding, cyanosis, and, if there is CNS involvement, irritability, bulging fontanelle, seizures, opisthotonos, and coma.

  (2) Congenital transmission: early vesicular rash, small for gestational age, low birth weight, chorioretinitis, diffuse brain damage, microcephaly, and intracranial calcification.

  e. Diagnosis. Positive culture result with specimen obtained from vesicular fluid, blood, or CSF results in a diagnosis. The diagnostic yield of CSF culture for neonates with CNS disease is less than 50%. The polymerase chain reaction (PCR) test has a much higher yield in CSF and should be performed if available. Other rapid identification tests include direct fluorescent antibody staining of vesicle scrapings and enzyme immunoassay antigen detection in vesicles or body fluids.

  f. Treatment.

  (1) Systemic infection: acyclovir, 10 mg/kg per dose every 8 hours for 2–3 weeks (Young and Mangum, 1998). Side effects are rare. Phlebitis may occur at the IV site because of alkaline pH of 10.

  (2) Ocular involvement: topical ophthalmic drug such as 3% vidarabine in addition to parenteral antiviral therapy. An ophthalmology consultation should be obtained.

  g. Prognosis. Approximately half of all infants with untreated infection die, with high morbidity rates in survivors. Morbidity and mortality rates are highest in infants with CNS or disseminated disease. Antiviral therapy improves prognosis, especially in infants with localized disease.

  h. Prevention.

  (1) Maternal history of HSV infection.

  (a) Weekly virologic and clinical screening beginning at 32 weeks.

  (b) Cesarean delivery if lesions are present or a culture result is positive at the time of delivery.

      (c) For known exposure to active recurrent infection at vaginal delivery or cesarean delivery, culture specimens should be obtained from the neonate 24–48 hours after birth. Treatment should be considered especially if the infant has symptoms, was born prematurely, acquired open wounds during delivery, or has other high-risk factors.

      (d) Delivery can be vaginal if no clinical or virologic evidence is present. Neonatal surface cultures can be considered but are not routinely recommended.

    (2) Primary infection. For infants born vaginally to women with suspected or documented active primary HSV infection at the time of delivery, give prophylactic acyclovir pending neonatal culture results. If delivery is cesarean, acyclovir administration should be considered, especially if rupture of membranes occurred more than 6 hours before delivery or if the neonate has symptoms.

    (3) Follow-up of at-risk infants. Infants who are at risk of HSV infection, even if culture result was negative after birth, should be followed up closely for a minimum of 6 weeks.

  i. Isolation procedures.

    (1) Mothers with HSV infections need to use strict hand-washing techniques before touching their infant.

    (2) Infants born to mothers with active lesions should be physically separated from other infants and managed with "transmission precautions," in addition to "standard precautions."

    (3) Infants born to mothers with a history of infection but without lesions at delivery do not require isolation. Good hand-washing technique should be stressed.

    (4) Infants with HSV infection should be isolated and managed with "transmission precautions."

5. Hepatitis B.

  a. DNA double-shelled virus.

  b. Transmission: vertical. The virus is also found in any bodily secretion, including human milk. There is no added risk to the infant of acquiring HBV infection when the mother is hepatitis B surface antigen (HBsAg) positive; therefore breast-feeding is not contraindicated if immunoprophylaxis recommendations are followed (Thureen et al., 1999).

  c. Presentation. Infants infected in utero are free of symptoms at birth. Infants infected at delivery or after birth do not have HBsAg present for at least 2–5 months. Infants who become chronically infected are at risk of having chronic hepatitis, cirrhosis, and/or other hepatocellular carcinoma.

  d. Prevention. Routine screening is used for all pregnant women and universal screening for all infants and children. Routine neonatal immunization is with hepatitis B vaccine: Engerix-B, 10 µg, or Recombivax-HB, 5 µg (AAP, 1999).

    (1) Term infant is immunized at discharge and again at 2 months and 6 months of age (AAP, 1999).

    (2) Preterm infant is immunized at discharge if weight is greater than 2 kg or at 2 months of age.

  e. Treatment. In the infant born to a HBsAg positive mother, treatment is 85–95% effective in preventing the development of the hepatitis B carrier state and should include the following:

    (1) Careful bathing of the neonate to remove blood and secretions that may be contaminated.

    (2) Administration of hepatitis B immune globulin (HBIG), 0.5 mL intramuscularly, as soon as possible within 12 hours of birth, in addition to a hepatitis B vaccine: Engerix-B, 10 µg, or Recombivax-HB, 5 µg (AAP, 1999).

f. Isolation procedures. Infants born to mothers with HBsAg should be cared for with "standard precautions." No isolation is required. Immediately after birth the infant should be handled with gloves until all maternal blood is removed.
6. Human immunodeficiency virus (HIV).
   a. Cytopathic human retrovirus.
   b. Use of reverse transcriptase enzyme. HIV uses the enzyme to produce viral DNA and integrates this into the DNA of the T-helper cells.
   c. Suppression of T-helper lymphocytes. This results in B-cell and suppressor T-cell dysfunction, with subsequent defects in cell-mediated immunity and development of opportunistic infections.
   d. Infection of monocytes and macrophages—also possible.
   e. Symptom-free infection. An infant can have an HIV infection with an absence of symptoms, suggesting that other factors (e.g., genetic predisposition, nutritional status) may contribute to the development of infection.
   f. Transmission.
      (1) Transmission is through blood or blood products.
      (2) Vertical transmission is thought to be the most common method of transfer, although time of transmission is uncertain.
         (a) Transplacental transmission has been demonstrated.
         (b) Intrapartum transmission during drug exposure to infected maternal blood or genital tract secretions is presumed.
         (c) HIV may be transmitted through human milk.
         (d) Risk of infection to an infant born to an HIV-infected mother who did not receive antiretroviral therapy during pregnancy is estimated to be between 13% and 39% (Hutto et al., 1991).
   g. Presentation. Signs and symptoms are rare in the neonatal period but may be seen in infancy.
      (1) Failure to thrive.
      (2) Generalized lymphadenopathy, hepatomegaly, and splenomegaly.
      (3) Recurrent mucosal infections.
      (4) Systemic bacterial infections.
      (5) Recurrent candidiasis.
      (6) Lymphoid interstitial pneumonitis.
      (7) Parotitis, hepatitis, nephropathy, cardiomyopathy.
      (8) Recurrent diarrhea.
      (9) Opportunistic infections.
      (10) Neurodevelopmental delay.
      (11) Malignancies.
   h. Diagnosis—current assays.
      (1) Antibody-based tests.
         (a) Enzyme-linked immunosorbent assay.
         (b) Western blot.
         (c) Indirect immunofluorescence assay.
      (2) Viral antigen detection: used to detect HIV antigen, usually the p24 antigen.
      (3) Viral nucleic acid detection. PCR and branched-chain DNA assays are used to monitor disease progression and therapy efficacy.
      (4) Viral culture.
      (5) Combination of tests (usually PCR and/or viral isolation). A diagnosis can be made in more than 90% of infants by 2 months of age, and in nearly 100% by 4 months of age (AAP, 1997b; Rossi et al., 1992).
   i. Management.
      (1) Prompt intervention during bacterial and treatable opportunistic infections.
      (2) Adequate nutrition.

(3) Antiretroviral therapy (CDC, 1994).
   (a) Zidovudine (ZDU; formerly azidothymidine, or AZT).
      (i) Nucleotide analog thought to function by inhibition of reverse transcriptase and/or by chain termination.
      (ii) Demonstrated toxic side effects in the neonate include macrocytosis, anemia, and neutropenia.
   (b) Ribavirin and dideoxycytidine are undergoing clinical trials.
(4) Perinatal prophylaxis (Connor et al., 1994; DeVita et al., 1997).
   (a) ZDU, 100 mg by mouth 5 times a day, initiated at 14–34 weeks' gestation and continued throughout the pregnancy.
   (b) Intrapartum loading dose of ZDU is 2 mg/kg IV over 1 hour, followed by continuous infusion of 1 mg/kg per hour until delivery.
   (c) Neonatal administration is 2 mg/kg per dose by mouth every 6 hours for 6 weeks, beginning at 8–12 hours of age (Young and Mangum, 1998).
(5) Prevention.
   (a) Cesarean delivery has not been shown to prevent transmission of HIV to the infant.
   (b) Breast-feeding concerns (AAP, 1995).
      (i) Transmission of HIV infection to infants from breast-feeding occurs at rates of 27–40% in women with primary infection post partum (Palasanthiran et al., 1993; Van de Perre et al., 1991).
      (ii) In developed countries with access to safe feeding alternatives, breast-feeding is contraindicated. In developing countries where breast-feeding is protective against a variety of infections and adequate nutritional substitutes may not be available, the current recommendation by the World Health Organization is that HIV-infected mothers continue to breast-feed (Dunn et al., 1992).
(6) Isolation procedures. "Standard precautions" should be strictly followed.

OTHER INFECTIONS

A. **Toxoplasmosis.**

1. Caused by intracellular protozoan parasite, *Toxoplasma gondii,* which is an important human pathogen.
2. Maternally acquired from consumption of poorly cooked meat or by exposure to infected cat feces. Only women who become acutely infected during pregnancy can give birth to a newborn infant with congenital toxoplasmosis. Estimated incidence of acute maternal infection in pregnancy is 1.1 in 1000 (Sever et al., 1988).
3. Congenitally acquired disease in the newborn infant by vertical transmission. Approximate neonatal incidence is 0.1 to 1 in 1000 live births.
4. Manifestations may include maculopapular rash, hepatomegaly, splenomegaly, jaundice, and thrombocytopenia
5. CNS involvement includes microcephaly or hydrocephalus accompanied by convulsions; cerebral calcifications may be seen on radiographs.
6. Sequelae include mental retardation, learning disabilities, impaired vision, and blindness.
7. Toxoplasmosis may be asymptomatic at birth but may be manifested as intellectual impairment in late infancy or childhood.

8. Diagnosis may be made by a number of methods: isolation or histologic demonstration of the organism, detection of *Toxoplasma* antigens in tissues and body fluids, detection of *Toxoplasma* nucleic acid by PCR, and serologic tests.
9. Treatment consists of pyrimethamine, trisulfapyrimidines, and a folic acid supplement to prevent bone marrow suppression.
10. Isolation procedures consist of "standard precautions."

B. **Syphilis.**

1. Cause: *Treponema pallidum*, a thin, motile spirochete.
2. Incidence of congenital syphilis: increased from 264 in 1985 to 3850 in 1992 (Evans and Frenkel, 1994).
3. Transmission: through sexual contact or by maternal-fetal transmission.
4. Presentation.
   a. Sometimes asymptomatic.
   b. Petechiae.
   c. Skin lesions: copper-colored maculopapular rash that is most severe on the hands and feet and appears at 1–3 weeks of age, with subsequent desquamation. Lesions present at birth may be bullous.
   d. Hepatosplenomegaly.
   e. Respiratory distress.
   f. CNS involvement.
   g. Rhinitis.
   h. Periostitis of long bones, with guarding of extremities.
5. Diagnosis.
   a. U.S. Public Health Service recommendation: all pregnant women screened with Venereal Disease Research Laboratory (VDRL) or rapid plasma reagin (RPR) test early in pregnancy and at the time of delivery.
   b. Diagnosis of active disease in the neonate.
      (1) High VDRL titer (four times higher than maternal titer).
      (2) Reactive RPR.
      (3) Serum IgM level greater than 20 mg/dL.
      (4) Confirmation with a positive result on fluorescent treponemal antigen-antibody absorption (FTA-ABS) test.
   c. Prevention. Uninfected infants possess maternally acquired antibodies at concentrations similar to those of infected infants. It may be difficult to interpret neonatal laboratory data; therefore it is important to determine adequacy of maternal treatment, possibility of reexposure, and family compliance with follow-up.
6. Treatment.
   a. Penicillin.
      (1) Benzathine penicillin G, 50,000 units/kg given intramuscularly once if infection is asymptomatic and CSF is normal (Bhatt et al., 1997).
      (2) Procaine penicillin G, 50,000 IU/kg per dose given intramuscularly once daily for 10–14 days if infection is symptomatic and CSF is abnormal (Young and Mangum, 1998); alternatively, aqueous crystalline penicillin G, 50,000 IU/kg per day divided every 8–12 hours (interval based on gestational age and postnatal age) and administered IV for 10–14 days (Young and Mangum, 1998).
      (3) Procaine and benzathine penicillins are administered intramuscularly only, providing tissue depots from which drug is absorbed for hours or days.
   b. Neonatal therapy: should be instituted if maternal treatment is uncertain or if treatment was given within the last 4 weeks of pregnancy.
7. Isolation procedures: "standard precautions."

Infection Control

A. In 1996 the Hospital Infection Control Practices Advisory Committee of the Centers for Disease Control and Prevention issued new guidelines for isolation practices for hospitalized patients (Garner, 1996).

B. Two major categories of infection control practices were designated (Garner, 1996; AAP, 1997c):

1. Standard precautions: expanded set of previously designated "universal precautions." Developed to protect patients and health care workers from blood-borne and other body fluid–borne infections; designed to prevent cutaneous and mucous membrane exposure to blood and body fluids. Guidelines include:
   a. Immediate hand washing or washing of other body surfaces if contaminated with blood and body fluids. This applies even if gloves are used, and hands should be washed immediately after glove removal. Hands should be thoroughly washed after all patient contact regardless of whether or not there was obvious contact with body fluids.
   b. Barrier precautions to prevent cutaneous and mucous membrane exposure to blood, body fluids, secretions, excretions, and contact with any items that might be contaminated with these fluids. Barriers include:
      (1) Gloves: should be worn when contacting blood and body fluids, mucous membranes, open skin, or items soiled by blood and body fluids. Hands should be washed immediately after glove removal. New gloves should be used with new patient contact and before touching noncontaminated items or surfaces.
      (2) Masks, face shields, and protective eye wear: should be used when patient contact or procedures can potentially generate splashes, sprays, or droplets of blood, body fluids, secretions, or excretions which might come in contact with the mucous membranes of the eyes, nose, or mouth.
      (3) Nonsterile gowns or aprons, should be worn when patient contact or procedures likely to generate splashes, sprays or droplets of blood, body fluids, secretions which may contaminate the caregiver's skin or clothing.
   c. Cleaning of patient care equipment that might be contaminated, to prevent skin and mucous membrane exposure and clothing contamination.
   d. Correct handling, transport, and cleaning of soiled linen to prevent skin and mucous membrane exposure and clothing contamination.
   e. "Sharps program" in place to prevent exposure by needle stick and other sharp object injuries during cleaning, using, or disposing of these items.
   f. Avoidance of mouth-to-mouth resuscitation; replacement by readily available resuscitation and ventilation equipment.
2. Transmission-based precautions: guidelines for the care of patients infected with specific pathogens or with syndromes in which the pathogenic organism may be spread by airborne, droplet, or contact routes. Measures additional to "standard precautions" are needed to prevent spread of infection. They are based on preventing transmission by one of three types of infection:
   a. Airborne transmission. Prevention requires special air handling and ventilation.
      (1) Private room with negative air pressure ventilation.
      (2) Masks.
      (3) Not required: gowns or gloves.
   b. Droplet transmission. Droplets do not remain suspended, so special air handling and ventilation measures are not required.

(1) Private room preferred but not required; cohorting of infants with same infection is acceptable.
(2) Masks.
(3) Not required: gowns and gloves.
  c. Contact transmission. Contact is the most common type of transmission of hospital-acquired infections.
    (1) Direct contact: person-to-person transmission. This frequently involves transmission that occurs during patient care.
    (2) Indirect contact: contact with a contaminated object such as gloves, dirty dressings, dirty linen, or instruments, or transmission by personnel from one patient to another because of failure to wash hands thoroughly between patients.
    (3) Preferred but not required: private room. Cohorting of infants with same infection is acceptable.
    (4) Not required: masks.
    (5) Required: gowns and gloves.
  d. Nursery infection control measures (AAP and American College of Obstetricians and Gynecologists [ACOG], 1997).
    (1) Routine, thorough hand washing: initially on entering the nursery, between patient contacts, and after touching contaminated objects.
    (2) Clothing worn by nursery personnel: short-sleeved hospital attire laundered in hospital. A long-sleeved gown should be worn over clothing when infant is held by nursing staff, other personnel, or parents.
    (3) Cover gowns: to be worn when caring for infants with known or suspected infection. Gowns should be discarded before another patient is handled.
    (4) Sterile, long-sleeved gowns, caps, bear masks, and masks for surgical procedures.
    (5) Hand jewelry should not be worn in nursery while caring for patients.
    (6) Disposable, nonsterile gloves: use, if desired, for care of patients in isolation or to protect caregiver from contamination during procedures.
    (7) Dirty diapers: handle with gloved hands.
  e. Screening of visitors for contagious infections before admission to the nursery.
3. Linen and trash disposal (AAP and ACOG, 1997).
  a. Linen provided does not need to be sterile but should be clean.
  b. Cloth or disposable diapers are acceptable.
  c. Soiled linen should be placed in plastic bags in hampers.
  d. Linen and all diapers should be removed from the nursery at least once every 8 hours.
  e. Nursery linens and cloth diapers should be laundered separately from other hospital linen.
4. Intravascular flush solutions (AAP and ACOG, 1997).
  a. Sterile, unpreserved flush solution should be provided by the pharmacy.
  b. Flush solution containers should be timed and dated and kept no longer than 8 hours at room temperature before being discarded.

REFERENCES

American Academy of Pediatrics: Herpes simplex. *In* Peter, G. (Ed.): 1997 Red Book: Report of the Committee on Infectious Diseases, 24th ed. Elk Grove Village, Ill., Author, 1997a, pp. 266–276.

American Academy of Pediatrics. HIV infection. *In* Peter, G. (Ed.): 1997 Redbook: Report of the Committee on Infectious Diseases, 24th ed. Elk Grove Village, Ill., Author, 1997b, pp. 279–304.

American Academy of Pediatrics: Infection control for hospitalized children. *In* Peter, G. (Ed.): 1997 Red Book: Report of the Committee on Infectious Diseases, 24th ed. Elk Grove Village, Ill., Author, 1997c, pp. 100–107.

American Academy of Pediatrics: Respiratory syncytial virus immune globulin intravenous: Indications for use. Pediatrics, 99:645–651, 1997d.

American Academy of Pediatrics Advisory Committee on Immunization Practices: Recommended Childhood Immunization Schedule—United States, January–December 1999. Elk Grove Village, Ill., Author, 1999.

American Academy of Pediatrics Committee on Pediatric AIDS: Human milk, breast feeding and transmission of human immunodeficiency virus in the United States. Pediatrics, 96:977–979, 1995.

American Academy of Pediatrics, American College of Obstetricians and Gynecologists: Infection control. In Hauth, J.C., and Merenstein, G.B. (Eds.): Guidelines for Perinatal Care, 4th ed. Elk Grove Village, Ill., Author, 1997, pp. 251–277.

American Academy of Pediatrics Committee on Infectious Diseases: Recommended Childhood Immunization Schedule—United States January–December 1999. Pediatrics, 103(1):182, 1999.

Bhatt, D.R., Reber, D.J., Wirtschafter, D.D., et al.: Neonatal Drug Formulary, 4th ed. Los Angeles, N.D.F. Los Angeles Publishers, 1997.

Blackburn, S.T., and Loper, D.L.: Maternal, Fetal, and Neonatal Physiology: A Clinical Perspective. Philadelphia, W.B. Saunders, 1992, pp. 470–490.

Centers for Disease Control: Rubella vaccination during pregnancy—United States, 1971–1986. MMWR Morb. Mortal. Wkly. Rep., 36:457–461, 1987.

Centers for Disease Control: Recommendations of the U.S. Public Health Service Task Force on the Use of Zidovudine to Reduce Perinatal Transmission of Human Immunodeficiency Virus. MMWR Morb. Mortal. Wkly Rep., 45(RR-11):1–20, 1994.

Centers for Disease Control and Prevention: Prevention of perinatal group B streptococcal disease: A public health perspective. MMWR Morb. Mortal. Wkly Rep., 45(R-7):1–24, 1996.

Christensen, R.D., Rothstein, G., Anstall, H.B., et al.: Granulocyte transfusions in neonates with bacterial infection, neutropenia and depletion of mature marrow neutrophils. Pediatrics, 70:1–6, 1982.

Conner, E.M., Sperling R.S., Gelber R., et al.: Reduction of maternal-infant transmission of human immunodeficiency virus type 1 with zidovudine treatment. N. Engl. J. Med., 331:1173–1180, 1994.

Cooper, L.Z., Preblud, S.R., and Alford, C.A., Jr.: Rubella. In Remington, J.S., and Klein, J.O. (Eds.): Infectious Diseases of the Fetus and Newborn Infant, 4th ed. Philadelphia, W.B. Saunders, 1995, pp. 268–311.

DeVita, V.T., et al.: AIDS: Etiology, Treatment and Prevention. Philadelphia, Lippincott-Raven, 1997.

Dunn, D.T., Newell, M.L., Ades, A.E., et al.: Risk of human immunodeficiency virus type 1 transmission through breastfeeding. Lancet, 340:585–588, 1992.

Evans, H.E., and Frenkel, L.D.: Congenital syphilis. In Evans, H.E. (Ed.): Perinatal AIDS. (Clinics in Perinatology.) Philadelphia, W.B. Saunders, 1994, pp. 149–162.

Garner, J.S.: Hospital Infection Control Practices Advisory Committee: Guidelines for isolation precautions in hospitals. Infect. Control Hosp. Epidemiol., 17:53–80, 1996.

Gerdes, J.S.: Clinicopathologic approach to the diagnosis of neonatal sepsis. Clin. Perinatol., 18:361–381, 1991.

Guerina, N.G.: Bacterial and fungal infections. In Cloherty, J.P., and Stark, A.R. (Eds.): Manual of Neonatal Care, 4th ed. Philadelphia, Lippincott-Raven, 1998, p. 271.

Hall, D.M., Thureen, P.J., and Abzug, M.J.: Infectious diseases. In Thureen, P.J., Deacon, J.M., O'Neill, P.A., and Hernandez, J. Assessment and Care of the Well Newborn. Philadelphia, W.B. Saunders, 1998, pp. 301–321.

Haque, K.N., Zaidi, M.H., and Bahakim, H.: IgM-enriched intravenous immunoglobulin therapy in neonatal sepsis. Am. J. Dis. Child., 142:1293–1296, 1988.

Harris, M.C., Deuber, C., Polin, R.A., et al.: Investigation of apparent false-positive urine latex particle agglutination tests for the detection of group B streptococcus antigen. J. Clin. Microbiol., 27:2214–2217, 1989.

Hutto, C., Parks, W.P., Laik, S., et al.: A hospital-based prospective study of perinatal infection with HI modifier virus type 1. J. Pediatr., 118:347–353, 1991.

Lott, J.W.: Neonatal Infection: Assessment, Diagnosis and Management. Petaluma, Calif., NICU Ink, 1994, p. 127.

Lott, J.W., and Kilb, J.R.: The selection of antibacterial agents for treatment of neonatal sepsis, or which drug kills which bug? Neonatal Pharmacology Quarterly. 1(1):19–29, 1992.

Manroe, B.L., Weinberg, A.G., Rosenfeld, C.R., et al.: The neonatal blood count in health and disease. Pediatrics, 95:89–98, 1979.

Mathers, N.J., and Polhandt, F.: Diagnostic audit of C-reactive protein in neonatal infection. Eur. J. Pediatr., 146:147–151, 1987.

Merenstein, G.B., Adams, K., and Weisman, L.E.: Infection in the neonate. In Merenstein, G.B., and Gardner, S.L. (Eds.): Handbook of Neonatal Intensive Care, 4th ed. St. Louis, Mosby–Year Book, 1998, pp. 413–436.

Oski, F., and Naiman, J.: Hematologic Problems in the Newborn. Philadelphia, W.B. Saunders, 1966.

Overall, J.C., Jr.: Viral infections of the fetus and neonate. In Feigin, R.D., and Cherry, J.E. (Eds.): Textbook of Pediatric Infectious Diseases, 3rd ed. Philadelphia, W.B. Saunders, 1992, pp. 924–959.

Palasanthiran, P., Ziegler, J.B.V., Stewart, G.J., et al.: Breastfeeding during primary maternal human immunodeficiency virus infection and risk of transmission from mother to infant. J. Infect. Dis., 167:441–444, 1993.

Philip, A.G.S., and Hweitt, J.R.: Early diagnosis of neonatal sepsis. Pediatrics, 65:1036–1041, 1980.

Polak, J.D., Lott, J.W., and Kenner, C.: Overview of the fetal/neonatal immune system. In Lott, J.W. (Ed.): Neonatal Infection: Assessment, Diagnosis, and Management. Petaluma, Calif., NICU Ink, 1994, pp. 11–20.

Rossi, P., et al.: Early diagnosis of HIV infection in infants: Report of a consensus workshop. J. Acquir. Immune Defic. Syndr., 5:1169–1178, 1992.

Schwersenski, S., McIntyre, L., and Bauer, C.R.: LP frequency and CSF fluid analysis in the neonate. Am. J. Dis. Child., 145:54–58, 1991.

Sever, J.L., Ellenberg, J.H., Ley A.C., et al.: Toxoplasmosis: Maternal and pediatric findings in 23,000 pregnancies. Pediatrics, 82:181–192, 1988.

Sever, J.L., South, M.A., and Shaver, K.A.: Delayed manifestations of congenital rubella. Rev. Infect. Dis. 7(suppl):5164–5169, 1985.

Stagno, S.: Cytomegalovirus. In Remington, J.S., and Klein, J.O. (Eds.): Infectious Diseases of the Fetus-Newborn Infant, 4th ed. Philadelphia, W.B. Saunders, 1995, pp. 312–353.

Stagno, S., Pass, R.F., Dworsky, M.E., et al.: Congenital and perinatal cytomegaloviral infections. Semin. Perinatol., 7:31–42, 1983.

Stagno, S., and Whitley, R.J.: Herpesvirus infections of pregnancy. I. Cytomegalovirus and Epstein-Barr virus infections. N. Engl. J. Med., *313*:1270–1274, 1985.

Stoll, B.J., Gordon, T., Korones, S.B., et al.: Early-onset sepsis in very low birth weight infants: A report from the National Institute of Child Health and Human Development Neonatal Research Network. J. Pediatr., *129*:72–80, 1996a.

Stoll, B.J., Gordon, T., Korones, S.B., et al.: Late-onset sepsis in very low birth weight neonates: A report from the National Institute of Child Health and Human Development Neonatal Research Network. J. Pediatr., *129*:63–71, 1996b.

Subramanian, K.N., Weisman, L.E., Rhodes, T., et al.: Safety, tolerance, and pharmacokinetics of a humanized monoclonal antibody to respiratory syncytial virus in premature infants and infants with bronchopulmonary dysplasia. Pediatr. Infect. Dis. J., *17*(2):110–115, 1998.

Thureen, P.J., Deacon, J.M., O'Neill, P.A., and Hernandez, J.: Assessment and Care of the Well Newborn. Philadelphia, W.B. Saunders, 1999.

Todd, J.K.: Tips on blood cultures. Contagious? Comments, *10*:1, 1991.

Vain, N.E., Naziumian, J.R., and Swarner, O.W.: Role of exchange transfusion in neonatal septicemia. Pediatrics, *66*:693–697, 1980.

Van de Perre, P., Simonon, A., Msellati, P., et al.: Postnatal transmission of human immunodeficiency virus type I from mother to infant. N. Engl. J. Med., *325*:593–598, 1991.

Vinal, D.F., and Huffman, S.G.: Perinatal infections. *In* Nichols, F.H., and Zwelling, E. (Eds.): Maternal-Newborn Nursing: Theory and Practice. Philadelphia, W.B. Saunders, 1997, pp. 1473–1519 (1478–1479 GBS).

Wald, E.R., Bergman, I., Taylor, H.G., et al.: Long-term outcome of group B streptococcal meningitis. Pediatrics, *94*:1, 1986.

Weiss, M.G., Ionides, S.P., and Anderson, C.L.: Meningitis in premature infants with respiratory distress: Role of admission lumbar puncture. J. Pediatr., *119*:973–975, 1991.

Welsh, J.K., and May, J.T.: Anti-infective properties of breast milk. J. Pediatr., *94*:1, 1979.

Whitley, R.J., and Arvin, A.M.: Herpes simplex virus infections. *In* Remington, J.S., and Klein, J.O. (Eds.): Infectious Diseases of the Fetus and Newborn Infant, 4th ed. Philadelphia, W.B. Saunders, 1995, pp. 354–376.

Young, T.E., and Mangum, O.B.: Neofax, 11th ed. Raleigh, N.C., Acorn Publishing, 1998.

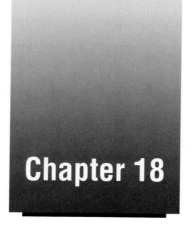

Chapter 18

Renal and Genitourinary Disorders

Janice Bernhardt

Objectives

1. Relate congenital renal/genitourinary disorders to embryologic development.

2. Apply knowledge of normal renal anatomy and physiology to renal pathophysiology that presents in the neonatal period.

3. Explain the etiology of selected neonatal renal/genitourinary disorders.

4. Describe clinical manifestations and complications that may be associated with selected neonatal renal/genitourinary disorders.

5. Determine the appropriate management of each disorder discussed.

6. Formulate an appropriate plan of care for each disorder discussed.

The genitourinary system has the highest percentage of anomalies, congenital or genetic, of all the organ systems (Bonilla-Felix, Brannon, and Portman, 1998). Prenatal diagnosis of some renal/genitourinary disorders is possible with the use of ultrasonography. Amniotic fluid volume, which may be an indication of renal function, can also be assessed by ultrasonography. The primary benefits of prenatal detection are the timely evaluation and treatment of the neonate, although in utero treatment may be an option in selected cases (Elder, 1997; Harrison, 1996; Housely and Harrison, 1998; Jona, 1998; Sullivan and Adzick, 1994). The most common urinary tract anomalies identified by prenatal ultrasonography are hydronephrosis, multicystic renal dysplasia, bladder outlet obstruction, and duplications of the collecting system (Gloor et al., 1995).

Knowledge of embryologic development and of anatomy and physiology is helpful in understanding and managing renal/genitourinary disorders. This chapter presents information on embryology and on anatomy and physiology of the kidney as a base from which to discuss selected neonatal renal/genitourinary disorders.

Embryology

A. Introduction.

1. Embryologic development of the urinary system begins within the first weeks after conception and progresses through three stages.
2. Both the urinary and the genital systems develop from the same germ layer of the embryo.

B. Kidney.

1. The kidneys develop in three sequential stages.
   a. Pronephros.
      (1) Plays a primary role in normal organogenesis.
      (2) Appears during 3–4 weeks' gestation.
      (3) Degenerates by the fifth week.
   b. Mesonephros.
      (1) Originates during 4–5 weeks' gestation, just before degeneration of the pronephros, and is fully developed by 37 days.
      (2) Consists of 30–40 glomerulotubular units.
      (3) Capsule and glomerulus form the mesonephros (renal) corpuscle.
      (4) Develops into genital glands.
      (5) Regresses at the end of the second month.
   c. Metanephros.
      (1) Develops early in the fifth week and functions within a few weeks.
      (2) Permanent kidney develops from the metanephric diverticulum (ureteric bud) and the metanephric mesoderm (metanephrogenic blastema).
      (3) Normal differentiation of the ureteric bud is essential for initiation of branching, which leads to formation of the urinary collecting system (ureter, pelvis, calyces, and collecting ducts) and to the start of nephron formation within the metanephric blastema.
      (4) Nephroblastic cells of the blastema differentiate into the glomerulus, proximal convoluted tubule, loop of Henle, and distal convoluted tubule.
      (5) Nephrons form from the proximal end of the renal/metanephric tubules, beginning at about 8 weeks and continuing until approximately 34–36 weeks. Approximately 800,000 nephrons result.
      (6) Minor calyces and their communicating papillary ducts are well delineated and resemble those of a mature kidney by 13–14 weeks' gestation.
      (7) By 4 months the kidney contains 14–16 lobes, equivalent to the mature kidney.
      (8) The kidney begins urine production and glomerular filtration at 9–10 weeks' gestation.

C. Urinary tract.

1. Differentiation of the urinary tract occurs synchronously with the early stages of metanephric development.
2. Urinary bladder develops at approximately 6 weeks' gestation.
3. Formation of the urethra is completed by the end of the first trimester.
4. Fetal ureter does not open functionally into the bladder until the ninth week.

D. Development of vascular supply.

1. The vascular pattern of the fetal kidney resembles that of the mature kidney by 14–15 weeks' gestation.

2. Renal blood flow in the fetus is low due to high renal vascular resistance and low systemic blood pressure.

Renal Anatomy

A. Gross anatomy.

1. **Cortex:** outermost portion of the kidney, which contains the glomeruli, proximal and distal convoluted tubules, and collecting ducts of the nephron.
2. **Medulla:** middle section of the kidney, which contains renal pyramids, straight portions of tubules, loops of Henle, vasa recta, and terminal collecting ducts.
3. **Renal sinus and pelvis:** innermost portion of the kidney. The renal sinus contains the uppermost part of the renal pelvis and calyces, surrounded by some fat in which branches of the renal vessels and nerves are embedded.
4. **Ureter:** excretory duct of the kidney, which transports urine from kidney to bladder.

B. Microscopic renal anatomy: the nephron.

1. Structural and functional unit of the kidney.
2. Composed of glomerulus, Bowman's capsule, and the tubules.
3. All nephrons are present by 32–34 weeks' gestation; functional maturation and hypertrophy continue into infancy (Bissinger, 1995; Blackburn, 1994; Bonilla-Felix et al., 1998).
4. Functional component of the nephron is the renal corpuscle/malpighian body, which consists of the glomerulus and the glomerular (Bowman's) capsule.
   a. Glomerulus is formed by a capillary network.
   b. Glomerular/Bowman's capsule is a membrane surrounding the glomerulus, which serves as a filter mechanism through which nonprotein components of blood plasma can enter the renal tubules.
5. Tubular system consists of proximal convoluted tubule, loop of Henle, distal convoluted tubule, and collecting duct.

Renal Hemodynamics

A. Renal blood flow.

1. Renal blood flow comprises 4–6% of the cardiac output during the first 12 hours of life and 8–10% of the cardiac output during the first week of life.
2. The rate of renal blood flow is determined by the cardiac output and the ratio of renal to systemic vascular resistance. Developmental changes in these parameters contribute to the postnatal increase in renal blood flow.
3. The primary factor responsible for maturational increase in renal blood flow and redistribution of intrarenal blood flow from the inner cortex to the outer cortex is decreased renal vascular resistance (Brion, Satlin, and Edelmann, 1994).
4. Renal plasma flow.
   a. Flow is 150 mL/min per 1.73 m^2 at term and increases to 200 mL/min per 1.73 m^2 in the first weeks of life.
   b. The low renal plasma flow in the neonate is due mainly to high renal vascular resistance but also to low perfusion pressure.

B. Regulation of renal blood flow.

1. Autoregulation of renal blood flow.
   a. Autoregulation refers to the ability of the kidney to maintain a relatively

constant glomerular filtration rate (GFR) over a range of systemic blood pressures (Seeley, Stephens, and Tate, 1995).
   b. Mechanisms (Bissinger, 1995).
      (1) Myogenic mechanism is the dilation or constriction of the afferent arteriole in response to changes in vascular wall tension for the purpose of maintaining normal blood flow.
      (2) Tubuloglomerular feedback mechanism consists of afferent and efferent feedback mechanisms.
         (a) Afferent arteriolar vasodilator feedback mechanism is activated by decreased glomerular filtrate in the tubules, which results in dilation of the afferent arteriole and increased GFR. When renal blood flow increases, the afferent arterioles constrict and return GFR to normal.
         (b) Efferent arteriolar vasodilator feedback mechanism is activated by decreased volume. This stimulates renin release and causes constriction of the efferent arteriole to a greater degree than constriction of the afferent arteriole and thus maintains the GFR.
2. Hormonal regulation of renal blood flow.
   a. Renin-angiotensin-aldosterone system (Bissinger, 1995).
      (1) Major renal hormonal system.
      (2) Well developed in the newborn infant; renin is present from 3 months' gestation onward.
      (3) Responsible for regulation of systemic blood pressure, sodium, potassium, and regional blood flow.
   b. Prostaglandins.
      (1) Synthesized in both cortex and medulla, and by glomerulus and tubules (Bailie, 1992).
      (2) Renal medulla seems to be the major site of prostaglandin synthesis in the kidney.
      (3) Most important prostaglandins in the kidney are prostaglandins E_2 and $F_{2\text{-alpha}}$, prostacyclin (prostaglandin I_2), and thromboxane A_2 (Bailie, 1992).
      (4) Role in regulation of renal function and control of systemic blood pressure.
         (a) Vasodilation.
         (b) Natriuresis.
         (c) Inhibition of the distal tubule's response to antidiuretic hormone.

Renal Physiology

A. **Postnatal changes.**

1. GFR doubles in the first 2 weeks of life in term and preterm neonates to 30–40 mL/min per 1.73 m^2 and increases to adult values of 100–120 mL/min per 1.73 m^2 between 1–2 years of life (Bissinger, 1995; Bonilla-Felix et al., 1998; Chevalier, 1996). Factors responsible for this increase (Chevalier, 1996) are:
   a. Increasing mean arterial blood pressure.
   b. Increasing renal blood flow.
   c. Increasing glomerular permeability and filtration surface area.
2. Fractional excretion of sodium decreases due to increasing tubular reabsorption.
3. Infant has an increasing ability to concentrate urine.
4. Renal vasoactive hormones are initially increased.
5. Renal vascular resistance decreases.
6. Renal blood flow increases.

B. Glomerular filtration.

1. As blood passes through the capillaries, plasma is filtered through the glomerular capillary walls. Filtrate is collected in Bowman's space and enters the tubules, where composition is modified until it is excreted as urine.
2. Glomerular filtration rate.
    a. Factors that may contribute to decreased GFR at birth are:
        (1) Small glomerular capillary area available for filtration.
        (2) Structural immaturity of glomerular capillary, which is associated with decreased water permeability.
        (3) Decreased blood pressure.
        (4) Increased hematocrit.
        (5) Renal vasoconstriction, which results in decreased glomerular plasma flow.
    b. Neonates born at less than 34 weeks' gestation have low GFR (0.5 mL/min) until nephrogenesis is completed (Blackburn, 1994).
3. Three primary factors determine GFR.
    a. Glomerular capillary hydrostatic pressure.
    b. Hydrostatic pressure in Bowman's capsule.
    c. Capillary colloid osmotic pressure.
4. Glomerular capillary hydrostatic pressure is the major controller of GFR (Blackburn, 1994).
5. Additional factors that affect GFR are:
    a. Capillary surface area.
    b. Permeability of capillary basement membrane.
    c. Rate of renal plasma flow.
    d. Changes in renal blood flow.
    e. Changes in blood pressure.
    f. Vasoactive changes in afferent or efferent arterioles.
    g. Ureteral obstruction.
    h. Edema of kidney.
    i. Changes in the concentration of plasma proteins.
        (1) Dehydration.
        (2) Hypoproteinemia.
    j. Increased permeability of the glomerular filter.
    k. Decrease in total area of glomerular capillary bed.

C. Tubular function.

1. Components of tubular system include proximal tubule, loop of Henle, distal tubule, and collecting ducts.
2. Tubules modify glomerular ultrafiltrate, leading to production of urine, which is accomplished by the process of tubular reabsorption and secretion.
    a. Tubular reabsorption is the movement of substances into the peritubular capillary plasma from the tubular epithelium, which occurs by diffusion and active transport. The proximal tubule is the major site of reabsorption (Bissinger, 1995).
    b. Tubular secretion is the movement of substances into the tubular epithelium from the peritubular capillary plasma. Tubular secretion is necessary for regulation of fluid and electrolyte balance, along with other renal processes (Blackburn, 1994).
3. Regulation of fluids and electrolytes is an important tubular function.
4. Tubular function is altered in the neonate due to decreased renal blood flow and GFR (Bissinger, 1995).
5. Tubular portions of the neonatal nephron are smaller and less functionally mature, resulting in an altered ability to transport sodium, urea, chloride, and glucose, with decreased renal thresholds for many substances (Blackburn, 1994).

6. Rapid maturation of proximal tubular cells occurs between 32 and 35 weeks' gestation (Jones and Chesney, 1992).
7. Significant maturation of tubular function occurs postnatally, especially in preterm infants born at less than 34 weeks' gestation (Jones and Chesney, 1992).
8. The tubular handling of various substances may reach adult levels at various postnatal ages (Jones and Chesney, 1992).

D. Concentration and dilution mechanism.

1. Maintenance of osmolality. The term and preterm infant's ability to dilute urine is fully developed, but concentrating ability is limited (Bissinger, 1995). A major function of the kidney is to maintain osmolality of extracellular fluid within the narrow range compatible with optimal cellular function.
2. Sites of urinary concentration and dilution.
    a. Loop of Henle.
    b. Collecting duct.
3. Factors responsible for the limited ability of the neonatal kidney to concentrate urine (Chevalier, 1996).
    a. Anatomic immaturity of the renal medulla.
    b. Decreased medullary concentration of sodium chloride and urea.
    c. Diminished responsiveness of the collecting ducts to arginine vasopressin.
4. Normal range of neonatal specific gravity: 1.002–1.010.
5. Maximum concentrating ability.
    a. Term infants: 700 mOsm of water per kilogram of body weight.
    b. Preterm infants: 600–700 mOsm of water per kilogram of body weight.
6. Capacity for urine dilution.
    a. 30–50 mOsm/kg of water.
    b. Ability of neonate to excrete a hypotonic load is limited, presumably due to the low GFR (Brion et al., 1994).

E. Acid-base balance.

1. Regulation of acid-base balance by the kidneys occurs in conjunction with the lungs and blood buffers. The role of the kidneys in regulating acid-base balance involves regulating the plasma bicarbonate by reabsorbing filtered bicarbonate and affecting hydrogen ion secretion through the formation of titratable acids and ammonium (Askin, 1997; Hanna, Scheinman, and Chan, 1995).
2. Renal response to acidosis.
    a. Reabsorption of bicarbonate in the proximal tubule.
    b. Increased secretion of hydrogen ions in the distal convoluted tubule.
    c. Production of ammonia.
3. Renal response to alkalosis.
    a. Excretion of bicarbonate.
    b. Decreased production of ammonia.
    c. Decreased hydrogen ion secretion in the distal tubule.
4. Neonatal limitations in maintaining acid-base homeostasis.
    a. Decreased ability to handle an acid load and compensate for acid-base abnormalities.
    b. Decreased renal threshold for bicarbonate, and decreased capacity to reabsorb bicarbonate results in slightly lower serum bicarbonate and pH.
    c. Decreased GFR.
    d. Decreased production of ammonia.
    e. Decreased ability to secrete organic acids.

Acute Renal Failure

A. **Definition:** acute deterioration in the ability of the kidneys to maintain homeostasis of the body fluids (Brion, Bernstein, and Spitzer, 1997.)

B. Etiology.

1. Prerenal: results from renal hypoperfusion and is the most common cause of acute renal failure in the neonate (Stewart and Barnett, 1997).
    a. Hypotension.
    b. Hypoperfusion caused by hemorrhage.
    c. Sepsis.
    d. Dehydration.
    e. Hypoxia.
    f. Respiratory distress syndrome.
    g. Congestive heart failure.
    h. Renal artery thrombosis.
2. Intrinsic: renal cellular damage involving functional compromise to the glomerular, tubular, and collecting system due to prolonged prerenal insult or use of nephrotoxic agents.
    a. Perinatal asphyxia: most common cause of intrinsic acute renal failure in newborn infants (Stewart and Barnett, 1997).
    b. Classification (McCourt, 1996).
        (1) Congenital.
            (a) Hypoplasia.
            (b) Dysplasia.
            (c) Polycystic kidney disease.
            (d) Nephrotic syndrome.
        (2) Inflammatory.
            (a) Congenital infection.
            (b) Pyelonephritis.
        (3) Vascular.
            (a) Cortical-medullary necrosis.
            (b) Arterial or venous thrombosis.
            (c) Intravascular coagulation.
        (4) Ischemic necrosis.
            (a) Asphyxia/hypoxia.
            (b) Dehydration.
            (c) Hemorrhage.
            (d) Sepsis.
            (e) Respiratory distress syndrome.
        (5) Nephrotoxic drugs (McCourt, 1996; Stewart and Barnett, 1997).
            (a) Aminoglycoside antibiotics.
            (b) Indomethacin.
            (c) Amphotericin B.
            (d) Radiologic contrast media.
3. Postrenal: obstruction to urinary flow distal to the kidney.
    a. Posterior urethral valves.
    b. Bilateral ureteropelvic junction obstruction.
    c. Imperforate prepuce.
    d. Urethral stricture.
    e. Urethral diverticulum.
    f. Megaureter.
    g. Ureterocele.
    h. Ureteropelvic/ureterovesical obstruction.
    i. Neurogenic bladder.

C. Incidence. The incidence of acute renal failure in the NICU has been reported to range from 1.5% to 23% (Brion et al., 1997).

D. Clinical presentation.

1. Oliguria/anuria: urinary excretion less than 0.5–1.0 mL/kg per hour after the first 24–48 hours of life (Bonilla-Felix et al., 1998; Brion et al., 1997).

2. Azotemia: blood urea nitrogen (BUN) greater than 20 mg/dL or rising more than 10 mg/dL per day.
3. Elevated serum creatinine: greater than 1 mg/dL or rising more than 0.2 mg/dL per day.

E. Clinical assessment.

1. Perinatal history.
   a. Low Apgar score.
   b. Perinatal asphyxia.
   c. Renal abnormalities on antenatal sonogram.
   d. History of oligohydramnios.
2. Urine output: less than 0.5–1.0 mL/kg per hour after the first 24–48 hours of life (Bonilla-Felix et al., 1998; Brion et al., 1997).
3. Daily weight: increase in daily weight greater than that predicted on basis of infant's condition and caloric intake.
4. Edema.
5. Blood pressure.
   a. Hypotension may be a factor in the development of acute renal failure.
   b. Hypertension may be observed in established cases of acute renal failure.

F. Diagnostic studies.

1. Urine.
   a. Urinalysis.
      (1) pH often greater than 6.
      (2) Specific gravity usually decreased.
      (3) Hematuria.
      (4) Casts.
      (5) Tubular cells.
      (6) Proteinuria.
   b. Sodium: increased with intrinsic renal failure.
   c. Osmolality: decreased.
   d. Creatinine: decreased.
   e. Culture: to rule out urinary tract infection/sepsis.
2. Blood.
   a. BUN: greater than 20 mg/dL or rise greater than 1.0 mg/dL per day.
   b. Creatinine concentration: greater than 1 mg/dL or rise greater than 0.2 mg/dL per day.
   c. Osmolality: increased.
   d. Electrolytes.
      (1) Hyperkalemia.
      (2) Hyponatremia.
      (3) Hypocalcemia.
      (4) Hyperphosphatemia.
   e. Glucose: increased.
   f. Total protein: decreased.
   g. Albumin: decreased.
3. Ultrasonography: to determine intrinsic or postrenal cause and to rule out urinary tract obstruction, renal vein thrombosis, congenital renal abnormality, and cystic disease.
4. Voiding cystourethrography: to rule out obstructive disease and reflux.
5. Radionuclide renal scans: to evaluate renal perfusion and function.

G. Differential diagnosis.

1. Prerenal acute renal failure.
2. Intrinsic acute renal failure.
3. Postrenal acute renal failure.

4. Differentiation between types.
  a. Assessment for specific etiologic factors.
  b. Prerenal versus renal parenchymal type.
    (1) Renal failure index

$$\frac{\text{Urine Na} \times \text{Plasma creatinine}}{\text{Urine creatinine}}$$

or fractional excretion of Na (Urine Na/Plasma Na × Plasma creatinine/Urine creatinine × 100). Value greater than 3 suggests intrinsic failure.
      (a) These values will have limited significance in neonates born at less than 32 weeks' gestation because of these infants' limited ability to conserve sodium.
      (b) Urinary indices lose their diagnostic usefulness after therapy for oliguria has begun, particularly with diuretics.
    (2) BUN/creatinine ratio. A disproportionate rise in the BUN/creatinine ratio suggests a prerenal etiology, whereas a proportionate rise indicates a renal parenchymal etiology.
    (3) Fluid challenge: crystalloid or colloid (5–20 mL/kg IV) over 1 hour. If oliguria persists, follow with furosemide (1–2 mg/kg IV) (Bonilla-Felix et al., 1998; Kenner, 1998; McCourt, 1996).
      (a) Rapid and sustained diuresis within 1–2 hours indicates a prerenal cause.
      (b) Urine output of less than 2 mL/kg per hour after furosemide administration suggests a parenchymal or postrenal cause.
    (4) Presence of casts, tubular cells, and proteinuria suggests parenchymal renal failure.
  c. Renal parenchymal versus postrenal.
    (1) Ultrasonography.
    (2) Voiding cystourethrography.

H. Complications.
1. Electrolyte imbalance.
2. Hyperproteinemia.
3. Anemia.
4. Thrombocytopenia.
5. Hemorrhagic diathesis.
6. Metabolic acidosis.
7. Edema.
8. Hypertension.
9. Congestive heart failure.

I. Patient care management.
1. Treat primary cause.
2. Strict management of intake and output. Restrict fluids to insensible water loss, urine output, and other losses with failure to respond to a fluid-diuretic challenge test (Brion et al., 1997).
3. Monitor specific gravity.
4. Monitor urine pH.
5. Monitor urine for hematuria, proteinuria, and glucosuria.
6. Monitor urine osmolality and sodium.
7. Monitor body weight once or twice daily.
8. Monitor serum glucose and electrolytes; treat imbalances. Sodium and potassium intake may need to be restricted.
9. Treat acidosis.

10. Restrict protein to 1–2 g/kg per day (McCourt, 1996).
11. Provide adequate nutrition.
12. Monitor blood pressure and treat hypertension. Hypertension secondary to fluid overload may be treated with restriction of sodium and fluid or with antihypertensive agents (Kenner, Amlung, and Flandermeyer, 1998).
13. Observe for signs and symptoms of congestive heart failure.
14. Assess for bleeding diathesis.
15. Avoid nephrotoxic medications and those with a high sodium content (e.g., carbenicillin, penicillin G, ampicillin, and cephalothin) (Kenner, 1998).
16. Peritoneal dialysis or continuous arteriovenous hemofiltration/continuous venovenous hemodialysis. The latter is a slow, continuous process of extracorporeal filtration that maintains hemodynamic status and electrolyte balance, making it suitable for hemodynamically unstable, critically ill newborn infants (Bonilla-Felix et al., 1998; McCourt, 1996).

J. Outcome.

1. Factors affecting outcome include etiology, extent of other organ damage, and whether anuria or oliguria is associated with the renal failure (McCourt, 1996).
2. Reversal of underlying condition is the most important factor in determining prognosis (Bonilla-Felix et al., 1998; Kenner et al., 1998).
3. Best prognosis is for patients with nonoliguric acute renal failure (Bonilla-Felix et al., 1998).
4. Long-term sequelae include chronic renal failure, decreased GFR, impaired tubular function, chronic hypertension, renal tubular acidosis, impaired ability to concentrate urine, nephrocalcinosis, and impaired renal growth (McCourt, 1996).

Hypertension

Hypertension is considered to be blood pressure at greater than the 95th percentile. (Bonilla-Felix et al., 1998).

A. Etiology.

1. The most common causes of neonatal hypertension include renovascular anomalies and intrinsic renal disease (Brion et al., 1997).
2. Additional causes include endocrine disorders, medications, and various other disease states.

B. Incidence.

1. Incidence of neonatal hypertension is approximately 0.2% (Brion et al., 1997).
2. Incidence of neonatal hypertension has been reported to be 1.2–5% of NICU admissions (Bonilla-Felix et al., 1998).

C. Disease states (Bonilla-Felix et al., 1998; Goble, 1993).

1. Renal.
   a. Renal dysplasia/hypoplasia.
   b. Polycystic kidney disease.
   c. Renal failure.
   d. Obstructive uropathy.
   e. Reflux nephropathy.
   f. Pyelonephritis.
   g. Glomerulonephritis.
   h. Tumors.
2. Vascular.
   a. Renal artery stenosis.

    b. Renal artery thrombosis.

    c. Coarctation of the aorta.

    d. Hypoplastic abdominal aorta.

    e. Arterial calcification

3. Endocrine.

    a. Adrenogenital syndrome.

    b. Cushing's disease.

    c. Hypoaldosteronism.

    d. Thyrotoxicosis.

4. Medications.

    a. Corticosteroids.

    b. Ocular phenylephrine.

    c. Theophylline.

    d. Deoxycorticosterone.

    e. Vitamin D.

    f. Pancuronium.

5. Other.

    a. Closure of abdominal wall defect.

    b. Fluid overload.

    c. Genitourinary surgery.

    d. Hypercalcemia.

    e. Increased intracranial pressure.

    f. Renal infection.

    g. CNS disorders.

    h. Seizures in preterm infants.

    i. Bronchopulmonary dysplasia.

    j. Pneumothorax.

    k. Drug-dependent mother.

D. Clinical presentation.

1. Presenting symptoms: may be nonspecific; mild to moderate hypertension may be asymptomatic (Brion et al., 1997).
2. Term infants.

    a. At birth: blood pressure (BP) greater than 90/60 mm Hg (mean BP >70 mm Hg).

    b. At 7 days: BP greater than 92/60 mm Hg (mean BP >70 mm Hg).

    c. At 8 days to 1 month: BP greater than 106/40 mm Hg (mean BP >85 mm Hg).

3. Premature infants weighing less than 1 kg.

    a. At birth: BP greater than 60/40 mm Hg.

    b. At 7 days: mean BP greater than 57 mm Hg.

    c. At 1 month: mean BP greater than 63 mm Hg.

4. Premature infants weighing greater than 1 kg.

    a. At birth: BP greater than 80/50 mm Hg (mean BP >60 mm Hg).

    b. At 7 days: mean BP greater than 65–70 mm Hg.

    c. At 1 month: mean BP greater than 71–76 mm Hg.

E. Clinical assessment.

1. Arterial blood pressure: persistent elevation of BP to greater than 90/60 mm Hg in term infant and 80/50 mm Hg in preterm infant (Rasoulpour and Marinelli, 1992).
2. Serum creatinine: may be within normal limits or elevated.
3. BUN: elevated with renal involvement.
4. Serum electrolytes: to determine whether values indicate renal involvement.
5. Urine output: may be decreased.
6. Urinalysis: may show normal results or hematuria or proteinuria.

7. Urine culture: to rule out renal infection.
8. Presence of unilateral/bilateral abdominal mass: rule out tumor or polycystic kidneys.
9. Cardiac status: size, rate, rhythm, murmur, signs and symptoms of congestive heart failure.
10. Assess femoral pulses: to rule out coarctation of the aorta.
11. Perinatal history: to identify history of umbilical artery catheter, renal disease, or congenital heart disease; maternal history of medications or illicit drug use during pregnancy; family history of renal or endocrine disease.
12. Failure to thrive.
13. Special endocrinologic studies: possibly necessary to establish definitive diagnosis (e.g., plasma renin activity, serum aldosterone, serum cortisol, urinary metanephrines, cathecholamines, and vanillylmandelic acid) (Goble, 1993).
14. Effects of hypertension, including fundoscopic examination and cardiac evaluation (Bonilla-Felix et al., 1998).

F. Diagnostic studies.

1. Renal ultrasonography with Doppler flow study: to rule out renovascular hypertension.
2. Echocardiography: to assess cardiac sequelae.
3. Renal scan: to detect renal thrombosis and surgically amenable lesions (e.g., ureteropelvic junction obstruction).
4. Magnetic resonance imaging or CT scan: to detect tumors or masses.

G. Complications.

1. Congestive heart failure.
2. Left ventricular hypertrophy.
3. Hypertensive retinopathy.
4. Intracranial hemorrhage.
5. Cerebrovascular accident.
6. Encephalopathy.

H. Patient care management.

1. Treat primary cause.
2. Measure resting blood pressure, using a cuff of the appropriate size.
3. Measure blood pressure in all four extremities.
4. Restrict sodium alone or in combination with diuretic therapy, to attempt to control hypertension in patients with sodium or volume overload (Brion et al., 1997).
5. Administer medications. Pharmacologic management should be considered for a sustained systolic pressure of greater than 90 mm Hg and diastolic pressure of 60 mm Hg in term infants, and 80 mm Hg systolic and 45 mm Hg diastolic in preterm infants (Goble, 1993).
   a. Diuretics (Goble, 1993).
      (1) Chlorothiazide: 20 mg/kg per day by mouth, divided into two doses.
      (2) Hydrochlorothiazide: 2 mg/kg per day by mouth, divided into two doses.
      (3) Furosemide: 1–2 mg/kg per dose IV; 2–3 mg/kg per day by mouth, divided into two doses.
      (4) Spironolactone: 1–3 mg/kg per day by mouth, divided into two doses.
   b. Antihypertensive agents (Bonilla-Felix et al., 1998).
      (1) Hydralazine: 0.4–0.8 mg/kg per dose every 6 hours, IV; or 0.25–1.5 mg/kg per dose twice to four times a day, by mouth (maximum dose, 4.5 mg/kg per day).

    (2) Propranolol: 0.025–1 mg/kg per dose twice a day, IV; or 1–4 mg/kg per dose twice to four times a day, by month.

    (3) Captopril: 0.1–2.0 mg/kg per dose three times a day, by mouth.

    (4) Sodium nitroprusside: 0.5–10 µg/kg per minute by continuous infusion.

I. Outcome.

1. Prognosis depends primarily on the etiology; however, time of diagnosis, presence of neurologic complications, and response to therapy are also factors (Brion et al., 1997).

2. Poor renal growth may ensue on the side with renal artery pathologic changes, and renal scans may show abnormalities (Bonilla-Felix et al., 1998).

Potter's Syndrome

A. **Bilateral renal agenesis with Potter's facies (Fig. 18–1).**

B. **Etiology:** Failure of ureteric bud to divide and develop (Kenner, 1998).

C. **Incidence.**

1. Approximately 1:4800 to 1:10,000 births (Brion et al., 1997; Housley and Harrison, 1998).

2. Male predominance.

D. **Clinical presentation.**

1. Anuria.
2. Potter's facies.
    a. Blunted nose.
    b. Receded chin.
    c. Prominent depression between lower lip and chin.
    d. Low-set ears.

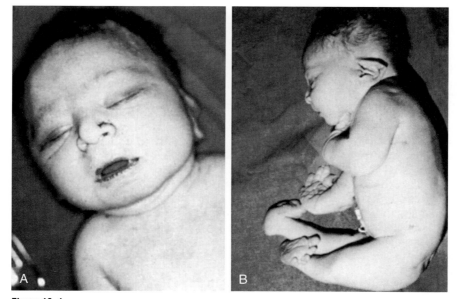

Figure 18–1
A and *B*, Potter's syndrome. (From Avery, G.B. [Ed.]: Neonatology: Pathophysiology and Management of the Newborn, 3rd ed. Philadelphia, J.B. Lippincott, 1987, p. 1045.)

　　e. Widely spaced eyes.
　　f. Depressed nasal bridge.
　　g. Prominent skinfold arising from epicanthus, progressing interiorly, and
　　　 extending laterally beneath the eyes.
3. Small for gestational age.
4. Pulmonary hypoplasia.
5. Excessively dry skin.
6. Relatively large and clawlike hands.
7. Bell-shaped chest.
8. History of oligohydramnios.
9. Bowed legs and clubbed feet possible.

E. **Clinical assessment.**

1. Urinary output: anuria after the first 24 hours without bladder distention.
2. Potter's facies.
3. Signs and symptoms of respiratory distress.
4. Perinatal history of oligohydramnios.
5. Presence of other associated anomalies.
　　a. Abnormal genitalia.
　　b. Gastrointestinal malformations.

F. **Physical examination:** palpation of abdomen for presence of kidneys.

G. **Diagnostic studies.**

1. Renal ultrasonography: to rule out renal agenesis.
2. Renal scan: if ultrasonography is inconclusive.
3. Umbilical artery angiography: to rule out presence of renal arteries.

H. **Differential diagnosis.**

1. Bilateral polycystic kidney disease.
2. Bilateral multicystic dysplastic kidney disease.

I. **Complications.**

1. Respiratory distress.
2. Pneumothorax.
3. Complications associated with acute renal failure.

J. **Patient care management.**

1. Comfort measures for neonate.
2. Support for the grieving family.

K. **Outcome.** Death usually occurs within hours to several days (Bonilla-Felix
et al., 1998; Kenner et al., 1998).

Autosomal Recessive Polycystic Kidney Disease

A. **Etiology:** Autosomal recessive.

B. **Incidence:** 1:6000 to 1:55,000 (Becker and Avner, 1995; Levine et al., 1997;
Martinez, 1995).

C. **Clinical presentation.**

1. History of oligohydramnios.
2. Bilateral flank masses.
3. Oliguria.
4. Abdominal distention.
5. Respiratory distress.

6. Increased serum creatinine after a few days.
7. Hypertension.
8. Hematuria.
9. Renal insufficiency.
10. Decreased glomerular filtration rate.
11. Potter's facies

D. **Clinical assessment.**

1. Urine output: decreased.
2. Urinalysis.
   a. Proteinuria.
   b. Hematuria.
   c. Decreased specific gravity.
3. Serum creatinine: elevated.
4. BUN: elevated.
5. Serum electrolytes.
   a. Hyperkalemia.
   b. Hyperphosphatemia.
   c. Hypocalcemia.
6. Serum pH: decreased.
7. Serum urea: elevated.
8. Blood pressure: elevated.
9. Respiratory distress.
10. Congestive heart failure.

E. **Physical examination:** bilateral flank masses.

F. **Diagnostic studies.** Renal ultrasonography shows symmetrically enlarged hyperechoic kidneys with loss of corticomedullary junction (Levine et al., 1997).

G. **Differential diagnosis.**

1. Multicystic dysplasia.
2. Hydronephrosis.
3. Renal vein thrombosis.
4. Renal tumor.
5. Autosomal dominant polycystic kidney disease.
6. Tuberous sclerosis.

H. **Complications.**

1. Renal failure.
2. Hepatic failure.
3. Hypertension.
4. Portal hypertension with palpable liver and esophageal varices.
5. Congestive heart failure.

I. **Patient care management.**

1. Genetic counseling for parents.
2. Supportive care.
   a. Treat hypertension.
   b. Treat congestive heart failure.
   c. Give adequate nutrition to support normal growth and development.
3. Infants surviving neonatal period: close monitoring for inevitable decrease in renal function (Becker and Avner, 1995).
4. Consideration of renal transplant once renal failure develops (Martinez, 1995).

J. Outcome.

1. Those who survive the perinatal period have varying degrees of renal insufficiency, and some develop hypertension (Levine et al., 1997).
2. Death usually results from a combination of renal and respiratory failure (Levine et al., 1997).
3. Survival time varies: 86% of affected children survive to 3 months; 79% to 1 year; 51% to 10 years; and 46% to 15 years (Martinez, 1995).

Multicystic Dysplastic Kidney Disease

A. Definition: renal dysplasia appearing as grapelike clusters. The abnormal parenchyma contains multiple cysts and a decreased number of nephrons. The proximal ureter is stenotic or nonpatent.

B. Etiology.

1. Developmental anomaly.
2. Nongenetic.

C. Incidence.

1. Reported as 1:4300 (Brion et al., 1997).
2. Males and females equally affected (Levine et al., 1997).
3. Most common form of renal cystic disease in neonates: unilateral multicystic dysplasia (Brion et al., 1997).

D. Clinical presentation.

1. Abdominal mass.
2. History of oligohydramnios.
3. Frequently associated with contralateral renal and extrarenal abnormalities, including cardiac, gastrointestinal, and CNS abnormalities, and several malformation syndromes (Becker and Avner, 1995; Brion et al., 1997; Levine et al., 1997).

E. Clinical assessment: signs and symptoms of renal failure.

F. Physical examination: abdominal palpation.
1. Irregular mass.
2. Usually unilateral.
   a. More often on left side.
   b. Possible hypertrophy of contralateral kidney; also risk of other abnormality, most commonly vesicoureteral reflex or ureteropelvic junction obstruction (Brion et al., 1997).

G. Diagnostic studies (Becker and Avner, 1995; Brion et al., 1997; Kenner, 1998).

1. Renal ultrasonography: noncommunicating cysts of varying size; lack of normal renal parenchyma.
2. Renal scan: absence of renal function.
3. Voiding cystourethrogram to rule out reflux.

H. Differential diagnosis.

1. Polycystic kidney disease.
2. Hydronephrosis.
3. Renal vein thrombosis.
4. Renal tumor.

I. Complications.

1. Hypertension.
2. Hematuria.
3. Infection.

J. Patient care management.

1. Nonoperative approach.
   a. Serial ultrasonography.
   b. Monitoring of blood pressure.
   c. Monitoring for infection.
   d. Monitoring for hematuria.
   e. Assessment for signs and symptoms of renal failure.
2. Operative approach: nephrectomy. Performance of nephrectomy is not necessary during neonatal period (Welch, 1994).

K. Outcome.

1. Bilateral involvement is incompatible with life.
2. There is an increased risk of the development of Wilms' tumor (Kenner et al., 1998).
3. Prognosis for multicystic dysplastic kidney disease is directly dependent on severity of kidney damage (Kenner, 1998).

Hydronephrosis

A. Definition: dilation of the pelvis and calyces of one or both kidneys, resulting from obstruction of urine flow (Spraycar, 1995).

B. Etiology. The etiology of most types of hydronephrosis is unclear (Bonilla-Felix et al., 1998); however, a urinary tract obstruction causes a retrograde increase in hydrostatic pressure and dilation above the lesion, resulting in impaired renal structure and function (Brion et al., 1997).

C. Incidence.

1. As many as 1% of newborn infants have a prenatal diagnosis of hydronephrosis or significant renal pelvic dilation (Elder, 1997).
2. The abnormality occurs predominantly in males and most often on the left side (Becker and Avner, 1995; Housely and Harrison, 1998; Reddy and Mandell, 1998).

D. Clinical presentation.

1. Palpable abdominal mass.
2. Decreased urinary output.
3. Poor urinary stream.
4. Urinary tract infection: common.

E. Clinical assessment.

1. Urinalysis.
   a. Findings possibly within normal limits.
   b. Proteinuria.
   c. Hematuria.
   d. Leukocyturia.
2. Serum creatinine: may be elevated.
3. BUN: may be elevated.
4. Antenatal ultrasonography: evidence of hydronephrosis.

F. **Physical examination.**

1. Abdominal palpation reveals enlarged kidney.
2. Observe for other genitourinary or associated anomalies that may occur outside the urinary tract.
    a. Imperforate anus.
    b. Congenital vertebral anomalies.
    c. Facial and skeletal anomalies.
    d. Malformed ears.
    e. Myelodysplasia.
    f. Absent or decreased abdominal musculature.
    g. Unexplained pneumonia.
    h. Absence or dysplasia of the radius.
    i. Hypoplasia of the pelvis.
    j. Unexplained septicemia.

G. **Diagnostic studies (Brion et al., 1997; Elder, 1997; Kenner, 1998; Reddy and Mandell, 1998).**

1. Ultrasonography.
2. Voiding cystourethrography.
    a. Rule out obstruction.
    b. Rule out vesicoureteral reflux.
3. Renal scan.

H. **Differential diagnosis (Reddy and Mandell, 1988).**

1. Obstructive.
    a. Ureteropelvic junction obstruction: most common cause of hydronephrosis in neonates (Ward, Kay, and Ross, 1998).
    b. Ureterovesical junction obstruction.
    c. Multicystic dysplastic kidney disease.
    d. Ureterocele/ectopic ureter.
    e. Duplicated collecting system.
    f. Posterior urethral valves: most common cause of severe obstructive uropathy in children (Elder, 1997).
    g. Urethral atresia.
    h. Sacrococcygeal teratoma.
    i. Hydrometrocolpos.
2. Nonobstructive.
    a. Physiologic dilation.
    b. Vesicoureteral reflux.
    c. Prune-belly syndrome.
    d. Renal cyst.
    e. Megacalycosis.

I. **Complications.**

1. Urinary tract infection.
2. Hypertension.
3. Damage to renal parenchyma.

J. **General patient care management.**

1. Strict intake and output.
2. Urinalysis.
    a. Hematuria.
    b. Proteinuria.
    c. Leukocyturia.

3. Monitoring of specific gravity.
4. Monitoring of urine for hematuria and proteinuria.
5. Urine culture.
6. Antibiotic prophylaxis (Belman, 1997; Elder, 1997).
7. Monitoring of serum electrolytes.
8. Serum creatinine.
9. BUN.

K. Specific patient care management.

1. Ureteropelvic junction obstruction (Shalaby-Rana, 1997).
   a. Management depends on age and affected kidney's function.
   b. Evidence of obstruction on diuretic renogram and preserved renal function may not require immediate pyeloplasty. Treat with antibiotics and follow up with a diuretic renogram in 3 months to determine any change in drainage pattern or deterioration in function of affected kidney.
   c. Pyeloplasty (excision of stenotic segment; normal ureter and renal pelvis are reattached) is indicated for obstruction with compromised renal function.
2. Posterior urethral valves.
   a. Catheterize initially.
   b. Correct fluid-and-electrolyte or other metabolic imbalances.
   c. Neonates whose diagnosis was made after 24 weeks' gestation or postnatally are treated in the neonatal period with endoscopic fulguration of the posterior urethral valves or decompression by various methods (i.e., percutaneous nephrostomy drainage, vesicostomy, or ureterostomies with later valve ablation) (Housely and Harrison, 1998).
3. Vesicoureteral reflux (Belman, 1997).
   a. Catheterize initially.
   b. Nonsurgical treatment.
      (1) Antibiotic prophylaxis: amoxicillin for first 2 months, followed by trimethoprim-sulfamethoxazole or nitrofurantoin daily.
      (2) Cystography should be repeated every 12–18 months to determine resolution of reflux.
      (3) Circumcision is recommended for male neonates to decrease the risk of urinary tract infection (Elder, 1997).
      (4) It is the treatment of choice for all infants regardless of reflux grade.
   c. Surgical repair is indicated for higher reflux grade and breakthrough infection, lack of compliance, and unlikely resolution (Greenfield, Manyan, and Wan, 1997).
4. For obstruction at ureterovesical junction, management is similar to that for obstruction of the ureteropelvic junction (Shalaby-Rana, Lowe, Black, and Majd, 1997). It consists of excision of the stenotic segment and ureteric reimplantation.

L. Outcome.

1. Success rates for pyeloplasty: reported as 91–98% (Elder, 1997).
2. Posterior urethral valves. Neonates identified after 24 weeks' gestation or postnatally have a 5% mortality rate; fewer than 25% of patients progress to chronic renal failure (Housely and Harrison, 1998).
3. Vesicoureteral reflux.
   a. Most reflux resolves; 60–80% of grades 1–3 cases resolve spontaneously (Belman, 1997).
   b. The generally accepted rate for complication-free correction of reflux, including all grades, is more than 95% when carried out by an experienced urologist (Belman, 1997).

Renal Vein Thrombosis

A. **Precipitating factors.**

1. Maternal diabetes.
2. Toxemia.
3. Maternal thiazide therapy.
4. Polycythemia.
5. Placental insufficiency.
6. Congenital heart disease.
7. Birth asphyxia.
8. Respiratory distress syndrome.
9. Sepsis.
10. Dehydration.
11. Hypovolemia.
12. Hyperosmolality.
13. Umbilical arterial catheter or umbilical venous catheter.

B. **Incidence.**

1. Accounts for 1.9–2.7% of neonatal deaths (Arneil et al., 1973).
2. Occurs more frequently in males.

C. **Clinical presentation.**

1. Hematuria.
2. Proteinuria.
3. Oliguria or anuria.
4. Anemia.
5. Thrombocytopenia.
6. Increased fibrin split products.
7. Decreased fibrinogen.
8. Decreased factors V and VII.
9. Azotemia.

D. **Clinical assessment.**

1. Perinatal history.
   a. Maternal diabetes.
   b. Asphyxia.
2. Decreased urine output.
3. Variable blood pressure.
4. Urinalysis.
   a. Hematuria.
   b. Proteinuria.
   c. Leukocyturia.
5. Urine culture: to rule out urinary tract infection.
6. Complete blood cell count: to rule out microangiopathic hemolytic anemia.
7. Platelet count: decreased.
8. BUN: increased.
9. Serum electrolytes.
   a. Hyponatremia.
   b. Hyperkalemia.
10. Serum pH: decreased.
11. Blood culture result: positive in cases of sepsis.

E. **Physical examination: palpation of smooth, enlarged kidney.**

F. Diagnostic studies.

1. Renal ultrasonography: enlarged kidney with a disordered central collection of echoes.
2. Intravenous pyelography: decreased urinary function.
3. Renal scan: nonfunctioning kidney.

G. Differential diagnosis.

1. Hydronephrosis.
2. Cystic disease.
3. Tumors of renal or adrenal origin.

H. Complications.

1. Renal tubular dysfunction.
2. Hypertension.
3. Some degree of renal atrophy.
4. Chronic renal infection.

I. Patient care management.

1. Treat underlying illness.
2. Correct electrolyte imbalances.
3. Administer antibiotics for positive culture result.
4. Treat symptoms.
   a. Hydration: assess volume and correct deficits.
   b. Oliguria: treat as for acute renal failure.
   c. Treat intravascular coagulation.
   d. Provide peritoneal dialysis or hemofiltration for fluid overload, severe electrolyte imbalance, acidosis, or bilateral thrombosis with anuria.

J. Outcome.

1. Kidney may recover or show signs of damage; depends in part on severity of underlying medical condition.
2. Long-term consequences can include low GFR, tubular dysfunction, and systemic hypertension (Brion et al., 1997).

Urinary Tract Infections

A. Etiology.

1. Abnormality of the urinary tract.
2. Sepsis.
3. Most common organisms are gram negative, predominantly *Escherichia coli*; common gram-positive organisms include staphylococci and enterococci (Ahmed and Swedlund, 1998; Brion et al., 1997; Kenner, 1998; Rushton, 1997).

B. Incidence (Ahmed and Swedlund, 1998; Brion et al., 1997).

1. Reported to range from 0.1% to 1.0% in all newborn infants and to be as high as 10% in low birth weight infants.
2. Occurs more frequently in males than females.

C. Disease states.

1. Sepsis.
2. Urinary tract anomalies.

D. Clinical presentation (Kenner et al., 1998; Rushton, 1997).

1. May be asymptomatic.

2. Symptomatic manifestations.
   a. Abnormal weight loss during the first days of life.
   b. Poor feeding.
   c. Irritability.
   d. Lethargy.
   e. Cyanosis.
   f. Jaundice.
   g. Septicemia.
   h. Dehydration.

E. **Diagnostic studies.**

1. Urine culture. Urine specimen should be obtained for culture via suprapubic aspiration or bladder catheterization.
2. Urinalysis.
   a. Leukocyturia.
   b. Hematuria.
   c. Casts, which suggest renal involvement.
3. Blood culture.
4. Complete blood cell count with differential cell count.
5. Renal ultrasonography: to rule out obstruction and determine kidney size.
6. Renal scan: to detect renal inflammation and scarring.
7. Cystourethrography: to rule out reflux.

F. **Differential diagnosis.**

1. Sepsis.
2. Urinary tract obstruction.

G. **Complications.**

1. Renal scarring.
2. Recurrence of urinary tract infection.
3. Bacteremia.
4. Urinary tract obstruction.
5. Vesicoureteral reflux.

H. **Patient care management.**

1. Administer antibiotic therapy for 14 days (Bonilla-Felix et al., 1998.)
   a. Use broad-spectrum antibiotics (e.g., ampicillin and aminoglycoside) during the first week of life (Brion et al., 1997).
   b. Vancomycin and cefotaxime should be administered for urinary tract infections occurring later (Brion et al., 1997).
2. Collect specimen for follow-up urine culture 3 days after antibiotic therapy is discontinued (Bonilla-Felix et al., 1998).
3. Cystourethrography should be done as soon as infection has resolved, to assess for reflux.
4. Antibiotic prophylaxis may be instituted in infants with an abnormal urinary tract after an initial urinary tract infection (Brion et al., 1997).

I. **Outcome:** excellent with prompt and adequate treatment.

Patent Urachus

A. **Definition:** a communication between the bladder and the umbilicus.

B. **Etiology:** failure of normal closure of epithelialized urachal tube, resulting in patent urachus.

C. **Incidence:** more common in males than in females (Gonzalez, 1996).

D. Clinical presentation.

1. Discharge of urine from umbilicus at birth or later.
2. Wet umbilicus.
3. Enlarged/edematous umbilicus.
4. Delayed sloughing of cord.

E. Physical examination: observation of umbilicus.

F. Diagnostic studies (Atala and Retik, 1997).

1. Analysis of fluid for urea and creatinine.
2. Bladder ultrasonography.
3. Voiding cystourethrography.
4. Transurethral injection of methylene blue.

G. Differential diagnosis.

1. Patency of vitelline/omphalomesenteric duct.
2. Omphalitis.
3. Simple granulation of a healing umbilical stump.
4. Infected umbilical vessel.
5. External urachal sinus.

H. Complications.

1. Urinary tract infection.
2. Excoriation.
3. Infection.

I. Patient care management.

1. Nonintervention: spontaneous closure may occur if defect is small and drainage is intermittent.
2. Operative intervention.
   a. Treatment of distal obstructive uropathy, if present, before surgical closure of urachal duct.
   b. Extraperitoneal surgical excision of urachal tract with bladder cuff (Atala and Retik, 1997).

J. Outcome: good with surgical procedure.

Hypospadias

A. Definition: urethral meatus on ventral surface of penis (Fig. 18–2). The condition varies in severity from a slightly malpositioned meatus still within the glans and without chordee to extreme genital ambiguity with hypoplastic phallus, bifid scrotum, and scrotal or perineal meatus.

B. Etiology.

1. Deficient anterior urethral development.
2. Delay or arrest in normal sequence of development, causing the urethra to open proximally and the prepuce to be incomplete ventrally.
3. Probably multifactorial mode of inheritance.

C. Incidence: reported as approximately 1:300 newborn boys (Baskin, Duckett, and Lue, 1996; Dawson and Whitfield, 1996).

D. Clinical presentation.

1. Urinary meatus located on undersurface of penis.
2. Deviation of urinary stream.

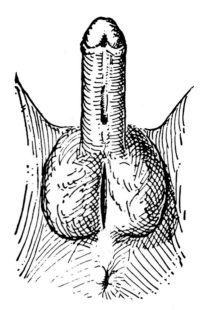

Figure 18–2
Hypospadias, showing in one drawing a composite of all three locations. (From Koyle, M.A., and Anand, S.K.: *In* Taeusch, H.W., Balland, R.A., and Avery, M.E. [Eds.]: Schaffer and Avery's Diseases of the Newborn, 6th ed. Philadelphia, W.B. Saunders, 1991, p. 885.)

E. **Clinical assessment.**

1. Direction of urinary stream.
2. Voiding pattern.

F. **Physical examination.**

1. Observation of external genitalia.
   a. Meatal location.
   b. Quantity of ventral shaft skin and dorsal foreskin; usually incomplete formation of ventral prepuce.
   c. Chordee: downward curving of penis.
      (1) Association with chordee variable.
      (2) Severity of chordee generally proportional to degree of hypospadias.
   d. Assess for presence of associated anomalies (e.g., inguinal hernia, cryptorchidism, hydrocele, and meatal stenosis) (Danish and Dahms, 1997). Undescended testes and inguinal hernias are the most commonly associated anomalies (Zaontz and Packer, 1997).
2. Palpation.
   a. Descent of testes.
   b. Presence of inguinal hernia.

G. **Complications.**

1. Without repair.
   a. Difficulty in voiding while standing.
   b. The presence of chordee may cause painful erection.
2. With postsurgical repair.
   a. Urethrocutaneous fistula.
   b. Balanitis xerotica obliterans.
   c. Meatal stenosis.
   d. Urethral stricture.
   e. Urethral diverticulum.

H. **Patient care management.**

1. Avoidance of circumcision.

2. Genotypic evaluation if only one gonad is palpated; congenital adrenal disease must be ruled out when no gonads are palpable (Belman, 1997).
3. Surgical repair.
   a. Move meatus distally.
   b. Improve cosmetic appearance of genitalia.
   c. Straighten curved penis.
   d. Most cases can be corrected with single-stage repair (Atala and Retik, 1997).
   e. Repair between 6 and 12 months of age is generally recommended (Belman, 1997).
   f. Multistage repair may be necessary for severe forms of hypospadias (Atala and Retik, 1997; Brion et al., 1997).

I. **Outcome:** good for surgical correction of simple hypospadias.

Exstrophy of the Bladder

A. **Definition: bladder exposed and protruding onto abdominal wall** (Fig. 18–3). The umbilicus is displaced downward, and the pubic rami are widely separated in the midline. The rectus muscles are separated.
1. Virtually all affected infants have associated epispadias (opening of the urinary meatus onto the dorsal aspect of the penis).
2. The remainder of the urinary tract is usually normal.

B. **Etiology.**

1. Part of the spectrum of conditions resulting from abnormal development of the cloacal membrane.

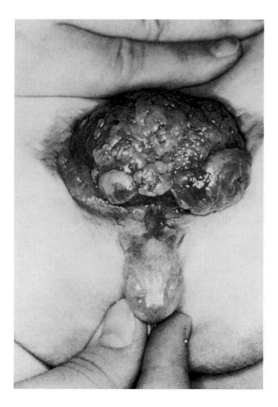

Figure 18–3
Patient with exstrophy of the bladder, associated with complete epispadias. The prominent cystic changes in the bladder mucosa are typical but are of no clinical significance. (From Avery, G.B. [Ed.]: Neonatology: Pathophysiology and Management of the Newborn, 3rd ed. Philadelphia, J.B. Lippincott, 1987, p. 996.)

2. Failure of the mesoderm to invade cephalad extension of the cloacal membrane.
3. Variant of exstrophy-epispadias complex determined by the position and timing of rupture of the cloacal membrane.

C. **Incidence.**

1. Approximately 1:10,000 to 1:50,000 live births (Ben-Chaim and Gearhart, 1996).
2. More common in males.

D. **Disease states:** exstrophy-epispadias complex.

E. **Clinical presentation:** external presentation of bladder.

F. **Clinical assessment.**

1. Signs and symptoms of infection.
2. Urine output.

G. **Physical assessment.**

1. Observation of external presentation of bladder.
2. Assessment of associated anomalies.
   a. Epispadias.
   b. Bifid clitoris.
   c. Anteriorly located vagina.
   d. Anteriorly located anus.
3. Palpation.
   a. Testes: to assess descent.
   b. Groin: to assess for presence of inguinal hernias.
   c. Symphysis pubis: to assess widening.

H. **Differential diagnosis:** complete exstrophy-epispadias complex.

I. **Complications.**

1. Infections.
2. Postoperative hydronephrosis.
3. Vesicoureteral reflux after bladder closure.
4. Swelling and edema in the bladder wall after surgery, which obstructs ureteral drainage and can lead to anuria, hypertension, or hydroureteronephrosis.
5. Urinary incontinence.
6. Anal incontinence.
7. Malignancy occurring 10 or more years later.

J. **Patient care management (Ben-Chaim and Gearhart, 1996).**

1. Prevent cord clamp from damaging bladder by using cord tie.
2. Cover exposed bladder with clear plastic wrap.
3. Irrigate bladder surface with sterile saline solution and replace the plastic wrap at each diaper change.
4. Surgical closure is needed within 72 hours.
5. Administer antibiotic therapy.
6. Renal ultrasonography or radionuclide scan is performed to determine presence or absence of upper tract abnormalities.
7. Assess for possible hydronephrosis and infections postoperatively.
8. Modified Bryant's traction for immobilization is used for 4 weeks in patients who have undergone closure without osteotomy or with only a posterior osteotomy; light Buck's traction, with legs supported on a pillow, is used if the approach was anterior.
9. Bladder is drained with a 10F suprapubic Malecot catheter for 4 weeks and with 3.5F ureteral stents for 2 weeks to prevent ureteral obstruction hypertension.

10. Antispasmodics, analgesics, and sedatives are administered to prevent bladder spasm and excessive crying, which may disrupt closure.
11. Intravenous pyelography or ultrasonography is performed to assess the upper tracts, and catheterization is performed to obtain residual urine and urine culture specimens before discharge.
12. If initial intravenous pyelogram shows good drainage, the condition of the upper tracts is followed up with ultrasonography every 6 months.
13. Subsequent repair of epispadias is performed at about 2–3 years of age.
14. Bladder neck reconstruction is performed at approximately 4–5 years of age.

K. **Outcome (Ben-Chaim and Gearhart, 1996).**

1. Results of functional closure of bladder exstrophy can be expected to be as high as a 75–85% continence rate with preservation of renal function.
2. Precise prognosis is directly related to the presence of other deformities (Kenner, 1998).

Inguinal Hernia

A. **Etiology:** failure of the proximal part of the processus vaginalis to close, producing a hernia sac.

B. **Incidence.**

1. Reported as 10–20 per 1000 live births (Skoog, 1997; Shochat, 1996).
2. Higher incidence of inguinal hernia reported in premature infants (Kenner, 1998; Shochat, 1996).
3. Occurs more frequently in males (Kenner, 1998; Shochat, 1996).
4. Location: 60% on right side; 30% on left side; 10% bilateral (Shochat, 1996).

C. **Disease states.**

1. Cryptorchidism.
2. Presence of multiple congenital anomalies, particularly those involving the lower abdomen, pelvis, or perineum; frequently associated with inguinal hernias.

D. **Clinical presentation:** swelling/lump in the inguinal area and/or scrotum.

E. **Physical examination.**

1. Palpation.
   a. Inguinal area and scrotum to determine herniation.
   b. Scrotum to determine testicular descent.
2. Observation: transillumination to rule out hydrocele.
3. Gestational age assessment: more common in premature infants because premature birth precedes closure of the processus vaginalis.

F. **Differential diagnosis.**

1. Hydrocele.
2. Testicular torsion.
3. Testicular tumor.
4. Undescended testicle.
5. Varicocele.

G. **Complications.**

1. Incarceration of hernia.
2. Venous infection of the testicle.
3. Testicular complications associated with hernia repair: vas deferens injury and testicular atrophy.

H. Patient care management.

1. Herniorrhaphy. Surgical repair of premature infants should be performed close to the time of discharge, after the infant is stable and has gained weight. The hernia may be monitored and reduced manually until that time.
2. Postoperative management. Maintain neonate in side-lying or supine position, with the head turned to the side to maintain integrity of suture line (Kenner, 1998).

I. Outcome: excellent after surgical repair (Kenner, 1998; Shochat, 1996).

Undescended Testicles (Cryptorchidism)

A. Etiology.

1. Endocrine dysfunction of the hypothalamic-pituitary-gonadal axis.
2. Abnormal epididymal development, with failure to induce testicular descent.
3. Anatomic abnormality preventing descent.

B. Incidence (Danish and Dahms, 1997).

1. Reported as 3.7% of term male infants.
2. Increased incidence in preterm infants.
3. At 1 year of age: 0.8%.

C. Disease states.

1. Specific types of cryptorchidism.
   a. Abdominal: testes located inside the internal inguinal ring.
   b. Canalicular: testes located between the internal and external inguinal rings.
   c. Ectopic: testes located away from the normal pathway of descent, between the abdominal cavity and the base of the scrotum.
2. Genetic syndromes.
   a. Klinefelter's syndrome.
   b. Noonan's syndrome.
   c. Prader-Willi syndrome.
3. Vasal and/or epididymal abnormalities.
4. Prune-belly syndrome.

D. Clinical presentation: absence of the testes in the scrotum.

E. Clinical assessment. Associated abnormalities may be present. There is an increased incidence of CNS abnormalities and hypospadias.

F. Physical examination.

1. Palpation of scrotum for presence of testes or associated hernia.
2. Palpation of inguinal area for presence of hernia.

G. Diagnostic studies.

1. Ultrasonography: identification of intra-abdominal testes.
2. Magnetic resonance imaging: identification of intra-abdominal testes.
3. Laparoscopy: identification of intra-abdominal testes.
4. Complete endocrine and electrolyte evaluation and chromosome analysis to rule out hypothalamic-pituitary insufficiency, female adrenogenital syndrome, and anorchism in phenotypic male infants with bilateral impalpable gonads (Gill and Kogan, 1997).

H. Differential diagnosis.

1. Specific type of cryptorchidism.
   a. Abdominal.

  b. Canalicular.
  c. Ectopic or maldescended.
 2. Anorchia: absence of testes.

I. **Complications (Danish and Dahms, 1997; Gill and Kogan, 1997; Lee, 1995).**

1. Testicular torsion.
2. Hernia.
3. Infertility.
4. Postoperative complications.
 a. Obstruction of the testicular vascular supply by direct injury.
 b. Compression from twisting of the vascular supply resulting from direct injury.
 c. Tight closure of the abdominal musculature.
 d. Narrowing of vessels by placing them under significant tension as the testis is brought into the scrotum.
 e. Transient testicular swelling from partial obstruction of lymphatic and venous drainage.
5. Increased risk of testicular cancer.

J. **Patient care management.**

1. Orchiopexy.
 a. Surgical procedure that alters the course of the spermatic artery and creates a direct line from the renal pedicle to the scrotum.
 b. Surgical repair is to be performed at 1–2 years of age (Rozanski and Bloom, 1995).
2. Hormonal treatment.
 a. Consists of administration of human chorionic gonadotropin (hCG), and/or gonadotropin-releasing hormone (GnRH), also referred to as luteinizing hormone-releasing hormone (LH-RH).
 b. May be attempted in an effort to avoid orchiopexy.
 c. May make technical aspects of orchiopexy easier.
3. Reevaluation of testicular location, size, and viability after 1 year.

K. **Outcome.**

1. Success rates for orchiopexy by anatomic testicular position have been reported as 74% for abdominal, 87% for canalicular, and 92% for those located beyond the external ring (Docimo, 1995).
2. Fertility may be impaired (Danish and Dahms, 1997; Gill and Kogan, 1997; Lee, 1995).

Circumcision

A. **Indications.** There are no absolute medical indications for routine circumcision in the newborn period, although the advantages, disadvantages, and risks of the procedure have been reviewed in the literature (Canadian Paediatric Society Fetus and Newborn Committee, 1996; Niku, Stock, and Kaplan, 1995; American Academy of Pediatrics Task Force on Circumcision, 1989).

B. **Incidence.** National Center for Health Statistics reported that 60.7% newborn boys were circumcised in 1992 (Holman, Lewis, and Ringler, 1995).

C. **Physical examination.**

1. Observation. Assess for the presence of abnormalities of the glans, foreskin, or urethral meatus.
2. Gestational age assessment. Circumcision should not be performed on premature infants until they meet discharge criteria.

D. Complications.

1. Hemorrhage.
2. Infection.
3. Injury to the glans.
4. Meatal stenosis.
5. Urethrocutaneous fistula.
6. Formation of skin bridge.
7. Adhesions.
8. Phimosis.
9. Concealed penis.
10. Inflammation of the meatus or meatal ulcer.
11. Chordee.
12. Inclusion cysts.
13. Lymphedema.
14. Necrosis.

E. Patient care management.

1. Circumcision should not be performed on infants with bleeding disorders or on those with abnormalities of the glans, foreskin, or urethral meatus.
2. Vitamin K should be administered within 1 hour after birth.
3. Local anesthesia and dorsal penile nerve block have been shown to alleviate the discomfort associated with the procedure (Mohan, Risucci, Casimir, and Gulrajani-LaCorte, 1998; American Academy of Pediatrics and American College of Obstetricians and Gynecologists, 1997; Taddio et al., 1997, Canadian Paediatric Society Fetus and Newborn Committee, 1996).
4. Risks and benefits should be discussed with parents and informed consent obtained.
5. Postoperative care.
   a. Check the site for bleeding, redness, or pus.
   b. Check for voiding.
   c. Avoid supine position.
   d. Change diapers frequently.
   e. Apply petroleum gauze to the site for 24 hours.
   f. Apply petroleum to site until healed.
6. Teach parent how to care for circumcision before discharge.

F. Outcome.
The precise incidence of complications after circumcision is unknown; however, data indicate that the rate is low and that the most common complications are local infection and bleeding (American Academy of Pediatrics and American College of Obstetricians and Gynecologists, 1997).

REFERENCES

Ahmed, S.M., and Swedlund, S.K.: Evaluation and treatment of urinary tract infections in children. Am Fam Physician 57(1):1573–1580, 1998.

American Academy of Pediatrics Committee on Fetus and Newborn and American College of Obstetricians and Gynecologists Committee on Obstetric Practice: Guidelines for Perinatal Care, 4th ed. Elk Grove Village, Ill., and Washington, D.C., American Academy of Pediatrics and American College of Obstetricians and Gynecologists, 1997.

American Academy of Pediatrics Task Force on Circumcision: Report of the Task Force on Circumcision. Pediatrics, 84:388–391, 1989 (erratum in Pediatrics, 1989;84:761).

Arneil, G.C., MacDonald, A.M., Murphy, A.V., et al.: Renal venous thrombosis. Clin. Nephrol., 1:119, 1973.

Askin, D.F.: Interpretation of neonatal blood gases. I. Physiology and acid-base homeostasis. Neonatal Network, 16(5):17–21, 1997.

Atala, A., and Retik, A.B.: Congenital urologic anomalies. In Schrier R.W., and Gottschalk, C.W. (Eds.): Diseases of the Kidney, vol. III. Boston, Little, Brown, 1997.

Bailie, M.D.: Development of the endocrine function of the kidney. Clin. Perinatol., 19(1):59–68, 1992.

Baskin, L.S., Duckett, J.W., and Lue, T.F.: Penile curvature. Urology, 48:347–356, 1996.

Becker, N., and Avner, E.D.: Congenital nephropathies and uropathies. Pediatr. Clin. North Am., 42:1319–1341, 1995.

Belman, A.B. Hypospadias update. Urology, 49:166–172, 1997.

Ben-Chaim, J., and Gearhart, J.P.: Current management of bladder exstrophy. Tech. Urol., 2(1):22–33, 1996.

Bissinger, R.L.: Renal physiology. I. Structure and function. Neonatal Network, 14(4):9–20, 1995.

Blackburn, S.T.: Renal function in the neonate. J. Perinat. Neonat. Nurs., 8(1):37–47, 1994.

Bonilla-Felix, M., Brannan, P., and Portman, R.J.: Neonatal nephrology. In Merenstein, G., and Gardner, S. (Eds.): Handbook of Neonatal Intensive Care, 4th ed. St. Louis, Mosby, 1998.

Brion, L.P., Bernstein, J., and Spitzer, A.: Kidney and urinary tract. In Fanaroff, A., and Martin, R.J. (Eds.): Neonatal-Perinatal Medicine: Diseases of the Fetus and Infant, vol. 2, 6th ed. St. Louis, Mosby–Year Book, 1997.

Brion, L.P., Satlin, L.M., and Edelmann, C.M., Jr.: Renal disease. In Avery, G.B., Fletcher, M.A., and MacDonald, M.G. (Eds.): Neonatology: Pathophysiology and Management of the Newborn, 4th ed. Philadelphia, J.B. Lippincott, 1994.

Canadian Paediatric Society Fetus and Newborn Committee. Neonatal circumcision revisited. Can. Med. Assoc. J., 154:769–780, 1996.

Chevalier, R.L.: Developmental renal physiology of the low birth weight preterm infant. J. Urol., 156:714–719, 1996.

Danish, R.K., and Dahms, W.T.: Abnormalities of sexual differentiation. In Fanaroff, A.A., and Martin, R.J. (Eds.): Neonatal-Perinatal Medicine: Diseases of the Fetus and Infant, 6th ed., vol 2. St. Louis, Mosby, 1997.

Dawson, C., and Whitfield, H.: Common paediatric problems. B.M.J., 312:1291–1294, 1996.

Docimo, S.G.: The results of surgical therapy for cryptorchidism: A literature review and analysis. J. Urol., 154:1148–1152, 1995.

Elder, J.S.: Antenatal hydronephrosis: Fetal and neonatal management. Pediatr. Clin. North Am. 44:1299–1321, 1997.

Gill, B., and Kogan, S.: Cryptorchidism. Pediatr. Clin. North Am., 44:1211–1227, 1997.

Gloor, J.M., Ogburn, P.L., Breckle, R.J., et al.: Urinary tract anomalies detected by prenatal ultrasound examination at Mayo Clinic Rochester. Mayo Clin. Proc., 70:526–531, 1995.

Goble, M.M.: Hypertension in infancy. Pediatr. Clin. North Am., 40:105–122, 1993.

Gonzalez, R.: Urologic disorders. In Behrman, R.E., Kliegman, R.M., and Arvin, A.M. (Eds.): Nelson's Textbook of Pediatrics, 15th ed. Philadelphia, W.B. Saunders, 1996.

Greenfield, S.P., Manyan, N.G., and Wan, J.: Experience with vesicoureteral reflux in children: Clinical characteristics. J. Urol., 158:574–577, 1997.

Hanna, J.D., Scheinman, J.I., and Chan, J.C.M.: The kidney in acid-base balance. Pediatr. Clin. North Am., 42:1365–1395, 1995.

Harrison, M.R.: Fetal surgery. Am. J. Obstet. Gynecol., 174:1255–1264, 1996.

Holman, J.R., Lewis, E.L., and Ringler, R.L.: Neonatal circumcision techniques. Am. Fam. Physician, 52:511–518, 1995.

Housley, H.T., and Harrison, M.R.: Fetal urinary tract abnormalities: Natural history, pathophysiology and treatment. Urol. Clin. North Am., 25(1):63–73, 1998.

Jona, J.Z.: Advances in fetal surgery. Pediatr. Clin. North Am., 45:599–604, 1998.

Jones, D.P., and Chesney, R.W.: Development of tubular function. Clin. Perinatol., 19(1):33–57, 1992.

Kenner, C.: Assessment and management of genitourinary dysfunction. In Kenner, C., Lott, J.W., and Flandermeyer, A.A. (Eds.): Comprehensive Neonatal Nursing: A Physiologic Perspective, 2nd ed. Philadelphia, W.B. Saunders, 1998.

Kenner, C., Amlung, S.R., and Flandermeyer, A.A.: Protocols in Neonatal Nursing. Philadelphia, W.B. Saunders, 1998.

Lee, P.A.: Consequence of cryptorchidism: Relationship to etiology and treatment. Curr. Probl. Pediatr. 25:232–236, 1995.

Levine, E., Hartman, D.S., Meilstrup, J.W., et al.: Current concepts and controversies in imaging of renal cystic diseases. Urol. Clin. North Am., 24:523–543, 1997.

Martinez, J.R., and Grantham, J.J.: Polycystic kidney disease: Etiology, pathogenesis and treatment. Dis. Mon., 41:693–765, 1995.

Masciello, A.L.: Anesthesia for neonatal circumcision: Local anesthesia is better than dorsal penile nerve block. Obstet. Gynecol., 75:834–838, 1990.

McCourt, M.: Acute renal failure in the newborn. Crit. Care Nurs., 16(5):84–94, 1996.

Mohan, C., Risucci, D.A., Casimir, M., and Gulrajani-LaCorte, M.: Comparison of analgesics in ameliorating the pain of circumcision. J. Perinat., 18(1):13–19, 1998.

Niku, S.D., Stock, J.A., and Kaplan, G.W.: Neonatal circumcision. Urol. Clin. North Am., 22:57–65, 1995.

Rasoulpour, M., and Marinelli, K.A.: Systemic hypertension Clin. Perinat., 19(1):121–137, 1992.

Reddy, P.P., and Mandell, J.: Prenatal diagnosis: Therapeutic implications. Urol. Clin. North Am., 25:171–180, 1998.

Rozanski, T.A., and Bloom, D.A.: The undescended testis: Theory and management. Urol. Clin. North Am., 22:107–118, 1995.

Rushton, H.: Urinary tract infections in children. Pediatr. Clin. North Am., 44:1133–1169, 1997.

Seely, R.R., Stephens, T.D., and Tate, P.: Anatomy and Physiology, 3rd ed. St. Louis, Mosby–Year Book, 1995.

Shalaby-Rana, E., Lowe, L.H., Blask, A.N., and Majd, M.: Imaging in pediatric urology. Pediatr. Clin. North Am., 44:1065–1089, 1997.

Shochat, S.J.: Inguinal hernias. In Behrman, R.E., Kliegman, R.M., and Arvin, A.M. (Eds.): Nelson's Textbook of Pediatrics, 15th ed. Philadelphia, W.B. Saunders, 1996.

Skoog, S.J.: Benign and malignant pediatric scrotal masses. Pediatr. Clin. North Am., 44:1229–1250, 1997.

Spraycar, M. (Ed.): Stedman's Medical Dictionary, 26th ed. Baltimore, Williams & Wilkins, 1995.

Stewart, C.L., and Barnett, R.: Acute renal failure in infants, children and adults. Crit. Care Clin., 13:575–590, 1997.

Sullivan, K.M., and Adzick, N.S.: Fetal surgery. Clin. Obstet. Gynecol., 37:355–371, 1994.

Taddio, A., Stevens, B., Craig, K., et al.: Efficacy and safety of lidocaine-prilocaine cream for circumcision. N. Engl. J. Med., 336:1197–1201, 1997.

Ward, A.M., Kay, R., and Ross, J.H.: Ureteropelvic junction obstruction in children. Urol. Clin. North Am., 25:211–217, 1998.

Welch, V.W.: The management of urologic disorders in the neonate. J. Perinat Neonat. Nurs., 8(1):48–58, 1994.

Zaontz, M.R., and Packer, M.G.: Abnormalities of the external genitalia. Pediatr. Clin. North Am., 44:1267–1297, 1997.

ADDITIONAL READINGS

American Academy of Pediatrics: Timing of elective surgery on the genitalia of male children with particular reference to the risks, benefits, and psychological effects of surgery and anesthesia. Pediatrics, *97*:590–594, 1996.

Avery, G.B., Fletcher, M.A., and MacDonald, M.G.: Neonatology: Pathophysiology and Management of the Newborn, 4th ed. Philadelphia, J.B. Lippincott, 1994.

Behrman, R.E., Kliegman R.M., and Arvin, A.M. (Eds.): Nelson's Textbook of Pediatrics, 15th ed. Philadelphia, W.B. Saunders, 1996.

Davenport, M.: Inguinal hernia, hydrocele, and the undescended testis. B.M.J., *312*:564–567, 1996.

Duffy, P.G.: Bladder exstrophy. Semin. Pediatr. Surg. *5*:129–132, 1996.

Guillery, E.N., and Robillard, J.E.: The renin-angiotensin system and blood pressure regulation during infancy and childhood. Pediatr. Clin. North Am., *40*:61–79, 1993.

Gutierrez, C.S.: Cryptorchidism. West. J. Med.,*163*(1):67–68, 1995.

Hellerstein, S.: Urinary tract infections old and new concepts. Pediatr. Clin. North Am., *42*:1433–1457, 1995.

Husmann, D.A., and Levy, J.B.: Current concepts in the pathophysiology of testicular undescent. Urology, *46:* 267–276, 1995.

King, L.R.: Hydronephrosis: When is obstruction not obstruction? Urol. Clin. North Am., *22*(1):31–42, 1995.

Koff, S.A.: Neonatal management of unilateral hydronephrosis. Urol. Clin. North Am., *25*:181–186, 1998.

Moore, K.L.: The Developing Human: Clinically Oriented Embryology, 5th ed. Philadelphia, W.B. Saunders, 1993.

Paulozzi, L.J., Erickson, J.D., and Jackson, R.J.: Hypospadias trends in two US surveillance systems. Pediatrics, *100*:831–834, 1997.

Reynolds, R.D.: Use of the Mogen clamp for neonatal circumcision. Am. Fam. Physician, *54*:1177–1182, 1996.

Ritchey, M.D., and Bloom, D.: Summary of the urology section. Pediatrics, *96*:138–143, 1995.

Scherer, L.R., III, and Grosfeld, J.L.: Inguinal hernia and umbilical anomalies. Pediatr. Clin. North Am., *40*:1121–1131, 1993.

Skoog, S.J., and Conlin, M.J.: Pediatric hernias and hydroceles the urologist's perspective. Urol. Clin. North Am., *22*:119–130, 1995.

Stock, J.A., Scherz, H.C., and Kaplan, G.W.: Distal hypospadias. Urol. Clin. North Am., 22:131–138, 1995.

Chapter 19

Neurologic Disorders

Mary McCulloch

Objectives

1. Identify the six primary stages of neurodevelopment and the congenital anomalies that result from defective development at each stage.

2. Define autoregulation.

3. Review a complete neurologic examination.

4. Examine birth injuries and patient care management.

5. Differentiate between the different types of intracranial hemorrhages and their origins, clinical presentation, and outcomes.

6. Recognize neonatal seizures, their distinguishing characteristics, and issues in patient care management.

7. Describe hypoxic-ischemic encephalopathy, including periventricular leukomalacia.

8. Distinguish pathophysiologic factors, clinical presentation, and patient care management of early- and late-onset meningitis.

The human brain is an intricate, fragile organ requiring precise development from the moment of conception. Several crucial developmental landmarks pinpoint major events in the development of the human brain. If the process is interrupted, malformation results.

Neurologic problems account for a significant number of admissions into the neonatal intensive care unit each year. These problems range from simple, easily treatable problems to major neurologic malformations.

This chapter provides a comprehensive review of neurodevelopment, neurophysiology, and neuromalformations. A greater understanding of these concepts may remove some of the mystery and complexity of the brain.

Anatomy of the Neurologic System

A. **Embryologic development (Table 19–1).**

1. Primary neurulation (dorsal induction).

Table 19–1
MAJOR EVENTS IN HUMAN BRAIN DEVELOPMENT AND PEAK TIMES OF OCCURRENCE

Major Developmental Event	Peak Time of Occurrence
Primary neurulation	3–4 weeks of gestation
Prosencephalic development	2–3 months of gestation
Neuronal proliferation	3–4 months of gestation
Neuronal migration	3–5 months of gestation
Organization	5 months of gestation—years postnatal
Myelination	Birth—years postnatal

From Volpe, J.J.: Neurology of the Newborn, 3rd ed. Philadelphia, W.B. Saunders, 1995.

    a. Occurs within the first month of life, ending between 24 and 28 days' gestation.
    b. Neural tube is formed by the invagination and curling of the neural plate distally.
    c. Closure of the neural tube gives rise to the central nervous system, including the cranial nerves.
    d. This evolution results in the formation of the skull and vertebrae.
    e. Inaccuracies of primary neurulation result in anencephaly, occipital encephalocele, myelomeningocele, and Arnold-Chiari malformation.
2. Prosencephalic development.
    a. Peak development is in the second and third months of gestation.
    b. This influences the formation of the face, forebrain, corpus callosum and septum pallucidum, optic nerves/chiasm, the hypothalamic structures (thalamus and hypothalamus [diencephalon]), and the cerebral hemispheres (telencephalon).
    c. Absence of olfactory bulbs and tracts is not uncommon.
    d. Disturbance in prosencephalic development causes facial and forebrain alterations.
      (1) Holoprosencephaly (abnormal formation of telencephalon and diencephalon).
      (2) Midline and midfacial defects.
        (a) Hypotelorism (less common: hypertelorism).
        (b) Cyclopia.
        (c) Cleft lip with or without cleft palate.
    e. Most common karyotype is normal (chromosomal disorder is possible).
3. Neuronal proliferation.
    a. Occurs between 3 and 4 months' gestation.
    b. Toxins and inherited diseases can significantly alter the number of neurons.
    c. Chemical and environmental substances can reduce the number of neurons, causing microcephaly vera.
    d. Excess neurons can produce macrencephaly.
    e. Disorders of proliferation of small veins cause Sturge-Weber syndrome (6% unilateral, 24% bilateral facial lesions).
4. Neuronal migration.
    a. Can occur as early as 2 months; peaks between 3 and 5 months.
    b. By 6 months' gestation, the neurons have migrated to their final, permanent place in the cortex.
    c. Neurons follow glial paths outward.
    d. Cells migrate and differentiate into six cortical layers (Finkel, 1984).
    e. Migration is critical for development of the cerebral cortex and the deeper nuclear structures.
      (1) Basal ganglia.

          (2) Hypothalamus.

          (3) Thalamus.

          (4) Brain stem.

          (5) Cerebellum.

          (6) Spinal cord.

    f. Dysfunction at this stage results in cortical malformation with abnormalities of neurologic function.

    g. Seizures may be the first clinical manifestation in the early postnatal period.

    h. Defects associated with abnormal migration range in severity and may be associated with other neurologic development.

    i. Abnormal development of gyrus denotes a neuronal migration disorder.

    j. Disorders include lissencephaly ("smooth brain"), agenesis of the corpus callosum, and schizencephaly (clefts found in the cerebral wall).

  5. Neuronal organization.

    a. Peaks at 5 months' gestation to several years after birth.

    b. Provides the basis for brain function and its complex circuitry.

    c. Includes cell differentiation, cell death, synaptic development, neurotransmitters, and myelination.

    d. Achieves stabilization of cell connections.

    e. Disorders due to organizational deficits and detrimental retardation (as with Down syndrome, Fragile-X syndrome, and Duchenne's muscular dystrophy [mild]) (Volpe, 1995).

  6. Myelination.

    a. Begins in the second trimester and continues into adult life.

    b. Involves myelin deposition around axons.

    c. Myelin, a fatty covering, insulates the circuitry; prevents leakage of current and enables rapid, efficient transmission of nerve impulses.

    d. Enhances intercellular communication.

    e. Deficiencies occur in some acquired and inherited diseases.

B. **Brain anatomy (Fig. 19–1).**

1. Cerebellum.

    a. Promotes integrative muscle function.

    b. Maintains balance.

    c. Enables smooth, purposeful movements.

2. Cerebrum: main components of cerebral hemisphere.

    a. Contains four lobes: parietal, frontal, occipital, and temporal.

    b. Corpus callosum: fiber bundles connecting the cerebral hemispheres.

    c. Cerebral cortex.

        (1) Encompasses the mind, the intellect.

        (2) Gray matter.

    d. Third ventricle: fluid-filled space.

    e. Thalamus: integrates sensory input.

    f. Hypothalamus: regulates body temperature.

3. Brain stem.

    a. Relays input and output signals between higher brain centers and the spinal cord.

    b. Three main components.

        (1) Medulla.

          (a) Implicated within cranial nerves VIII, IX, X, XI, and XII.

          (b) Controls areas of the abdomen, thorax, throat, and mouth.

        (2) Pons: carries information between the brain stem and the cerebellum.

        (3) Midbrain: involved in **eye** movements.

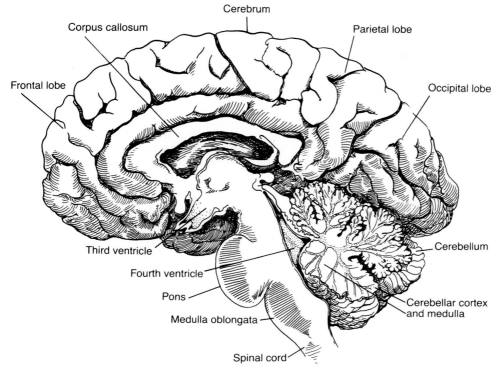

Cerebrum

Corpus callosum

Parietal lobe

Frontal lobe

Occipital lobe

Cerebellum

Third ventricle

Fourth ventricle

Pons

Cerebellar cortex
and medulla

Medulla oblongata

Spinal cord

Figure 19–1
Anatomy of the brain.

Physiology of the Neurologic System

A. Glucose metabolism.

1. Cerebral metabolism is influenced by the availability of glucose and oxygen.
2. Glucose is transported from blood to brain by a glucose transporter found in capillaries (De Vivo et al., 1991).
3. Serum glucose provides the brain with a glucose pool.
4. The neonatal brain is glucose dependent. The CNS is quickly and significantly affected by hypoglycemia (Volpe, 1995).
5. Glycogen stores are minimal or nonexistent in the premature baby.
6. The brain depends on adequate circulation to supply both oxygen and glucose to create enough energy for normal growth and metabolism.
7. Anaerobic metabolism causes lactic acid buildup.
8. Anaerobic metabolism produces significantly smaller amounts of energy.
9. Newborn blood glucose levels less than 30 mg/dL are associated with significant increases in cerebral blood flow.
10. Defining the lower limit of the neonatal blood glucose level is difficult because the infant's ability to present overt symptoms of hypoglycemia is not developed.

B. Cerebral blood flow.

1. Cerebral blood flow is affected by pH (controlled by hydrogen ions and carbon dioxide levels), potassium, hypoxemia, osmolarity, and calcium ion concentrations.
   a. The brain increases cerebral blood flow to spare itself inadequacies.

b. As pH decreases, cerebral blood flow increases.
c. As potassium levels increase, cerebral blood flow increases.
d. Hypoxemia causes an increase in cerebral blood flow to provide adequate oxygenated blood to the brain.
e. Increased osmolarity causes increased cerebral blood flow.
f. An increase in calcium ions causes a decrease in cerebral blood flow.
g. Cerebral blood flow increases when blood glucose levels fall to less than 30 mg/dL; the hypoglycemic brain recruits previously unperfused capillaries to maintain glucose levels (Volpe, 1995).
h. Degree and duration of hypoglycemia are significant (Volpe, 1995).
i. Studies have shown that neonatal neurologic signs can be minimal or absent with subsequent abnormal cognitive development.

2. Autoregulation.
a. Maintains steady-state cerebral blood flow despite systemic blood pressure changes.
b. Premature infants have attenuated cerebral autoregulation (Papile, 1997b).
c. Attenuated cerebral autoregulation occurs and cerebral vasculature vasodilates maximally in response to hypoxemia and hypercapnia (Papile, 1997b).
  (1) Hypotension leads to ischemia.
    (a) Ischemia damages blood vessels and surrounding elements supporting the blood vessels.
    (b) Once adequate blood supply resumes, hemorrhage can occur into ischemic areas.
  (2) Hypertension leads to hemorrhage.

Neurologic Assessment

A. History.

B. Observation.

1. Determine state (Table 19–2).
2. Note posture.
  a. Gestational age determines posture.
    (1) Premature infants: open, extended position reflecting diminished tone.
    (2) Term infants: flexed position reflecting adequate tone.
  b. Sequelae of intrauterine position may be evident.
  c. Abnormal findings are:
    (1) Hyperextension.
    (2) Asymmetry.
    (3) Flaccidity.

Table 19–2
SUMMARY OF NEUROLOGICAL STATES

Neurologic State	Physical Findings
Deep sleep	No observable movement
REM sleep	Eye movement, body movement, and irregular respiratory activity
Drowsy	
Quiet-alert	
Active	
Crying	

REM, Rapid eye movement.

Table 19-3
CRANIAL NERVES

Cranial Nerve	Bedside Testing Mechanisms
I. *Olfactory* (smell)	Place ammonia under nose; response is startle, grimace
II. *Optic*	Check PERL
III. *Oculomotor* (muscles of the eye)	PERL, EOM full and conjugate
IV. *Trochlear* (superior oblique muscle of the eye)	
V. *Trigeminal* (sensory to face, motor to jaw)	Touch cheek; should turn cheek toward stimulus
VI. *Abducens* (lateral gaze, abducts eyeball)	Rotate infant; eyes look in the direction of travel
VII. *Facial*	Asymmetric facial movements
VIII. *Auditory*	Infant quiets to voice; blinks to clap of hand
IX. *Glossopharyngeal* (taste)	Strong gag response
X. *Vagus* (pharynx, larynx, esophagus)	Cry is not hoarse
XI. *Accessory* (sternocleidomastoid muscles)	Turn supine infant's head to one side; infant attempts to bring head to midline
XII. *Hypoglossal* (muscles of tongue)	Insert finger in mouth while sucking; note force of tongue; note vesiculations or quivering tongue (uncommon)

PERL, Pupils equal and reactive to light; *EOM,* extraocular movements.
Adapted from Scanlon, J.W., Nelson, T., Grylack, L.J., and Smith, Y.F.: A System of Newborn Physical Examination. Baltimore, University Park Press, 1979; and Whaley, L.F., and Wong, D.L.: Nursing Care of Infants and Children, St. Louis, C.V. Mosby, 1979.

3. Note movements.
   a. Symmetric or asymmetric body movements.
   b. Note movement quality (jitteriness, seizures, tremors, and clonus).
   c. Quantity (absent or pronounced).
4. Note respiratory activity.
   a. Signs of distress.
   b. Hypoventilation (apnea).
   c. Quality of cry.
      (1) High pitched (consider meningitis, drug withdrawal, neurologic abnormalities).
      (2) Stridor (consider vocal cord damage).
5. Observe skin.
   a. Lesions (note number, size, shape, and color and texture).
      (1) Café-au-lait spots (6 or more lesions of ≥1.5 cm; may be neurofibromatosis).
      (2) Port-wine facial hemangioma (consider Sturge-Weber syndrome).
      (3) Areas of depigmentation.
   b. Abrasions, lacerations, bruises, and forcep marks.

C. **Physical examination.**

1. Check the skull size, shape, symmetry, hair whorls, fontanelles, and sutures.
2. Measure occipital frontal circumference (OFC).
   a. At less than the 10th percentile (symmetric vs asymmetric).
   b. At greater than the 90th percentile (symmetric vs asymmetric).
3. Examine the face for abnormalities in structure.
   a. Placement of ears.
   b. Neck skinfolds.
4. Spine (intact, openings, masses).
5. Cranial nerve function.
   a. Refer to Table 19-3.
   b. Blink reflex requires intact cranial nerves III and VII.
   c. Corneal reflex requires intact cranial nerves V and VII.
      (1) Generally elicited only if one suspects brain or eye damage (Whaley and Wong, 1995).
      (2) Cranial nerves IX, X, and XII regulate the tongue, swallow, gag, and cry.

6. Muscle tone.
   a. Evaluate head lag, ventral suspension, clonus, and recoil from extension.
   b. Check symmetry; briskness versus flaccidity.
7. Reflexes.
   a. Check grasp (bilaterally), Babinski, Moro, gag, suck, root, and tonic neck.
   b. Evaluate symmetry and strength of response.
   c. Abnormal Moro reflex: consider clavicular or humeral fractures or brachial plexus injury.
   d. Grasp varies with gestational age; if grasp is absent, consider nerve damage (refer to Birth Injuries, below).

Neurologic Disorders

A. **Anencephaly.**

1. Pathophysiology.
   a. Absent anterior neural tube closure, exposing neural tissue.
   b. Malfunction of the first stage of neurologic development, primary neurulation.
   c. Lack of brain above the brain stem.
   d. Partial absence of skull bones, with absent cerebrum and with or without missing cerebellum, brain stem, and spinal cord.
2. Clinical presentation.
   a. Exposed neural tissue with little definable structure.
   b. The anomalous skull has a froglike appearance when viewed face-on.
   c. Amniotic fluid reveals high levels of alpha-fetoprotein late in the first trimester (Sarnat, 1997).
3. Outcome.
   a. Stillbirth occurs in 75% (Volpe, 1995).
   b. Survival is unlikely beyond the neonatal period.
4. Patient care management.
   a. Provide comfort measures for the infant.
   b. Obtain genetic consultation; encourage parents to seek genetic counseling.
   c. Support the grieving process.
   d. Encourage the family to see their baby, because the family's imaginary impressions may be worse than reality.
   e. Clinicians must maintain a delicate balance between benefit and harm.

B. **Microcephaly.**

1. Definition.
   a. Small brain.
   b. OFC at less than the 3rd percentile for gestational age (Vannucci, 1997a).
2. Pathophysiology.
   a. Neuronal proliferation defect.
   b. Occurs between 3 and 4 months' gestational age (Volpe, 1995).
   c. The most severe microcephaly occurs earlier in utero.
3. Etiology.
   a. Teratogens.
      (1) Irradiation.
      (2) Maternal alcoholism or cocaine abuse.
   b. Maternal hyperphenylalaninemia.
   c. Genetic (usually autosomal recessive; can be X-linked) (Avery, Fletcher, and MacDonald, 1994).
   d. TORCH infections (*t*oxoplasmosis, *o*ther, *r*ubella, *c*ytomegalovirus, and *h*erpes) are associated.

e. Human immunodeficiency virus, although usually after the neonatal period.

f. Unknown causes (most common).

4. Clinical presentation.

a. Small head, backward sloping of the forehead, small cranial volume.

b. Neurologic deficits rarely evident at birth.

5. Diagnostic evaluation.

a. Perform a complete physical examination including neurologic assessment.

b. Elicit a thorough maternal history.

c. Use tests to confirm or rule out etiologic factors aligned with maternal history.

d. Computed tomography (CT) or magnetic resonance imaging (MRI) is performed.

6. Patient care management.

a. Record accurate measurement of OFC, length, and weight weekly.

b. Note percentiles and alert physician to abnormalities.

c. Document clearly any deviations from normal.

d. Obtain tests as ordered; note dates to follow up results.

e. Ensure that the family is informed.

f. Obtain consultations as needed: genetics, infectious diseases.

7. Outcome.

a. Dependent on severity.

b. May be associated with developmental delays.

C. **Hydrocephalus.**

1. Definition: excess cerebrospinal fluid (CSF) in the ventricles of the brain due to a decrease in reabsorption or overproduction.

a. CSF is in balance between formation and absorption.

b. CSF is produced at a rate of 0.33 mL/min from brain parenchyma, cerebral ventricles, areas along the spinal cord, and the choroid plexus (60% is from the choroid plexus).

2. Pathophysiology.

a. Excessive CSF production (rare).

b. Inadequate CSF absorption secondary to abnormal circulation.

c. Excess ventricular CSF secondary to aqueductal outflow obstruction causes obstructive, noncommunicating hydrocephalus (refer to Fig. 19–2 for a simplified diagram of the brain).

(1) The condition is most common in newborn infants.

(2) Obstructive hydrocephalus may progress rapidly.

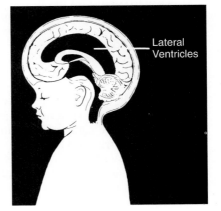

Figure 19–2
Hydrocephalus. (Used and reprinted with permission of the Ross Laboratories, Columbus, OH 43216, from *New Perspectives on Intraventricular Hemorrhage.* © 1988, Ross Laboratories.)

    d. Excess ventricular CSF with flow between the lateral ventricles and the subarachnoid space results in communicating, nonobstructive hydrocephalus.

3. Congenital hydrocephalus.
    a. Precipitating factors.
      (1) Aqueductal stenosis.
      (2) Dandy-Walker cyst (cystic transformation of ventricle IV).
      (3) Myelomeningocele with Arnold-Chiari malformation (herniation of the hindbrain, usually causing obstructive hydrocephalus).
      (4) Congenital masses and tumors.
      (5) Congenital infection (toxoplasmosis, cytomegalovirus [CMV] infection).
    b. Associated congenital defects.
      (1) Spina bifida.
      (2) Encephalocele.
      (3) Holoprosencephaly.
    c. Clinical presentation.
      (1) Large head.
      (2) Widened sutures.
      (3) Full (bulging) and tense fontanelles.
      (4) Increasing OFC.
      (5) Setting-sun eyes (may signify brain tissue damage).
      (6) Visible scalp veins.
    d. Diagnostic studies.
      (1) Positive transillumination.
      (2) Cranial ultrasonography.
      (3) Cranial CT scan.
    e. Patient care management.
      (1) Intrauterine diagnosis affords the family more options and allows time for preparation and anticipation.
      (2) Perform a thorough physical examination, assessing for further anomalies.
      (3) Obtain neurosurgery and genetics consultation.
      (4) Confirm diagnosis and cause.
      (5) Consider the possible need for reservoir placement versus ventriculoperitoneal (VP) shunt placement.
      (6) Support the infant by decreasing noxious stimuli (dim lights, minimal handling).
      (7) Position the head carefully.
      (8) Water-pillow beds diminish skin breakdown and may provide a source of comfort.
      (9) Provide normal infant care as much as possible.
     (10) Involve parents in infant's care as soon as family is ready.
     (11) Position the infant prone for oral feedings.
     (12) Allow parents to view an infant with a VP shunt or review pictured handouts.
     (13) Review VP shunt with parents preoperatively and postoperatively.
     (14) Prevent skin breakdown by not allowing the infant to put his or her head on the shunt side postoperatively.
     (15) Relieve the infant's probable stiff neck by holding the child's neck on the shunt side during feedings.
     (16) Review signs of infection or blocked shunt with the family.
        (a) Irritability.
        (b) Vomiting.
        (c) Increasing head size.
        (d) Lethargy.

(e) Changes in feeding patterns.

(f) Bulging fontanelle.

(17) If incision site reddens, position infant on opposite side to relieve pressure from this area.

4. Posthemorrhagic hydrocephalus (PHH).

a. Pathophysiology.

(1) Progressive dilation of the ventricles after intraventricular hemorrhage (IVH) caused by injury to the periventricular white matter.

(2) Two types: acute and chronic.

(a) Acute.

(i) Rapidly appears—within days of the initial hemorrhage.

(ii) Probably occurs secondary to malabsorption of CSF secondary to a blood clot.

(b) Subacute, chronic.

(i) Inhibition of CSF flow.

(ii) Blood from IVH.

b. Incidence.

(1) Approximately 45% of infants with IVH have no evidence of hydrocephalus (Volpe, 1995).

(2) Acute ventricular dilation develops in approximately 50% of surviving infants with hemorrhage; in the majority, it resolves spontaneously or remains static (Papile, 1997a).

c. Clinical presentation: severe ventricular dilation.

(1) Rapid increase in head size (begin days to weeks after ventricular dilation present).

(2) Apnea.

(3) Lethargy.

(4) Increased intracranial pressure.

(5) Tense, bulging anterior fontanelle.

(6) Cranial sutures separating.

d. Diagnostic studies.

(1) Graph of weekly OFC measurements.

(2) CT scan.

(3) Cranial ultrasonography.

e. Patient care management.

(1) Obtain daily OFC measurements.

(2) Perform serial cranial ultrasonography.

(3) Request a neurosurgical consultation.

(4) Perform serial lumbar taps (accelerate removal of protein and blood in CSF) (Kreusser et al., 1985).

(5) Administer drugs that diminish CSF production rates: furosemide (Lasix), 1 mg/kg per day, and acetazolamide (Diamox), up to 100 mg/kg per day (Kovnar and Volpe, 1982b).

(6) Consider an osmotic agent: glycerol, starting with 1 g/kg by mouth every 6 hours and slowly increasing for a week to 2 g/kg every 6 hours (Kovnar and Volpe, 1982b). Kovnar and Volpe (1982b) suggested that, with the use of any of these drug agents, blood urea nitrogen (BUN) and electrolytes should be monitored. Monitoring of serum glucose levels when glycerol is prescribed is also recommended.

(7) Consider placing a reservoir or VP shunt.

(8) Observe the infant for signs of increasing intracranial hemorrhage and hydrocephalus.

(9) Support the family.

(10) Maintain open communication among all team members and the family.

5. Outcome.
   a. Poor outcomes are likely when cerebral decompression does not occur after VP shunt placement.
   b. Initial IVH severity is the major determining factor in PHH development.
   c. In slightly more than 50% of the cases, severe hemorrhage results in progressive ventricular dilation (Volpe, 1995).
   d. Without therapy, a considerable number of infants exhibit halted progression, with or without resolution (Volpe, 1995).
   e. Deficits are motor and/or cognitive.

D. **Myelomeningocele.**
1. Definition.
   a. Neural tube defect.
      (1) Spina bifida occulta involves vertebral bone.
      (2) Defect is invisible (may be found if problems develop in later infancy or in childhood).
      (3) Meningocele is the protrusion of the meninges lying directly under the skin.
      (4) Myelocele is the exposure of the internal surface of the spinal cord or the nerve roots.
   b. In myelomeningocele, the spinal cord and meninges are exposed through the skin and onto the surface of the back.
   c. In myeloschisis, large areas of the spinal cord are without dermal or vertebral covering.
2. Pathophysiology.
   a. Results from failure of posterior neural tube to close.
   b. Eighty percent of cases occur in the lumbar region (the last region of the neural tube to close).
   c. Environmental factors, maternal nutrition, genetics, and teratogens, including maternal hyperthermia, are implicated.
3. Clinical presentation.
   a. The majority of cases occur in the thoracolumbar, lumbar, and lumbosacral regions.
   b. A herniated sac, sealed or leaking, protrudes from the back.
   c. Defects include vascular networks surrounding abnormal neural tissue.
   d. Most lesions have incomplete skin coverage.
4. Associated disease states.
   a. Hydrocephalus.
      (1) With OFC at greater than the 90th percentile, 95% of infants will have hydrocephalus.
      (2) All newborn infants with myelomeningocele should be evaluated for hydrocephalus with CT scan and cranial ultrasonography shortly after birth.
   b. Arnold-Chiari malformation.
      (1) Hindbrain malformation with or without aqueductal atresia.
      (2) Almost always present with myelomeningocele (Goddard-Finegold, 1998; Noetzel, 1989).
      (3) Many affected infants develop hydrocephalus.
      (4) Common features.
          (a) Reflux and aspiration.
          (b) Laryngeal stridor.
          (c) Central hypoventilation, apnea.
5. Patient care management.
   a. Prenatal diagnosis helpful.
   b. Examine lesion and measure size.
   c. Culture specimen from lesion if sac is open.

d. Wrap lesion with sterile gauze moistened with warm sterile saline solution; place a sterile feeding tube within the gauze mesh for intermittent infusion of warm saline solution.

e. Maintain the infant in a prone kneeling position, and protect the knees from skin breakdown.

f. Place a drape over the buttocks below the lesion; utilize the drape's adhesive backing to secure the drape to the body.

g. Obtain immediate consultation.
   (1) Neurosurgery.
   (2) Urology.

h. Perform a thorough physical examination to assess the level of the injury, sensory involvement, and anal wink; include an OFC measurement.

i. Encourage an open discussion among the family, the consultants, and the primary care team, providing the following:
   (1) Underlying physiology.
   (2) Physical examination findings.
   (3) Consultant reports.
   (4) Prognosis.
   (5) Complications.
   (6) Long-term care.
   (7) Options.

j. Begin preparing the family for discharge.
   (1) Suggest that the parents contact a support group.
   (2) Involve the parents in their infant's care.

k. Postoperatively, follow positioning instructions from the neurosurgeon.

l. Spend time making eye contact with the infant.

m. Watch for signs of hydrocephalus (refer to section C, Hydrocephalus, above).

n. Watch for development of Arnold-Chiari malformation that may present with feeding problems (reflux, aspiration), laryngeal stridor (due to vocal cord paralysis), or central hypoventilation or apnea.

o. Maintain meticulous hygiene by clearing stool and urine quickly.

p. Provide adequate nutrition.

q. Orthopedic consultation is appropriate for maximal function of lower extremities.

r. Physical therapy encourages maximal range of motion.

6. Outcome.
   a. Survival in 90%, with 80% or more having normal intelligence and 85% being ambulatory with or without special aids (McLone, 1992).
   b. Good outlook with meningocele because of normal spinal cord.
   c. Varying degrees of paralysis: commonly in the lower extremities (Volpe, 1995)
      (1) Lesions below the first sacral vertebra: infants can learn to walk unaided.
      (2) Lesions between the fourth and fifth lumbar vertebrae: infants may be able to walk with crutches or braces.
      (3) Lesions above the second lumbar vertebra: infants usually become wheelchair dependent.
   d. If surgery for defect closure is not performed, 80% die by 8 weeks and 100% are dead by 10 months (Fenichel, 1990).

E. Encephalocele.

1. Definition.
   a. Neural herniation.
   b. May or may not contain meninges or brain parenchyma.

2. Pathophysiology (Volpe, 1995).
   a. Precise pathogenesis is unknown.
   b. About 70–80% of encephaloceles occur in the occipital region.
   c. About 10–20% of lesions in the occipital region contain no neural elements.
3. Precipitating factors.
   a. Environmental and genetic factors.
   b. May be multifactorial.
4. Clinical presentation.
   a. Protruding midline skin-covered sac from the head or base of neck.
   b. Majority of sacs occur in the occipital region.
5. Diagnostic studies.
   a. Second-trimester intrauterine ultrasonography.
   b. Cranial ultrasonography.
   c. CT scan.
   d. MRI.
6. Patient care management.
   a. Examine the infant closely.
   b. Obtain neurosurgery consultation.
   c. Educate and support the family.
   d. Treat seizure activity.
7. Outcome.
   a. Early surgery recommended.
   b. Prognosis based on brain involvement.
   c. Possible motor deficits.
   d. Possible impaired intellectual function.
   e. May be complicated by hydrocephalus.

Craniosynostosis

A. Definition.

1. Premature closure of cranial sutures.
2. Occurs along one or more suture lines (see Fig. 19–3 for names and placement of cranial sutures).

B. Pathophysiology.

1. Cause unclear.
2. Hypothesized that the craniosynostosis results from lack of normal brain growth.
3. May be a result of metabolic disorders such as idiopathic hypercalcemia.

C. Incidence.

1. Reported as 0.4:1000 to 1:1000 births (Chadduck, 1994).
2. Sagittal craniosynostosis most common.

D. Clinical presentation.

1. Asymptomatic.
2. Cranial suture line reveals bony prominence; even and smooth bilaterally.
3. Inability to move the suture.
4. Abnormal cranial shape.
5. Later signs.
   a. Increased intracranial pressure.
   b. Increased irritability.
   c. Possible separation of other sutures.

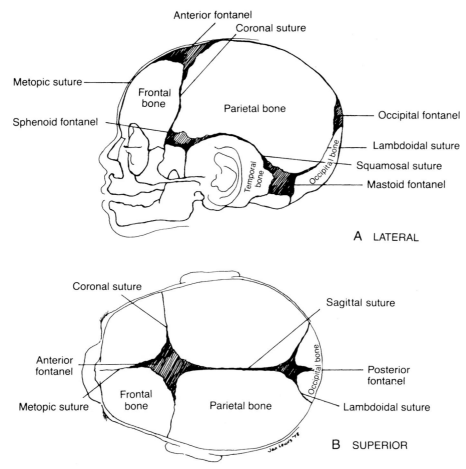

Figure 19–3
A and *B,* Two views of neonatal skull, showing clinically important fontanelles and sutures. (Reprinted with permission from Scanlon, J.W., Nelson, T., Grylack, L.J., and Smith, Y.F.: A System of Newborn Physical Examinations. Baltimore, University Park Press, 1979, p. 47.)

E. Diagnostic studies.

1. Skull x-ray examination.
2. CT scan.
3. Weekly graph of OFCs.

F. Patient care management.

1. Thorough physical examination.
2. Obtain neurosurgery consultation.
3. Educate and support the family.
4. Watch for signs of increased intracranial pressure.
    a. Irritability.
    b. Lethargy.
    c. Vomiting.
    d. Bulging fontanelle.
5. Early surgical treatment is recommended (Chadduck, 1994).

G. Outcome.

1. Surgically correctable.

   2. Good outcome; possible absence of sequelae.
   3. Cosmetically pleasing outcome.
   4. Multiple craniosynostoses associated with numerous syndromes (Vannucci, 1997a).

Birth Injuries

A. **Definition.** Most widely used definition of birth injury: any injury that occurs during the entire phase of the birth process, comprising labor and delivery (Schullinger, 1993). Occurrence of the injury may be natural or iatrogenic.

B. **Etiology.**
1. Abnormal labor time (long or short).
2. Large size for gestational age.
3. Cephalopelvic disproportion.
4. Prematurity.
5. Birth dystocia.
6. Abnormal presentation (transverse, breech, face, and brow).
7. Instrument-assisted extraction (vacuum or forceps).

C. **Incidence.**
1. Ranges from less than 2% of live births to about 6:1000 to 8:1000 (Schullinger, 1993).
2. Ranked eleventh in major causes of neonatal death (3.7 deaths per 100,000 live births) in 1993 (Mangurten, 1997).

D. **Disease states.**
1. Cephalohematoma.
   a. Pathophysiology.
     (1) Subperiosteal hemorrhage.
     (2) Does not extend across the cranial suture lines.
     (3) Usually unilateral.
   b. Incidence: 0.4–2.5% of deliveries (Mangurten, 1997).
   c. Clinical manifestations.
     (1) Enlarges during the first few days after birth.
     (2) Feels firm.
     (3) Does not transilluminate.
   d. Patient care management.
     (1) Provide supportive care to the family and their baby.
     (2) Watch for hyperbilirubinemia.
     (3) If sudden enlargement occurs, question infection.
     (4) Educate the family.
     (5) Assess neurologic status.
   e. Outcome.
     (1) Bony calcified ring may develop; usually disappears within 6 months.
     (2) Usually takes 2 weeks to 3 months for resolution (Hernandez, 1984).
     (3) Essentially all cases resolve (Volpe, 1995).
2. Caput succedaneum.
   a. Pathophysiology.
     (1) Hemorrhagic edema crossing cranial suture lines.
     (2) Commonly seen after vaginal delivery.
   b. Clinical manifestations.
     (1) Evident at birth.
     (2) Hemorrhagic scalp edema, causing discoloration at the site.
     (3) Does not grow in size after birth.

    c. Patient care management.
       (1) No treatment is given.
       (2) Educate and counsel the family.
    d. Outcome: resolution occurs during first few days of life.
3. Subgaleal hemorrhage.
    a. Pathophysiology.
       (1) Hemorrhage beneath the scalp.
       (2) Possible entry of blood into the subcutaneous tissue of the neck.
       (3) Hematoma may cross suture lines in sufficient quantities to lead to exsanguination of the infant.
    b. Incidence.
       (1) Reported as approximately 4:10,000 deliveries (Mangurten, 1997).
       (2) Occurs much less often than caput succedaneum.
       (3) Usually associated with a difficult delivery requiring mid-forceps or vacuum extraction (Mangurten, 1997).
    c. Clinical presentation.
       (1) Often a fluctuant mass of the scalp.
       (2) May increase in size postnatally.
       (3) Hypotonia, pallor, lethargy, seizures.
    d. Patient care management.
       (1) Close observation required.
          (a) Observe for indications of bleeding.
          (b) Observe for shock.
          (c) Monitor blood pressure.
       (2) Infant may need blood transfusion on an emergent basis.
       (3) Observe for hyperbilirubinemia.
       (4) Ensure that infant receives vitamin K promptly.
    e. Outcome: Once the infant has survived the acute phase, recovery occurs in 2–3 weeks (Volpe, 1995).
4. Skull fractures.
    a. Pathophysiology.
       (1) Linear fracture can occur.
       (2) Depressed fractures occur secondary to excessive force used with forceps and extreme molding.
    b. Incidence.
       (1) Unknown.
       (2) Linear fracture fairly common finding.
       (3) Depressed fracture much less common than linear.
    c. Clinical presentation.
       (1) Linear fracture: asymptomatic.
       (2) Depressed fracture.
          (a) Presents with depressed surface of skull; indented, without craniotabes.
          (b) Does not cross the suture lines.
          (c) Possible marked separation of adjacent sutures.
          (d) Most often occurs in right parietal bone.
    d. Diagnostic studies.
       (1) X-ray examination.
       (2) CT scan.
    e. Patient care management.
       (1) Obtain neurosurgery consultation.
       (2) Assess closely for neurologic deficits.
       (3) If lesion is less than 2 cm and patient is without neurologic deficits, follow clinically; spontaneous resolution expected within a few weeks.
    f. Outcome.
       (1) Linear fractures usually heal completely within 3 months.

        (2) Depressed fracture outcome is dependent on degree of cerebral injury and success of therapy.

    5. Brachial nerve plexus injuries.

      a. Pathophysiology.

        (1) Excessive stretching of brachial plexus during delivery.

        (2) Duchenne-Erb paralysis, involving cervical nerves 5 and 6 (upper arm paralysis).

        (3) Klumpke's paralysis, involving cervical nerve 6 to thoracic nerve 1 (lower arm paralysis).

        (4) Combination of Duchenne-Erb and Klumpke's paralysis, involving the entire arm from cervical nerve 5 to thoracic nerve 1 (entire-arm paralysis).

      b. Risk factors (Laurent et al., 1993).

        (1) Multiparous mother.

        (2) Prolonged labor.

        (3) Large size for gestational age.

        (4) Shoulder dystocia.

      c. Clinical presentation.

        (1) Duchenne-Erb palsy.

          (a) Affected arm is abducted and internally rotated.

          (b) The elbow is extended, with arm pronation and wrist flexion (waiter's tip position).

          (c) Asymmetric Moro's reflex (absent in the affected arm), with a normal grasp.

        (2) Klumpke's paralysis.

          (a) Extremely rare.

          (b) Involves intrinsic muscles of the hand.

          (c) No grasp in the affected hand.

        (3) Entire-arm paralysis.

          (a) A combination of the above.

          (b) Occurs more often than isolated Klumpke's paralysis.

          (c) Entire affected arm is flaccid.

          (d) Moro and grasp reflexes are absent.

      d. Diagnostic studies.

        (1) Obtain x-ray examination of affected arm and shoulder.

        (2) Obtain serial electromyographic studies.

        (3) Rule out fracture of the clavicle or humerus.

        (4) Rule out shoulder dislocation.

        (5) Rule out cerebral injury.

      e. Patient care management.

        (1) Obtain neurology consultation.

        (2) Obtain serial electromyographic examinations to note improvements.

        (3) Begin passive range-of-motion exercise, beginning after the swelling and inflammation subside.

        (4) Exercise the arm with every diaper change.

        (5) Request a physical therapy consultation (infant may be able to benefit from splints at some point).

        (6) Educate and support the entire family.

      f. Outcome.

        (1) Generally spontaneous recovery occurs (Smith, 1989).

        (2) About 88% fully recover by 4 months, and 92% fully recover by 12 months (Volpe, 1995).

        (3) If no appreciable recovery is noted by 3 months, surgical exploration may be warranted (Volpe, 1995).

(4) Avulsion of the brachial plexus with permanent paralysis is uncommon (Gordon et al., 1973).

(5) Mild Erb's palsy may be seen.

    (a) May last only 1 day.

    (b) Majority of cases resolve during the first 3 weeks after birth.

6. Phrenic nerve paralysis.

  a. Pathophysiology.

    (1) Diaphragmatic paralysis involving overstretching of cervical nerves 3, 4, and 5.

    (2) Results from torn nerve sheaths with edema and hemorrhage.

    (3) Often associated with brachial plexus injury.

  b. Clinical presentation.

    (1) Variable, depending on severity.

    (2) Episodes of cyanosis.

    (3) Decrease in breath sounds on affected side.

    (4) Irregular, labored breathing.

    (5) Usually unilateral.

    (6) Possible association with Erb's palsy on same side.

  c. Diagnostic studies.

    (1) Chest x-ray examination.

    (2) Fluoroscopy.

    (3) Ultrasonography (especially for serial evaluation).

  d. Patient care management.

    (1) Administer oxygen and ventilatory support as needed.

    (2) Place the infant affected side down (splint the affected side).

    (3) Follow physical examination closely to note improvements.

    (4) Counsel and teach the family.

7. Traumatic facial nerve palsy.

  a. Pathophysiology.

    (1) Trauma causes hemorrhage and edema into the nerve sheath, rather than a true disruption of the nerve fiber (Volpe, 1995).

    (2) Weakness of the facial muscles results.

  b. Incidence: between 2:1000 and 8:1000 births (Falco and Eriksson, 1990).

  c. Clinical manifestations.

    (1) Varies with the degree of nerve involvement.

    (2) Usually presents the first 2 days after birth.

    (3) Persistently open eye on the affected side.

    (4) Suck with drooling.

    (5) Mouth drawn to normal side during crying.

    (6) Corner of mouth does not pull down on affected side.

    (7) Eyeball may roll up behind open eyelid.

    (8) Usually does not increase in severity.

  d. Patient care management.

    (1) Artificial tears for the open eye.

    (2) Possible need to tape or patch affected eye to protect cornea.

    (3) Support of parents.

    (4) Necessary to watch for signs of improvement.

  e. Outcome.

    (1) High rate of spontaneous recovery by 7–10 days, especially between 1 and 3 weeks of age.

    (2) Detectable deficits rarely evident after several months.

    (3) For persistence beyond a few weeks, pediatric neurology referral (Goddard-Finegold, Mizrahi, and Lee, 1998).

Intracranial Hemorrhages

A. Subdural hemorrhage.

1. Definition.
   a. Tears of cerebral veins over cerebral hemispheres (most common).
   b. Tears of venous sinuses in posterior fossa.
   c. Occurrence with or without laceration of the dura.
2. Etiology (Volpe, 1995).
   a. Large fetal head in comparison with size of birth canal and with rigid pelvic structures.
   b. Vaginal breech delivery.
   c. Malpresentation (breech, face, brow, foot).
3. Incidence.
   a. Uncommon occurrence.
   b. Usually affects term infants.
4. Clinical presentation.
   a. Often normal presentation (minimal to no clinical symptoms).
   b. On day 2 or 3: seizures (usually focal), hemiparesis, and deviation of the eyes.
   c. Dilated, poorly reactive pupil on the same side as the hemorrhage.
   d. Doll's-eye reflex: normal to abnormal.
5. Chronic subdural effusion: present within the first 6 months of life with enlarging OFC.
6. Diagnostic studies.
   a. CT scan.
   b. MRI scan.
7. Outcome.
   a. If tear or rupture is large, outlook is poor.
   b. If condition worsens, outlook is poor.
   c. Hydrocephalus occasionally develops.
   d. High percentage of infants do well.

B. Subarachnoid hemorrhage (primary).

1. Pathophysiology.
   a. Bleeding of venous origin in the subarachnoid space (not secondary to extension).
   b. May be precipitated by trauma (especially in term infants) or hypoxia (especially in premature infants) (Volpe, 1995).
2. Incidence: common type of neonatal intracranial hemorrhage.
3. Clinical presentation.
   a. Ranges from normal to seizure activity beginning on day 2 of life.
   b. Infant looks healthy between seizures: "well baby with seizures" (Volpe, 1995).
   c. Recurrent apnea (more common in preterm infants).
4. Diagnostic studies.
   a. CT scan.
   b. Diagnosis of exclusion. Other forms of intracranial bleeding are eliminated by CT scan.
5. Outcome.
   a. Good.
   b. Sequelae very uncommon (Kovnar and Volpe, 1982b).

C. Intracerebellar hemorrhage.

1. Pathophysiology.
   a. Hemorrhages within the cerebellum.

   b. Results from primary bleeding or extension of intraventricular or subarachnoid hemorrhage into the cerebellum.

   c. Association exists with respiratory distress, hypoxic events, prematurity, and traumatic delivery.

   d. Intravascular, vascular, and extravascular factors (Volpe, 1995).

     (1) Breech presentation and difficult forceps delivery secondary to a compliant skull, with external pressure causing occipital pressure.

     (2) Vitamin K deficiency, thrombocytopenia.

     (3) Vulnerable cerebral capillaries exposed to rapid colloid infusion, causing hypertensive spikes.

     (4) Richly vascularized subpial and subependymal locations.

     (5) Poor vascular support for subependymal and subpial germinal matrices.

     (6) Extension of blood into the cerebellum associated with:

       (a) Large volume of blood present with IVH.

       (b) Increased intracranial pressure.

       (c) Incomplete myelination of the cerebellum.

2. Incidence (Volpe, 1995).

   a. About 5–10% of neonatal deaths studied by autopsy.

   b. Higher in preterm infants than in term.

   c. Occurrence of 15–25% in premature infants born at less than 32 weeks' gestation or weighing less than 1.5 kg at birth.

3. Clinical presentation.

   a. Apnea.

   b. Respiratory irregularities.

   c. Bradycardia possible.

   d. Decreasing hematocrit and bloody CSF.

4. Diagnostic studies.

   a. Cranial ultrasonography (lack of symmetric echogenicity may be important).

   b. Autopsy.

5. Outcome.

   a. More favorable in term infant than in premature infant.

   b. Poor outcome in premature infant.

   c. Probable neurologic deficits.

D. **Periventricular-intraventricular hemorrhages.**

1. Pathophysiology.

   a. Prematurity: birth at less than 34 weeks' gestation; respiratory failure requiring mechanical ventilation.

   b. Associated with increasing arterial blood pressure and perinatal asphyxia.

   c. Associated clinical factors.

     (1) Prematurity.

     (2) Maternal general anesthesia (hemorrhage is probably due to indication for anesthesia, rather than anesthesia itself) (Bada et al., 1990).

     (3) Low 5-minute Apgar score.

     (4) Asphyxia.

     (5) Low birth weight.

     (6) Acidosis.

     (7) Hypotension or hypertension.

     (8) Low hematocrit (Bada et al., 1990).

     (9) Respiratory distress requiring mechanical ventilation.

     (10) Rapid administration of sodium bicarbonate.

     (11) Rapid volume expansion.

     (12) Infusion of hyperosmolar solution.

     (13) Coagulopathy.

       (14) Pneumothorax.

       (15) Ligation of patent ductus arteriosus.

       (16) Transport.

  d. Occurs once subependymal germinal matrix hemorrhage extends into lateral ventricles.

  e. Most extensive periventricular-intraventricular hemorrhage is a parenchymal intracerebral hemorrhage (Papile, 1997a).

       (1) Involves bleeding into the periventricular (i.e., intracerebellar) white matter and may also precipitate cerebral infarction.

       (2) Only 10–15% of infants with hemorrhages.

       (3) With time, on follow-up scans, may see formation of porencephalic cyst at original hemorrhage site.

  f. See Figure 19–4 for description and grading system.

       (1) Small hemorrhage: grade I or II (Papile, 1997a).

       (2) Moderate hemorrhage: grade III (Papile, 1997a).

       (3) Severe hemorrhage: grade IV (Papile, 1997a).

2. Incidence.

  a. In 1993, incidence was 19–45% of infants with birth weight less than 1500 g (Papile, 1997b).

  b. Infants born at less than 28 weeks' gestation have three times higher risk than infants born at 28–31 weeks' gestation (Papile, 1997b).

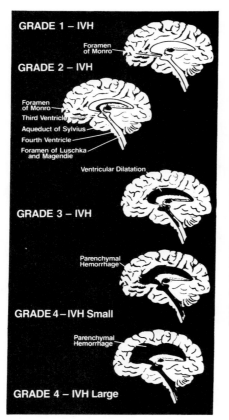

Grade I IVH: Subependymal hemorrhage in the Periventricular Germinal Matrix. Often localized at the Foramen of Monro.

Grade 2 IVH: Partial filling of lateral ventricles without ventricular dilatation.

Grade 3 IVH: Intraventricular hemorrhage with ventricular dilatation.

Grade 4 IVH (small and large): Parenchymal involvement or extension of blood into the cerebral tissue itself. Can be present to a lesser degree.

Correlation between the severity or extent of involvement and subsequent impairment is not absolute. Because outcomes are so varied, assessment of early symptoms and the practice of purposeful interventions are extremely important.

Figure 19–4

Quantification of extent of intraventricular hemorrhage (IVH). Four grades of hemorrhagic involvement categorized IVH as differentiated by Papile and Burstein. (Used and reprinted with permission of Ross Laboratories, Columbus, OH 43216, from New Perspectives on Intraventricular Hemorrhage. © 1988, Ross Laboratories.)

c. Only 2–3% normal term infants have a periventricular-intraventricular hemorrhage (Heibel et al., 1993).
   (1) More than half of these hemorrhages originated at the subependymal germinal matrix.
   (2) The remainder originated at the choroid plexus.
3. Timing of onset (Papile, 1997b).
   a. About 40% occur before 12 hours of age in infants weighing less than 1250 g (three times higher risk of being more severe if early occurrence).
   b. About 50% occur by 24 hours of age.
   c. About 80% occur by 48 hours of age.
   d. About 90% occur by 72 hours of age.
   e. By 10 days of age, all have occurred.
   f. By 7 days of age, 99.5% have occurred.
4. Clinical presentation.
   a. Presentation ranges from unnoticeable to dramatic.
      (1) Sudden deterioration.
      (2) Oxygen desaturation.
      (3) Bradycardia.
      (4) Metabolic acidosis.
      (5) Significant decrease in hematocrit.
      (6) Hypotonia.
      (7) Shock.
      (8) Hyperglycemia.
      (9) Tense anterior fontanelle.
   b. Symptoms of worsening hemorrhage.
      (1) Full, tense fontanelles.
      (2) Increased ventilatory support.
      (3) Seizures.
      (4) Apnea.
      (5) Decrease in level of consciousness and/or activity.
5. Diagnostic studies.
   a. Optimal time to screen: 7 days of age, because 90% of all hemorrhages have occurred (Papile, 1997a).
      (1) If test result is normal, there is no need to recheck.
      (2) If test result is positive for periventricular-intraventricular hemorrhage, repeat test in 2 weeks.
   b. Cranial ultrasonography.
   c. CT scan.
   d. Lumbar puncture (CSF studies show elevated red blood cells, increased protein concentration, xanthochromia, and decreased glucose concentration) (Kovnar and Volpe, 1982b).
   e. Rule out septic shock or meningitis.
6. Outcome.
   a. Mortality rate is 50% with severe hemorrhage, 15% with moderate hemorrhage, and 5% with small hemorrhage.
   b. These hemorrhages are an important cause of morbidity and death in low birth weight infants.
   c. Hemorrhage alone does not account for all neurologic deficits.
   d. Approximately 50% of premature infants are free of neurologic symptoms (Papile, 1997a).
   e. Approximately 25–30% very low birth weight infants discharged from a level III NICU have a periventricular-intraventricular hemorrhage without major neurodevelopmental sequelae. (Papile, 1997a).
   f. Conditions involving infarction, porencephaly (the ventricles of the brain and the subarachnoid space are connected by a small opening), and parenchymal damage most closely account for neurologic deficits (Enzmann, 1989).

    g. Outcome depends on degree of severity of hemorrhage.
      (1) Small hemorrhage (Papile, Munsick-Bruno, and Schaefer, 1983).
        (a) Neurodevelopmental disability similar to that in premature infants without hemorrhage.
        (b) Major neurodevelopmental disability in 10%.
      (2) Moderate hemorrhage.
        (a) Major neurodevelopmental disability in 40% during infancy (Papile et al., 1983).
        (b) Mortality rate 10%, with progressive hydrocephalus in fewer than 20% (Hill and Volpe, 1992b).
      (3) Severe hemorrhage.
        (a) Major neurodevelopment disability in 80% (Papile et al., 1983).
        (b) Mortality rate 50–60%, with hydrocephalus common in survivors (Hill and Volpe, 1992b).

7. Prenatal pharmacologic interventions (Papile, 1997a).
    a. Phenobarbital.
      (1) Unsupported postnatal use at this time to prevent periventricular-intraventricular hemorrhage.
      (2) May worsen condition.
    b. Vitamin K: unclear benefit.
    c. Indomethacin: further studies necessary.
    d. Ethamsylate: unavailable in the United States.
    e. Vitamin E: further studies needed to clarify efficacy.
    f. Pancuronium.
      (1) Safety and risk/benefit rate need to be proved.
      (2) Serious side effects, including edema and renal failure, are associated.

8. Patient care management.
    a. Prevent preterm birth, perinatal asphyxia, and birth trauma.
    b. Promote in utero transport.
    c. Promote nonstressful intrapartum course.
    d. Provide efficient, expedient intubation.
    e. Minimize handling; cluster scheduled patient-care measures.
    f. Minimize noxious stimuli (dim the lights, quiet the environment).
    g. Avoid noxious procedures when possible.
    h. Avoid events associated with wide swings in arterial and venous pressures.
      (1) Seizures.
      (2) Excess motor activity.
      (3) Apnea.
      (4) Crying.
      (5) Pneumothorax.
    i. Avoid administration of hyperosmolar solutions.
    j. Prevent blood pressure swings: give volume replacement slowly.
    k. Avoid overventilation leading to pneumothorax.
    l. Use two people for endotracheal suctioning.
    m. Use noninvasive monitoring of oxygen and carbon dioxide levels (maintain within normal limits).
    n. Monitor and maintain normal pH.
    o. Correct abnormal clotting.
    p. Be alert to signs of a hemorrhage.
    q. Educate and support the parents.

Seizures

A. **Definition:** symptom of neurologic dysfunction (not a disease).

B. Pathophysiology.

1. Seizures result from excessive simultaneous electrical discharge or depolarization of neurons.
2. Metabolic encephalopathies.
   a. Decreased production of adenosine triphosphate.
      (1) Ischemia.
      (2) Hypoxemia.
      (3) Hypoglycemia.
   b. Hyponatremia or hypernatremia.
   c. Hypocalcemia, hypomagnesemia.
   d. Inborn errors of metabolism.
   e. Pyridoxine dependency.
   f. Hyperammonemia.
3. Structural.
   a. Intraventricular hemorrhage (IVH).
   b. Intrapartum trauma.
   c. Cerebral cortical dysgenesis: result of abnormal neuronal migration.
   d. Hypoxic-ischemic encephalopathy, the most common diagnosis of neonatal seizures (Yager and Vannucci, 1997).
4. Intracerebral meningitis.
   a. Bacterial infection.
      (1) Group B beta-streptococci and *Escherichia coli*: 65% of the cases (Hill and Volpe, 1992c).
      (2) *Listeria monocytogenes*.
   b. Nonbacterial infection: TORCH.
5. Withdrawal from maternal drugs.
   a. Uncommon cause of seizures (may cause jitteriness).
   b. Onset during first 3 days of life.
   c. Drugs.
      (1) Narcotic-analgesics.
      (2) Sedative-hypnotics.
      (3) Alcohol.
6. Familial (genetic).
   a. Onset in second and third days of life.
   b. Infant appears well between seizures.
   c. Self-limiting: within 1–6 months, seizures stop.
   d. Autosomal dominant inheritance.

C. Clinical presentation.

1. Subtle.
   a. Most frequent of neonatal seizures.
   b. Present at some degree in most term and premature newborn infants having seizures.
   c. Often unrecognized.
   d. Presentation varies.
      (1) Horizontal deviation of the eyes.
      (2) Pedaling movements.
      (3) Rowing, stepping movements.
      (4) Eye blinking or fluttering.
      (5) Nonnutritive sucking.
      (6) Smacking of lips.
      (7) Drooling.
      (8) Apnea (convulsive apnea usually does not occur by itself).
2. Tonic.
   a. Characteristic in premature infants weighing 500 g.

b. Often seen with severe IVH.

c. Generalized tonic extension of all extremities or flexion of upper limbs with extension of lower extremities.

d. Often mimics decorticate posturing.

3. Multifocal clonic.

a. Characteristic in term infants with hypoxic-ischemic encephalopathy.

b. Clonic movements migrating from one limb to another without a specific pattern.

4. Focal clonic.

a. Uncommon.

b. Presents as localized clonic jerking.

5. Myoclonic.

a. Very rare in neonatal period.

b. Multiple jerks of upper or lower limb flexion.

D. Diagnostic studies.

1. Perform physical examination.

a. Rule out jitteriness.

(1) Characterized by trembling of hands and feet.

(2) No involvement of eye movements.

(3) Stopped by gentle, passive flexion of affected extremity.

b. Note infant's history, which may provide a predisposed underlying etiology.

2. Laboratory work.

a. Serum glucose level.

b. Electrolyte levels (sodium, potassium, chloride, calcium, magnesium).

c. Arterial blood gas analysis.

d. Urea, ammonia.

3. Diagnostic study for sepsis.

a. Lumbar puncture.

b. Culture of blood, urine, and CSF specimens; bacterial and viral.

c. Complete blood cell count and platelet count.

4. Electroencephalography, CT scan, cranial ultrasonography, MRI.

5. Skull films if etiology is trauma.

6. Twelve-lead electrocardiography.

7. Consideration of following laboratory tests:

a. Blood pyruvate.

b. Lactate.

c. TORCH.

d. Urinary drug screen.

8. Neurology consultation.

E. Patient care management.

1. Determine underlying etiology.

2. Resuscitate as necessary.

3. Obtain diagnostic studies as ordered.

4. Provide pharmaceutical therapy (Young and Mangum, 1997).

a. Phenobarbital.

(1) Load: 20 mg/kg slow IV for 10–15 minutes.

(2) Close monitoring of respiratory status.

(3) Maintenance dosage: 3–5 mg/kg per day, beginning 12–24 hours after the loading dose.

(4) Therapeutic range: 15–30 μg/mL.

(5) Excretion.

(a) Metabolized by liver: 50–70%.

(b) Unchanged in urine: 20–30%.

(6) Consider as the drug of choice (Yager and Vannucci, 1997).

b. Phenytoin. *Many facilities are replacing phenytoin with fosphenytoin. Check with your physician or pharmacist.*
   (1) Load: 15–20 mg/kg IV (for 30 minutes or longer).
   (2) Maintenance.
       (a) Dosage: 4–8 mg/kg per day.
       (b) Recommended administration routes.
           (i) By IV slow push.
           (ii) By mouth.
   (3) Therapeutic range.
       (a) 6–15 mg/mL.
       (b) 10–20 mg/mL.
   (4) Excretion.
       (a) Protein bound (approximately 90%).
       (b) Displaced by bilirubin, increasing free drug levels.
c. Fosphenytoin.
   (1) Load: approximately 20 mg/kg (phenytoin equivalents) for status epilepticus and 10–20 mg/kg (phenytoin equivalents) for correction of subtherapeutic levels (Pellock, 1996). Continuous electrocardiographic, blood pressure, and respiratory status monitoring with loading doses (Boucher, 1996).
   (2) Maintenance.
       (a) Dosage: 4–6 mg/kg per day (phenytoin equivalents) (Pellock, 1996).
       (b) Rate of administration: up to 3 mg/kg per minute for children (Cloyd, 1996).
       (c) Recommended administration routes (Pellock, 1996).
           (i) IM: not an option for neonates due to lack of muscle tissue.
           (ii) IV: complicated for neonates due to fragile skin.
           (iii) Water soluble and thus compatible with common IV solutions.
       (d) Therapeutic range and excretion.
           (i) Peak plasma concentrations: about the time that IV infusion is complete; half-life is 6–21 minutes (Cloyd, 1996).
           (ii) Rapidly converted by the body to generate therapeutic levels of phenytoin (Runge and Allen, 1996).
           (iii) See section b, Phenytoin, above.
d. Lorazepam.
   (1) Administer: 0.05–0.1 mg/kg slow push IV (for status epilepticus).
   (2) Repeat dose based on clinical response.
   (3) Note routes of excretion.
       (a) By kidneys.
       (b) Lipid soluble.
   (4) Lorazepam produces anticonvulsant effect in minutes after administration.
   (5) Monitor oxygenation and vital signs.
   (6) Document precisely.
   (7) Educate and inform the family.
   (8) Provide support as needed.

E. Outcome.

1. Related to underlying etiology.
2. Refer to Table 19–4.

Hypoxic-Ischemic Encephalopathy

A. Definitions of hypoxic-ischemic encephalopathy (HIE).

1. Hypoxemia and anoxia (diminished oxygen in blood supply; partial or complete). Moderate to severe hypoxia leads to metabolic acidosis.

Table 19–4
PROGNOSIS FOR INFANT WITH NEONATAL SEIZURES: RELATION TO NEUROLOGIC DISEASE

Neurologic Disease*	Normal Development (%)†
Hypoxic-ischemic encephalopathy	50
Intraventricular hemorrhage‡	10
Primary subarachnoid hemorrhage	90
Hypocalcemia	
Early onset	50§
Later onset	100
Hypoglycemia	50
Bacterial meningitis	50
Developmental defect	0

*Prognosis is for those cases with the stated neurologic disease when seizures are a manifestation (thus, value usually will differ from *overall* prognosis for the disease).
†Values are rounded off to nearest 5%.
‡Usually severe intraventricular hemorrhage associated with major periventricular hemorrhagic infarction.
§Represents primarily the prognosis of complicating illness; prognosis approaches that of later-onset hypocalcemia if no or only minor neurologic illness is present.
From Volpe, J.J.: Neurology of the Newborn, 3rd ed. Philadelphia, W.B. Saunders, 1995.

  2. Ischemia (diminished blood supply perfusing the brain).
    a. Systemic hypotension.
    b. Occlusive vascular disease.
  3. Hypoxia and ischemia, which lead to neurologic dysfunction.
  4. Asphyxia.
    a. Impairment of gas exchange of respiratory gases—oxygen and carbon dioxide.
    b. Mixed respiratory and metabolic acidosis.
    c. Failure of systemic multiorgan systems, including heart, lungs, liver, and kidneys.

B. **Incidence of HIE (Vannucci, 1997b).**

  1. About 2–4% of term infants.
  2. Approximately 60% of very low birth weight infants.
  3. Timing of occurrence.
    a. Antepartum occurrence: 20%.
    b. Intrapartum occurrence: 30%.
    c. Antepartum-intrapartum occurrence: 35%.
    d. Postpartum occurrence: 10%.

C. **Clinical staging (Sarnat and Sarnat, 1976).**

  1. Stage I (mild encephalopathy): characteristic features.
    a. Hyperalert state.
    b. Normal muscle tone, active suck, strong Moro reflex, normal/strong grasp, and normal doll's-eye reflex.
    c. Increased tendon reflexes.
    d. Myoclonus present.
    e. Hyperresponsiveness to stimulation.
    f. Tachycardia possible.
    g. Dilation of pupils, reactive.
    h. Sparse secretions.
    i. No convulsions (unless due to hypoglycemia or preexisting conditions that predisposed the infant to the perinatal distress).
    j. Electroencephalographic findings: within normal limits.

2. Stage II (moderate encephalopathy).
   a. Characteristic features.
      (1) Lethargy.
      (2) Hypotonia.
      (3) Increased tendon reflexes.
      (4) Myoclonus.
      (5) Seizure activity frequent.
      (6) Weak suck.
      (7) Incomplete Moro reflex.
      (8) Strong grasp.
      (9) Overactive doll's-eye reflex.
      (10) Pupils constrictive and reactive.
      (11) Respirations variable in rate and depth; respirations may be periodic.
   b. Critical period: infant's condition either improves or deteriorates.
   c. Indications of deterioration.
      (1) No signs of improvement.
      (2) Development of:
         (a) Seizures.
         (b) Cerebral edema.
         (c) Lethargy.
         (d) Abnormalities on electroencephalogram.
   d. Recovery.
      (1) No further seizure activity.
      (2) Electroencephalographic findings return to normal.
      (3) Transient jitteriness.
      (4) Improvement in level of consciousness.
3. Stage III (severe encephalopathy).
   a. Clinical course.
      (1) Level of consciousness deteriorates from obtunded to stuporous to comatose.
      (2) Mechanical ventilation is required to sustain life.
   b. Clinical features.
      (1) Apnea/bradycardia.
      (2) Seizures appearing within the first 12 postnatal hours. Seizures occur in 50–60% of patients who do ultimately seize within the first 6–12 hours. Premature infants present with generalized seizures. Term infants demonstrate multifocal clonic seizures. All these infants display subtle seizures (Volpe, 1995).
      (3) Severe hypotonia and flaccidity. Suck, Moro, and grasp reflexes absent.
      (4) Stuporous to comatose.
      (5) Absent or depressed reflexes.
      (6) Doll's-eye reflex weak or absent.
      (7) Pupils often unequal; variable reactivity and poor light reflex.
   c. Deterioration (Volpe, 1995).
      (1) Deterioration occurs within 24–72 hours.
      (2) Severely affected infants often worsen, sinking into deep stupor or coma.
      (3) Death may ensue.
   d. Survivors.
      (1) Infants who survive to this point often improve in the next several days to months.
      (2) Feeding difficulties often develop secondary to abnormalities of suck and swallow. These are due to the poor muscle tone connected to involvement of cranial nerves for these functions.
      (3) Generalized hypotonia is common; hypertonia is uncommon.
      (4) Severe neurologic disabilities may ensue.

D. Diagnostic studies (Vannucci, 1997b).

1. Valuable in assessing the nature of the brain insult and the extent of the brain injury.
2. Used to track the evolution of HIE.
   a. Precise history.
   b. Complete neurologic examination.
   c. Electroencephalography.
      (1) Confirm or deny clinical diagnosis of seizures.
      (2) Provide prognostic information regarding severity of permanent brain damage.
   d. Evoked potentials.
   e. Creatinine kinase and other biochemical/enzyme markers.
   f. Lumbar puncture, CSF analysis.
   g. CT scan.
   h. Cranial ultrasonography.
   i. Technetium scan.
   j. MRI.
   k. Intracranial pressure monitoring.

E. Patient care management.

1. Prevent perinatal hypoxia, ischemia, and asphyxia (anticipation of risk factors, appropriate intervention).
2. Perform prompt, efficient resuscitation by trained staff.
3. Maintain physiologic oxygenation and acid-base balance.
4. Correct fluid, electrolyte, and caloric abnormalities.
5. Monitor blood volume; avoid blood pressure swings and hypotension.
6. Maintain optimal perfusion.
7. Treat seizures.
8. Perform a thorough neurologic examination.
9. Monitor and manage disturbances of other body organs.
   a. Pulmonary.
   b. Cardiac.
   c. Hepatic.
   d. Renal.
10. Educate and support the family.
11. Obtain neurology consultation.

F. Outcome (Volpe, 1995).

1. Based on severity of brain insult; selective neuronal necrosis.
2. Death within newborn period in 20–50% of asphyxiated infants who exhibit HIE.
3. Overall neurologic sequelae with HIE at 3½ years of age: approximately 17%.
4. Factors associated with poor outcome.
   a. Apgar score.
      (1) If score is 0–3 for 20 minutes or more, approximately 60% die.
      (2) If score is less than 3 at 1 minute and less than 5 at 5 minutes, with abnormal neurologic signs (feeding difficulties, apnea, hypotonia, seizures):
         (a) About 20% die.
         (b) About 40% are normal.
         (c) About 40% have neurologic sequelae.
   b. Encephalopathy.
      (1) Mild: no subsequent deficits.
      (2) Severe: 75% die, 25% have sequelae.
      (3) Term infants: 60% normal, 30% abnormal, and 10% die.

(4) Premature infants: 50% normal, 20% abnormal, and 30% die.
(5) Duration of abnormal neurologic signs: good indicator of severity of HIE injury.
(6) Disappearance of abnormal neurologic signs by 1–2 weeks: good chance of being normal (possibility of learning disabilities not ruled out).
5. Seizures early (first 12 hours of life) and/or difficult to control: associated with poorer prognosis.
6. Hyperactivity and attention difficulties: in infants with less severe encephalopathy (Kovnar and Volpe, 1982a).
7. Rapid initial improvement indicative of better outcomes.
8. Long-term sequelae based on:
   a. Site.
   b. Extent of cerebral injury.
   c. Duration of abnormal clinical presentation.

Periventricular Leukomalacia

A. Definition of periventricular leukomalacia (PVL).

1. Ischemic, necrotic periventricular white matter.
2. Principally ischemic lesion of arterial origin.
3. Multicystic encephalomalacia with or without secondary hemorrhage into ischemic area.

B. Pathophysiology.

1. Predisposition.
   a. Systemic hypotension severe enough to impair cerebral blood flow (Volpe, 1992).
   b. Occurrence of focal cerebral infarction and cerebral ischemia.
   c. Major systemic hypotension.
   d. Episodes of apnea and bradycardia.
2. Occurrence secondary to inadequate cerebral perfusion.
3. Manifestation of hypoxic-ischemic encephalopathy in preemies.

C. Incidence.

1. Unknown.
2. About 80–90% of PVL in premature infants (Papile, 1997a).
3. Often manifested beyond first week of life (Papile, 1997a).

D. Clinical presentation.

1. Possibly asymptomatic.
2. Weakness of lower extremities (Hill and Volpe, 1992a).

E. Diagnostic studies.

1. Cranial ultrasonography.
2. CT scan.
3. MRI.

F. Outcome.

1. Spastic dysplegia (major motor deficit common in premature infants with PVL).
2. Motor deficits in premature infants; possible spontaneous resolution in first several years of life.
3. Significant upper arm involvement associated with intellectual deficits.
4. Visual impairment.
5. Lower limb weakness.

6. Outcome based on:
   a. Location.
   b. Extent of injury.

Meningitis

A. Definition.

1. Infection of CNS.
2. Early-onset infection from pathogens in vaginal flora (e.g., group B beta-streptococci and *Escherichia coli*).
3. Late-onset infection from environmental microbes found in nursery environment (e.g., *Pseudomonas aeruginosa* and *Staphylococcus aureus*).

B. Pathophysiology.

1. Organisms reach the fetus.
   a. Transplacental organisms lead to congenital infection.
   b. Ascending organisms from the vagina or cervix lead to early-onset infection.
   c. Late-onset infection develops in infants infected by passage through birth canal.
   d. Organism introduction after birth from surrounding environment leads to iatrogenic infection.
2. Precipitating factors include:
   a. Maternal infection.
   b. Prolonged ruptured membranes.
   c. Prematurity.
3. Organisms.
   a. Bacteria.
      (1) Aerobic.
         (a) Group B beta-streptococci (most common).
         (b) *E. coli* (second most common).
         (c) *Listeria monocytogenes* (third most common).
      (2) Anaerobic.
   b. Viruses.
      (1) TORCH infection.
      (2) Enterovirus.
   c. Fungi.

C. Congenital presentation.

1. Congenital viral infection.
   a. Preterm delivery.
   b. Possible low birth weight.
   c. Blueberry-muffin rash.
   d. Inflammation of other affected organs.
   e. Microcephaly.
2. Early-onset bacterial meningitis.
   a. Presentation with shock in first 24 hours.
   b. Possible rapid progression to shock.
   c. Respiratory distress.
   d. Hypotension.
   e. Apnea.
   f. Seizures.
   g. Temperature instability.
   h. Diarrhea.

     i. Hepatomegaly.
     j. Jaundice.
  3. Late-onset meningitis.
     a. Nonspecific symptoms.
     b. Lethargy.
     c. Feeding intolerance.
     d. Irritability.
     e. Posturing.
     f. Temperature instability.
     g. Apnea.
     h. Bradycardia.
     i. Bulging fontanelles.
     j. Nuchal rigidity.

D. **Diagnostic studies.**

  1. CSF.
     a. Organism found on Gram stain.
     b. Low glucose level.
     c. Elevated protein concentration and white blood cell count.
     d. Culture for specific identification of organism.
     e. Counterimmune electrophoresis.
  2. Complete diagnostic study for sepsis.

E. **Patient care management.**

  1. Promote prevention.
  2. Detect early and treat.
  3. Perform thorough physical examination.
  4. Observe for seizure activity.
  5. Obtain infectious disease consultation.
  6. Provide pharmaceutical agents (Nelson, 1996).
     a. Initial therapy.
       (1) Ampicillin or penicillin G (IV).
       (2) *In addition,* aminoglycoside (IV or IM).
       (3) Ampicillin and cefotaxime recommended for aminoglycoside-resistant organism.
       (4) Treatment 7–10 days for sepsis without a focus; minimum of 21 days for gram-negative meningitis.
     b. Group B beta-streptococcus.
       (1) Ampicillin or penicillin G (IV or IM).
       (2) *In addition:* gentamicin (IV or IM) (discontinue if sensitivities warrant).
     c. Coliform bacteria (e.g., *E. coli*).
       (1) Cefotaxime (IM or IV).
       (2) *In addition,* aminoglycoside as a suitable alternative.
     d. *L. monocytogenes* and enterococci.
       (1) Ampicillin (IV or IM).
       (2) *In addition,* aminoglycoside (IV or IM).
     e. *Staphylococcus epidermidis.*
       (1) Vancomycin (IV or IM).
       (2) Methicillin resistance in many strains.
     f. *S. aureus.*
       (1) Methicillin (IV or IM).
       (2) Vancomycin if methicillin-resistant strain.
       (3) Rarely cause of meningitis in the newborn infant (vancomycin for meningitis).
     g. *P. aeruginosa.*
       (1) Mezlocillin or ticarcillin (IV or IM).
       (2) *In addition:* aminoglycoside (IV or IM).

    h. *Bacteroides fragilis* (anaerobic).

      (1) Metronidazole, clindamycin, mezlocillin, or ticarcillin (IV or IM).

      (2) For CNS infection, metronidazole recommended.

7. Sample CSF at specific intervals until sterile.
8. Treat at least 2 weeks after sterilization of CSF.
9. Obtain and test CSF sample 48 hours after antibiotic therapy has been discontinued.
10. Educate and support the family.

F. **Outcome.**

1. Dependent on rapidity of detection and initiation of adequate drug therapy.
2. Survivors of bacterial meningitis: 50% have significant neurologic sequelae.
   a. Hydrocephalus.
   b. Seizures.
   c. Sensorineural hearing loss.
   d. Visual losses.
   e. Mental and motor disabilities.

REFERENCES

Avery, G.A., Fletcher, M.A., and MacDonald, M.G.: Neonatology: Pathophysiology and Management of the Newborn, 4th ed. Philadelphia, J.B. Lippincott, 1994.

Boucher, B.A.: Fosphenytoin: A novel phenytoin prodrug. Pharmacotherapy, *16*:777–791, 1996.

Chadduck, W.M.: Craniosynostosis. *In* Cheek, W.R. (Ed.): Pediatric Neurosurgery: Surgery of the Developing Nervous System. Philadelphia, W.B. Saunders, 1994, pp. 111–123.

Cloyd, J.: Pharmacologic considerations of fosphenytoin therapy. Pharmcol. Ther., *21*(5S):13S–20S, 1996.

De Vivo, D.C., Trifiletti, R.R., Jacobson, R.I., et al.: Defective glucose transport across the blood-brain barrier as a cause of persistent hypoglycorrhachia, seizures, and developmental delay. N. Engl. J. Med., *325*:703–709, 1991.

Enzmann, D.R.: Imaging of hypoxic-ischemic cerebral damage. *In* Stevenson, D.K., and Sunshine, P. (Eds.): Fetal and Neonatal Brain Injury: Mechanisms, Management and the Risks of Practice. Philadelphia, B.C. Decker, 1989, pp. 196–220.

Falco, N.A., Eriksson, E.: Facial nerve palsy in the newborn: Incidence and outcome. Plast. Reconstr. Surg., *85*(1):1–4, 1990.

Fenichel, G.M.: Neonatal Neurology, 3rd ed. New York, Churchill Livingstone, 1990.

Goddard-Finegold, J.: The intrauterine nervous system. *In* Taeusch, W.H., and Ballard, R.A. (Eds.): Avery's Diseases of the Newborn, 7th ed. Philadelphia, W.B. Saunders, 1998, pp. 802–832.

Goddard-Finegold, J., Mizrahi, E.M., and Lee, R.T.: The newborn nervous system. *In* Taeusch, W.H., and Ballard, R.A. (Eds.): Avery's Diseases of the Newborn, 7th ed. Philadelphia, W.B. Saunders, 1998, pp. 839–891.

Gordon, M., Rich, H., Deutschberger, J., et al.: The immediate and long-term outcome of obstetric birth trauma. Am. J. Obstet. Gynecol., *117*:51–56, 1973.

Heibel, M., Heber, R., Bechinger, D., et al.: Early diagnosis of perinatal cerebral lesions in apparently normal full-term newborns by ultrasound of the brain. Neuroradiology, *35*:85–91, 1993.

Hill, A., and Volpe, J.J.: Hypoxic-ischaemic cerebral injury. *In* Roberton, N.R.C. (Ed.): Textbook of Neonatology. New York, Churchill Livingstone, 1992a, pp. 1061–1075.

Kovnar, E., and Volpe, J.J.: Current concepts in neonatal neurology. I. Hypoxic-ischemic brain injury. Perinatology-Neonatology, *6*(4):51–63, 1982a.

Kreusser, K.L., Tarby, T.J., Kovnar, E., et al.: Serial lumbar punctures for at least temporary amelioration of neonatal posthemorrhagic hydrocephalus. Pediatrics, *75*:719–723, 1985.

Laurent, J.P., Lee, R., Shenaq, S., et al.: Neurosurgical correction of upper brachial plexus birth injuries. J. Neurosurg., *79*:197–203, 1993.

Mangurten, H.H.: Birth injuries. *In* Fanaroff, A.A., and Martin, J.R. (Eds.): Neonatal-Perinatal Medicine: Diseases of the Fetus and Infant, 6th ed. St. Louis, Mosby–Year Book, 1997, pp. 425–454.

McLone, D.G.: Continuing concepts in the management of spina bifida. Pediatr. Neurosurg., *18*:254–256, 1992.

Nelson, J.D.: Pocketbook of Pediatric Antimicrobial Therapy, 12th ed. Baltimore, Williams & Wilkins, 1996.

Papile, L.: Intracranial hemorrhage. *In* Fanaroff, A.A., and Martin, R.J. (Eds.): Neonatal-Perinatal Medicine Diseases of the Fetus and Infant, 6th ed. St. Louis, Mosby–Year Book, 1997a, pp. 891–899.

Papile, L.: Prevention of IVH: Pharmacologic strategies. Paper presented at a meeting of the National Association of Neonatal Nurses, Phoenix, September 1997b.

Papile, L., Munsick-Bruno, G., and Schaefer, A.: Relationship of cerebral intraventricular hemorrhage and early childhood neurologic handicaps. J. Pediatr., *103*:273–277, 1983.

Pellock, J.M.: Seizure therapy in the pediatric setting. Pharmacol. Ther., *21*(5S):21S–23S, 1996.

Runge, J.W., and Allen, F.H.: Emergency treatment of status epilepticus. Neurology, *46*(6):S20–S23, 1996.

Sarnat, H.B., and Sarnat, M.S.: Neonatal encephalopathy following fetal distress. Arch. Neurol., *33*:696–705, 1976.

Sarnat, H.S.: Embryology and malformations of the CNS. *In* Fanaroff, A.A., and Martin, R.J. (Eds.): Neonatal-Perinatal Medicine: Diseases of the Fetus and Infant, 6th ed. St. Louis, Mosby–Year Book, 1997, pp. 826–856.

Schullinger, J.N.: Birth trauma. Pediatr. Clin. North Am., *40*:1351–1358, 1993.

Shinnar, S., Molteni, R.A., Gammon, K., et al.: Intraventricular hemorrhage in the premature infant. N. Engl. J. Med., *306*:1464–1468, 1982.

Smith, S.A.: Peripheral neuropathies in children. *In* Swaiman, K.F. (Ed.): Pediatric Neurology: Principles and Practice, vol. 2. St. Louis, C.V. Mosby, 1989, pp. 1105–1123.

Vannucci, R.C.: Disorders of head size and shape. *In* Fanaroff, A.A., and Martin, R.J. (Eds.): Neonatal-Perinatal Medicine: Diseases of the Fetus and Infant, 6th ed. St. Louis, Mosby–Year Book, 1997a, pp. 924–931.

Vannucci, R.C.: Hypoxia-ischemia: Clinical aspects. *In* Fanaroff, A.A., and Martin, R.J. (Eds.): Neonatal-

Perinatal Medicine: Diseases of the Fetus and Infant, 6th ed. St. Louis, Mosby–Year Book, 1997b, pp. 877–891.

Volpe, J.J.: Brain injury in the premature infant: Current concepts of pathogenesis and prevention. Biol. Neonate, *62*:231–242, 1992.

Volpe, J.J.: Neurology of the Newborn, 3rd ed. Philadelphia, W.B. Saunders, 1995, pp. 3, 68.

Whaley, L.F., and Wong, D.L.: Nursing Care of Infants and Children, 5th ed. St. Louis, Mosby, 1995.

Yager, J.Y., and Vannucci, R.C.: Seizures in neonatal period. *In* Fanaroff, A.A., and Martin, R.J. (Eds.): Neonatal-Perinatal Medicine: Diseases of the Fetus and Infant, 6th ed. St. Louis, Mosby–Year Book, 1997, pp. 899–911.

Yen, I.G., Khoury, M.J., Erickson, D., et al.: The changing epidemiology of neural tube defects. Neural Tube Defects, *146*:857–861, 1992.

Young, T.E., and Mangum, O.B.: Neofax: A Manual of Drugs Used in Neonatal Care, 10th ed. Raleigh, N.C., Acorn Publishing, 1997.

ADDITIONAL READINGS

Allan, W.C., and Volpe, J.J.: Periventricular-intraventricular hemorrhage. Pediatr. Clin. North Am., *36*(1):47–63, 1986.

Altman, D.S., Perlman, J.M., Volpe, J.J., et al.: Cerebral oxygen metabolism in newborns. Pediatrics, *92*:99–104, 1993.

Ashwal, S.: Brain death in the newborn. Clin. Perinatol., *16*:501–518, 1989.

Ashwal, S., and Schneider, S.: Brain death in the newborn. Pediatrics, *84*:429–437, 1989.

Barone, M.A. (Ed.): The Harriet Lane Handbook, 14th ed. St. Louis, Mosby, 1996.

Bartoshesky, L.E., Haller, J., Scott, M., and Wojick, C.: Seizures in children with meningomyelocele. Am. J. Dis. Child., *139*:400–402, 1985.

Beeby, P.J., Elliott, E.J., Henderson-Smart, D.J., et al.: Predictive value of umbilical artery pH in preterm infants. Arch. Dis. Child., *71*:F93–F96, 1994.

Blackburn, S.T., and Loper, D.P.: Maternal, Fetal and Neonatal Physiology. Philadelphia, W.B. Saunders, 1992.

Bralet, J., Schreiber, L., and Bouvier, C.: Effect of acidosis and anoxia on iron delocalization from brain homogenates. Biochem. Pharm., *43*:979–983, 1992.

Brann, A.W.: Hypoxic-ischemic encephalopathy (asphyxia). Pediatr. Clin. North Am., *33*:451–464, 1986.

Carey, B.E.: Neurologic assessment. *In* Trappero, E.P., and Honeyfield, M.E. (Eds.): Physical Assessment of the Newborn. Petaluma, Calif., NICU Ink, 1993, pp. 121–138.

Carter, B.S., Portman, R.J., Gaylord, M.S., and Merenstein, G.B.: Prospectively predicting asphyxial severity. Clin. Res., *35*(1):75A,1987.

Carter, B.S., Portman, R.J., Gaylord, M.S., et al.: Prediction of perinatal asphyxial severity [abstract]. Pediatr. Res., *20*:376A, 1986.

Casaer, P., Eggermont, E., and Volpe, J.J.: Neonatal clinical neurological assessment. *In* Roberton, N.R.C. (Ed.): Textbook of Neonatology. New York, Churchill Livingstone, 1992, pp. 1035–1041.

Charney, E.B., Weller, S.C., Sutton, L.N., et al.: Management of the newborn with myelomeningocele: Time for a decision-making process. Pediatrics, *75*:58–64, 1985.

Cotten, J.M.: A comprehensive nursing approach to the neonate with myelomeningocele. Neonatal Network, *2*(4):7–16, 1984.

Coulter, D.M.: Birth trauma. *In* Cloherty, J.P., and Stark, A.R. (Eds.): Manual of Neonatal Care. Boston, Little, Brown, 1980, pp. 251–255.

de Courten-Myers, G.M., Kleinholz, M., Wagner, K.R., et al.: Normoglycemia (not hypoglycemia) optimizes outcome from middle cerebral artery occlusion. J. Cereb. Blood Flow Metab., *14*:227–236, 1994.

De Praeter, C., Vanhaesebrouck, P., Govaert, P., et al.: Creatine kinase isoenzyme BB concentrations in the cerebrospinal fluid of newborns: Relationship to short-term outcome. Pediatrics, *88*:1204–1210, 1991.

DeVries, S.L., Dubowitz, L.M.S., Dubowitz, V., et al.: Predictive value of cranial ultrasound in the newborn baby: A reappraisal. Lancet, *137*(2):137–140, 1985.

Diebler, C., and Dulac, O.: Pediatric Neurology and Neuroradiology: Cerebral and Cranial Diseases. Berlin, Springer-Verlag, 1987.

Drugs and Therapeutics: A Medical Letter on Drugs for Viral Infections. The Medical Letter, 1000 Main St., New Rochelle, NY 10801; vol. 32 (ISSN 824), 1990.

Dubowitz, L.M.S., Dubowitz, V., Palmer, P.G., et al.: Correlation of neurologic assessment in the preterm newborn infant with outcome at 1 year. J. Pediatr., *105*:452–456, 1984.

Ellison, P.H., Largent, J.A., and Bahr, J.P.: A scoring system to predict outcome following neonatal seizures. J. Pediatr., *99*:455–459, 1981.

Emery, J.R., and Peabody, J.L.: Head position affects intracranial pressure in newborn infants. J. Pediatr., *103*:950–953, 1983.

Fishman, R.A.: The glucose-transporter protein and glucopenic brain injury. N. Engl. J. Med., *325*:731–732, 1991.

Freeman, J.M.: Neonatal seizures: Diagnosis and management. Fetal Neonatal Med., *77*:701–708, 1970.

Freitag-Koontz, M.J.: Parents' grief reaction to the diagnosis of their infants' having severe neurologic impairment and static encephalopathy. J. Perinatal Neonatal Nurs., *2*(2):45–57, 1988.

Gaudier, F.L., Goldenberg, R.L., Nelson, K.G., et al.: Acid-base status at birth and subsequent neurosensory impairment in surviving 500 to 1000 gm infants. Am. J. Obstet. Gynecol., *170*:48–53, 1994.

Govaert, P., Vanhaesebrouck, P., De Praeter, C., et al.: Vacuum extraction, bone injury and neonatal subgaleal bleeding. Eur. J. Pediatr., *151*:532–535, 1992.

Guyton, A.C.: Textbook of Medical Physiology, 8th ed. Philadelphia, W.B. Saunders, 1991.

Hambleton, G., and Wigglesworth, J.S.: Origin of intraventricular hemorrhage in the preterm infant. Arch. Dis. Child., *51*:651–659, 1976.

Hans, C.L.: Perinatal hypoxic-ischemic brain damage and intraventricular hemorrhage. Arch. Neurol., *37*:585–587, 1980.

Hayden, P.W.: Adolescents with meningomyelocele. Pediatr. Rev., 6:245–252, 1985.

Ho, E.: Neural tube defects. Nurs. Mirror, *156*(9):iv–vi, 1983.

Hoffman, H.J., and Raffel, L.: Craniofacial surgery. *In* McLaurin, R.L., Schut, L., Venes, J.L., and Epstein, F. (Eds.): Pediatric Neurosurgery: Surgery of the Developing Nervous System, 2nd ed. Philadelphia, W.B. Saunders, 1989, pp. 120–144.

Horn, M., and Scholte, W.: Delayed neuronal death and delayed neuronal recovery in the human brain following global ischemia. Acta Neuropathol., *85*:79–87, 1992.

Kalbus, B.H., and Neal, K.G.: A Laboratory Manual and Study Guide for Human Anatomy. Long Beach, Calif., ELOJ Publishing, 1978.

Kinney, M.R., Dear, C.B., Packa, D.R., and Voorman, D.M.N. (Eds.): AACN's Clinical References for Critical Care Nursing. New York, McGraw-Hill, 1981.

Kurtzke, J.F., Goldberg, I.D., and Kurland, L.T.: The distribution of death from congenital malformations of the nervous system. Neurology, *23*:483–496, 1973.

Labson, L.H.: Newborn exam: Neurologic evaluation. Patient-Care, March 1983, pp. 121–123, 127, 130–132.

Laurent, J.P., and Check, W.R.: Craniosynostosis. *In* McLaurin, R.L., Schut, L., Venes, J.L., and Epstein, F. (Eds.): Pediatric Neurosurgery: Surgery of the Developing Nervous System, 2nd ed. Philadelphia, W.B. Saunders, 1989, pp. 107–133.

Legido, A., Clancy, R.R., and Berman, P.H.: Neurologic outcome after electroencephalographically proven neonatal seizures. Pediatrics, *88*:583–596, 1991.

Lemire, R.J.: Neural tube defects. J.A.M.A., *259*:558–561, 1988.

Levine, M.G., Holroyde, J., Woods, J.R., et al.: Birth trauma: Incidence and predisposing factors. Obstet. Gynecol., *63*:792–795, 1984.

Leviton, A., Kuban, K.C., Pagano, M., et al.: Antenatal corticosteroids appear to reduce the risk of postnatal germinal matrix hemorrhage in intubated low birth weight newborns. Pediatrics, *91*:1083–1087, 1993.

Lienhard, G.E., Slot, J.W., and James, D.E.: How cells absorb glucose. Sci. Am., *266*(1):86–91, 1992.

Lou, H.C.: Perinatal hypoxic-ischemic brain damage and intraventricular hemorrhage. Arch. Neurol., *37*:585–587, 1980.

Lou, H.C., Lassen, N.A., and Friis-Hansen, B.: Impaired autoregulation of cerebral blood flow in the distressed newborn infant. J. Pediatr., *94*:118–121, 1979.

Lou, H., Pryds, O., and Greisen, G.: Pathogenesis of hypoxic-ischaemic encephalopathy and germinal matrix haemorrhage. *In* Robertson, N.R.C. (Ed.): Textbook of Neonatology. New York, Churchill Livingstone, 1992, pp. 1057–1060.

Low, J.A., Froese, A.B., Galbraith, R.S., et al.: The association between preterm newborn hypotension and hypoxemia and outcome during the first year. Acta Paediatr., *82*:433–437, 1993.

Low, J.A., Panagiotopoulos, C., and Derrick, E.J.: Newborn complications after intrapartum asphyxia with metabolic acidosis in the term fetus. Am. J. Obstet. Gynecol., *170*:1081–1087, 1994.

Luciano, D.S., Vander, A.J., and Sherman, J.H.: Human Function and Structure. New York, McGraw-Hill, 1978.

Lupton, B.A., Hill, A., Roland, E.H., et al.: Brain swelling in the asphyxiated term newborn: Pathogenesis and outcome. Pediatrics, *82*:139–146, 1988.

McFarland, L.V., Raskin, M., Daling, J.R., et al.: Erb/ Duchenne's palsy: a consequence of fetal macrosomia and method of delivery. Obstet. Gynecol., *68*:784–788, 1986.

McLaughlin, J.F., Shurtleff, D.B., Lamers, J.Y., et al.: Influence of prognosis on decisions regarding the care of newborns with myelodysplasia. N. Engl. J. Med., *312*:1589–1594, 1985.

Menkes, J.H.: Perinatal central nervous system asphyxia and trauma. *In* Taeusch, H.W., Ballard, R.A., and Avery, M.E. (Eds.): Schaffer's Diseases of the Newborn, 6th ed. Philadelphia, W.B. Saunders, 1991, pp. 406–421.

Ment, L.R., Duncan, C.C., Ehrenkranz, R.A., et al.: Intraventricular hemorrhage in the preterm neonate: Timing and cerebral blood flow changes. J. Pediatr., *104*:419–425, 1984.

Ment, L.R., Oh, W., Ehrenkranz, R.A., et al.: Low-dose indomethacin therapy and extension of intraventricular hemorrhage: A multicenter, randomized trial. J. Pediatr., *124*:951–955, 1994.

Ment, L.R., Oh W., Philip, A.G.S., et al.: Risk factors for early intraventricular hemorrhage in low birth weight infants. J. Pediatr., *121*:776–783, 1992.

Ment, L.R., Scott, D.T., Ehrenkranz, R.A., and Duncan, C.C.: Neurodevelopmental assessment of very low birth weight neonates: Effect of germinal and intraventricular hemorrhage. Pediatr. Neurol., *1*:164–168, 1985.

Ment, L.R., Stewart, W.B., Ardito, T.A., et al.: Indomethacin promotes germinal matrix microvessel maturation in the newborn beagle pup. Stroke, *23*:1132–1137, 1992.

Mizrahi, E.M.: Consensus and controversy in the clinical management of neonatal seizures. Clin. Perinatol., *16*:485–500, 1989.

Moorcraft, J., Bolas, N.M., Ives, N.K., et al.: Spatially localized magnetic resonance spectroscopy of the brains of normal and asphyxiated newborns. Pediatrics, *87*:273–282, 1991.

Nocon, J.J., McKenzie, D.K., Thomas, L.J., et al.: Shoulder dystocia: An analysis of risks and obstetric maneuvers. Am. J. Obstet. Gynecol., *168*:1732–1739, 1993.

Painter, M.J., Bergman, I., and Crumrine, P.: Neonatal seizures. Pediatr. Clin. North Am., *33*:91–109, 1986.

Painter, M.J., Pippenger, C., Wasterlain, C., et al.: Phenobarbital and phenytoin in neonatal seizures: Metabolism and tissue distribution. Neurology, *31*:1107–1112, 1981.

Papile, L.: Neonatal brain injury and its assessment. Paper presented at a meeting of The Fetus and Newborn: State of the Art Care, San Diego, September 1987.

Papile, L.: Hypoxic/ischemic encephalopathy: Diagnosis and management. Paper presented at a meeting of the National Association of Neonatal Nurses, Phoenix, September 1990.

Papile, L., Burstein, J., Burstein, R., and Koffler, H.: Incidence and evolution of subependymal and intraventricular hemorrhage: A study of infants with birth weights less than 1,500 grams. J. Pediatr., 92:529–534, 1978.

Partridge, J.C., Babcock, D.S., Steichen, J.J., et al.: Optimal timing for diagnostic cranial ultrasound in low-birth-weight infants: Detection of intracranial hemorrhage and ventricular dilation. J. Pediatr., 102:281–287, 1983.

Passo, S.: Positioning infants with myelomeningocele. Am. J. Nurs., 74:1658–1660, 1974.

Passo, S.: Malformations of the neural tube. Nurs. Clin. North Am., 15(1):5–21, 1980.

Paternak, J.F.: Hypoxic-ischemic brain damage in the term infant. Pediatr. Clin. North Am., 40:1061–1072, 1993.

Percy, A.K.: Neonatal asphyxia and static encephalopathies. In Fishman, M.A. (Ed.): Pediatric Neurology. Orlando, Grune & Stratton, 1986, pp. 57–70.

Perlman, J.M.: Systemic abnormalities in term infants following perinatal asphyxia: Relevance to long-term neurologic outcome. Clin. Perinatol., 16:475–484, 1989.

Perlman, J.M., Goodman, S., Kreusser, K.L., and Volpe, J.J.: Reduction in intraventricular hemorrhage by elimination of fluctuating cerebral blood-flow velocity in preterm infants with respiratory distress syndrome. N. Engl. J. Med., 312:1353–1357, 1985.

Phelan, J.P., and Ahn, M.O.: Perinatal observations in forty-eight neurologically impaired term infants. Am. J. Obstet. Gynecol., 171:424–431, 1994.

Pryds, O.: Control of cerebral circulation in the high-risk neonate. Ann. Neurol., 30:321–329, 1991.

Raimondi, A.J.: Cystic transformation of the IV ventricle (the Dandy-Walker cyst). In Hoffman, H.J., and Epstein, F. (Eds.): Disorders of the Developing Nervous System: Diagnosis and Treatment. Boston, Blackwell Scientific Publications, 1986, pp. 235–246.

Reproductive Toxicology, a medical letter on environmental hazards to reproduction [Reproductive Toxicology Center, 2524 L St., Washington, D.C. 20037], ISSN 0736-5098, 1987.

Rhoads, G.G., and Mills, J.L.: Can vitamin supplements prevent neural tube defects? Current evidence and ongoing investigations. Clin. Obstet. Gynecol., 39:569–578, 1986.

Rubin, A.: Birth injuries: Incidence, mechanisms and end results. Obstet. Gynecol., 23:218–221, 1964.

Scher, M.S., Aso, K., Beggarly, M.E., et al.: Electrographic seizures in preterm and full-term neonates: Clinical correlates, associated brain lesions, and risk for neurologic sequelae. Pediatrics, 91:128–134, 1993.

Scher, M.S., and Painter, M.J.: Controversies surrounding neonatal seizures. Pediatr. Clin. North Am., 36:281–310, 1989.

Seidman, D.S., Laor, A., Gale, R., et al.: Long-term effects of vacuum and forceps deliveries. Lancet, 337:1583–1585, 1991.

Shankaran, S., Cepeda, E., Muran, G., et al.: Antenatal phenobarbital therapy and neonatal outcome. I. Effect on intracranial hemorrhage. Pediatrics, 97:644–648, 1996.

Shaver, D.C., Bada, H.S., Korones, S.B., et al.: Early and late intraventricular hemorrhage: The role of obstetric factors. Obstet. Gynecol., 80:831–837, 1992.

Socol, M.L., Garcia, P.M., and Riter, S.: Depressed Apgar acores, acid-base status, and neurologic outcome. Am. J. Obstet. Gynecol., 170:993–999, 1994.

Steer, C.R.: Barbiturate therapy in the management of cerebral ischemia. Dev. Med. Child Neurol., 24:219–231, 1982.

Svenningsen, N.W., Blennow, G., Lindroth, M., et al.: Brain-oriented intensive care treatment in severe neonatal asphyxia. Arch. Dis. Child., 57:176–183, 1982.

Sykes, G.S., Molloy, P.M., Johnson, P., et al.: Do Apgar scores indicate asphyxia? Lancet, 1:494–496, 1982.

Thorns, S.: Controversy, treatment and care. Nurs. Mirror, 154(24):32–33, 1982.

Thorp, J.A., Parriott, J., Ferrette-Smith, D., et al.: Antepartum vitamin K and phenobarbital for preventing intraventricular hemorrhage in the premature newborn: A randomized, double-blind, placebo-controlled trial. Obstet. Gynecol., 83(1):70–76, 1994.

Torrence, C.: Neonatal seizures. I. A developmental and clinical understanding. Neonatal Network, 4(1):9–16, 1985.

Traystman, R.J., Kirsch, J.R., and Koehler, R.C.: Oxygen radical mechanisms of brain injury following ischemia and reperfusion. J. Appl. Physiol., 71:1185–1195, 1991.

van Bel, F., Dorrepaal, C.A., Benders, M.J.N.L., et al.: Changes in cerebral hemodynamics and oxygenation in the first 24 hours after birth asphyxia. Pediatrics, 92:365–372, 1992.

Vandar, A.J., Sherman, J.H., and Luciano, D.S.: Human Physiology: The Mechanisms of Body Function, 2nd ed. New York, McGraw-Hill, 1970.

Vannucci, R.C.: Embryology and malformations of the CNS. In Fanaroff, A.A., and Martin, R.J. (Eds.): Neonatal-Perinatal Medicine: Diseases of the Fetus and Infant, 6th ed. St. Louis, Mosby–Year Book, 1997, pp. 826–856.

Volpe, J.J.: Perinatal hypoxic-ischemic brain injury. Pediatr. Clin. North Am., 23:383–397, 1976.

Volpe, J.J.: Intraventricular hemorrhage and brain injury in the premature: Neuropathology and pathogenesis. Clin. Perinatol., 16:361–386, 1989a.

Volpe, J.J.: Intraventricular hemorrhage and brain injury in the premature infant: Diagnosis, prognosis and prevention. Clin. Perinatol., 16:387–411, 1989b.

Wilder, B.J. (Ed.): The use of parenteral antiepileptic drugs and the role for fosphenytoin. Neurology, 46(6):S1–S28, 1996.

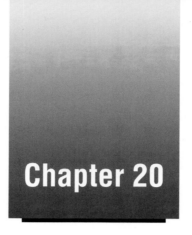

Chapter 20

Neonatal Pain Management

Judy Bildner

Objectives

1. Discuss maturation of the pain pathway in the neonate.

2. Discuss the historical events that led to pain research in the neonate.

3. Describe behavioral and physiologic responses to pain in the neonate.

4. Review care strategies and procedures in the NICU that cause pain.

5. Describe various pain assessment tools available to the NICU nurse to evaluate pain in the neonate.

6. Describe nonpharmacologic and pharmacologic pain relief and discuss the risks and benefits of each.

Since the mid-1980s, caregivers in neonatal intensive care have become more aware of the need to treat pain in neonates. Previously, it was believed that infants did not experience pain because the level of myelinization prevented reception of pain. It was also believed that infants have no memory of painful procedures and that pharmacologic agents to control pain might be dangerous to the developing neonate, so that the risks would outweigh the benefits. Numerous researchers have since demonstrated that neonates are mature enough for pain perception and to have memory of painful procedures (Andrews and Fitzgerald, 1994; Craig et al., 1993; Franck, 1987; Stevens et al., 1994 and 1995). Progress has been made in identifying pain in the neonate and interventions to alleviate neonatal pain. This chapter will review pain pathways, identification of pain, and interventions to alleviate pain in the neonate.

Neuroanatomy of Pain

A. **Nervous system development.** Neural pathways for pain can be followed from sensory receptors in the skin to the cerebral cortex.
1. Cutaneous sensory perceptions (Humphrey, 1964).
    a. Seventh week of gestation: appear in the perioral region of the fetus.
    b. Week 11: appear in the rest of the face, hands, and soles of the feet.

c. Week 15: progress toward the trunk, proximal portion of the arms, and soles of the feet.

d. Week 20: appear in all cutaneous and mucous surfaces.

2. Transmission through the CNS (Humphrey, 1964).

   a. Development of synapses between sensory fibers and interneurons in the dorsal horn of the spinal cord occurs at week 6.

   b. Various cells in the dorsal horn start forming before week 13 and are complete by 30 weeks' gestation.

   c. The cerebral cortex begins to develop by week 8 and has a full compliment of neurons by 20 weeks.

   d. Higher-center pain perception via cortical connections with the thalamus are complete by 24 weeks.

   e. Recognition of most pain occurs in the cerebral cortex, although some pain perception may occur at subcortical levels such as at the thalamus (Clancy, Anand, and Lally, 1992).

B. **Nociception.** Nociceptors are free nerve endings found throughout the body: the skin, blood vessels, subcutaneous tissue, muscle, fascia, periosteum, viscera, and joints (Anand and Hickey, 1987).

1. Lack of myelin in the nerve tracts does not mean lack of function, but slower conduction.

2. Nociceptive nerve tracts in the spinal cord and CNS undergo complete myelination up to the brain stem and thalamus by 30 weeks.

3. Nociceptive impulses are carried through unmyelinated and thinly myelinated fibers even in adult peripheral nerves.

4. Transmission of nociception (Deshpande and Anand, 1996; Fitzgerald and Anand, 1993). Transmission of nociceptor impulses occur along two types of afferent sensory fibers.

   a. A-delta fibers: thinly myelinated, rapid conducting fibers associated with sharp pain or "first pain" (e.g., sharp, localized, pricking).

   b. C fibers: polymodal, unmyelinated, slow conducting fibers associated with aching, burning, poorly localized, or "second pain."

   c. Peripheral sensory fibers, both A and C, enter the spinal cord through the dorsal roots of a spinal nerve.

   d. Synapse occurs in the dorsal horn and ascends to the cerebral cortex by way of the dorsal column system and the spinothalamic tract.

   e. Neurotransmitters (epinephrine, norepinephrine, dopamine, acetylcholine, and serotonin) are responsible for the transmission of impulses across synaptic clefts. These are first expressed at 34–38 weeks (Deshpande and Anand, 1996).

   f. The thalamus is the principal relay station to the cerebral cortex for sensory impulses from the spinal cord, brain stem, and cerebellum. Thalamocortical pain fibers are myelinated by 37 weeks (Deshpande and Anand, 1996).

C. **Cerebral cortex.** Maturity of the cerebral cortex is suggested by:

1. Fetal and neonatal electroencephalogram (EEG) patterns. Intermittent EEG bursts are seen in both cerebral hemispheres at 20 weeks and sustained bursts at 22 weeks. At 26–27 weeks the bursts are bilaterally synchronous, and by 30 weeks wakefulness and sleep are identified by EEG patterns (Deshpande and Anand, 1996).

2. Behavioral development. Well-defined periods of quiet sleep, active sleep, and wakefulness are seen in utero by 28 weeks. Cognitive, coordinative, and associative capabilities indicate a mature cortex in response to visual and auditory stimuli (Clancy et al., 1992).

History

For many years, neonates did not receive anesthesia either for surgery or for postoperative analgesia. It was believed that neonates did not feel pain because of their immature CNS and unmyelinated pain fibers.

A. **Myths regarding neonatal pain.**

1. Neonates have no memory of pain.
2. Objective assessment is impossible.
3. Analgesics cannot be administered safely.
4. Pain is a subjective experience that cannot be communicated by neonates (Agarwal, Hagedorn, and Gardner, 1998).

B. **In the mid to late 1980s, pain in neonates began to receive recognition.** Literature discussed anesthesia in the neonate to include infant circumcision, patent ductus arteriosus ligations, and outcomes. The studies demonstrated that infants experience pain (Anand and Hickey, 1987; Grunau and Craig, 1987; Johnston and Strada, 1986; Porter, Miller, and Marshall, 1986).

C. **In 1986 a mother, angry that her infant did not receive anesthesia during minor surgical procedures, took her complaint to the Washington press.** The publicity was phenomenal and heightened the awareness of the public and professionals. This led the American Academy of Pediatrics (AAP) and the American Society of Anesthesiologists to make a public statement that most infants need pain medications (AAP, 1987).

D. **In February 1992 the Agency for Health Care Policy and Research published clinical practice guidelines for infants, children, and adolescents regarding both operative and medical procedures.** The purpose of these guidelines is to assist health services in establishing and providing consistent, cost-effective, high-quality care. (U.S. Department of Health and Human Services, 1992).

1. The guidelines divide the institutions' responsibility into four aspects:
   a. Education of families regarding pain relief and their role as part of the team.
   b. Clear documentation of assessment and pain management.
   c. Adoption of a standard of care for pain relief.
   d. Quality assessment and improvement programs to establish pain relief effectiveness.
2. In 1995 both the National Association of Neonatal Nurses and the Association of Women's Health, Obstetric, and Neonatal Nurses published position statements on pain in neonates (AWHONN, 1995; NANN, 1995).
3. Stevens, Johnston, and Grunau (1995) presented important principles for pain management of the neonate:
   a. Pain can be minimized by careful assessment of the infant's response before, during, and after painful procedures. Careful reassessment at regular intervals provides more effective analgesia and management.
   b. Tools evaluating neonatal pain must have established validity and reliability.
   c. Because pain is multidimensional, both physiologic and behavioral parameters must be evaluated. Health status, behavioral state, and gestation must also be considered.
   d. Parents should be involved as advocates for their infant. Their input should be taken seriously and used in their assessment. (Stevens et al., 1995)
4. Since these publications, research on pain management is growing. Neonatal pain tools are being developed, tested, and published. Analgesic intervention is being used in infants.

Pain: Definition

A. **There are many sources available that define pain.** The definition may differ slightly, but all carry a common theme of discomfort. The International Association for the Study of Pain defines pain as "an unpleasant sensory and emotional experience associated with actual or potential tissue damage or described in terms of such damage. Pain is always subjective" (Merskey et al., 1979). Though this standard definition reflects the general aspect of pain, the latter part of the definition implies that nonverbal infants and neonates do not feel pain. Measurement of neonatal pain must be evaluated objectively.

B. **It is proposed that behavioral alterations caused by pain be the infant's self-report and not be assumed to be only "surrogate measures" of pain (Anand and Craig, 1996).**

NICU Procedures and Care Strategies That Cause Pain

A. **Many activities and interventions in the NICU will cause pain.** Of these activities, procedures are the most prevalent and include heel sticks; IV insertion; peripheral central line insertion; arterial punctures; intubation; lumbar puncture; chest tube insertion; insertion of a nasogastric tube; insertion of umbilical artery and venous catheters; removal of supernumerary digits; tape removal; circumcision; surgery; and immunizations. Research evaluating invasive procedures in NICUs found, in one study, 3000 procedures performed on 54 infants during their hospitalization (Barker and Rutter, 1995).

B. **The NICU environment (light and sound) is also an overwhelming place that can cause stress to the neonate.** Overstimulation may cause the infant to shut down and thus prevent the infant from exhibiting behavioral responses to pain (Agarwal et al., 1998).

C. **Adverse outcomes of NICU interventions may also contribute to the pain experience.** These include, but are not limited to, IV infiltrates and extravasation; chemical burns; epidermal stripping from tape removal; irritation caused by chest tube movement during positioning; chest physiotherapy; and fractures.

D. **Infants with chronic lung disease often have multisystem complications that cause pain.** These complications may include inguinal hernia, rickets, and nephrolithiasis (Sherf and Park, 1990).

Infant Pain Response

The elaborate nervous system in the neonate exhibits a multiplicity of responses to environmental stimuli. The infant's responses to pain can therefore be described as behavioral and physiologic.

A. Behavioral responses.

1. Motor responses include but are not limited to limb withdrawal, swiping, thrashing, increased tone such as rigidity and fist clenching, and decreased tone such as flaccidity. Both premature and term infants react and communicate their response to pain. Regardless of gestational age, infants show greater body activity in response to invasive procedures, in comparison with noninvasive procedures (Craig et al., 1993).
2. Facial expression includes facial grimacing, consisting of lowered brows, eyes squeezed shut, furrowing of the brow, open lips, and quivering of the chin (Agarwal et al., 1998; Grunau and Craig, 1990; Krechel and Bildner, 1995;

Shapiro, 1989). Gestational age is a powerful modifier of pain expressions in the neonate. Infants born at younger gestational ages have less baseline facial activity and less reactivity to both innocuous and noxious stimuli than do term infants (Craig et al., 1993).

3. Crying has been found to be significant as a behavioral aspect of pain.
    a. Increases in peak fundamental frequency (pitch), peak spectral energy, cry duration, and intensity are reported features (Grunau and Craig, 1990; Stevens, Johnston, and Horton, 1994).
    b. Cry is modified by severity of illness. Severely ill infants' cry response to pain has a higher peak fundamental frequency, shorter cry duration, and longer latency than that of healthy infants (Stevens et al., 1994).

4. Complex responses in the neonate relate to changes in the state system. Sleep-wake cycles change, activity levels change, and the neonate may become extremely fussy or listless. Behavior state may modify the facial expression of pain. Infants in active awake states have a greater proportion of facial activity than do infants in sleep states in response to a noxious stimulus (Grunau and Craig, 1987; Stevens et al., 1994).

B. **Physiologic responses.** As with behavioral responses, there are also physiologic responses. The literature reveals several physiologic parameters associated with pain.

1. These include decreased oxygenation, measured as a decreased transcutaneous oxygen saturation (Rawlings, Miller, and Engle, 1980; Williamson and Williamson, 1983), and increases in vital signs such as heart rate and blood pressure (Franck, 1987; Johnston and Strada, 1986; Purcell-Jones, Dormon, and Sumner, 1988).

2. Physiologic outcomes are objective and precise measurements that can be used to evaluate the pain response.

3. Physiologic parameters cannot always be interpreted as signifying pain and thus must be evaluated along with behavioral parameters (Craig et al., 1993).

C. **Hormonal and metabolic responses.**

1. Not always readily assessed and/or associated with pain.

2. Insulin secretion may decrease. Catecholamines, cortisol levels, glucagon, aldosterone, and other corticosteroids may increase (Anand, 1990).

3. The increase in glucose can be detrimental to the growing immature brain. These hormonal changes directly affect fat, protein, and carbohydrate stores, resulting in a delay in healing. This is significant in the postsurgical period (Anand et al., 1985; Anand and Hickey, 1992).

D. **Decompensatory response.**

1. When pain stimuli or pain persists for hours or days without intervention, the infant exhibits a decompensatory response. The sympathetic nervous system, or the "fight or flight" mechanism, can no longer compensate. As a result, the physiologic parameters return to baseline (Shapiro, 1989).

2. "Return to baseline" does not indicate that pain is no longer felt or is tolerated, but it does make the infant's pain more difficult to evaluate.

E. **Pain behaviors versus irritability/agitation behaviors.** Pain is often evaluated as irritability and agitation. These indicators are similar but can be distinguished from those of pain. Indicators that are similar and yet distinct are shown in Table 20–1.

Table 20–1
PAIN VERSUS IRRITABLE BEHAVIORS

	Pain Behavior	Irritable Behavior
Cry	Sudden, high pitched	Whining
Facial expression	Grimace, lowered brows, eyes shut tight, furrowing of brow, open lips, quivering of chin	Frown, gaze aversion, worried faces
Motor response	Withdrawal, swiping, thrashing, increased tone, decreased tone	Rigid posture: arching, flailing of extremities, random head and body movement, tremulous
Complex response	Sleep/wake cycle changes: wakeful, increased irritability, listlessness, change in activity level, feeding difficulties, bonding interruption	Easily aroused, fuss/cry interchangeable, high level of persistence, ineffective in self-consoling, hyperalert
Physiologic	Increased HR up to 30%, increased RR up to 30%, increased BP up to 30%; shallow respiration, pallor, flushing, diaphoresis, palmar sweating, decreased transcutaneous PO_2, dilated pupils	Increased HR and BP with activity only, duskiness only after prolonged, transcutaneous PO_2 decreases after prolonged, no diaphoresis, increased respiratory rate and effort
Hormonal/metabolic	Decreased insulin secretion and thus hyperglycemia; increased catecholamines, cortisol levels, glucagon, aldosterone; decreased fat, protein, carbohydrate stores	

HR, Heart rate; *RR*, respiratory rate; *BP*, blood pressure.
Data from Agarwal et al., 1998; Shapiro, 1989; Broome and Tanzillo, 1990; Craig et al., 1993.

Pain Assessment

Pain assessment can be influenced by past experience with pain relief, knowledge base of the medical professional, attitude toward pain assessment, fear of addiction, and communication among team members providing care to the infant.

A. Pain assessment is usually based on subjective assessment of behavioral responses.

B. Neonatal pain tools have been developed and tested with the use of behavioral indices only (Craig et al., 1993; Ekman and Friesen, 1978; Grunau and Craig, 1990; Lawrence et al., 1993; Taddio et al., 1995), whereas others have incorporated both behavioral and physiologic indices (Krechel and Bildner, 1995; Norden et al., 1991a, 1991b; Stevens et al., 1996). These pain tools have also been developed to include various types of pain, such as procedural or acute pain (Krechel and Bildner, 1995; Lawrence et al., 1993).

C. "The 'golden rule' of pain assessment must be: What is painful to an adult is painful to an infant until proven otherwise" (Franck, 1989). This rule, along with the use of valid and reliable tools, must be used for the assessment and intervention of pain.

Pain Assessment Tools

A. **CRIES:** a postoperative pain tool (Table 20–2) (Krechel and Bildner, 1995).
1. Acronym for five behavioral and physiologic parameters: C = crying; R = requires oxygen to maintain saturation at greater than 95%; I = increased vital signs; E = expression; and S = sleeplessness.

Table 20–2
CRIES: NEONATAL POSTOPERATIVE PAIN MEASUREMENT SCORE

	Score			Tips for Scoring CRIES
	0	**1**	**2**	
Crying	No	High pitched	Inconsolable	Score 0: no cry or cry not high pitched Score 1: cry high pitched, but consolable Score 2: high-pitched cry, inconsolable
Requires O$_2$ for saturation >95%	No	<30%	>30%	Score 0: no oxygen required from baseline Score 1: oxygen requirement <30% from baseline Score 2: oxygen requirement >30% from baseline
Increased vital signs	HR and BP ≤preoperative values	HR or BP ↑ <20% of preoperative values	HR or BP ↑ >20% of preoperative values	Score 0: HR and BP are both unchanged or at less than baseline Score 1: HR or BP is increased by <20% Score 2: HR or BP is increased by >20% NOTE: Measure BP last so as not to wake the infant.
Expression	None	Grimace	Grimace/grunt	Score 0: no grimace Score 1: grimace only is present Score 2: grimace and nonaudible grunt present NOTE: Grimace consists of lowered brow, eyes squeezed shut, deepening nasolabial furrow, and open lips and mouth.
Sleepless	No	Wakes at frequent intervals	Constantly awake	Score 0: continuously asleep Score 1: awakens at frequent intervals Score 2: awake constantly NOTE: Based on infant's state during previous hour.

HR, Heart rate; *BP,* blood pressure.
Neonatal pain assessment tool developed at the University of Missouri—Columbia.
From Krechel, S., and Bildner, J.: CRIES: A new neonatal post-operative pain measurement score: Initial testing of validity and reliability. Paediatr. Anaesth., *5*(1):53–61, 1995.

2. Demonstrates beginning validity and reliability for use in infants born at 32 weeks' gestation and later. It was tested against the objective pain scale, previously validated in abstract only.
3. Tool scoring system, 0 to 10, is structured in the same fashion as the Apgar score and was designed to make the tool easy to use and remember.
4. Score is used postoperatively.
5. Pain is assessed hourly for a period of not less than 24 hours. A score of 4 or above indicates pain, and any assessment of 4 or above should receive pain intervention. The neonate should then be reevaluated 15–30 minutes after analgesia to assess for pain relief.

B. **The Premature Infant Pain Profile (PIPP) (Stevens et al., 1996) (Table 20–3).**

1. Seven-item, four-point scale for assessment of pain in premature infants.
2. Multidimensional; includes heart rate, oxygen saturation, brow bulge, eye squeeze, and nasolabial furrow.
3. Unique in that it includes two contextual modifiers (e.g., gestational age and behavioral state).
4. Beginning construct validity was established by using extreme groups or situations (pain vs no pain).
5. Initial validity has been established.

C. **Though CRIES and PIPP have their weaknesses, they can be used until more specific tools are developed.** NICUs should adopt a formal method of evaluating neonatal pain.

Nursing Care of the Infant in Pain

Skilled observation, assessments, and interventions are the responsibility of the care providers. Pain intervention may be provided by both nonpharmacologic and pharmacologic methods.

A. **Nonpharmacologic comfort measures: can be used for mild pain or distress.** Individualized nursing care interventions decrease infant pain and stress. By decreasing the pain and stress, short- and long-term outcomes (i.e., physiologic, behavioral, and developmental) are improved (Als et al., 1994).
1. Minimal handling protocols can decrease stress and increase sleep periods.
2. Comfort measures.
    a. Nonnutritive sucking (Marchetti et al., 1991).
        (1) Use of a pacifier soothes infant to reduce level of arousal.
        (2) Sucrose on a pacifier can calm much more quickly and is used for pain reduction during circumcision (Blass and Hoffmeyer, 1991).
    b. Body containment. Improper body position contributes to discomfort and pain. Promoting flexion can decrease gross motor movement and arousal. This can be accomplished by holding, swaddling, nesting, and providing grasping opportunities (Gardner, 1994; Broome and Tanzillo, 1990)

Table 20-3
PREMATURE INFANT PAIN PROFILE

Infant Study Number: _____
Date/time: _____
Event: _____

Process	Indicator	0	1	2	3	Score
Chart	Gestational age	36 weeks and more	32–35 weeks, 6 days	28–31 weeks, 6 days	less than 28 weeks	
Observe infant 15 s	Behavioral state	active/awake eyes open facial movements	quiet/awake eyes open no facial movements	active/sleep eyes closed facial movements	quiet/sleep eyes closed no facial movements	
Observe baseline Heart rate __ Oxygen saturation __						
Observe infant 30 s	Heart rate Max __	0–4 beats/min increase	5–14 beats/min increase	15–24 beats/min increase	25 beats/min or more increase	
	Oxygen saturation Min __	0–2.4% decrease	2.5–4.9% decrease	5.0–7.4% decrease	7.5% or more decrease	
	Brow bulge	None 0–9% of time	Minimum 10–39% of time	Moderate 40–69% of time	Maximum 70% of time or more	
	Eye squeeze	None 0–9% of time	Minimum 10–39% of time	Moderate 40–69% of time	Maximum 70% of time or more	
	Nasolabial furrow	None 0–9% of time	Minimum 10–39% of time	Moderate 40–69% of time	Maximum 70% of time or more	
					Total score	

From Stevens, B., Johnston, C., Petryshen, P., and Taddia, A.: Premature infant pain profile: Development and initial validation. Clin. J. Pain, *12*(1):13-22, 1996.

   c. Facilitated tucking. Gentle motor containment of the infants' extremities in a flexed midline position close to the trunk of the body, while the infant is in a side-lying or supine position, may provide comfort (Corff et al., 1995).

B. **Pharmacologic pain control (Fitzgerald and Anand, 1993).**

1. Narcotic analgesics: morphine and fentanyl. Analgesics are recommended when moderate to severe pain is assessed. Sedatives reduce agitation precipitated by painful events but do not provide pain relief.

   a. Systemic opioids induce analgesia by acting at various levels of the CNS.
     (1) Spinal cord. Opioids impair or inhibit the transmission of nociceptive input from the periphery to the CNS.
     (2) Basal ganglia. Opioids activate a descending inhibitory system.
     (3) Limbic system. Opioids alter the emotional response to pain, making it more tolerable (Deshpande and Anand, 1996).

   b. Special considerations in neonates are as follows:
     (1) A wide variation in both metabolism and clearance of analgesia can be expected in the neonatal population (McClain and Anand, 1996).
     (2) Decreased protein binding results in an increase in the free fraction of the drug available and an increase in permeability of the blood-brain barrier (McClain and Anand, 1996).

   c. Fentanyl is used as follows:
     (1) Bolus dose: 1–4 µg/kg every 2–4 hours (Young and Mangum 1998).
     (2) Continuous infusion: 1–5 µg/kg per hour (Deshpande and Anand, 1996).
     (3) Onset is almost immediately after IV administration.
     (4) Duration of action is 30–60 minutes.
     (5) Complications include respiratory depression, bradycardia, feeding intolerance, and diminished clearance with increased intra-abdominal pressure.
     (6) Assess for signs of tolerance (changes in vital signs and oxygen saturation, tachycardia, and hypertension) that require an increase in the dosage (Young and Mangum, 1998; Deshpande and Anand, 1996).
     (7) For weaning, decrease the dose by 10% every 6 hours (Maguire and Maloney, 1988). Assess for signs of withdrawal: irritability, hypertonicity, diaphoresis, increased temperature, and vomiting after initiation of feeding (Norton, 1988).

   d. Morphine is used as follows:
     (1) Bolus dose: 0.05 mg/kg to 0.2 mg/kg per dose by IV slow push, intramuscular route, or subcutaneous route. Repeat as required, usually every 4 hours (Young and Mangum, 1998; Deshpande and Anand, 1996).
     (2) Continuous infusion: 10–15 µg/kg per hour (Young and Mangum, 1998; Deshpande and Tobias, 1996).
     (3) Onset of action: beginning a few minutes after IV administration, with peak analgesia occurring at 20 minutes.
     (4) Duration: 2–4 hours (Young and Mangum, 1998; Deshpande and Anand, 1996).
     (5) Complications: respiratory depression, hypotension, bronchoconstriction, decreased gastrointestinal motility/constipation, and urinary retention (Young and Mangum, 1998; Deshpande and Tobias, 1996).
     (6) Weaning: with prolonged use, decrease of dose by 10% per day (Maguire and Maloney, 1988). Observe for signs of withdrawal: irritability, hypertonicity, diaphoresis, fever, and vomiting after initiation of feeding (Norton, 1988).

e. Infants demonstrating narcotic withdrawal need to be closely observed. The neonatal abstinence score is recommended for use with infants receiving prolonged opioid therapy (Deshpande and Anand, 1996).
2. Nonnarcotic analgesia: acetaminophen.
   a. Short-term use for mild to moderate pain.
   b. Wide margin of safety when used in the appropriate dose range.
   c. Peak serum concentration: approximately 60 minutes after an oral dose (Young and Mangum, 1998).
   d. Dose: 10–15 mg/kg per dose every 6–8 hours by mouth; 20–25 mg/kg per dose every 6–8 hours by rectum (Young and Mangum, 1998; Deshpande and Anand, 1996).
3. Topical pain control: EMLA (*e*utetic *m*ixture of *l*ocal *a*nesthetics).
   a. Cream containing prilocaine and lidocaine.
   b. Used for circumcisions, IV sticks.
   c. Must be applied and then covered with an occlusive dressing for a minimum of 60 minutes before the procedure.
   d. Slow systemic absorption; low serum levels.
   e. Not approved for use in preterm infants.
   f. Effective interruption of nociceptive input from the epidermis and from deeper structures (McClain and Anand, 1996).
   g. Complication. One of the metabolites of prilocaine (*o*-toluidide) can cause methemoglobinemia (Bonini, Johnston, Faucher, and Amanda, 1993).
4. Local pain control: lidocaine.
   a. Local anesthesia for procedures such as circumcision, chest tube insertion, and cutdown.
   b. Dose: 0.5% solution. Infiltration of less than 0.5 ml/kg is recommended to prevent toxic effects (McClain and Anand, 1996).
5. Hypnotics and sedatives. These drugs do not provide pain relief. They are used to complement the management of pain in conjunction with analgesics, and may calm the infant, enhance sleep, reduce stress, and break hyperanxiety states. Common sedatives used in the NICU are chloral hydrate, phenobarbital, and two benzodiazepines: lorazepam (Ativan), and midazolam (Versed).
6. Neuromuscular blocking agents. Chemical paralysis is often used for severely ill neonates. Because the use of paralytic agents masks the behavior signs of pain, sedatives or analgesics should be used in conjunction with paralytics (Shapiro, 1989).

Pain Control Using Regional Anesthesia

For regional anesthesia, an opioid and a local anesthetic are administered via the spinal or epidural (caudal) route. The opioids bind to the receptors in the dorsal horn of the spinal cord and can affect sensory neurons without affecting motor or sympathetic activities (Rasmussen, 1996). Morphine, because of its hydrophilic nature, tends to stay in the cerebrospinal fluid longer and to travel toward the brain (Rasmussen, 1996).

A. **Spinal route:** the space within the spinal canal.

B. **Epidural (caudal) route:** the space just outside the spinal canal where the nerve roots are located. Provides a route for anesthesia and analgesia during operative procedures and can be used for postoperative pain management and for operative procedures below the umbilicus, such as inguinal hernia repair, repair of low imperforate anus, and placement of central venous catheters (Valley, 1997). Spinal and epidural routes can be used with a one-time injection of an agent or a continuous infusion through a catheter.
1. Agents used include morphine and fentanyl.

a. Morphine (Duramorph): always used without a preservative.
   (1) Spinal dose: 5–20 µg/kg as one-time administration; can provide analgesia for as long as 26–36 hours without the administration of any other analgesia (Rasmussen, 1996).
   (2) Epidural dose: 3–8 µg/kg per hour.
b. Fentanyl.
   (1) Spinal dose: 0.2–0.5 µg/kg.
   (2) Epidural dose: single dose of 0.5–1 µg/kg, with an infusion of 2–5 µg/ml at a rate of 0.3–0.4 ml/kg per hour (Rasmussen, 1996).
2. Absolute and relative contraindications to regional anesthesia include:
   a. Systemic infection: septicemia, meningitis.
   b. Bleeding disorders: coagulopathy, thrombocytopenia.
   c. Allergy to local anesthetics.
   d. Parent/guardian refusal.
   e. Hypovolemia.
   f. Degenerative CNS diseases.
   g. Other: malformation of the spinal column, hydrocephalus with increased intracranial pressure, poorly controlled seizures.

REFERENCES

Agarwal, R., Hagedorn, M.I., and Gardner, S.L.: Pain and pain relief. *In* Merenstein, G.B., and Gardner, S.L.: Handbook of Neonatal Intensive Care, 4th ed. St. Louis, Mosby, 1998, pp. 173–196.

Als, H., Lawhorn, G., Duffy, F.H., et al.: Individualized developmental care for the very low birth weight preterm infant: Medical and neurofunctional effects. J.A.M.A., 272:853–858, 1994.

American Academy of Pediatrics Committee on Fetus and Newborn, Committee on Drugs, Section on Anesthesiology, and Section on Surgery. Neonatal anesthesia. Pediatrics, 80:446, 1987.

Anand, K.J.S.: The biology of pain perception in newborn infants. *In* Tyler, D., and Krane, J. (Eds.): Advances in Pain Research Therapy, vol 15. New York, Raven Press, 1990.

Anand, K.J.S., Brown, M.F., Causon, R.C., et al.: Can the human neonate mount an endocrine and metabolic response to surgery? J. Pediatr. Surg., 20:41–48, 1985.

Anand, K.J.S., and Craig, K.D.: New perspectives on the definition of pain [editorial]. Pain 67:3–6, 1996.

Anand, K., and Hickey, P.: Pain and its effects in the human neonate and fetus. N. Engl. J. Med., 317:1321–1329, 1987.

Anand, K.J.S., and Hickey, P.R.: Halothane-morphine compared with high-dose sufentanil for anesthesia and postoperative analgesia in neonatal cardiac surgery. N. Engl. J. Med., 326:1–9, 1992.

Andrews, K., and Fitzgerald, M.: The cutaneous withdrawal reflex in human neonates: Sensitization receptive fields, and the effects of contralateral stimulation. Pain, 56(1):95–102, 1994.

Association of Women's Health, Obstetrics, and Neonatal Nurses. Position Paper: Pain in Neonates. Washington, D.C., Author, 1995.

Barker, D., and Rutter, N. Exposure to invasive procedures in neonatal intensive care unit admissions. Arch. Dis. Child., Fetal Neonatal ed., 72:F47–48, 1995.

Benini, F., Johnston, C.C., Faucher, D., and Amanda, F.V.: Topical anesthesia during circumcision in newborn infants. J.A.M.A., 270:850–853, 1993.

Blass, E.M., Hoffmeyer, L.B.: Sucrose as an analgesic for newborn infants. Pediatrics, 87:215, 1991.

Broome, M.E., and Tanzillo, H.: Differentiating between pain and agitation in premature neonates. J. Perinat. Neonat. Nurs. 4(1):53–62, 1990.

Clancy, G.O., Anand, K.J.S., and Lally, P.: Neonatal pain management. Crit. Care Clin. North Am., 4:527–535, 1992.

Corff, K., Seideman, R., Venkataraman, P.S., et al.: Facilitated tucking: A nonpharmacologic comfort measure for pain in preterm neonates. J. Obstet. Gynecol. Neonat. Nurs., 24(2):143–147, 1995.

Craig, K.D., Whitfield, M.F., Grunau, R., et al.: Pain in the preterm neonate: Behavioral and physiological indices. Pain, 52:287–289, 1993.

Deshpande, J.K., and Anand, J.S.: Basic aspects of acute pediatric pain sedation. *In* Deshpande, J.K., and Tobias, J.D. (Eds.): The Pediatric Pain Handbook. St. Louis, Mosby–Year Book, 1996, pp. 1–48.

Ekman, P., and Friesen, W.V.: Facial Action Coding System: A technique for the measurement of facial movement. Palo Alto, Calif., Consulting Psychologists Press, 1978.

Fitzgerald, M., and Anand, K.J.S.: Developmental neuroanatomy and neurophysiology of pain. *In* Schechter, N.L., Berde, C.B., and Yaster, M. (Eds.): Pain in Infants, Children, and Adolescents. Baltimore, Williams & Wilkins, 1993.

Franck, L.S.: A national survey of the assessment and treatment of pain and agitation in the neonatal intensive care unit. J. Obstet. Gynecol. Neonat. Nurs., 16:387–393, 1987.

Franck, L.S.: Pain in the nonverbal patient: Advocating for the critically ill neonate. Pediatr. Nurs., 15(1):65–68, 90, 1989.

Gardner, S.L.: Pain and pain relief in the neonate. Matern. Child Nurs., 19(March/April):85–90, 1994.

Gardner, S.L.: The neonate and the environment: Impact on development. *In* Merenstein, G.B., and Gardner, S.L. (Eds.): Handbook of Neonatal Intensive Care, 4th ed. St. Louis, Mosby–Year Book, 1998, pp. 197–241.

Grunau, R.V.E., and Craig, K.D.: Pain expression in neonates: Facial action and cry. Pain, 28:395–410, 1987.

Grunau, R.V.E., and Craig, K.D.: Facial activity as a measure of neonatal pain expression. Adv. Pain Res. Ther., 15:147–155, 1990.

Grunau, R.V.E., Johnston, C.C., and Craig, K.D. Neonatal facial and cry responses to invasive and non-invasive procedures. Pain, 42:295–305, 1990.

Humphrey, T.: Some correlations between the appearance of human fetal reflexes and the development of the nervous system. Prog. Brain Res., 4:93–135, 1964.

Johnston, C.C., and Strada, M.E.: Acute pain response in infants: A multidimension description. Pain, 24:373–382, 1986.

Krechel, S., and Bildner, J. CRIES: A new neonatal post-operative pain measurement score: Initial testing of validity and reliability. Paediatr. Anaesth., 5(1):53–61, 1995.

Lawrence, L., Alcock, D., McGrath, P., et al.: The development of a tool to assess neonatal pain. Neonatal Network, 12(6):59–66, 1993.

Maguire, D.P., and Maloney, P.: A comparison of fentanyl and morphine use in neonates. Neonatal Network, 7:27–32, August 1988.

Marchetti, L., Main, R., Redick, E., et al.: Pain reduction interventions during neonatal circumcision. Nurs. Res., 40:241–244, 1991.

Merskey, H., Albe-Fessard, D.G., Bonica, J.J., et al.: Pain terms: A list with definitions and notes on usage. Pain 6:249–252, 1979.

McClain, B.C., and Anand, K.J.S.: Neonatal pain management. In Deshpande, J., and Tobias, J. (Eds.): The Pediatric Pain Handbook. St Louis, Mosby–Year Book, 1996, pp. 197–234.

National Association of Neonatal Nurses. Position statement on pain management in infants. Neonatal Network, 14:54, 1995.

Norden, J., Hannallah, R., Getson, P., et al.: Concurrent validation of an objective pain scale for infants and children. Anesthesiology, 75:A935, 1991a.

Norden, J., Hannallah, E., Getson, P., et al.: Reliability of an objective pain scale in children. Anesth. Analg., 72:S199, 1991b.

Norton, S.J.: After effects of morphine and fentanyl analgesia: A retrospective study. Neonatal Network, 7(3):25–28, 1988.

Porter, F.L., Miller, R.H., and Marshall, R.: Neonatal pain cries: Effect of circumcision on acoustic features and perceived urgency. Child Dev., 57:790–802, 1986.

Purcell-Jones, G., Dormon, F., and Sumner, E.: Pediatric anesthetist's perceptions of neonatal and infant pain. Pain, 33:181–187, 1988.

Rasmussen, G.E.: Epidural and spinal anesthesia and analgesia. In Deshpande, J., and Tobias, J. (Eds.): The Pediatric Pain Handbook. St. Louis, Mosby–Year Book, 1996, pp. 81–112.

Rawlings, D.J., Miller, P.A., and Engle, R.D.: The effect of circumcision on transcutaneous PO_2 in infants. Am. J. Dis. Child., 134:76–78, 1980.

Shapiro, C.: Pain in the neonate: Assessment and intervention. Neonatal Network, 8(1):7–19, 1989.

Sherf, R.F., and Park, S.A.: Complications in infants with bronchopulmonary dysplasia. Bronchopulmonary Dysplasia: Strategies for Total Patient Care. Neonatal Network, 9:35–55, 1990.

Stevens, B.I., Johnston, C.C., and Grunau, R.V.E.: Issues of assessment of pain and discomfort in neonates. J. Obstet. Gynecol. Neonatal Nurs., 24:849–855, 1995.

Stevens, B., Johnston, C., and Horton, L.: Factors that influence the behavioral responses of premature infants. Pain, 51:101–109, 1994.

Stevens, B., Johnston, C., Petryshen, P., and Taddio, A.: Premature infant pain profile: Development and initial validation. Clin. J. Pain, 12(1):13–22, 1996.

Taddio, A., Nulman, I., Koren, B.S., et al.: A revised measure of acute pain in infants. J. Pain Symptom Manage., 10:456–463, 1995.

U.S. Department of Health and Human Services, Public Health Service, Agency for Health Care Policy and Research: Acute pain management in infants, children, and adolescents: Operative and medical procedures. In Quick Reference Guide for Clinicians (DHHS publication No. (AHCPR) 92-0019.) Silver Springs, Md., AHCPR Clearinghouse, 1992, pp. 3–22.

Valley, R.D.: Anesthesia and postoperative pain management. In Nakayama, D.K., Bose, C.L., Chesheir, N.C., and Valley, R.D. (Eds.): Critical Care of the Surgical Newborn. New York Futura, 1997, pp. 148–157.

Williamson, E.S., and Williamson, M.L.: Physiologic stress reduction by a local anesthetic during newborn circumcision. Pediatrics, 71:36–40, 1983.

Young, T.E., and Mangum, O.B.: Neofax: A Manual of Drugs Used in Neonatal Care, 11th ed. Raleigh, N.C., Acorn Publishing, 1998.

Chapter 21

Developmental Support in the Neonatal Intensive Care Unit

Susan Koch

Objectives

1. Identify intervention strategies to maximize an infant's capacity for behavioral organization.

2. Identify intervention strategies to promote parent-infant interaction.

3. Describe predictable, sequential patterns of neuromotor maturation.

4. Demonstrate supportive positioning-handling strategies to encourage the development of normal motor patterns in an infant.

5. List four common feeding problems encountered in high-risk infants.

6. Design a developmental care plan to communicate an infant's unique needs with regard to environmental modifications, positioning techniques, and promotion of self-quieting behaviors.

Developmental support in the NICU integrates the developmental needs of infants with intensive medical care. Development occurs along a continuum, with the usual course of development being interrupted by the birth of a preterm or ill newborn. Care providers now recognize that an infant responds to and interacts with the environment by using various "cues" and is able to communicate on many different levels. Understanding an infant's developmental needs and learning how to provide the interventions necessary to support development are essential in providing optimal care for these infants.

The second but equally important component of developmentally supportive care is the recognition of the family as an equal and highly respected member of the health care team. Whether the family is able to "reside" in the NICU or must communicate with their child and his caregivers over long distances, every caregiver must strive to facilitate the parental role of the family from the time of admission and must not treat family members as "visitors."

Infants at high risk who are assisted in maintaining physiologic and behavioral organization will conserve energy for growth, exhibit clearer behavioral cues, facilitate parent-infant attachment, and develop self-consoling or habituating behaviors. As a result, they will be better equipped to deal with the complex and dynamic environment in the NICU, as well as to interact with their parents, providing for a mutually satisfying parent-infant relationship. This chapter provides information on the developmental needs of the newborn and discusses strategies for providing this care.

Developmentally Supportive Care

Provision of developmentally supportive care involves the following:

A. **Implementing appropriate intervention strategies to foster parent-infant interaction and enhance parents' understanding of their infant as an individual.**

B. **Assessing infant behavior according to the synactive theory of development (Als et al., 1982).** The framework for premature infant behavior work by Als et al. is subdivided into three subsystems: autonomic, motor, and state. However, it is often described as having five areas of emphasis.
1. Physiologic or autonomic system: behaviorally observable in color changes, respiratory pattern, and visceral responses (emesis, gagging, hiccups, bowel movements).
2. Motor system: behaviorally observable in posture, tone, and overall movements.
3. State organizational system: behaviorally observable in a range of states, pattern of state transitions, and clarity of states.
4. Attention and interactional system: observable in the ability to be attentive and take in cognitive and social information from the environment.
5. Self-regulatory system: behaviorally observable in strategies the infant uses to maintain or return to state of balance and relaxation.

C. Assessing an infant's *unique* behavioral style and providing individualized intervention programs.

D. Facilitating an infant's neurosocial behavioral organization by:
1. Organizing care in a contingent manner by *recognizing* and *responding to* the infant's behavioral cues.
2. Effecting change within the physical and social environment of the NICU.

Behavioral Organization

A. **Behavioral organization** is the ability to maintain a balance among autonomic, motor, state, attention-interactional, and self-regulatory subsystems of behavioral maturation as the infant deals with a variety of sensory and postural demands imposed on him or her (Als et al., 1982). An infant's capacity for behavioral organization is reinforced and enhanced by caregivers who recognize and respond to the infant's behavioral cues by:
1. Providing "time-out" when an infant demonstrates *avoidance* behaviors (Als et al., 1982; Fig. 21–1).
2. Supporting and enhancing the infant's own attempts at balance between *approach* behaviors (Als et al., 1982; Fig. 21–1).

B. **Points to consider when assessing** an infant's levels of behavioral stability or organization.
1. How does the infant respond to the daily caregiving routine? How can the family be as involved in daily caregiving as they are comfortable?
2. Does a particular position agitate the infant more than another?
3. What, if anything, in the environment has a negative impact on the infant?

SELF REGULATION PARAMETERS									
	CATALOG OF REGULATION MANEUVERS					CATALOG OF REGULATION MANEUVERS			
	Spit-ups	Gags	Hiccoughs	Bowel Mvt		Tongue Extension	Hand on Face	Sounds	
	Grimace	Arching	Finger Splay	Airplane		Hand Clasp	Foot Clasp	Fingerfold	Tuck
WITHDRAWAL OR AVOIDANCE BEHAVIOR	Salute	Sitting on Air			APPROACH OR GROPING BEHAVIOR	Body Movement	Hand to Mouth	Grasping	Leg/Foot Bracing
	Sneezing	Yawning	Sighing	Coughing		Mouthing	Suck Search	Sucking	Hand Hold
	Averting	Frowning				Ooh Face	Locking	Cooing	

Figure 21–1
Approach and avoidance behaviors. (From Als, H., Brazelton, T.B., Lester, B.M., and Tronick, E.Z.: Manual for the assessment of preterm infants' behavior (APIB). *In* Fitzgerald, H.E., Lester, B.M., and Yogman, M.W. [Eds.]: Theory and Research in Behavioral Pediatrics. New York, Plenum Press, 1982, p. 70.)

4. How much stimulation can the infant tolerate before losing the ability to stay organized?
5. What support is necessary to help the infant maintain stability?
6. Can the timing and organization of medical and nursing procedures be altered to help decrease the infant's level of stress and increase his or her organization?

C. State system.

1. Provides context for any interaction between infant and environment; used by the infant to control the amount and kind of input received from the environment.
2. Six sleep-awake states.
   a. Sleep states.
      (1) *State 1A:* infant in deep sleep with momentary regular breathing, eyes closed, and no eye movements under closed lids; relaxed facial expression; no spontaneous activity, oscillating fairly rapidly with isolated startles, jerky movements or tremors and other behavior characteristics of State 2 (light sleep).
      (2) *State 1B:* infant in deep sleep with predominantly regular breathing, eyes closed, no eye movements under closed lids, relaxed facial expression; no spontaneous activity except isolated startles.
      (3) *State 2A:* light sleep with eyes closed; rapid eye movements can be observed under closed eyelids; low activity level with diffuse or disorganized movements; irregular respirations, with many sucking and mouthing movements, whimpers, facial twitching, and much grimacing; the impression of a "noisy" state is given.
      (4) *State 2B:* light sleep, with eyes closed; rapid eye movements observable under closed lids; low activity level, with movements and dampened startles; movements likely to be of lower amplitude and more monitored than in State 1. Infant responds to various internal stimuli with dampened startle. Respirations are more irregular; mild sucking and mouthing movements can occur off and on; and one or two whimpers, as well as an isolated sigh or smile, may be observed.
   b. Transitional states.
      (1) *State 3A:* drowsy or semidozing; eyes may be open or closed, eyelids fluttering or exaggerated blinking; if eyes open, infant has glassy, veiled

look. Activity level is variable, with or without interspersed, mild startles from time to time. Diffuse movement occurs, with fussing and/or much vocalization, with whimpers, facial grimacing, and so forth.

(2) *State 3B:* Drowsy; same as above but with less discharge of vocalization, whimpers, facial grimacing, and so forth.

c. Awake states.
   (1) *State 4:* alert.
      (a) *State 4AL:* awake and quiet, with minimal motor activity; eyes half open or open but with glazed or dull look, giving impression of little involvement and distance; or eyes focused, yet infant seems to look through, rather than at, object or examiner; or the infant is clearly awake and reactive but has eyes open intermittently.
      (b) *State 4AH:* awake and quiet, minimal motor activity, eyes wide open, "hyperalert" or giving the impression of panic or fear; may appear to be hooked by the stimulus, seems to be unable to modulate or break the intensity of the fixation.
      (c) *State 4B:* alert with bright, shiny look; seems to focus attention on source of stimulation and appears to process information actively and with modulation; motor activity is at a minimum.
   (2) *State 5:* active.
      (a) *State 5A:* eyes may or may not be open, but infant clearly awake and aroused, as indicated by motor arousal, tonus, and mildly distressed facial expression, grimacing, or other signs of discomfort; diffuse fussing.
      (b) *State 5B:* Eyes may or may not be open, but infant is clearly awake and aroused, with considerable, well defined motor activity. Infant is also clearly fussing but not crying.
   (3) *State 6:* crying.
      (a) *State 6A:* intense crying, as indicated by intense grimace and cry face; yet cry sound may be very strained or very weak or even absent.
      (b) *State 6B:* rhythmic, intense crying that is robust, vigorous, and strong in sound.

D. **Signs of stress.**
1. Autonomic system: changes in vital signs (e.g., increase or decrease in heart rate, blood pressure, respiratory rate, or temperature); changes in color; hiccups, gagging, straining, spitting up, and sneezing.
2. Motor system: generalized hypotonia, frantic flailing, finger splaying, hyperextension of extremities or trunk.
3. Sleep states: diffuse sleep states (twitching, grimacing, glassy-eyed look, gaze aversion, panicked look, irritability), rapid transitions between states, or inappropriate state for the circumstances.

E. **Intervention strategies:** to help the infant manage stress and organize behavior.
1. An infant is capable of demonstrating the most competent behavior when in an organized, quiet, alert state (Biber et al., 1989b). Techniques to help the infant reach an organized state include swaddling, nonnutritive sucking, decreasing or modifying visual and auditory stimulus, and trying to elicit grasping or rooting reflexes.
2. Handling is any touch, movement, or caregiving activity requiring contact (e.g., during medical procedures, diapering). With physiologically unstable high-risk infants, handling must be kept to a minimum to avoid further medical compromise and to help the infant conserve energy. However, with

infants who are physiologically stable and behaviorally organized, parental stroking can be a technique that encourages closeness with the newborn. Several studies (Adamson-Macedo, 1985; Kramer, 1975; Oehler, 1985) suggest that gentle supplemental stroking of physiologically stable infants may be beneficial, or at least have no adverse effects. Harrison et al. (1996) described a stroking technique that involves touching of the buttocks and lower back but avoids the chest or the abdomen.

3. Provision of developmentally supportive positioning interventions may promote a calm state and physiologic stability in the high-risk infant. If the infant is motorically stressed, help him or her to reorganize by holding extremities in flexion close to body until infant is calm, thereby decreasing unnecessary energy expenditure and encouraging self-regulation.

4. Providing a momentary time-out from incoming stimuli when a baby is stressed and disorganized allows him or her time to draw fully on self-regulatory abilities.

5. Observe for avoidance behaviors (e.g., gaze aversion, regurgitation, crying, increased extension patterns) in response to movement transitions or particular positions.

6. When repositioning an infant, contain the limbs to help the infant maintain stability and stay in control; use slow, gentle movements.

7. Encourage positions that allow the infant to place his or her hands near the mouth.

8. Knowledge of an infant's individual sensitivities and responses will facilitate the caregiver's selection of the most effective consoling technique. Communication of this information can be enhanced through primary nursing and the use of a developmental care plan.

9. "Kangaroo care," also known as skin-to-skin care, is an intervention that not only promotes parental involvement but also improves pulmonary function. The improved pulmonary function appears to be related to the vertical position, which increases oxygen saturation. The major controversy with kangaroo care involves its use with extremely premature infants. Another issue for caregivers to be aware of is the necessity of maintaining physiologic and behavioral stability during transfer from bed to parents and back again (Gale and VandenBerg, 1998).

Fostering Parent-Infant Interaction

A. Parental support strategies. The key to supporting mutually satisfying parent-infant interaction is to establish a family-centered approach on admission that will empower the parents to assume the natural parental role of advocating for their child's needs and desires. Supporting the parents' ability to understand their infant's level of communication through the infant's behavior will place the parents in a better position to respond to and interact with their infant in a developmentally supportive manner.

B. Intervention strategies.

1. Establish an atmosphere in the NICU that is welcoming to parents and does not treat them as "visitors" but as parents.

2. Help parents identify the most effective techniques for interacting with their infant (e.g., recognizing stress and time-out signs).

3. Place parents in situations where they will succeed in interacting positively with their infant.

4. Help parents identify both the consoling measures unique to their infant and how their child is providing feedback concerning the consoling measures.

5. Have the caregiving team work with the parents to plan specific activities (i.e., verbal interaction, eye contact, use of toys, recorded tapes of parent's voice, stroking) for parental interaction when appropriate.
6. Encourage parents to assume caregiving responsibilities when appropriate.
7. Discuss parents' expectation and goals for themselves and their infant. Encourage families to write down these expectations and goals. Writing down these dreams and goals will be the beginning of a lifelong care plan.
8. Encourage the parents to use their child's medical record as a communication tool.
9. Be aware of and involve the family's support system. Encourage parent-to-parent support if possible, either in a formal or an informal manner.
10. Always treat parents with the respect that is due to the most important member of the health care team.
11. Recognize that the parents are the constant in the child's life and that the various health professionals will come and go.

Neuromotor Development

A. **Neuromotor maturation** follows a predictable sequence as the premature infant progresses to 40 weeks of postconceptional age. Because the typical NICU environment is incompatible with the neurodevelopmental needs of the preterm infant, the caregiver is challenged to provide an appropriate environment for neuromaturation. However, with developmental attention the following progression can be attained within an NICU environment:
1. Generalized hypotonia progresses to flexion.
2. Random movements become purposeful and controlled.
3. Primary reflexes become consistent and complete.
4. Gradual perfection of primary reflexes proceeds cephalocaudally.
5. Muscle tone proceeds caudocephally.

B. **Sequential patterns of maturation** are identified by examining the following:
1. Resting postures (Amiel-Tison, 1968).
   a. Generalized hypotonia.
   b. Thigh flexion.
   c. Hip flexion.
   d. Froglike position.
   e. Total body flexion.
   f. Hypertonia.
2. Resistance to passive movement (Amiel-Tison, 1968).
   a. Full, passive range of motion.
   b. Extreme head lag, with attempt to right the head when pulled to sit.
   c. Some weight placed on feet when held in a supported stand.
   d. Stepping and placing responses are complete.
3. Active movements (Amiel-Tison, 1968).
   a. Spasmodic, random movements.
   b. Reflexive movements.
   c. Reciprocal movements.
   d. Wide variety of smooth and purposeful movements.
4. Sequence of development is predictable. However, *timing is individual* and may be affected by variables such as acuity of the infant's condition, postnatal complications, and certain medications.

C. **Positioning strategies** (Biber et al., 1989b).
1. A variety of positioning options are available. The benefits of positioning options must be measured in terms of impact on entire infant, not just on one subsystem. It is essential to monitor the infant's physiologic and behavioral

responses to various positioning strategies; gains in motor and state control systems may be offset by destabilizing effects to heart rate, respiratory rate, blood pressure, and so forth.

2. Counteract emerging stereotypical or abnormal postures. Promote newborn physiologic flexion. Physiologic flexion develops in the last trimester of pregnancy in response to decreased space in utero and as an active process in neurologic development (Moore and Nilsson, 1966); infants born prematurely do not have the opportunity to develop physiologic flexion. Supine positioning should be avoided. Flexion in a side-lying position is preferred to avoid a "frogleg" position.

3. Premature infants often engage in intentional movements aimed at making and maintaining contact with a stable surface in their immediate environment (Newman, 1981). This is a coping strategy used to maintain organizational balance through containment. Provide these infants with "boundaries" at their head, side, and feet (i.e., "nesting").

4. Provide positive input during the time spent without direct physical contact (Biber et al., 1989b).
   a. Facilitate midline orientation (hand-to-mouth activity) and symmetric positioning.
   b. Enhance self-quieting skills and behavioral organization.
   c. Encourage relaxation and improve digestion.
   d. Prevent bony deformities and skin breakdown.
   e. Increase awareness of body in space.
   f. Facilitate visual and auditory skill development.
   g. Facilitate development of head control.
   h. Avoid extremity restraints, especially four-point restraints.

5. Prone position.
   a. Benefits.
      (1) Facilitates flexion (Connally and Montgomery, 1987).
      (2) Facilitates development of early head control (Bobath and Bobath, 1972).
      (3) May improve oxygenation because of mechanical advantages on chest wall expansion (Martin et al., 1979).
   b. Principles.
      (1) Hips and knees should be flexed, with knees under hips and hips higher than shoulders.
      (2) Arms flexed, with hands near head and hand on face side near mouth.

6. Side-lying position: benefits.
   a. May facilitate flexion.
   b. May encourage hand-to-mouth activity, a self-quieting behavior.
   c. May be used to discourage arching or opisthotonus by providing boundaries to support.

7. Flexion: principles.
   a. Hips and knees flexed.
   b. Arms "cuddled" forward at shoulders and softly flexed.
   c. Head in line with body or slightly flexed.

8. Supine position.
   a. Frequently necessary due to medical interventions (e.g., ventilator, arterial lines, chest tubes); however, it is important to avoid having the infant in a supine position. Infants maintained in this position may have difficulty developing flexor patterns because:
      (1) Supine position facilitates extension.
      (2) Difficult for infant to flex against gravity.
   b. Principles.
      (1) Hips and knees slightly flexed upward, toward abdomen.

(2) Shoulders flexed forward, with hands on chest or abdomen.

(3) Arms and legs symmetric, with head in midline or comfortably turned to one side.

9. The American Academy of Pediatrics (AAP) issued positioning guidelines in 1992 and modified them in 1996. These guidelines recommended the supine position as the preferred sleep position during infancy. The AAP stressed that the supine and side-lying positions place an infant at less risk of sudden infant death syndrome (SIDS). The AAP reaffirmed that these guidelines were intended for healthy neonates only (Lockridge, 1997).

D. **Occupational and physical therapists can offer treatment** to the infant in these areas (Biber et al., 1989b; Fig. 21–2).

1. Normalizing muscle tone.
2. Increasing infant's tolerance for touch and/or handling.
3. Improving oral-motor control for sucking.
4. Preventing limitations in movement.
5. Developing normal movement patterns.
6. Developing more mature movement patterns.
7. Integrating normal infant movement patterns into caregiver's daily activities.
8. Developing more normal righting and equilibrium reactions.
9. Promoting relaxation.

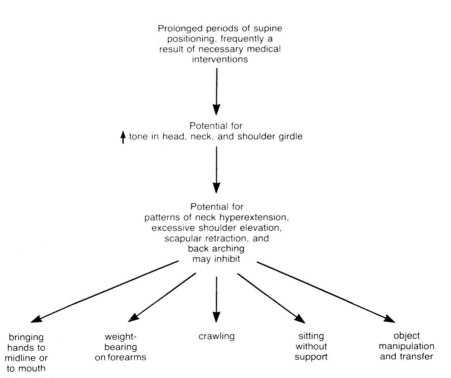

Figure 21–2

"Red alert" indicators for consultation and follow-up. (From Biber, P., Creger, P., Kolar, D., et al.: Developmentally supportive positioning and therapeutic handling strategies. *In* Creger, P. [Ed.]: Infant Interaction Program, Module 5: Developmentally Supportive Positioning and Therapeutic Handling of the Hospitalized Infant. Denver, The Children's Hospital Association, 1989, p. 36.)

Nutritive and Nonnutritive Sucking and Feeding Abilities

A. Sucking response.

1. Simple, rhythmic motor reflex (Wolff, 1968).
2. Composed of a pattern of bursts and pauses that allow infant to rest, regroup, socialize, and process cognitive information (Brazelton, 1987).
3. Neurodevelopmental progression of sucking response.
   a. At 9½ weeks' postconceptional age (PCA): perioral stimulation produces opening of mouth; lips do not protrude as in the sucking reflex (Humphrey, 1964).
   b. At 14 weeks' PCA: basic taste bud morphologic features and nerve supply are established (Bradley, 1972).
   c. At 17 weeks' PCA: sucking response (Dubignon, Campbell, and Patington, 1969) and swallowing (Heird and Anderson, 1977) have been observed.
   d. At 24 weeks' PCA: ganglion cells have innervated entire gastrointestinal system, allowing for motility (Heird and Anderson, 1977).
   e. At 28 weeks' PCA: rooting, sucking, and swallowing reflexes are well established, but response may be slow and imperfect (Amiel-Tison, 1968).
   f. At 32 weeks' PCA: gag reflex is present and serves as a protective mechanism for feeding (Fanaroff and Klaus, 1986).
   g. At 34 weeks' PCA: coordination of suck-swallow-breathe at 32–34 weeks (Bu'lock, Woolridge, and Baum, 1990; Bragdon, 1983) is possible because of myelinization of the medulla (Logan and Bosma, 1967). Two studies (Als, 1986 and 1988) demonstrated that infants who had had developmentally supportive care were able to effectively coordinate suck, swallow, and breathing at 45 days earlier than 34 weeks' gestation and progressed to bottle or breast feeding. Als showed that the infant may need to practice sucking or receive oral stimulation to be more successful in later feeding.

B. Successful oral feeding experiences.

1. Safe: caregiver should believe that infant's risk of aspiration is minimal (Biber, Creger, and Kolar, 1989a).
2. Pleasurable: feeding interaction should provide positive reinforcement to infant and caregiver (Biber et al., 1989a).
3. Functional: infant should consume enough formula in reasonable amount of time to ensure adequate caloric intake and growth (Biber et al., 1989a).
4. The most important variable affecting the success of oral feedings is the consistency of caregivers/primary nursing team who are able to establish a relationship with the baby and the family and to assess progress over time (Deloian, 1998).
5. Other variables to assess: the infant's gestational age and weight, muscle tone, ability to achieve and maintain an alert state, and ability to coordinate a rhythmic suck/swallow.
6. Nonnutritive sucking: exposing the preterm infant to nonnutritive sucking is an important component that enhances later success in oral feeding (McCain, 1995 and 1997). Benefits include:
   a. Simple intervention for the nursing staff.
   b. Rate of sucking: 1 suck per second.
   c. Fewer behavioral changes during feedings.
   d. More success in bringing the infant to an alert state, which improves feeding success.
   e. Transition to oral feedings is often more successful when opportunities for nonnutritive sucking are given during tube feedings.
   f. Provides an opportunity for parental interaction and involvement.

C. **Nutritive sucking.**

1. Greater coordination of the suck-swallow-breathe sequence required than in nonnutritive sucking.
2. To encourage as normal a suck-swallow pattern as possible while infant maintains physiological, motor, and state stability, it is very important to hold the nipple still and stimulate the infant with voice and touch. Allow rest between suck bursts.
3. Four nutritive sucking patterns.
   a. Mature sucking pattern: two sucks per second, with simultaneous swallowing occurring during the sucking bursts (Palmer, 1989; Harris 1986).
   b. Immature sucking bursts: one to four sucks per burst, with swallowing occurring before and after the sucks. At less than 40 weeks' gestation, this sucking pattern is considered normal. A mature sucking pattern, after 40 weeks, is 10 or more sucks per burst (Palmer, 1993; Palmer, Crawley, and Blink, 1993).
   c. Disorganized pattern: reflects lack of symmetry in total sucking response, rather than lack of coordination (Palmer, 1993; Palmer et al., 1993).
   d. Dysfunctional pattern: refers to interruption of feeding process by abnormal movements of tongue and jaw, such as lack of rate change between nutritive and nonnutritive sucking, wide jaw excursion, or flaccid tongue movement (Palmer, 1993; Palmer et al., 1993).

D. **Assessment:** variables to assess before initiation of nutritive sucking (VandenBerg and Goderez, 1987).

1. Ability to organize physiologic, motor, and state systems.
2. Receptivity to nonnutritive sucking opportunities.
3. Ease with which rooting reflex is elicited.
4. Coordination of suck and swallow during nonnutritive sucking.
5. Presence or absence of "hunger" behaviors (crying, rooting, hand-to-mouth activity). Satiation may inhibit sucking behavior (Satinoff and Stanley, 1963).
6. Physical demands of infant's daily routine, where energy reserves may be limited.
7. Growth curve: gaining weight consistently over time while on gavage feeds.
8. General muscle tone. Infant with truncal hypotonia may also have decreased oral-motor tone.
9. Oxygen requirement. Supplemental oxygen may make a difference between success and failure.

E. **Interventions.**

1. Setting the scene for nutritive sucking (VandenBerg and Goderez, 1987).
   a. Research studies have shown that premature infants feed better on a demand schedule.
   b. Observe infant's subtle hunger cues: state change to drowsy, lip licking, finger chewing, hands to mouth, and so forth.
   c. Allow sufficient time to give infant "undivided attention."
   d. Plan to assess infant's color, heart rate, respiratory rate and effort, muscle tone, and state; apnea or bradycardia during feeding may indicate that infant is not ready for nutritive sucking.
   e. Be aware of environmental factors (sounds, lights, movements) that may contribute to the infant's disorganization.
   f. Use infant's cues to determine timing of feedings. For example, does the infant become more aroused, root, get hands to mouth, or try to suck?
   g. Consider swaddling infant to minimize extraneous movements and to provide external stability; swaddling encourages flexion, which facilitates sucking (Connally and Montgomery, 1987). Be sure that the swaddling is

not restricting the availability of the infant's hands. If the hands are available, the infant may then be able to get them to the mouth.

h. Begin preparing the infant for nutritive sucking by using nonnutritive sucking: hold the infant during gavage feedings and use a pacifier. Assess the infant's ability to come to an alert state.

i. Primary nursing facilitates consistency of caregiver and feeding techniques.

2. Mechanical considerations that should be consistent with each feeding (VandenBerg and Goderez, 1987).

   a. Size of nipple.
      (1) Affects infant's ability to close mouth around nipple.
      (2) Affects how far back into throat formula is ejected.
   b. Shape of nipple.
      (1) Affects seal of infant's lips around nipple.
      (2) Affects how far back into throat the formula is ejected.
      (3) Determines "fit" inside infant's mouth.
   c. Firmness of nipple.
      (1) Affects strength of suck required to extract formula.
      (2) Affects amount of formula ejected per suck.
   d. Size of hole in nipple.
      (1) Affects amount of formula ejected per suck.
      (2) Affects rate of flow for formula.
      (3) Affects strength of suck required to extract formula.

3. Documentation of feeding.
   a. Infant state.
   b. Type of nipple.
   c. Volume.
   d. Problems: fatigue, endurance, coordination, and leakage.
   e. Duration of feeding.

4. Common feeding problems (VandenBerg, 1990).
   a. State disorganization.
      (1) Feeding behavior is affected by infant state, or level of arousal (Meier and Pugh, 1985). Infants pursue feedings more eagerly and demonstrate more organized nutritive sucking pattern if awake and active first.
      (2) Cue-based feeding may be more profitable than feeding on a rigid schedule. With a fragile infant, the first feeding may last only 30 seconds; subsequent feedings would then be increased in duration. Remember that the infant is in charge of duration with cue-based feedings and to stop *before* the infant loses control.
      (3) Clinical conditions that affect infant state (e.g., anemia, hypoglycemia, jaundice) may influence feeding behavior (Meier and Pugh, 1985).
   b. Poor coordination of suck-swallow-breathe pattern. A nursing intervention would be to pace feedings and shorten sucking bursts to encourage the infant to breathe and swallow.
   c. Fatigue.
      (1) Feeding process can be tiring for preterm or disorganized infant. Sucking is composed of a pattern of bursts and pauses. Help parents distinguish between fatigue and pauses (rest periods), which are a normal part of sucking activity.
      (2) Limit number of bottle feedings per day until organization and endurance improve. Assess infant's feeding regimen. Consider decreasing the volume and feeding more frequently, or decreasing the frequency and providing a larger volume. Another strategy would be to increase the caloric content and decrease both the volume and the frequency. Note that a feeding lasting longer than 30 minutes for an infant beyond 1 month of corrected age or one who is fragile is not recommended.

d. Inability to shift from nonnutritive to nutritive sucking.
   (1) The nonnutritive suck is faster and causes too much formula to be ejected per suck.
   (2) Infants who cannot change their rate of suck may have a neurologically based problem (Palmer, 1989).

F. **Evaluation: "stop" signs.**
1. Infants with significant feeding difficulties are at risk for speech and language abnormalities (Illingworth, 1969). The same muscles necessary for successful nutritive sucking activity are used in speech production.
2. "Stop" sign behaviors. (NOTE: Short rest period may reduce or eliminate behaviors.)
   a. State change to sleep.
   b. Increased biting, tongue thrusting, lack of jaw closure.
   c. Subtle or patent disengagement, such as gagging and hiccuping repeatedly, desaturations, head turn, back arch, and salute.
   d. Inability to suck.
   e. Eager sucking on pacifier but weak or arrhythmic nutritive suck.
   f. Aversive behavior (squirming, hyperextension, turning head away, pursing of lips, crying) that occurs consistently after the infant takes a few nutritive sucks.

G. **Breast-feeding of the preterm infant.**

1. Indicators of readiness (Meier and Pugh, 1985).
   a. Postconceptional age of 34–35 weeks (to allow for mature suck-swallow reflex).
   b. Ability to maintain infant's body temperature while being held.
   c. Mother's readiness to breast-feed.
2. Improvement of chances for success.
   a. Assess infant state.
      (1) Level of arousal is associated with infant's ability and eagerness to breast-feed (Meier and Pugh, 1985).
      (2) Preterm infants pursue the breast more eagerly and demonstrate more organized nutritive sucking pattern if awake and active first.
      (3) Feed the infant on the basis of cues rather than according to a rigid schedule.
   b. Provide assistance.
      (1) Provide privacy.
      (2) Assist mother with finding a comfortable position.
      (3) Guide infant's head onto breast; simultaneously encourage wider opening of infant's mouth to encompass areola.
   c. Assess daily fluid balance and weight gain.
      (1) Must allow the infant to consume more volume in one feeding than another when using cue-based schedule (Meier and Pugh, 1985).
      (2) Monitor daily fluid balance and weight gain over time, rather than specific volume intake every 3–4 hours. Consider before-and-after weights to monitor ingested milk intake and required supplements once the infant has established a pattern of some consistent suckling.
   d. Allow total feeding time flexibility.
      (1) Breast-feeding sessions frequently last longer than bottle-feeding sessions: infant independently paces breast-feeding session, sucking and pausing as individually necessary.
      (2) Breast-feeding infants integrate nutritive sucking, rest periods, and social behaviors, thereby lengthening overall feeding time (Meier and Anderson, 1987).

(3) Help the preterm infant control breast-feeding experiences by monitoring physiologic and/or clinical indicators to prevent fatigue.

e. Provide anticipatory guidance.

(1) Mothers are easily disappointed and discouraged when infant will not awaken to breast-feed (Meier and Pugh, 1985).

(2) Offer consultation with lactation specialist to address any foreseeable problems.

(3) Some infants may be able consistently to organize nutritive sucking and interactional periods; others demonstrate more variable feeding patterns, ranging from organized sucking to little nutritive feeding activity.

f. Apply breast-feeding recommendations to preterm infant and family on an individual basis.

Auditory Assessment and Follow-up of Infant at Risk of Impairment

A. Background.

1. Hearing loss. Estimates vary widely on the prevalence of hearing loss in neonates, from 0.9:1000 to 2.4:1000 (Mauk et al., 1991). The 1993 National Institutes of Health (NIH) Consensus Statement estimated hearing loss to be 1:1000 (NIH Statement, 1993).

2. Hearing impairment. Reported as 3:1000 in otherwise healthy newborn infants (Coplan, 1987; Feinmesser and Tell, 1976).

   a. Limited speech production skills (Osberger et al., 1986).

   b. Reduced academic achievement, especially in language-related areas (Allen, 1986).

3. Noise level. The typical NICU often has noise levels in the range of 65–85 decibels. Noises are often of high intensity and low frequency (Gottfried and Hodgman, 1984; Weibly, 1989). The sound of the closing of an incubator's porthole can reach 117–135 decibels (Bess, Peek, and Chapman, 1979; Weibly, 1989). These levels exceed the 58-decibel maximum safe level recommended by the AAP (1974). Premature infants are particularly sensitive to loud noises because of the immaturity of the sensitive cochlea and organ of Corti (Beckham and Mishoe, 1982). In 1997 the AAP Committee on Environmental Health recommended that any noise within the NICU exceeding 45 decibels is best avoided. Simple strategies, such as no tapping on incubators, the wearing of soft-soled shoes, and careful closing of portholes, were suggested. Overall, the AAP encouraged NICUs to evaluate noise levels when purchasing new equipment or when renovating nursery space.

B. Types of hearing loss (Biber et al., 1989c).

1. Conductive hearing loss.

   a. Caused by interference in sound transmission from external auditory canal to inner ear.

   b. Inner ear capable of normal function.

   c. Associated with frequent ear infections.

   d. Sounds muffled or faint.

   e. Loss of air-conducted sounds; sounds transmitted in inner ear by bone conduction (skull and temporal bones) are heard normally.

   f. May resolve spontaneously; most can be corrected medically or surgically.

2. Sensorineural hearing loss.

   a. Caused by damage to sensory end organ (cochlear hair cells) or by dysfunction of auditory nerve.

   b. Sounds distorted or muffled.

    c. Air and bone conduction thresholds usually equal.
    d. High tones inaudible.
    e. Loss usually irreversible.
    f. Loss treated with hearing aid and speech therapy.
3. Mixed hearing loss.
    a. Combination of conductive and sensorineural loss.
    b. Bone-conduction thresholds below normal, and air conduction even more so.
    c. Gap between air- and bone-conduction threshold levels should disappear after conductive loss is treated.
    d. Hearing levels not likely to return to normal.
4. Central auditory dysfunction.
    a. Sounds are transmitted normally but interpreted incorrectly by the brain.
    b. Manifested by decreased auditory comprehension.
5. Ototoxic hearing loss.
    a. Damage to cochlea and/or vestibular part of inner ear, resulting in permanent sensorineural hearing loss; loss is usually bilateral and symmetric.
    b. Drugs implicated in ototoxicity.
        (1) Aminoglycoside antibiotics.
            (a) Streptomycin.
            (b) Neomycin.
            (c) Gentamicin.
            (d) Kanamycin.
            (e) Tobramycin.
            (f) Amikacin
            (g) Vancomycin
        (2) Diuretics.
            (a) Ethacrynic acid (Edecrin).
            (b) Furosemide (Lasix).
    c. Factors that may enhance risk of ototoxic effects.
        (1) Increased serum drug level.
        (2) Decreased renal function.
        (3) Use of more than one ototoxic drug simultaneously or in consecutive courses.
        (4) Use of ototoxic drug in increased daily doses for an extended period.

C. **Three major tools** used to screen neonatal hearing.
1. High-risk register (HRR): A.B.C.D.'s of deafness (Downs and Silver, 1972); an infant with any of the following seven risk factors in prenatal, perinatal, or neonatal history has an increased chance of hearing impairment.
    a. *A:* asphyxia (may include infants with Apgar scores of 0–3 who do not exhibit spontaneous respirations by 10 minutes, and those with hypotonia existing to 2 hours of age.
    b. *B:* bacterial meningitis (especially *Haemophilus influenzae*).
    c. *C:* congenital perinatal infection (cytomegalovirus, rubella, herpes, toxoplasmosis, syphilis).
    d. *D:* defects of head or neck.
    e. *E:* elevated bilirubin exceeding indications for exchange.
    f. *F:* family history of childhood hearing impairment.
    g. *G:* gram birth weight: ≤500 g.

Retrospective studies (Mauk et al., 1991; Shimizu et al., 1990) have shown that only about 50% of children who have later hearing loss had any of these risk factors. Therefore the HRR has been shown to have limited value as a screening tool but is useful in maintaining awareness among professionals of those infants who are at higher risk of hearing loss.

2. Auditory brain-stem response (ABR) (Spivak, 1998).
   a. ABR test is a noninvasive measurement of electrophysiologic response of brain-stem auditory pathways to an acoustic stimulus.
   b. ABRs can be recorded in infants at very low stimulus levels: reduces possibility of missing infant with mild to moderate hearing loss.
   c. ABRs can be used to identify unilateral or asymmetric hearing impairment.
3. Evoked otoacoustic emissions (EOAEs). EOAE tests are quick, reliable, safe, efficient, and cost-effective, and they demonstrate excellent performance characteristics. EOAEs are sounds that are generated in the cochlea in response to stimulation presented to the ear. EOAE tests are noninvasive and require no electrode preparation or placement; responses can be elicited easily from well babies and infants in the NICU (Gravel and Tocci, 1998).

D. **Universal newborn screening.** The 1993 NIH Consensus Statement strongly endorsed universal newborn hearing screening. Many other conferences and consensus statements have recommended the need to identify hearing loss early in life, but the consensus statement coming from the NIH has been the springboard for the introduction of the screening of all newborn infants. The NIH consensus statement recommends the screening of all infants by 3 months of age with an initial screen by EOAE test, followed by rescreening with an ABR test at 3–6 months (Orlando and Prieve, 1998).

E. **Implications for caregivers (Biber et al., 1989c).**

1. "Listen" to the environment from the infant's viewpoint; assess appropriateness of existing or additional auditory stimulation.
2. Points to consider when designing care plan. (*Note:* Not every item will be appropriate for every infant, and no single item will be appropriate for a particular infant all the time.)
   a. High-frequency sounds usually arouse attention.
   b. Low-frequency sounds may produce sleep.
   c. Sudden loud noises may induce agitation and/or crying, producing physiologic signs of stress.
   d. Simulate diurnal noise levels.
   e. Provide auditory stimulation from different locations: Does infant quiet? Anticipate sounds when repeated? Document observations.
   f. Behavioral assessment of infant and evaluation of interventions must be ongoing.

F. **Follow-up and management (Biber et al., 1989c).**

1. Parents of all newborns.
   a. Should receive information about normal auditory, speech, and language development.
   b. Benefit from information about expected milestones in communication development, enhancing their ability to detect abnormal auditory, speech, and language development.
   c. Should be informed of the importance of early audiologic evaluation of suspected hearing problems.
2. Hearing of at-risk infants should be evaluated by an audiologist prior to discharge or no later than 3 months of age (Fig. 21–3).

Developmental Care Plan

A. **Written communication** developed between the family and health care providers that outlines the plan to support an individual infant's capacity for behavioral organization. It is based on the infant and family's strengths, needs, and goals.

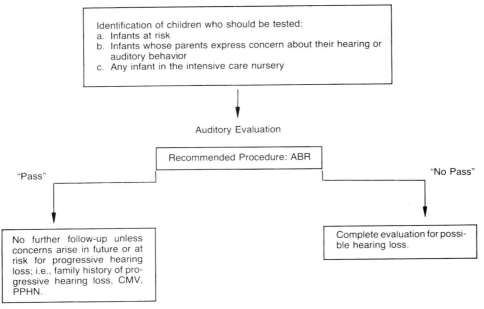

Figure 21–3
Identification and assessment of infants at risk of hearing impairment. *ABR*, Auditory brain-stem response; *CMV*, cytomegalovirus; *PPHN*, persistent pulmonary hypertension of the newborn. (From Hayes, D.: Identification and assessment of infants at risk for hearing impairment. *In* Creger, P. [Ed.]: Infant Interaction Program, Module 4: Assessment of the Auditory System and Follow-up of the Infant at Risk for Hearing Loss. Denver, The Children's Hospital Association, 1989, p. 29.)

B. **Should coordinate input** from multidisciplinary team: parents, medicine, nursing, occupational therapy, physical therapy, respiratory therapy, and social services.

C. **Allows infant's family and primary nurse to make specific recommendations** regarding environmental modifications, positioning techniques, calming measures, and the promotion of self-quieting abilities.

REFERENCES

Adamson-Macedo, E.N.: Effects of tactile stimulation of preterm infants. Neonatal Network, *31*(6):330–336, 1985–1986.

Allen, T.: Patterns of academic achievement among hearing impaired students: 1974 and 1983. *In* Schildroth, A., and Karchmer, M. (Eds.): Deaf Children in America. San Diego, College-Hill Press, 1986, pp. 161–206.

Als, H.: Individualized behavioral and environmental care for the VLBW preterm infant at high risk for bronchopulmonary dysplasia: NICU and developmental outcome. Pediatrics, *78*:1123–1132, 1986.

Als, H.: ICU stress for the high-risk preterm infant. Paper presented at Developmental Interventions in Neonatal Care, San Diego, November 1988, Contemporary Forums Syllabus, p. 7.

Als, H., Brazelton, T.B., Lester, B.M., et al.: Manual for the assessment of preterm infants' behavior (APIB). *In* Fitzgerald, H.E., Lester, B.M., and Yogman, M.W. (Eds.): Theory and Research in Behavioral Pediatrics. New York, Plenum Press, 1982, pp. 65–132.

Amiel-Tison, C.: Neurological evaluation of the maturity of newborn infants. Arch. Dis. Child., *43*:89–93, 1968.

Becker, P.T., Grunwald, P.C., Moorman, J., and Stuhr, S.: Outcomes of developmentally supportive nursing care for very low birth weight infants. Nursing Research, *40*:150–155, 1991.

Beckham, R.W., and Mishoe, S.C.: Sound levels inside incubators and oxygen hoods used with nebulizers and humidifiers. Respir. Care, *35*:1272–1279, 1982.

Bess, F.H., Peek, B., and Chapman, J.: Further observations on noise levels in infant incubators. Pediatrics, *63*:100–106, 1979.

Biber, P., Creger, P., and Kolar, D.: The promotion of positive feeding experiences. *In* Creger, P. (Ed.): Infant Interaction Program, Module 6: Neurodevelopmental Assessment of Feeding Abilities and Follow-up of the Disorganized Feeder. Denver, Children's Hospital Association, 1989a, pp. 7–8.

Biber, P., Creger, P., Kolar, D., et al.: Developmentally supportive positioning and therapeutic handling strategies. *In* Creger, P. (Ed.): Infant Interaction Program, Module 5: Developmentally Supportive Positioning and Therapeutic Handling of the Hospitalized Infant. Denver, Children's Hospital Association, 1989b, pp. 11–28.

Biber, P., Creger, P., Mediavilla, K., et al.: Four basic types of hearing impairments: General implications for care-givers. *In* Creger, P. (Ed.): Infant Interaction Program, Module 4: Assessment of the Auditory System and Follow-up of the Infant at Risk for Hearing Loss. Denver, Children's Hospital Association, 1989c.

Bobath, B., and Bobath, K.: The neurodevelopmental approach to treatment. *In* Pearson, P., and Williams, C. (Eds.): Physical Therapy Services in the Developmental Disabilities. Springfield, Ill., Charles C Thomas, 1972.

Bradley, R.N.: Development of the tastebuds on gustatory papillae in human fetuses. *In* Bosma, J.F. (Ed.): Third Symposium on Oral Sensation and Perception: The Mouth of the Infant. Springfield, Ill., Charles C Thomas, 1972, pp. 137–162.

Bragdon, D.B.: A basis for the nursing management of feeding the premature infant. J. Obstet. Gynecol. Neonat. Nurs., 12:515–575, 1983.

Brazelton, T.B.: Behavioral competence of the newborn infant. *In* Avery, G.B. (Ed.): Neonatology: Pathophysiology and Management of the Newborn, 3rd ed. Philadelphia, J.B. Lippincott, 1987, pp. 379–399.

Bu'lock, F., Woolridge M.W., and Baum J.D.: Development of coordination of sucking, swallowing and breathing: Ultrasound study of term and preterm infants. Dev. Med. Child Neurol., 32:669–678, 1990.

Collinge, J.M., Bradley, K., Perks, C., et al.: Demand vs. scheduled feedings for premature infants. J. Obstet. Gynecol. Neonatal Nurs., November/December:362–367, 1982.

Connally, B.H., and Montgomery, P.C. (Eds.): Therapeutic Exercise in Developmental Disabilities. Chattanooga, Chattanooga Corporation, 1987.

Coplan, J.: Deafness: Ever hear of it? Delayed recognition of permanent hearing loss. Pediatrics, 79:206–213, 1987.

Deloian, B.: Caring Connections: Nursing Support Transitioning Premature Infants and Their Families Home From the Hospital. Denver, University of Colorado Health Sciences Center, 1998.

Downs, M.P., and Silver, H.K.: The "A.B.C.D.'s" to H.E.A.R.: Early detection in nursery, office and clinic of the infant who is deaf. Clin. Pediatr., 11:563–566, 1972.

Dubignon, J.M., Campbell, D., and Patington, M.W.: The development of nonnutritive sucking in premature infants. Biol. Neonate, 14:270–278, 1969.

Fanaroff, A., and Klaus, M.: Feeding and selected disorders of the gastrointestinal tract. *In* Klaus, M., and Fanaroff, A. (Eds.): Care of the High-Risk Neonate. Philadelphia, W.B. Saunders, 1986, pp. 113–146.

Feinmesser, M., and Tell, L.: Neonatal screening for detection of deafness. Arch. Otolaryngol., 102:297–299, 1976.

Gale, G., and VandenBerg, K.A.: Kangaroo Care. *Neonatal Network*, 17(5):69–70, 1998.

Gottfried, A., and Hodgman, J.: How intensive is newborn intensive care? An environmental analysis. *Pediatrics*, 74:292–294, 1984.

Gravel, J.S., and Tocci, L.L.: Setting the stage for universal hearing screening. *In* Spivak, L.G. (Ed.): Universal Newborn Hearing Screening. New York, Thieme, 1998, pp. 7, 17–20.

Harris, M.B.: Oral motor management of the high-risk infant. *In* Sweeny, J.K. (Ed.): The High-Risk Neonate: Developmental Therapy Perspectives. New York, Haworth Press, 1986, pp. 231–251.

Harrison, L., Olivet, L., Cunningham, K., et al.: Effects of gentle human touch on preterm infants: Pilot study results. Neonatal Network, 15(2):35–37, 1996.

Heird, W., and Anderson, T.: Nutritional requirements of the low birth weight infant. *In* Behrman, R.E. (Ed.): Neonatal Perinatal Medicine: Diseases of the Fetus and Infant. St. Louis, C.V. Mosby, 1977.

Humphrey, T.: Embryology of the central nervous system with some correlations with functional development. Ala. J. Med. Sci., 1:60–64, 1964.

Illingworth, R.: Sucking and swallowing difficulties in infancy: Diagnostic problem of dysphagia. Arch. Dis. Child., 44:655–665, 1969.

Kramer, M. Extra tactile stimulation of the premature infant. Nursing Research, 24:324–334, 1975.

Lockridge, T.: Now I lay me down to sleep: SIDS and infant sleep positions. *Neonatal Network*, 16(7):25–31, 1997.

Logan, W.J., and Bosma, J.F.: Oral and pharyngeal dysphasia in infancy. Pediatr. Clin. North Am., 14:47–61, 1967.

McCain, G.C.: Promotion of preterm infant feeding with non-nutritive sucking. J. Pediatr. Nurs., 10(1):3–8, 1995.

McCain, G.C.: Behavioral state activity during nipple feedings for preterm infants. *Neonatal Network*, 16(5):43–47, 1997.

Martin, R.J., Hereof, N., Rubin, D., et al.: Effect of supine and prone positions on arterial oxygen tension in the preterm infant. Pediatrics, 63:528–531, 1979.

Mauk, G.W., White, K.R., Mortensen, L.B., et al.: The effectiveness of screening programs based on high-risk characteristics in early identification of hearing impairment. Ear Hear., 12(3):12–19, 1991.

Meier, P., and Anderson, G.C.: Responses of small preterm infants to bottle and breastfeeding. Matern. Child Nurs. J., 12:97–105, 1987.

Meier, P., and Pugh, E.J.: Breastfeeding behavior of small preterm infants. Matern. Child Nurs. J., 10:396–401, 1985.

Moeller, M., Osberger, M., and Eccarius, M.: Receptive language skills. *In* Osberger, M. (Ed.): Language and learning skills in hearing impaired students. ASHA Monogr., 23:41–53, 1986.

Moore, K.L., and Nilsson, L.: A Child is Born. New York, Dell Publishing, 1966.

Morris, S.E.: Oral-motor development: Normal and abnormal. *In* Wilson, J.M. (Ed.): Oral-motor Function and Dysfunction in Children. Chapel Hill, University of North Carolina at Chapel Hill, 1977, pp. 114–122.

National Institutes of Health Consensus Statement: Early Identification of Hearing Impairment in Infants and Young Children. Rockville, Md., Author, 1993 (March 1–3).

Newman, L.F.: Social and sensory environment of low birth weight infants in a special care nursery. J. Nerv. Ment. Dis., 169:448–455, 1981.

Oehler, J.M.: Examining the issue of tactile stimulation of preterm infants. Neonatal Network, 31:330–336, 1985.

Orlando, M.S., and Prieve, B.A.: Models for universal newborn hearing screening programs. *In* Spivak, L.G. (Ed.): Universal Newborn Hearing Screening. New York: Thieme, 1998, p. 52.

Osberger, M., Moeller, M., Eclairs, M., et al.: Expressive language skills. *In* Osberger, M. (Ed.): Language and Learning Skills of Hearing Impaired Students. ASHA Monogr., 23:54–56, 1986.

Palmer, M.: Feeding problems and treatment strategies for infants with BPD, drug addiction, tracheostomies, and neuromuscular disorders. Presented at Contemporary Forums Conference: Developmental Interventions in Neonatal Care, New Orleans, 1989.

Palmer, M.M.: Identification and management of the transitional suck pattern in premature infants. J. Perinatal Neonatal Nurs., 7(1):66–75, 1993.

Palmer, M.M., Crawley, K., and Blink, I.A.: Neonatal oral-motor assessment scale: A reliability study. J. Perinatol., 8(1):28–35, 1993.

Palmer, M.M., and Heyman, M.B.: Assessment and treatment of sensory- versus motor-based feeding problems in very young children. Infants and Young Children, 6(2):67–73, 1993.

Satinoff, E., and Stanley, W.C.: Effect of stomach loading on sucking behavior in neonatal puppies. J. Comp. Physiol. Psychol., 56:66–68, 1963.

Shimizu, H., Walters, R.J., Proctor, L.R., et al.: Identification of hearing impairment in the neonatal intensive care unit population: Outcome of a five-year project at the Johns Hopkins Hospital. Semin. Hearing, 11:150–160, 1990.

Spivak, L.G. (Ed.): Universal Newborn Hearing Screening. New York, Thieme, 1998.

VandenBerg, K.A.: Nippling management of the sick neonate in the NICU: The disorganized feeder. Neonatal Network, 9:9–15, 1990.

VandenBerg, K.A., and Goderez, L.: Neurodevelopmental assessment of feeding problems and interventions for the disorganized feeder in NICU and follow-up. (Handout: "Feeding Variables," conference syllabus, Developmental Interventions in Neonatal Care Conference.) San Francisco, Contemporary Forums, July 1987.

Weibly, T. Inside the incubator. Matern. Child Nurs. J., 14:96–100, 1989.

Wolff, P.H.: The serial organization of sucking in the young infant. Pediatrics, 42:943–956, 1968.

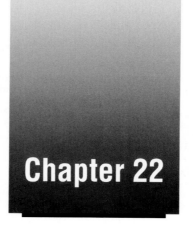

Chapter 22

Genetics and Fetal Anomalies

Julieanne Schiefelbein

Objectives

1. Define birth defects and possible causes.

2. Become familiar with genetic terminology.

3. Identify the number of chromosomes in a normal human cell.

4. Describe the characteristics and causes of structural and numeric chromosomal abnormalities, modes of inheritance of single-gene disorders, and multifactorial inheritance.

5. Describe what prenatal diagnostic tests are available and which anomalies they detect.

6. Describe the components and benefits of genetic counseling.

7. Identify three patient care management issues in genetic counseling.

8. Verbalize the systematic process used to evaluate the malformed infant.

9. List common congenital malformations and possible mechanisms of cause.

The neonate born with a genetic defect or fetal anomaly presents a challenge to the NICU team. A definitive diagnosis is essential for management and care of the neonate and the neonate's family.

Congenital malformations commonly have multiple causes. This chapter includes information on basic genetics, characteristics and causes of some common fetal anomalies, and a systematic process for evaluation of the malformed infant. Commonalities of patient care management issues are addressed, with the understanding that every family requires individualized care.

Basic Genetics

TERMINOLOGY

A. **Birth defect:** an abnormality of structure, function, or metabolism, whether genetically determined or a result of environmental interference during embryonic or fetal life. A congenital defect may cause disease from the time of conception through birth or later in life (*March of Dimes*).

B. **Chromosome:** structural elements in cell nucleus that carry the genes and convey genetic information.

1. Each cell (except erythrocytes) in the body contains all the chromosomes received from both parents within its nucleus.
2. There are 23 pairs of chromosomes, for a total of 46 chromosomes, with one maternal and one paternal chromosome creating each pair.

C. **Gene:** the smallest unit of inheritance of a single characteristic, responsible for a physical, biochemical, or physiologic trait and located with other genes in linear sequence along the chromosome.

D. **Genotype:** hereditary composition of an individual.

E. **Autosome:** one of 22 chromosomes that do not determine the sex of the individual.

F. **Sex chromosomes:** the X and Y chromosomes, which are responsible for sex determination—XX for female and XY for male.

G. **Diploid:** containing a set of maternal and a set of paternal chromosomes, for a total of 46 chromosomes.

H. **Gamete:** one of two cells, containing 23 chromosomes (haploid number), with the union of a male gamete and a female gamete required during sexual production to create a new individual (with the diploid number of chromosomes).

I. **Haploid:** having half the number of chromosomes found in the person's cells; characteristic of the gametes.

J. **Locus:** the position that the gene occupies on a chromosome.

K. **Karyotype:** pictorial representation of the chromosomal characteristics of an individual or species.

L. **Allele:** one of a series of alternate forms of a gene at the same locus on a chromosome (Jones, 1997; Jorde, Carey, and White, 1996; Gelehrter, Collins, and Ginsburg, 1998).

DOMINANCE AND RECESSIVENESS

A. **Phenotype:** observable characteristics of an individual.

B. **Heterogeneous chromosomes:** differing pair of chromosomes, one from each parent, arraying differing genes for specific traits. When there are unlike genes on a locus, one gene dominates.

C. **Homologous chromosomes:** a matched pair of chromosomes, one from each parent, carrying the genes for the same traits.

D. **Dominant gene:** a gene that is expressed in the heterozygous state. In a dominant disorder, the mutant gene overshadows the normal gene. A dose of this gene is needed for expression.

E. **Recessive gene:** a gene whose effect is masked or hidden unless both genes of a set of homologous chromosomes at a given locus are abnormal, thus showing the disease. In a heterozygote (carrier) the normal gene overshadows the mutant gene.

F. Possible combinations of chromosomes:

1. Both genes can be dominant—AA (homozygous).

2. Both genes can be recessive—aa (homozygous).
3. One gene can be dominant and one can be recessive—Aa (heterozygous).

G. **Autosomal dominant disorders:** more than 1218 identified disorders.
1. Characteristics of autosomal dominant disorders.
    a. Males and females are both affected equally; either parent can pass the gene on to sons or daughters.
    b. An affected offspring has an affected parent if the mutation is not new.
    c. Half the sons and half the daughters of an affected parent can be anticipated to have the disorder. There is a 50% chance with each pregnancy.
    d. Unaffected offspring of an affected parent will have all normal offspring if the mate is an unaffected person (assuming complete penetrance).
    e. If two affected persons mate, three fourths of their offspring will be affected. A double dose of the mutant gene in any of the offspring will result in a lethal anomaly (except in the case of Huntington's disease).
    f. Family history of an anomaly indicates a vertical route of transmission through successive generations on one side of the family (if not a new mutation).
2. Examples of autosomal dominant disorders: myotonic dystrophy, neurofibromatosis, and coronary artery disease (Jones, 1997; Nora et al., 1994).

H. **Autosomal recessive disorders:** approximately 947 identified disorders.
1. Characteristics of autosomal recessive disorders.
    a. Both males and females are affected equally.
    b. Parents of affected offspring are rarely affected and are usually heterozygous carriers.
    c. After the birth of an affected offspring, there is a 25% chance, with each pregnancy, of having another affected offspring and a 50% chance that the offspring will be a carrier.
    d. There may be a distant relative with the disorder.
    e. Affected persons who mate with unaffected persons will have offspring who will be heterozygous carriers.
    f. If two affected persons mate, all offspring will be affected.
    g. No family history indicates a horizontal route of transmission in the same generation.
    h. There can be a difference in expression of the disorder: very mild in one member and extremely severe in another.
2. Examples of autosomal recessive disorders: cystic fibrosis, sickle cell anemia, Tay-Sachs disease, thalassemia major (Connor and Ferguson-Smith, 1993).

I. **X-linked dominant disorders:** 171 known disorders.
1. Characteristics of X-linked dominant disorders.
    a. Both sexes can be affected; because females have a double chance of receiving the mutant X chromosome, they have twice the risk of being affected.
    b. Affected males will have all affected daughters and no affected sons.
    c. Affected females will transmit the disorders in the same manner as with autosomal dominant patterns.
    d. Two thirds of the time, affected females have an affected mother; one third of the time, they have an affected father.
    e. Family history shows no father-to-son transmissions.
2. Example: vitamin D–resistant rickets (Davies, 1993).

J. **X-linked recessive disorders.**

1. Characteristics of X-linked recessive disorders.
    a. Only male offspring are affected, with rare exceptions. A female offspring will be affected if she has both a carrier mother and an affected father.

b. Carrier females transmit the disorder.

c. All sons of affected males will be normal.

d. All daughters of affected males will be carriers (with each pregnancy).

e. Heterozygous females transmit the gene to half their sons, who will be affected, and to half their daughters, who will be carriers.

f. Transmission is horizontal among males in the same generation; in addition, a generation will be skipped, and second-generation males will be affected.

2. Examples: Duchenne's muscular dystrophy, hemophilia, color blindness, and glucose-6-phosphate dehydrogenase deficiency (Pickler and Munroe, 1995).

Chromosomal Defects

ABNORMAL NUMBER

A. **Polyploidy:** more than two sets of homologous chromosomes, showing multiples of the haploid number.

B. **Nonmultiples** are designated by the suffix "somy"; monosomy is one less than the diploid number (45), and trisomy is one more than the diploid (47).

C. **Causes.**

1. Nondisjunction: failure of paired chromosomes to separate during cell division.

2. Chromosome lag: failure of a chromosome to travel to the appropriate daughter cell.

3. Anaphase lag: chromosome lag during third state of division of a cell nucleus in meiosis and mitosis.

D. **Mosaicism:** nondisjunction of an anaphase lag that occurs during mitosis after fertilization, resulting in two different cell lines in the same person (Davies, 1993; Jones, 1997).

ABNORMAL STRUCTURE

A. **Deletion:** loss of a chromosomal segment.

B. **Translocation:** occurrence of a chromosome segment at an abnormal site, either on another chromosome or in the wrong position on the same chromosome (i.e., an inversion).

C. **Polygenic defects:** type of inheritance in which a trait is dependent on many different gene pairs with cumulative effects.

D. **Environmental influences.** Inadequate nutritional intake, certain drugs, irradiation, and viruses are examples that could alter the genetic makeup of an offspring while in vitro. Multifactorial: genes plus environment.

E. **Basic generalizations.**

1. Loss of an entire autosome is usually incompatible with life.

2. One X chromosome is necessary for life and development.

3. If the male-determining Y chromosome is missing, life and development may continue but will follow female pathways.

4. Extra entire chromosomes, the translocation of extra chromatin material, and the insertion of extra chromatin material are often compatible with life and development.

5. Multiple congenital structural defects are present when gross aberrations are present (Gelehrter et al., 1997).

F. Incidence.

1. Autosomal aberrations: 5:1000 births.
2. Sex chromosome aberrations: 2:1000 births.
3. Spontaneous abortions: 60% are associated with chromosomal aberration (Jorde et al., 1996).

Prenatal Diagnosis

Recent technologic advances and marked progress in the understanding of the etiology and pathogenesis of many common disorders have allowed many families a prenatal diagnosis.

INDICATIONS AND ADVANTAGES OF PRENATAL DIAGNOSIS

A. Indications.

1. Advanced maternal age.
2. Prior child with a chromosome disorder.
3. Family history of neural tube defects.
4. Previous child with multiple malformations.
5. Carriers of X-linked diseases.
6. Carriers of chromosome translocation.
7. Couples at risk of having a child with a specific inborn error of metabolism (previous child or by carrier testing).
8. Ultrasonographic identification of major malformation, polyhydramnios, and/or intrauterine growth restriction (Jorde et al., 1996).

B. Advantages.

1. Knowledge that the fetus is unaffected.
2. Time to explore options and prepare for an affected newborn infant.
3. Opportunity electively to choose either to avoid starting a pregnancy or to abort an affected fetus.
4. Opportunity for the physician to plan delivery, management, and care of the infant when the disease is diagnosed in the fetus (Jorde et al., 1996).

PRENATAL TESTS

Maternal Serum Alpha-Fetoprotein (MSAFP) Test

A. **Screening test** done at 16–18 weeks' gestation to determine amount of protein produced by fetus and normally found in amniotic fluid. Smaller amounts normally cross the placenta and enter the mother's blood. This test is uninterpretable after 22 weeks' gestation.

B. **Preparation.** Explain to client that this is a screening test, *not* a diagnostic test. Explain that an abnormal result does not indicate an abnormality but will indicate the possible need for a diagnostic test to rule out abnormalities.

C. **Reasons for high maternal serum alpha-fetoprotein (MSAFP)** (≥ 2 multiples of the median).

1. Greater gestational age than expected (incorrect due date).
2. Multiple gestation.
3. Risk of fetal complications, including spontaneous abortion, premature labor, or baby who will not attain full birth weight.

4. Fetal structural defect: neural tube, abdominal wall, esophageal or intestinal obstruction, or renal anomalies.
5. Undetermined reason, with subsequent normal outcome of newborn infant.

D. **Reasons for low MSAFP** (≤0.5 multiples of the median).
1. Younger gestational age than expected (incorrect due date).
2. Chromosomal birth defect, Down syndrome being the most common.
3. Undetermined reason, with subsequent normal outcome of newborn infant.

E. **If abnormal MSAFP:** perform ultrasonography to confirm estimated gestational age and assess for anomalies.

F. **If overestimated or underestimated gestational age:** recalculate MSAFP on basis of corrected age; provide client with preliminary revised due date and recalculated MSAFP concentration. Reschedule follow-up ultrasonography in 2–3 weeks to confirm new due date.

G. **If confirmation of gestational age by ultrasonography subsequent to** *high* **MSAFP:** repeat MSAFP determination, schedule genetic counseling and offer amniocentesis for fetal chromosomes, amniotic fluid alpha1-fetoprotein, and acetylcholinesterase.

H. **If confirmation of gestational age by ultrasonography subsequent to** *low* **MSAFP:** schedule genetic counseling and offer client amniocentesis for chromosomes and alpha-fetoprotein. This ultrasonography should include Down-syndrome screening for frontal lobe findings, mild ventriculomegaly, nuchal edema, cardiac defects, mild renal pelvis dilation, and abnormalities of the fetal hand (Thompson, McInnes, and Willard, 1991).

Ultrasonography

A. **Preparation for ultrasonography:** explain to the client that a transducer coated with ultrasonic gel will be placed on her abdomen, with high-frequency sound waves used to display sectional planes of the uterine contents on a monitor. Explain that ultrasonography cannot detect all anomalies and cannot guarantee fetal outcome.

B. **Initial assessment:** recommended by 16–20 weeks for gestational age verification and evaluation.

C. **Ultrasonography:** to detect abnormalities of fetus, placenta, amniotic fluid, and uterus; to monitor changes in anatomy and growth with serial ultrasonography.

D. **Diagnostic capability:** only as good as the person's training—not just contingent on the equipment.

E. **No known harmful effects.**

F. **Critical to safety of amniocentesis:** chorionic villus sampling and percutaneous blood sampling.

G. **Anatomic landmarks commonly observed:** fetal spine, kidneys, bladder, stomach, three-vessel cord, cord insertion, four-chambered heart, face, upper lip, biparietal diameter, head circumference, abdominal circumference, femur length, transcerebellar diameter, placenta, amount of amniotic fluid, uterus, and adnexa.

H. **Detectable anomalies:** many, including those indicative of various syndromes.

I. **Examples:** anencephaly, atrial septal defect, cardiac anomalies, choroid plexus cyst, cleft lip, craniosynostosis, cystic hygroma, cystic kidneys, encephalocele, gastroschisis, hydrocephalus, microcephaly, myelomeningocele, omphalocele, skeletal dysplasia (Ewigman, Crane, and Frigoletto, 1994; Gelehrter et al., 1998; Jorde et al., 1996).

Amniocentesis ("amnio")

A. **Removal of 10–30 mL of amniotic fluid** through a needle placed into the woman's abdomen, for the purpose of chromosomal analysis and other biochemical tests as indicated.

B. **Preparation.** Review risks and benefits of the procedure, discuss options based on current information, and arrange to obtain results of amniocentesis. Explain that normal results of amniocentesis do not guarantee a good fetal outcome. Obtain written consent for this procedure. Obtain client's blood type before procedure. If she is Rh negative, obtain father's blood type.

C. **Usual timing of procedure:** 16–18 gestational weeks, but amniocentesis can be performed later in gestation and as early as 14 weeks.

D. **Indications.**

1. Woman of advanced maternal age (>35 years at time of expected delivery).
2. Previous fetus with Down syndrome.
3. Previous fetus with neural tube defect.
4. Both parents known as heterozygous carriers of autosomal recessive chromosome.
5. Both parents known as carriers of sex-linked recessive disorder.
6. Client or partner with balanced chromosomal translocation of his or her chromosomes.
7. High or low MSAFP with accurate gestational age.

E. **Fluid analysis:** requires 2–3 weeks for cells to grow adequately for accurate analysis.

F. **Risks:** overall risk to mother or fetus is 1%.
1. Spontaneous abortion: approximately 0.5% of cases.
2. Hemorrhage.
3. Infection.
4. Premature labor.
5. Rh sensitization from fetal bleeding into maternal circulation.
6. Trauma to fetus or placenta.

G. **Analysis.**

1. Fetal sex: determined through special staining techniques, karyotype, or amniotic fluid testosterone levels, providing risk information for X-linked disorder.
2. Alpha-fetoprotein: abnormally high or low levels raise concern (see earlier section on MSAFP test, under Prenatal Tests).
3. Biochemical: metabolism disorders, including Tay-Sachs disease (a lipid disorder) and amino acid, carbohydrate, and mucopolysaccharide metabolism disorders, can be discovered by 20 weeks' gestation.
4. Chromosomes: abnormalities, including Down syndrome, other trisomies, and other chromosomal abnormalities, can be detected at 16 weeks' gestation by karyotyping.

H. **Postamniocentesis care.**

1. Assess fetal heart activity.
2. Cleanse insertion site and apply protective cover.
3. Instruct client to rest for 24 hours, to lift no more than 10 pounds (approximately 4.5 k), and to avoid straining.

4. Administer immune globulin (RhoGAM) if client is Rh negative and if father of fetus is either Rh positive or of unknown blood type. Do not give RhoGAM if Rh sensitization.
5. When results are available, explain their implications (Gelehrter et al., 1997).

Chorionic Villus Sampling

A. **Transvaginal or transabdominal sampling** of the chorionic villi. Obtain fetal cells for the purpose of chromosomal analysis and other biochemical tests. Chorionic villus sampling (CVS) cannot identify neural tube defects.

B. **Preparation.** Review risks and benefits of the procedure, discuss options, and arrange to obtain CVS results. Obtain written consent for this procedure.

C. **Timing of procedure:** usually 8–10 weeks of gestation.

D. **Indications.**

1. Client prefers to make decisions regarding pregnancy in first trimester.
2. Severe oligohydramnios.

E. **Contraindications.**

1. Multiple gestation.
2. Uterine bleeding during this pregnancy.
3. Active genital herpes infection or other cervical infection.
4. Uterine fibroids.

F. **Fetal cell analysis:** requires 24–28 hours for initial results.

G. **Risks:** overall, 2–3%.
1. Infection.
2. Bleeding.
3. Cervical lacerations.
4. Miscarriage: 1–5%.

H. **Techniques of CVS.**

1. Vaginal CVS. Catheter is inserted through the vagina and cervix into the chorion outer tissue of the embryonic sac, and a tiny amount of the chorionic villi is aspirated by suction or cut with forceps.
2. Abdominal CVS. Needle is inserted through the abdomen into the chorion to obtain a sample of the chorionic villi.

I. **Post-CVS care.**

1. Same recommendations as for postamniocentesis care.
2. Nothing in the vagina (tampon, douche, intercourse) for 24 hours.
3. If transvaginal sample, instruct client to use sanitary napkins as needed for 24–48 hours.

Percutaneous Umbilical Blood Sampling (PUBS)

A. **Sampling:** removal of fetal blood through a needle placed into the woman's abdomen and into the umbilical vein.

B. **Preparation:** same as that recommended for CVS.

C. **Timing:** 18 weeks to term.

D. **Indications.**

1. Client wants fast results to support her decision making regarding pregnancy.
2. Abnormality is identified by ultrasonography late in pregnancy.

3. Client has been exposed to infectious disease that could affect development of fetus.
4. Blood incompatibility (Rh disease).
5. Drug or chemical level in fetal blood needs to be assessed.

E. **Risks.**

1. Same as amniocentesis: infection, bleeding, isoimmunization, miscarriage, trauma to the fetus—for overall 1–5% risk factor.
2. Perforation of uterine arteries, clotting in fetal cord.
3. Premature delivery.

F. **Results:** fetal blood analysis takes 3 days.

G. **Postsampling care:** same as postamniocentesis care (Avery, 1994; Nora et al., 1994).

Future Developments

HUMAN GENOME PROJECT

A. What is the Human Genome Project?

1. The project started in mid-1980s and is the single most important coordinated medical research initiative in the history of biomedical research.
2. The goals of the project are to map genes on chromosomes and to determine the sequence of the nucleotides that make up human DNA, which is the basic genetic material. It is expected that genome research will produce a ream of new information about the genes involved in inherited disorders, birth defects, and common conditions influenced by genetic factors.
3. Though the outcome of the Human Genome Project itself is not ethically problematic, the use of the data generated presents major ethical questions that must be addressed. The future, then, presents the challenges of addressing the project's implications (Collins and Galas, 1993).

B. Ethical, Legal, and Social Issues program.

1. Study is now under way on the ethical, legal, and social issues related to increasingly rapid progress in the field of human genetics. Four areas were identified for initial emphasis: privacy of genetic information, safe and effective introduction of genetic information in the clinical setting, fairness in the use of genetic information, and professional and public education.
2. The program also emphasizes the importance of understanding the cultural, ethnic, social, and psychologic influences that must inform policy development and service delivery issues.
3. With time, these issues must be addressed to ensure that the maximal benefit is gained from the project (Collins and Galas, 1993; Gelehrter et al., 1997; Geller, 1995).

GENETIC COUNSELING

A. **Definition:** a communication process that deals with the human problems associated with the occurrence, or the risk of occurrence, of genetic disorders in a family. This process involves collaboration of persons from multiple disciplines (physician, sonographer, nurse, genetic counselor, social worker, neonatologist, and pediatric specialist, as indicated) and family support (adapted from Epstein and Ad Hoc Committee on Genetic Counseling, 1975). Genetic counseling is a nondirective communication process that deals with the human problems associated with the occurrence, or the risk of occurrence, of a genetic disorder in a family.

B. **Principles of genetic counseling.**

1. Based on correct diagnosis and pattern of inheritance.
2. Nondirective.
3. Reinforcement of information previously presented.
4. Emphasis on communication with the primary care physician.

C. **Goal of genetic counseling** is to assist the family in comprehending:
1. Diagnosis.
2. Role of heredity.
3. Recurrence risks and options.
4. Possible courses of action.
5. Methods of ongoing adjustment.

D. **Indications (Gelehrter et al., 1997).**

1. Previously affected child, parent, grandparent.
   a. Congenital malformation.
   b. Sensory defect.
   c. Metabolic disorder.
   d. Mental retardation.
   e. Known or suspected chromosome abnormality.
   f. Neuromuscular disorder.
   g. Degenerative CNS disease.
2. Previously affected cousins.
   a. Muscular dystrophy.
   b. Hemophilia.
   c. Hydrocephalus.
3. Consanguinity.
4. Hazards of ionizing radiation.
5. Recurrent miscarriages.
6. Concern for teratogenic effect.
7. Advanced maternal age.
8. High or low MSAFP.

E. **Methods of obtaining information needed.**

1. Questionnaire.
2. Pedigree.
3. Medical records.
4. Physical examination.
5. Laboratory tests.
6. Carrier detection.

F. **Provision of medical facts.**

1. Differential diagnosis.
2. Risks to fetus and mother.
3. Probable course of disorder.
4. Recommended management for prenatal course.
5. Type and timing of delivery.
6. Neonatal, pediatric, and long-term care requirements.

G. **Explanation of hereditary factors** that contribute to the disorder.

H. **Discussion with parents** regarding all alternatives.
1. Home care of newborn infant.
2. Institutionalization.
3. Adoption.
4. Appropriate method of termination for gestational age.

5. Objective information regarding fetus/neonate status. Provide statistical risk factors as they relate to this individual fetus.
6. Identification of which normal characteristics can exist in the affected fetus. Point these out in pictures to promote awareness of total condition of fetus.
7. Assistance to parents: understanding of causes, risks of recurrence, and limits of current treatments.
8. Discussion of options available for dealing with risk of recurrence.
9. Written information for parents and information regarding support groups.
10. Explanation of recommended obstetric care, mode and timing of delivery, and neonatal care (Gelehrter et al., 1997; Jones, 1997).

Newborn Care

DIAGNOSIS

A. **Complete diagnosis:** important in planning care. Consideration for the infant's overall problems, in addition to the defect, is essential.

B. **Evaluation of infant with birth defect.** A birth defect is a structural or functional abnormality of the body that is present from birth. The effects of a birth defect may be either immediate or delayed until later in life.

C. Syndrome.

1. Definition: a constellation of anomalies that cannot be explained otherwise and that result in similar patterns of expression.
2. Examples: fetal alcohol syndrome, trisomy 21.

D. Sequence.

1. Definition: a primary event or anomaly that sets a pattern of other events (anomalies).
2. Example: Pierre Robin sequence.

E. Malformation.

1. Definition: an abnormality of morphogenesis due to intrinsic problems within the developing structures.
2. Examples: neural tube defects, cleft lip and palate.

F. Deformation.

1. Definition: an abnormality of morphogenesis due to intrinsic problems within the developing structures.
2. Examples: Pierre Robin sequence, uterine position defects, oligohydramnios sequence.

G. Disruption.

1. Definition: an abnormality of morphogenesis due to disruptive forces acting on the developing structure. Can be due to pressure on developing structures.
2. Examples: amniotic bands, vascular accidents, infections.

H. Genetic heterogeneity.

1. Definition: different causes may produce similar characteristics.
2. Examples: hydrocephalus, cleft lip and palate.

HISTORY

A. Family history.

1. History of three generations.

2. Defects in the family history related to the problem in the child.
3. Medical records and/or photos of similarly affected relatives.
4. History of consanguinity.
5. Reproductive history, such as frequent spontaneous abortions.
6. Pattern of inheritance of the problems.

B. Prenatal history.

1. Length of gestation.
2. Fetal activity level.
3. Maternal exposures: to infections, illness, high fevers, medications, x-ray examinations, known teratogens, alcohol, smoking, and use of street and prescription drugs.
4. Obstetric factors: uterine malformations, complications of labor, presenting fetal part.
5. Neonatal factors: birth weight, length, head circumference, Apgar scores.

EXAMINATION AND CARE

A. Physical examination.

1. General: asymmetry, problems of relationship, inappropriate size and strength.
2. Face: configuration; centered features with normal spacing; round, triangular, flat, birdlike, elfin, coarse, or expressionless characteristics.
3. Head: size of anterior fontanelle, prominence of frontal bone, flattened or prominent occiput, abnormalities in shape (proportionally large or small).
4. Skin: intact, or presence of skin tags, open sinuses, tracts.
5. Hair: texture, hairline, presence of whorls.
6. Eyes: structure and color of iris, presence of colobomas, centering and spacing of epicanthal folds (hypotelorism or hypertelorism), ptosis, slanting, eyelash length.
7. Ears: protruding or prominent shape, location, low set, unilateral or bilateral defect, presence and/or degree of rotation.
8. Nose: beaked, bulbous, pinched, upturned, misshapen, two nares, flattened bridge, patency, centered on face.
9. Oral: intact palate, presence of smooth philtrum, natal teeth; shape and size of tongue, mouth, jaw (micrognathia).
10. Neck: short and/or webbed, redundant folds.
11. Chest: symmetric; presence of accessory nipples.
12. Abdomen: number of cord vessels, presence of abdominal wall defects and abdominal musculature, prune belly.
13. Genitourinary system (male): hypospadias—4 degrees, dependent on placement of meatus; chordee; ambiguous genitalia; testes descended.
14. Anus: position, patency.
15. Spine: intact, scoliosis, lordosis, kyphosis.
16. Extremities: length, shape, absence of bones.
17. Hands and feet: broad, square, or spadelike shape, polydactyly, clinodactyly, syndactyly, abnormal creases in the palm of the hand (simian or Sydney creases), contractures, abnormally large or small size, overriding fingers, proximally placed thumb, rocker-bottom feet.

B. Causation of defect.

1. Identify the primary abnormality.
2. Recognize etiologic heterogeneity (a defect having more than one cause).
3. Determine category of congenital malformation, according to etiology.
   a. Malformation.

    b. Deformation.
    c. Disruption.
    d. Syndrome.
    e. Sequence.
    f. Genetic heterogeneity.

C. **Family care management for all genetic syndromes or disorders.**

1. Provide grief counseling. Acknowledge short- and long-term grief; promote awareness that each of the parents may be in a different stage of the grief process, creating additional stress. Recommend that parents communicate their needs to each other and ask for support when needed.
2. Encourage genetic counseling.
3. Facilitate family use of support systems: social services, Aid to Families with Dependent Children, Women-Infant-Children (WIC) program, March of Dimes, clergy, mental health services, support groups.
4. Provide unconditional emotional support. Allow parents and siblings to verbalize feelings.
5. Identify normal aspects of neonate that can coexist with the syndrome or disorder.
6. Promote parent involvement in care; offer choices in care and interventions.
7. Discuss treatment options and their risks and benefits.
8. Provide literature.
9. Obtain legal and ethical counsel when parents prefer not to pursue medical interventions (Connor and Ferguson-Smith, 1993; Davies, 1993).

SPECIFIC DISORDERS

Beckwith-Wiedemann Syndrome

A. **Etiology and precipitating factors.**

1. Unknown cause.
2. Gender predominance: 60% are female.

B. **Incidence:** 1:14,000.

C. **Clinical presentation.**

1. Large muscle mass with subcutaneous tissue; birth weight greater than 3200 g.
2. Head: microcephaly.
    a. Prominent occiput.
    b. Large fontanelle.
    c. Malocclusion with mandibular prognathism (forward projection of the jaw).
    d. Unusual linear fissures in lobe of external ear.
    e. Prominent eyes.
    f. Strabismus.
3. Omphalocele or other umbilical anomaly.
4. Cryptorchidism.
5. Large tongue (macroglossia).
6. Other major manifestations.
    a. Accelerated osseous maturation.
    b. Mild to moderate mental deficiency; normal intelligence possible.
    c. Large kidneys with renal medullary dysplasia.
    d. Pancreatic hyperplasia.
    e. Fetal adrenocortical cytomegaly.
    f. Interstitial cell hyperplasia.
    g. Pituitary hyperplasia.

    h. Neonatal polycythemia.

    i. Hypoglycemia, usually after the first day of life.

7. Care management.

    a. Airway support as indicated.

    b. Place infant on side to facilitate breathing; may need oral airway.

    c. Facilitate feeding with use of a large, soft nipple.

    d. Treat hypoglycemia.

    e. Consider partial exchange for polycythemia greater than 65%.

8. Complications and outcome.

    a. Hypoglycemia: may be severe enough to cause death or slow development.

    b. Feeding difficulties because of large tongue.

    c. Polycythemia.

    d. Pneumonia.

    e. Possible failure to thrive.

    f. Healthy outcome in individuals who survive infancy (Avery, 1994; Hooshang, 1998).

Cleft Lip With or Without Cleft Palate

A. **Etiology and precipitating factors.**

1. Defective development of embryonic primary palate may cause clefts of the lip and of the anterior portion of the maxilla.
2. Defective development of the embryonic secondary palate may cause clefts of the hard and soft palates and often appear in persons with cleft lip.
3. There are at least 50 recognized syndromes that involve cleft lip and/or cleft palate as a characteristic.
4. Cleft lip and/or cleft palate may be caused by mutant genes, chromosomal aberrations, teratogen, or multifactorial inheritance.

B. **Incidence:** cleft lip and/or cleft palate.

1. White population: 1:1000 to 1:2500 births.
2. Japan: 2:1000 births.
3. American black population: 0:1000 births.
4. About twice as frequent in males as in females.
5. Associated with phenytoin (Dilantin) use during pregnancy (Hooshang, 1998; Jones, 1993).

C. **Clinical presentation.**

1. Cleft lip with or without cleft palate is usually apparent at birth.
2. There may be variations in the degree of the malformations.

    a. Cleft lip may be unilateral or bilateral.

    b. If cleft lip is unilateral, two thirds are on the left side.

    c. If cleft lip is bilateral, it is often accompanied by a cleft palate.

3. Varying degrees of nasal distortion, with deformed or absent teeth, may be present.
4. Cleft palate may occur as a single defect and is less apparent at birth.
5. Assessment can be made by placing the examiner's fingers on the palate.
6. Infant may have difficulty in feeding because of the inability to create suction (Avery, 1994; Jones, 1993).

D. **Complications and outcome.**

1. Impaired hearing caused by upper respiratory tract infections and recurrent otitis media due to inefficient function of the eustachian tube.
2. Impaired social adjustment: minimal if surgery is successful.
3. Impaired speech and hearing.

4. Aspiration.
5. Orthodontic problems.
6. Good outcome with surgical correction.

E. **Care management.**

1. Feeding: special nipples, such as cleft palate nipples, split nipples, and squeeze bottles.
2. Surgical correction: depends on abnormality and surgeon's preference.

Cornelia de Lange Syndrome

A. **Etiology and precipitating factors: unknown.**

B. **Incidence:** 1:150,000 births.

C. **Clinical presentation and physical examination.**

1. Very small in stature, but not because of skeletal dysplasia.
2. Irregular hairline.
3. Narrow forehead.
4. Thick eyebrows that meet at midline.
5. Long eyelashes.
6. Flat nasal bridge.
7. Short, upturned nose with anteverted nares.
8. Prominent philtrum.
9. Small mandible.
10. Short, tapering extremities.
11. Short, tapering digits with incurved fifth finger.
12. Hirsutism.
13. Congenital heart disease.
14. Microcephaly.
15. Growling cry.

D. **Complications and outcome.**

1. Aspiration in infancy.
2. Increased susceptibility to infections.
3. Failure to thrive.
4. High mortality rate during infancy because of poor feeding and growth.
5. Usually severe mental defects in survivors (Gelehrter et al., 1997; Jones, 1997).

Crouzon's Syndrome

A. **Etiology and precipitating factors: autosomal dominant.**

B. **Incidence:** unknown.

C. **Clinical presentation.**

1. Ocular proptosis, due to shallow orbits.
2. Possible divergent strabismus, hypertelorism.
3. Hypoplasia of maxilla.
4. Possible curved, parrotlike nose.
5. Craniosynostosis of coronal, lambdoid, and sagittal sutures, leading to short anterior, posterior, and wide lateral dimensions of the cranium.

D. **Complications and outcome: normal life possible.**

E. **Patient care management.**

1. Provide emotional support for patients.

2. Surgery may be done if craniosynostosis is present with increased intracranial pressure (Hooshang, 1998; Jorde et al., 1996).

Trisomies

Trisomy 21

A. **Incidence and etiology.**

1. Incidence by maternal age is as follows:
   a. 15–29 years: 1:1500.
   b. 30–34 years: 1:800.
   c. 35–39 years: 1:270.
   d. 40–44 years: 1:100.
   e. 45 years or older: 1:50.
2. Accounts for 15–20% of cases of severe mental retardation.
3. Risk increases with maternal age.
4. Twenty-five percent of Down syndrome infants receive an extra chromosome from their father.
5. Person has 47 chromosomes (3 of chromosome 21).
6. Extra chromosome fits into group G 21, 22. Extra chromosome results from nondisjunction during meiosis. May occur unrelated to mother's age and appear as follows:
   a. Chromosomes: 46.
   b. Translocation of chromosome 21.
   c. Familial transmission: autosomal dominant.
   d. No abnormalities if chromosomes are balanced. There is one No. 21 and one No. 14 chromosome.
   e. Production of unbalanced gametes by balanced carriers; should consider prenatal diagnosis.
7. Some infants have mosaicism for trisomy 21 or translocation 14/21 or 21/22.
   a. Some have all the defects.
   b. Some have only a few of the defects.
   c. Some of this group may have normal intellectual ability.

B. **Clinical presentation.**

1. Size: small; 20% are premature.
2. Skull: short and round with a flat occiput.
3. Eyes: slant upward and outward.
4. Prominent epicanthal fold.
5. Flat face.
6. Brushfield's spots: iris may be speckled with ring of round, grayish spots or flecks of gold in light-colored eyes.
7. Cheeks: red.
8. Palate: narrow and short.
9. Nose: short with flat bridge.
10. Tongue: protrudes; can become dry and wrinkled.
11. Skin: loose around lateral and dorsal aspects of neck.
12. Hands.
    a. Fingers: short.
    b. Hands: square.
    c. Thumb: low set; separated more than usual from second finger.
    d. Fifth finger: short; curves inward.
    e. Single or bilateral simian crease (present in 40% of Down syndrome).
13. Umbilicus: herniated.
14. Feet.

    a. Wide space between great toe and second toe.

    b. Deep crease that starts between the great toe and the second toe and curves toward the medial edge of the sole.

15. Muscular hypotonia.
16. Narrow acetabular angle.
17. Narrow iliac index.
18. Broadened iliac bones.
19. Retarded psychomotor development.
20. Heart: ventricular septal defect or other congenital heart defects in 50%.
21. Duodenal atresia (Hooshang, 1998; Jones, 1997).

C. **Complications and outcome.**

1. Congestive heart failure due to congenital heart disease.
2. Upper respiratory tract infections.
3. Developmentally delayed.
4. Mildly to severely mentally retarded: IQ ranges from 25 to 70.

Trisomy 18

A. **Etiology and precipitating factors.**

1. Nondisjunction most frequent but possible partial trisomy, translocation, or mosaicism.
2. Advanced parental age.

B. **Incidence:** 1:3500 births.

C. **Clinical presentation:** Nos. 1–7 (below) appear in most cases; Nos. 8–14 (below) may also appear.
1. Weight: low birth weight in term infant.
2. Ears: low set and/or abnormal shape.
3. Micrognathia and microstomia.
4. Mental retardation.
5. Hands.
    a. Clenched hand with flexed fingers.
    b. Flexion contraction of the two middle digits.
    c. Underfolded thumb.
6. Heart: usually ventricular septal defect with patent ductus arteriosus.
7. Feet: rocker bottom.
8. Eyes: ptosis of one or both eyelids.
9. Syndactyly.
10. Head: abnormally prominent occiput.
11. Genitourinary defects.
12. Hernias, especially umbilical.
13. Simian crease appears in 25%.
14. Arches on seven or more fingers in 80% of cases.

D. **Complications and outcome.**

1. Mortality rate: 30% die within 2 months of birth, usually of heart failure.
2. Survival: 10% survive the first year with severe mental retardation.

E. **Care management.**

1. No treatment beyond supportive care.
2. Gavage feeding as needed for poor feeding.
3. Oxygen as needed for respiratory distress.
4. Parental support (Avery, 1994; Gelehrter et al., 1997; Jones, 1997).

Trisomy 13

A. **Etiology:** unknown; may be related to older maternal age.

B. **Incidence:** 1:5000 births.

C. **Clinical presentation.**

1. Psychomotor retardation.
2. Ears: malformed.
3. Hands: flexion deformities of hand, fingers, and wrist; postaxial polydactyly, simian creases, clenched hands.
4. Heart: usually ventricular septal defect, patent ductus arteriosus, or rotational anomalies such as dextroposition.
5. Feet: rocker bottom.
6. Eyes: microphthalmos, colobomas of iris, cataracts.
7. Nose: broad and flattened, cleft lip and palate.
8. Umbilicus: hernia, omphalocele.
9. Genitalia.
   a. Female: bicornate or septate uterus.
   b. Male: cryptorchidism, small scrotum with anterior placement.
10. Kidneys: polycystic.
11. Skin: cutaneous hemangiomas.
12. Brain: gross defects, grand mal seizures, myoclonic jerks.
13. Hematologic abnormalities, such as increased frequency of nuclear projections in neutrophils and/or persistence of embryonic and/or fetal type of hemoglobin.

D. **Complications and outcome.**

1. Mortality rate: 44% die within the first month.
2. Survival: 18% survive the first year.
3. Severe mental retardation.

E. **Care management.**

1. No treatment beyond supportive care.
2. Parental support (Avery, 1994; Jones, 1997; Wong, 1995).

Turner's Syndrome XO

A. **Etiology and precipitating factors:** absence of X chromosomes, caused by nondisjunction, which results in 45 chromosomes.

B. **Incidence:** 1:2000 to 1:5000 live-born females.

C. **Clinical presentation and physical examination.**

1. Short stature, mean birth weight 2900 g.
2. Webbed neck.
3. Low posterior hairline.
4. Micrognathia.
5. Low-set and sometimes malformed ears.
6. Widely spaced hypoplastic nipples on a shield-shaped chest.
7. Increased carrying angle at the elbow.
8. Cardiac anomalies: coarctation of the aorta or aortic valvular stenosis.
9. Learning difficulties: intelligence is normal.
10. Abnormal growth patterns.
11. Congenital lymphedema of hands and feet.
12. Broad nasal bridge.

13. Ptosis of the eyelids.
14. Epicanthal folds.
15. Lack of secondary sexual characteristics.
16. Gonadal dysplasia.
17. Horseshoe kidney.
18. Unilateral renal agenesis.

D. **Complications and outcome:** most raised as females, with good outcome despite failure of sexual development.

E. **Care management.**

1. Early.
   a. Supportive.
   b. Surgery to correct treatable defects.
2. Late.
   a. Estrogen treatment.
   b. Counseling and psychiatric support (Avery, 1994; Hooshang, 1998).

VATER Association

VATER is an acronym for *v*ertebral anomalies, *a*nal atresia, *t*racheo*e*sophageal fistula, and *r*adial and renal dysplasia.

A. **Etiology and precipitating factors:** unknown.

B. **Incidence:** unknown.

C. **Clinical presentation.** Three or more of the following defects are present:
1. Vertebral anomalies.
2. Anal atresia with or without fistula.
3. Tracheoesophageal fistula with esophageal atresia.
4. Radial dysplasia, including thumb or radial hypoplasia, polydactyly, and syndactyly.
5. Renal anomaly.
6. Single umbilical artery.

D. **Complications and outcome.**

1. Failure to thrive.
2. Possibility of normal life after slow mental development during infancy.

E. **Care management.**

1. Supportive: prognosis and management depend upon extent and severity of the anomalies.
2. Surgery: surgical correction of anomalies.

VACTERL Association

VACTERL is an acronym for an association characterized by the sporadic, nonrandom association of specific abnormalities: *v*ertebral abnormalities, *a*nal atresia, *c*ardiac abnormalities, *t*racheo*e*sophageal fistula and/or esophageal atresia, *r*enal agenesis and dysplasia, and *l*imb defects.

A. **Etiology and precipitating factors.**

1. Unknown.
2. Injury between 4 and 6 weeks to a specific mesodermal area may produce simultaneous anomalies of the hindgut, lower vertebral column, lower urinary tract, and developing kidney.
3. Abnormalities: average of 7 or 8 per patient.

B. **Incidence:** rare (about 250 reported cases worldwide).

C. **Clinical presentation (Avery, 1994; Hooshang, 1998; Jones, 1997; Wong, 1995).**

1. Vertebral anomalies.
2. Anal atresia with or without fistula.
3. Cardiac anomalies: commonly ventricular septal defects.
4. Tracheoesophageal fistula with or without esophageal atresia.
5. Radial dysplasia, including thumb or radial hypoplasia, polydactyly, and syndactyly.
6. Renal anomaly.
7. Single umbilical artery.

D. **Complications and outcome.**

1. Failure to thrive.
2. Normal Life: minimal CNS anomalies with only occasional mental retardation.

E. **Care management (Wong, 1995).**

1. Supportive: prognosis and management depend on extent and severity of the anomalies.
2. Surgery: Surgical correction of anomalies.

ACKNOWLEDGMENT

I wish to acknowledge the contribution of Sharon Kuhrt and Lynn Hornick, whose work in the first edition provided the basis of this chapter.

REFERENCES

Avery, G.: *Neonatology, Pathophysiology and Management of the Newborn, 4th ed.* Philadelphia, J.B. Lippincott, 1994.

Collins, F., and Galas, D.: A five-year plan for the U.S. Human Genome Project. *Science,* 262:43–46, 1993.

Connor, J.M., and Ferguson-Smith, M.A.: *Essential Medical Genetics. 4th ed.* Oxford, Blackwell Scientific Publications, 1993.

Davies, K.E. (Ed.): *Genetic Disease Analysis: A Practical Approach, 2nd ed.* Oxford, Oxford University Press, 1993.

Epstein C.J., Chairman, and Ad Hoc Committee on Genetic Counseling. Report of the Committee on Genetic Counseling. *Am. J. Hum. Genet.,* 27:240–242, 1975.

Ewigman, B.G., Crane, J.P., and Frigoletto, F.E.: Effect of prenatal ultrasound screening on perinatal outcome. *N. Engl. J. Med.* 330:1114, 1994.

Gelehrter, T.D., and Collins, F.S.: *Principles of Medical Genetics.* Baltimore, Williams & Wilkins, 1990.

Gelehrter, T.D., Collins, F.S., and Ginsburg, G.: *Principles of Medical Genetics, 2nd ed.* Baltimore, Williams & Wilkins, 1997.

Geller, G: Cystic fibrosis and the pediatric caregiver: Benefits and burdens of genetic technology. *Pediatr. Nurs.,* 21(1):57–61, 1995.

Hooshang, T.: *Handbook of Syndromes and Metabolic Disorders: Radiologic and Clinical Manifestations.* St. Louis, Mosby, 1998.

Jones, K.: *Smith's Recognizable Patterns of Human Malformation, 5th ed.* Philadelphia, W.B. Saunders, 1997.

Jones, M.C.: Facial clefting: Etiology and developmental pathogenesis. *Clin. Plast. Surg.,* 20:599, 1993.

Jorde, L.B., Carey, J.C., and White, R.L.: Medical Genetics. St. Louis, Mosby, 1996.

March of Dimes Foundation, White Plains, New York.

Nora, J.J., Clarke Fraser, F., Bear, J., et al.: Medical Genetics: Principles and Practice, 4th ed. Philadelphia, Lea & Febiger, 1994.

Pickler, R.H., and Munro, C.L.: Gene therapy for inherited disorders. J. Pediatr. Nurs., 10(1):40–47, 1995.

Thompson, M.W., McInnes, R.R., and Willard, H.F.: Thompson and Thompson Genetics in Medicine, 5th ed. Philadelphia, W.B. Saunders, 1991.

Williams & Lesick, 1994.

Wong, D.L.: Whaley and Wong's Nursing Care of Infants and Children, 5th ed. St. Louis, Mosby, 1995.

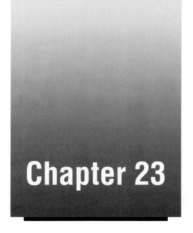

Chapter 23

Neonatal Orthopedic Conditions

Leann Sterk

Objectives

1. Recognize the need for accurate, comprehensive musculoskeletal examination of the newborn infant.
2. Discuss developmental and perinatal factors that place the neonate at risk of having orthopedic abnormalities.
3. Identify common neonatal orthopedic conditions, assessment, and interventions.
4. Review the influence of the family environment on the neonate with an orthopedic condition.

The process of the development and maturation of the musculoskeletal system is dynamic and vulnerable to injury throughout gestation. Abnormalities within the system range from minor to devastating. Assessment and care of the infant with an orthopedic condition must be based on an understanding of anatomy and function. This chapter will review development of the musculoskeletal system and the assessment and treatment of pathologic findings.

Skeletal System

A. **Morphologic development:** dependent on the formation of the notochord, the first skeletal structure.
1. Formation begins during the second week of gestation.
2. During the third week of gestation, development of the notochord induces formation of the neural plate. Further maturation results in formation of the neural tube.
3. Differentiation of the neural tube results in the formation of the axial musculoskeleton from paraxial mesoderm. Further development results in somite formation. Somites mature, giving rise to specific cell types: dermatomes, myotomes, and sclerotomes.

B. **Congenital defects:** abnormal cellular formation and growth. Failure to form needed cells or to produce cell-inducing mediators results in progressive changes that end in abnormality. If cellular development is normal, alterations may develop as a result of abnormal biochemical synthesis and growth failure. A high degree of interdependence among segments of the developing musculoskeletal system leads to complex and associated anomalies.

C. Skeletal development.

1. Axial skeleton. Formation of the vertebral column, sternum, ribs, and skull begins in the fourth week of gestation as aggregation and differentiation of the somites occur.
2. Appendicular skeleton. Limb bones and the pelvic and pectoral girdles develop from ectoderm and mesoderm during the fourth week of gestation.
3. Joints. Formation occurs from mesenchyme chondrification. Joints are identified as synovial, hyaline, or fibrous. Simultaneous development of the joint capsule occurs, ensuring contact with soft tissues and adjacent bone.

Muscular System

Muscle development occurs in conjunction with notochord and neural tube development. As paraxial columns and somites are formed, specific cell myotomes develop and then undergo progressive differentiation, resulting in specialized muscle groups: skeletal, smooth, and cardiac.

Clinical and Physical Assessment

The infant is a reflection of genetic interplay and the uterine environment, which contribute to significant variability in musculoskeletal expression. Each neonate should receive a comprehensive musculoskeletal examination to facilitate early recognition and treatment of problems.

A. Perinatal factors.

1. Altered growth patterns evident on prenatal ultrasound.
2. Uterine bleeding during the pregnancy.
3. Exposure to teratogenic agents: irradiation, drugs, industrial chemicals.
4. Fetal position: dependent on uterine and fetal factors, specifically breech.
5. Infection: onset during pregnancy, causative agent, course, treatment received.
6. Oligohydramnios: time of occurrence within the pregnancy.
7. Patterns of fetal movement.
8. Delivery: difficult, shoulder dystocia, breech.

B. Family history.

1. Familial musculoskeletal disorders.
2. Maternal uterine abnormalities.
3. Maternal disease or nutritional factors.

C. Medication history.

1. Current use of sedatives, anticonvulsants, neuromuscular agents.
2. Maternal exposure to recreational drugs, alcohol, tranquilizers, anticonvulsant drugs.

D. Physical examination.

1. Assessment achieved through inspection, palpation, and auscultation.
   a. General assessment of position, body symmetry, range of motion, level of responsiveness.
   b. Accurate measurements of body parts: occipital frontal circumference, limb length, body length.

2. System assessment.
   a. Head and neck.
      (1) Skull: configuration, proportion to body, position and size of fonta- nelles, suture lines.
      (2) Neck: proportion, range of motion, symmetry, bony abnormalities, webbing (excessive skin on the back of the neck).
   b. Trunk and spine.
      (1) Anterior chest.
         (a) Symmetry, shape, movement, obvious masses, bruising.
         (b) Clavicles: size, contour, masses, fractures.
         (c) Rib cage: shape, obvious bony deformities.
      (2) Posterior chest.
         (a) Spinal column integrity: neural tube defect, bony abnormali- ties.
         (b) Spinal curvature: kyphosis, scoliosis, lordosis.
         (c) Trunk: symmetric passive flexion, extension, lateral bending.
         (d) Rib cage: shape, obvious bony deformity.
      (3) Upper extremities.
         (a) Limbs: number, completeness, length, obvious positional or bony abnormality, contour, proportion to the body.
         (b) Hands: shape, size, position to the limb, number of digits.
         (c) Nails: shape, presence, surface defect.
         (d) Movement: spontaneous or passive, contractures, hyperextension, joint abnormality.
         (e) Digits: webbing, position to hand, spacing, number of digits, mo- tion, creases.
      (4) Lower extremities.
         (a) Hips: presence, range of motion, spontaneous movement.
         (b) Limb: number, completeness, length, proportion to body, positional abnormality, fractures, obvious bony abnormalities, contour of bone.
         (c) Knees: contour, presence, range of motion, presence and location of patella, joint function.
         (d) Ankles: spontaneous movement, range of motion, joint abnormali- ties.
         (e) Feet: presence, position to the limb, bony abnormalities, number and position of toes, range of motion.
         (f) Digits: number, position to foot, spacing and number, webbing, sole creases, range of motion of forefoot and heel, position of heel to forefoot.

Pathologic Conditions

NECK ABNORMALITIES

Defects of the neck can be either muscular or bony. Causes of abnormalities are either congenital or acquired.

A. **Klippel-Feil syndrome:** congenital fusion of variable numbers (two or more) of the cervical vertebrae (Epps and Salter, 1996; Guille et al., 1995).
1. Syndrome consists of a deformity triad of low posterior hairline, short neck, and limitation of neck movement (Loder, 1996; Thomsen, Schneider, and Weber, 1997). Physical findings are directly related to degree of cervical involvement and are present in fewer than 50% of patients (Guille et al., 1995).
   a. Cause is uncertain, with the exception of rare cases of inherited defect.
   b. Abnormality effect may not be limited to cervical spine.

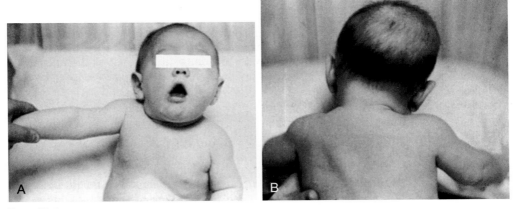

Figure 23–1
A, Congenital torticollis affecting the right sternocleidomastoid muscle in a 3-month-old baby. *B*, Note flattening of left occiput and right head tilt. (From Avery, G.B. [Ed.]: Neonatology: Pathophysiology and Management of the Newborn, 3rd ed. Philadelphia, J.B. Lippincott, 1987, p. 1163.)

   c. Three types exist, showing specific morphologic features.
     (1) Type I: massive fusion of many cervical and upper thoracic vertebrae with synostosis.
     (2) Type II: fusion at only one or two interspaces with hemivertebrae, occipitoatloid fusion, and other abnormalities in the cervical spine.
     (3) Type III: cervical fusions associated with lower thoracic or lumbar fusion.
   d. Minor cervical lesions must be evaluated for hidden abnormalities of the genitourinary, cardiopulmonary, nervous, and auditory systems. Upper extremity anomalies and Sprengel's deformity (congenital elevated scapula) must also be considered. Scoliosis is an associated anomaly, occurring in 60% of patients (Epps and Salter, 1996; Guille et al., 1995; Loder, 1996).
  2. Diagnosis is made through physical examination and radiographic studies.
   a. The most common physical sign is limitation in range of motion of the neck.
   b. Flexion-extension x-ray films of the cervical spine, computerized tomography (CT) scans, and magnetic resonance imaging (MRI) studies assist in defining the abnormality, assessing cervical stability, and discovering whether neural compression is present.
  3. Treatment is dependent on the level and extent of cervical fusion. Prognosis for an active life is good for those infants minimally as well as more severely affected if early diagnosis and treatment are provided (Theiss, Smith, and Winter, 1997).
  4. Early parental involvement is essential and must be supported because infants with Klippel-Feil syndrome frequently require ongoing treatment as a result of their orthopedic and associated anomalies.

  B. **Torticollis ("wry neck"):** a condition in which the infant holds the head in a rotated, tilted position (Epps and Salter, 1996). Two types have been identified: muscular and bony.
  1. Congenital muscular torticollis presents as a nontender, mobile mass or tumor that is palpable and is attached to or located within the body of the sternocleidomastoid muscle (Fig. 23–1). Development of a muscle contracture within the next several weeks causes the child to hold his or her head in the characteristic position of flexion, lateral bend, and contralateral rotation.

    a. Etiology is secondary to tearing of muscle and subsequent bleeding into the muscle which later forms a mass which is first palpable within 2–4 weeks of age. Resolution of the mass generally occurs over 8–10 weeks following birth.

    b. May be associated with breech, primiparous, or difficult birth, although it has been reported after both normal and operative deliveries. The lesion may be secondary to uterine factors, because there are a greater number of right-sided lesions (Loder, 1996).

    c. Hip dysplasia and clubfoot are associated conditions and should be identified if present.

    d. Other etiologic theories include antenatal myositis, neurogenic disorders, ischemia resulting from decreased arterial inflow or congested venous outflow, perinatal compartment syndrome, or a neuropathy (Walsh and Morrissy, 1998).

    e. Radiographs may be helpful but difficult to obtain because of the head position. Laminograms and flexion-extension films may be helpful. Cervical spine abnormalities must be ruled out.

    f. Treatment is with conservative measures such as passive exercise, stretching, and positioning in neutral and hyperextended positions. Ninety percent of cases of muscular torticollis can be managed with a stretching program (Epps and Salter, 1996).

    g. Parents need to take an active role in the exercise programs, including environmental modification such as positioning the crib and toys to encourage stretching. Surgical remedy (release of the sternocleidomastoid muscle) is recommended if the deformity persists after 1 year of age.

    h. Nursing care for infants with this deformity is centered around accurate assessment of the defect and prevention of further injury. An active role in the education of those individuals providing care and exercises is vital to the success of the treatment.

2. Congenital bony torticollis is a combined head tilt and rotary deformity. It indicates a problem with the cervical spine at C1-C2 as 50% of cervical spine rotation occurs at this joint (Loder, 1996).

    a. Osseous types of torticollis: basilar impressions, atlanto-occipital anomalies, congenital cervical fusion, and unilateral absence of the first cervical vertebra.

    b. Etiology of these anomalies is multifactorial.

    c. Characteristic presentation: short, broad neck; low hairline; and torticollis. Asymmetry of the face and skull may be present.

    d. Physical examination: no contractures or shortening of the muscle. No mass is palpable. Range of motion is dependent on underlying pathologic condition.

    e. Radiographs may be useful in defining bony abnormalities but may be difficult to obtain secondary to the deformity, shadows of the mandible and difficulty in positioning the infant. MRI studies are useful to detail neuroanatomy.

    f. Treatment: dependent on individual and specific defect. Operative and nonsurgical remedies are used. Treatment of these anomalies is often complex and requires a multidisciplinary approach. Defects often progress with time and can result in serious neurologic compromise and pain. Immobilization with bracing may provide relief. If neurologic symptoms are present, cervical fusion may be indicated.

    g. Nursing support for these lesions rests with a clear understanding of the underlying defect. Assessment of cervical stability is an ongoing task for medical staff as well as family members if further injury is to be prevented.

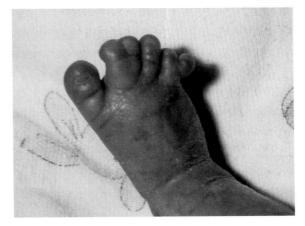

Figure 23–2
Syndactyly of second and third toes and polydactyly. (Courtesy of Jane Deacon, RNC, MS, NNP, The Children's Hospital, Denver, Colorado.)

LIMB ABNORMALITIES

Minor limb abnormalities are common and usually correctable and may serve as an indicator of more serious abnormalities. Causes have been linked to genetic, environmental, and chromosomal factors.

A. **Syndactyly:** webbing or fusion of any portion of two or more digits. Described as complete if webbing exists along the entire length of the digit or incomplete if webbing occurs only distally—usually to the middle of the proximal phalanx (Bayne, Costas, and Laurie, 1996). The defect is further classified as single if the skin alone is affected, or as complex if the bones of adjacent fingers are fused (Fig. 23–2).

1. Incidence: 1:2000 to 1:2500 births (Eaton and Lister, 1990). Males are affected twice as often as females, with approximately half of the cases manifested bilaterally. Feet are more commonly affected than hands. Familial incidence may be as high as 20–40%.
2. Etiology: believed to be sporadic in 80% of affected infants (Bayne et al., 1996).
3. Associated conditions: a variety of syndromes (e.g., Apert's syndrome and congenital constriction band syndrome), as well as visceral, skin, and other skeletal anomalies.
4. Physical examination: webbing or fusion of two or more digits, with both physical and functional impairment.
5. Radiographs: assist in classification of the abnormality as simple or complex.
6. Treatment: dependent on physical findings; highly individualized. If surgical treatment is undertaken, the timing is vital to later functional capacity.
    a. Surgery is generally performed between 6 months and 1 year of age—especially if the affected digits have a greater discrepancy in size and growth rates. Delay in surgery may result in bowing of the longer digit. Surgical correction should be completed by a few years of age to allow for development of independent movement and dexterity (Tolo and Wood, 1993).
    b. Surgical remedy is not without risk because of the potential for damage to the neurovascular bundle, the underlying condition of joints and tendons, and underlying bony abnormalities.
    c. Skin grafting is frequently necessary because the sum of the circumference of two adjacent fingers is always greater than the circumference of isolated digits (Bayne et al., 1996).
7. Genetic counseling: extended to parents in light of described patterns of inheritance and the frequency of associated anomalies. Risk assessment must include previous occurrence within the family.

8. Nursing care: support and information for the parents of the infant. These lesions are highly visible, and acceptance of the defect by family members is vital for their active participation in therapy.

B. **Polydactyly:** development of supernumerary digits, usually involving the ulnar aspect of the hand. The affected digits are often incomplete and are lacking in muscular development. The anomaly results from a duplication error in which a stimulus induces excessive limb bud formation. Bilateral defects are common (Fig. 23–2).
1. Incidence: common.
2. Etiology: inherited as an autosomal dominant trait.
3. Associated conditions: other abnormalities of the skeletal system, including syndactyly of the hands and polydactyly of the toes.
4. Physical examination: extra digits on either hands or feet. The abnormality is divided into three classifications: soft tissue mass connected by a tissue pedicle; partial duplication involving the phalanges; and complete duplication of the finger, with formation of the metacarpal bone (Bayne et al., 1996). Defects are further classified according to their anatomic placement.
   a. Preaxial, or duplicate, thumbs occur most commonly as an isolated lesion in 0.08:1000 births. It occurs with greater frequency in Native American and Asian populations. This defect has been associated with Holt-Oram and Fanconi syndromes.
   b. Triphalangeal thumb is also referred to as a thumbless, five-fingered hand. The defect occurs in 1:25,000 live births, demonstrated equally between the sexes, and is bilateral in 80% of affected children (Bayne et al., 1996). This defect is thought to be autosomal dominant. Multiple syndromes are associated with this lesion: trisomies 13 to 15, and Blackfan-Diamond and Fanconi syndromes.
5. Radiographs: useful in identifying bony defects and guiding treatment.
6. Treatment: dependent on specific defect. Therapy is aimed toward preservation of function and motion, as well as provision of cosmetic remedy. Surgical intervention is commonly used.
7. Nursing care: support of parents through discovery of the lesion and throughout treatment. Care of the affected digit includes observation of circulatory status and prevention of infection and further injury.

C. **Absent radius:** partial or total absence of parts involving the radial or preaxial border of the arm (Bayne et al., 1996). The radius is either absent, shortened, thin, or of little usefulness.
1. Incidence: 1:30,000 to 1:100,000 births.
2. Etiology: believed to be mixed. An autosomal dominant pattern has been described. Environmental factors such as viral infections, chemicals, and drugs may exert an effect that alters limb formation.
3. Associated conditions: other defects involving the heart, genitourinary, and gastrointestinal systems (e.g., Holt-Oram syndrome and trisomy 17).
4. Classification (Bayne et al., 1996): short distal radius, hypoplastic radius, partial absence of the radius, and total absence.
5. Physical examination: radial deviation of the hand. The degree of deviation is dependent on the underlying anatomy—the greater the degree of absence, the greater are the deviation and subsequent bowing of the extremity. The limb is often two-thirds the length of the opposite, unaffected extremity. Muscle and neurovascular deficiencies vary in proportion to the skeletal defect. Thumbs may be absent or, if present, defective to some extent. Bilateral involvement is more commonly associated with associated syndromes.
6. Radiographic evaluation: helpful if the defect is part of a syndrome.
7. Treatment: based on accurate functional assessment before any surgical intervention is undertaken (Lloyd-Roberts and Fixsen, 1990). Management goals are

centered on improving alignment, function, and stability. The range of options for management are wide, including no treatment, plaster correction and splinting, and surgical centralization of the wrist on the ulna. Early diagnosis and intervention are needed to prevent loss of function (Bayne et al., 1996).
8. Genetic counseling: especially relevant when associated anomalies exist. Parental involvement and support are vital for either treatment option, because long-term, active participation is needed for splinting, casting, and exercise remedies.
9. Nursing care: based on an understanding of the pathologic condition behind the lesion. Treatment is often complex and long term, requiring the nurse to participate actively in case management.

D. **Talipes equinovarus** (also known as clubfoot): a developmental deformity of the hind foot that results from multiple anatomic factors (Thompson et al., 1992). Deformities of muscle, tendon sheaths, ligaments, joint capsules, and bones affect the development of the abnormality. Equinovarus deformity accounts for 97% of clubfoot anomalies, occurring bilaterally in 44% of infants (Sullivan, 1996).
1. Incidence: 1:1000 births, males being affected twice as often as females (Wong, 1997).
2. Etiology: believed to be a combination of factors.
   a. Extrinsic: related to changes within the uterine environment, such as rupture of membranes resulting in oligohydramnios and possibly amniotic bands, or to the effects of uterine pressure exerted during a critical developmental period.
   b. Mendelian: part of a syndrome from a genetic basis. Both autosomal dominant and recessive inheritance patterns, as well as X-linked recessive inheritance patterns, have been identified. Clubfoot is part of Freeman-Sheldon, Larsen's, and Smith-Lemli-Opitz syndromes (Sullivan, 1996).
   c. Multifactorial inheritance: high incidence of idiopathic clubfoot in subsequent siblings of an affected infant—strong evidence of multifactorial inheritance as a major cause of the deformity.
   d. Neural origin: neuromuscular pathologic condition, resulting in in-utero muscle imbalance as a cause of the deformity. Changes in innervation may cause an increase in muscle fibrosis, leading to shortening of muscles and development of joint contractures and affecting the embryonic development of the talus, causing the deformity (Khermosh and Wientroub, 1998).
3. Physical examination: forefoot adduction, varus deformity of the hind foot, and equinus of the ankle (Fig. 23–3).
4. Radiographs: vital for identification of bony defect, but it is difficult to draw valid conclusions about bony structure because of the late appearance of the tarsals. Measurement of the anteroposterior and lateral talocalcaneal angles after treatment indicates the degree of correction achieved (Sullivan, 1996).
5. Treatment: highly individualized according to the severity of the defect. Goal of treatment is a functional, pain-free, plantigrade foot with good mobility. Manipulation and serial castings are often used initially to stretch tight muscles and ligaments. Plaster is used to maintain the position of the manipulated part. Serial castings are often required, and surgical treatment will eventually be required to restore normal bony architecture and to balance muscle forces. Surgery is indicated for failure to achieve results by closed methods (Drvaric, Kuivilla, and Roberts, 1989). A variety of surgical procedures exist for correction of this deformity. Outcome of surgical treatment is dependent on early intervention and the specific defect.
6. Nursing care: recognition and assessment of the defect. With nonsurgical casting, care also includes observation of skin and circulation. Parent education and support are important because follow-up care is generally handled on an

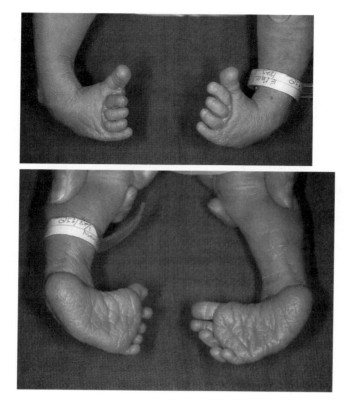

Figure 23–3
Bilateral talipes equinovarus. Note structural deformity of hind part of foot. (Courtesy of Jane Deacon, RNC, MS, NNP, The Children's Hospital, Denver, Colorado.)

outpatient basis. The importance of family involvement in the treatment plan must be clearly communicated by the nurse to the family.

E. **Talipes calcaneovalgus:** common, relatively benign, flexible deformity. It occurs as a result of the foot position in utero, when the foot is positioned with the sole against the uterine wall and the dorsal skin of the foot resting against the anterior surface of the tibia.

1. Incidence: 30:1000 live births (Silvani, 1992).
2. Etiology: uncertain but believed to be extrinsic in relation to an abnormal intrauterine position with excessive internal limb rotation. Oligohydramnios is frequently an associated condition (Silvani, 1992).
3. Physical examination: free mobility of the foot to passive manipulation; marked dorsiflexion and eversion of the foot with a valgus of the heel (Silvani, 1992). Ankle dorsiflexion is normal. The fibula is prominent as a result of excessive dorsiflexion in utero.
4. Radiographs: not usually needed because the condition is generally easily differentiated from a structural defect. If needed, an MRI will differentiate talipes calcaneovalgus from congenital convex pes valgus (rigid, rocker-bottom flatfoot) (Silvani, 1992).
5. Treatment: primarily passive exercise or plaster casting, depending on the severity of the lesion. The goal is to obtain a plantar-flexed varus position to stretch those tendons that have been positionally shortened in utero.
   a. Mild cases: stretching exercises that move the foot into equinus and varus positions—15–20 times in four or five sessions daily (Griffin, 1994).
   b. Resistant deformities: corrective casts, changed as needed for growth (Churgay, 1993).

6. Parent education: awareness that deformity is not serious and the long-term prognosis is good with appropriate therapy. The parents' support in exercise and casting is important to the outcome.
7. Nursing care: accurate assessment to differentiate the defect from more serious structural defects. The nurse should also assist the parents in providing needed exercises to the affected extremity. If casting is needed, instruct the family on cast care and observation of the feet while casted.

F. **Metatarsus adductus, or metatarsus varus** (terms used synonymously in practice): medial deviation of the metatarsals as a result of either positional or structural abnormality (Fig. 23–4).
1. Incidence: 2:1000 births (Salter, 1983).
2. Etiology: related to interplay between environmental and genetic predisposition. Intrauterine position of the fetal foot against the uterine wall can result in the deformity (Morcuende and Ponseti, 1996).
3. Associated anomalies: muscular torticollis and congenital hip dysplasia.
4. Physical examination: dependent on the type of defect. The most significant finding is the presence or absence of rigidity of the forefoot.
   a. Structural defects demonstrate inability of the forefoot to be abducted beyond the midline. The base of the fifth metatarsal is prominent, creating a crease on the medial side of the foot. The heel is maintained in a varus position. The sole is kidney shaped.
   b. Positional defects demonstrate greater flexibility, and the forefoot is easily abducted. The foot is turned in, with the heel in a neutral position. Ankle motion is normal.
5. Radiographs: define the defect and rule out other associated anomalies.

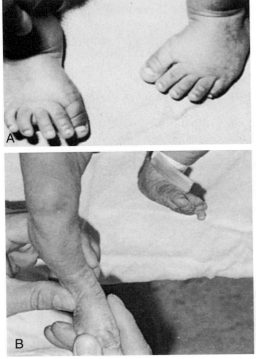

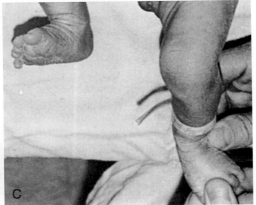

Figure 23–4
A, Structural metatarsus adductus. *B,* Structural metatarsus adductus. The forefoot does not abduct beyond neutral. *C,* Positional metatarsus; the forefoot abducts beyond the midline. (From Avery, G.B. [Ed.]: Neonatology: Pathophysiology and Management of the Newborn, 3rd ed. Philadelphia, J.B. Lippincott, 1987, p. 1061.)

    6. Treatment: guided by the deformity.
      a. Positional. Majority of infants require no treatment, and resolution occurs with growth. Gentle, passive range-of-motion exercises may assist with resolution.
      b. Casting. Structural defects may require serial castings for 3–6 weeks until the forefoot can be placed passively in the valgus position and the lateral foot border is straight. If no treatment has been undertaken by 1 year of age, casting has little effect and surgery is needed.
    7. Nursing care: assistance with diagnosis; education of parents regarding exercise techniques and the need for continued follow-up. If casting is needed, instruct the family on cast care and observation of the feet while casted.

    G. **Developmental dysplasia of the hip (DDH)** (formerly known as congenital dislocation of the hip): wide spectrum of abnormalities affecting the femoral head and the acetabulum. In the newborn infant, hip dysplasia refers to a hip that can be manipulated to subluxation and to dislocation or reduced from either of these positions (Aronsson, Goldberg, Kling, and Ray, 1994; Weinstein, 1996). Developmental dysplasia and dislocation encompass embryonic, fetal, and infant periods. Several reports have described the occurrence of dislocation, or dysplasia, of the hip after a normal neonatal screening examination (Davies and Walker, 1984).
    1. Incidence: 1:1000 to 2:1000 live births. Females are affected more than males, at a ratio of 6:1 (Bennet and MacEwen, 1989). The defect is more common in Native American populations, Japanese, and central and southern Europeans. There is a decreased incidence in African, Korean, and Chinese populations.
    2. Etiology: multifactorial. Environmental, genetic, and ethnic factors appear to be significant.
      a. Prenatal positioning provides a significant risk factor. Breech positioning, especially frank breech with hips flexed and knees extended, increases the risk. Sixteen percent of infants with DDH have had a breech presentation, versus 3% in the general population (Aronsson et al., 1994).
      b. Ligamentous laxity is also a factor in DDH. The laxity can result from a circulating maternal hormone (relaxin) that exerts an effect resulting in hip dislocation. Familial ligamentous laxity has also been identified.
      c. Genetic predisposition is also a factor in development. Recurrence rates for siblings of an affected infant are significantly greater than the general incidence of the defect.
    3. Associated anomalies: torticollis, talipes equinovarus, metatarsus adductus, and firstborn (Novacheck, 1996).
    4. Physical examination: history of breech positioning, family history of hip dislocation, or ligamentous laxity. Manipulation of the hip utilizing Ortolani's or Barlow's maneuver is meant to elicit dislocation and reduction of the unstable hip (see Chapter 5, Physical Assessment of the Newborn Infant). Differences in abduction of the hip, apparent shortening of the affected femur, and extra skinfolds are present. Not all hip dislocations are observed on neonatal examination and are believed to develop from neonatal hip instability (Weinstein, 1996). Anatomic changes are minimal in the newborn infant, but as the hip becomes permanently dislocated, pathologic changes of the acetabulum, femoral head, hip capsule, joint, and ligaments become progressive. The end result is a degenerative change of the femoral head and acetabulum.
    5. Radiographs: may be difficult to obtain because of problems in positioning the infant; usually diagnostic of dysplasia or subluxation of the hip. Ultrasonography is also useful in detection of DDH and in monitoring the response of the hip to treatment (Bailik, Wiener, and Benderly, 1992).
    6. Treatment: initiated when hip instability is discovered during the neonatal period. The first goal of treatment is to obtain concentric reduction of the hip

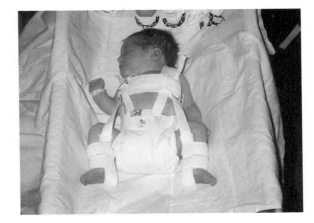

Figure 23–5
Infant with dislocated hips in a Pavlic harness.
(Courtesy of Jane Deacon, RNC, MS, NNP, The
Children's Hospital, Denver, Colorado.)

and to maintain that reduction while supporting femoral head and acetabular development (Weinstein, 1996; Aronsson et al., 1994).

   a. Flexion and some degree of abduction are achieved with a harness. This is preferred over casting or rigid bracing. A Pavlik harness is commonly used (Fig. 23–5) (Grill et al., 1988). The harness needs to be closely monitored because failure of reduction within 2–3 weeks may cause erosive changes in the superior lateral acetabulum (Atar, Lehman, and Grant 1993).

   b. Serial radiographs follow up the response to treatment. Duration of use is individual—usually 4–6 weeks. During this time, proper fit and adjustment of the harness are vital to ensure hip stability and to avoid secondary pathologic changes in the femoral head and acetabular cartilage and secondary impairment of bone growth.

7. Parent education: understanding of the importance of parents in maintaining the prescribed harness or splint; vital to resolution of the problem. The importance of follow-up must be communicated to ensure that further dislocation or complications are recognized.

8. Nursing care: assessment of abnormality, patient advocacy, nurturing of infant, parent education. The nurse is often the first to recognize a potential subluxation or dislocation as part of the initial neonatal assessment (Wong, 1997). The ability to perform examination maneuvers accurately is a vital skill for all nurses. Once the defect is identified, the nurse becomes a patient advocate—providing protection from further injury and serving as a resource for information on issues related to treatment and maintenance of the device used for correction. The nurse must also adapt nurturing activities to meet the needs of the infant or child and must also teach the parents to apply and maintain the reduction device.

H. **Amniotic bands:** upper or lower limb abnormalities resulting from bands of fibrous tissue encircling body parts (Fig. 23–6). Congenital constriction bands occur in any part of any extremity but are most commonly seen in the distal portion of limbs, with upper extremities twice as often affected as lower extremities (Bayne et al., 1996).

1. Incidence: approximately 1:5000 to 1:15000 births (Bayne et al., 1996).

2. Etiology: unclear but thought to be related to the interplay between germ plasm defects and constriction band formation (Bayne et al., 1996). Premature rupture of membranes is often associated with this condition (Tolo and Wood, 1993). Localized rupture of the amniotic sac results in entanglement of the body parts in amniotic threads.

3. Associated anomalies: syndactyly, brachydactyly, clubfoot, cleft lip, cleft palate, and cranial vault defects.

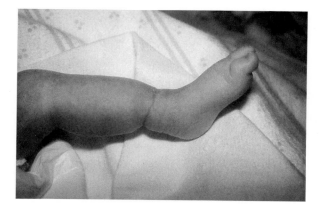

Figure 23–6
Amniotic band constriction of lower leg. (Courtesy of Jane Deacon, RNC, MS, NNP, The Children's Hospital, Denver, Colorado.)

4. Defects, classified into four types: simple ring constriction; ring constrictions with bony fusion distally; ring constrictions with fusion of soft tissue parts; and intrauterine amputations.
5. Physical examination: careful evaluation of the vascular supply and pattern of swelling distal to the constriction. Joints may be motionless or stiff if severe lymphedema is present.
6. Radiographs: assist with clarification of the type of defect and associated defects.
7. Treatment: dependent on severity of involvement. Incomplete and complete ring deformities are generally treated for improvement in cosmetic effect. Surgical procedures are aimed at releasing constrictions and improving contour of the affected part. Defects with greater constrictive force are aimed at improving venous and lymphatic drainage. Associated syndactyly is also released. Timing of repair is dependent on lesion severity. Severe constriction may require emergent care, whereas less involved deformity can be corrected at 1–2 years of age.
8. Nursing focus: ongoing assessment of the affected extremity. Circulatory competency must be monitored and preserved as the infant grows despite the initial therapy offered.

I. **Arthrogryposis multiplex congenita:** nonprogressive, multiple, congenitally rigid joints (Goldberg, 1996). The major form of arthrogryposis multiplex congenita is amyoplasia, a term that refers to the classic syndrome, in which there is involvement of the upper and lower extremities (Sarwark et al., 1990; Shapiro et al., 1993). If only two extremities are affected, it is most often the lower extremities. No sensory or intelligence loss is associated.
1. Incidence: 1:3000 live births.
2. Etiology: uncertain; related to abnormalities of the central nervous system, intrauterine environment, infection, and environmental factors. No genetic disorder is known.
   a. Deformities appear to be the result of diminished intrauterine movement (Tolo and Wood, 1993). Joint formation occurs, but the soft tissue structures surrounding the joint become fibrotic. These infants are known to have a decreased number of anterior horn cells within the spinal cord. The end result is a lack of fetal movement and abnormal amniotic fluid circulation, which may in turn affect fetal position.
   b. May occur as a component of heterogeneous, neurogenic, and myopathic disorders (Goldberg, 1996).
3. Physical examination: symmetric joint contractures with marked limitation of active and passive motion of the involved joints.

    a. Upper extremities: internal rotation and adduction of the shoulder, extension at the elbow, and flexion of the wrist and fingers. Fingers are slender and held close together.

    b. Lower extremities: flexion at the hips and knees; foot deformity—usually clubfoot or vertical talus.

    c. Skin: waxlike appearance with absence of creases at the joints. Capillary hemangiomas of the face are common.

4. Radiographs: obtained to rule out associated problems such as congenital hip dysplasia, spinal dysraphism, and fractures of the femur.

5. Treatment: aimed toward maximizing potential and prevention of further deformity. Early initiation of passive range-of-motion exercise of shoulders, elbows, and knees has been found to improve function. Serial casting of peripheral joints may be needed. Associated abnormalities of talipes equinovarus and hip dysplasia require similar treatment as if arthrogryposis were not present. Surgical relief is individualized and often delayed until functional assessment of the hands and arms is obtained (Goldberg, 1996).

6. Nursing care: careful assessment of range-of-motion and other associated abnormalities; parent education. The nature of this defect requires long-term support from the family, and nurses are in an ideal position to assist parents with information about the normal intelligence and favorable functional prognosis for their child.

SKELETAL DISORDERS

A. **Osteogenesis imperfecta:** a group of heterozygous inherited disorders of connective tissue characterized by defects of connective tissue and bone (Wong, 1997).

1. Incidence: uncommon (Thomas and Harvey, 1992).

2. Etiology: autosomal dominant, with recessive forms described. There is a wide range of phenotypic expression for the disease.

3. Four classifications (Sillence, 1981):

    a. Type I: autosomal dominant inheritance; characterized by bone fragility, blue sclerae, possible hearing loss, and onset of fractures after birth.

    b. Type II: autosomal recessive inheritance; lethal in perinatal period; sclerae are dark blue, concertina femurs and beaded ribs are present, and there is extreme bone fragility.

    c. Type III: autosomal recessive inheritance; fractures are present at birth, deformities are progressive, and sclerae and hearing are normal.

    d. Type IV: autosomal dominant inheritance; bones are fragile, and sclerae and hearing are normal.

4. Physical findings and characteristics: vary with disease type.

    a. Abnormalities of bones, fractures, changes in bone shape and contour: skull is often misshapen because of wormian bone development. Vertebrae fracture easily, and scoliosis may result.

    b. Skin: thin, translucent, and easily distensible.

    c. Teeth: dentition delayed and defective; teeth are soft, translucent.

    d. Ocular: sclerae have bluish tint because of a lack of collagen.

    e. Joints: easily dislocated.

    f. Neurologic findings: hydrocephalus and intracranial hemorrhage.

    g. Metabolic effects: sweating, increased body temperature, resting tachycardia and tachypnea.

5. Radiographs: assist in defining the defect. Presence of new or healed fractures, angular deformities, and bowing of the extremities assist in defining disease type.

6. Treatment goals: centered around management of new fractures to prevent malalignment and around long-term support to attain ambulation. Fractures

may be difficult to treat because of structural bone abnormalities and ligament laxity. For severe or progressive deformities, surgical fixation may be needed. Scoliosis is difficult to treat because of the advancement of spinal curvature and poor bone quality. Early segmental fusion may improve function and prevent respiratory compromise.

7. Parent education. Families must learn to cope with this complex disorder, which places a significant burden on the family irrespective of the disease type identified. Long-term management of all aspects of this disease is essential. Parents must work toward prevention of fractures and must be reassured that spontaneous fractures occur despite the best of care.

8. Nursing-care focus: family support and provision of information regarding type of defect present. Infants with this disorder require careful handling to prevent fractures. They must be supported when turned or positioned. Methods of preventing new fractures must be identified, and the nurse must work with the family to achieve resources to support ambulation and long-term follow-up.

B. Osteochondrodysplasia: dwarfing conditions that involve abnormalities in development of the skeleton. The expression of these abnormalities are observed in the limbs, trunk, and skull.

1. Achondroplasia is the most commonly seen form of short-limb dwarfism. Primary defect is abnormal endochondrial bone formation.
   a. Incidence: 1:10,000 live births (Thomas and Harvey, 1992).
   b. Etiology: transmission of defect as an autosomal dominant trait. Eighty percent of cases occur as a new mutation. Most parents of affected infants are average in size and have no family history of osteochondrodysplasia.
   c. Associated conditions: generally multiple, long-term problems that include maxillary hypoplasia, speech problems, recurrent otitis media, poor head control, and gait abnormalities.
   d. Physical findings: large head with unusual-appearing facies, normal trunk height with rhizomelic shortening of extremities, and associated excessive or restricted motion of joints (Bassett, 1996).
   e. Radiographs: films of skull, spine, and extremities to reveal characteristic features and aid diagnosis (see also Chapter 29, Radiologic Evaluation of the Newborn Infant).
   f. Treatment: accurate diagnosis and genetic counseling to begin. A geneticist knowledgeable in skeletal dysplasias is needed to provide the basis of care. Parents should be counseled regarding further risks of transmission for themselves and the affected infant.
   g. Parent education: ongoing needs of infant. Family understanding of the need for continued evaluation and support as the infant matures is essential.
   h. Nursing care: holistic, because multiple systems can be affected. As the newborn infant matures, careful assessment of physical and developmental parameters is essential.

2. Thanatophoric dwarfism (type I): uniformly fatal in perinatal period (see also Chapter 29).

C. Osteomyelitis: inflammation of a long bone, caused by a microorganism (Lott, Kenner, and Polak, 1994). Osteomyelitis can lead to destruction of bone and to life-threatening illness.

1. Factors that predispose the neonate to osteomyelitis.
   a. Vascular supply to the bone allows for penetration of capillaries through the epiphyseal plates of the long bones. End result is communication between metaphysis and the joint space (Freij and McCracken, 1994). Spread of infection from site to site may occur with both bone and joint involvement.

  b. Neonatal bone is soft; when infection is present, pus is rapidly formed on subperiosteal surfaces. Periosteum may be lifted off the bone, and abscess formation occurs. Bone destruction results from bacterial toxins and products of inflammation.
  c. Neonates have a limited ability to respond to bone and joint sepsis because of impairment in cellular and humoral functions.
  d. Synovial lining of joints provides a good environment for bacterial growth. Synovial necrosis and cartilage destruction can result within days of the initial infection.
2. Bacterial agents identified as causative in the newborn period include group b Streptococcus, *Haemophilus influenzae*, coliforms, *Candida albicans*, and *Staphylococcus aureus*.
3. Symptoms: pain on motion, redness, swelling, and paralysis of the affected limb (Lott et al., 1994).
4. Diagnosis: sepsis workup, needle aspiration of skin, subcutaneous tissue, and affected bone or joint (Klein and Marcy, 1990).
5. Radiographs: can be diagnostic, showing nonspecific soft tissue swelling and metaphyseal and epiphyseal areas of rarefaction that resemble punched-out areas of the bone and may require serial examinations for progression or resolution of the infection.
6. Treatment: prolonged antibiotic therapy (3–4 weeks) after systemic and local signs are gone. Therapy is based on identity of infecting organism. A spinal tap is suggested because the infant may have a concurrent meningitis but no obvious symptoms of meningeal infection (Freij and McCracken, 1994). Supportive measures are aimed at preserving motion and preventing loss of joint function.
7. Nursing care: ongoing monitoring of vital signs, assessment of the affected extremity, antibiotic administration, and assessment of motion and function. Moving and turning should be carried out carefully and gently to minimize pain. Pain medication should be administered to provide comfort.

METABOLIC BONE DISEASE

  See Chapter 14, Metabolic Disorders.

FRACTURES

  Fractures can occur during the birthing process and are related to a combination of maternal and fetal conditions. The most common fractures involve the clavicle, humerus, and femur. Fractures may not be readily evident because of the absence of deformity and problems in pain recognition.

A. **Clavicle:** the bone most frequently injured at birth (Wong, 1997).
1. Etiology: most often diagnosed at the time of delivery when a snap is heard, followed by absence of movement of the arm.
2. Physical findings: vary with fracture type. Asymptomatic fractures are detected as a lump over the clavicle 7–10 days after delivery. Displaced fractures reveal decreased or absent motion of the arm, discoloration over the fracture site, crepitus (the crackling sound produced by the rubbing together of fractured bone fragments), tenderness, and irregularity along the clavicle. Asymmetric Moro's reflex, focal swelling or tenderness, or cries in pain when the arm is moved may also be present (Wong, 1997).
3. Radiograph: confirms fracture (see Chapter 29).
4. Treatment: careful handling, especially when dressing; no other special treatment. Shoulder immobilization and arm abduction may be considered if the infant exhibits pain symptoms.

5. Parental involvement: centered on education and infant care issues.
6. Nursing care: education of parents regarding the fracture and regarding careful handling (i.e., support the upper and lower back, rather than pulling the infant up from under the arms), dressing, support of the infant, and recognition of pain.

B. Humerus.

1. Etiology: difficult delivery.
2. Radiographs: differentiation from septic arthritis.
3. Physical findings: loss of spontaneous arm movement, followed by swelling and by pain on passive motion. Assessment of the status of soft tissue and nerve involvement must be accomplished as an ongoing process.
4. Treatment: immobilization of the arm at the side, the elbow at 90-degree flexion for 10–14 days to allow formation of callus and pain control.
5. Parent education: information about the normal progression of bone growth, to ensure appropriate follow-up care.
6. Nursing care: providing parents with information about the fracture and methods to immobilize the arm and to provide comfort measures and pain control. The importance of follow-up care must also be reinforced.

C. Femur.

1. Etiology: difficult delivery.
2. Physical findings: loss of motion or limited motion, edema, irritability with movement.
3. Radiographs: for differentiation from septic arthritis.
4. Treatment: splinting and pain control. Callus formation occurs within 2–4 weeks. Complete recovery is expected.
5. Parent education: information about the normal progression of bone growth, to ensure appropriate follow-up care.
6. Nursing care: education of the parents regarding the fracture and methods to splint the leg, as well as the importance of follow-up care. Provide comfort measures and pain control as needed.

REFERENCES

Aronsson, D.D., Goldberg, M.J., Kling, T.F., Jr., and Ray, D.R.: Developmental dysplasia of the hip. Pediatrics, 94:201–208, 1994.

Atar, D., Lehman, W.B., and Grant, A.D.: Pavlik harness pathology. J. Pediatr. Orthop. Part B, 2:75–77, 1993.

Bailik, V., Wiener, F., and Benderly, A.: Ultrasonography and screening in developmental displacement of the hip. J. Pediatr. Orthop. Part B, 1:51–54, 1992.

Bassett, G.: The osteochondrodysplasias. In Morrissy, R.T. (Ed.): Lovell and Winter's Pediatric Orthopedics, 4th ed. Philadelphia, Lippincott-Raven, 1996, pp. 203–255.

Bayne L., Costas, B., and Laurie, G.: The upper limb. In Morrissy, R.T. (Ed.): Lovell and Winter's Pediatric Orthopedics, 4th ed. Philadelphia, Lippincott-Raven, 1996, pp. 781–848.

Bennet, J.T., and MacEwen, G.D.: Congenital dislocation of the hip. Clin. Orthop., 247:15–21, 1989.

Churgay, C.A.: Diagnosis and treatment of pediatric foot deformities. Am. Fam. Physician, 47:883–889, 1993.

Davies, S.J., and Walker, G.: Problems in the early recognition of hip dysplasia. J. Bone Joint Surg., 66:479–484, 1984.

Drvaric, D.M., Kuivilla, T.E., and Roberts, J.M.: Congenital clubfoot: Etiology, pathoanatomy, pathogenesis and the changing spectrum of early management. Orthop. Clin. North Am., 20:641–647, 1989.

Eaton, C.J., and Lister, G.D.: Hand Clin., 6:555–575, 1990.

Epps, H.R., and Salter, R.B.: Orthopedic conditions of the cervical spine and shoulder [Common Orthopedic Pediatric Problems]. Pediatr. Clin. North Am., 43:919–929, 1996.

Freij, B., and McCracken, G.: Acute infections. In Avery, G., Fletcher, M.A., and MacDonald, M. (Eds.): Neonatology: Pathophysiology and Management of the Newborn, 4th ed. Philadelphia, J.B. Lippincott, 1994, pp. 1082–1114.

Goldberg, M.: Syndromes of orthopaedic importance. In Morrisy, R.T. (Ed.): Lovell and Winter's Pediatric Orthopedics, 4th ed. Philadelphia, Lippincott-Raven, 1996, pp. 255–304.

Griffin, P.: Orthopaedics. In Avery, G., Fletcher, M.A., and MacDonald, M. (Eds.): Neonatology: Pathophysiology and Management of the Newborn, 4th ed. Philadelphia, Lippincott-Raven, 1994, pp. 1179–1194.

Grill, F., Behsahel, H., Candell, J., et al.: The Pavlik harness and the treatment of the congenitally dislocating hip: Report on a multicenter study of the European Pediatric Orthopedic Society. J. Pediatr. Orthop., 8:1–8, 1988.

Guille, J.T., Miller, A., Bowen, J.R., et al.: The natural history of Klippel-Feil syndrome: Clinical roentgenographic and MRI findings at adulthood. J. Pediatr. Orthop., 15:617–626, 1995.

Khermosh, O., and Wientroub, S.: Clubfoot: What have we learned in the last quarter century? J. Pediatr. Orthop., 18:137–138, 1998.

Klein, J.O., and Marcy, S.M.: Bacterial sepsis and meningitis. In Remington, J.S., and Klein, J.O. (Eds.): Infectious Diseases of the Fetus and Newborn Infant, 3rd ed. Philadelphia, W.B. Saunders, 1990, pp. 601–656.

Lloyd-Roberts, G., and Fixsen, J.: The forearm and hand. In Lloyd-Roberts, G., and Fixen, J. (Eds.): Orthopaedics in Infancy and Childhood, 2nd ed. London, Butterworth-Heinmann, 1990, pp. 108–120.

Loder, R.: The cervical spine. In Morrissy, R.T. (Ed.): Lovell and Winter's Pediatric Orthopedics, 4th ed. Philadelphia, Lippincott-Raven, 1996, pp. 703–739.

Lott, J.W., Kenner, C., and Polak, J.D.: Common neonatal infections and complications. In Lott, J.W. (Ed.): Neonatal Infection: Assessment, Diagnosis, and Management. Petaluma, Calif., NICU Ink, 1994, pp. 45–46.

Morcuende, J.A., and Ponseti, I.V.: Congenital metatarsus adductus in early human fetal development. Clin. Orthop. 33:261–266, 1996.

Novacheck, T.F.: Developmental dysplasia of the hip. Pediatr. Clin. North Am., 43:829–848, 1996.

Salter, R.B.: Textbook of disorders and injuries of the musculoskeletal system, 2nd ed. Baltimore, Williams & Wilkins, 1983, pp. 101–144.

Sarwark, J.F., MacEwen, G.D., Scott, C.I., Jr.: Current concepts review: Amyoplasia (a common form of arthrogryposis). J. Bone Joint Surg., 72A:465–469, 1990.

Shapiro, F., and Specht, L.: Current concepts review: The diagnosis and orthopaedic treatment of childhood spinal muscular atrophy, peripheral neuropathy, Fried-reich ataxia, and arthrogryposis. J. Bone Joint Surg., 75A:1699–1714, 1993.

Sillence, D.: Osteogenesis imperfecta: An expanding panorama of variants. Clin. Orthop., 159:11–25, 1981.

Silvani, S.H.: Congenital pes valgus in foot and ankle. In Valentine, S.J. (Ed.): Foot and Ankle Disorders in Children. New York, Churchill Livingstone, 1992, pp. 170–174.

Sullivan, J.: The child's foot. In Morrissy, R.T. (Ed.): Lovell and Winters' Pediatric Orthopedics, 4th ed. Philadelphia, Lippincott-Raven, 1996, pp. 1077–1136.

Theiss, S.M., Smith, M.D., and Winter, R.B.: The long-term follow-up of patients with Klippel-Feil syndrome and congenital scoliosis. Spine, 22:1219–1222, 1997.

Thomas, R., and Harvey D.: Neonatology colour guide. New York, Churchill Livingstone, 1992, pp. 71, 77.

Thompson, G.H., and Simons, G.W.: Congenital talipes equinovarus (clubfeet) and metatarsus adductus. In Drennan, J.C. (Ed.): The Child's Foot and Ankle. New York, Raven Press, 1992, pp. 97–133.

Thomsen, M.N., Schneider, U., and Weber, M.: Scoliosis and congenital anomalies associated with Klippel-Feil syndrome types I–III. Spine, 22:396–401, 1997.

Tolo, T., and Wood, B.: Orthopaedic concerns in neuromuscular disease. In Tolo, T., and Wood, B. (Eds.): Pediatric Orthopaedics in Primary Care. Baltimore, Williams & Wilkins, 1993, pp. 263–277.

Walsh, J.J., and Morrissy, R.T.: Torticollis and hip dislocation. J. Pediatr. Orthop., 18:219–221, 1998.

Weinstein, S.: Developmental hip dysplasia and dislocation. In Morrissy, R.T. (Ed.): Lovell and Winter's Pediatric Orthopedics, 4th ed. Philadelphia, Lippincott-Raven, 1996, pp. 903–950.

Wong, D.L.: The child with musculoskeletal or articular dysfunction. In Whaley and Wong's Essentials of Pediatric Nursing, 5th ed. St. Louis, C.V. Mosby, 1997.

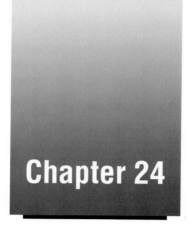

Chapter 24

Neonatal Dermatology

Catherine L. Witt

Objectives

1. Name three functions of the skin.

2. Describe two ways in which the skin of a newborn or preterm infant differs from that of an adult.

3. Identify three factors that affect the appearance of the neonate's skin.

4. Identify two nursing interventions that provide protection for the preterm infant's skin.

5. Recognize three common skin lesions that are normal variations in the newborn infant. Describe their appearance and treatment, if any.

6. Describe three common vascular lesions in the neonate, their appearance, and appropriate treatment.

7. Identify two syndromes associated with vascular lesions.

8. Evaluate two pigmented lesions occurring in the newborn infant and list implications associated with each.

9. Name two types of infectious skin lesions and select the appropriate treatment.

Careful assessment of the skin is an important element of the neonatal physical examination. The appearance of the skin gives the nurse important clues regarding gestational age, nutritional status, function of organs such as the heart and liver, and the presence of cutaneous or systemic disease. It is important for the clinician to be familiar with normal variances in the skin of the newborn infant, as well as those variances that signify disease.

Proper care of the neonate's skin can directly affect mortality and morbidity, especially in the preterm infant. The skin is the first line of defense against infection. Proper skin care can protect the integrity of the skin and prevent breakdown.

Anatomy and Physiology of the Skin

A. Anatomy of the skin—three main layers (Fig. 24–1):

1. Epidermis: outermost layer, which functions as a barrier from outside penetration. The epidermis is subdivided into five layers.

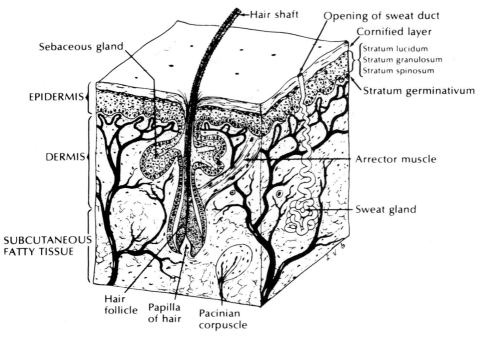

Figure 24–1
Several layers and structures of human skin. (From Francis, C.C., and Martin, A.H.: Introduction to Human Anatomy, 7th ed. St. Louis, C.V. Mosby, 1975.)

    a. Stratum corneum: outermost layer, consisting of closely packed dead cells that are consistently brushed off and replaced by lower levels of the epidermis. These cells are flatter and have thicker walls than other cells. The cells are held together by intracellular lipids, which aid in forming the protective barrier of the skin.

    b. Lower layers of epidermis: contain keratin-forming cells that create the outer layer of skin; as well as melanocytes, which produce melanin, or pigment. Despite racial differences in pigmentation, the number of melanocytes in a given surface area of skin is the same (Weston, Lane, and Morelli, 1996).

2. Dermis: directly under the epidermis; 2-4 mm thick at birth.

    a. Composed of collagen and elastic fibers that connect the epidermis and dermis and provide the skin with the ability to stretch and then to return to normal shape.

    b. Contains a rich supply of blood vessels and nerves that carry sensations of heat, touch, pain, and pressure from the skin to the brain and provide protection against injury, infections, or other invasions.

    c. Sweat glands, sebaceous glands, and hair shafts are also found in the dermis.

3. Subcutaneous layer: fatty tissue functions as insulation, protection of internal organs, and calorie storage.

B. Functions of the skin.

1. Physical protection.

    a. Mechanical.

        (1) Tightly packed, thick-walled cells, held together by intercellular lipids, provide a protective barrier against transepidermal water loss and external invasions.

(2) Process of constant sloughing and replacement of stratum corneum prevents colonization of the skin surface by bacteria and other organisms.

b. Chemical/bacterial.
   (1) Acidic surface of skin (pH < 5.0) provides defense against bacteria and other microorganisms.
   (2) Production of melanin protects against damage from ultraviolet-light radiation.

2. Heat regulation.
   a. Production and evaporation of sweat.
   b. Dilation and constriction of blood vessels.
   c. Insulation of body by subcutaneous fat.

3. Sense perception: heat, touch, pain, and pressure.

C. **Differences in newborn/preterm skin.**

1. Basic structure is same as that of the adult; the less mature the infant, the less mature is the functioning of the skin.

2. The earlier the gestational age, the more thin and gelatinous is the skin, with fewer layers in the stratum corneum and a thinner dermis with fewer elastic fibers. The epidermis matures quickly after birth in the preterm infant and resembles that of a term infant within 2-3 weeks of age (Evans and Rutter, 1986).

3. Subcutaneous fat is accumulated predominantly during the third trimester.
   a. Preterm babies have little fat, resulting in an inability to maintain body temperature and blood glucose level.
   b. Brown fat, which is important for temperature regulation in the newborn infant, begins to differentiate during the seventh month of gestation (Moore and Persaud, 1993).

4. Immature skin is thinner and therefore more permeable.
   a. An infant, especially a preterm infant, quickly absorbs topically applied drugs and chemicals (Choonara, 1994; Harpin and Rutter, 1983).
   b. Greater permeability allows for greater insensible water loss in the preterm infant.
   c. Higher surface area/body weight ratio allows for greater absorption of chemicals and greater transepidermal water loss.

5. Fewer fibrils connect the dermis and epidermis, and they are more fragile in term and preterm skin than in the skin of an adult. The stratum corneum is thinner in the term and preterm infant. Risk of injury from tape, monitors, and handling is increased, especially in the preterm infant; this type of injury includes removal of the outermost layer of the dermis with removal of tape or electrodes (Lund et al., 1997).

6. Sweat glands are present at birth, but full adult functioning is not present until the second or third year of life. Sweating may occur in the term infant but is not present in infants born at less than 36 weeks' gestation.
   a. The newborn infant has limited ability to tolerate excessive heat.
   b. Vasodilation to increase heat loss can result in hypotension and dehydration caused by increased insensible water loss.

Care of the Newborn Infant's Skin

A. **Term newborn infant.**

1. Initial bath with water and a mild soap.
   a. Avoid strong alkaline soaps to minimize alteration of surface pH.
   b. Soaps containing hexachlorophene should not be used. The hexachlorophene has been shown to be absorbed through the skin (Kopelman, 1973).

c. Safety of other bacteriostatic soaps has not been determined. These should be used with caution and rinsed off completely.

d. As soon as the body temperature is stable (>36.5° C) it is advisable to bathe the healthy term infant to decrease the caregiver's risk of exposure to blood-borne pathogens (Penny-MacGillivray, 1996). Standard precautions, including the use of gloves, should be adhered to when handling the infant who has not been bathed after delivery and during any invasive procedure in which the caregiver may be exposed to body fluids.

2. Parents may prefer to give the first bath themselves.

3. Vernix caseosa contains large amounts of fats, which protect the skin from the amniotic fluid and bacteria in utero. It insulates the stratum corneum and should not be scrubbed off during the initial bath (Peters, 1996).

4. When possible, avoid puncturing the skin of babies with suspected maternal infections.

5. Routine use of emollients is not recommended in the term infant. Creams and emollients that contain perfumes are drying and may irritate the infant's skin. Products that change the pH of the skin decrease the bacteriostatic properties (National Association of Neonatal Nurses [NANN], 1997). If cracking or fissures develop in the skin, a nonperfumed product should be used.

B. Preterm infant.

1. Keep skin clean with water. Mild, nonalkaline soap may be used. Preterm infants should be bathed infrequently during the first 2 months of life to avoid excessive drying of the skin and to avoid overstimulation, stress, and fatigue (NANN, 1997; Peters, 1996).

2. Handle infant gently and minimally to avoid trauma.

3. Minimize use of tape as much as possible. Use care when removing tape to avoid stripping the epidermis (Gordon and Montgomery, 1996).
   a. Safety of adhesive solvents is uncertain. Cotton balls soaked with warm water can be used effectively for removing tape and other adhesives.
   b. Gelled adhesives and pectin-based barriers have been found to be helpful in avoiding trauma to the skin during their removal (Lund et al., 1997).
   c. Pectin or hydrocolloid layers applied before adhesives may protect the skin from damage when endotracheal tubes or catheters are secured.
   d. Benzoin and other adhesive bonding agents form a strong bond between the adhesive and the epidermis, increasing the risk of stripping the epidermis when the adhesive is removed. Use of these agents with preterm infants should be avoided.
   e. Increased permeability of the skin allows absorption of some medications and products such as alcohol and povidone-iodine (Betadine) (Linder et al., 1997). When these substances are used for an invasive procedure, it is recommended that they be removed completely with water as soon as possible to prevent absorption or chemical burns.

4. Emollient creams that are free of preservatives and perfumes may be of benefit to the preterm infant by decreasing transepidermal water loss and skin breakdown (Lane and Drost, 1993; Nopper et al., 1996).

5. A tent with warm mist may protect the skin and decrease insensible water loss in the very low birth weight infant.

6. Transparent adhesive dressings can be used over wounds and abrasions and to secure IV catheters and central lines. They can also be placed over bony prominences such as the knees to prevent skin abrasions (Kuller and Lund, 1998).

C. Umbilical cord care.

1. Sterile cutting of cord at delivery and rapid drying of umbilical cord appear to be most effective in preventing umbilical infections (Schuman and Oksol, 1985).

2. Isopropyl alcohol and triple dye (a solution containing gentian violet, brilliant cresyl green, and proflavine hemisulfate) are the agents most commonly used for cord care. Schuman and Oksol (1985) showed no difference in infection rate between the two methods.
3. Tub bath should be delayed until cord has fallen off, generally 10–14 days.

Assessment of the Newborn Infant's Skin

A. Factors affecting the appearance of the skin.

1. Gestational age.
2. Postnatal age.
3. Nutritional status and hydration.
4. Racial origin.
5. Type and amount of available light.
6. Hemoglobin and bilirubin levels.
7. Environmental temperatures.
8. Oxygenation status.

B. Definitions used to describe skin lesions (Weston et al., 1996).

1. Macule: a pigmented, flat spot that is visible but not palpable. Macules greater than 1 cm in diameter may be referred to as a patch.
2. Papule: a solid, elevated, palpable lesion, with distinct borders less than 1 cm in diameter.
3. Nodule: a papule larger than 1 cm in diameter.
4. Vesicle: an elevated lesion or blister filled with serous fluid and less than 1 cm in diameter.
5. Bulla: a fluid-filled lesion larger than 1 cm.
6. Pustule: a vesicle filled with cloudy or purulent fluid.
7. Petechiae: subepidermal hemorrhages, pinpoint in size. They do not blanch with pressure.
8. Ecchymosis: a large area of subepidermal hemorrhage.
9. Wheal: area of edema in the upper dermis, creating a palpable, slightly raised lesion.

Common Skin Lesions

A. Normal variations in newborn skin.

1. Cutis marmorata (Fig. 24–2).
   a. Bluish mottling or marbling effect of the skin.
   b. Physiologic response to chilling, caused by dilation of capillaries and venules.
   c. Disappears when infant is rewarmed.
   d. May be sign of stress or overstimulation in newborn infant.
   e. Common in infants with trisomies 18 and 21.
   f. If condition persists in infants 6 months of age or older, it may be a symptom of hypothyroidism or a vascular abnormality such as cutis marmorata telangiectasia.
2. Harlequin color change (Fig. 24–3).
   a. A sharply demarcated red color seen in the dependent half of the body when the infant is lying on its side. When the infant's position is reversed, the color changes to the other side. This condition may also be seen when the infant is lying flat.
   b. Caused by immaturity or temporary disturbance of the autonomic regulation of the cutaneous vessels.

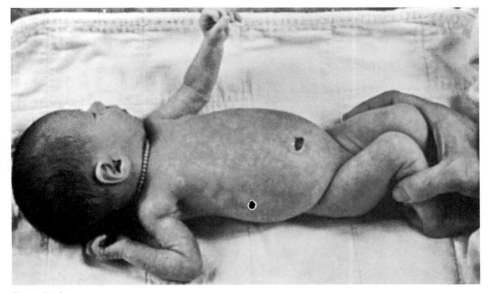

Figure 24–2
Cutis marmorata. (Courtesy of Jacinto Hernandez, M.D., The Children's Hospital, Denver, Colorado.)

Figure 24–3
Harlequin color change. (Courtesy of Jane Deacon,
RNC, MS, NNP, The Children's Hospital, Denver,
Colorado.)

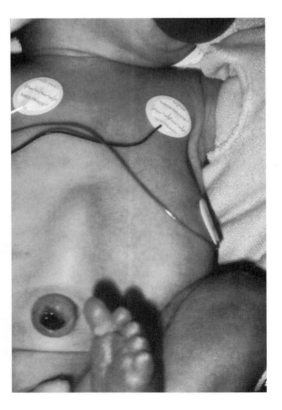

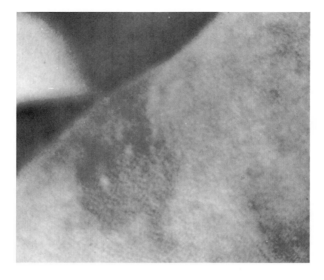

Figure 24–4
Erythema toxicum. (Courtesy of Jacinto Hernandez, M.D., The Children's Hospital, Denver, Colorado.)

3. Erythema toxicum (newborn rash) (Fig. 24–4).
   a. Small white or yellow pustules surrounded by an erythematous base (erythematous base caused by a histamine release).
   b. Benign, found in up to 70% of newborn infants (Margileth, 1994).
   c. Seen in neonates and infants up to 3 months of age.
   d. Lesions come and go on various sites of face, trunk, and limbs, although they are never seen on the palms of the hands or soles of the feet.
   e. Cause unknown, but condition may be exacerbated by handling or by chafing of linen.
   f. Differential diagnosis: may resemble a staphylococcal infection. Diagnosis can be confirmed by smear of aspirated pustule showing numerous eosinophils.
   g. No treatment is necessary. Lotions or creams may exacerbate condition.
4. Milia (Fig. 24–5).
   a. Multiple yellow or pearly white papules about 1 mm in size; epidermal inclusion cysts composed of laminated, keratinous material. They occur on the brow, cheeks, and nose.
   b. Milia are observed in about 40% of term infants (Margileth, 1994).

Figure 24–5
Milia. (Courtesy of Jacinto Hernandez, M.D., The Children's Hospital, Denver, Colorado.)

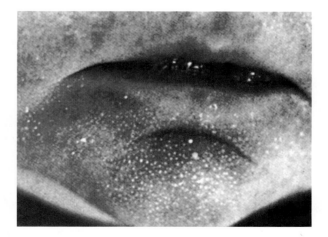

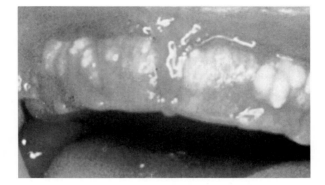

Figure 24–6
Epstein's pearls. (Courtesy of Jacinto Hernandez, M.D., The Children's Hospital, Denver, Colorado.)

    c. No treatment is necessary. They resolve spontaneously during the first few weeks after birth.

5. Epstein's pearls (Fig. 24–6).
    a. Oral counterpart of facial milia. They can be seen on the midline of the palate or on the alveolar ridges.
    b. Epstein's pearls occur in approximately 60% of neonates (Weston et al., 1996).

6. Sebaceous gland hyperplasia.
    a. Tiny (<0.5 mm) white or yellow papules found on the nose, cheeks, and upper lips of newborn infants.
    b. Common in term infants but rarely seen in preterm infants.
    c. Represents overactivity of the sebaceous follicles and are a manifestation of maternal androgen stimulation.
    d. They resolve without treatment within a few weeks.

7. Miliaria. Caused by occlusion of sweat ducts by keratin, resulting in retention of sweat. There are four types of miliaria.
    a. Miliaria crystallina: clear, thin vesicles, 1–2 mm in diameter, that develop in the epidermal portion of the sweat glands. They are seen over the head, neck, and upper aspect of the trunk in newborn infants.
    b. Miliaria rubra: commonly referred to as prickly heat; results from prolonged occlusion of pores, leading to release of sweat into the lower epidermis. Condition appears as pink or white papules and vesicles 2–4 mm in diameter, with an erythematous base. The lesions are generally found in the flexure areas, such as the neck, groin, and axillae, as well as on the face and the upper aspect of the chest.
    c. Miliaria pustulosa: resulting from continued exposure to heat, which leads to infiltration of the vesicles with leukocytes. This is rare in most climates and resolves with change to a dry, cool environment.
    d. Miliaria profunda: rare in infants; infection of lower portion of sweat glands in the dermis. Treatment consists of avoidance of further sweating and keeping the skin cool and dry.

8. Diaper dermatitis.
    a. May be caused by chafing from diapers, by prolonged contact with urine or feces, or by a sensitivity to chemicals in disposable diapers or in detergent used in laundering cloth diapers.
    b. The best treatment is prevention by frequent diaper changes and by protection of the skin with a barrier product containing zinc oxide. The skin should be cleansed with warm water after voiding or stooling. Avoid diaper wipes that contain alcohol.
    c. Cornstarch and baby powder should not be used. They provide a medium

for growth of bacteria and yeast, and inhaled particles are irritating to the respiratory tract (NANN, 1997).
  d. *Candida* diaper dermatitis: see item 2 under section E, Infectious Lesions, p. 591.

B. Lesions resulting from trauma.

1. Forceps marks:
    a. Forceps marks are red or bruised areas seen over the cheek, scalp, or face of infants after forceps delivery.
    b. The infant should be examined for underlying tissue damage or other signs of birth trauma such as scalp abrasions, fractured clavicles, or facial palsy.
2. Subcutaneous fat necrosis.
    a. A hard, circumscribed, red or purple nodule under the dermis in the subcutaneous tissue. Nodules appear on the trunk, extremities, or face, usually during the first 2 weeks of life. They may grow larger initially and then resolve spontaneously within several weeks.
    b. Subcutaneous fat necrosis has been attributed to trauma, cold stress, shock, and asphyxia and is caused by crystallization of the subcutaneous fat cells.
    c. Hypercalcemia may be associated with subcutaneous fat necrosis in infants with multiple nodules. Serum calcium levels should be monitored (Cunningham and Paes, 1991).
3. Scalp lacerations.
    a. Scalp lacerations may be caused by trauma during delivery, placement of scalp electrodes, or fetal blood pH sampling.
    b. Treatment consists of keeping the area clean and dry and assessing the area for infection.
4. Intravenous infiltrations.
    a. Vascular access sites in the infant should be assessed hourly for assessment of patency and detection of infiltrates. The IV catheter should be removed immediately if patency is not certain or if signs of infiltration are apparent.
    b. Hyaluronidase can be used subcutaneously at the site of the infiltrate to increase absorption of the infiltrated fluid (NANN, 1997).

C. Pigmented skin lesions.

1. Hyperpigmented macules (mongolian spots) (Fig. 24–7).
    a. Large macules or patches, gray or blue green, seen most commonly over the buttocks, flanks, or shoulders.
    b. Most common pigmented lesion seen at birth, occurring in 90% of black, Asian, and Hispanic infants and in 1–5% of white infants (Margileth, 1994).
    c. Hyperpigmented macules are caused by the increased presence of melanocytes dispersed in the dermis.
    d. The spots fade somewhat during the first few years after birth, particularly as surrounding skin darkens, but may persist into adulthood.
    e. It is important to document size and location to avoid question of nonaccidental trauma.
2. Congenital melanocytic nevi (pigmented nevi).
    a. Dark brown or black macules that may or may not be hairy. Nevi may occur anywhere on the body, with the "bathing trunk" area being the most common site.
    b. Most are small, less than 2 cm, with smooth surfaces. Large nevi (>10 cm) are rare (Weston et al., 1996).
    c. Pigmented nevi are generally benign, but malignant changes occur in approximately 10% of larger lesions (Margileth, 1994).
    d. Close observation for changes in size or shape is indicated, with possible surgical excision. Large, unusually shaped nevi may be difficult to assess for

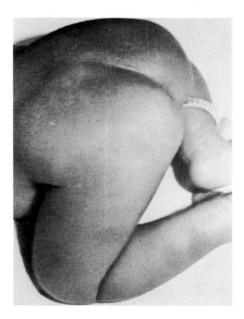

Figure 24–7
Hyperpigmented macules (mongolian spots). (Courtesy of Jacinto Hernandez, M.D., The Children's Hospital, Denver, Colorado.)

changes and should be followed closely, with removal at or before puberty (Weston et al., 1996).
  e. A hairy nevus present over the spine may be associated with spina bifida or meningocele.
  f. Pigmented nevi may also be associated with neurofibromatosis or tuberous sclerosis.
3. Transient neonatal pustular melanosis (Fig. 24–8).
  a. Superficial vesiculopustular lesions that rupture during the first 12–48 hours after birth, leaving small, brown, hyperpigmented macules. The macules may be surrounded by very fine white scales. They may rupture before delivery, presenting as macules.
  b. Benign; found in up to 5% of black infants and in about 0.2% of white babies (Ramamurthy et al., 1976).

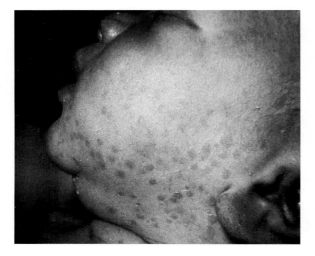

Figure 24–8
Neonatal pustular melanosis. (Courtesy of Jane Deacon, RNC, MS, NNP, The Children's Hospital, Denver, Colorado.)

    c. No treatment is necessary. The macules generally fade during the first few weeks or months after birth.

    d. Aspirating the contents of the vesicles will reveal a variable number of neutrophils and few or no eosinophils.

4. Café-au-lait spots (Fig. 24–9).

    a. Tan or light brown patches with well-defined borders.

    b. When less than 3 cm in length and fewer than 6 in number, they are of no pathologic significance.

    c. Six or more spots may be an indication of neurofibromatosis (Arnsmeier, Riccardi, and Paller, 1994).

       (1) Neurofibromatosis is a condition in which tumors form on cutaneous nerves and along the thoracic, brachial, and lumbar nerve trunks. Cranial nerves may also be affected.

       (2) It is an autosomal dominant disorder.

       (3) Café-au-lait spots may be the only finding of this disease in the neonatal period.

5. Ash leaf macules.

    a. White macules in the shape of an ash leaf or thumbprint; seen primarily over the trunk or buttocks.

    b. Found in 90% of infants with tuberous sclerosis (Margileth, 1994).

    c. May be difficult to see in fair-skinned infants. Use of a Wood (ultraviolet) lamp will aid in examination.

    d. Infants with unexplained seizures should be examined for these macules.

    e. May also be a normal finding or may be associated with neurofibromatosis.

D. Vascular lesions.

1. Nevus simplex.

    a. Nevus simplex (storkbite) refers to macular pink areas of distended capillaries found on the nape of the neck, the upper eyelids, the nose, or the upper lip. They have diffuse borders, blanch with pressure, and become pinker with crying.

    b. These are the most common of vascular birthmarks, seen in 30–50% of newborn infants (Weston et al., 1996).

    c. The lesions tend to fade by the first or second year, with the exception of those on the nape of the neck, which may persist.

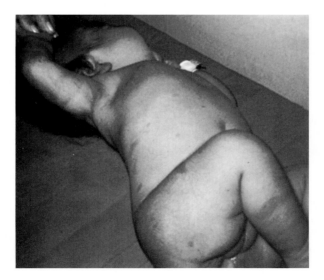

Figure 24–9
Café-au-lait spots. (Courtesy of Jacinto Hernandez, M.D., The Children's Hospital, Denver, Colorado.)

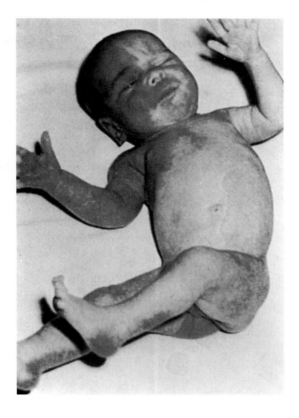

Figure 24–10
Sturge-Weber syndrome. (Courtesy of Jacinto Hernandez, M.D., The Children's Hospital, Denver, Colorado.)

2. Port-wine stain.
   a. A flat vascular nevus is present at birth. It is usually pink in infancy, but it may be red or purple. The nevus may be small or may cover almost half of the body. It is flat, is sharply delineated, and blanches minimally. Facial lesions are the most common.
   b. Port-wine stains consist of mature capillaries that are dilated and congested directly below the epidermis. The cause is unknown.
   c. The nevus does not grow in area or size. It will not resolve and should be considered permanent.
   d. The pulsed-dye laser has been successful in lightening most port-wine stains by up to 50%. The laser works by causing intravascular coagulation (Goldman, Fitzpatrick, and Ruiz-Esparza, 1993; Kane et al., 1996). Light-colored facial lesions have the best results; red or purple lesions that are thick and nodular respond less well. Most infants require three or four treatments. Other methods of surgical excision have been largely unsatisfactory (Ashinoff and Geronemus, 1991).
   e. Sturge-Weber syndrome (Fig. 24–10).
      (1) Port-wine stains confined to a pattern similar to that of the branches of the trigeminal nerve may be associated with Sturge-Weber syndrome.
      (2) Central feature of this syndrome is disordered proliferation of endothelial cells, particularly in the small veins. It is associated with atrophic changes in the cerebral cortex and calcium deposits in the walls of small vessels and areas of affected cortex (Margileth, 1994).
      (3) Sturge-Weber syndrome is manifested by glaucoma, focal seizures, hemiparesis, and mental retardation.

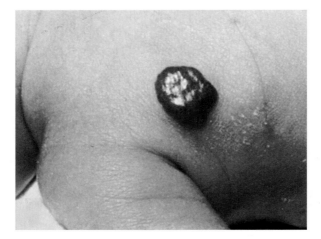

Figure 24–11
Strawberry hemangioma. (Courtesy of Jacinto Hernandez, M.D., The Children's Hospital, Denver, Colorado.)

3. Strawberry hemangioma (Fig. 24–11).
   a. Strawberry hemangioma is a raised, lobulated, soft, bright red tumor located on the head, neck, trunk, or extremities. These lesions may also occur in the throat, where they can cause airway obstruction, requiring a tracheostomy in extreme cases.
   b. Lesions are caused by dilated capillaries occupying the dermal and subdermal layers, in association with endothelial proliferation.
   c. About 20–30% are present at birth, and 90% are evident by 2 months of age (Margileth, 1994). The lesions occur in approximately 1–2% of newborn infants and are more common in preterm infants with females predominating (Blei, Walter, Orlow, and Marchuk, 1998; Freiden et al., 1997). The lesions may also be familial (Blei, 1998).
   d. Strawberry hemangiomas will generally increase in size during the first 6 months, and then become stable in size before undergoing gradual spontaneous regression, with most leaving no trace. This may take several years. Infants will often have more than one lesion.
   e. Treatment of choice is to allow the lesion to regress spontaneously. If the lesion is interfering with vision, is bleeding or ulcerating, or is impinging on other vital functions, treatment should be considered.
      (1) Systemic corticosteroid therapy is the treatment of choice for most hemangiomas (Freiden et al., 1997).
      (2) Flash-lamp pumped pulsed-dye laser may be effective on some lesions.
      (3) Cryosurgery may be helpful, but concerns about scarring have prevented this option from becoming widespread (Freiden et al., 1997).
      (4) Interferon alfa-2b may be effective in treating steroid-resistant lesions (Tamayo, L. 1997).
   f. The infant should be monitored for signs of impingement on vital organs or functioning, such as stridor, poor feeding, and difficulty in swallowing.
   g. The cosmetic concerns of parents require a caring, supportive approach. Pictures illustrating spontaneous regression may be helpful.
4. Cavernous hemangioma.
   a. This lesion is composed of large venous channels and vascular elements lined by endothelial cells.
   b. It involves the dermis and subcutaneous tissue and appears as a bluish-red discoloration under the overlying skin.
   c. The cavernous hemangioma has poorly defined borders and may feel cystic, like a "bag of worms," when palpated (Ruiz-Maldonado, Parish, and Beare, 1989).

d. Like the strawberry hemangioma, the cavernous hemangioma will increase in size during the first 6–12 months and then involute spontaneously.

e. Treatment is not indicated unless the lesion is interfering with vital functions, including airway obstruction, in which case systemic corticosteroid treatment may be helpful.

f. Kasabach-Merritt syndrome:
   (1) Giant cavernous hemangiomas may be associated with sequestration of platelets and thrombocytopenia.
   (2) Treatment consists of systemic corticosteroid therapy. Transfusions of platelets and blood are frequently necessary (Weston et al., 1996). The lesions may resolve spontaneously.
   (3) It has been suggested that infants with Kasabach-Merritt syndrome do not have true cavernous hemangiomas but, rather, a different type of vascular malformation (Enjolras et al., 1997).

g. Klippel-Trenaunay-Weber syndrome.
   (1) Syndrome consists of hypertrophy of a limb with associated vascular nevi and hypertrophy of underlying bone and soft tissue.
   (2) Rare congenital abnormality, seen mostly in males (Margileth, 1994).
   (3) No specific treatment for the disease. Severe limb hypertrophy may require orthopedic consultation, with possible amputation of affected limb.

E. **Infectious lesions.**

1. Thrush.
   a. A fungal infection of the mouth or throat, caused by *Candida albicans*.
   b. Very common in infants.
   c. Manifested as patches of adherent white material scattered over the tongue and mucous membranes.
   d. Treated with an oral antifungal preparation such as nystatin (Mycostatin).

2. *Candida* diaper dermatitis.
   a. Fungal infection of skin in the diaper area; may include buttocks, groin, thighs, and abdomen.
   b. Caused by organism *C. albicans*.
   c. Manifested as a moist, erythematous eruption, often with white or yellow satellite pustules.
   d. Treatment consists of an antifungal creme or ointment preparation such as nystatin (Mycostatin), applied to the rash several times per day. Oral antifungal treatment may be recommended in cases of persistent *Candida* dermatitis.

3. Systemic *Candida* infection.
   a. Very low birth weight infants are at risk of having systemic, invasive fungal infections, with invasion of the fungus beyond the stratum corneum. *C. albicans* is the most common fungus, but other species have been identified (Rowen et al., 1995).
   b. Improving the barrier function of the skin by minimizing trauma and maintaining a sterile environment may help prevent onset of this infection.

4. Herpes.
   a. Neonatal herpes simplex infection is one of the most serious viral infections in the neonate.
   b. Rash appears as vesicular or pustular rash (Fig. 24–12).
   c. Seventy percent of infants with herpes will have subsequent rash, but not necessarily before other signs and symptoms of illness develop. Therefore the absence of vesicles does not eliminate the possibility of disease.
   d. Treatment with an antiviral agent such as acyclovir should begin immediately. The earlier treatment is begun, the better the outcome (Weston et al., 1996).

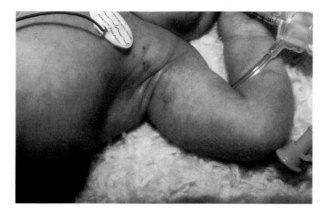

Figure 24–12
Herpes simplex vesicles. (Courtesy of Jane Deacon, RNC, MS, NNP, The Children's Hospital, Denver, Colorado.)

5. "Scalded skin" syndrome (also known as bullous impetigo, toxic epidermal necrolysis, Ritter's disease, and nonstreptococcal scarlatina).
   a. An inflammatory skin disorder generally caused by the phage strain of group II staphylococcus. May follow an upper respiratory tract infection or otitis media.
   b. Manifested as a widespread, tender erythema, followed by blisters ranging from small vesicles to large bullae. Caused by the release of an endotoxin that acts on the stratum granulosa of the epidermis. The blisters, which frequently begin in the diaper area and spread to the rest of the body, rupture, leaving large, raw, scaldlike areas.
   c. Treatment includes isolation and aseptic handling to prevent further infection in the infected infant and the spread of bacteria to others. The infant is treated systemically with methicillin because of the number of penicillin-resistant strains in the phage strain of group II staphylococcus. A topical antibiotic ointment such as bacitracin may be applied locally.
6. Congenital viral infection.
   a. Petechiae and purpuric macules on the head, trunk, and extremities of affected infants. The lesions are often described as "blueberry muffin" spots and are caused by dermal erythropoiesis (Fig. 24–13).

Figure 24–13
Blueberry muffin rash. (Courtesy of Jacinto Hernandez, M.D., The Children's Hospital, Denver, Colorado.)

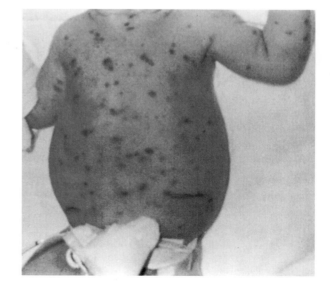

b. The lesions generally disappear in 2–3 weeks. Treatment is based on the underlying disorder.

c. Although the lesions are most often associated with rubella, they are also seen in association with other congenital infections such as cytomegalovirus, toxoplasmosis, syphilis, and herpes.

d. Affected infants may also have growth restriction, jaundice, hepatosplenomegaly, and thrombocytopenia.

F. Hereditary and miscellaneous lesions.

1. Epidermolysis bullosa.
   a. Disease characterized by the formation of vesicles and bullae over various parts of the body. The underlying genetic defect may be autosomal dominant or recessive.
   b. Vesicles may appear spontaneously or in response to minor trauma such as routine handling.
   c. Lesions may appear at birth or a few weeks later.
   d. Three types of vesicles that may appear at birth.
      (1) Simple, nonscarring: bullae form in small numbers throughout childhood and heal without scarring. Often disappear at puberty. Prevention of trauma and infection is important.
      (2) Dystrophic, scarring: more severe form of the disease, with lesions forming scars, loss of nails, and contractures. Death may result from secondary infections.
      (3) Epidermolysis bullosa lethalis: most severe form, with large, numerous lesions, usually present at birth. Large areas of epidermis are lost, leaving red, weeping erosions. Esophageal lesions may also occur. The life span of these patients is generally short. Treatment is supportive care, minimizing trauma and infection (Weston et al., 1996).

2. Collodion baby.
   a. Term describes an appearance rather than a disease. These babies are born covered with a tight, shiny, transparent membrane that cracks and peels off after a few days. A few infants will have no underlying disorder, but many will have some form of ichthyosis (Weston et al., 1996) (Fig. 24–14).
   b. Treatment consists of liberal application of sterile olive or mineral oil several times a day to hydrate and lubricate the skin, careful handling, and prevention of infection.

3. Ichthyosis.
   a. Ichthyosis is a disease involving excessive scaling of the skin, caused by excessive production of stratum cornuem cells or faulty shedding of the stratum corneum (Weston et al., 1996). There are four types of ichthyosis.
      (1) Ichthyosis vulgaris: an autosomal dominant disease, usually appearing after 3 months of age. This is the most common and most benign of the ichthyosis disorders, occurring in approximately 1 in 250 infants (Margileth, 1994). It consists of fine white scales and excessively dry skin (Rand and Baden, 1983).
      (2) X-linked ichthyosis: appears at birth or during the first year of life. It occasionally occurs in a collodion baby. The disorder consists of large, thick, dark-brown scales over the entire body, with the exception of the palms and soles. It occurs in males only.
      (3) Lamellar ichthyosis: an autosomal recessive trait that is manifested at birth as bright red erythema and universal desquamation. Some infants resemble collodion babies. Scales are large, flat, and coarse and may be less prominent in infancy than later in childhood. Eversion of the lips and eyelids may occur, and the palms and soles may be thickened. Hyperkeratosis may be seen on skin biopsy, although this is not diagnostic of the disorder (Weston et al., 1996).

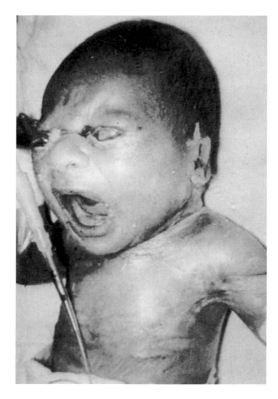

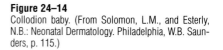

Figure 24–14
Collodion baby. (From Solomon, L.M., and Esterly, N.B.: Neonatal Dermatology. Philadelphia, W.B. Saunders, p. 115.)

(4) Bullous ichthyosis: autosomal dominant disorder characterized by recurrent formation of bullous lesions, erythroderma, and excessive dryness and peeling. As the child grows, the involvement generally becomes limited to small, thick, hard scales, most often found in the flexure regions. Hyperkeratosis may be seen on the palms and soles (Rand and Baden, 1983). Infection in the neonatal period with *Staphylococcus aureus* is of primary concern because of the widespread skin breakdown.

b. Treatment of ichthyosis is limited to use of topical preparations to hydrate and lubricate the skin. Daily baths with a water-dispersible bath oil, with use of alpha hydroxy acid ointments, may be helpful (Weston et al., 1996).

c. Drying soaps and detergents should be avoided (Sybert, 1990).

d. Care must be taken to prevent infection of dry or cracked skin.

4. Harlequin fetus.

a. The harlequin fetus previously was considered to have a severe form of ichthyosis but may in fact have a separate rare autosomal recessive disease (Weston et al., 1996). The harlequin fetus has hard, thick, gray or yellow scales that cause severe deformities of skeletal and soft tissues.

b. The condition is untreatable, and most infants die within a few hours or days of life.

5. Cutis aplasia.

a. Term refers to congenital absence of skin, either as a midline defect, a posterior scalp defect, or several small or large defects involving the upper and lower extremities (Fig. 24–15).

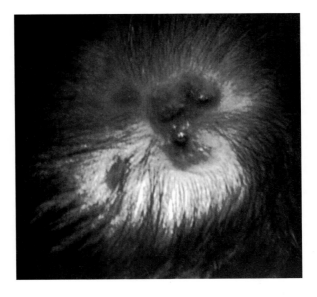

Figure 24–15
Cutis aplasia. (Courtesy of Jacinto Hernandez, M.D., The Children's Hospital, Denver, Colorado.)

    b. Lesions heal slowly over several months, leaving a hypertrophic or atrophic scar.

    c. May be associated with other defects such as cleft lip and palate, heart disease, tracheoesophageal fistula, and other midline defects. It is commonly seen in infants with trisomy 13.

REFERENCES

Arnsmeier, S.L., Riccardi, V.M., and Paller, A.S.: Familial multiple café au lait spots. Arch. Dermatol., *130*:1425–1427, 1994.

Ashinoff, R., and Geronemus, R.G.: Capillary hemangiomas and treatment with flash-lamp pumped pulsed dye laser. Arch. Dermatol., *127*:202, 1991.

Blei, F., Walter, J., Orlow S.J., and Marchuk, D.A.: Familial segregation of hemangiomas and vascular malformations as an autosomal dominant trait. Arch. Dermatol., *134*:718–742, 1998.

Choonara, I.: Percutaneous drug absorption and administration. Arch. Dis. Child., *71*:73–74, 1994.

Cunningham, K., and Paes, B.A.: Subcutaneous fat necrosis of the newborn with hypercalcemia: A review. Neonatal Network, *10*(3):7–14, 1991.

Enjolras, O., Wassef, M., Mazoyer, E., et al.: Infants with Kasabach-Merritt syndrome do not have "true" hemangiomas. J. Pediatr., *130*:631–640, 1997.

Evans, N.J., and Rutter, N.: Development of the epidermis in the newborn. Biol. Neonate, *49*(2):74–80, 1986.

Francis, C., and Martin, A.H.: Introduction to Human Anatomy, 7th ed. St. Louis, C.V. Mosby, 1975, pp. 413–437.

Freiden, I.J., Eichenfield L.F., Esterly N.B., et al.: Guidelines for care of hemangiomas of infancy. J. Am. Acad. Dermatol., *37*:631–637, 1997.

Goldman, M.P., Fitzpatrick R.E., and Ruiz-Esparza, J.: Treatment of port-wine stains (capillary malformation) with the flashlamp-pumped pulsed dye laser. J. Pediatr., *122*:71–77, 1993.

Gordon, M., and Montgomery L.A.: Minimizing epidermal stripping in the very low birth weight infant: Integrating research and practice to affect infant outcome. Neonatal Network, *15*(1):1996.

Harpin V., and Rutter, N.: Barrier properties of the newborn infant's skin. J. Pediatr., *120*:419, 1983.

Kane S.K., Smoller, B.R., Fitzpatrick, R.E., et al.: Pulsed dye laser–resistant port-wine stains. Arch. Dermatol., *132*:839–841, 1996.

Kopelman, A.E.: Cutaneous absorption of hexachlorophene in low birth weight infants. J. Pediatr., *82*:972–975, 1973.

Kuller, J.M., and Lund, C.H.: Assessment and management of integumentary dysfunction. *In* Kenner, C., Lott, J.W., and Flandermeyer, A.A. (Eds.): Comprehensive Neonatal Nursing: A Physiologic Approach, 2nd ed. Philadelphia, W.B. Saunders, 1998, pp. 648–681.

Lane, A.T., and Drost, S.S.: Effects of repeated application of emollient cream to premature neonate's skin. Pediatrics, *92*:415–419, 1993.

Linder N., Davidovitch, N., Reichman, B., et al.: Topical iodine-containing antiseptics and subclinical hypothyroidism in preterm infants. J. Pediatr., *131*:434–439, 1997.

Lott, J.W., Kenner, C.L., and Polack, J.D.: Common neonatal infections and complications. *In* Lott, J.W. (Ed.): Neonatal Infection: Assessment, Diagnosis, and Management. Petaluma, Calif., NICU Ink, 1994, pp. 47–48.

Lund, C.H., Nonato, L.B., Kuller, J.M., et al.: Disruption of barrier function in neonatal skin associated with adhesive removal. J. Pediatr., *131*:367–372, 1997.

Margileth, A.: Dermatologic conditions. *In* Avery, C.B. (Ed.): Neonatology: Pathophysiology and Management of the Newborn, 4th ed. Philadelphia, J.B. Lippincott, 1994, pp. 1229–1268.

Moore, K.L., and Persaud, T.V.N.: The Developing Human: Clinically Oriented Embryology. Philadelphia, WB Saunders, 1993, pp. 443–457.

National Association of Neonatal Nurses. Guidelines for Practice: Neonatal Skin Care. Petaluma, Calif., Author, 1997.

Nopper, A.J., Horii, K.A., Sookdeo-Drost, S., et al.: Topical ointment therapy benefits premature infants. J. Pediatr., *128*:660–669, 1996.

Penny-MacGillivray, T.: A newborn's first bath: When? J. Obstet., Gynecol., Neonatal Nurs., 25:481–486, 1996.

Peters, K.L.: Dinosaurs in the bath. Neonatal Network, *15*(1):71–73, 1996.

Ramamurthy, R.S., Reveri, M., Esterly, N.B., et al.: Transient neonatal pustular melanosis. J. Pediatr., *88*:831–835, 1976.

Rand, R.E., and Baden, H.P.: The ichthyoses: A review. J. Am. Acad. Dermatol., *88*:285, 1983.

Rowen, J.L., Atkins, J.T., Levy M.L., et al.: Invasive fungal dermatitis in the <1000 gm neonate. Pediatrics, *95*:682–687, 1995.

Ruiz-Maldonado, R., Parish, L.C., and Beare, J.M.: Textbook of Pediatric Dermatology. Philadelphia, Grune & Stratton, 1989.

Schuman, A.J., and Oksol, B.A.: The effect of isopropyl alcohol and triple dye on umbilical cord separation time. Milit. Med., *150*(1):49–51, 1985.

Sybert, V.P.: Guide to information for families with inherited skin disorders. Pediatr. Dermatol., 7:214, 1990.

Tamayo, L., et al.: Therapeutic efficacy of interferon alfa-2b in infants with life-threatening giant hemangiomas. Arch. Dermatol., *133*:1567–1571, 1997.

Weston, W.L., Lane, A.T., and Morelli, J.T.: Color Textbook of Pediatric Dermatology, 2nd ed. St. Louis, Mosby, 1996.

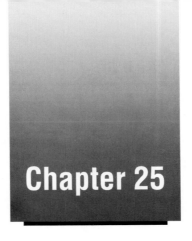

Chapter 25

Ophthalmologic Disorders

Carla Shapiro and Debbie Fraser Askin

Objectives

1. Describe the normal anatomy of the eye.

2. Identify the major function(s) of each structure.

3. Describe the components of a nursing assessment of the eyes in the neonate.

4. Describe the nurse's role in assisting the physician with neonatal eye examinations.

5. Describe one process of objectively measuring visual acuity in neonates.

6. For each of six types of eye disorders in the neonatal period—traumatic injuries to the eye, conjunctivitis, nasolacrimal duct obstruction, cataracts, infections ("TORCH" diseases), and retinopathy of prematurity—(a) provide an overview of the pathogenesis and (b) describe commonly used treatment modalities, outlining the specific nursing care measures designed to meet the needs of neonates with these disorders.

An examination of the neonate's eyes is an important, though often neglected, portion of a physical assessment. There is a great deal of clinically significant information that the astute nurse can glean from a thorough evaluation of the neonate's eyes. Evidence of intrauterine infection, birth trauma, congenital malformations, disease, and a variety of genetic abnormalities can be detected during the course of the nurse's assessment of the neonate's eyes.

This chapter provides the neonatal nurse with a review of normal eye anatomy, together with the major function(s) of each structure; the essential components of an assessment of the newborn's eyes; an overview of the most common eye disorders in the neonate; and common treatment modalities and nursing measures used in the treatment of various ocular disorders in the newborn infant.

Anatomy of the Eye (Fig. 25–1)

PROTECTIVE STRUCTURES

A. **Eyelids:** shade the eyes during sleep; protect from excessive light or foreign objects; spread lubricating secretions over the eyeball.

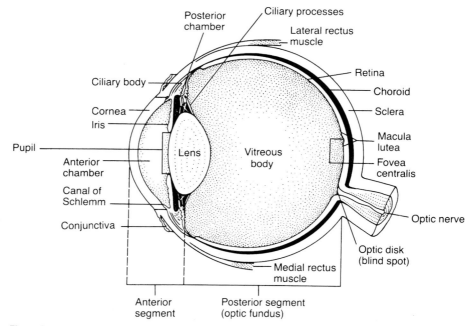

Figure 25–1
Cross section of the eyeball. (From J. Ophthal. Nurs. Technol., *6*(5):178, 1987. With permission of Burroughs Wellcome Co.)

B. **Conjunctiva:** mucous membrane lining the inner aspect of the eyelids (palpebral) and onto the eyeball to the periphery of the cornea (bulbar).

C. **Lacrimal system:** manufactures and drains away tears; cleans, lubricates, and moistens the eyeball.

D. **Bony orbit or socket:** surrounds and protects the eyeball. Most important opening within the orbit is the optic foramen, through which the optic nerve, ophthalmic artery, and ophthalmic vein from each eye pass through en route to the brain.

THE EYEBALL

A. **Outer layer (fibrous tunic).**

1. Cornea: transparent; reflects light rays.
2. Sclera: the "white" of the eye; normal bluish appearance in newborn infants; gives shape to the eyeball and protects the inner parts.

B. **Middle layer (vascular tunic): the uveal tract.**

1. Iris and pupil: a circular pigmented diaphragm with a central hole; controls the amount of light entering the eye.
2. Ciliary body: the anterior portion of the choroid.
3. Choroid: a vascular, pigmented membrane that lines most of the internal surface of the sclera, absorbs light rays, and nourishes the retina.

C. **Inner layer: the retina.**

1. Extends from the ora serrata to the optic nerve.
2. Functions in image formation.
   a. Photoreceptors: rods and cones.

b. Bipolar cells.

c. Ganglion cells.

3. Optic disc: retinal blood vessels enter the eye, and optic nerve exits the eye. Blind spot in field of vision because optic disc has no photoreceptors.

4. Optic nerve: second cranial nerve.

5. Macula: exact center of the retina and location of sharpest vision.

D. **Anterior cavity (filled with aqueous humor).**

1. Anterior chamber: behind the cornea, in front of the iris.

2. Posterior chamber: behind the iris, in front of the suspensory ligament and lens.

E. **The lens:** a biconvex, transparent capsule that refracts light; the most important focusing mechanism of the eye.

F. **Posterior cavity (filled with vitreous humor):** lies between the lens and the retina. Contributes to intraocular pressure, gives shape to the eyeball, and holds the retina in place.

EXTRAOCULAR MUSCLES

A. **Musculature.** Six muscles move each globe. The muscles of each eye work in conjunction with each other.

B. **Innervation.** The extraocular muscles are innervated by the oculomotor (third cranial) nerve, the abducens (sixth cranial) nerve, and the trochlear (fourth cranial) nerve.

Patient Assessment

HISTORY

A. **Pregnancy:** first-trimester infections (e.g., rubella), unknown rashes, fever, venereal disease, vaginal discharge, medications.

B. **Birth history:** gestational age, duration of labor, use of forceps.

C. **Family history:** incidence of ocular disorders, especially retinoblastoma; systemic diseases.

EXAMINATION

The examination is performed with the baby in a quiet, alert state. To facilitate the examination, have the baby suckle during the procedure (Green and Stevens, 1993).

A. **External assessment.**

1. General facial configuration: should be symmetric. Note distance between the eyes; an abnormal width between the eyes is referred to as hypertelorism.

2. Spontaneous eye movements: note range of motion and conjugation (the ability of the eyes to move together). Infants can track and follow objects with both eyes. Erratic or purposeless movements may be observed during the first few weeks of life. Median focal distance for the neonate is about 8 inches (20 cm).

B. **Reaction to light or visual stimuli:** strong blink reflex to bright light or stimulation of the lids, lashes, or cornea. A somewhat unsteady gaze can be observed shortly after birth, with ability to fixate on a stimulus for 4–10 seconds and refixate every 1.0–1.5 seconds. Ability to maintain fixation and to follow does not occur until 5–6 weeks of age.

C. **Pupils:** shape should be round and reaction to light should be equal; constriction to both direct and contralateral stimulation should occur. The red reflex should be elicited bilaterally; normally appears as a homogeneous bright red-orange color. Opacities or interruptions may indicate cataracts or retinoblastoma.

D. **Eyelids:** note symmetry, epicanthal folds, bruising or edema, lacerations, ptosis, presence of lacrimal puncta.

E. **Conjunctiva:** should be pink and moist; redness or exudate is abnormal.

F. **Cornea:** may be somewhat less than transparent or slightly hazy in the first few days of life in both premature and term infants. Sclerae may be bluish in premature or small babies as a result of thinness.

G. **Irises:** should be similar in appearance; note pigmentation. A coloboma, or keyhole pupil, may be associated with congenital anomalies. Brushfield's spots are silvery-gray spots scattered around the circumference of the iris. Strongly associated with Down syndrome.

H. **Lens:** should be clear and black with direct illumination. Examination of the anterior vascular capsule of the lens is a useful adjunct to determination of gestational age in preterm infants between 27 and 34 weeks.

I. **Doll's-eye reflex:** as head is turned *toward* each shoulder, eyes move in opposite direction.

Visual Acuity Testing

The visually evoked response is a simple, noninvasive, objective way to determine visual acuity in a neonate or infant (Taylor, 1992; Taylor and McCulloch, 1992).

A. **Visually evoked response measures electrical response of the brain's primary visual cortex to a visual stimulus.**

B. **Three electrodes are placed on the neonate's scalp:** one electrode is placed over the primary visual cortex, at the back of the head; another electrode is placed at a reference location, typically on an ear; and the third electrode, for grounding, goes on the forehead.

C. **The neonate is positioned in front of a pattern stimulator, which presents alternating black and white stripes of different sizes.**

D. **An electrodiagnostic test system measures the electrical response of the visual cortex to the rapidly reversing stripes.** The relative size of the brain's response to the reversing striped stimulus depends on the size of the stimulus and the patient's visual acuity. By measuring the response to several stripe sizes, one can predict the stripe size at which the brain will no longer respond. This measurement is directly related to visual acuity.

E. **Entire test takes approximately 10 minutes.** This includes time to apply and remove electrodes, position neonate, record data, and analyze and print test results.

F. **Early quantification of vision loss or impairment allows for correction or referral to early intervention programs, which can ameliorate long-term consequences of disability.**

Pathologic Conditions and Management

BIRTH TRAUMA

Pathophysiology

A. Direct result of duration and difficulty of delivery.

B. Improperly applied forceps.

C. Compression of cranial nerves.

Clinical Presentation

A. Petechiae; ecchymoses; edema; and/or lacerations of lids, conjunctiva, or globe.

B. Bright red patches on conjunctiva (subconjunctival hemorrhage).

C. Droopy eyelids.

Complications

These injuries are generally mild and transient, often resolving spontaneously.

CONJUNCTIVITIS

Conjunctivitis is an inflammatory reaction resulting from invasion of conjunctiva by pathologic organisms.

Etiology

A wide variety of infectious agents are capable of producing conjunctivitis in the newborn infant. The most common causes in North America include the following:

A. *Neisseria gonorrhoeae:* peripartum transmission.

B. *Chlamydia trachomatis:* peripartum transmission.

C. *Staphylococcus aureus:* acquired during the neonatal period.

D. Enteric pathogens.

Neisseria gonorrhoeae

A. Incidence. Reported as less than 0.03%. May be higher in areas with poor perinatal care or irregular antibiotic eye prophylaxis after birth.

B. Onset of infection: onset of symptoms usually between days 2 and 5 of life.

C. Clinical presentation.

1. Edema of the eyelids.
2. Purulent discharge.
3. Redness/hyperemia of the conjunctiva.

D. Diagnostic findings.

1. History.
   a. Maternal history of sexually transmitted disease.
   b. Age at onset of infection.

2. Physical examination.
   a. Clinical signs of inflammation.
   b. Purulent discharge.
3. Laboratory.
   a. Gram stain shows gram-negative diplococci.
   b. Culture positive for gonococci from conjunctival surface or exudate.

E. Nursing care.

1. Isolate infant in accordance with infection control guidelines.
2. Irrigate eyes with sterile normal saline solution hourly until discharge is eliminated.
3. Promptly administer appropriate systemic therapy. Topical antimicrobial therapy is *not* required.
   a. Penicillin-sensitive *N. gonorrhoeae:* aqueous crystalline penicillin G, IV or IM, 50,000–100,000 U/kg per day in two or three divided doses for 7 days based on postconceptional and postnatal age (consult a drug manual such as Neofax for specific information).
   b. Penicillin-resistant *N. gonorrhoeae:* ceftriaxone, 50 mg/kg (maximum 125 mg) IV or IM in a single dose (Young and Mangum, 1998).
4. Parents of infected infant should be referred for evaluation and treatment.

F. Complications.

1. Infants with gonococcal conjunctivitis are at risk of having corneal ulceration, perforation, and subsequent visual impairment.
2. Systemic complications involving the blood, joints, or CNS may occur in a small number of infants.

Chlamydia trachomatis

A. Incidence.

1. The most common cause of conjunctivitis in the neonatal period, especially in areas with poor perinatal care or irregular administration of erythromycin eye prophylaxis after delivery.
2. About 50% of babies born to mothers who are colonized with *C. trachomatis* will develop the disease.
3. Prevention of infection in the newborn infant is dependent on prenatal detection and treatment of the mother or on the use of an effective form of eye prophylaxis at birth (e.g., erythromycin ointment).

B. Onset. Symptoms are usually observed between 5 and 14 days of age.

C. Clinical presentation. Symptoms vary from mild conjunctivitis to intense edema of the lids with purulent discharge.

D. Diagnostic findings.

1. Identification of *Chlamydia* antigen.
2. Stains of conjunctival scrapings.
3. Culture of conjunctival scrapings.

E. Patient management.

1. Therapy of choice is ophthalmic and oral erythromycin (estolate preparation), 12.5 mg/kg per dose by mouth every 6 hours for 14 days (Young and Mangum, 1998).
2. Topical therapy alone is *inadequate* to eradicate the organism from the upper respiratory tract.
3. Parents of infected infants should be referred for evaluation and therapy.

F. **Complications.** Infection is spread via the nasolacrimal system to the nasopharynx, leading to *Chlamydia*-related pneumonia.

NASOLACRIMAL DUCT OBSTRUCTION

Pathophysiology

A. **Lacrimal apparatus** consists of structures that produce tears (lacrimal glands) and structures responsible for drainage of tears (upper and lower puncta, canaliculi, lacrimal sac, and nasolacrimal duct). System functions to clean, lubricate, and moisten the eyeball.

B. **Term and preterm newborn infants have the capacity to secrete tears** (reflex tearing to irritants) but usually do not secrete emotional tears until 2–3 months of age.

C. **Congenital obstruction** is usually caused by an imperforate membrane at the distal end of the nasolacrimal duct.

D. **Congenital nasolacrimal obstruction is the most common abnormality of the neonate's lacrimal apparatus.** Incidence of this condition ranges between 2% and 6% of all newborn infants.

Clinical Presentation

A. **Usually within the first few weeks of life.**

B. **Persistent tearing (epiphora).** Need to rule out congenital glaucoma.

C. **Crusting or matting of the eyelashes:** "sticky eye."

D. **Spilling of tears over the lower lid and cheek;** a "wet look" in the involved eye(s).

E. **Absence of conjunctival infection.**

F. **Mucopurulent material** refluxing from either punctum when gentle pressure is applied over the involved nasolacrimal sac.

Complications

A. **Acute dacryocystitis:** inflamed, swollen lacrimal sac.

B. **Fistula formation.**

C. **Orbital or facial cellulitis.**

Nursing Care

A. **Conservative management,** with daily massage of the nasolacrimal sac in an attempt to rupture the membrane at the lower end of the duct.

B. **Technique.** Technique consists of placing the index finger over the common canaliculus to block the exit of material through the puncta, and stroking downward firmly.

C. **Digital pressure increases hydrostatic pressure in the nasolacrimal sac,** which may cause a rupture of the membranous obstruction.

D. **If a mucopurulent discharge is present,** antibiotic eyedrops (sodium sulfacetamide) or ointment (erythromycin) may be required.

E. **Cleansing of eyes.** Eyes should be cleaned with moist compresses, with secretions mechanically removed.

F. **Duration of conservative management.** Conservative management is advocated for the first year of life.

G. **Resolution.** The majority of nasolacrimal obstructions resolve spontaneously or with massage by 1 year of age.

H. **Surgical treatment.** Unresolved obstructions can be successfully treated surgically: tear duct probing is done, with the infant under general anesthesia, after the first year of life.

CATARACTS

Congenital cataracts are the main treatable cause of visual impairment in infancy. The sooner in life the cataracts are removed surgically and proper optics are restored, the better the child's visual prognosis.

Pathophysiology

A. **Lens.** The lens is a biconvex, transparent capsule that refracts light. It is the most important focusing mechanism of the eye.

B. **Cataract.** A cataract is an opacity of any size or degree in the lens of the eye.

C. **Path of light.** Normally the light from an object passes directly through the lens to a focal point on the retina, producing a sharp image. Cataracts result in a degraded image or no image at all.

D. **Visual impairment.** Cataracts lead to varying degrees of visual impairment, from blurred vision to blindness, depending on the location and extent of the opacity. In neonates, cataracts are often transient, disappearing spontaneously within a few weeks.

Etiology or Precipitating Factors

A. **Idiopathic:** developmental variation, not associated with other abnormalities.

B. **Genetically determined:** most common mode of inheritance—autosomal dominant.

C. **Congenital rubella:** cataracts in 50% of newborn infants with congenital rubella syndrome.

D. **Other congenital infections.**
1. Toxoplasmosis.
2. Cytomegalovirus infection.
3. Herpes simplex.
4. Varicella.

E. **Metabolic disorders (e.g., galactosemia).**

F. **Chromosomal abnormalities (e.g., Down syndrome).**

G. **Clinical syndromes (e.g., Crouzon's disease, Pierre Robin syndrome).**

H. **Prematurity.**

Clinical Presentation

A. **White pupil** (leukocoria).

B. **Searching nystagmus** (at 1–2 months of age).

Diagnostic Findings

A. History

1. Family history of ocular disease or systemic disorders.
2. Pregnancy, especially first-trimester TORCH infections (see explanation of acronym under Congenital Infections, below).

B. Physical examination.

1. Normally, the pupils look black to the bare eye of the examiner when light is directed at them.
2. Examine to detect a white pupil by shining a light into each eye, with the light source held to one side.
3. If the opacity is small, it may be identified only when the pupils are dilated, and with the use of an ophthalmoscope.
4. Consider other diseases of the eye that may produce a white pupil (e.g., retinoblastoma).

Complications

A. **Varying degrees of visual impairment,** leading to developmental delay.

B. **Presence and/or severity of associated ocular defects,** such as microphthalmos and glaucoma.

Nursing Care

A. **Eye examination.** Assist the physician in carrying out a thorough eye examination of the newborn infant. This includes administering drops to dilate the pupils before the examination and supporting the infant's head to facilitate examination.

B. **Parental education.** In collaboration with the physician, assist parents in understanding the nature, possible cause, and treatment of cataracts in the newborn infant, together with the prognosis for future vision. Surgery is indicated whenever the cataract is likely to interfere with vision.

C. **Explore any feelings of guilt the parents may have** in relation to the cause of the cataracts; provide appropriate support.

D. **Encourage parent-infant attachment.** Baby may not be able to see the parents but can learn to know their voices, smell, and touch.

E. Care for the patient postoperatively.

1. Prevent increased intraocular pressure. Keep the baby comfortable, well fed, and free of pain to decrease crying.
2. Administer eyedrops or ointments as ordered postoperatively.
3. Apply clean eye patches or protective shields to protect the eye from rubbing or bumping and to prevent irritation from light.
4. Monitor for complications of cataract surgery. These are relatively infrequent but include infection within the eye, glaucoma, and retinal detachment. Note any increased redness or haziness of the eye, increased tearing, photophobia, or cloudiness of the cornea. Increased crying, irritability, disruption in sleeping patterns, or rubbing of the eye may indicate pain.
5. Assist the parents in understanding the essential role of optical correction devices, such as glasses or contact lenses, on their infant's vision and development.
6. Promote appropriate visual stimulation and foster normal infant development

by teaching parents about newborn visual preferences (e.g., black-and-white contrast or medium-intensity colors; the human face; geometric shapes; checkerboards designs).

Outcome

Visual prognosis depends not only on the extent of cataracts, age at removal, surgical outcome, and rapid optical correction but also on the nature of other associated anomalies of the eye or syndromes.

Congenital Infections

The developing eyes are highly vulnerable to the damaging effects of prenatal infection (Matoba, 1984; Samson, 1988), and ocular abnormalities may in fact be the predominant manifestation of the disease. A number of the congenitally acquired infections are associated with abnormal ocular conditions, including cataracts, chorioretinitis, corneal opacities, and glaucoma.

The most common of these infections are referred to by the acronym TORCH: *t*oxoplasmosis, *o*ther (e.g., congenital syphilis and viral infections), *r*ubella, *c*ytomegalovirus, and *h*erpes. (See also Chapter 17, Neonatal Infections.)

CONGENITAL RUBELLA SYNDROME

Pathophysiology

A. **Timing of infection.** Consequences of the transplacental infection are determined primarily by the timing of the viral insult.

B. **Infection in the first trimester of pregnancy presents the greatest hazard to organogenesis, including that of the eyes.**

Incidence

Ocular abnormalities are the cardinal manifestations of congenital rubella, occurring in 40–60% of patients.

Clinical Presentation

A. **Gestational age.** Findings in the infant exposed to rubella in utero depend on the gestational age at which the infection occurred.

B. **Ocular manifestations.**

1. Cataracts: in approximately 50% of patients.
2. Pigmentary retinopathy.
3. Microphthalmos.
4. Glaucoma: in 10–25% of patients.

C. **Other common manifestations include intrauterine growth restriction, hepatomegaly, thrombocytopenia, and cardiac anomalies (see also Chapter 17, Neonatal Infections).**

Nursing Care

A. **Virus shedding may continue for months after birth. Infants with suspected congenital rubella should be isolated from other newborn infants and from pregnant women (both in the hospital and at home after discharge).**

B. Parents need to understand the immediate and long-term effects of this disease.

C. See Nursing Care section, under Cataracts, above.

Outcome

A. **Prognosis:** depends on severity of symptoms and number of organ systems involved.

B. **Mortality rate:** in first year of life may approach 80% when multisystem involvement occurs.

C. **Multiple disabilities:** common in surviving infants.

D. **Consequences of congenital rubella:** may not be evident at birth but may become apparent in subsequent months.

E. **Follow-up:** ongoing follow-up and evaluation after discharge of infant from hospital. Major problems after the neonatal period include communication disorders, hearing defects, and mental or motor retardation.

CYTOMEGALOVIRUS

Pathophysiology

A. **Cytomegalovirus (CMV) can cause a perinatal viral infection.**

B. **Congenital illness is most severe if infection occurs early in pregnancy,** the period of greatest susceptibility of the developing fetus.

Etiology

A. **Ubiquitous virus.** CMV can cause infection in all age groups.

B. **Route of transmission.** Infection may be acquired transplacentally, during birth (via the cervix), or through breast milk.

C. **Transfusion.** An important possible cause of morbidity in premature infants is transfusion-acquired CMV. All premature infants should receive seronegative blood products.

Incidence

A. The *most common* congenital viral infection.

B. In the presence of primary acute maternal infection, 25–50% of fetuses are affected.

Clinical Presentation

A. **A diagnosis of congenital CMV infection can rarely be made on the basis of clinical findings alone.** Only 5–10% of neonates infected with CMV will have symptoms at birth.

B. **Laboratory diagnostic methods** (e.g., isolation of the virus from the urine) must be employed if this condition is suspected.

C. **Chorioretinitis** is present in 10–20% of infants with symptoms and is the *single most common finding* in congenitally infected infants.

D. **Other eye abnormalities** include conjunctivitis, corneal clouding, cataracts, and optic atrophy.

E. Other manifestations include intrauterine growth restriction, hepatosplenomegaly, and bleeding disorders (see also Chapter 17, Neonatal Infections).

Complications

A. Cytomegalic inclusion disease.

B. Sensorineural hearing loss, the most important late sequela.

Nursing Care

A. No effective treatment exists. Supportive nursing care measures, aimed at specific symptoms, are employed.

B. Use of gowns and good hand-washing technique are essential to prevent the spread of infection.

C. Seronegative pregnant women should not care for infants with known or suspected infection.

D. These infants require long-term follow-up.

Outcomes

A. Mortality rate. Overall mortality rate for symptomatic congenital infection is up to 30%.

B. Few survivors are normal. In 10–20% of infants who are free of symptoms at birth, neurologic sequelae, such as mental retardation or sensorineural deafness, may develop in the first years of life.

TOXOPLASMOSIS

Pathophysiology

Fetal damage occurs as a direct result of inflammation caused by the presence of cysts in the tissues, including the eyes.

Etiology

A. Maternal infection by the protozoan *Toxoplasma gondii* in the first and second trimesters of pregnancy is often associated with transplacental infection of the fetus.

B. Infection is acquired through contact with the excrement of infected cats and ingestion of improperly cooked meat.

Incidence

A. The incidence of maternal infection ranges from 0.15 to 0.64%.

B. Fetal infection occurs in about 0.07–0.13% of all pregnancies.

Clinical Presentation

A. Chorioretinitis is the most common manifestation.

B. Other manifestations include hepatosplenomegaly, jaundice, and bleeding disorders (see also Chapter 17, Neonatal Infections).

Specific Nursing Care

A. Nursing care includes pharmaceutical treatment of *Toxoplasma* infection by administering *sulfadiazine* and *pyrimethamine*. These agents will eradicate the cysts but will not reverse damage already done.

B. Give supportive care to the family, with sensitivity to feelings of guilt they might have.

C. Teach parents to recognize the signs of visual impairment in infancy (e.g., failure to fix and focus on objects or faces).

Outcome

A. Prognosis for infants with congenital infection: poor.

B. Mortality rate: roughly 10–15% of infected infants.

C. Psychomotor retardation: severe in 85% of survivors.

D. Visual disturbances: develop in 50% of surviving infants.

Retinopathy of Prematurity

Formally referred to as retrolental fibroplasia, retinopathy of prematurity (ROP) is a vasoproliferative retinopathy that occurs primarily in premature infants.

Pathophysiology

A. Human retina is avascular until 16 weeks' gestation. After this time, a capillary network begins to grow, starting at the optic nerve and branching outward toward the ora serrata (edge of the retina).

B. Nasal periphery is vascularized by about 32 weeks' gestation, but the process is not complete in the more distant temporal periphery until 40–44 weeks.

C. After premature birth, this process of normal vasculogenesis may be arrested as a result of injury from some noxious agent(s) or stressor(s).

D. Vasoproliferation. This arrest of normal vasculogenesis is later followed by a phase of rapid, excessive, irregular vascular growth and shunt formation (vasoproliferation), stimulated by a "vasoactive factor."

E. Area of new growth generally forms an abrupt ridge between the vascular and avascular retina, particularly in the temporal periphery.

F. ROP may resolve if the vasculature in the area recovers and resumes advancing normally, allowing the retina to become completely vascularized.

G. If the new vasculature proceeds to develop abnormally, these capillaries may extend into the vitreous body and/or over the surface of the retina (where they do not belong). Leakage of fluid or hemorrhage from these weak, aberrant blood vessels may occur.

H. Blood and fluid leakage into various parts of the eye can result in scar formation and traction on the retina.

I. Traction may pull the macula out of its normal position, thus affecting visual acuity. If the macula is slightly out of position, vision will be mildly affected.

J. Tractional exudative retinal detachment results in blindness.

Etiology

A. Complex multifactorial disorder.

B. Possible risk factors (Hagedorn, Gardner, and Abman, 1998).

1. Prematurity/low birth weight: *most important clinical factor associated with ROP.*
2. Hyperoxia.
3. Hypoxia.
4. Multiple birth.
5. Blood transfusions.
6. Intraventricular hemorrhage.
7. Apnea/bradycardia episodes.
8. Sepsis.
9. Hypercapnia/hypocapnia.
10. Patent ductus arteriosus.
11. Vitamin E deficiency.
12. Lactic acidosis.
13. Prenatal complications: maternal hypertension; diabetes; bleeding; smoking.
14. Duration of mechanical ventilation and oxygen therapy.
15. Exposure to bright light.

Incidence

A. Incidence of ROP appears to increase significantly as birth weight and gestational age decrease.

B. Risk of ROP rises dramatically from 47% for infants of 1.0–1.250 kg birth weight to 70% for those weighing 750–999 g and to 90% in infants weighing less than 750 g at birth (Oellerich, 1997 [p. 168]).

Stages of Retinopathy

A. Standardized approach for describing ROP, developed by the Committee for the Classification of Retinopathy of Prematurity (1984) according to five stages.

1. Stage 1: demarcation line within the plane of the retina separating the avascular and vascular retinal regions.
2. Stage 2: ridge or elevation extending out of the plane of the retina.
3. Stage 3: ridge with extraretinal fibrovascular proliferation, either:
   a. Continuous with the posterior edge of the ridge.
   b. Posterior but disconnected from the ridge.
   c. Into the vitreous.
4. Stage 4: subtotal retinal detachment.
   a. Extrafoveate.
   b. Involving the foveae.
5. Stage 5: total retinal detachment.

B. "Plus" disease: an indicator of activity. Signs (in increasing severity) include:

1. Engorgement and tortuosity of the posterior pole retinal vessels.
2. Iris vessel engorgement.
3. Pupil rigidity.
4. Vitreous haze.

C. Rush disease, an aggressive type of ROP. Rush disease develops between 3 and 5 weeks after delivery and may progress rapidly to severe ROP.

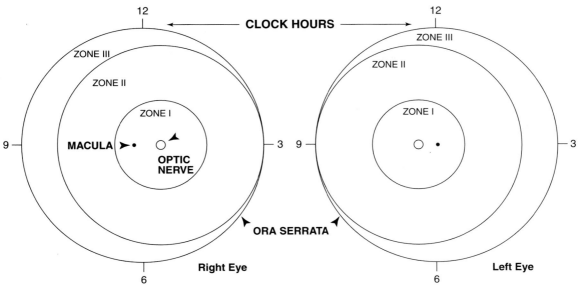

Figure 25–2
Zones in retinopathy of prematurity. (From George, D.S.: The latest in retinopathy of prematurity. M.C.N.: American Journal of Maternal Child Nursing, *13*(July/Aug):254–258, 1988.

D. **Zones for classification of ROP (Fig. 25–2).**

1. Zone 1: extends from the optic disc to twice the disc-foveal distance—a radius of 30 degrees.
2. Zone 2: extends from the periphery of the nasal retina (ora serrata) in a circle around the anatomic equator.
3. Zone 3: anterior to zone 2; present temporally, inferiorly, and superiorly but not in the nasal retina.

Physical Examination

A. **Examination of the high-risk neonate.** All newborn infants born at *less than 30 weeks' gestation or with a birth weight of less than 1500 g* should have their eyes examined by a trained pediatric ophthalmologist when in stable clinical condition, 4–6 weeks after birth (approximately 32–34 weeks' postconceptional age) (American Academy of Pediatrics, 1997; Canadian Pediatric Society, 1998; Fielder and Levene 1992; Joint Working Party of the Royal College of Ophthalmologists and the British Association of Perinatal Medicine, 1996).

B. **Dilation of pupils.** Infant's pupils should be dilated with a mydriatic agent before examination, to facilitate optimal evaluation. Cycloplegic mydriatic agents (e.g., cyclopentolate, tropicamide) have rapid onset of action, with peak ophthalmic effects between 20 and 60 minutes. It is necessary to protect eyes from bright light after mydriasis. Assess for symptoms of systemic absorption (e.g., tachycardia, restlessness) and notify physician immediately if symptoms are present.

C. **Documentation.** Location and extent of any retinopathy should be precisely documented and classified according to the guidelines developed by the international Committee for the Classification of Retinopathy of Prematurity (1984).

D. **Follow-up.**

1. Infants who are found to have areas of retinal immaturity on initial examination should have repeated examinations every other week and, subsequently, every 3–4 weeks until vascularization has reached the ora serrata.

2. If ROP is present during the initial examination, the infant should be examined weekly or every other week, depending on the severity of clinical findings.

Prevention

A. **Precautions while using oxygen.** Although the role of oxygen in the pathogenesis of ROP is unclear, cautious and judicious administration and monitoring of oxygen remains one possible preventative measure.
1. Continuous assessment and monitoring of the infant receiving oxygen to control arterial oxygenation. Cautious administration of oxygen while carrying out nursing procedures such as suctioning.
2. Ongoing assessment of the oxygen delivery system, including calibration of oxygen analyzers, monitoring fractional inspired oxygen, checking/recording ventilator settings, circuit, and oxygen saturation monitors.
3. Use of oxygen blenders to deliver precise oxygen concentrations.

B. **Results.** At present, no data are available demonstrating a definitive reduction in the incidence of ROP as a result of improved oxygen monitoring.

C. **Sensory stimulation.** Provide a variety of forms of sensory stimulation to the infant, appropriate to level of development and behavioral cues.

D. **Assessment.** Assess newborn infant's ability to fix and focus.

E. **Assistance.** Assist the physician in carrying out a safe, minimally stressful eye examination of the newborn infant.

F. **Protection against bright light.** Protect the infant's eyes from bright light by shielding the incubator with a blanket and reducing the light in the nursery. The use of eye pads should be evaluated according to the principles of developmental care.

G. **Parent education.** Provide accurate parent education about the possibility of ROP (when parents are ready to receive information about potential non–life-threatening complications). Ensure that parents understand that ROP is essentially a problem of immaturity whose cause is yet unknown.

Treatment

A. **Timing of treatment.** Treatment is indicated when ROP reaches threshold stage, defined as stage 3+ disease—involving 5 or more contiguous clock hours or 8 or more total clock hours or being associated with "plus" disease.

B. **Laser photocoagulation.**
1. Uses either an argon or diode laser to coagulate the avascular periphery of the retina.
2. With results similar to cryotherapy results, laser surgery can be performed in the nursery without general anesthesia.
3. Has fewer systemic and ocular side effects and carries less risk of damage to adjacent structures (Knight-Nanan and O'Keefe, 1996; Noonan and Clark, 1996).
4. Complications: cataracts; burns to the cornea, iris, or lens; retinal, periretinal or vitreous hemorrhage; photocoagulation of the fovea; and late-onset retinal detachment (Christiansen and Bradford, 1995; McNamara, Tasman, Brown, and Federman, 1991).

C. **Nursing care for the infant undergoing laser photocoagulation.**
1. Preoperatively, the infant should be given nothing by mouth for 4–6 hours;

phenylephrine with cyclopentolate (Cyclomydril) and sedation should be given as ordered.
2. Intraoperatively, monitor the baby and give medications as indicated.
3. After laser photocoagulation, the infant's respiratory status, oxygen saturation, and vital signs should be monitored.
4. Assess the eyes for drainage and edema.
5. Medications such as Cyclomydril and the combination dexamethasone, neomycin, and polymyxin B sulfate (Maxitrol) may be ordered to reduce postoperative complications (Hunsucker, King, Stamm, and Cisneros, 1995).

D. Cryotherapy.

1. Although the use of cryotherapy is decreasing, it continues to be used in some centers.
2. Super-cooled probe is used to freeze the avascular retina, preventing vessel proliferation.
3. Invasive procedure requires anesthesia.
4. Complications include scarring of the retina; periorbital edema; conjunctival hematoma or laceration; elevation of intraocular pressure; retinal, periretinal, or vitreous hemorrhage; central renal artery occlusion; freezing of the optic nerve; and late-onset retinal detachment (Vander, 1994; McNamara et al., 1991).

E. Nursing care of the infant undergoing cryotherapy.

1. Monitor the infant closely for possible risks of the procedure.
   a. Risks of undergoing general anesthesia.
   b. Arrhythmias induced from the use of lidocaine (Xylocaine).
   c. Bradycardia caused by vagal stimulation created by pressure on the eyeball.
   d. Edema of the eyelids.
   e. Infection.
   f. Intraocular bleeding.
2. Ensure patient safety and comfort during the treatment.
   a. Place baby in supine position.
   b. Maintain adequate heat source throughout the procedure.
   c. Monitor vital signs and oxygenation status throughout the procedure.
   d. Provide comfort measures and analgesia as needed.
3. Provide postoperative care after the treatment.
   a. Administer eyedrops or ointments as ordered.
   b. Shield infant from unnecessary direct light.
   c. If mydriatic agents were used, observe infant for signs of feeding intolerance, gastric distention, and/or aspirates when feedings are resumed.

F. Vitreoretinal surgery aimed at salvaging vision after retinal detachment remains controversial. To date vision results are poor (Quinn, 1994; Trese, 1992).

G. Provide emotional support and appropriate community referrals for parents whose infant will have significant visual impairment.

Complications

A. Mydriatic eyedrops and eye examinations can produce hypertension, reflex bradycardia, and apnea as a result of drug effects and vagal stimulation.

B. Varying degrees of visual impairment (e.g., myopia) may require corrective lenses to improve visual acuity.

C. Additional complications include:

1. Strabismus.
2. Glaucoma.
3. Cataracts.
4. Amblyopia.
5. Retinal detachment and blindness.

Outcome

A. Ninety percent (or more) cases of acute ROP resolve spontaneously, with little or no visual loss.

B. Laser and cryotherapy have been shown to decrease the risk of blinding complications of ROP by 50%. A significant number of visual impairments may result, especially in the presence of disease in zone 1.

REFERENCES

American Academy of Pediatrics, American Association for Pediatric Ophthalmology and Strabismus, and American Academy of Ophthalmology: Screening examination of premature infants for retinopathy of prematurity. Pediatrics, *100*:273, 1997.

Canadian Pediatric Society: Retinopathy of prematurity: Recommendations for screening. Pediatr. Child Health, *3*(3):173–180, 1998.

Christiansen, S.P., and Bradford, J.D.: Cataracts in infants treated with argon laser photocoagulation for threshold retinopathy of prematurity. Am. J. Opthalmol., *119*:175–180, 1995.

Committee for the Classification of Retinopathy of Prematurity. An international classification of retinopathy of prematurity. Arch. Opthalmol., *102*:1130–1134, 1984.

Fielder, A.R., and Levene, J.D.: Screening for retinopathy of prematurity [review]. Arch. Dis. Child., *67*:860–867, 1992.

Green, H.L., and Stevens, C. Here's how I do it: Newborn eye examination. Physician Assistant, *17*(6): 69, June 1993.

Hagedorn, M.I., Gardner, S., and Abman, S. Respiratory diseases. In: Merenstein, G., and Gardner, S. (Eds.): Handbook of Neonatal Intensive Care, 4th ed. St. Louis, Mosby, 1998.

Hunsucker, K., King, C., Stamm, S., and Cisneros, N.: Laser surgery for retinopathy of prematurity. Neonatal Network, *14*(4):21–26, 1995.

Joint Working Party of the Royal College of Ophthalmologists and the British Association of Perinatal Medicine. Retinopathy of prematurity: Guidelines for screening and treatment. Early Hum. Dev., *46*:239–258, 1996.

Knight-Nanan, D.M., and O'Keefe, M.: Refractive outcomes in eyes with retinopathy of prematurity treated with cryotherapy or diode laser: 3-year follow-up. Br. J. Ophthalmol., *80*:998–1011, 1996.

Matoba, A.: Ocular viral infections. Pediatr. Infect. Dis., *3*:358–368, 1984.

McNamara, J.A., Tasman, W., Brown, G.C., and Federman, J.L.: Laser photocoagulation for stage 3+ retinopathy of prematurity. Ophthalmology, *98*:576–580, 1991.

Noonan, C.P., and Clark, D.I.: Trends in the management of stage 3 retinopathy of prematurity. Br. J. Ophthalmol. *80*:278–281, 1996.

Oellerich, R.: Complications of positive-pressure ventilation. In Askin, D. (Ed.): Acute Respiratory Care of the Neonate. Petaluma, Calif., NICU Ink, 1997, pp. 168.

Quinn, G.E.: Screening and outcome of retinopathy of prematurity. Curr. Opin. Ophthalmol., *5*:66–71, 1994.

Samson, L.F.: Perinatal viral infections and neonates. J. Perinat. Neonat. Nurs., *1*(4):56–65, 1988.

Taylor, M.J.: Visual evoked potentials. Clin. Dev. Med., *120*:93–111, 1992.

Taylor, M.J., and McCulloch, D.L.: Visual evoked potentials in infants and children. J. Clin. Neurophysiol., *9*:357–372, 1992.

Trese, M.T.: Surgery for retinopathy of prematurity. Int. Ophthalmol. Clin., *32*(2):105–111, 1992.

Vander, J.: Retinopathy of prematurity: Diagnosis and management. J. Ophthalmic Nurs. Technol., *13*:207–212, 1994.

Young, T.E., and Mangum, O.B.: Neofax: A Manual of Drugs Used in Neonatal Care, 11th ed. Raleigh, N.C., ACORN PUBLISHING, 1998.

ADDITIONAL READINGS

Atkinson, J., and Van Hof–van Duin, J.: Visual assessment during the first years of life. Clin. Dev. Med., *128*:9–29, 1993.

Baily, D.: Retinopathy of prematurity: Screening, treatment, counselling—whose responsibility? J. Neonatal Nurs., *3*(5):5–8, 1997.

Boyd-Monk, H.: The structure and function of the eye and its adnexa. J. Ophthalmic Nurs. Technol., *6*(5):176–183, 1987.

Calhoun, J.H.: Problems of the lacrimal system in children. Pediatr. Clin. North Am., *34*:1457–1465, 1987.

Calhoun, J.H.: Cataracts in children. Pediatr. Clin. North Am., *30*:1061–1069, 1993.

Chew, E., and Morin, J.D.: Glaucoma in children. Pediatr. Clin. North Am., *30*:1043–1060, 1983.

Cohen, K., and Byrne, S.: The role of the nurse in assisting with examinations on premature infants. Neonatal Network, *8*(2):31–35, 1989.

Crawford, J.S., and Morin, J.D. (Eds.): The Eye in Childhood. New York, Grune & Stratton, 1983.

Cryotherapy for Retinopathy of Prematurity Cooperative Group: Multicenter trial of cryotherapy for retinopathy of prematurity: Preliminary results. Pediatrics, 81:697–706, 1988.

Deglin, J., and Vallerand, A.: Davis's Drug Guide for Nurses, 5th ed. Philadelphia, F.A. Davis, 1997.

Dennehy, P.J., Warman, R., Flynn, J., et al.: Ocular manifestations in pediatric patients with acquired immunodeficiency syndrome. Arch. Ophthalmol., 107:978–982, 1989.

Dobson, V., and Quinn, G.: Retinopathy of prematurity. Optometry Clin., 5(2):105–124, 1996.

Fisher M.: Conjunctivitis in children. Pediatr. Clin. North Am., 34:1447–1455, 1987.

Flynn, J.: Retinopathy of prematurity. Pediatr. Clin. North Am., 34:1487–1516, 1987.

Friendly, D.: Eye disorders. In: Avery, G.B., Fletcher, M.A., and MacDonald, M.G. (Eds.): Neonatology: Pathophysiology and Management of the Newborn, 4th ed. Philadelphia, J.B. Lippincott, 1994, pp. 1195–1210.

Gold, R.S.: Cataracts associated with the treatment for retinopathy of prematurity. J. Ophthalmol. Strabismus, 34(2):123–124, 1997.

Gordin, P.C.: Retinopathy of prematurity, NAACOG Update Series, 6:26, 1989. (Princeton, N.J., Continuing Professional Education Center.)

Isenberg, S., and Everett, S.: Cardiovascular effects on mydriatrics in low-birth weight infants. J. Pediatr., 105(1):111–112, 1984.

Long, C.A.: Cryotherapy: A new treatment of retinopathy of prematurity. Pediatr. Nurs., 15(3):269–272, 1989.

Ludington-Hoe, S.: What can newborns really see? Am. J. Nurs., 83:1286–1289, 1983.

Lueder, G.T.: Neonatal lacrimal system anomalies. Semin. Ophthalmol., 12(2):109–116, 1997.

Nelson, L.B.: Congenital nasolacrimal duct obstruction. J. Ophthalmol. Nurs. Technol., 6(2):57–60, 1987.

Nucci, P., Capoferri, C., Alfarano, R., and Brancato, R.: Conservative management of congenital nasolacrimal duct obstruction. J. Pediatr. Ophthalmol. Strabismus, 26(1):39–43, 1989.

Palmer, E.A., Flynn, J.T., Hardy, R.J., et al.: Incidence and early course of retinopathy of prematurity. Ophthalmology, 98:1628–1640, 1991.

Phelps, D.L.: The eye. In Fanaroff, A.A., and Martin, R.J. (Eds.): Neonatal-Perinatal Medicine, 5th ed. St. Louis, C.V. Mosby, 1992, pp. 1391–1392.

Pike, M.G., Jan, J., and Wong, P.K.: Neurological and developmental findings in children with cataracts. Am. J. Dis. Child., 143:706–710, 1989.

Preslan, M.W. Laser therapy for retinopathy of prematurity. J. Pediatr. Ophthalmol. Strabismus, 30(2):80–83, 1993.

Shapiro, C.: Retrolental fibroplasia: What we know and what we don't know. Neonatal Network, 4(6):33–45, 1986.

Silverman, W.A., and Flynn, J.T. (Eds.): Retinopathy of Prematurity. Boston, Blackwell Scientific Publications, 1985.

Symanski, M.E., Newman, C., and Bachinski, B.: Treating congenital cataracts. M.C.N. Am. J. Matern. Child Nurs., 19:335–338, 1994.

Teplin, S.: Visual impairment in infants and young children. Infants Young Child., 8(1):18–51, 1995.

Yetman, R.J., and Coody, D.K.: Conjunctivitis: A practice guideline. J. Pediatr. Health Care, 11:238–241, 1997.

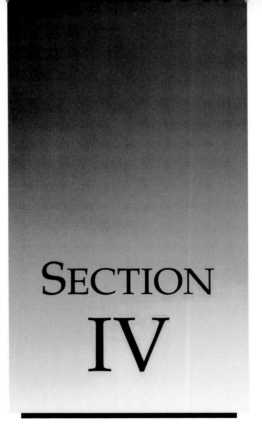

SECTION IV

SOCIAL TRENDS AND FAMILY CARE

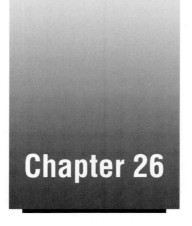

Chapter 26

Perinatal Substance Abuse

Sue Botham

Objectives

1. Describe three physiologic or behavioral signs of an infant exposed to cocaine in utero.

2. Describe the effects of cocaine during pregnancy.

3. Discuss three physiologic characteristics of an infant with a diagnosis of fetal alcohol syndrome.

4. List three nursing interventions (nonpharmacologic) appropriate for withdrawing infants.

5. List two psychologic characteristics of women who abuse drugs and alcohol.

6. Discuss two nursing interventions applicable when working with mothers who abuse drugs and alcohol.

The use and abuse of licit and illicit drugs in society have increased alarmingly during the past 25–30 years. Patterns of drug abuse have also changed, and polydrug use has become more prevalent. Data collected from the National Hospital Discharge Survey in the United States, between 1979 and 1990, identified a 576% increase in the number of drug-using parturient women. The study estimated that, as a result of substance abuse in pregnancy, 48,000 drug-affected infants are born each year. They commented that, although an epidemic of drug use among pregnant women in the 1980s occurred, the size and severity had been overstated (Dicker and Leighton, 1994).

Perinatal exposure is associated with high morbidity and mortality rates, and as a consequence, drug abuse in pregnancy is a problem with devastating social, medical, and economic implications. Prenatal care and drug treatment programs can make a significant difference and greatly improve pregnancy outcomes. Treatment programs must focus on both licit and illicit drugs. Because drug abuse extends across different regions and different age, ethnic, and socioeconomic groups (Rogers and Werner, 1995), a drug history should be taken for all pregnant women to ensure that they receive the care necessary for optimal pregnancy outcome. This chapter examines the licit and illicit drugs commonly used in pregnancy and the adverse effects they have on pregnancy, the fetus, and the newborn infant. Reports on outcomes for these infants are often conflicting. A contributing factor may be that neurologic development is multifactoral and influenced by biologic and environmental factors and by the interaction between the two (Brooks-Gunn, McCarton, and Hawley, 1994). Polydrug use may be another confounder. Management recommendations and nursing interventions, which are appropriate for all illicit drugs, are then detailed. This discussion is followed by psychologic and social profiles of drug-dependent mothers and some ethical and legal issues for consideration.

Cigarette Smoking

A. **Reported incidence of smoking in pregnancy:** ranges from 14.6% to 29% (Forrest, Horsley, Roberts, and Barrow, 1995; Kendrick and Merritt, 1996). This wide variation appears dependent on how the data were collected and the population was studied. An increased incidence of smoking has been reported for women of:
1. Low social class.
2. Low educational level.
3. Unemployed status.
4. Younger age.
5. Marital status: single, separated, or divorced (Forrest et al., 1995).

B. **Pharmacology.**
1. Cigarettes act as CNS stimulants.
2. The active constituents of cigarette smoke are nicotine, tar, carbon monoxide, and cyanide.
3. Nicotine is water and lipid soluble and crosses the placenta; effects on the fetus are secondary to placental vasoconstriction and reduced oxygen availability.
4. Carbon monoxide combines with hemoglobin to form carboxyhemoglobin. This impairs oxygenation for both the mother and fetus, resulting in fetal hypoxia (Zuckerman, 1988).
5. There is a dose-related response between the number of cigarettes smoked and neonatal effects.

C. **Effects on pregnancy (increased incidence).**
1. Spontaneous abortion.
2. Placenta previa.
3. Abruptio placentae.
4. Preterm labor.

D. **Effects on the fetus and newborn infant.**
1. Increase in intrauterine growth retardation.
   a. Decrease in birth weight.
   b. Decrease in head circumference.
   c. Decrease in length.
2. Small increased risk of congenital malformations, including CNS malformations, hypospadias, inguinal hernia, and eye and ear malformations.
3. Cigarette smoking, in combination with other variables: possible contributing factor (Zuckerman, 1988).
4. Neurobehavioral effects suggesting that children exposed to prenatal nicotine do less well on tests of cognitive, psychomotor, language, and general academic achievement.
5. Sudden infant death syndrome (SIDS).
   a. Increased risk of SIDS.
   b. Household exposure to tobacco smoke before or after birth: increased risk of SIDS.
   c. Sixty percent of these deaths attributed to effects of tobacco smoke before and after birth (Blair et al., 1996).

E. Nursing considerations.

1. Documentation of growth parameters.
2. Education regarding risk factors associated with SIDS; advise:
   a. Supine position for sleep.
   b. Head to remain uncovered during sleep.
   c. Smoke-free environment for infant.
   d. Avoidance by smokers of sharing bed with infant (Henderson-Smart, Ponsonby, and Murphy, 1998).

Alcohol

A. **Estimated incidence of any alcohol consumption** in 1995 by pregnant women in the United States: 16.3%. The incidence of frequent alcohol consumption was 3.5%, a significant increase from 0.8% in 1991 (Centers for Disease Control and Prevention, 1997).

B. **Incidence of fetal alcohol syndrome (FAS).**

1. Worldwide incidence of FAS is estimated at 0.97:1000 live births.
2. United States has the highest rate, at 1.95:1000 live births, compared with 0.08:1000 live births in other countries (Abel, 1995).
3. Combined rate of FAS and alcohol-related neurodevelopment disorder may be as high as 9.1:1000 live births (Sampson et al., 1997).
4. FAS occurs in all ethnic groups, with the highest incidence in African American and Native American groups.
5. FAS occurs in all socioeconomic groups, with a higher incidence in low socioeconomic groups (Abel, 1995).
6. Firstborn children appear less likely to have FAS than subsequent offspring.
7. There is a significant risk of a sibling's having FAS, given another case in the family (Abel, 1990).

C. **Pharmacology.**

1. Alcohol is a CNS depressant.
2. Alcohol is absorbed rapidly from the stomach and the intestines.
3. Ethanol and its metabolite, acetaldehyde, are critical components of alcohol.
4. Alcohol is a teratogen. The midline CNS is a developmental field especially susceptible to these effects, and the severity of facial anomalies is associated with midline brain anomalies (Swayze et al., 1997).
5. Variability in infants is related to factors such as dose levels, chronicity of alcohol use, gestational stage and duration of exposure, and sensitivity of fetal tissues.
6. Ethanol reaches the fetus through diffusion across the placental membranes bidirectionally at a rate dependent on the concentration gradient.
7. Ethanol impairs normal placental function and alters the transfer of essential nutrients to the fetus, which may already be reduced because of a suboptimal maternal diet.
8. Fetal ethanol concentration is eliminated by maternal hepatic biotransformation.

D. **Dosage of alcohol.**

1. No safe level of alcohol consumption has been established for pregnant women.
2. Risk to the fetus appears greatest with:
   a. Consumption of more than 3 ounces of absolute alcohol per day: 6 standard drinks.
   b. Binge drinking: 5 ounces or more at one sitting.

3. With lower levels of alcohol consumption, some infants are affected and others are not.
4. Outcome is associated with chronicity, as well as amount. The most affected children are born to women in the chronic stages of alcoholism.

E. Effects on pregnancy.

1. Spontaneous abortion is increased approximately twofold to fourfold in moderate and heavy drinkers.
2. There is an increased risk of abruptio placentae.
3. Breech presentation: FAS is strongly associated with breech presentation for both moderate and heavy drinkers.
4. When heavy drinking ceases during pregnancy, abnormalities and growth restriction that develop in later stages will be prevented.

F. Effects on the fetus and neonate.

1. FAS is the leading cause of mental retardation and the only preventable cause. Diagnostic criteria include:
   a. History of maternal alcohol consumption.
   b. Characteristic facial anomalies, which include short palpebral fissure, flat midface, smooth philtrum, and thin vermillion of the upper lip.
   c. Evidence of growth restriction in at least one of the following:
      (1) Low birth weight for gestational age.
      (2) Decelerating weight with time, unrelated to nutrition.
      (3) Disproportional low weight to height.
   d. CNS neurodevelopmental abnormalities in at least one of the following:
      (1) Decreased cranial size at birth.
      (2) Structural brain abnormalities (e.g., microcephaly, agenesis of corpus callosum, cerebellar hypoplasia).
      (3) Neurologic signs—as age appropriate (e.g., impaired fine motor skills, neurosensory hearing loss, poor eye-hand coordination).
2. Alcohol-related birth defects. Congenital anomalies may include:
   a. Cardiac: atrial or ventricular septal defects, tetralogy of Fallot.
   b. Skeletal.
   c. Renal: aplastic or dysplastic kidneys; hydronephrosis.
   d. Ocular: strabismus.
   e. Auditory: conductive or neurosensory hearing loss.
3. Alcohol-related neurodevelopmental disorder.
   a. CNS neurodevelopmental abnormalities in one of the following:
      (1) Decreased cranial size at birth.
      (2) Structural brain abnormalities (e.g., microcephaly, agenesis of corpus callosum, cerebellar hypoplasia).
      (3) Neurologic signs: as age appropriate (e.g., impaired fine motor skills, neurosensory hearing loss, poor eye-hand coordination).
   b. Evidence of behavior or cognitive abnormalities that are inconsistent with developmental level and unexplained by hereditary or environmental factors alone (Stratton, Howe, and Battaglia, 1996).
4. Withdrawal from alcohol.
   a. Withdrawal symptoms from alcohol are relatively mild in comparison with infant narcotic withdrawal.
   b. Onset is between birth and 12 hours after birth.
   c. Symptoms include the following:
      (1) Hypertonia.
      (2) Tremors.
      (3) Opisthotonos.
      (4) Weak suck and poor feeding pattern.
   d. Infants sleep little, cry more, and engage in exaggerated mouthing behavior.

G. Nursing considerations.
1. Careful assessment.
2. Documentation of growth parameters, including head circumference, length, and birth weight.
3. Careful examination of facial features.
4. Neurologic assessment for symptoms of neonatal withdrawal patterns.
5. Genetics consultation is indicated if FAS is suspected.
6. Family counseling and assessment of parenting skills.

H. **Ten-year follow-up study** of children with a reported diagnosis of FAS.
1. Characteristic craniofacial malformations decreased with time and became less obvious but did not disappear.
2. Microcephaly persisted.
3. Mental retardation persisted.
4. Male children remained underweight and had short stature; female adolescents were of normal weight (Spohr, Willms, and Steinhausen, 1993).

Cocaine

A. **Reported incidence of cocaine use in pregnancy:** 2.6–17% (Bell and Lau, 1995).

B. **Pharmacology.**
1. Cocaine is a CNS stimulant and taken for its mood-altering properties.
2. It is described as one of the most powerfully addicting substances of human abuse.
3. It may be taken orally, sublingually, intranasally, or intravenously or may be inhaled.
4. Cocaine is derived from the leaves of the South and Central American plant *Erythroxylon coca.*
5. "Crack" cocaine is made by mixing cocaine powder with water and baking soda. The resulting pellets crack when heated and release the cocaine vapor, which is inhaled.
6. Cocaine is fat soluble and of relatively low molecular weight, so it readily passes the blood-brain barrier and also moves across the placenta by diffusion.
7. Cocaine is metabolized and made water soluble by plasma and liver cholinesterases for excretion in the urine. Cocaine metabolism appears slower in the fetus and newborn infant, and metabolites may persist in the infant's urine 4–7 days after delivery.
8. Cocaine blocks the presynaptic reuptake of norepinephrine and dopamine, producing an excess of these neurotransmitters at the postsynaptic receptor sites.
9. This results in peripheral vasoconstriction, tachycardia, hypertension, and hyperthermia. Acute myocardial infarction, cerebrovascular accident, pulmonary edema, and renal and bowel infarction may then occur.
10. Cocaine use is frequently associated with polydrug use.

C. **Effects in pregnancy.** Cocaine use in pregnancy is associated with little or no prenatal care, which contributes to the poor pregnancy outcomes.
1. Pregnant addicts may present with a number of medical complications related to their drug use.
   a. Anorexia.
   b. Anemia.
   c. Cardiac disease.

2. Sexually transmitted diseases or infections may also be present.
   a. Gonorrhea.
   b. Syphilis.
   c. Hepatitis B and C.
   d. Human immunodeficiency virus (HIV) infection.
3. Vasoconstriction and hypertension resulting from cocaine use are mainly responsible for the adverse outcomes of use in pregnancy.
   a. Spontaneous abortion.
   b. Abruptio placentae.
   c. Fetal hypoxia and stillbirth.
   d. Pregnancy-induced hypertension.
   e. Preterm labor.
   f. Precipitate delivery.

D. Effects on the fetus and neonate.

1. An increase in congenital anomalies has been reported, and it has been suggested that cocaine may be a teratogen. The vasoconstrictive or hyperthermic properties of cocaine may be responsible (Bingol et al., 1987). Anomalies reported are:
   a. Genitourinary tract.
   b. Cranial defects.
   c. Cardiac anomalies, particularly ventricular septal defect.
   d. Bowel atresia.
   e. Terminal limb defects.
2. Intrauterine growth restriction includes:
   a. Low birth weight.
   b. Decreased head circumference.
   c. Decreased length.
3. Fetal depression in labor may result in meconium aspiration or persistent pulmonary hypertension after delivery.
4. Cerebrovascular accident and infarction may occur.
5. Risk ratio for SIDS in cocaine-exposed infants is 1.6 (Kandall et al., 1993).
6. After birth, these infants may have signs of CNS irritability, considered to be an effect of cocaine rather than withdrawal. The infants may be restless, irritable, tremulous, and hypertonic.
7. After this hyperirritability phase, the infant may become drowsy and lethargic, similar to the cocaine withdrawal experienced by adults (D'Apolito and McRorie, 1996).
8. The following changes in behavioral state are based on the Brazelton Neonatal Behavioral Assessment Scale:
   a. Difficulty in responding to the human voice and face.
   b. Depressed interactive behaviors and poor responses to environmental stimuli.
   c. Maintenance of alert states with difficulty, alternating between periods of sleep and agitation.
   d. Poor response to comforting by caregivers.
   e. Startle that is easily elicited.
   f. Rapid change in state.
   g. By 1 month of age, improvement in state control abilities but with continuation of less competence than drug-free newborn infants.
   h. Distress easily aroused, as manifested by rapid respirations, frantic gaze aversion, color changes, and disorganized motor activity.
   i. Possibly permanent findings, resulting in later difficulties in concentration, abnormal play patterns, and flat, apathetic moods (Hurt, 1990).
9. Neuromotor deficits may include:
   a. Hypertonic or hypotonic muscle tone.

b. Abnormal movements.

c. Abnormal suck-swallow pattern, resulting in poor feeding (Huffman, Price, and Langel, 1994).

E. **Limited follow-up studies but suggest that:**

1. Hypertonia may persist for up to 2 years.
2. Infants with cocaine-related hypertonia exhibit lower cognitive scores.
3. Weight and length normalize at 1 year of age, but head circumference remains smaller throughout first 2 years of life.
4. Speech and language deficits may be present (Kenner and D'Apolito, 1997).

Amphetamines

A. **Incidence of amphetamine use in pregnancy in California:** reported as 0.66% (Noble et al., 1997).

B. **Pharmacology.**

1. Amphetamines are a group of drugs that act as CNS stimulants.
2. Group consists of amphetamine, dextroamphetamine, methamphetamine, and methylenedioxymethamphetamine (MDMA, "ecstasy").
3. Amphetamines may be taken for appetite suppression, narcolepsy, or illicit abuse purposes.
4. They can be inhaled, injected, smoked, or taken orally.
5. Amphetamines act by enhancing the release of the neurotransmitters noradrenaline and dopamine, stored in the nerve endings of the CNS and the periphery and causing vasoconstriction and hypertension.
6. A sense of intense physical and psychologic exhilaration is produced, lasting from 2–14 hours, depending on the dosage.
7. Effects are similar to those of cocaine.

C. **Reports of the effects on pregnancy are limited but include increased incidence of:**

1. Prematurity.
2. Abruptio placentae.

D. **Effects on the fetus and newborn infant.**

1. Intrauterine growth restriction.
2. Neonatal withdrawal, characterized by:
   a. Abnormal sleep patterns.
   b. Poor feeding.
   c. Tremors.
3. Increase in aggressive behavior and peer-related problems at 4 and 8 years of age, as reported in Swedish study (Eriksson and Zetterstrom, 1994).

Marijuana

A. **Reported incidence of marijuana use in pregnancy:** variable; ranges from 9.5% to 27% (Bell and Lau, 1995). However, marijuana consistently rates as the most commonly used illicit drug.

B. **Pharmacology.**

1. Marijuana has both depressant and mild hallucinogenic effects on the CNS.
2. Drug is usually smoked in cigarette or pipe; alternatively, can be cooked in biscuits or cakes.

3. Marijuana comes from dried leaves and flowering tops of the plant *Cannabis sativa.*
4. Hashish is more potent and is prepared by drying and compressing resin of flowering tops and leaves of female cannabis plant.
5. Psychoactive ingredient is tetrahydrocannabinol (THC), which has high affinity for lipids and accumulates in the fatty tissues throughout the body.
6. Placental transfer is highest in the first trimester of pregnancy.
7. Smoking marijuana increases the blood carbon monoxide level and may result in hypoxia.

C. **Reported effects of marijuana on pregnancy:** limited, inconsistent, and conflicting. Marijuana use is often associated with the use of tobacco, alcohol, and other illicit drugs, which may contribute to these findings. Controversial issues relate to:
1. Length of gestation.
2. Duration of labor and outcome.

D. **Reported effects on the fetus and neonate:** also controversial and relate to:
1. Congenital anomalies.
2. Intrauterine growth retardation.
3. Neurobehavioral function: short and long term.

Opiates

A. **Incidence of opiate use in pregnancy:** reported as 1.6% in California (Noble et al., 1997).

B. **Pharmacology.**
1. Opiates are CNS depressants.
2. They are derived from the opium poppy, *Papaver somniferum.*
3. Heroin is a semisynthetic opiate that may be sniffed, smoked, or injected.
4. Heroin is quick acting and produces a sense of euphoria within 10 seconds after injection.
5. Methadone, a synthetic opiate, is usually taken orally but can be injected.
6. Methadone is absorbed slowly and has a long duration of action, making it suitable for treatment of heroin addicts.
7. Methadone in pregnancy is preferred to heroin because:
   a. Drug level delivered to the fetus is more stable and reduces the risk of fetal withdrawal.
   b. There is less risk of infection from the use of contaminated needles.
8. Opiates interfere with the normal menstrual cycle, thereby reducing fertility. Many addicted women do not realize they are pregnant until between the fifth and seventh months.

C. **Effects in pregnancy.**
1. Pregnant addicts may present with a number of medical complications related to their drug use:
   a. Anorexia.
   b. Anemia.
   c. Cardiac disease.
   d. Thrombosis.
   e. Abscesses.
2. Sexually transmitted diseases or infections may also be present:
   a. Gonorrhea.
   b. Syphilis.

     c. Hepatitis B and C.

     d. HIV.

3. Many of the effects of opiate use in pregnancy are correlated directly to the amount of prenatal care received and the maternal lifestyle, rather than to the drug itself.

4. Morbidity and mortality rates are lower in infants born to methadone-dependent women who have adequate prenatal care.

5. Spontaneous abortions are common.

6. Obstetrical complications include:

     a. Toxemia.

     b. Abruptio placentae.

     c. Premature labor.

     d. Shorter-than-average labor.

     e. Precipitous delivery.

     f. Breech delivery.

     g. Fetal distress.

D. **Effects on the fetus and neonate.**

1. Hypoxia due to an unstable intrauterine environment and reduction in placental blood flow.

2. Lower Apgar scores, with a need for resuscitation. Concern about the administration of naloxone, a narcotic antagonist for respiratory depression, has been raised. Rapid withdrawal and seizures may result, and urgent treatment for withdrawal may be needed (American Academy of Pediatrics Committee on Drugs, 1998).

3. Meconium aspiration and aspiration pneumonia.

4. Intrauterine growth retardation.

5. Lower incidence of respiratory distress syndrome.

6. Lower degrees of physiologic jaundice.

7. Congenital infections.

8. Increased incidence of SIDS:

     a. Risk ratio 3.6 for methadone.

     b. Risk ratio 2.3 for heroin.

     c. Risk ratio 3.2 for methadone and heroin (Kandall et al., 1993).

9. Neonatal abstinence syndrome (NAS).

E. **Results of follow-up studies:** not consistent, but some have suggested that there may be alterations in physical growth and in neurologic, behavioral, and cognitive functioning in early infancy and childhood (Kenner and D'Apolito, 1997).

F. **Comparison of methadone with heroin.**

1. With adequate prenatal care in a low-dose methadone program, perinatal outcome is improved in terms of prematurity, fetal loss, and medical complications.

2. Both groups of infants present with low birth weight; however, methadone infants are larger.

3. Infants exposed to both methadone and heroin may exhibit signs of NAS. However, NAS usually occurs later in infants exposed to methadone because it is stored in the fetal lung, liver, and spleen and metabolized after birth. Very little heroin is stored by the fetus (Weiner and Finnegan, 1998).

4. Methadone may be associated with a greater likelihood of neonatal seizures and with more intense and longer withdrawal. However, these findings may be based on doses of methadone that are higher than now recommended.

G. NAS.

1. More than two thirds of babies born to opiate-dependent women will exhibit signs of NAS.
2. Time of onset varies from shortly after birth to 2 weeks of age and relates to:
   a. Drugs used.
   b. Timing and dose of drug(s) before delivery.
   c. Nature of labor.
   d. Type of anesthesia/analgesia given during labor.
   e. Maturity and nutritional status of infant.
3. Signs appear within 72 hours after birth in the majority of infants.
4. Duration ranges from 8 to 16 weeks or longer.
5. Presentation of NAS is variable. It may be mild and transient, intermittent, or delayed in onset, or it may begin acutely, show improvement, and then revert to subacute withdrawal.
6. Withdrawal is more severe in infants whose mothers are chronic drug users.
7. The closer to delivery that a mother takes the drug, the greater is the delay of onset and the more severe are the signs (Weiner and Finnegan, 1998).
8. NAS is usually milder in the preterm infant, and sweating is not seen (Doberczak, Kandall, and Wilets, 1991).
9. Neonatal abstinence is described as a generalized disorder characterized by 21 signs most commonly seen in withdrawing infants (Finnegan, 1990).
   a. Neurologic signs.
      (1) Hypertonia.
      (2) Tremors.
      (3) Hyperreflexia.
      (4) Irritability and restlessness.
      (5) High-pitched cry.
      (6) Sleep disturbances.
      (7) Seizures.
   b. Autonomic nervous system dysfunction.
      (1) Yawning.
      (2) Nasal stuffiness.
      (3) Sweating.
      (4) Sneezing.
      (5) Low-grade fever.
      (6) Skin mottling.
   c. Gastrointestinal abnormalities.
      (1) Diarrhea.
      (2) Vomiting.
      (3) Poor feeding.
      (4) Regurgitation.
      (5) Dysmature swallowing.
      (6) Excessive sucking.
   d. Respiratory signs: tachypnea.
   e. Miscellaneous.
      (1) Skin excoriation.
      (2) Behavioral irregularities.

H. Use of neonatal abstinence scoring system. (See Appendix C.)

1. Neonatal Abstinence Scoring System assists in the detection of the onset of withdrawal symptoms and charts the progression and response to therapeutic intervention.
2. Scoring system can be used to assess withdrawal from opiods and nonopiod CNS depressants (Weiner and Finnegan, 1998).

3. Assess high-risk infants 2 hours after birth and then every 4 hours.
4. If, at any point, the score is 8 or greater, the scoring should be initiated every 2 hours and should be continued for at least 24 hours.
5. If pharmacotherapy is not needed, the infant is scored for the first 96 hours of life.
6. If the infant scores 8 or higher on three consecutive scoring times, the infant should be evaluated for pharmacotherapy.
7. Because NAS symptoms simulate common neonatal metabolic conditions such as hypoglycemia, hypocalcemia, sepsis, and meningitis, a complete blood cell count and calcium and glucose levels should be obtained before therapy is initiated.

I. Pharmacologic treatment of NAS.

1. Approximately 50–60% of infants exposed in utero to opiates will require pharmacologic intervention to control withdrawal (Weiner and Finnegan, 1998).
2. Pharmacologic treatment is commenced only if withdrawal is not controlled by supportive measures.
3. Pharmacologic agents used to treat NAS include phenobarbital, paregoric, tincture of opium, oral morphine, diazepam, and chlorpromazine (D'Apolito and McRorie, 1996).
4. Experts suggest that opiates are used for the management of NAS due to opiate exposure and as sedatives for infants with NAS due to nonopiate or polydrug exposure (Franck and Vilardi, 1995).
5. An oral morphine solution is now the opiate of choice because of the high alcohol content of paregoric and tincture of opium. Paregoric also contains camphor, anise oil, and benzoic acid (Franck and Vilardi, 1995).
6. Opiates do not make the infant drowsy or interfere with infant feeding, and they are effective in controlling gastrointestinal disturbances.
7. Once withdrawal is under control, pharmacologic treatment can be gradually withdrawn.
8. Control is defined as meeting the following conditions:
   a. Scores of 8 or less.
   b. Easily consolable infant.
   c. Rhythmic sleep and feeding cycle.
   d. Steady weight gain.

J. Iatrogenic NAS.

1. Opiates are now used extensively in the care of critically ill neonates and infants as analgesias and sedatives to assist in ventilation.
2. After prolonged use, abrupt cessation of these drugs may result in signs of withdrawal.
3. The infant should be weaned from opiate; the neonatal abstinence scoring system may be adapted to assist in this process (Franck and Vilardi, 1995).

Management Recommendations

A. Document maternal drug use and prenatal care patterns.

B. Obtain toxicology screening for all infants with a moderate index of suspicion. For urine, obtain the earliest urine possible. Consent may be needed in some states.

C. Consider HIV testing pending the mother's consent and your hospital's policy.

D. **If a careful physical examination reveals any malformations,** growth retardation, or microcephaly, evaluate for cause and consider screening for congenital infections (see Chapter 17, Neonatal Infections, for management).

E. **Obtain cranial ultrasound, renal ultrasound, EEG,** visual evoked response, and brainstem auditory evoked response, based on clinical indications prior to discharge.

F. **Observe carefully** for signs of feeding intolerance.

G. **Evaluate for signs of withdrawal,** using an abstinence score (see earlier section on NAS).

H. **Counsel mother regarding breast-feeding.**

I. **Initiate careful discharge planning,** with attention to maintaining surveillance after discharge, including evaluation of neurodevelopmental status.

J. **Consult with social services:** referral to agencies or for foster care, as dictated by the case (this includes cases of FAS). The mother must be informed of all medical, social, and legal circumstances regarding the baby. This process needs to be documented in the medical record.

Nursing Intervention

A. **The infant.**
1. Make careful, ongoing physical assessments, including use of the neonatal abstinence score.
2. Observe the infant for seizure activity.
3. Assess the infant's tolerance of environmental stimuli.
4. Minimize environmental and physical stimulation.
   a. Provide dim lighting.
   b. Speak quietly around the baby.
   c. Consider bed placement to avoid high-traffic areas.
5. Provide pacifiers.
6. Swaddle tightly with a cotton sheet in a flexed position, taking care not to overheat the infant.
7. The prone position is often used for preterm or sick infants with respiratory distress; however, it has been associated with SIDS and should be used with caution in this population with an already increased incidence of SIDS (Kenner and D'Apolito, 1997).
8. Sheepskin may be useful in protecting skin from excoriation. Any excoriated areas should be kept clean.
9. Relaxation baths may assist in settling and comforting the infant.
10. Provide gentle rocking in a vertical position to decrease irritability and restlessness.
11. Do not talk to the infant when rocking or feeding.
12. Cluster activities to allow for extensive rest periods, but take care not to overload and exhaust the infant.
13. Consider occasional gavage feeding without awakening for infants who have difficulty in sleeping.
14. For feeding difficulties, offer small, frequent feedings with frequent burping.
15. Monitor fluid balance and daily weight. High-caloric, low-volume feedings may be effective; however, diarrhea and general feeding intolerance may prohibit this approach.
16. Administer sedation as indicated.

B. **Mother-nurse interactions.**

1. The nurse must confront her own feelings regarding these issues.
2. Addiction is an illness requiring treatment, and all patients should be treated in a professional manner.
3. Develop a therapeutic relationship with the mother by establishing trust.
4. Provide consistency in caregivers, preferably with a primary nurse.
5. Provide clear information and specific guidelines for expected behavior.
6. Presenting truthful information and education in a nonjudgmental manner is the most effective approach.
7. Assist mothers to attach emotionally with their infants by encouraging touch and caretaking.
8. Provide positive reinforcement and immediate feedback for all caretaking activities.
9. Parent education should be goal directed. Outline clearly the caretaking and clinical milestones toward discharge.
10. Explain the infant's behavior. Discuss the baby's sensitivity to the environment and to excessive handling.
11. Explain to the mother that the infant's behavior is not a rejection of her.
12. Teach the mother to intervene early with a crying baby; explain that the mother's response does not "spoil" the infant but that the infant is not yet able to quiet himself or herself.
13. Provide kangaroo care opportunities, whereby the infant is placed on the mother's chest, skin to skin.
14. Acknowledge to oneself that these mothers and infants require flexibility, high energy, patience, and a nonjudgmental attitude.

Breast-feeding and the Drug-dependent or Virus-infected Woman

A. **Smoking.** The long-term effects of breast-feeding while smoking are unclear. If mothers smoke, it is recommended that they do not smoke at any time when actually nursing or in the infant's presence. If it is not possible to stop smoking, mothers should be encouraged to decrease the number of cigarettes and also consider low-nicotine cigarettes.

B. **Alcohol.** Moderate to heavy drinking has been shown to interfere with oxytocin release, causing inhibition of the letdown reflex. Alcohol crosses into the breast milk, and changes in the infant's sleep-wake patterning have been demonstrated. Infants fall asleep sooner but sleep for shorter periods (Mennella and Gerrish, 1998). Use of alcohol during lactation should be discouraged.

C. **Cocaine and amphetamines.** Breast-feeding is contraindicated. Cocaine remains for up to 60 hours after maternal ingestion.

D. **Marijuana.** Impairment of DNA and RNA formation and of use of essential proteins has been reported. Breast-feeding is not recommended for these mothers.

E. **Heroin.** Heroin-dependent women should not breast-feed.

F. **Methadone.**

1. It is unclear how much methadone is present in breast milk and at what levels it is safe to breast-feed.
2. All women who are taking methadone and also breast-feeding should be educated about the effects of high doses of methadone and the use of illicit drugs.

3. They should be familiar with the signs of infant withdrawal and know where to seek treatment if signs develop (D'Apolito, 1994, 1995).
4. Breast-feeding by a woman using methadone should not be stopped abruptly; the infant should be weaned gradually to prevent withdrawal.

G. **Hepatitis B.** Hepatitis B virus has been detected in breast milk of women who have tested positive for hepatitis B surface antigen; however, breast-feeding is not a contraindication (Gardner, Snell, and Lawrence, 1998). Hepatitis B immunoglobulin and vaccine should be given to infants at birth and vaccination completed as scheduled.

H. **Hepatitis C.**

1. Data concerning the presence of hepatitis C virus in breast milk are limited, and further research in this area is needed.
2. Although RNA from the hepatitis C virus has been detected in human milk, breast-feeding is not seen as a major risk for maternal-infant transmission of hepatitis C. Breast-feeding is not contraindicated, but the benefits and risks of breast-feeding should be explained to the mother to allow her to make an informed decision (American Academy of Pediatrics Committee on Infectious Diseases, 1998).
3. However, neonatal exposure to blood from cracked nipples should be avoided.

I. **HIV.**

1. The HIV antigen has been isolated in breast milk. It is recommended that women who are HIV-seropositive be counseled not to breast-feed.
2. Women who are HIV-seronegative but at high risk for seroconversion should be given information concerning the transmission of HIV through breast milk and methods to reduce the risk of becoming infected (American Academy of Pediatrics Committee on Pediatric AIDS, 1995).

Problems Associated With Maternal Drug Use

A. General information regarding drug-dependent women.

1. Drug-dependent women often have never experienced a positive relationship with their own parents.
2. They often come from dysfunctional families.
3. As children, many of the women were exposed to domestic violence, physical abuse, and sexual abuse.
4. As adults, they are often abused by their spouses.
5. Many have never observed positive parenting.
6. Many lack knowledge of normal child development and of child care skills necessary for effective parenting.

B. Psychologic profile of the drug-dependent woman.

1. Has multiple psychosocial problems.
2. Usually has an enduring pattern of drug use.
3. Demonstrates periods of serious depression, a sense of powerlessness, and low self-esteem.
4. Is often homeless and/or lacks social supports.
5. Maintains satisfactory personal relationships with difficulty.
6. Is unable to modify her behavior from past experience.
7. Is unable to anticipate the consequences of her behavior.
8. Is single; the father is often drug dependent or not involved in parenting.
9. Is in unstable, even dangerous living conditions.

10. Lacks the coping mechanisms, skills, and support to assist her during a crisis, such as the birth of a sick infant.
11. Experiences intense guilt after the birth of her infant.

C. **Maternal-infant relationships.**

1. The attachment process between mother and infant, like all relationships, is one of reciprocity.
2. Factors in the infant that contribute to poor parenting include behavior that is characteristic of prenatal drug exposure:
    a. Exhibits extreme irritability, with arching and writhing behavior.
    b. Resists comforting.
    c. Rarely reaches an alert state.
    d. Has low threshold for stimulation and is easily disturbed.
    e. Has erratic sleep patterns.
    f. Is difficult to feed and has poor weight gain.
3. The drug-dependent mother may be unskilled and may lack experience in mothering.
4. A high-risk profile exists because of the severity of the mother's addiction, coupled with her own psychologic profile and lifestyle, the infant's behavior, and the mother's lack of knowledge and experience in dealing with infants.

Ethical and Legal Considerations

A. **Three ethical principles** are of major importance when one is considering issues relating to substance abuse in women (Tiedje, 1998).
1. Justice: equitable allocation of health, social resources, and treatment for substance abusers.
2. Autonomy: maternal autonomy versus fetal rights.
3. Beneficence: advocacy for what is best for the mother and child.

B. **Legal implications** for substance abuse in pregnancy vary from country to country and from state to state. In several states the rights of the fetus are primary, and women who abuse drugs in pregnancy are imprisoned or placed on mandatory drug testing and treatment programs. However, most countries have mandatory laws for health care providers to report child abuse and neglect. Thus notification to the authorities may be necessary after delivery if staff are concerned about the parents' ability to care for the infant. These infants have a higher-than-expected risk of abuse than infants in the general population (Jaudes, Ekwo, and Van Voorhis, 1995).

C. **In the criminal model versus the harm-reduction model,** experts in the field of perinatal substance abuse believe that substance abuse is an illness and do not support prosecution of mothers (Catlin, 1997). Fear of prosecution may deter women from seeking prenatal care and treatment for their drug problems. Lack of prenatal care is one of the major preventable factors that contribute to adverse pregnancy outcomes among pregnant drug users (Garcia, 1997). The harm-reduction model balances what is best for each individual with protection of the public good (Tiedje, 1998).

D. **When the rights and needs of the mother are separated** from those of the fetus, the resultant solutions appear adversarial. When the rights and needs of the mother and those of fetus are viewed as interrelated, solutions may be developed to support both.

E. **For clearly identified high-risk infants,** the greatest impact may be possible only by protecting the child. Sometimes, children need to be removed from an addicted family and an unstable home environment and placed in a protected environment until the mother can receive help with her addiction and lifestyle.

Identification and notification of infants exposed to substances during pregnancy can have beneficial outcomes for the mother and her infant and should not be viewed in a negative manner by health care professionals (MacMahon, 1997).

E **Primary prevention is always suggested** to be the key in the health care framework, and neonatal drug withdrawal is preventable. Unfortunately, licit and illicit drug use is becoming more prevalent in today's society, and pregnant women are no exception. Prenatal care and early intervention programs are essential in an attempt to reduce or eliminate the consequences of substance abuse in pregnancy (Weiner and Finnegan, 1998). Chapters 33 and 34, on ethical and legal issues, will provide more detailed information.

REFERENCES

Abel, E.L.: Fetal alcohol syndrome. Oradell, N.J., Medical Economic Books, 1990.

Abel, E.L.: An update on incidence of FAS: FAS is not an equal opportunity birth defect. Neurotoxicol. Teratol., 17:437–443, 1995.

American Academy of Pediatrics Committee on Drugs: Neonatal drug withdrawal. Pediatrics, 101:1079–1088, 1998.

American Academy of Pediatrics Committee on Infectious Diseases: Hepatitis C virus infection. Pediatrics, 10:481–485, 1998.

American Academy of Pediatrics Committee on Pediatric AIDS: Human milk, breastfeeding, and transmission of human immunodeficiency virus in the United States. Pediatrics, 96:977–979, 1995.

Bell, G.L., and Lau, K.: Perinatal and neonatal issues of substance abuse. Pediatr. Clin. North Am., Substance Abuse, 42(2):261–281, 1995.

Bingol, N., Fuchs, M., Diaz, V., et al.: Teratogenicity of cocaine in humans. J. Pediatr., 110:93–96, 1987.

Blair, P.S., Fleming, P.J., Bensley, D., et al.: Smoking and the sudden infant death syndrome: Results from 1993–5 case-control study for confidential inquiry into stillbirths and deaths in infancy. B.M.J., 313:195–198, 1996.

Brooks-Gunn, J., McCarton, C., and Hawley, T.: Effects of in utero drug exposure on children's development: Review and recommendations. Arch. Pediatr. Adolesc. Med., 148:33–39, 1994.

Catlin, A.J.: Commentary on Deborah L. Burns' article "Positive Toxicology Screening in Newborns: Ethical Issues in the Decision to Legally Intervene." Pediatr. Nurs., 23(1):76–78, 1997.

Centers for Disease Control and Prevention: Alcohol consumption among pregnant and childbearing-aged women—United States, 1991 and 1995: Behavioral Risk Factor Surveillance System. M.M.W.R. Morb. Mortal. Wkly Rep., 46(16):346–350, 1997.

D'Apolito, K.: Methadone maintenance and breast feeding: Do they mix?. Neonatal Network, 13(8):64, 1994.

D'Apolito, K.: Methadone maintenance and breast feeding continued.... Neonatal Network, 14(4):77–78, 1995.

D'Apolito, K.C., and McRorie, T.I.: Pharmacologic management of neonatal abstinence syndrome. J. Perinat. Neonatal Nurs., 9(4):70–80, 1996.

Dicker, M., and Leighton, E.A.: Trends in the U.S. prevalence of drug-using parturient women and the drug-affected newborns, 1979 through 1990. Am. J. Public Health, 84:1433–1438, 1994.

Doberczak, T.M., Kandall, S.R., and Wilets, I.: Neonatal opioid abstinence syndrome in term and preterm infants. J. Pediatr., 118:933–937, 1991.

Eriksson, M., and Zetterstrom, R.: Amphetamine addiction during pregnancy: 10-year follow-up. Acta Paediatr. Suppl., 404:27–31, 1994.

Finnegan, L.P.: Neonatal abstinence syndrome. In Nelson, N. (Ed.): Current Therapy in Neonatal Perinatal Medicine. Toronto, B.C. Decker, 1990, p. 314.

Forrest, D., Horsley, S., Roberts, E., and Barrow, S.: Factors relating to smoking and pregnancy in the North Western Region. J. Public Health Med., 17:205–210, 1995.

Franck, L., and Vilardi, J.: Assessment and management of opioid withdrawal in ill neonates. Neonatal Network, 14(2):39–48, 1995.

Garcia, S.: Ethical and legal issues associated with substance abuse by pregnant and parenting women. J. Psychoactive Drugs, 29(1):101–111, 1997.

Gardner, S.L., Snell, B.J., and Lawrence, R.A.: Breast feeding the neonate with special needs. In Merenstein, G.B., and Gardner, S.L. (Eds.): Handbook of Neonatal Intensive Care, 4th ed. St. Louis, Mosby, 1998.

Henderson-Smart, D.J., Ponsonby, A.-L., and Murphy, E.: Reducing the risk of sudden infant death syndrome: A review of the scientific literature. J. Paediatr. Child Health, 34:213–219, 1998.

Huffman, D.M., Price, B.K., and Langel, L.: Therapeutic handling techniques for the infant affected by cocaine. Neonatal Network, 13(5):9–13, 1994.

Hurt, H.: Medical controversies in evaluation and management of cocaine-exposed infants. In Special Currents (M404). Columbus, Ohio, Ross Laboratories, May 1990.

Jaudes, P.K., Ekwo, E., and Van Voorhis, J.: Association of drug abuse and child abuse. Child Abuse Negl., 19:1065–1075, 1995.

Kandall, S.R., Gaines, J., Habel, L., et al.: Relationship of maternal substance abuse to subsequent sudden infant death syndrome in offspring. J. Pediatr., 123:120–126, 1993.

Kendrick, J.S., and Merritt, R.K.: Women and smoking: an update for the 1990s. Am. J. Obstet. Gynaecol., 175(3 pt 1):528–535, 1996.

Kenner, C., and D'Apolito, K.: Outcomes for children exposed to drugs in utero. J. Obstet. Gynecol. Neonatal Nurs., 26:595–603, 1997.

MacMahon, J.R.: Perinatal substance abuse: The impact of reporting infants to child protective services. Pediatrics, 100(5):e1, 1997.

Mennella, J.A., and Gerrish, C.J.: Effects of exposure to alcohol in mother's milk on infant sleep. Pediatrics, *101*(5):e2, 1998.

Noble, A., Vega, W.A., Kolody, B., et al.: Perinatal substance abuse in California: Findings from the Perinatal Substance Exposure Study. J. Psychoactive Drugs, *29*(1):43–53, 1997.

Rogers, P.D., and Werner, M.J.: The Pediatric Clinics of North America: Substance Abuse. Philadelphia, W.B Saunders, *42*(2):259, 1995.

Sampson, P.D., Streissguth, A.P., Bookstein, F.L., et al.: Incidence of fetal alcohol syndrome and prevalence of alcohol-related neurodevelopmental disorder. Teratology, *56*:317–326, 1997.

Spohr, H.L., Willms, J., and Steinhausen, H.C.: Prenatal alcohol exposure and long-term developmental consequences. Lancet, *341*:907–910, 1993.

Stratton, K., Howe, C., and Battaglia, F. (Eds.): Fetal alcohol syndrome. Washington, D.C., National Academy Press, 1996.

Swayze, V.W., Johnson, V.P., Hanson, J.W., et al.: Magnetic resonance imaging of brain anomalies in fetal alcohol syndrome. Pediatrics, *99*:232–240, 1997.

Tiedje, L.B.: Ethical and legal issues in the care of substance-using women. J. Obstet. Gynecol. Neonatal Nurs., *27*(1):92–98, 1998.

Weiner, S.M., and Finnegan L.P.: Drug withdrawal in the neonate. *In* Merenstein, G.B., and Gardner, S.L. (Eds.): Handbook of Neonatal Intensive Care, 4th Ed. St. Louis, Mosby, 1998.

Zuckerman, B.: Marijuana and cigarette smoking during pregnancy: Neonatal effects. *In* Chasnoff, I. (Ed.): Drugs, Alcohol, Pregnancy and Parenting. Boston, Kluwer, 1988.

ADDITIONAL READING

Adams, C., Eyler, F.D., and Behnke, M.: Nursing interventions with mothers who are substance abusers. J. Perinat. Neonat. Nurs., 3(4):43, 1990.

Alder, M.: Scientific perspectives on cocaine abuse. Pharmacology, 29:20–27, 1987.

Atkins, W.: Cocaine: The drug of choice. *In* Chasnoff, I. (Ed.): Drugs, Alcohol, Pregnancy and Parenting. Boston, Kluwer, 1988, p. 91.

Briggs, G.G., Freeman, R.K., and Yaffe, S.J.: Drugs in Pregnancy and Lactation. Baltimore, Williams & Wilkins, 1990.

Chasnoff, I.J., Hunt, C.E., Kletter, R., et al.: Prenatal cocaine exposure is associated with respiratory pattern abnormalities. Am. J. Dis. Child., 143:583–587, 1989.

Clarren, S.K., and Smith, D.W.: The fetal alcohol syndrome. N. Engl. J. Med., 298:1063–1067, 1978.

Coles, C.D., Smith, I., Fernhoff, P.M., et al.: Neonatal ethanol withdrawal: Characteristics in clinically normal, nondysmorphic neonates. J. Pediatr., 105:445–450, 1984.

Deren, S.: Children of substance abusers: A review of literature. J. Subst. Abuse Treat., 3:77–94, 1986.

Dixon, S.: Effects of transplacental exposure to cocaine and methamphetamine on the neonate. West. J. Med., 150:436–442, 1989.

Dixon, S., Bresnahan, K., and Zuckerman, B.: Cocaine babies: Meeting the challenge of management. Contemp. Pediatr., March 1990.

Eliason, M., and Williams, J.: Fetal alcohol syndrome and the neonate. J. Perinat. Neonat. Nurs., 3(4):64, 1990.

Ernhart, C.B., Wolf, A.W., Linn, P.L., et al.: Alcohol-related birth defects: Syndromal anomalies, IUGR, and neonatal behavioral assessment. Alcoholism, 9:447–453, 1985.

Finnegan, L.P.: Substance abuse. Perinatol.-Neonatol., 6(4):17–23, 1982.

Flandermeyer, A.: A comparison of the effects of heroin and cocaine abuse upon the neonate. Neonatal Network, 6(3):42–48, December 1987.

Flandermeyer, A.A.: The drug-exposed neonate. *In* Kenner, C.A., Lott, J.W., and Flandermeyer, A.A. (Eds.): Comprehensive Neonatal Nursing: A Physiologic Perspective, 2nd ed. Philadelphia, W.B. Saunders, 1998.

Fried, P.A.: Marijuana use by pregnant women: Neurobehavioral effects on neonates. Drug Alcohol Depend., 6:415, 1980.

Griffith, D.: The effects of perinatal cocaine exposure on infant neurobehavior and early maternal infant interactions. *In* Chasnoff, I., Ed.: Drugs, Alcohol, Pregnancy and Parenting. Boston, Kluwer, 1988, p. 105.

Halliday, H.C., MacReid, M., and McClure, G.: Results of heavy drinking in pregnancy. Br. J. Obstet. Gynecol., 89:892–895, 1982.

Harrison, G.G., Branson, R.S., and Vaugher, Y.E.: Association of maternal smoking with body composition of the newborn. Am. J. Clin. Nutr., 38:757, 1983.

Hingson, R., Alpert, J., and Day, N.: Effects of maternal drinking and marijuana use on fetal growth and development. Pediatrics, 70:539, 1982.

Householder, J., Hatcher, R., Burns, W.M., et al.: Infants born to narcotic-addicted mothers. Psychol. Bull., 92:453, 1982.

Lynch, M., and McKeon, V.: Cocaine use during pregnancy: Research findings and clinical implications. J. Obstet. Gynecol. Neonatal Nurs., 19(4):285, 1990.

National Institute on Drug Abuse: Cocaine use in America. Prevention Networks, Department of Health and Human Services (publication No. ADM 86-1433). Washington, D.C., U.S. Government Printing Office, 1986.

Oro, A., and Dixon, S.: Perinatal cocaine and methamphetamine exposure: Maternal and neonatal correlates. J. Pediatr., 111:571–578, 1987.

Perinatal Advisory Council of Los Angeles: Perinatal protocol: Maternal substance use and neonatal drug withdrawal. J. Perinatol., 8:387–392, 1988.

Robe, L.B., Gromisch, D.S., and Iosub, S.: Symptoms of neonatal ethanol withdrawal. Curr. Alcohol., 8:485–493, 1981.

Russell, M.: The impact of alcohol-related birth defects in New York State. Neurobehav. Toxicol., 2:277–283, 1980.

Sokol, R.J., Miller, S.I., and Reed, G.: Alcohol abuse during pregnancy: An epidemiologic study. Alcoholism, 4:135–145, 1980.

Staisy, N., and Fried, P.: Relationships between moderate maternal alcohol consumption during pregnancy and infant neurological development. J. Studies Alcohol, 44:262–270, 1983.

Sullivan, K.: Maternal implications of cocaine use during pregnancy. J. Perinat. Neonat. Nurs., 3(4):12, 1990.

Ward, S., Schutz, S., and Kirshria, V.: Abnormal sleeping ventilatory patterns in infants of substance-abusing mothers. Am. J. Dis. Child., 140:1015, 1986.

Wegman, M.E.: Annual summary of vital statistics, 1986. Pediatrics, 80:817–827, 1987.

Weiss, R.: Subtypes of cocaine abuse. Psychiatr. Clin. North Am., 9:3–10, 1986.

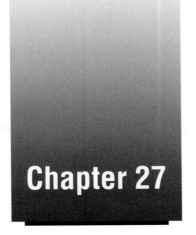

Chapter 27

Families in Crisis

Carole Kenner and Stephanie Amlung

Objectives

1. Define the concept of crisis.

2. Recognize the psychologic tasks that the mother and family must accomplish to establish a healthy parent-child relationship after the crisis of the birth of a premature or sick infant.

3. Describe assessment strategies for identifying a family in crisis.

4. Identify the risks of teenage parenting on the adolescent and the infant.

5. Identify nursing interventions to support a family coping with stressful events surrounding the birth of their infant.

6. Evaluate maternal behaviors found to be predictive of specific parenting outcomes.

7. Recognize emotional characteristics related to grief.

8. Describe nursing interventions to support the parents experiencing a perinatal loss.

9. Identify specific behaviors to be assessed in determining parental attachment to their infant.

10. Describe nursing strategies to promote parental acquaintance and attachment.

With the current technologic advances, even the most acutely ill or most premature infant has a good chance of going home. Neonates born as prematurely as 23 weeks' gestation are surviving. For parents, though these advances are increasing the odds of having a live baby, they also have brought on tremendous stress (Miles, Holditch-Davis, and Shepherd, 1998).

When an infant requires health care at birth because of prematurity, illness, or congenital malformations, or when an infant dies, the effects of these unexpected events on the parents can be overwhelming. The families of these infants may experience multiple crisis events during the infant's hospitalization (Kenner and Bagwell, 1998). Assessment skills are critical for the neonatal nurse who is caring for an infant and family at this period of crisis. The parents usually display signs of anxiety, fear, and powerlessness. It is the nurse who is viewed as the advocate for the family and who has the most continuous interactions with them. Nursing care is generally concerned with both the physiologic and psychosocial needs of the patient and the family. However, the focus of this chapter is the psychosocial aspects of supporting parents who must cope with stressful events surrounding the birth of their infant. It will highlight various types of families who may experience a crisis when their infant requires an NICU stay. Many of the strategies or interventions are the same for all groups of parents because they represent parenting needs.

Crisis and the Birth of the Sick or Premature Infant

Pregnancy and transition to parenthood have been recognized as periods of stress and change during which mothers and fathers are attempting to master the normal developmental process of parenthood. These major life changes have been referred to as *developmental or maturational stressors*. In contrast, the birth of a premature or sick infant and the death of an infant are unexpected stressful life events for which a person or family is often physiologically unprepared. Such events are referred to as *situational or accidental stressors*. When such maturational and situational stressors occur simultaneously, the resulting pressure can overwhelm a person's usual coping resources and support systems. Ineffective coping causes personal and family psychologic disequilibrium or crisis, which continues until new ways of coping can be developed and maintained. Coping, however, is intimately tied to cultural values and beliefs, so these must be taken into account.

A. **Several psychologic tasks** have been identified that the mother and family must accomplish to cope with the crisis of a premature birth or of the birth of a sick infant and to establish a basis for a healthy parent-child relationship (Krebs, 1998).
1. *Preparation for the possible loss of the infant.* Parents must consider the possibility of disability or death of the infant while simultaneously hoping for the infant's survival.
2. *Acknowledgment of failure to deliver a term infant.* The mother struggles with feelings of guilt and failure and searches for causes of the infant's condition.
3. *Adaptation to the intensive care environment.* Parents must be helped to develop secure relationships in an unfamiliar and stress-provoking setting.
4. *Resumption of interaction with the infant once the threat of loss has passed.* Parents must participate in the infant's care and gain confidence in their abilities.
5. *Preparation for taking the infant home.* Parents must understand the special needs and characteristics of the premature or sick infant and the necessary precautions that must be taken and yet maintain a positive relationship with the infant, realizing that these needs are only temporary. Failure to resolve these tasks can contribute to such maladaptive parenting as overprotectiveness, resulting in the "vulnerable child syndrome" and in other negative child outcomes such as failure to thrive, emotional deprivation, and battering (Miles et al., 1998).

B. **Definition of *crisis:*** a temporary disequilibrium that occurs when people face an important problem or transitional phase so stressful that they are unable to cope by using their customary problem-solving resources (Wereszczak, Miles, and Holditch-Davis, 1997). It usually lasts from 4 to 6 weeks. This period is the optimal time for effective interventions with the family.

C. **Discussion.** During early stages of a crisis, parents are more receptive to overtures of help from other family members, friends, and the health care team. Nurses are in a key position because they work so directly with the parents to anticipate a family crisis and to promote positive coping and effective use of social supports (Moore and Freda, 1998). A family in crisis cannot effectively interact with their newly born infant because all their energies are going toward the crisis. When interventions are put into place to promote effective coping and positive social support, the crisis will resolve and psychologic equilibrium, a necessary step toward the establishment of a healthy parent-child relationship, will be restored. Factors that influence a family's return to equilibrium include the following:

1. Understanding of the infant's problem and the need for NICU care and understanding of their parental role.
2. Resolution of the family's grief reaction to the need for NICU care.
3. Use of positive coping and social supports (Kenner and Bagwell, 1998).

Specific Population of Parents: Adolescents

Parents who are adolescent have some unique needs. They undergo the crises of parenthood and of having an infant in the NICU. In addition, these parents are dealing with the normal developmental tasks of adolescence. Sometimes these tasks seem in conflict with their needs as new parents. The nurse must be aware of these conflicts and realize their unique blending needs of taking on a new role and being at their developmental stage.

Adolescence is a turning point, or change period. It moves a child from childhood toward the maturation of the adult. Many physiologic changes are occurring, first at puberty and then in the move toward adulthood. Physical appearance changes, and the adolescent becomes capable of childbearing. Maturation of the reproductive system now occurs much earlier than in the past. In the United States, girls are reaching menarche as young as 8 years of age. Adolescence is the time when childbearing becomes a potential reality for most individuals.

Development of the personality is tied to role attainment, much as for parents and the parenting role. Adolescents strive to have an identity unique from those of other family members. They are developing their self-concept and self-esteem. The peer group becomes important for validation of attitudes, values, and beliefs (Koshar et al., 1998). Adolescence is a time of constant change and usually turmoil—a period of maturational crisis.

A. **Some developmental tasks of this period are:**

1. Independence from adults.
2. Preparation for financial security.
3. Gender identification.
4. A stable, realistic, positive sense of self.

B. **In addition, adolescence:**

1. Is characterized by high anxiety.
2. Can be anticipated; therefore preparation can be made.
3. Requires normal social support for a successful transition.
4. Is relatively easy to resolve because the individual's values usually do not conflict with societal expectations for the outcome, which is adult behavior.
5. Is a period of vulnerability to a crisis occurrence if a traumatic event is added to the transitional state.

The Family in Crisis

ASSESSMENT

A. **Determine parents' understanding of the situation** (i.e., realistic vs distorted). The parents' ability to resolve the crisis depends on their realistic perception of their situation: they need to be fully informed about their infant's condition and expected progress. An inability to understand the crisis may be related to low socioeconomic status or cultural values and beliefs. Parents of a lower socioeconomic status may not fully understand what to expect of their infant or their role because they may lack good role models for themselves or the financial means to provide adequate, safe care for themselves or their infant. Cultural values and beliefs also may play a role because different cultures view the infant in relationship to parents in different ways. In some cultures, such as in India or China, only male offspring are valued and girl babies are dismissed as nonessential.

B. **Determine parents' grief response.** The extent to which they are experiencing a grief reaction must be determined. This grief may be in the form of anticipatory grief because they fear the infant might die, even though the physical condition does not appear to warrant this fear.

C. **Determine parents' adaptation to and coping** with the stressful event.
1. Are the parents maintaining responsibilities related to activities of daily living (e.g., eating, personal grooming)?
2. To what degree has the family's normal lifestyle been affected by the crisis? (Are they able to return to work? keep house? care for other children in the household?)
3. Are the parents exhibiting positive coping skills?
4. To what extent has the financial status of the family been affected?

D. **Determine what support systems exist** for the parents and whether they are being used. It is also important to determine whether these supports are positive. The parents may have several people in their support network, but if these people are critical of how the parents are conducting themselves, then they may not be viewed as positive supports.
1. Who are the significant others in the lives of the parents? Consider biological kinship (family) and/or emotional kinship (friends).
2. What professional supports are available?
3. Is a parent support group available?

E. **Understanding the origins of a crisis, and their links with the normal "ups and downs" of life, is crucial to successful assessment and intervention. Events that stimulate the occurrence of a crisis, such as those of the teenage parent in the NICU, can originate from:**
1. Being in a transitional state, such as:
   a. Adolescence to adulthood.
   b. Childhood to parenthood.
2. Being a part of a social-cultural structure and:
   a. Violating customs embedded in that structure, such as a teenager's becoming pregnant and having a baby, *or*
   b. Behaving outside the accepted teenage social norms, as the role of parent would demand (although these examples are culture specific): for example, being tied down to taking care of a baby or having to arrange for child care at a time when peers are freely going to sports games and dances and having fun.
   c. Being exposed to hazardous or disturbing situations, such as:
      (1) Birth of a first child. This is a disturbing situation because no one knows exactly what to expect of parenthood—a role never before experienced.
      (2) Lack of experience with parenthood.
      (3) Bearing of a sick newborn infant.

PROBLEMS ASSOCIATED WITH ADOLESCENT PREGNANCY

When teens become pregnant, they often experience the following problems:

A. **Loss of peer group.** Adolescents' peers often disappear, leaving them without support and feeling socially isolated. Their self-concept changes as they approach parenthood because, before the pregnancy, the peer group helped shape their self-perception (Alpers, 1998).

B. **Disruption of family ties.** The pregnant adolescent and her boyfriend often bring on direct conflict with their parents. The rationale for this conflict is that the parents of the adolescents often believe that adolescence is an inappropriate time to start a family and that the adolescents need to live by the parental house rules. At the same time, the adolescent parents may be trying to take on adult responsibilities while feeling that they are being treated as children. This conflict removes a possible positive social support. It also disrupts the effort to assume a parental role if the adolescents' parents try to make decisions regarding the coming infant.

C. **Maternal health problems.** The pregnant female adolescent often has engaged in risky behaviors besides being sexually active. She may smoke, drink, or use drugs. She is at risk of having human immunodeficiency virus (HIV) infection and other sexually transmitted infections (STIs). This risk is not unique to adolescents but is possible because of the feelings of invincibility that accompany this age. The pregnant adolescent may be emotionally immature and may have to interrupt her education to bear the child. She may be forced into a marriage she does not want or is not ready for at this time. She may lack knowledge about normal fetal and infant growth and development. She may have very unrealistic expectations of a baby and of herself as a parent. She may have sought pregnancy as a way to have someone need her. She may not seek prenatal care or may try to hide the pregnancy by limiting weight gain. These actions may put her health and her infant's health at risk. She also often lacks parenting skills.

D. **Paternal problems.** The adolescent father may have engaged in risky sexual behaviors. He may have been smoking or used alcohol or drugs. He also may be at risk of having HIV infection or other STIs. If he is infected, the pregnant adolescent and the fetus are also at risk because these infections can be passed on to the maternal-fetal unit. The male adolescent may be generally stable psychologically, but he may not be thinking about future consequences of his sexual behavior, such as his inability to fulfill his parenting role. For example, because of his risky behaviors, he may have contracted HIV, which will take him away from the pregnant adolescent and his future child. If his behaviors are viewed by his family, his significant other, or her family as irresponsible, he may be isolated from an active role in future parenting. He may feel excluded from decisions regarding the continuation of the pregnancy or the placement of the child after birth. He may interrupt his own education to provide financial support to his new "family." He may be forced into a marriage he neither wants nor is ready for at present.

E. **Risks to the infant.** The infant is at risk of having a faulty, or negative, parent-infant interaction, generally because of the parents' lack of understanding of the normal growth and development process. The parents also often have unrealistic expectations of the child and their role as parents and may lack parenting skills. The infant may be small for gestational age or premature and may require an expensive hospitalization that the parents are not ready financially or cognitively to accept. The infant may be less responsive or organized in cues for care by the parents. He or she may be more at risk of having slowed or delayed growth because of the parents' lack of understanding of normal infant care and feeding practices. The infant may not receive the type and amount of stimulation necessary for positive cognitive or behavioral development. An infant who is premature tends to be more irritable, to feed poorly, to have poor self-regulatory behaviors, and to be difficult to console. This seeming lack of responsiveness to parenting efforts often reinforces the adolescent parents' poor self-esteem and poor self-concept, which often accompany adolescent pregnancy. The infant may also be at risk of experiencing abuse or neglect.

1. Prematurity, birth between 23 and 27 weeks, is more common among infants of adolescent mothers. The risk factors for delivering early are (Bartram, Joffe, and Perry, 1998):
   a. Low pregnancy weight.
   b. Lower socioeconomic status.
   c. Marital status: single.
   d. Tobacco use (smoking).
   e. Narcotic use.
   f. Anemia (hemoglobin concentration <11 g/dL).
   g. First child.
   h. Poor prenatal care.
2. Low birth weight (<2500 g) is also a risk factor for an adolescent's offspring. The risk can be as much as six times greater for 14-year-old and younger mothers (Bartram et al., 1998).

INTERVENTION

A. **Be present with the physician or nurse practitioner** at the initial meeting with the parents.

B. **Talk with the mother and father** together whenever possible. Consider cultural values of each family. In some cultures the father must receive the information first (Kenner and Bagwell, 1998).

C. **Determine and address the parents' perceptions** of the infant's condition (Kenner and Bagwell, 1998).

D. **Be consistent with information** given to parents by the staff. If in an academic health care setting where the physicians or nurse practitioners rotate frequently, be sure that any changes in care that are reflective only of these staff changes are explained within that context. If parents do not understand the basis of these changes or are not told when their infant's condition really changes, then mistrust begins. Then the chance that the crisis will escalate is highly probable (Kenner and Bagwell, 1998; Miles et al., 1998).

E. **Do not overload parents with detailed information** about their infant during their initial visits to the NICU; provide basic facts and allow the parents time to process the information.

F. **Assess the grief response.** Males and females express their grief in different ways. However, most, if not all, parents experience some form of grief by just having an infant who requires specialize care (Kenner and Bagwell, 1998). This reaction must be assessed throughout the hospital stay. Sometimes this response is directly tied to their understanding of the infant's condition.

G. **Acknowledge any feeling of guilt that might be expressed** about the unexpected birth outcome. Let the parents know that these feelings are normal (Siegel, Gardner, and Merenstein, 1998).

H. **Facilitate adaptation of the parents' new role** by being very good listeners, by observing body language, and by helping them to verbalize their feelings (Siegel, Gardner, and Merenstein, 1998).

I. **Periodically assess the parents' understanding** of their infant's condition and their interpretation of the information that has been given to them. Information must be reinforced throughout the hospital stay. Whenever anyone is anxious, little information is actually heard or retained.

J. **Write notes from the infant to the parents** concerning current status (e.g., equipment, feedings, oxygen concentration) and take pictures of the infant periodically. A notebook containing the notes and pictures can be kept at the infant's bedside for the parents. This intervention should be individualized because not all parents want this form of "communication." It is one strategy, however, for some parents that promotes positive attachment.

K. **Allow parents the freedom to express negative ideas without being judged.** Fear and frustration over the inability to control their infant's circumstances are often the basis for parental anger displaced to staff.

L. **Encourage parents to participate in the care as they desire.** Parents need to understand and develop their roles as parents. If professionals provide all the care, a clear message is conveyed to the parents that they are not capable of helping their infant. They must understand all the things they have to contribute to the team approach to care.

M. **Do not refer to parents as visitors.** Parents are not visitors. They are parents and are partners in the care of the infant. They are an integral part of the infant's care and should be a focus of nursing care.

N. **Promote a developmentally supportive environment for the family.** Use of kangaroo care (skin-to-skin contact, done by placing the naked infant next to the parent's naked chest, with a blanket or gown drapped over the parent and infant), dimmed lights or cycled lights, private areas for parent interaction with the infant, and swaddling or cuddling of the infant promote positive development of the infant and family (Gray, Dostal, Ternullo-Retta, and Armstrong, 1998, Gretebeck, Shaffer, and Bishop-Kurylo, 1998; Griffin, 1998).

O. **Determine parents' network of social support.** The social support network may include family, friends, clergy, and health professionals. Also determine whether the level of support is adequate from the parents' and the health professionals' standpoint.

P. **Encourage parents to share their concerns and fears** with each other. Often it is not until the infant is discharged that parents share their feelings with each other.

Q. **Assist parents in maintaining their relationship with one another.** Reinforce with them that they must take time for themselves as a couple. If the mother is alone, encourage her to maintain ties with other family members and her friends.

R. **Assist parents in maintaining their relationship with the infant's siblings** by helping them to recognize the needs of the other children and identify how the needs can be met.

S. **Assist the adolescent parents in defining their role with their own parents** by helping them to learn how to talk with their parents.

T. **Encourage parents to attend a parent support group.** Involvement in a parent support group has been demonstrated to facilitate parental grieving, reduce fears, and increase feelings of parental competence (Bracht, Ardal, Bot, and Cheng, 1998; Levin, 1998; Raines, 1998). This intervention must be culture specific. In some cultures, it is not acceptable to discuss family problems openly.

EVALUATION OF MATERNAL PARENTING OUTCOMES

A. **Predictors of good maternal parenting outcomes (Kenner and Bagwell, 1998).**

1. Anxiety level is moderate to high: she worries about the infant's chances of surviving, the possibility of abnormality, and her competence as a mother.
2. Seeks information about the infant.
3. Demonstrates warmth toward infant and in other relationships.
4. Has a support system (i.e., father of the infant, her mother, friends).
5. Has had a previous successful experience with a premature infant (i.e., previous child, a sibling, other relative), which enables her to feel more experienced and confident.
6. Recognizes positive attributes of the child (i.e., smiling) (Johnson-Crowley, 1998).
7. Views self positively.
8. For an adolescent, has a centralized locus of behavioral control.
9. Exhibits effective caregiving.
10. Makes positive eye contact with the infant.

B. **Predictors of poor maternal parenting outcomes (Kenner and Bagwell, 1998).**

1. Exhibits an inappropriately low anxiety level.
2. Demonstrates passivity—does not actively seek out information related to infant's condition.
3. Has limited verbal interaction.
4. Visits infrequently and for short periods in the NICU. (Remember that sometimes infrequent visits are due to a lack of transportation and not true parenting problems).
5. Is unaware of the infant's needs.
6. Has unrealistic expectations of the infant or the parenting role.
7. Personalizes the infant's behavior as a failure of her ability to parent or that the baby is "bad."
8. During pregnancy, expressed little desire to have a child.
9. Is more likely to express disappointment about the sex of the infant.
10. Has no support system.
11. Is an adolescent with little or no social support system.
12. Exhibits role confusion.

GRIEF AND LOSS

A. **Introduction.** Unfortunately, not all pregnancies result in a healthy term infant. When adverse neonatal events occur, often the parents are overwhelmed by grief. As the parents realize that their newborn baby is "less than perfect" and not the infant of their fantasies, acute grief reactions occur. One of the early tasks of parenting is to resolve the discrepancy between the idealized infant and the real infant. In the case of neonatal death, the parents also grieve for the lost opportunity to parent the child. To assist parents therapeutically in working through the feelings associated with loss, nurses working with high-risk infants must understand the grief process, recognize typical parental behaviors associated with grief, and provide appropriate nursing interventions.

B. **Definitions.**

1. *Grief:* the response of sadness and sorrow to the loss of a valued object (Siegel et al., 1998).

2. *Anticipatory grief:* grieving that occurs before an actual loss. If the outcome for the infant is healthy, then anticipatory grieving can lead to difficulties in attachment and problems in the parent-infant relationship.
3. *Chronic grief:* unresolved or blocked grief; frequently seen in parents of a disabled child, who is a constant reminder of loss.

C. Assessment.

1. Grief responses to death, premature birth, or the birth of an infant with a malformation are similar. These responses do not necessarily occur in the same sequence for all people. In addition, the responses may overlap and recur. Stages of grief (Siegel et al., 1998) are:
   a. Shock.
   b. Denial and/or panic: refusal to accept reality; intense anxiety.
   c. Anger, guilt, and shame; awareness of loss suffered becomes acute.
   d. Acceptance, adaptation, and reorganization; grief continues, but the individual is able to reestablish a state of equilibrium.
2. One of the goals of the staff working with parents is to encourage the development of attachment, or an affectional tie, between the parent and infant. However, because the birth of a premature or a physically or psychologically challenged infant creates a sense of loss, the parents must first resolve their grief before attachment can be fully achieved (Nurses Association of the American College of Obstetricians and Gynecologists, 1991; Siegel et al., 1998).

Interventions for Facilitating Grief

A. Listen: parents need to be given the opportunity to express their feelings.

B. Acknowledge the pain of their loss: gives the parents permission to talk about their loss and provides support for acknowledging and working through their grief (Kenner and Bagwell, 1998).

C. Convey an attitude of acceptance, openness, and availability to the family: grieving people need permission to experience their feelings, regardless of how uncomfortable or unpleasant (Siegel et al., 1998).

D. Help the parents to understand the individuality of the grieving process. Mothers and fathers usually have "incongruent grieving": they do not grieve at the same pace (Peppers and Knapp, 1980). This incongruence frequently leads to marital discord because of misconceptions about feelings and an inability to communicate.

Interventions for Parents Experiencing a Perinatal Loss

A. Encourage the family to see, hold, and spend time with the infant before and after death (Kleingbeil, 1986).
1. Be sensitive to individual and cultural differences in rituals of saying goodbye.
2. Physically bring the family together and offer privacy. Some hospitals have a neonatal hospice program in which the family is involved with the infant's care (Butler, 1986; Landon-Malone, Kirkpatrick, and Stull, 1987; Siegel, Rudd, and Cleveland, 1985).

B. Provide the parents with the following mementos: photograph of the infant, identification bracelet, footprints, completed crib card, blanket, wisp of hair, and birth certificate. Keep these mementos in a file in the nursery for future retrieval should parents choose not to take the items at the time of the infant's death. This intervention must be individualized according to the needs and desires of each family.

C. Provide information about support groups and/or grief counseling.

D. Encourage the parents to name the infant.

E. Provide a booklet about perinatal loss for the parents.

F. Discuss options for autopsy, disposition of the body, and a memorial or funeral service.

G. Offer the option for the infant to be baptized.

H. Assist parents in understanding the importance of informing siblings about the death of the infant. Suggest that they use simple statements based on the children's level of understanding (Siegel et al., 1998).

I. Talk with parents about possible responses from family and friends, who often minimize the infant's death in an attempt to offer comfort.

Interventions for Parents With a Preterm or Physically or Psychologically Challenged Infant

These interventions have been incorporated into the interventions listed in the previous section, The Family in Crisis, and in the following section, Family-Infant Bonding.

Family-Infant Bonding

Parents who have an infant who is born ill, prematurely, or physically or psychologically challenged are potentially at risk of having parenting difficulties. These stressful events around the time of the infant's birth generate feelings of anxiety, disappointment, and grief in the parents. Moreover, early disruptions in the acquaintance and attachment process between parent and infant place these parents in a state of increased vulnerability for establishing a nurturing relationship with their infant. Opportunities for parents to learn to interpret their infant's unique needs and to develop reciprocal interaction through sensitivity to behavioral cues are also interrupted (Krebs, 1998; Kenner and Bagwell, 1998). The relationship between parent-infant attachment and later parenting behaviors has been well established. In addition, the parent-infant attachment is the basis for all the infant's subsequent attachments and is the relationship through which a sense of self is developed (Kennell and Klaus, 1982, pp. 151–226; Kenner and Bagwell, 1998). Therefore an important component of nursing care of the high-risk infant is facilitation of parent-infant interaction and attachment.

A. Definitions.

1. *Bonding:* a gradual, reciprocal process that begins with acquaintance. It is a unique and specific relationship between two people and endures across time (Jenkins and Tock, 1986; Kennell and Klaus, 1982, pp. 151–226). Bonding occurs on a different timetable for mothers than for fathers. Although mothers experience a sharp increase in bonding around the fifth month of pregnancy and have intensifying feelings throughout the pregnancy, the father's feelings usually tend to develop more slowly than the mother's and become congruent after birth, when infant caretaking begins (Peppers and Knapp, 1980; Kenner and Bagwell, 1998; Krebs, 1998).
2. *Attachment:* the quality of the bond, or affectional tie, between parents and their infant, which begins early in the prenatal period, appears to increase when fetal movement is felt and is intensified with interaction between the parent and the infant after birth (Siegel et al., 1998).

B. **Discussion.** The development of a warm, nurturing, and reciprocal relationship between infant and parent is essential for a healthy physiologic outcome to the crisis of the birth of a premature, sick, or malformed infant (Kenner and Bagwell, 1998). "The parent 'at risk' cannot resolve a crisis surrounding birth of their infant and simultaneously establish warm attachment bonds while retaining his or her self-esteem without the support of others in the social system" (Mercer, 1977, p. 5). Neonatal nurses can provide this support by assessing the parents' responses to their infant and facilitating their acquaintance and attachment process with the infant.

C. **Assessment.**

1. Note pattern of parental visiting to the NICU, duration of visits, and frequency of phone calls. This pattern, if abnormal, is predictive of maternal parenting difficulties (Kennell and Klaus, 1982). If parents are not visiting frequently, be careful to determine the reasons (i.e., cultural practices after childbirth, conflicting obligations between work and family roles, or lack of transportation to the hospital) before assuming that the parents are unconcerned or that parenting difficulties exist.
2. Identify the development of attachment behaviors. Mothers' activity with their infants has been found to be indicative of the initial adjustment to the infant, important past and present interpersonal relationships, and involvement in taking care of the infant (Siegel et al., 1998). Examples of attachment behaviors include:
   a. Touching: typical maternal progression of touching the premature infant is from fingertip touching of the infant's extremities to palmar stroking of the infant's trunk, to holding and embracing the infant. This progression of touch usually occurs during a period of several visits to the NICU.
   b. Looking "en face": aligning head with infant's head in the same plane to make eye-to-eye contact with the infant.
   c. Talking to the infant, calling the infant by name.
   d. Bringing pictures, toys, and/or clothes to the hospital.
   e. Participating in caretaking activities, such as feeding, bathing, and clothing the infant.

INTERVENTIONS TO ENCOURAGE FAMILY-INFANT BONDING

A. **If at all possible, show the infant to the parents in the delivery room and allow them to touch the infant, if only for a few moments.** This helps to establish the reality of the infant for the parents (Kennell and Klaus, 1982; Kenner and Bagwell, 1998; Litchfield, 1983).

B. **Encourage the parents to visit** their infant in the intensive care nursery as soon as possible.

1. Before the first visit to the nursery, prepare the parents for what to expect by giving them written information about the unit, describing the atmosphere of the nursery (i.e., noise, high activity level, infants attached to various kinds of equipment) and discussing the normal aspects of their infant as well as deviations.
2. If the mother is unable to visit because of conditions such as ordered bed rest or transport of the infant to another hospital, the father can be given pictures of the infant for the mother. In addition, the mother should be given the phone number of the nursery and encouraged to call as often as desired.
3. For the parents of an infant born with a malformation, encourage the parents to see the infant together as soon as possible, but do not force them to interact. Point out to the family the normal qualities of the infant as well as the abnormalities (Kenner and Bagwell, 1998; Krebs, 1998).

C. Ensure that, during the family's first visit, the nurse assigned to the infant stays at the bedside to explain equipment and the infant's condition, as well as to answer questions, provide emotional support, and encourage touching of the infant.

D. Convey a positive, realistic attitude about the infant rather than a negative or fatalistic viewpoint, which may alienate the parents and impair attachment (Kenner and Bagwell, 1998).

E. Assist the parents with holding and cuddling their infant as soon as possible, taking into consideration the infant's condition and the parents' readiness (e.g., assist in managing respiratory and monitoring equipment and IV lines). Some nurseries are implementing skin-to-skin care (also called kangaroo care) by parents as an alternative to the traditional modes of providing care to stable, hospitalized premature infants. This care consists of positioning the infant, dressed only in diapers, upright and prone between the mother's breasts. This vertical position in skin-to-skin contact provides tactile stimulation and warmth from the mother, as well as opportunities for eye-to-eye contact, auditory stimulation, and breast-feeding. Mothers usually wear their own front-opening blouses or dresses that are loosely fitted. Fathers can also be encouraged to engage in kangaroo care (Luddington-Hoe, Hadeed, and Anderson, 1991; Blackburn and VandenBerg, 1998).

F. Encourage the parents to participate in caretaking activities as warranted by the infant's condition and tolerance for input. Explain to parents of very premature infants the relationship between neurologic maturity and the capacity for handling stimulation (Blackburn and VandenBerg, 1998).

G. Model nurturing parenting behavior such as stroking, touching, and talking to the infant for parents who may need assistance in developing positive parenting behaviors.

H. Give positive reinforcement to parents as they interact with their infant. For example, say that "he seems to calm down when you talk with him," or "he really seems to sleep better after you have held him" (Kenner and Bagwell, 1998). Assisting parents to recognize positive changes in the infant in response to their caretaking has a strong impact on the parents and increases their feelings of success (Kenner and Bagwell, 1998).

I. Use consistent caregivers for the premature or sick infant to establish a rapport with the parents.

J. Role-model caregiving techniques—one on one, if possible—especially for adolescent parents.

K. Avoid power struggles with parents by defining their role and recognizing that they are the parents and that the infant is theirs, not the staff's.

L. Suggest that the parents or siblings bring something for the infant, such as a small toy, pictures of the family members to be taped on the infant's bed, and/or a tape recording of the parents' voices to be played for the infant. Share personalized information about the infant with the parents, such as "she really enjoys sucking on her pacifier" or "she was really active while I was giving her a bath," to assist the parents in individualizing and accepting the infant.

M. Encourage sibling visitation in the unit or window observation of the infant (Broughton, 1998).

N. Promote developmental care that includes the family unit in the plan of care and an environment that supports the parents. Provide a private area, or a transitional care area, to encourage parental stays within a more homelike environment, and encourage developmental care that includes parents as an integral part of the health care team.

O. **After the mother's discharge from the hospital, maintain communication** with the parents by providing them with the phone number of the unit. For parents of transported infants, sending pictures and cards from their infant to show current status, arranging for transportation assistance through social service agencies for parents who lack means of travel (Kenner and Bagwell, 1998), and maintaining frequent phone contact with parents can be helpful in promoting parent-infant attachment (Brown et al., 1989).

P. **Give the mother the opportunity to provide breast milk** for the baby should she so desire, and support her in this endeavor. However, be careful not to overemphasize the importance of breast-feeding. The rationale is that if she should be unsuccessful or decide to stop breast-feeding, feelings of guilt or disappointment may occur if breast-feeding has been touted as the ideal infant feeding method (Kennell and Klaus, 1982, pp. 151–226).

Q. **Identify situations in which there are difficulties in parent-infant interaction or problems in the family's functioning** (Siegel et al., 1998).

R. **Be sensitive to cultural practices** that may influence parent-infant behaviors while bonding and attachment remain strong.

S. **Identify infants who are at risk of having developmental difficulties** (Siegel et al., 1998).

T. **Identify the unique needs of the parent with lower socioeconomic status.** This parent may want to provide the best possible care to the infant but either may not know how to do so (poor role models) or may not have the means to provide for the infant's perceived needs.

U. **Assess the cultural needs of minority parents.** This means to be culturally sensitive to what the parenting role means in that culture and then gear the interventions toward these cultural values and beliefs.

EVALUATION OF PARENT-INFANT BONDING

Evaluation of parental behaviors should be based on ongoing patterns rather than on isolated incidents (Mercer, 1977).

A. **Positive attachment behaviors (Kennell and Klaus, 1982).** The parent:
1. Visits frequently.
2. Has named the infant.
3. Makes positive comments when talking to or about the infant.
4. Demonstrates increasing skill in holding the infant.
5. Displays increasing eye and body contact between parent and infant (i.e., kissing, fondling, stroking, nuzzling).

B. **Behaviors of concern (Kennell and Klaus, 1982).** The parent:
1. Is overly optimistic.
2. Appears unconcerned about the infant's condition.
3. Does not ask questions.
4. Is passive or indifferent.
5. Avoids close body contact by holding the infant at a distance; props the bottle whether or not the infant is held; positions the bottle in such a way that milk is unable to flow from the nipple.
6. Is unable to describe any physical or behavioral features unique to the infant.
7. Attributes inappropriate characteristics to the infant, such as "she's lazy and stubborn just like her father" (Wallisch, 1983).

C. Make sure these areas of concern are considered within the context of the culture of the parents. Different cultures approach parenthood and parent-infant interaction in different ways.

Summary of Parental Needs to Be Met by NICU Staff

A. Help mother reconceptualize image of "ideal" infant to image of her premature, acutely ill, or malformed infant (Klaus and Kennell, 1982).

B. Help mother deal with feelings of guilt.

C. Help parents develop affectionate ties with infant through the infant's features (e.g., soft eyes; pretty, soft skin) and learn to read infant's behavioral cues.

D. Assist parents in gaining confidence in holding the infant by encouraging them to participate in caretaking tasks.

E. Promote communication between the parents.

F. Be sensitive to the unique needs of the individual families.

G. Assist families in preparing for the transition to home care after discharge (Kenner and Bagwell, 1998).

H. Provide support for parents during the transition phase after discharge of their infant from the NICU (Brooten et al., 1986; Butts et al., 1988; Gennaro and Stringer, 1991; Kenner and Bagwell, 1998).

I. Assist parents in dealing with neonatal death in a personally meaningful way.

J. Assist the parents in describing their cultural values and beliefs, if applicable, to understand their view of their infant and their role as parents.

Summary

A nurse who can remember what it was like to walk into an NICU the first time, and the feelings of helplessness, inadequacy, and powerlessness in that situation, can gain insight into the parents' perspective. In addition to the feelings that a health professional might have, however, the parents have the added burden of being emotionally attached to the infant, which adds to their fears. A positive resolution to the crisis of having a sick or premature neonate is seen if the parents have returned to their precrisis state of functioning, if they have grown from the experience, and if they are exhibiting positive coping behaviors. The nurse is pivotal in recognizing the family in crisis, anticipating the crisis, and preventing it from being a long-term problem.

REFERENCES

Alpers, R.R.: The changing self-concept of pregnant and parenting teens. J. Prof. Nurs., 14(2):111–118, 1998.

Bartram, J., Joffe, G.M., and Perry, L.: Prenatal environment: Effect on neonatal outcome. In Merenstein, G.B., and Gardner, S.L. (Eds.): Handbook of Neonatal Intensive Care, 4th ed. St. Louis, Mosby, 1998, pp. 9–29.

Blackburn, S.T., and VandenBerg, K.A.: Assessment and management of neonatal neurobehavioral development. In Kenner, C.A., Lott, J.W., and Flandermeyer, A.A. (Eds.): Comprehensive Neonatal Care: A Physiologic Perspective, 2nd ed. Philadelphia, W.B. Saunders, 1998, pp. 939–968.

Bracht, M., Ardal, F., Bot, A., and Cheng, C.M.: Initiation and maintenance of a hospital-based parent group for parents of premature infants: Key factors for success. Neonatal Network, 17(3):33–37, 1998.

Brooten, D., Kumar, S., Brown, L., et al.: A randomized clinical trial of early discharge and home follow-up of very low birthweight infants. N. Engl. J. Med., 315:934–939, 1986.

Broughton, S.M.: Sibling adaptation to the neonate. *In* Kenner, C., Lott, J.W., and Flandermeyer, A.A. (Eds.): Comprehensive Neonatal Care: A Physiologic Perspective, 2nd ed. Philadelphia, W.B. Saunders, 1998, pp. 69–72.

Brown, L.P., York, R., Jacobsen, B., et al.: Very low birth-weight infants: Parental visiting and telephoning during initial infant hospitalization. Nurs. Res., 38:233–236, 1989.

Butler, N.C.: The NICU culture versus the hospice culture: Can they mix? Neonatal Network, 5(2):35–42, 1986.

Butts, P.A., Brooten, D., Brown, L., et al.: Concerns of parents of low birthweight infants following hospital discharge: A report of parent-initiated telephone calls. Neonatal Network, 7(2):37–42, 1988.

Caplan, G.: Principles of Preventive Psychiatry. New York, Basic Books, 1964.

Gennaro, S., and Stringer, M.: Stress and health in low birthweight infants: A longitudinal study. Nurs. Res., 40(5):308–311, 1991.

Gray, K., Dostal, S., Ternullo-Retta, C., and Armstrong, M.A.: Developmentally supportive care in a neonatal intensive care unit: A research utilization project. Neonatal Network, 17(2):33–38, 1998.

Gretebeck, R.J., Shaffer, D., and Bishop-Kurylo, D.B.: Clinical pathways for family-oriented developmental care in the intensive care nursery. JPNN, 12(1):70–80, 1998.

Griffin, T.: The visitation policy. Neonatal Network, 17(2):75–76, 1998.

Jenkins, R.L., and Tock, M.K.S.: Helping parents bond to their premature infant. M.C.N.: Am. J. Matern. Child Nurs., 11:32–34, 1986.

Johnson-Crowley, N.: Systematic assessment and home follow-up: A basis for monitoring the neonate's integration into the family unit. *In* Kenner, C., Lott, J.W., and Flandermeyer, A.A. (Eds.): Comprehensive Neonatal Care: A Physiologic Perspective, 2nd ed. Philadelphia, W.B. Saunders, 1998, pp. 905–920.

Kennell, J.H., and Klaus, M.H.: Caring for the parents of premature or sick infants. *In* Klaus, M.H., and Kennell, J.H. (Eds.): Parent-Infant Bonding, 2nd ed. St. Louis, C.V. Mosby, 1982, pp. 151–226, 259–292.

Kenner, C., and Bagwell, G.A.: Assessment and management of the transition to home. *In* Kenner, C., Lott, J.W., and Flandermeyer, A.A. (Eds.): Comprehensive Neonatal Care: A Physiologic Perspective, 2nd ed. Philadelphia, W.B. Saunders, 1998, pp. 969–979.

Kleingbeil, C.G.: Extended nursing care after a perinatal loss: Theoretical implications. Neonatal Network, 5(3): 21–28, 1986.

Koshar, J.H., Lee, K.A., Goss, G., et al.: The Hispanic teen mother's origin of birth, use of prenatal care, and maternal and neonatal complications. J. Pediatr. Nurs., 13(3):151–157, 1998.

Krebs, T.L.: Clinical pathway for enhanced parent and preterm infant interaction through parent education. J. Pediatr. Nurs., 12:38–49, 1998.

Landon-Malone, K.A., Kirkpatrick, J.M., and Stull, S.P.: Incorporating hospice care in a community hospital NICU. Neonatal Network, 6(1):13–19, 1987.

Levin, B.: Grief counseling. Am. J. Nurs., 98(5):69–72, 1998.

Litchfield, M.D.: Family-infant bonding. *In* Vestal, K.W., and Mackenzie, C.A.M. (Eds.): High risk perinatal nursing. Philadelphia, W.B. Saunders, 1983, pp. 64–79.

Luddington-Hoe, S.M., Hadeed, A.J., and Anderson, G.C.: Physiologic responses to skin-to-skin contact in hospitalized premature infants. J. Perinatol., 11(1):19–24, 1991.

Mercer, R.T.: Nursing care for parents at risk. Thorofare, N.J., Charles B. Slack, 1977.

Miles, M.S., Holditch-Davis, D., and Shepherd, H.: Maternal concerns about parenting prematurely born children. M.C.N., Am. J. Matern. Child Nurs., 23(2):70–75, 1998.

Moore, M.L., and Freda, M.C.: Reducing preterm and low birthweight births: Still a nursing challenge. M.C.N.: Am. J. Matern. Child Nurs., 23(4):200–208, 1998.

Nurses Association of the American College of Obstetricians and Gynecologists: NAACOG Standards for the Nursing Care of Women and Newborns, 4th ed. Washington, D.C., Author, 1991.

Peppers, L.G., and Knapp, R.J.: Motherhood and Mourning: Perinatal Death. New York, Praeger, 1980.

Raines, D.A.: Values of mothers of low birth weight infants in the NICU. Neonatal Network, 17(6):41–64, 1998.

Siegel, R., Gardner, S.L., and Merenstein, G.B.: Families in crisis: Theoretical and practical considerations. *In* Merenstein, G.B., and Gardner, S.L. (Eds.): Handbook of Neonatal Care, 4th ed. St. Louis, Mosby, 1998, pp. 647–672.

Siegel, R., Rudd, S.H., Cleveland, C., et al.: A hospice approach to neonatal care. *In* Corr, C.A., and Corr, D.M. (Eds.): Hospice Approaches to Pediatric Care. New York, Springer, 1985, pp. 127–152.

Wallisch, S.: Stress: The infant, family, and nurse. In Vestal, K.W., and McKenzie, C.A.N. (Eds.): High Risk Perinatal Nursing. Philadelphia, W.B. Saunders, 1983, pp. 97–117.

Wereszczak, J., Miles, M.S., and Holditch-Davis, D.: Maternal recall of neonatal intensive care unit. Neonatal Network, 16(4):33–40, 1997.

Whitfield, J.M., Siegel, R.E., Glicken, A.D., et al.: The application of hospice concepts to neonatal care. Am. J. Dis. Child., 136:421–424, 1982.

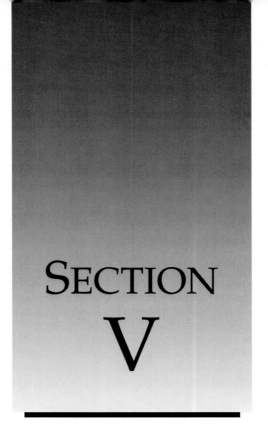

SECTION V

CLINICAL PRACTICE

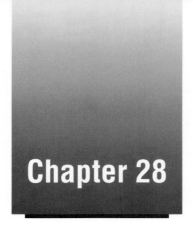

Chapter 28

Pharmacology in Neonatal Care

Roger G. Martin

Objectives

1. Describe nursing responsibilities and interventions when administering medications to the neonate.

2. Define the concepts of (a) pharmacotherapy, (b) drug, and (c) pharmacokinetics.

3. Describe the variables that may contribute to the response of a drug in the neonate.

4. Describe differences of absorption, distribution, metabolism, and excretion between an adult and a neonate.

5. Identify specific considerations when one is administering drugs of the following types to a neonate: (a) antimicrobial agents, (b) cardiovascular agents, (c) diuretics, and (d) central nervous system agents.

The study and clinical application of neonatal pharmacology can facilitate safe medication administration in the neonate. The application of pharmacologic principles involves evaluating existing knowledge related to the pharmaco-dynamic and pharmacokinetic responses of the neonate to specific drugs. This knowledge must be considered relative to gestational and chronologic age, weight, fluid status, and the health-illness state of individual organ systems. The decision to administer a medication should be evaluated for desired response and potential for undesirable reaction. The nurse is in the ideal position to observe and evaluate both response and reaction and to intervene if necessary.

This chapter provides pharmacologic information specific to the neonate. Information on drug dosages and implications for drug administration is provided in individual clinical chapters. Additional current reference materials should also be available in the neonatal intensive care unit.

Principles of Pharmacology

TERMINOLOGY

A. Pharmacology.

1. The science studying the actions of chemicals on living systems and molecules.

2. The study of the origins, nature, and effects of drugs on human beings or animals.

B. Pharmacotherapy.

1. A branch of pharmacology that focuses on the study of drugs or chemicals used to prevent, diagnose, or treat disease.
2. The administration of a drug or drugs to a patient with the intent of achieving a specific response. This response is limited to augmentation, abolition, or modulation of a normal physiologic process.

C. Drug.

1. Any substance or mixture of substances intended to be used for the cure, mitigation, or prevention of disease in human beings or animals.
2. A nonfood substance that affects living protoplasm.

D. Pharmacodynamics: the study of how chemicals produce their biologic effects on living tissue.

E. Pharmacokinetics.

1. The specialized study of the mathematical relationship between a drug dosage regimen and the resulting serum concentration.
2. The study of the time course of absorption, distribution, metabolism, and excretion of a drug in human beings or animals.

F. Bioavailability: the portion of the administered dose that reaches the systemic circulation.

G. Therapeutic index: the range of drug concentration between a beneficial drug effect or response and a toxic or overdose response.

H. Half-life: the time necessary for a measured drug concentration to fall to half its original value at the start of the interval.

PHARMACODYNAMICS

A. Receptor concept: the principle that drugs act by forming a complex with a specific macromolecule in a way that alters that molecule's function. This alteration in function may include inhibition or potentiation of the macromolecule's activity to create the desired drug effect. Receptor effects are as follows:

1. The drug's affinity for binding to the receptor plays a large part in the determination of the concentration of the drug required to achieve the desired response.
2. The individual characteristics of the receptor are responsible for the selective nature of drug response.
3. Receptor theory of drug action allows an explanation of drug antagonists. The antagonist drug may alter the characteristics of the receptor molecule in a way that then limits or inhibits the response to the original drug.
4. Some drugs do not appear to act through receptors. Their action is related to a direct response in the recipient.

B. General mechanisms of drug action.

1. Based on the nature of the receptor/drug complex.
2. Types of receptor/drug complexes.
   a. Receptor/drug complexes that regulate gene expression.
      (1) One common class of drugs acts by mediating a response that ultimately involves gene expression and new protein synthesis.
      (2) These drugs generally do not have a rapid effect after initial administration.

   b. Some receptor/drug complexes change cell membrane permeability.
      (1) Many clinically useful drugs act by changing the cell membrane permeability and therefore altering all membrane characteristics.
      (2) These drugs may have a very short time lag between administration and response.
   c. Some receptor/drug complexes increase the intracellular concentration of a second messenger molecule.
      (1) These drugs increase production and activity of enzyme systems within the cell.
      (2) These drugs may stimulate a rapid response in changing cell characteristics.

C. **Relationship between drug dose and clinical response.**

1. Individuals in a population receiving a medication may have a wide range of responses to a drug dose. An idiosyncratic drug response is an abnormal response to a drug that is not usually observed. These unpredictable responses include the following:
   a. Low sensitivity: a patient who, on receiving the usual drug dose, exhibits a clinical or biologic response that is less intense than is usually observed.
   b. Extreme sensitivity: a patient whose response to a drug is more intense than is usually observed.
   c. Unpredictable adverse reaction: a patient whose drug reaction is substantially different from what would have been predicted; for example, the patient's physiologic response to a particular drug may differ from the usual response in most patients.
   d. Tolerance: a diminished response to a given drug dosage that is related to long-term administration of a drug.
   e. Tachyphylaxis: a rapidly diminished drug response without a drug dosage change. This may be caused by any of a number of factors, including a limited number of receptor sites or limited numbers of transmitter chemicals.

2. Factors that may affect individual drug response are:
   a. Alterations in drug concentration: a change from the expected norm in the amount of drug that reaches the receptor molecule.
   b. Variation in amounts of antagonistic substances: an unusually large or limited amount of antagonistic substances that alter receptor molecule response.
   c. Alterations in numbers or function of receptor molecules: an increased or diminished number of receptor molecules changes the number of potential drug/receptor complexes.
   d. Changes in concentration of molecules other than receptor molecules: if drug response is ultimately dependent on an effect on molecules other than those of the drug/receptor complex, drug response may be limited by the amount of the third molecule type.

D. **Desired versus undesired effects of medications.**

1. No drug causes only one effect: all drugs have several effects, which can be divided into three groups.
   a. Desired, or therapeutic, effects: those effects that are the desired outcome of the drug administration.
   b. Side effects: those drug effects that result from drug administration and that are in addition to the desired effects. All drugs have some side effects, varying from minor and clinically insignificant to major side effects that are sufficiently adverse to require discontinuation of the drug therapy.
   c. Toxic effects: drug response that results from a drug overdose or unexpected high serum drug concentrations.

2. It is the responsibility of the health care provider to weigh the benefits of the therapeutic effect against the undesirable side effects and the risk of toxic effects and make adjustments accordingly.

PHARMACOKINETICS

A. Principles of drug absorption (Fig. 28–1).

1. General principles of drug absorption.
   a. The movement of a drug from the site of administration to the bloodstream or other site of action.
   b. Regardless of the route of administration, all drugs must cross cell membranes to reach their site of action.
      (1) Most drugs cross cell membranes by passive diffusion. Physicochemical properties of the drug molecule have a major impact on the ease of diffusion.
      (2) Drugs may also enter the cell through other mechanisms, such as active transport or facilited diffusion.
   c. The absorption of a drug is dependent, in large part, on the site of administration. The common sites of administration are:
      (1) Gastrointestinal (GI): commonly used because of convenience.

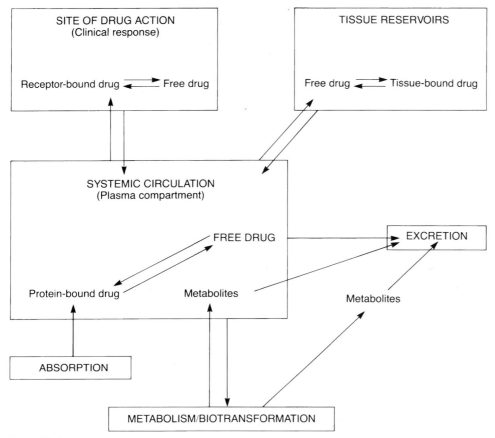

Figure 28–1
Components of drug movement, or pharmacokinetics—absorption, metabolism, and excretion—and diagrammatic indication of drug distribution.

(a) Large surface and large absorption area of the GI tract favor absorption.

(b) Presence of marked changes in pH from the stomach through the distal portion of the GI tract, pancreatic and other digestive enzymes, and intestinal bacterial flora may affect absorption.

(c) Oral administration of a drug may result in movement of the absorbed drug directly from the intestinal absorption site to the liver, where the drug may be metabolized and excreted in significant amounts. This "first pass" effect limits the bioavailability of the drug.

(d) Time of response varies, depending on drug absorption characteristics, but is generally delayed.

(2) Inhalation: useful for gaseous or easily vaporized drugs.

(a) Large surface area of the alveolar membranes and the generous blood flow favor absorption.

(b) Medications administered by this route have a particular advantage when the site of desired action is the tracheobronchial tree.

(c) Drug response may be very rapid.

(d) Inhalation of certain drugs (e.g., epinephrine, atropine, lidocaine) is useful in some emergency situations when IV access is not readily available.

(3) Topical: utility limited to drugs whose absorptive characteristics allow permeation through the skin or mucous membranes.

(a) Response may be limited to local area of application.

(b) Some topically applied medications (e.g., nitroglycerin) can have a systemic effect.

(c) Rate of absorption is inversely related to membrane thickness and directly related to membrane water content.

(d) Response time is variable.

(4) Intramuscular: administration into muscle body.

(a) Bypasses most absorptive barriers.

(b) Limited to drugs that do not cause tissue damage at administration site and are soluble at physiologic pH.

(c) Slower response because of time lag between administration and achievement of blood concentration.

(d) Response time is dependent on blood flow to muscle and may be greatly delayed in hypoperfused tissue.

(5) Subcutaneous: administration into the subcutaneous tissue.

(a) Bypasses most absorptive barriers.

(b) Slower response to achieve significant blood levels.

(c) Limited types and volumes of drug.

(d) Dependent on local blood flow; possible significant delay in hypoperfusion states.

(6) Intravenous: direct administration into the bloodstream.

(a) Bypasses all absorptive barriers.

(b) Hazardous. Large amount of drug may be delivered directly both to the target organs and to other tissues.

(c) Very rapid response.

2. Drug absorption in the neonate.

a. Oral absorption.

(1) GI surface area. Structurally the neonatal GI tract has a greater ratio of surface area to body mass. This provides a more absorptive surface area (Nagourney and Aranda, 1992).

(2) Immature GI system. Some substances may be absorbed at a higher rate. Few studies exist that quantify rates of GI absorption in neonates.

(3) Gastric emptying and intestinal transit times. These may be prolonged; they normally reach adult values at 6–8 months of age.
  (a) Gastric and intestinal motility is dependent on gestational age, illness state, oral intake, and composition of feeding. Gastroesophageal reflux is common, particularly in premature neonates; its net effect is the delay of gastric emptying time.
  (b) Net effect of prolonged GI transit times appears to be, in most cases, increased absorption, in comparison with that of adults (Nagourney and Aranda, 1992).
  (c) May also decrease bioavailability because of increased first-pass loss or increased GI destruction of drug.
  (d) Low transit times and enterohepatic recirculation may also increase the bioavailability and pharmacologic effect of some substances (Chemtob, 1992).
(4) Gastrointestinal tract acidity: a major determinant of drug absorption.
  (a) pH of GI tract nearly neutral at birth.
  (b) May not begin to reach normal adult values until 2 weeks of age and may not completely reach adult pH values of 1–3 until 6 to 8 months of age (Aranda, Hales, and Reider, 1992).
  (c) Gastric pH is dependent on extrauterine factors. In healthy term neonates, gastric pH is high in the first 12 hours. It then normalizes rapidly after the initiation of oral feedings (Nahata, 1996).
  (d) Premature neonates born at less than 32 weeks' gestation have diminished gastric acid secretion, which appears to increase as a function more of postnatal age than of gestational age (Nagourney and Aranda, 1992).
  (e) The net effect of GI acidity is dependant on pH characteristics of the drug and preparation. Drugs that normally may not be absorbed well in the stomach may be absorbed at a higher rate in the neonate because of decreased stomach acidity (e.g., oral insulin has been shown to be absorbed well in the first minutes of life, whereas phenytoin exhibits decreased GI absorption in neonates because of increased pH of the GI tract) (Roberts, 1984).
(5) Pancreatic enzyme function.
  (a) Neonates are deficient in pancreatic enzymes at birth.
  (b) This deficiency may inhibit absorption of some medications that require pancreatic enzymes for efficient absorption.
(6) Beta-glucuronidase: an enzyme in the neonatal GI tract that may be present up to seven times the adult amounts.
  (a) This enzyme deconjugates medications metabolized by the liver. Deconjugated drug may then become available for reabsorption.
  (b) May cause a prolonged drug effect through reabsorption and for that reason may delay excretion.
(7) Bacterial flora: composition and rate of colonization of the GI tract by the normal bacterial flora may affect both GI tract motility and the metabolism of some drugs (Nagourney and Aranda, 1992).
  (a) The significance of this effect is highly variable. It is dependent on oral intake and other factors such as antibiotic administration.
  (b) Normal colonization in vaginally born, well, term neonates occurs by 4–6 days of age.
(8) GI tract perfusion: in very ill neonates, hypoperfusion of the gut may decrease drug absorption.
(9) Illness states: some may significantly alter absorption. Diseases of genetic (e.g., cystic fibrosis) or circulatory (e.g., necrotizing enterocolitis) origin will alter intestinal mucosa and may either increase or decrease GI absorption.

b. Rectal absorption. May be a very efficient means of drug administration to a neonate.
   (1) Serum levels of some drugs may be as high as, or higher than, levels obtained through other routes of administration (Roberts, 1984).
   (2) Relative volume and fragility of the neonatal rectum must be considered.
c. Inhalation.
   (1) Good route for administration of medications (e.g., albuterol, terbutaline) whose desired site of action is the tracheobronchial tree.
   (2) May be less effective in a newborn infant with pulmonary hypertension and poor or abnormally distributed pulmonary blood flow.
   (3) Provides an excellent route for administration of some drugs (e.g., epinephrine) used for resuscitation when vascular access is not readily available.
   (4) Used with increasing frequency in neonatal intensive care for the administration of various surfactant preparations.
d. Topical absorption. Percutaneous absorption has particular advantages and risks in the newborn infant.
   (1) With increasing gestational age, skin thickness increases and water content decreases.
   (2) Maturation of the epidermis occurs between 23 and 33 weeks' gestation. In the extremely premature neonate, the stratum corneum is almost absent. It forms during the first 2–3 weeks after birth. Formation of this layer of the skin has a major impact on the permeability of the skin to water and other substances (Nagourney and Aranda, 1992).
   (3) With increasing gestational age, the ratio of skin surface area to weight decreases, providing relatively less absorptive surface in comparison with body mass.
   (4) This allows much more efficient percutaneous absorption of drugs in neonates of lower birth weight and younger gestational age.
   (5) Poses a particular hazard in care, because substances that may be safely applied to the skin of a more mature patient may be absorbed in dangerous amounts in the immature neonate (Nahata, 1996).
e. Intramuscular/subcutaneous absorption.
   (1) Absorption is dependent on local blood flow and muscle activity, which may be affected by many factors in the neonate.
      (a) Poor peripheral blood flow and low blood pressure are common in newborn infants. These problems become less common with increasing gestational age but can occur in the presence of many neonatal disease states.
      (b) Poor cardiac output frequently occurs with many illness states in the neonatal period.
      (c) Subsequent increases in peripheral perfusion after resolution of primary illness states may put the newborn infant at risk of having an increase in the rate and amount of drug absorption.
      (d) Diminished muscle activity in the ill neonate decreases muscle perfusion and consequently may limit absorption of drugs administered by this route.
   (2) Minimal subcutaneous tissue and muscle mass significantly limit these two routes of administration, particularly in the low birth weight newborn infant.
f. Intravenous absorption.
   (1) Bypasses all absorptive barriers.
   (2) Most effective and reliable method of drug administration. Drug is delivered directly to the circulating plasma volume. Most drugs administered to neonates during the acute phase of illness are given by this route.

(3) Significant serum drug concentrations reached rapidly, allowing for immediate potential drug response. This includes both desired and undesired or toxic reactions.

(4) Adequate and equal distribution to all organs or compartments is not guaranteed. Characteristics of some biologic membranes may limit drug distribution to body compartments (e.g., cerebrospinal fluid with meningitis).

(5) Rapid achievement of potentially dangerous serum drug concentrations may require administration of the intravenous medication over a prolonged period.

B. **Principles of drug distribution.**

1. Distribution: movement of the absorbed drug to and through various body compartments. The extent of this movement, the "size" of the compartment, the number and character of the binding sites, and the amount of the drug administered determine the amount of drug at the desired site of action. When drug movement reaches a steady state, the volume of distribution is defined as the hypothetical volume of body fluid that would be required to dissolve the total amount of drug as found in the serum. This volume is sometimes described as apparent volume of distribution. This volume may be larger than the total body volume if the drug is highly protein or tissue bound.

2. Body compartments.
   a. Total body water: approximately 0.70–0.75 L/kg (70–75% of body weight) in the well term neonate.
   b. Extracellular water: approximately 0.35 L/kg (35% of body weight) in the well term neonate (Nagourney and Aranda, 1992). Large water-soluble molecules are distributed through this space. Because most drugs have some water solubility, they can dissolve and be transported by blood and body fluids to their site of action. As a result, the changes in body water that commonly occur in the ill neonate have an effect on a wide range of medications given in the NICU.
   c. Intracellular water: space divided from the rest of the water compartments by the cell membrane.
   d. Intravascular water: approximately 0.10 L/kg (10% of body weight) in the well term neonate. Very large or tightly protein-bound molecules are distributed through this space.
   e. Fat: wide variability of neonatal values, based on gestational age and intrauterine/postnatal growth patterns. Body fat percentages also vary widely in neonates. This percentage increases from 1% of body weight at 28 weeks' gestation to approximately 15% in an appropriately grown term neonate (Chemtob, 1992; Nagourney and Aranda, 1992). Drugs with more lipid solubility have affinity for this space. If lipid solubility is less, drugs are not as readily distributed.
   f. Bone: neonatal values not available. Certain ions are distributed in this space, but most are not distributed in significant amounts.

3. Protein-binding sites.
   a. Drugs may also form a complex with other large circulating molecules (usually proteins). This binding to molecules may result in an undesirable drug response because only unbound drug can be distributed to active receptor sites.
   b. The amount of drug that binds to these sites has a direct effect on the amount of drug available for the desired pharmacologic effect. The more of the drug that is protein bound, the less it is available for the desired drug effect.
   c. Primary binding protein for acidic drugs in the serum is albumin. Albumin has several binding sites, a few with high affinity and several with low affinity (Nagourney and Aranda, 1992).

    d. The primary binding proteins for basic molecules are lipoproteins, glyco-proteins, and beta-globulins (Chemtob, 1992).

    e. This binding may also have the effect of displacing another drug or substance, freeing it for action with another receptor.

4. Drug movement: dependent on the following two factors:

    a. Blood flow: amount and distribution of blood flow to the target organ or cell affect the delivery of a drug absorbed into the bloodstream. Continued adequate blood flow is required to maintain an adequate concentration of the drug at the target organ.

    b. Drug solubility: in biologic tissues, the relative ability of the drug to dissolve in biologic fluids. Defined by how readily the drug dissolves into the specific tissue and/or body fluids.

      (1) Drugs with low lipid solubility are not distributed well through lipid membranes, though they may be distributed well through the body water spaces. Highly lipid-soluble drugs are distributed readily through most lipid membranes but are not distributed well through body water spaces.

      (2) The relative drug solubility may make some drug use inappropriate. A drug with low lipid solubility will not reach high concentrations in an organ that is primarily fat.

5. Drug distribution in the neonate.

    a. Body compartments: significant differences in distribution of body mass in the neonate.

      (1) Total body water. As gestational age increases, total body water, as a percentage of total body mass, decreases.

        (a) As body water, as a percentage of body mass, increases, water-soluble drugs have a larger volume of distribution.

        (b) Because of increased total body water, a less mature neonate may then require a larger per-kilogram dose to achieve the same drug concentration and effect as an older patient.

        (c) Changing amounts of body percentage of body fat may make the volume of distribution smaller for drugs distributed primarily through fatty tissue because of high lipid solubility.

      (2) Extracellular water. The percentage of this physiologic volume increases transiently in the first few days of life. This has an additive effect on the volume of distribution for some drugs.

      (3) Volume of distribution. In the first several days after birth, neonates may have rapid changes in volume of distribution for water-soluble drugs, in relation to normal physiology and illness states.

        (a) Healthy term and preterm neonates have marked decreases in total body water volume, in both absolute terms and in the percentage of total body weight (Heimann, 1992).

        (b) Body water loss is divided into two main categories: sensible and insensible. Sensible losses can be measured and quantified. In term neonates, insensible losses occur in a strong relationship to metabolism. In extremely premature neonates, insensible losses occur primarily through evaporative loss, independant of metabolic rate, and are difficult to quantify (Chemtob, 1992).

        (c) Drugs frequently administered to the neonate (e.g., diuretics) may have a major impact on body water volume and, as a side effect, may alter volume of distribution (Chemtob, 1992).

        (d) Neonates with disease states that alter water excretion (e.g., primary renal disease, secretion of inappropriate antidiuretic hormone [SIADH], congestive heart failure, capillary leak syndromes) may have expansion of body water as a result of this dysfunction.

    (e) The preceding alterations make drug dosing with medications that are primarily distributed in body water (e.g., aminoglycoside antibiotics such as gentamicin) difficult.

    (f) Frequent monitoring of drug levels may be required as the mentioned changes in body compartment volumes occur.

  b. **Protein binding.** Several factors influence protein binding.

    (1) In premature and ill neonates, total plasma protein levels are decreased.

      (a) This diminishes the potential for circulating plasma protein/drug complexes.

      (b) Serum albumin levels, as the primary serum binding protein, may be markedly decreased in the ill, extremely low birth weight neonate.

      (c) Binding sites are limited in number and affinity.

      (d) Net effect is to allow more free drug at the same serum concentration. May allow more drug action by formation of a receptor-drug complex.

      (e) May allow desired drug response at lower serum concentrations: Serum concentration = Protein-bound drug + Unbound drug.

    (2) Many neonates have increased plasma unconjugated bilirubin levels.

      (a) Unconjugated bilirubin has been shown to displace some drugs from albumin-binding sites, which allows more free drug for action.

      (b) In contrast, some drugs may displace unconjugated bilirubin from albumin-binding sites. This may promote kernicterus because of increased free, unconjugated bilirubin concentrations.

    (3) Increased serum free fatty acid concentrations have been shown to displace some drugs from plasma albumin-binding sites (Chemtob, 1992).

    (4) Blood pH.

      (a) Acidosis is a common finding associated with many neonatal disorders.

      (b) Changes in blood pH have been shown to change albumin-binding characteristics. This may cause drug displacement from albumin.

      (c) Changes in blood pH may also cause drugs to displace unconjugated bilirubin (see above).

    (5) Maternal drugs may cross the placenta and compete for albumin binding sites.

    (6) Some drugs have affinity to binding sites outside the vascular space (e.g., digoxin to myocardial and skeletal muscle proteins). This increases the volume of distribution (Chemtob, 1992).

  c. **Drug movement.** An important part of drug distribution involves drug movement from the site of administration to sites throughout the body.

    (1) Drug movement is dependent on local blood flow.

    (2) Several neonatal conditions affect blood flow.

      (a) Hypotension: may affect peripheral drug absorption and/or distribution.

      (b) Distributive shock: caused by inappropriate vasodilation; seen with septicemia. Drug distribution to specific organs may be limited by local underperfusion.

      (c) Pulmonary hypertension: may impede drug delivery to pulmonary vascular bed.

      (d) Patent ductus arteriosus: blood flow may be distributed preferentially to either the pulmonary or systemic circulation, depending on pressure differential.

      (e) Congestive heart failure: may affect peripheral drug absorption or distribution.

C. Principles of drug metabolism.

1. General principles of drug metabolism. Metabolism (biotransformation) is the *chemical change* of a drug into another form. This transformed drug may be pharmacologically active or inactive. Sites of metabolism include:
   a. Liver: the primary organ of drug metabolism.
      (1) Metabolic activity is divided into two main types.
         (a) Phase I (nonsynthetic) metabolism of drugs: primarily oxidation, reduction, hydrolysis, or hydroxylation reactions, which generally occur in the smooth endoplasmic reticulum of the hepatocyte.
         (b) Phase II (synthetic) metabolism of drugs: primarily involves conjugation of the drug with another substance.
      (2) Hepatic uptake of the drug is dependent on the concentration of the drug in the liver (dependent on hepatic blood flow) and the hepatocyte concentration of ligandin (Y-protein). This protein is responsible for substrate uptake by hepatic cells.
      (3) In the first-pass effect, hepatic biotransformation may markedly alter drug availability by directly metabolizing drugs absorbed from the GI tract, before those drugs reach other organs.
   b. Kidney, intestine, lung, adrenal gland, and skin are also tissues capable of biotransformation of certain compounds. These sites of metabolism are much more limited.

2. Metabolism/biotransformation in the neonate.
   a. Phase I enzyme systems. Concentration of enzymes appears to be adequate in the term neonate.
      (1) Function may be markedly reduced.
      (2) Maturation occurs as a function of chronologic rather than postconceptional age, with a wide range of variability.
      (3) Maturation of nonsynthetic enzyme systems during the first several days requires careful monitoring of serum levels of some classes of medications (e.g., anticonvulsants). At term gestation, neonates have approximately 30% of adult ability to metabolize phenytoin. Half-life is significantly prolonged. Within several weeks of drug exposure, metabolic enzyme activity for phenytoin surpasses adult activity.
      (4) Certain drugs (e.g., phenobarbital) are thought to induce enzyme maturity in the fetus and neonate. This is the basis for the administration of phenobarbital as an adjunct treatment or as prophylaxis for hyperbilirubinemia (Nagourney and Aranda, 1992).
   b. Phase II enzyme systems.
      (1) Also immature, according to data on clinical drug transformation and excretion.
      (2) May not reach adult levels in concentration and function until well after the neonatal period.
      (3) Both enzyme systems may be vulnerable to hypoxic-ischemic insult.
   c. Synthetic metabolism: unique aspects in the neonate.
      (1) The major metabolic pathway of theophylline in the neonate is methylation to caffeine. The caffeine is then eliminated slowly because its half-life is long.
      (2) The major metabolic pathway in the adult is demethylation of caffeine to theophylline. Theophylline is eliminated unchanged and therefore has a relatively short half-life.
      (3) Because caffeine elimination is slow, half-life in neonates is prolonged until several months of age, when the "adult" demethylation metabolic pathway develops (Aranda et al., 1992).

d. Ligandin (Y-protein): the protein responsible for substrate intake by the hepatocytes.
   (1) Concentrations low at birth.
   (2) May reach near adult values during the neonatal period (Roberts, 1984).
e. First-pass effect: poor GI motility may increase the potential for first-pass effect. Prolonged GI transit times may increase potential for hepatic metabolism and eventual excretion of orally administered drugs (see gastrointestinal absorption of drugs, subsection c, in section A, Principles of Drug Absorption, under Pharmacokinetics above).
f. Maturational changes in drug metabolism: major clinical significance. Careful monitoring of serum levels of some drug classes (e.g., anticonvulsants, methylxanthines) is necessary in the first weeks of life.

D. **Principles of drug excretion.**

1. General principles of drug excretion. Excretion is the final elimination of drug from the body. The process of excretion begins with administration of the drug and ends when the drug is completely eliminated from the body. There are several important organs of excretion:
   a. Minor organs. Small amounts of drugs may be excreted through salivary, sweat, and mammary glands.
   b. Lungs. The lungs are an important route of excretion of gaseous anesthetics but are relatively less important for other drugs.
   c. GI tract. The large, lipid-soluble surface of the GI tract allows diffusion of drugs from the bloodstream.
   d. Liver. The most important site of drug biotransformation also serves as an important site of drug excretion. The excretion of bile is an important means of drug elimination.
      (1) Conditions that limit bile flow may limit the efficacy of this elimination.
      (2) Metabolite or drug elimination in bile is dependent on solubility characteristics of that substance in bile.
   e. Kidneys. The primary method of drug elimination involves two processes:
      (1) Glomerular filtration: the removal, by passive filtration, of small unbound drug molecules at the glomerulus. Glomerular filtration is dependent on renal blood flow and the characteristics of the glomerular membranes.
      (2) Tubular secretion: the active secretion of large or protein-bound molecules into the tubular urine. Tubular secretion is dependent on the efficiency of tubular function.
      (3) Tubular reabsorption: significant renal tubular reabsorption, for some drugs, back into the circulating plasma. Renal clearance = (Filtration clearance + Secretion clearance) × (1 – Fraction reabsorbed).
2. Excretion in the neonate.
   a. Minor organs. Very limited sweat production makes excretion by this mode insignificant.
   b. Lungs.
      (1) Excretion by the lungs is not well studied in the neonatal population.
      (2) Lung disease common in newborn infants. Adult data indicate that this may affect or limit the ability to excrete medications by this method.
   c. GI tract. Limited motility affects excretion and increases the potential for reabsorption of drugs or metabolites back into the circulation.
   d. Liver.
      (1) Limited oral intake, long-term parenteral nutrition, or intrinsic hepatic disease may reduce bile flow.
      (2) Reduces the efficacy of this route.

e. Kidney.
  (1) Renal blood flow.
    (a) Clamping of the umbilical cord is a significant event that signals a major increase in renal blood flow, although, as a percentage of cardiac output, renal blood flow is limited in neonates in comparison with older children and adults.
    (b) Limited renal blood flow as an absolute value and as a percentage of cardiac output restricts drug or metabolite delivery to the kidney for excretion.
    (c) Renal blood flow increases with increasing gestational and postnatal age.
  (2) Glomerular filtration: extremely limited compared with adult values (30% of adult values, per unit of body surface area; reaches adult values by 3–5 months of age).
    (a) Significantly decreased in the neonate; rate is inversely related to gestational age.
    (b) Neonates born at less than 34 weeks' gestation have fewer glomeruli, with total glomerular mass inversely proportional to gestational age (John and Guignard, 1992).
    (c) Limited glomerular filtration reduces removal of drugs or metabolites at the glomerulus.
    (d) Glomerular filtration has been shown to mature with postnatal age, independent of gestational age at birth.
    (e) Drug excretion dependent on glomerular filtration includes aminoglycosides, indomethacin, and digoxin.
  (3) Tubular secretion.
    (a) Neonates have a relatively small mass of functional tubular cells, as well as immaturity of tubular function. This function limitation is thought to be caused in part by a decrease of renal blood flow to the renal tubular region and in part by shortened renal tubules (John and Guignard, 1992; Nagourney and Aranda, 1992).
    (b) This limitation in tubular mass and function causes poor excretion of drugs and metabolites removed by this method.
    (c) Tubular secretion matures much more slowly than glomerular filtration.
    (d) Tubular secretion is vulnerable to hypoxic-ischemic insult.
    (e) Drugs dependent on tubular secretion for excretion include penicillins, furosemide, and thiazide diuretics.
  (4) Tubular absorption.
    (a) May occur through either passive diffusion or active transport.
    (b) Passive diffusion appears to be the most important process.
    (c) Drugs dependent on tubular absorption for elimination include aminoglycosides and caffeine.
  (5) Urinary flow.
    (a) Because of changes in renal blood flow, glomerular filtration, and tubular secretion in the neonate, urinary output is not a reliable sign of renal excretion of drugs.
    (b) Blood level monitoring is required to ensure safe serum levels of renally excreted medications.

Drug Categories

ANTIMICROBIAL AGENTS

A. **Variety of antimicrobial drugs.** The use of a larger variety of antimicrobial agents in the newborn population has occurred in the last several years because of advancing clinical sophistication in the use of antimicrobial drugs as well as an expanding body of knowledge on the use of such agents in the newborn population.

B. Definitions.

1. Antimicrobial drugs: medications that inhibit the growth of or kill microorganisms; include antibacterial agents, antifungal agents, and antiviral agents.
   a. Bacteriostatic drugs: agents that inhibit the growth of microorganisms, preventing their growth and allowing normal body defense mechanisms to control spread of the organism.
   b. Bactericidal drugs: agents whose primary purpose is to kill microorganisms. At lower concentrations, they may be bacteriostatic.
2. Antibiotics are a class of antibacterial agents that are produced from other species of microorganisms (e.g., penicillin). Other antimicrobials are chemically altered or synthetic substances.
3. Minimal inhibitory concentration (MIC): the lowest concentration of a drug that stops visible spread of organism growth in a laboratory setting. In vivo, this cannot be directly measured and is dependent on achieved tissue concentration and numbers of bacteria present.
4. Minimal bactericidal concentration (MBC): lowest concentration of a drug that results in 99.9% or greater decline in microbial number, measured in laboratory setting. Useful, when compared with known potential toxic concentration levels, in choosing antimicrobial regimen that does the greatest good with minimal adverse or toxic effects.
5. Resistance: the ability of microorganisms to counteract the bacteriostatic or bactericidal effects of an antimicrobial agent.
   a. Resistance may occur when the chromosomal makeup of the organism has changed or mutated.
   b. Resistance interferes with drug action either through changes in the microorganism's cellular structure or through production of enzymes that reduce antimicrobial activity.

C. Basic principles of antimicrobial use.

1. Must reach target tissue in a concentration adequate to inhibit the growth of or to kill the desired microorganism.
   a. This concentration ideally would be such that it would have limited side effects or toxic effects on target tissues or the patient as a whole.
   b. This concentration must be readily achievable and sustainable for the desired duration of antimicrobial therapy.
2. Choice of antimicrobial regimen must take into account.
   a. Microorganism sensitivity to available antimicrobial agents.
   b. Relative permeability of the target tissue to agent of choice.
   c. Bioactivity of chosen antimicrobial agent in target tissue.
   d. Known MIC/MBC in relation to existing body of knowledge concerning side effects and toxic effects in the specific population.
   e. Specific characteristics of the individual patient in relation to the chosen antimicrobial's pharmacokinetics (e.g., in a patient with impaired renal function, a nephrotoxic antimicrobial should be avoided if possible).

D. Specific considerations in newborn population.

1. Pharmacodynamics.
   a. Tissue concentration of drug may be altered by clinical and physiologic conditions that may increase or decrease bioavailability of the drug in the target tissue. (For example, cerebrospinal fluid penetration by antibiotics

may be excellent early in meningitis. As meningeal inflammatory response subsides, penetration of the cerebrospinal fluid diminishes.)

b. Differences in response or potential for toxic effects may result from immaturity and/or illness state.

2. Pharmacokinetics.

a. In seriously ill neonates, greater consideration must be made for clinical status than for gestational or chronologic age.

b. Absorption.

(1) Changes in GI tract pH affect absorption of oral medication: may be increased or decreased (e.g., oral penicillin G is absorbed better in neonates than in older infants and children because of increased gastric pH).

(2) Changes in skin permeability in the extremely immature neonate may allow topically applied antimicrobial agents to be absorbed systemically.

c. Distribution.

(1) Decreasing body water and increasing body fat concentration in more mature neonates affect the volume through which the antimicrobial agent is distributed. This may make dosage adjustments necessary in the first days of life.

(2) Blood flow changes may affect absorption and distribution of antimicrobials administered intramuscularly or subcutaneously (e.g., repeated intramuscular administration of aminoglycosides to premature babies may result in local tissue damage and unacceptably variable rates of absorption).

d. Metabolism. Limited hepatic function, because of immaturity or an illness state, may affect dosage regimen of some antibiotics, requiring smaller or less frequent doses of some antibiotics (e.g., nafcillin, erythromycin).

e. Excretion. Limited renal function with lower gestational age may prolong half-life of antimicrobials (e.g., aminoglycosides, cephalosporins, penicillin) excreted by the kidneys. This limited renal function (glomerular filtration rate and tubular secretion) commonly improves significantly in the first few days of life and with advancing chronologic age. For this reason, serum antibiotic levels must be monitored closely and dosage adjustments made accordingly.

DIURETICS

A. Introduction.

1. Commonly used in both acute and long-term neonatal intensive care to promote the removal of excessive extracellular fluid.

2. Site of action of nearly all diuretic agents is the luminal surface of the renal tubular cell.

B. Basic principles of diuretic use.

1. Use must be based on a thorough understanding of function of the various segments of the nephron in the neonatal population.

2. Diuretic drugs whose primary purpose is to cause the excretion of excess extracellular fluid commonly cause a secondary or side effect of loss of electrolytes, along with the desired water loss. Knowledge of specific action for each diuretic drug will assist the clinician in monitoring electrolytes for undesirable losses.

3. Pharmacologic response is dependent on the existing level of renal function and on the drug's ability to reach the target tissue in amounts adequate to produce the desired diuretic effect.

4. Any drug or other therapy that increases glomerular filtration rate may have an indirect diuretic effect. Some drugs that act on the cardiovascular system to increase cardiac output or increase renal blood flow through vasodilation may cause diuresis. Maximal water and electrolyte excretion usually occurs in the first days of use. Later, decreased glomerular filtration rate and hyperaldosteronism resulting from diuretic-induced hypovolemia limit these losses.

C. **Specific considerations in the newborn population.**

1. Pharmacodynamics.
   a. Renal tubular function is limited in all neonates and is more limited in less mature neonates.
   b. Clinical response to diuretic agents is commonly affected because of existing poor renal tubular absorption. Limited tubular function potentiates electrolyte loss with many diuretic agents (e.g., furosemide, chlorothiazide).
2. Pharmacokinetics.
   a. Absorption. Oral absorption may be limited, requiring a larger per kilogram dose (e.g., of furosemide) to achieve the desired effect. Others (e.g., chlorothiazide) are absorbed well orally.
   b. Distribution. Some diuretic medications are strongly protein bound. Some concern has been raised over displacement of bilirubin from albumin (e.g., by furosemide, spironolactone).
   c. Excretion.
      (1) Many diuretic drugs are dependent on reaching the lumen of the proximal tubule to achieve diuresis.
      (2) Low renal blood flow and low glomerular filtration rate, along with limited renal tubular function, may delay excretion and limit effectiveness of the drug. (For example, plasma clearance of furosemide has been shown to be prolonged in extremely premature neonates and in neonates with renal failure) (John and Guignard, 1992).

CARDIOVASCULAR AGENTS

A. **Introduction.**

1. A broad group of drugs that affect the regulation, inhibition, or stimulation of the cardiovascular system.
2. Increasing use in acute and long-term care of the infant in neonatal intensive care.

B. **Types of cardiovascular drugs.**

1. Inotropic agents.
   a. A broad range of drugs that act to improve cardiac output by increasing the heart rate (chronotropic effect), increasing the force of myocardial contraction (inotropic effect), and increasing vascular tone.
   b. Most widely studied of cardiovascular drugs.
   c. Used both for cardiovascular resuscitation and long-term support of the myocardium.
   d. Specific inotropic agents.
      (1) Digitalis glycosides (e.g., digoxin).
      (2) Sympathomimetic amines (e.g., epinephrine, dopamine, dobutamine, isoproterenol).
         (a) Clinical responses stimulated by this group of drugs are classified according to effects on "receptors" in the body. These receptors are categorized as either alpha or beta types and are further subcategorized as alpha-1 or alpha-2 and beta-1 or beta-2.
            (i) Alpha-1-adrenergic receptor response: constriction and contractions of vascular smooth muscle.

          (ii) Alpha-2-adrenergic receptor response: decreased motility and tone of intestine and stomach.

          (iii) Beta-1-adrenergic receptor response: increased strength and rate of myocardial contraction.

          (iv) Beta-2-adrenergic receptor response: vascular smooth muscle dilation and bronchial muscle relaxation.

      (b) Response to each of these medications depends on relative amounts of alpha and beta effects.

      (c) Prolonged administration of sympathomimetic amines can cause a diminished response in alpha and beta receptors. The result is diminished clinical efficacy, referred to as tachyphylaxis.

  2. Antihypertensives.

    a. Used to normalize blood pressure in patients with hypertension or to reduce afterload in patients with poor myocardial function.

    b. May be used to inhibit pathophysiologic changes that cause increased blood pressure (e.g., captopril) or directly reduce blood pressure through changes in intravascular volume (e.g., diuretics) or vascular resistance (e.g., diazoxide, hydralazine).

  3. Vasodilators.

    a. May be used acutely to diminish blood pressure in hypertensive patients, alter vascular resistance or capacities in congestive heart failure, and reduce pulmonary vascular resistance in conditions associated with pulmonary hypertension.

    b. Include drugs such as diazoxide, hydralazine, nitroprusside, tolazoline, and propranolol.

  4. Antiarrhythmics.

    a. Used in drug therapy for cardiac arrhythmias causing adverse effects on cardiovascular stability.

    b. Group includes adenosine and lidocaine.

C. **Basic principles of cardiovascular drug use.**

1. Wide range of pharmacologic action of this class of medications requires specific, in-depth knowledge about each drug and about concurrent drug therapy before use.

2. Knowledge of the pathophysiologic basis of neonatal cardiovascular disease is necessary to ensure proper application of this class of drugs.

3. Many of these drugs have overlapping or synergistic effects. This overlap in clinical response makes optimal choice of a drug difficult.

4. Extensive knowledge and application of invasive and noninvasive cardiovascular monitoring techniques in the neonatal population are necessary to allow titration of medication administration to clinical response.

D. **Specific considerations in newborn population.**

1. Pharmacodynamics.

    a. Specific in-depth knowledge about neonatal cardiovascular physiology and pathophysiology is required to determine the need for these types of medications.

    b. Cardiovascular drugs are commonly used in conjunction with other medications that may affect the neonate's response to the drug regimen. (For example, the digoxin-furosemide combination (electrolyte loss with diuretic) may potentiate a toxic response to an inotropic agent.)

2. Pharmacokinetics.

    a. Absorption. Many cardiovascular drugs cannot be given effectively through any significant absorptive barrier. For this reason, IV administration is necessary in many cases.

b. Distribution.
   (1) Poor cardiac output/shock states may affect distribution of drug to all tissues.
   (2) Drug administered for a desired response to one target organ may cause an undesirable systemic response (e.g., systemic hypotension after administration of tolazoline as a pulmonary vasodilator).
   (3) Some cardiovascular drugs are highly albumin bound; raises the possibility of indirect bilirubin displacement from albumin.
c. Metabolism.
   (1) Hepatic metabolic activity may markedly affect bioavailability of drug (e.g., high rate of first-pass clearance with oral hydralazine administration) (Nagourney and Arnada, 1992).
   (2) Metabolites of drug may cause toxic response (e.g., cyanide liberation as a result of nitroprusside metabolism).
   (3) Rapid metabolism and serum clearance may require constant IV infusion (e.g., of dopamine or dobutamine).
d. Excretion. Impaired renal function will markedly affect excretion and bioavailability of some drugs. Requires particular attention to careful monitoring of clinical response and serum drug levels.

CENTRAL NERVOUS SYSTEM DRUGS

A. Introduction.

1. In adult patients, the most widely used group of medications.
2. Value of pain control and mood alteration in the neonatal population has only recently been recognized.
3. Recent increased interest in the use of CNS drugs in the newborn population has caused a recognition that the body of knowledge about these drugs is limited.
4. Use of these drugs is increasing as neurobehavioral assessment skills increase among neonatal caregivers.

B. Definitions.

1. Analgesic drug: a medication (e.g., morphine, meperidine, acetaminophen) that provides diminished sensation of pain. Helps to promote control of undesirable responses to a painful event.
2. Anesthetic drug: a medication that removes pain sensation either through peripheral nerve block (e.g., lidocaine) or through CNS effects (e.g., high-dosage fentanyl citrate).
3. Sedative/hypnotic drugs: medications that provide mood alteration in patients with anxiety. Divided into two groups: barbiturates (e.g., phenobarbital, secobarbital) and nonbarbiturates (e.g., chloral hydrate, chlorpromazine, lorazepam). These drugs do not provide relief from pain.
4. Addiction: a lifestyle change that occurs in a drug-dependent person. This lifestyle change involves a focus on drug use. Cannot occur in a neonate.
5. Tolerance: a condition that may occur with many types of drugs. Tolerance exists when larger doses and higher serum concentrations of the drug are required to achieve the desired response, and commonly occurs in conjunction with physical dependence.
6. Dependence: a physiologic state in which the individual requires regular drug administration for continued physiologic well-being. Can easily be remedied through a dosage-tapering regimen.

C. General principles.

1. Mechanism of action of CNS drugs is frequently not clearly understood.

2. Assessment of need for these drugs must be carefully performed as an ongoing process.
   a. Close attention must be paid to differentiation of need for sedation, pain relief, or both.
   b. These medications may cause the development of drug tolerance and/or dependence.
3. Consideration must be made for the risks and benefits of the medication in relation to potential side or toxic effects.
4. The science of the study of neonatal neurologic development is new, and much is yet to be learned. The effect that CNS drugs may have on that development is largely unknown.

D. Specific considerations in the newborn population.

1. Pharmacodynamics.
   a. Limited knowledge of CNS development in premature and term neonates mandates a special need for caution in the use of CNS-active medications.
   b. Specific physiologic characteristics in the neonatal population require careful observation for harmful side or toxic effects (e.g., blood pressure decreases with morphine administration).
   c. Narcotic analgesics may cause respiratory depression and may precipitate respiratory failure in newborn infants.
2. Pharmacokinetics.
   a. Absorption.
      (1) Poor GI motility and high first-pass clearance may make oral administration ineffective for many drugs (e.g., morphine, meperidine).
      (2) Oral or rectal absorption of mild analgesics and sedatives is often adequate.
      (3) Careful assessment of clinical response is necessary.
   b. Metabolism.
      (1) Slower hepatic metabolism may cause prolonged half-life and increase the potential for toxic effects caused by metabolites (e.g., meperidine).
      (2) Hepatic disease may markedly increase the risk of toxic effects (e.g., chloral hydrate).
   c. Excretion.
      (1) Limited renal function or failure may cause toxic effects as a result of accumulation of drug or metabolites (e.g., meperidine, chloral hydrate).
      (2) Drug may have a direct effect on renal function.
         (a) Blood flow to kidney may be diminished (e.g., morphine).
         (b) Urinary output may be diminished (e.g., morphine-caused changes in smooth muscle tone; chlorpromazine effect on renal tubular function).

Nursing Implications for Drug Administration in the Neonate

A. **Nurses' responsibility** involves primary moral, legal, and ethical duties in patient care, which places the primary responsibility for providing safe drug administration on nursing in most cases.

B. Specific, in-depth knowledge about the pharmacodynamics and pharmacokinetics of drugs administered in the NICU is absolutely necessary in the informed assessment of clinical response and potential for risk.

C. Careful assessment of vital sign parameters and clinical responses may assist in the evaluation of desirable or undesirable drug responses.

D. **Careful observation of the neonate for therapeutic and toxic drug effects** will allow safe drug administration, minimizing toxic responses while achieving maximal desired response.

E. **Monitoring renal function through intake and output measurements** may alert the care team to potential changes in drug metabolism and/or excretion.

F. **Meticulous drug dosing** involves giving the medication at the correct time and within the correct time interval, which is essential for the maximal desired effect by many drugs, with minimal undesired effects.

G. **Facilitation of drug serum level monitoring with absolute accuracy** makes safe administration of drugs, with a narrow margin between effective and toxic levels, possible.

H. **Cross-checking** on a regular basis is a nursing responsibility. Because of the very small volumes of medication commonly given to the NICU patient, a system for regular cross-checking of drug volume accuracy before administration should be established when possible.

I. **Drugs known to have specific recommendations for safe administration** should be given under a defined protocol for administration.

J. **Drug precautions** must be observed. Any drug or drug preparation known to have a high risk of adverse effects in the neonate should be removed from the patient care area or should be specifically labeled to avoid inadvertent administration.

K. **Facilitation of or participation in clinical trials** designed to evaluate a drug's efficacy does much to advance the body of knowledge related to neonatal pharmacology.

L. **Recognition of established clinical experience with individual drugs in the neonatal population is essential.** Because some drugs are introduced into the clinical area after only minimal study of specific drug response in the neonate, early observation of potential toxic effects may avert a later disaster.

REFERENCES

Aranda, J.V., Hales, B.F., and Reider, M.F.: Developmental pharmacology. *In* Fanaroff, A.A., and Martin, R.J. (Eds.): Neonatal-Perinatal Medicine, 5th ed. St. Louis, Mosby, 1992.

Chemtob, S.: Basic pharmacologic principles. *In* Polin, R.A., and Fox, W.W. (Eds.): Fetal-Neonatal Physiology. Philadelphia, W.B. Saunders, 1992.

John, E.G., and Guignard, J.P.: Development of renal excretion of drugs during ontogeny. *In* Polin, R.A., and Fox, W.W. (Eds.): Fetal-Neonatal Physiology. Philadelphia, W.B. Saunders, 1992.

Heimann, G.: Basic pharmacokinetic principles. *In* Polin, R.A., and Fox, W.W. (Eds.): Fetal-Neonatal Physiology. Philadelphia, W.B. Saunders, 1992.

McHenry, C.M., and Salerno, E.: Pharmacology in Nursing. St. Louis, Mosby, 1998.

Nagourney, B.A., and Aranda, J.V.: Physiologic differences of clinical significance. *In* Polin, R.A., and Fox, W.W. (Eds.): Fetal-Neonatal Physiology. Philadelphia, W.B. Saunders, 1992.

Nahata, M.C., Pediatrics. *In* Dipiro, J.T., Talbert, R.L., Gray, C.Y., et al. (Eds.): Pharmacotherapy: A Pathophysiologic Approach. Stamford, Conn., Appleton & Lange, 1996.

Roberts, R.J.: Drug Therapy in Infants: Pharmacologic Principles and Clinical Experience. Philadelphia, W.B. Saunders, 1984.

ADDITIONAL READINGS

Benet, L.Z., Mitchell, J.R., and Sheiner, L.B.: Pharmacokinetics: The dynamics of drug absorption, distribution, and elimination. *In* Gilman, A., Rall, T.W., Nies, A.S., and Taylor, P. (Eds.): The Pharmacological Basis of Therapeutics. New York, Pergamon Press, 1990.

Bourne, H.R., and Roberts, J.M.: Drug receptors and pharmacodynamics. *In* Katzung, B.G. (Ed.): Basic and Clinical Pharmacology. Norwalk, Conn., Appleton & Lange, 1995.

Briggs, G.G., Freeman, R.K., and Yaffe, S.J.: Drugs in Pregnancy and Lactation, 3rd ed. Baltimore, Williams & Wilkins, 1990.

Clark, J.B., Queener, S.F., and Karb, V.B.: Pharmacological Basis of Nursing Practice. St. Louis, C.V. Mosby, 1990.

Grant, D.M., and Spielberg, S.P.: Genetic regulation of drug metabolism. *In* Polin, R.A., and Fox, W.W. (Eds.): Fetal-Neonatal Physiology. Philadelphia, W.B. Saunders, 1992.

Gynyon, G.: Pharmacokinetic considerations in neonatal drug therapy. Neonatal Network, 7(5):9–12, 1989.

Katzung, B.G.: Basic principles of pharmacology. *In* Katzung, B.G. (Ed.): Basic and Clinical Pharmacology. Norwalk, Conn., Appleton & Lange, 1995.

Lagercrantz, H., and Marcus, C.: Sympathoadrenal mechanisms during development. *In* Polin, R.A., and Fox, W.W., (Eds.): Fetal-Neonatal Physiology. Philadelphia, W.B. Saunders, 1992.

Martin, R.G.: Drug disposition in the neonate. Neonatal Network, 4(4):15–19, 1986.

Powlak, R.P., and Herfert, L.A.T. (Eds.): Drug Administration in the NICU: A Handbook for Nurses. Petaluma, Calif., Neonatal Network, 1988.

Reid, M.D., and Besunder, J.B.: Developmental pharmacology: Ontogenic basis of drug disposition. Pediatr. Clin. North Am., 36:1053–1073, 1989.

Ward, R.M.: The use of therapeutic drugs: *In* Avery, G.B., Fletcher, M.A., and MacDonald, M.G. (Eds.): Neonatology: Pathophysiology and Management of the Newborn. Philadelphia, J.B. Lippincott, 1994.

Young, T.E., and Mangum, O.B.: Neofax: A Manual of Drugs Used in Neonatal Care, 9th ed. Raleigh, N.C., Acorn Publishing, 1996.

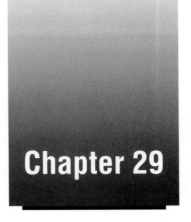

Chapter 29

Radiologic Evaluation of the Newborn Infant

Jane Deacon

Objectives

1. Define common radiologic terms used to describe an x-ray.

2. Differentiate various densities that are evident on an x-ray.

3. Describe radiologic findings that are commonly seen in neonatal disease states.

4. Differentiate normal from abnormal findings on a chest x-ray.

5. Recognize findings on an x-ray that are consistent with congenital heart disease.

6. Describe an x-ray consistent with necrotizing enterocolitis.

7. Review correct line and endotracheal tube placement on an x-ray.

Radiographic interpretation of abnormalities in a sick newborn infant is an established part of diagnostic evaluation. This evaluation assists the clinician in determining a diagnosis or formulating a differential diagnosis for treatment of the patient. Rarely is a newborn infant admitted to the NICU without having at least one x-ray taken, and frequently several additional films are needed during the course of treatment. Nurses need to become familiar with common radiographic findings to add to the knowledge base on which patient care is founded. This chapter reviews essentials of radiologic interpretation, discusses pathologic findings, and presents x-rays with common findings.

Basic Concepts

A. Radiographs are "composite shadowgrams" representing the sum of densities (white through black) interposed between the x-ray beam and the source (Squire and Novelline, 1988)

B. From the shadow forms, densities, and shapes, information can be deduced or inferred regarding anatomy, pathology, and function.

Terminology

A. **Air bronchogram:** air in the the bronchial tree visualized against a background of generalized alveolar atelectasis (Swischuk, 1997).

B. **Artifact:** an unnaturally occurring silhouette that is artificially reproduced on an x-ray and is not a part of the patient (e.g., EKG leads, temperature probes).

C. **Cardiothoracic ratio:** computed by dividing the maximum cardiac width by the maximum thoracic width to determine the heart size (Squire and Novelline, 1988).

D. **Carina:** bifurcation of the trachea, usually about the level of the third and fourth thoracic vertebrae (Wilmot and Sharko, 1987). Used in determining location of endotracheal tube.

E. **Expiratory film:** obtained when the infant is in expiration; appears to increase cardiac size, accentuate lung markings, and decrease normal lung expansion.

F. **Exposure:** amount of radiation used, producing a film ranging from light to dark. An underpenetrated (underexposed) film causes images to appear light and hazy. Overpenetration (overexposure) causes the film to be dark and to lack contrast, in comparison with an appropriately penetrated and exposed film.

G. **Hyperexpanded lungs:** lungs expanded to greater than the ninth rib.

H. **Hypoexpanded lungs:** lungs expanded to less than the seventh rib.

I. **Inspiratory film:** obtained when infant is in full inspiration and the lungs project to the eighth rib above the right diaphragmatic dome, with the trachea shown in a straight projection. This is the most desirable for chest film interpretation.

J. **Interlobar fissure:** accumulation of fluid in the pleural space between the lung lobes. The fissure may be fluid filled and may appear as a distinctive line.

K. **Perihilar:** pertaining to radiographic area bordering mediastinal structures.

L. **Pleural effusion:** abnormal collection of fluid in the pleural space (Wilmot and Sharko, 1987).

M. **Radiolucent:** pertaining to substances with varying degrees of transparency (Squire and Novelline, 1988).

N. **Radiopaque:** pertaining to substances that are dense and nonpenetrable to x rays (Squire and Novelline, 1988).

O. **Rad:** fundamental unit of radiation measurement.

P. **Roentgen:** unit of exposure.

Q. **Rotation:** turned from the midline. Chest structures closest to the beam are magnified, making their shadows appear enlarged and distorted (Squire and Novelline, 1988).

R. **Skinfold:** the most common artifact seen in the neonate. Manifests as a straight line of variable length that can travel across or outside the chest or across the diaphragm and into the abdomen. Results from folding of excessive skin; may mimic a pneumothorax. However, the obliquity of the line produced by a skinfold is opposite to that produced by the edge of the lung in pneumothorax (Swischuk, 1997).

S. **Proper technique:** signifies correct exposure, positioning, and timing in relation to inspiration and proper labeling of a film.

T. **X ray:** radiant energy of very short wavelength that penetrates substances opaque to light differently according to wavelength (Squire and Novelline, 1988).

X-ray Views Commonly Used in the Newborn Infant
(Fig. 29–1)

A. **Anteroposterior view.** X-ray tube is positioned above the infant's chest, with the x-ray beam passing through from front to back. Most common view used in the neonate for general assessment.

B. **Cross-table lateral view.** X-ray beam passes horizontally through infant in the supine position. Used to verify line placement, for assessment of free air in the chest, and for general assessment.

C. **Lateral decubitus view.** X-ray beam passes horizontally through the patient, who is positioned with suspect side uppermost. The film is placed on the infant's back, and the patient is placed perpendicular to the bed, facing the x-ray tube. The patient is usually elevated on diapers or blankets, with the arm positioned above the head and out of the field of view. Free air will rise to the highest portion of the thorax if a pneumothorax is present. If an abdominal perforation is present, free air will also rise above the liver when the patient is positioned with the left side down.

Radiographic Densities

A. **Radiodensities of various substances and tissues differ according to their composition (Squire and Novelline, 1988).**

1. The least dense (radiolucent) substance will radiograph black or dark gray because the sparse molecules offer no obstacle to the rays.
2. A very dense (radiopaque) object such as lead will radiograph gray or white because no rays or only a few rays will penetrate it, so the film underneath will remain unchanged.

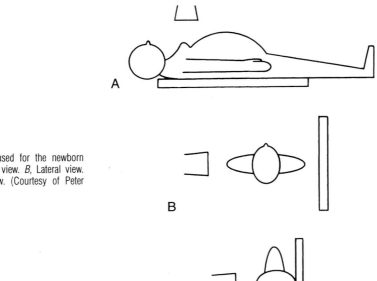

Figure 29–1
X-ray views commonly used for the newborn infant. *A,* Anteroposterior view. *B,* Lateral view. *C,* Lateral decubitus view. (Courtesy of Peter Honeyfield, M.D.)

3. Subcutaneous fat is very radiolucent and produces a dark gray shadow on x-ray film.
4. Blood, muscle, and liver are of similar densities and will be seen as white and medium gray. Moist solid or fluid-filled organs and tissue masses have about the same radiodensity—greater than air but less than bone or metal.
5. Bone is composed of an organic matrix into which the complex bone mineral (primarily calcium) is precipitated. Organic substances will reduce the radiodensity of bone and will be seen as white with a tinge of gray.
6. Metal such as the surgical clip used for patent ductus arteriosus ligation is very dense and radiopaque. All the x rays are absorbed by the metal, producing a white image on the film.

B. **Differentiation of densities is the basis for interpretation of an x-ray film.** For example, because of the contrast in densities between the fluid-filled heart, which radiographs white, and the air-filled lungs, which radiograph black, the heart can be seen against the lungs. Organs of the same density that are located side by side, such as the heart and the thymus, may be difficult to distinguish from each other. Changes in normal density can indicate a pathologic process, such as severe hyaline membrane disease, which will appear on the film completely white instead of black, which indicates air density.

Risks Associated with Radiographic Examination in the Neonate

A. Early radiation effects (Wagner and Dominguez, 1992).

1. Adverse effects of x rays do not occur unless a threshold amount of radiation is delivered.
2. Threshold amounts are far in excess of the radiation delivered during an x-ray examination.

B. **Delayed effects of x rays.** The risk of radiation-induced childhood leukemia after abdominal radiography of the premature neonate would not be likely to exceed 0.02% unless 100 or more studies are performed.

C. Risks to personnel.

1. Risks to personnel in the area where studies are properly done are too small to be of serious concern.
2. At 2 m from the patient, the risk to personnel from an abdominal radiograph of the neonate is much less than the equivalent risk from 1 day of natural background radiation.

Approach to Interpreting an X-ray

A. Develop a systematic approach and a definite order for assessing a film to ensure that no pathology is missed.

B. **Labeling.** Note name or identification of the patient, date and time of the film, and radiographic labeling on right or left side of the film.

C. Assess for correct exposure of the film.

D. **Note positioning.** Clavicles and ribs should be even on both sides of the chest. Rotation distorts structures.

E. Individually assess all anatomic and pathologic changes on each film.

1. Lung fields.

    a. Normal lung expansion: Eight ribs projecting above the right diaphragmatic dome, with the trachea in a straight position.

    b. Lung volume, determined by noting the number of ribs expanded on an inspiratory film.

    c. Pulmonary vascularity: vessels branching from the lung root (hilum) and decreasing in size, with extension into the lung fields. Vascularity will be increased or diminished depending on pathologic state.

    d. Presence of free air: pneumothorax, pneumoperitoneum, pneumopericardium, and pneumomediastinum.

2. Mediastinum.

    a. Heart.

      (1) Size.

      (2) Malposition: any inappropriate position of the heart—that is, any position other than the usual position in the hemithorax.

      (3) Contour: variable because of the influence of patient position and angulation of the x-ray beam.

      (4) Shape: may indicate pathologic change—for example, boot-shaped heart in tetralogy of Fallot and egg-shaped heart in transposition of the great vessels.

      (5) Pulmonary vascular markings: may be significantly diminished, as in pulmonary atresia, or increased, as in congestive heart failure (CHF).

    b. Trachea.

      (1) Normally located within the mediastinum.

      (2) Assessment on x-ray film for presence and position of endotracheal tube.

    c. Thymus.

      (1) Size.

      (2) Presence or absence.

      (3) Sail sign.

    d. Diaphragm.

      (1) General pattern: two smooth, curved shadows on either side of the heart, taking off from the midline at the origin of the tenth and eleventh ribs (Squire and Novelline, 1988; Swischuk, 1997).

      (2) Contour: possibly flattened with lung overdistention or elevated if there is abdominal distention.

      (3) Diaphragmatic hernia: abdominal contents passing through a hole in the diaphragm.

      (4) Eventration: herniation of bowel and liver against a weakened hemidiaphragm.

    e. Gastrointestinal (GI) tract.

      (1) Esophagus. Distended, air-filled esophageal pouch may be visible in esophageal atresia.

      (2) Tracheoesophageal fistula. Fistula is present if an esophageal atresia exists and if air is visible in the stomach and intestine.

      (3) Passage of air through stomach and intestines.

      (4) Location of stomach bubble.

      (5) Bowel gas pattern.

      (6) Presence of pneumatosis intestinalis.

      (7) Presence of calcifications as a result of bowel perforation in utero.

      (8) Fluid, seen as a gasless abdomen. It is necessary to distinguish fluid from masses.

      (9) Pneumoperitoneum. Free air is seen within the peritoneal cavity.

     (10) Obstructions. Gaseous distention of the bowel is seen at various levels, depending on the location of the obstruction.

    f. Skeletal system.

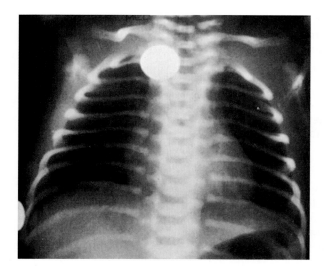

Figure 29–2
Normal appearance of the chest on an x-ray film.

    (1) General skeletal assessment. Assess for symmetry, size, continuity, intactness, and abnormalities.
    (2) Fractures of long bones, clavicles, ribs, and skull. A dark line is seen along any portion of a fractured bone because of the air or tissue that settles between the bone fragments (Hazinski and Snow, 1992).
  g. Tubes and catheters.
    (1) Position of endotracheal tube, gastric tube, or chest tube.
    (2) Umbilical catheter placement.
    (3) Central venous line placement.

Respiratory System

A. The normal chest (Fig. 29–2).

1. Complete aeration of the chest occurs within a few breaths after onset of respirations at delivery (Blickman, 1998).
2. Residual fluid may be present in the alveoli after delivery. Early films (<6 hours after delivery) may show increased bronchovascular markings because of this fluid.
3. Normal lung pattern.
  a. Uniform radiolucent appearance.
  b. Hilar and perihilar regions show some increased density because of vascular, bronchial, and hilar structures, which produce some increase in density.
  c. Periphery shows few, if any, markings.
  d. Fluid in the various interlobar fissures represents a normal variation.

B. Thymus.

1. Occupies the anterior part of the superior portion of the mediastinum and consists of right and left lobes (Hedlund et al., 1998).
2. Appears as a smoothly rounded outline superior to the cardiac shadow and blending imperceptibly with the cardiac silhouette.
3. Definite notch visible in some cases at the junction of the cardiac silhouette and the thymus.
4. Generally more prominent on the right.
5. Shape may alter markedly with degree of inspiration.

6. Rapid involution during times of stress.
7. Aplasia of the thymus (DiGeorge's syndrome).
8. Creation of "sail sign" when mediastinal air lifts the thymus upward.

C. Trachea.

1. Trachea is normally displaced slightly to the right by the left aortic arch.
2. Deviated trachea supports a mediastinal shift.
3. On inspiration, the trachea dilates and lengthens.
4. On expiration, the trachea constricts and shortens.
5. On deep inspiration, the trachea and major bronchi are well distended and are easily identifiable.

PULMONARY PARENCHYMAL DISEASE

A. Respiratory distress syndrome (hyaline membrane disease) (Fig. 29–3A).

1. Pronounced under aeration. Fewer than eight ribs expand on inspiration on anteroposterior, film with doming of the hemidiaphragms on lateral view.
2. Bilateral diffuse alveolar infiltrates. Reticulogranular (ground-glass) appearance is due to microatelectasis of the alveoli (Hedlund et al., 1998).
3. Homogeneous pattern throughout both lung fields.
4. Air bronchograms. Air-filled bronchi (black) are contrasted against the more radiopaque (whiter) lung fields (Blickman, 1998).
5. With severe disease a generalized opacity or frank "white out" appearance (Fig. 29–3 B).
6. Reticulogranular pattern and air bronchograms. May resemble those seen in group B streptococcal pneumonia and may be impossible to distinguish from hyaline membrane disease.
7. X-ray findings after surfactant administration (Fig. 29–4).
   a. Improvement in pulmonary aeration on x-ray.
   b. Asymmetric distribution of surfactant, showing areas of improved lung alternating with areas of unchanged respiratory distress syndrome (RDS) (Levine, Edwards, and Merritt, 1991).

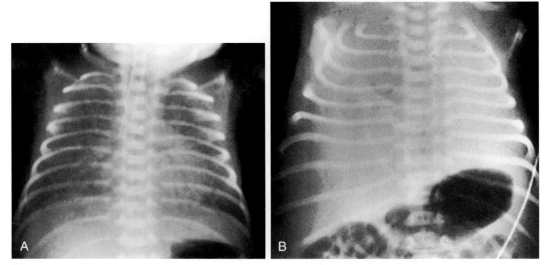

Figure 29–3
A, Hyaline membrane disease. Note reticulogranular lung pattern and air bronchograms. *B*, Severe hyaline membrane disease. Note "white out" appearance bilaterally with faint air bronchograms visible.

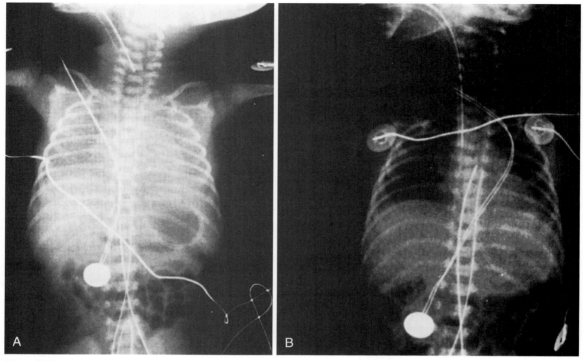

Figure 29–4
Hyaline membrane disease before administration of surfactant *(A)* and significant clearing after administration *(B)*.

    c. Poor prognosis with pulmonary interstitial emphysema after surfactant therapy (Blickman, 1998).

B. **Pulmonary interstitial emphysema (Fig. 29–5).**

1. Alveolar overdistention is due to assisted ventilation, visualized as multiple small, cystlike radiolucencies that are bilateral, unilateral, localized, or in a diffuse pattern (Emmanouilides and Bayeen, 1988).
2. Condition may lead to a pneumothorax or other air leak.

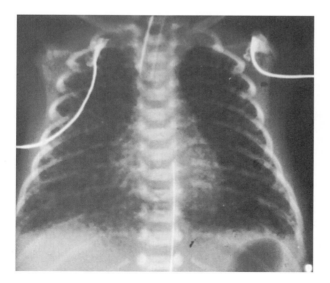

Figure 29–5
Pulmonary interstitial emphysema. Note hyperexpansion bilaterally and pinpoint dark bubbles throughout both lung fields.

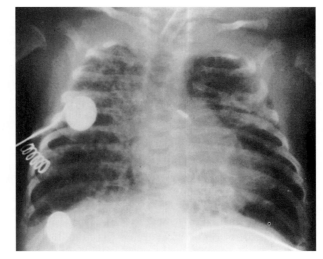

Figure 29–6
Bronchopulmonary dysplasia. Note ill-defined densities bilaterally. Also note fractured rib in the upper left portion of the chest and pale-appearing ribs.

C. **Bronchopulmonary dysplasia (BPD) (Fig. 29–6).**

1. Initial x-ray picture shows lung disease (e.g., hyaline membrane disease, meconium aspiration syndrome) (Hedlund et al., 1998).
2. Radiologic appearance and course of BPD have changed since Northway and Rosan (1968) described four stages (Northway, 1991; Leonidas and Berdon, 1993).
   a. By the end of the first or second week, there is a persistent haziness of vessel margins progressing to linear densities that persist into the third or fourth week of life.
   b. Subsequently there is gradual development of a bubbly appearance of the lungs in association with hyperaeration, which is more pronounced at the lung bases. This persists after 1 month of age and represents a modified form of stage IV BPD.

D. **Transient tachypnea of the newborn (TTN) (retained fetal lung fluid, wet lung disease) (Fig. 29–7).**

1. Bilateral, symmetric perihilar streakiness due to increased interstitial and alveolar fluid (Fanaroff and Martin, 1997).

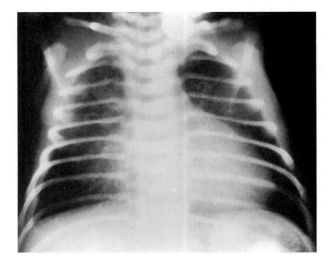

Figure 29–7
Transient tachypnea of the neonate. Note mild hyperexpansion and perihilar streakiness. A small pleural effusion is also present on the right side.

2. Mild to moderate overaeration of the lungs and occasionally pleural effusions (Swischuk, 1997).
3. Possible fluid in minor (or horizontal) fissure and major (or oblique) lobar fissure (Blickman, 1998).
4. Mildly enlarged cardiothymic silhouette (Blickman, 1998).
5. Lung fields begin to clear in 24–48 hours (Swischuk, 1997).

E. **Meconium aspiration syndrome (Fig. 29–8).**

1. Mild cases may show a normal lung pattern to mild infiltrates with over-expanded lungs.
2. Bilateral asymmetric areas of atelectasis; hyperaeration with flattened hemidiaphragms (Blickman, 1998; Hedlund et al., 1998).
3. Hyperaeration of the lungs and flattened hemidiaphragms (Hedlund et al., 1998).
4. Possible atelectasis if airway is obstructed because of debris.
5. Possible air leaks (pneumothorax or pneumomediastinum) resulting from overdistention and rupture of the alveoli.

F. **Pneumonia.**

1. Patchy, occasionally asymmetric, radiating, bilateral interstitial infiltrate. A nodular pattern may predominate in hazy lungs, and an effusion is a common occurrence (Blickman, 1998).
2. Reticulogranular pattern similar to that of hyaline membrane disease. Some alveoli contain inflammatory exudate, which will appear more opaque and reticulogranular on x-ray than those filled with air (Swischuk, 1997; Hedlund et al., 1998).
3. Group B streptococcal pneumonia, often indistinguishable from RDS (Swischuk, 1997; Hedlund et al., 1998) (Fig. 29–9).

PULMONARY AIR LEAKS

A. **Pneumothorax (Fig. 29–10A).**

1. Accumulation of air in the pleural space. Air can outline the lung circumferentially or can accumulate.

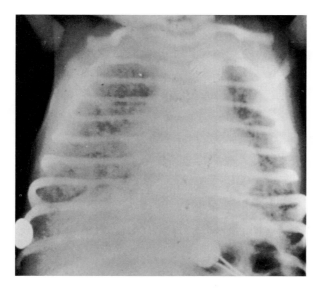

Figure 29–8
Meconium aspiration syndrome. Note the coarse, patchy infiltrates bilaterally.

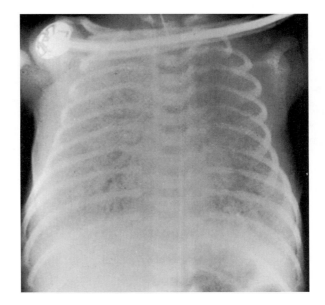

Figure 29–9
Group B streptococcal pneumonia. Note the reticulogranular appearance seen with hyaline membrane disease.

2. Mediastinal shift of structures away from the affected side as air accumulates (tension pneumothorax) (Jaquith, 1986).
3. Outline of the collapsed lung, with a band of hyperlucency between the chest wall and the underlying lung (Swischuk and John, 1995).
4. Other findings related to pneumothorax.
    a. Pneumothorax not under tension may not exhibit a mediastinal shift.
    b. Diaphragm on affected side of a pneumothorax under tension will be flattened because of tension placed on it by air accumulation superior to it (Hedlund et al., 1998).
    c. Skinfold may mimic a pneumothorax (Swischuk, 1997) (Fig. 29–10B).

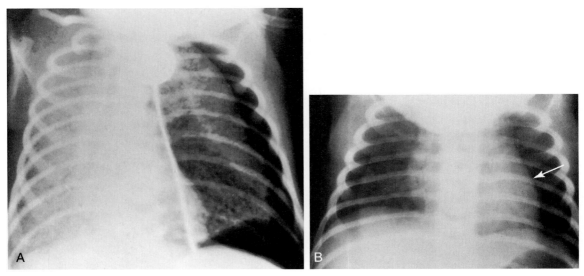

Figure 29–10
A, Left tension pneumothorax. Note the mediastinal shift toward the right side. B, Note skinfold on right *(arrow)*. It can be mistaken for a pneumothorax. It extends beyond the chest and crosses over the diaphragm.

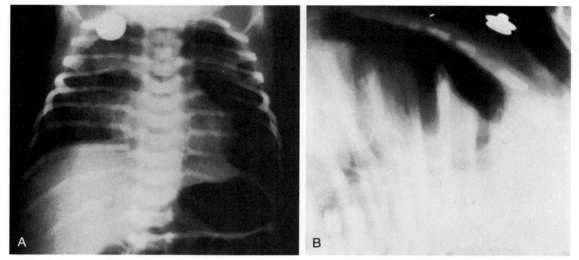

Figure 29–11
A, Pneumomediastinum with thymus lifted, demonstrating the "sail sign." *B,* Pneumomediastinum on lateral view. Note that air in anterior chest outlines the thymus.

B. Pneumomediastinum (Fig. 29–11).

1. Mediastinal air collection, which produces irregular gas collections within the soft tissues of the superior mediastinum, with air frequently outlining the undersurface of the thymus gland and thus creating a "sail sign" (Swischuk, 1997).
2. Can accompany a pneumothorax.
3. On lateral film, a radiolucent area of hyperlucency in the superior retrosternal space.

C. Pneumopericardium (Fig. 29–12).

1. Radiolucent halo of free air surrounds the heart as air accumulates within the pericardial space (Hedlund et al., 1998).
2. Width of air around the heart is proportional to the amount of air present. Air is limited to the pericardium and cannot extend beyond the origins of the aorta and pulmonary artery (Hedlund et al., 1998).
3. Decreased cardiac size may indicate cardiac tamponade.

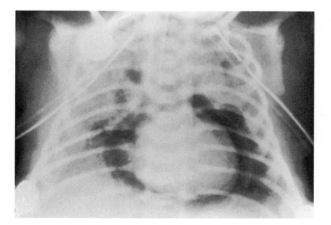

Figure 29–12
Pneumopericardium. Note that air completely encircles the heart. Bilateral chest tubes are also in place.

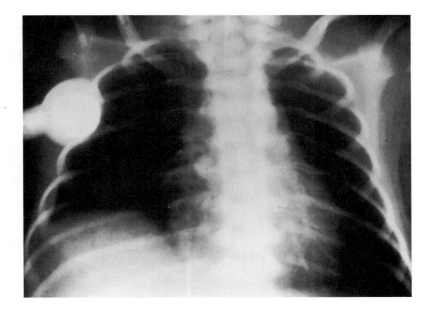

Figure 29–13
Paralysis of right side of diaphragm. Note that right side of diaphragm is markedly elevated in comparison with left side of diaphragm.

4. Other pulmonary air leaks and/or pulmonary interstitial emphysema are generally present.
5. Pneumopericardium is rare in the absence of assisted ventilation.

MISCELLANEOUS CAUSES OF RESPIRATORY DISTRESS

A. **Diaphragmatic paralysis (phrenic nerve injury) (Fig. 29–13).**

1. Elevation and fixation of a diaphragmatic leaflet (Swischuk, 1997).
2. More common on the right than the left side and usually unilateral.
3. Mediastinum may be shifted away from the affected side.
4. Most often results from obstetric injury to the brachial plexus (Swischuk, 1997).
5. Erb's palsy an associated finding.

B. **Eventration of the diaphragm (Fig. 29–14).**

1. Weakness of the hemidiaphragm, with abdominal organs pushing up against it but not entering the chest because no opening exists.
2. Either partial or complete; usually right-sided (Hedlund et al., 1998).

C. **Pulmonary edema (Fig. 29–15).**

1. Increased pulmonary permeability is common in premature infants with lung injury which can manifest as diffuse haziness of the lungs to a white-out appearance (Swischuk and John, 1995).
2. Significant association between high fluid intake and subsequent occurrence of a clinically significant patent ductus arteriosus and BPD.
3. Also common with certain congenital heart defects due to increased pulmonary blood flow (coarctation of the aorta, hypoplastic left heart syndrome).

THORACIC SURGICAL PROBLEMS

A. **Congenital diaphragmatic hernia (Fig. 29–16A).**

1. Herniation of abdominal contents through various portions of the diaphragm into the thoracic cavity, most commonly through the foramen of Bochdalek (Hedlund et al., 1998).

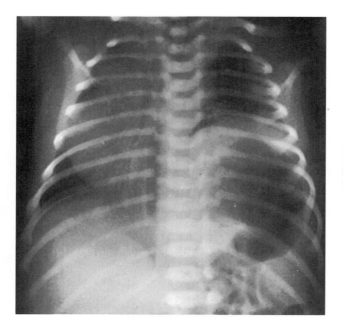

Figure 29–14
Eventration of the diaphragm. Note left side of diaphragm bulging upward, with the stomach pushing up against it.

2. Seventy-five percent occur on the left side (Swischuk, 1997).
3. Hemithorax filled with loops of bowel, stomach, and often liver; displaces the mediastinal structures away from the affected side (Swischuk, 1997).
4. Abdomen relatively gasless and may be scaphoid (Hedlund et al., 1998).
5. Contralateral pneumothorax possible with assisted ventilation or as a result of pulmonary hypoplasia on the unaffected side.
6. If the x-ray is obtained before the bowel is expanded with air, the affected hemithorax may appear entirely opacified with the mediastinal structures shifted to the opposite side (Swischuk, 1997) (Fig. 29–16B).

B. Congenital lobar emphysema (Fig. 29–17).

1. Most common cause of cystic malformation of the lung.
2. Air trapped within one or more lung lobes at birth, resulting in obstructive emphysema.

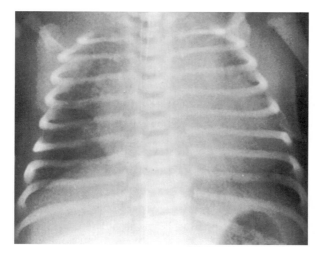

Figure 29–15
Pulmonary edema. Note congested lung fields and cardiomegaly.

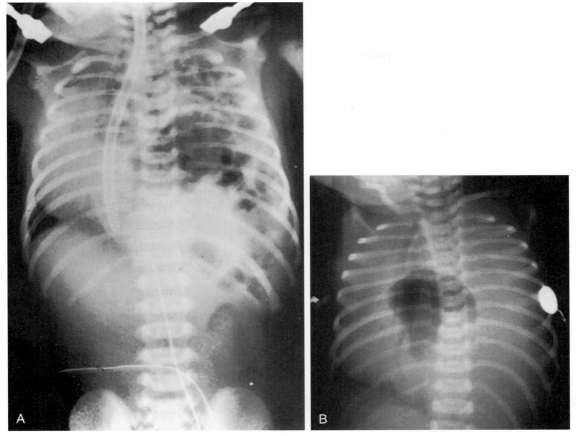

Figure 29–16
A, Left diaphragmatic hernia. Note presence of bowel in the left side of the chest, a mediastinal shift to the right, and a lack of bowel in the abdomen. *B,* Left diaphragmatic hernia before much air has expanded the bowel. Note that trachea and heart have shifted to the right.

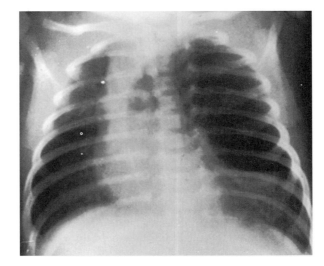

Figure 29–17
Congenital lobar emphysema. Note hyperlucency of the left upper lung lobe, with a mediastinal shift toward the right.

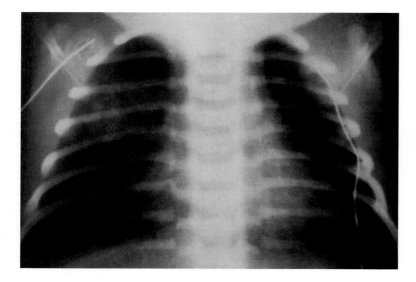

Figure 29–18
Cystic adenomatoid malformation in the right lung.

3. Overdistended affected lobe, with mediastinum shifted to contralateral side.
4. Possibly hyperlucent but may also be opaque because of fluid accumulation distal to the obstruction (Swischuk, 1997).
5. Generally limited to the upper lobes.

C. **Cystic adenomatoid malformation (Fig. 29–18).**

1. Overdistention of affected lobe, with mediastinal shift to contralateral side.
2. Lobar overdistention, caused by air and fluid.
3. Upper lobes most frequently affected (Swischuk, 1997).
4. X-ray findings: multiple air-filled cysts, mediastinal shift, and compression of opposite lung. Diaphragmatic hernia must be ruled out.

Cardiovascular System

A. **Size of the heart.**

1. Difficult to assess on anteroposterior film because of a large thymus. Lateral film assessing a specific chamber enlargement may be more useful (Swischuk, 1997).
2. Enlargement suggested by cardiothoracic ratio greater than 65% (Strife, Bissett, and Burrows, 1998) (Fig. 29–19).
3. Malpositioning: may represent cardiac displacement, developmentally abnormal cardiac position, or ambiguous rotation or site (Strife et al., 1998).
4. Possible transient enlargement as a result of polycythemia, perinatal anoxia, or normally increased fluid present at birth.

B. **Pulmonary vascularity.**

1. Normal vascular markings are seen in the middle one third of the lung fields (Fig. 29–20).
2. Decreased vascular markings occur with obstruction along the right ventricular outflow tract of the heart and are manifested as hyperlucency in both lung fields. (Fig. 29–21).
3. Increased pulmonary vascularity occurs when excess blood flow causes congestion in the blood vessels and is manifested as increased streakiness, hazy lung fields, and increased densities as the condition worsens.

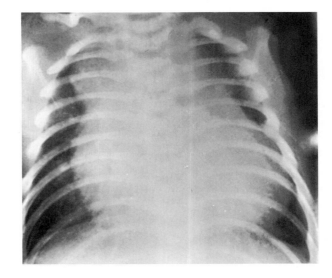

Figure 29–19
Cardiomegaly. Note that the enlarged heart occupies the majority of the thorax.

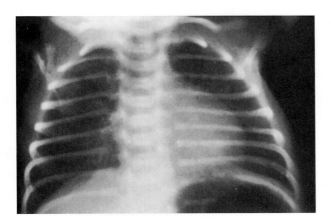

Figure 29–20
Normal pulmonary vascularity. Note the presence of vascularity radiating from the perihilar region.

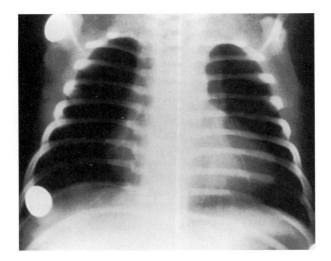

Figure 29–21
Hyperlucent lung fields because of decreased blood flow to the lungs.

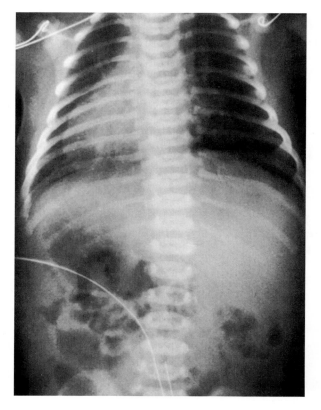

Figure 29-22
"Mirror image" dextrocardia. Note the apex of the heart pointing to the right, with the stomach located on the right and the liver on the left.

C. Positional anomalies of the heart.

1. Types of malposition are as follows:
   a. Dextrocardia: right-sided heart.
   b. Mesocardia: midline heart.
   c. Extrathoracic: ectopia cordis.
2. Position of other organs in relation to the heart is also incorporated into the definition of cardiac malposition. Positions of the abdominal organs are as follows:
   a. Situs solitus: normal abdominal organ position.
   b. Situs inversus: stomach and spleen on right, liver on left, and left atrium on right.
   c. Situs ambiguus: abdominal organs and atrial position are anatomically uncertain. The liver may be symmetric and at midline, and the stomach may be central. There may be duplication or absence of unilateral structures such as the spleen (asplenia or polysplenia).
3. "Mirror image" dextrocardia with situs inversus is the most common type of malposition; congenital heart disease is unlikely (Philip, 1996) (Fig. 29–22).
4. Dextrocardia with situs solitus—dextrocardia is an isolated finding with all other organs in their normal position. Incidence of congenital heart disease is 95–98% (Strife et al., 1998).
5. Cardiac malposition caused by shift of the heart within the thorax must be differentiated from extracardiac causes, such as pneumothorax, hypoplastic lung, diaphragmatic hernia, decreased lung volume, and lung mass.

D. Lesions with increased pulmonary vascularity.

1. Left-to-right shunt or intracardiac mixing.

a. Transposition of the great vessels. Plain film shows "egg on a string" appearance. Cardiac silhouette of normal size or mild cardiomegaly may be seen (Blickman, 1998). Pulmonary vascularity is variable, depending on the presence or absence of a ventricular septal defect or a patent ductus arteriosus.

b. Total anomalous pulmonary venous return. X-ray film shows cardiomegaly; increased pulmonary vascularity; and enlargement of the right atrium, right ventricle, and pulmonary artery. The "snowman" appearance of the heart, caused by a characteristic widening of the superior mediastinum due to the connecting blood vessels, is rarely seen in the neonate because of the slow development of excessive pulmonary blood flow (Swischuk, 1997).

c. Atrioventricular canal defect (A-V canal) (endocardial cushion defect). Pulmonary vascular resistance usually remains high enough to delay the onset of CHF until after the first 1–2 weeks, after which marked cardiomegaly and vascular congestion are evident.

d. Truncus arteriosus. Right and left ventricles are prominent, with left atrial dilation. As CHF develops, pulmonary vessels become indistinct and obscured by pulmonary edema.

e. Atrial septal defect. Chest x-ray may be normal, with small defects. With large left-to-right shunts, there are moderate cardiac enlargement and increased pulmonary vascularity. The right atrium and right ventricle are enlarged.

f. Ventricular septal defect. With small defects the heart size and vascularity may be normal. With moderate-sized defects, heart size may be enlarged, with increased pulmonary vascular markings. With large defects and increased blood flow, cardiomegaly is evident because of right and left ventricular enlargement. Pulmonary vascularity is markedly increased. CHF, interstitial edema, and alveolar fluid may be present.

g. Patent ductus arteriosus. Pulmonary vasculature and cardiac silhouette may be obscured by underlying lung disease of RDS. Lung fields may show pulmonary edema and increasing heart size compared with heart size on previous x-ray films.

2. Left-sided obstruction. Outflow of blood from the left side of the heart or return of blood from the lungs is obstructed, which will eventually cause CHF.

a. Hypoplastic left heart syndrome (aortic atresia, mitral atresia). Pulmonary vascularity may appear normal until significant cardiac decompensation is present, and then cardiomegaly and CHF become evident. Right atrial enlargement may also be seen (Swischuk, 1997). This is most common cause of CHF in the first few days of life.

b. Coarctation of the aorta. Heart size is normal, but left ventricular enlargement may subsequently be seen on lateral views (Swischuk, 1997). X-ray findings vary according to the degree of patency of the patent ductus arteriosus and the severity of the obstruction at the coarctation site. CHF occurs, with ductal closure resulting in cardiomegaly and pulmonary venous congestion.

c. Aortic stenosis. Normal cardiac size and vasculature may be seen, with mild stenosis of the aortic valve. Left ventricular enlargement occurs, with cardiac decompensation or associated aortic regurgitation resulting in cardiomegaly and venous congestion (Blickman, 1998).

3. Lesions with decreased pulmonary vascularity. All these lesions involve some form of obstruction to the normal flow of blood through the right outflow tract. They can be located anywhere from the tricuspid valve to the pulmonary artery.

a. Pulmonary valve atresia with intact ventricular septum. Pulmonary vascularity is reduced or normal, depending on alternative sources of pulmonary blood flow, such as a patent ductus arteriosus. A shallow or concave pulmonary artery is evident (Swischuk, 1997). Closure of the ductus arteriosus and obstruction of the right ventricular outflow tract cause decreased pulmonary blood flow. Pulmonary vessels are underfilled and appear small and thin, which results in dark, hyperlucent lung fields. Heart size is variable, but cardiomegaly is usually present because of right atrial and left ventricular enlargement (Swischuk, 1997).

  b. Tricuspid atresia Tricuspid valve has complete atresia, and the right ventricle and right outflow tract are underdeveloped. Chest x-ray shows a normal or small heart and diminished pulmonary blood flow (Strife et al., 1998).

  c. Tetralogy of Fallot. Cardiac size and shape are frequently normal. Pulmonary vascular markings are decreased. A "boot-shaped" contour may occur from a small, concave pulmonary artery and a prominent cardiac apex as a result of right ventricular hypertrophy (Strife et al., 1998).

  d. Pulmonary stenosis. Severe valvular obstruction is associated with hypoxemia because of a right-to-left shunt at the foramen ovale (Wechsler and Wernovsky, 1998). This is referred to as critical pulmonary stenosis. Neonate's chest x-ray is normal, but cardiomegaly with predominant right atrium and right ventricle, decreased pulmonary vascularity, and dilation of the pulmonary artery eventually occur.

Gastrointestinal System

A. **Characteristics of the normal abdomen (Fig. 29–23).**

1. Air is present in the stomach immediately after birth because of respiratory movement of the thorax and swallowing of air. By 24 hours of life, air should appear in the rectum (Blickman, 1998).
2. A gasless abdomen may be seen in infants with decreased swallowing, decreased GI motility (i.e., with intubation or chemical paralysis), vomiting, or gastric decompression from suctioning.
3. Resuscitation may increase the amount of bowel gas seen on an x-ray.

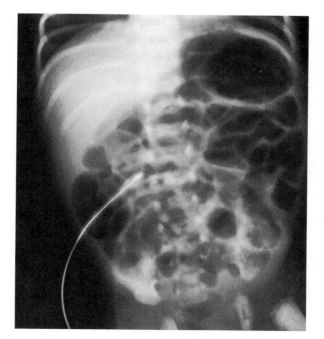

Figure 29–23
Normal bowel gas pattern. Note the presence of stomach bubble and air through the entire abdomen to the rectum.

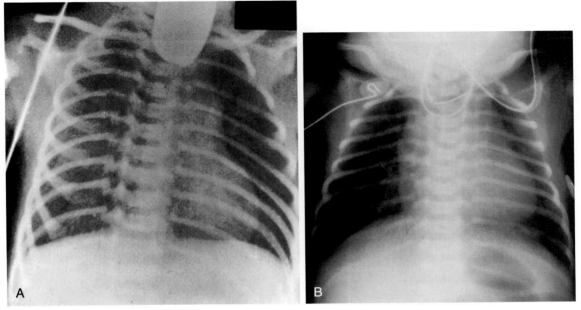

Figure 29–24
A, Esophageal atresia. Contrast medium outlines esophagus, which ends in a blind pouch. *B,* Esophageal atresia with tracheoesophageal fistula. A gastric tube cannot be advanced because of the esophageal atresia. Air is in the abdomen, confirming the presence of the tracheoesophageal fistula.

B. **The esophagus.**

1. May show indentations near the aortic arch and left main-stem bronchus.
2. May assume peculiar configurations because of flexibility during the respiratory cycle.
3. Air in the esophagus a normal finding on regular chest films.

C. **Esophageal abnormalities.**

1. Esophageal atresia (Fig. 29–24*A*). A portion of the esophagus is atretic, and both distal and proximal portions of the esophagus end in blind pouches.
   a. On x-ray a radiolucent, air-filled, distended proximal esophageal pouch is present. The abdomen is gasless because no air can enter (Swischuk, 1997). The proximal pouch can be identified by passing a radiopaque tube and obtaining a chest film. The tube will not advance beyond 9–11 cm (Blickman, 1998).
   b. Aspiration pneumonitis of the upper lobes, especially the right upper lobe, is a common finding.
2. Esophageal atresia with tracheoesophageal fistula (Fig. 29–24*B*).
   a. Esophageal atresia with fistulous connection to the distal esophageal pouch is the most common esophageal anomaly.
   b. Excessive dilation of the stomach and/or small bowel, resulting from distal fistula communication between the lungs and the stomach, may occur (Blickman, 1998).
   c. Chest film should be obtained with a radiopaque tube in place. The tube will not advance into the stomach, and air will be present in the GI tract.
3. Tracheoesophageal fistula with no esophageal atresia (H type of fistula).
   a. Difficult to identify without a contrast study.
   b. Fistula characteristically assumes an upwardly oblique configuration on contrast study.
   c. Widespread pulmonary infiltrates are commonly present because of constant aspiration through the fistula into the lungs.

D. **The stomach.**

1. Visible directly beneath the left diaphragm.
2. Often appears large in the neonate as a result of dilation with air.
3. Mucosal folds are absent. Stomach wall appears smooth (Swischuk, 1997).
4. Begins to empty moments after being filled.

E. **Abnormalities of the stomach.**

1. Pyloric stenosis.
   a. Symptoms develop 2 to 8 weeks after birth (Swischuk, 1997).
   b. Plain films demonstrate a distended stomach and duodenum, with disproportionately less gas in the small bowel (Swischuk, 1997).
   c. Ultrasonography is the study of choice for the diagnosis.
2. Gastric perforation.
   a. Uncommon, but may result from gastric ulcers, hypoxia-induced focal necrosis, gastric tubes, or indomethacin therapy for closure of ductus arteriosus.
   b. Possible overinflation due to distal obstruction, as with mechanical ventilation.
   c. Common finding of free air (pneumoperitoneum) with absence of gastric gas.

F. **Duodenal abnormalities (Fig. 29–25).**

1. Duodenal atresia and stenosis.
   a. Infants with duodenal atresia present with vomiting in the first few hours of life. Those with stenosis present at variable times, depending on the degree of stenosis.
   b. Duodenal atresia and stenosis are present in approximately 33% of infants with Down syndrome (trisomy 21) (Blickman, 1998).
   c. X-ray demonstrates dilation of the stomach and proximal duodenum, producing the characteristic "double bubble" pattern. No air is present distal to the duodenum (Swischuk, 1997).
2. Annular pancreas.
   a. Pancreas grows in the form of an encircling ring around the duodenum (Blickman, 1998).

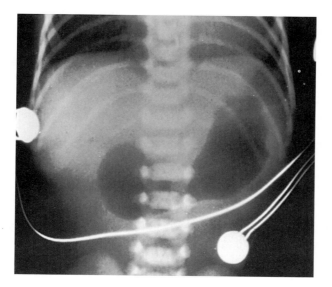

Figure 29–25
Duodenal atresia with characteristic "double bubble" pattern.

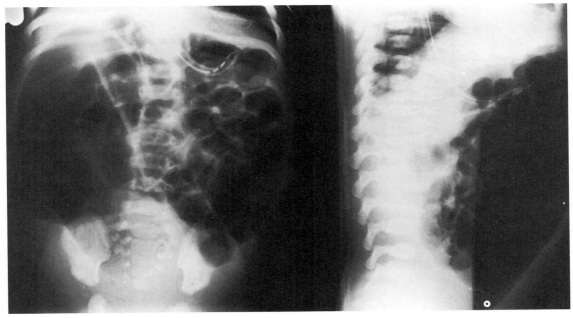

Figure 29–26
Meconium ileus with perforation and free air visible on lateral film.

b. Presentation is similar to that of duodenal atresia or stenosis.
c. X-ray findings are generally indistinguishable from duodenal atresia or stenosis (Swischuk, 1997). Identification is made with ultrasonography.

G. **Abnormalities of the small bowel.**

1. Small-bowel atresia and stenosis.
   a. Single or multiple areas of atresia or stenosis may exist.
   b. Clinically abdominal distention and bile-stained vomiting are apparent early on.
   c. Types of small-bowel atresia.
      (1) High jejunal obstruction. One or two loops of bowel are visible on x-ray.
      (2) Mid-jejunal obstruction. More dilated loops are visible on x-ray.
      (3) Distal ileal atresia. Many dilated loops are visible on x-ray.
2. Meconium ileus (Fig. 29–26).
   a. Twenty percent of infants with cystic fibrosis present with meconium ileus at birth (Blickman, 1998).
   b. Obstruction results from impaction of thick, tenacious meconium in the distal portion of the small bowel. Ileal atresia or stenosis, ileal perforation, meconium peritonitis, and volvulus are common complications (Buonomo, Taylor, Share, and Kirks, 1998).
   c. Clinical presentation includes bile-stained vomiting, abdominal distention, and failure to pass meconium.
   d. X-ray shows a low small-bowel obstruction with numerous, variably sized air-filled loops of bowel (Blickman, 1998). There is a "soap bubble" appearance in the right lower quadrant as a result of trapping of air in meconium.
   e. A contrast-enema study will demonstrate a microcolon. A water-soluble contrast agent draws large amounts of fluid into the intestine and lubricates the meconium, allowing it to pass without surgical intervention. This technique is successful 30–50% of the time (Blickman, 1998).

3. Midgut volvulus.
   a. Most common form of small-bowel volvulus.
   b. Twisting and spiraling of entire gut around the superior mesenteric artery, resulting in vascular compromise, necrosis, perforation, and gangrene.
   c. May present with bilious vomiting.
   d. May be difficult to determine on x-ray because findings are variable, from a normal abdomen to one suggesting a gastric outlet obstruction, partial obstruction of the duodenum, or small-bowel obstruction (Buonomo et al., 1998).
   e. Ultrasonography, barium enema, or x-ray of upper GI tract may be needed for diagnostic purposes or to demonstrate complete obstruction of third portion of duodenum (Buonomo et al., 1998).

H. **Abnormalities of the colon.**

1. Hirschsprung's disease (aganglionosis of the colon) (Fig. 29–27).
   a. Typical presentation is vomiting, obstruction, and failure to pass meconium within the first 24–36 hours of life.
   b. Commonly involves the distal colonic segment—rectal and rectosigmoid areas.
   c. Plain films show some degree of low small-bowel or colonic obstruction, air-fluid levels, and distention of the bowel (Blickman, 1998). Rectal gas may be absent or sparse.
   d. Barium enema will support the findings, and a rectal biopsy will show absence of ganglion cells.
2. Meconium plug syndrome/small left colon syndrome.
   a. Normal meconium becomes impacted in the distal portion of the colon. In meconium plug syndrome, the obstruction is generally in the sigmoid colon. In small left colon, the site of obstruction is the splenic flexure.
   b. Functional immaturity of the colon, especially in infants of diabetic mothers, is thought to be the cause of the initial inability to pass meconium (Blickman, 1998).

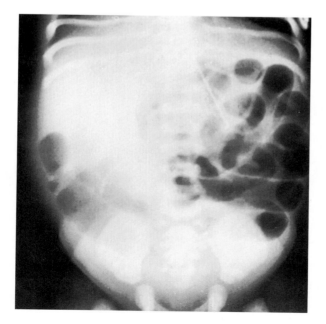

Figure 29–27
Hirschsprung's disease. Note abdominal distention with dilated loops of bowel and lack of air present in the distal portion of the bowel.

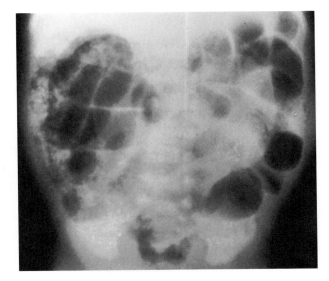

Figure 29–28
Necrotizing enterocolitis. Note presence of distended bowel loops and pneumatosis intestinalis.

    c. Condition is manifested within the first 23–36 hours of age with abdominal distention, bilious vomiting, and failure to pass meconium.

    d. Diagnosis is by contrast-enema examination. The examination may also be therapeutic by dislodgment of the meconium (Swischuk, 1997).

    e. Plain films are nonspecific and usually show a low small bowel with distention of the bowel obstruction.

3. Necrotizing enterocolitis (Fig. 29–28).

    a. X-ray findings include generalized distention caused by paralytic ileus, asymmetric distribution of bowel gas, and localized distention of bowel loops (Buonomo et al., 1998).

    b. X-ray films are obtained every 6–8 hours to follow the progression of the disease in the acute phase (Swischuk, 1997). A cross-table lateral view, along with plain film, should be obtained to detect free air (Swischuk, 1997). Most perforations occur in the first 2 days of the diagnosis (Buonomo et al., 1998).

    c. Subsequently, individual loops may become tubular, with thickened bowel walls.

    d. Persistently dilated loop may be evident on consecutive films.

    e. At any point, pneumatosis cystoides intestinalis can be seen. This represents gas formed in the intestinal wall by bacteria. The typical picture is linear or of a bubbly or foamy appearance. Air may be located in the submucosal or subserosal layer and can enter the GI tract or portal venous system (Blickman, 1998).

    f. Right segment of colon and terminal ileum are most likely to be affected, although the entire colon may be affected.

    g. Necrotizing enterocolitis, the most common cause of intestinal perforation, is seen as free abdominal gas on plain film or in left lateral decubitus view.

I. Pneumoperitoneum (Fig. 29–26).

1. Most commonly a result of perforation of the GI tract because of perinatal asphyxia, indomethacin therapy, gastric overdistention, iatrogenic perforation with a thermometer, and as a complication of necrotizing enterocolitis and GI obstruction (Swischuk, 1997).

2. Air may dissect from the neonate's chest during positive-pressure ventilation.

3. Presents with abdominal distention and respiratory distress, or abdominal wall erythema.

4. Supine x-ray may not reveal free air (Swischuk, 1997), necessitating lateral decubitus or cross-table view.
5. Abdomen is distended and radiolucent on x-ray (Swischuk, 1997). Individual loops of bowel are visible because of air inside and outside the bowel wall. Falciform ligament (an opaque stripe) may be visualized in the right upper quadrant or upper mid portion of the abdomen.

J. **Meconium peritonitis.**

1. Results from intrauterine GI perforation due to obstruction (atresia, stenosis, imperforate anus) and/or volvulus associated with meconium ileus (Swischuk, 1997).
2. Calcifications, which are easily identifiable on x-ray, assume a focal or diffuse, patchy, irregular pattern. Multiple white-speckled areas are seen in one area or throughout the abdomen and may be present in the scrotum (Swischuk and John, 1995).
3. Calcifications will slowly disappear.

K. **Abdominal ascites (Fig. 29–29).**

1. Twenty-five percent of cases result from urinary tract obstruction. Other cases include infants with fetal hydrops, GI obstruction with perforation, and peritonitis (Buonomo et al., 1998).
2. Uniform density to the distended abdomen is noted with a gasless or centralized bowel gas pattern. Body wall edema may also be present in infants with fetal hydrops.

Skeletal System

A. **Fractures:** occur most often during delivery with an increased incidence during breech deliveries. In breech deliveries, fractures can occur in both upper and lower extremities.

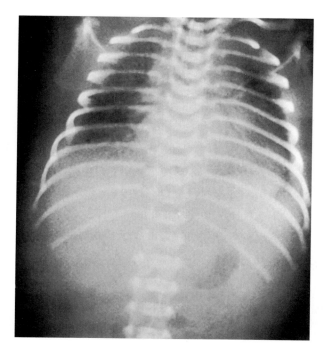

Figure 29–29
Abdominal ascites with bilateral pleural effusions.

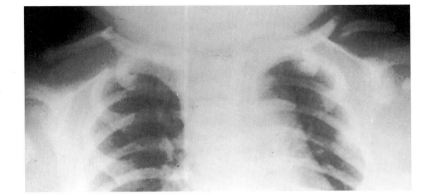

Figure 29–30
Fractured left clavicle.

1. Clavicle: fractured during delivery (Fig. 29–30). Fractures occur at the mid clavicle most commonly. Fractured clavicle is common in large infants during difficult vaginal delivery (Swischuk, 1997).
2. Rib fractures: may occur at delivery and be asymptomatic (Swischuk, 1997). With multiple fractures the infant may show signs of respiratory distress and pain. Premature infants may have rib fractures as a result of osteopenia of prematurity 8–16 weeks after birth (Fig. 29–31) (Swischuk, 1997). These bones are fragile and will fracture with handling and chest physiotherapy. Fractures may be preceded by a thin, "washed out" appearance to the ribs or extremities.
3. Skull fractures.
   a. Can be linear, buckled, or frankly depressed.
   b. Linear and buckling fractures most often occur in the parietal bone and may be suspected in the presence of cephalhematoma or other skull trauma.
   c. CT scan is more helpful than plain films for evaluation of skull fractures.

B. **Bony dysplasias.**

1. Osteogenesis imperfecta (see Chapter 23).
2. Dwarfism (common types) (Swischuk, 1997; Laor, Jaramillo, and Oestreich, 1998).
   a. Achondroplasia: short extremities and marked flaring of the metaphyses. Classic signs include spinal curvature and narrowed spinal canal; short, squared-off iliac wings; deep-set sacrum; flat acetabular roofs; and bulky proximal femurs.

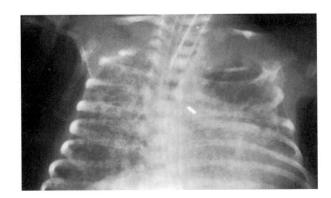

Figure 29–31
Fractured rib on left, with pale, "washed out" ribs.

b. Thanatophoric dwarfism (type I) (Fig. 29–32): marked underdevelopment of the skeleton; extremely short, bent, or curved long bones; and flaring of the metaphyses. Vertebral bodies are very flat and underdeveloped. Thorax is small and narrow, with pulmonary hypoplasia. Condition is uniformly fatal in the perinatal period.

Indwelling Lines and Tubes

A. Endotracheal tube.

1. Placement is 1.2 cm below the vocal cords and 2 cm above the carina, with the neonate's head in neutral position (Hedlund et al., 1998).
2. Placement beyond the carina results in occlusion of a bronchus (usually the right main-stem bronchus), with subsequent atelectasis and clinical deterioration (Fig. 29–33).

B. Umbilical artery catheter (Fig. 29–34A). Proceeds from the umbilicus down toward the pelvis, making an acute turn into the internal iliac artery and common iliac artery advancing into the aorta (Strife et al., 1998).

1. Low placement: at third and fourth lumbar vertebrae (Short-Bartlett, 1996).
2. High placement: at sixth through tenth thoracic vertebrae (Short-Bartlett, 1996).

C. Umbilical venous catheter (Fig. 29–34B). Passes cephalad to join the left portal vein.

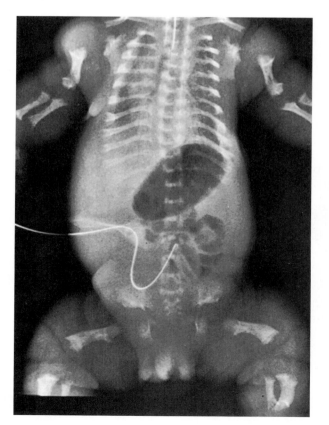

Figure 29–32
Thanatophoric dwarf. Note small, narrow thorax and shortness of long bones.

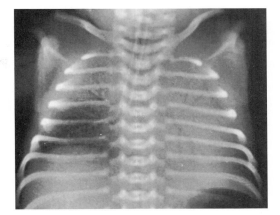

Figure 29–33
Endotracheal tube is down the right main-stem bronchus, causing atelectasis of the right upper lobe and entire left lung.

1. On lateral view the catheter is directly distal to the abdominal wall until it passes through the ductus venosus.
2. Correct placement is above the diaphragm at the junction of the right atrium (Strife et al., 1998).

D. Chest tube.

1. X-rays are obtained to determine placement and effectiveness in reinflating the lung.
2. Lateral chest x-ray film will determine anterior or posterior placement. For air evacuation, anterior placement is desirable. For fluid evacuation, posterior placement is most effective.
3. Correct placement will show the tube in the mid-clavicular line with the distal chest tube hole inside the thoracic space.

E. Central venous line. Tip should be located in the superior vena cava or right atrium above the tricuspid valve (Hughes, 1996).

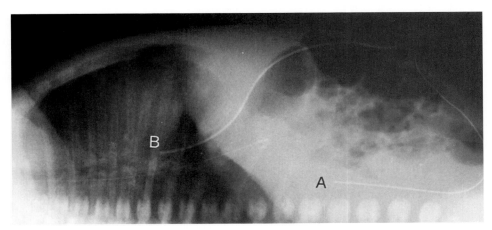

Figure 29–34
Umbilical artery catheter *(A)* enters abdomen and proceeds distally as it enters the aorta. Umbilical venous catheter *(B)* proceeds toward the head, passes through the ductus venosus, and lies in the inferior vena cava.

REFERENCES

Bick, U., Muller-Leisse, C., Troger, J., et al.: Therapeutic use of surfactant in neonatal RDS. Pediatr. Radiol., 22:169–172, 1992.

Blickman, H.: Pediatric Radiology: The Requisites, 2nd ed. St. Louis, Mosby, 1998.

Buonomo, C., Taylor, G.A., Share, J.C., and Kirks, D.R.: Gastrointestinal tract. In Kirks, D.R. (Ed.): Practical Pediatric Imaging: Diagnostic Radiology of Infants and Children. Philadelphia, Lippincott-Raven, 1998, pp. 822–996.

Emmanouilides, G.C., and Bayeen, G.B.: Neonatal Cardiopulmonary Distress. Chicago, Year Book Medical Publishers, 1988, pp. 5–6, 49–74, 324.

Fanaroff, A.A., and Martin, R.J.: Neonatal Perinatal Medicine: Diseases of the Fetus and Infant, 4th ed. St. Louis, Mosby, 1997, p. 1046.

Hazinski, M.F., and Snow, J.: Chest x-ray interpretation. In Hazinski, M.F. (Ed.): Nursing Care of the Critically Ill Child. St. Louis, C.V. Mosby, 1992, pp. 499–519.

Hedlund, G.L., Griscom, N.T., Cleveland, R.H., and Kirks, D.R.: Respiratory system. In Kirks, D.R. (Ed.): Practical Pediatric Imaging. Philadelphia, Lippincott-Raven, 1998, pp. 619–812.

Hughes, W.T.: Fluid and metabolic therapy. In Taeusch, H.W., Christiansen, R.O., and Buescher, E.S. (Eds.): Pediatric and Neonatal Tests and Procedures. Philadelphia, W.B. Saunders, 1996, pp. 275–276.

Jaquith, S.: Chest x-ray interpretation: Implications for nursing intervention. Dimensions of Critical Care Nursing, 5(1):8–17, 1986.

Laor, T., Jaramillo, D., and Oestreich, A.E.: Musculoskeletal system. In Kirks, D.R. (Ed.): Practical Pediatric Imaging: Diagnostic Radiology of Infants and Children. Philadelphia, Lippincott-Raven, 1998, pp. 350–354.

Leonidas, J.C., and Berdon, W.B.: The neonatal chest. In Silverman, F.N., and Kuhn, J.P. (Eds.): Caffey's Pediatric X-Ray Diagnosis: An Integrated Imaging Approach. St. Louis: Mosby–Year Book, 1993, pp. 1984–1989.

Levine, D., Edwards, D.K. III, and Merritt, T.A.: Synthetic vs. human surfactants in the treatment of respiratory distress syndrome: Radiographic findings. A.J.R. Am. J. Roentgenol., 157:371–374, 1991.

Northway, W.H. Jr.: Bronchopulmonary dysplasia and research in diagnostic radiology. A.J.R. Am. J. Roentgenol., 156:681–687, 1991.

Northway, W.H. Jr., and Rosan, R.C.: Radiographic features of pulmonary oxygen toxicity in the newborn: Bronchopulmonary dysplasia. Radiology, 91:49–58, 1968.

Philip, A.G.S.: Neonataology: A Practical Guide, 4th ed. Philadelphia, W.B. Saunders, 1996, p. 306.

Short-Bartlett, S.C.: Arterial catheterization. In Taeusch, H.W., Christiansen, R.O., and Buescher, E.S.: Pediatric and Neonatal Tests and Procedures. Philadelphia, W.B. Saunders, 1996, pp. 165–167.

Squire, L.F., and Novelline, R.A.: Fundamentals of Radiology, 4th ed. Cambridge, Mass., Harvard University Press, 1988.

Strife, J.L., Bissett, G.S., and Burrows, P.E.: Cardiovascular system. In Kirks, D.R. (Ed.): Practical Pediatric Imaging. Philadelphia, Lippincott-Raven, 1998, pp. 512–613.

Swischuk, L.E.: Imaging of the Newborn, Infant, and Young Child, 4th ed. Baltimore, Williams & Wilkins, 1997.

Swischuk, L.E., and John, S.D.: Differential Diagnosis in Pediatric Radiology, 2nd ed. Baltimore, Williams & Wilkins, 1995.

Wagner, L.K., and Dominguez, R.: Risks associated with diagnostic examinations in the neonate. In Dominguez, R. (Ed.): Diagnostic Imaging of the Premature Infant. New York, Churchill Livingstone, 1992, pp. 25–33.

Wechsler, S.B., and Wernovsky, G.: Cardiac disorders. In Cloherty, J.P., and Stark, A. (Eds.): Manual of Neonatal Care. Philadelphia, Lippincott-Raven, 1998, p. 419.

Wilmot, D.M., and Sharko, G.E.: Pediatric Imaging for the Technologist. New York, Springer-Verlag, 1987, pp. 258, 262.

ADDITIONAL READINGS

Abman, J.H., and Groothius, J.R.: Pathophysiology and treatment of bronchopulmonary dysplasia: Current issues. Pediatr. Clin. North Am., 41:277–289, 1994.

Carey, B.E.: Chest x-ray findings in respiratory distress syndrome. Neonatal Network, 13(1):67–72, 1994.

Carey, B.E., and Trotter, C.: The chest x-ray findings in retained lung fluid. Neonatal Network, 13(4):65–69, 1994.

Carey, B.F., and Trotter, C.: Bronchopulmonary dysplasia. Neonatal Network, 15(4):73–77, 1996.

Fletcher, E.W., Baum, J.D., and Draper, G.: The risk of diagnostic radiation of the newborn. Br. J. Radiol., 59:165, 1986.

Flores, M.T.: Understanding neonatal chest x-rays. Part II. Clinical and radiological manifestations of selected lung disorders. Neonatal Network, 12(8):9–15, 1993.

Harris, M.A., and Valmorida, J.N.: Neonates with congenital heart disease. Part I. Overview. Neonatal Network, 15(6):81–85, 1996.

Harris, M.A., and Valmorida, J.N.: Neonates with congenital heart disease. Part II. Congenital cardiac defects with increased pulmonary blood flow. Neonatal Network, 15(8):61–65, 1996.

Harris, M.A., and Valmorida, J.N.: Neonates with congenital heart disease. Part III. Congenital cardiac defects with decreased pulmonary blood flow. Neonatal Network, 16(2):59–63, 1997.

Jones, K.L.: Smith's Recognizable Patterns of Human Malformation, 5th ed. Philadelphia, W.B. Saunders, 1997, pp. 486–491.

Moore, C.S.: Meconium aspiration syndrome. Neonatal Network, 13(7):57–60, 1994.

Quinn, D., and Shannon, L.F.: Congenital anomalies of the gastrointestinal tract. Part I. The stomach. Neonatal Network, 14(8):63–66, 1995.

Quinn, D., and Shannon, L.F.: Congenital anomalies of the gastrointestinal tract. Part III. The colon and rectum. Neonatal Network, 15(2):63–67, 1996.

Shannon, L.F., and Quinn, R.: Congenital anomalies of the gastrointestinal tract. Part II. The small bowel. Neonatal Network, 15(1):57–61, 1996.

Trotter, C., and Carey, B.E.: Assessment of inspiratory effort. Neonatal Network, 11(8):61–63, 1992.

Trotter, C., and Carey, B.E.: How to evaluate lung fields on the neonatal chest x-ray film. Neonatal Network, 12(2):63–66, 1993.

Vargo, L.: Evaluation of cardiac size on the neonatal chest x-ray. Neonatal Network, 12(3):65–67, 1993.

Chapter 30

Neonatal Transport

S. Louise Bowen

Objectives

1. Identify the advantages and disadvantages of one-way versus two-way transport.

2. Discuss important considerations in the selection of transport vehicles.

3. Discuss the important factors to be considered in making a decision on team composition.

4. Describe the process of neonatal transport from the referring call to transport of the patient to arrival at the receiving hospital.

5. Identify potential risks associated with the transport environment.

6. Discuss legal and ethical considerations relating to neonatal transport.

In the late 1950s and early 1960s, intensive care for newborn infants first became available. As the scope of care for critically ill infants expanded, so did the number of hospitals offering this service. Unfortunately, because of the uneven distribution of these services, many areas remained without available resources. In the early 1970s the need to regionalize perinatal care was recognized by health care providers. In 1976 the National Foundation–March of Dimes released the report *Toward Improving the Outcome of Pregnancy,* which described regionalized care and identified criteria for level I, II, and III hospitals (Committee on Perinatal Health, 1976). This committee also recommended the establishment of formal relationships between hospitals delivering different levels of care within a region so that every baby could receive appropriate care. The concept of regionalization led naturally to the need for the development of neonatal transport. This chapter discusses various aspects of neonatal transport. Stabilization of the infant before transport is discussed in previous chapters.

Historical Aspects

A. **In 1899,** when most infants were born at home, the first ambulance incubator was developed to transport premature infants from home to Chicago's Lying-In Hospital (Butterfield, 1993; Cone, 1985).

B. In 1935 the Chicago Board of Health operated a special ambulance with incubator, oxygen, and humidity and staffed with public health nurses (Chou and MacDonald, 1989).

C. In 1948 the New York City Department of Health, Maternity and Newborn Division, established a well-organized transport service staffed with ambulance drivers, nurses, a pediatrician, and a transport clerk (Losty, Orlofsky, and Boles, 1950; Wallace, Losty, and Baumgartner, 1952).

D. In 1966 Dr. Sydney Segal published guidelines for neonatal transport (Segal, 1966), which were expanded in 1972 into a comprehensive transport manual (Segal, 1972).

Philosophy of Neonatal Transport

A. Neonatal transport is one component of an organized approach to regionalized care, which includes level I, II, and III nurseries; perinatal centers; maternal transport; and neonatal transport.

B. The concept of regionalization is changing in the current health environment because of the formation of health care and physician alliances and managed care contracts (McCormick and Richardson, 1995).

C. Maternal transport results in improved neonatal outcomes, in comparison with neonatal transport (Harding and Morton, 1993; Kollee et al., 1992).

1. Despite careful maternal screening, infants requiring intensive care will continue to be born in hospitals not equipped to provide that service.
2. Interfacility transport, such as neonatal transport, is inherently different from typical emergency medical services.
   a. Stabilization during interfacility transport is accomplished in the controlled setting of a medical facility, such as a hospital or medical clinic, in comparison with stabilization performed at the scene of an accident with limited support services.
   b. In interfacility transport, a patient is moved from a controlled setting (referring hospital) to the transport environment before arriving in the controlled setting of the receiving center. Scene-response systems move a patient from an uncontrolled setting to the controlled setting of a medical facility. The focus of emergency medical services (EMS) is on immediate, short-term stabilization to sustain the patient until arrival at the medical facility. Interfacility transport systems focus on providing intensive care services from the referral facility and throughout the transport; thus more time is spent in stabilization at the point of origin. The level of care should remain the same or increase during neonatal interfacility transport.

D. One-way versus two-way transport.

1. One-way transport uses services of personnel, equipment, and vehicles dispatched by the referral hospital to the receiving center. Two-way transport uses the services of personnel, equipment, and vehicles dispatched by the receiving center.
2. Advantages of one-way transport.
   a. Time saving in patient arrival at the receiving center.
   b. Knowledge of the patient by referring staff.
3. Disadvantages of one-way transport.
   a. Justification of the expense of maintaining experienced staff and equipment is difficult because of the small number of transports.

    b. One-way transport may deplete the resources of local EMS or the referring hospital for the duration of the transport.

    c. Referring hospital and local EMS may not have appropriate equipment or training for transport of neonates.

4. Advantages of two-way transport.

    a. More cost-effective use of expensive equipment.

    b. More experienced transport staff trained specifically in neonatal transport.

    c. Provide equipment specifically for neonatal transport.

5. Disadvantages.

    a. Time delay in moving patient from referring facility.

    b. Expense of maintaining transport program.

E. **Neonatal back/return transport (Chester, 1994; Croop and Kenner, 1990; Donovan and Schmitt, 1991; Kuhnly and Freston, 1993; Phibbs and Mortensen, 1992; Schwab and O'Dowd, 1994).**

1. Advantages.

    a. More efficient use of beds at tertiary care centers.

    b. Improved relations between community hospitals and tertiary care center.

    c. Greater opportunity for parental involvement.

    d. Familiarity of primary physician with infant before discharge home.

    e. Decreased cost during convalescence.

2. Disadvantages.

    a. Financial analysis of cost to keep infant at tertiary care center versus cost of transport. Transfer of neonate back to referring hospital may depend on managed-care or insurance contract.

    b. Potential need for transport back to tertiary care center if patient's condition deteriorates at community hospital.

Selection of Transport Vehicles

A. **General considerations (American Academy of Pediatrics [AAP], 1993; Association of Air Medical Services, 1990; Schneider et al., 1992; Thomas et al., 1990).**

1. Appropriate vehicle selection may be dictated by diagnosis, clinical condition of the patient, available resources at the referring hospital, location of referring hospital, distance and duration of transport, geographic characteristics of referral area (road conditions, traffic conditions, construction detours), weather, cost of the transport, and reimbursement.

2. Vehicles must be appropriately equipped, including power supplies, invertor, oxygen and compressed-air supply, suction, lighting, altitude pressurization where appropriate, means for securing incubators and all equipment, and room for adequate personnel.

3. An integrated system using multiple modes of transportation allows maximum flexibility to meet patient needs in a cost-effective manner.

4. Decisions regarding the appropriate vehicle for individual transport should be made by the medical control physician at the tertiary hospital, the transport team, and the referring physician in consideration of the impact on patient care and outcome, advantages and disadvantages of each vehicle, and cost.

B. **Specific vehicle considerations.**

1. Ambulance (Scott, Smith, and O'Connor, 1994).

    a. Advantages.

      (1) In general, most cost-effective means of transport.

> (2) Ability to carry equipment and personnel for twins in specially equipped ambulances.
>
> (3) Increased space and patient more accessible.
>
> (4) Ability to stop vehicle or divert to the closest hospital in an emergency.
>
> b. Disadvantages.
>
> > (1) Long response times as a result of distance, traffic, and geographic location.
> >
> > (2) Delay of admission to tertiary care center because of long-distance ground transport.

2. Helicopters (AAP, 1993).

   a. Advantages.

   > (1) Speed in response to calls and in returning patient to the receiving center for distances up to 100 miles (AAP, 1993).
   >
   > (2) Decreased response time to the referring facility possibly useful as a marketing tool.
   >
   > (3) Use of one-way helicopter transport to increase team's response time to referring hospital (Werman and Neely, 1996).

   b. Disadvantages.

   > (1) Impact of noise and vibration on the neonate, personnel, and transport equipment.
   >
   > (2) Difficulty in identifying problems when they occur because of noise and vibration (pneumothorax, extubation).
   >
   > (3) Safety concerns.
   >
   > (4) High operational costs.
   >
   > (5) Space and weight limitations.
   >
   > (6) Down time because of weather.

3. Fixed-wing aircraft (AAP, 1993).

   a. Advantages.

   > (1) Primarily beneficial for long-distance transports, usually greater than 100–150 miles.
   >
   > (2) Although fixed-wing transportation is expensive, possible favorable cost comparison over long distances when staff time is taken into consideration.

   b. Disadvantages.

   > (1) If no contractual agreements with aircraft vendors, possible inadequate equipment and unfamiliarity of team with the aircraft or with general vendor operation.
   >
   > (2) Requires coordination of ground transportation for both ends of the trip.
   >
   > (3) Space limitations.

Transport Personnel

A. Composition of a neonatal transport team varies, depending on federal and state regulations, budget, staff availability, professional standards, patient population, referral area, expectations and available resources at referral hospital, skill and educational level of team, diagnosis, clinical condition of the neonate, and volume of transports (Beyer, Land, and Zaritsky, 1992; McCloskey and Johnston, 1990; National Association of Neonatal Nurses [NANN], 1994). The team may be staffed by using various combinations, with a minimum of two individuals trained in the management of neonates. At least one team member should be a physician, registered nurse, or neonatal nurse practitioner. Team composition may vary according to individual transport or may remain the same for all transports (AAP, 1993; McCloskey and Orr, 1995). The following personnel may be used:

1. Registered nurses.

2. Neonatal nurse practitioners.
3. Respiratory therapists.
4. Physicians/neonatologists.
5. Emergency medical technicians/paramedics.
6. Fellows and residents.

B. Roles for transport personnel, including functions, responsibilities, qualifications, and competencies, must be clearly outlined in job descriptions.

C. Team composition considerations (NANN, 1998).

1. Physicians (McCloskey and Johnston, 1992; McCloskey, King, and Byron, 1989).
   a. Neonatologists provide highest level of clinical expertise. May strain resources available in a busy neonatal transport practice. May improve public relations with community physicians.
   b. Residents may provide less consistency as a result of rotations and lack of educational experience in neonatal intensive care.
   c. Fellows may provide more consistency and increasing levels of expertise as they advance through their fellowship.
   d. In some systems, physicians may be used on an as-needed basis for critically ill patients.
2. Registered nurses (Lee, 1991; National Flight Nurses Association, 1997) require advanced knowledge and procedural skills. Have been shown to provide expert, high-quality care in phone consultation with physicians. Educational requirements include in-service programs, national certifications and/or neonatal nurse practitioner programs, the American Heart Association–AAP Neonatal Resuscitation Program, and the American Heart Association–AAP Pediatric Advanced Life Support Course.
3. Respiratory therapists.
   a. Frequent team members because of the majority of neonates with a respiratory component.
   b. May assist with nursing functions as licensed by the state.
   c. Responsible for respiratory equipment, airway maintenance, participation in maintaining adequate oxygenation and ventilation during transport.
4. Emergency medical technicians/paramedics.
   a. Role varies, depending on experience and education in neonatal care.
   b. Functions may include assisting with nursing and respiratory therapy responsibilities.
5. Expertise required within the transport team.
   a. Assessment.
      (1) History taking.
      (2) Physical examination.
      (3) Interpretation of laboratory and x-ray findings.
   b. Knowledge of neonatal physiology and pathophysiology.
   c. Excellent communication and public relations skills.
   d. Clinical experience and expertise.
   e. Physical examination and fitness criteria (physical agility and stamina).
   f. Knowledge of aviation physiology.
   g. Transport safety.
   h. Knowledge of transport environment.
   i. Independence and flexibility.
   j. Procedures.
      (1) Endotracheal intubation.
      (2) Arterial access (umbilical artery catheters, percutaneous artery catheters, arterial sampling).
      (3) Needle thoracentesis.

(4) Chest tube insertion.
(5) Venous access (umbilical venous catheters, peripheral IV lines).
(6) Intraosseous insertion.
6. Justification for a neonatal team.
  a. Staffing: dedicated, unit based, on call.
  b. Use of personnel when there are no transports.
  c. Volume of transports.
  d. Review of other systems that could transport the neonate.
  e. Reimbursement.
  f. Continual search for opportunities to decrease cost and/or improve efficiency.
  g. Demonstration of improvement in patient outcome.

Transport Equipment (NANN, 1998)

A. **Transport equipment must be checked on a regular basis** to ensure that it is adequately stocked, functioning properly, and ready for immediate transport.

B. **Recommended equipment must be operable on battery power.**
1. Portable incubator.
2. Cardiorespiratory monitor with pressure tracing and recorder.
3. Transcutaneous oxygen and carbon dioxide monitor.
4. Pulse oximeter.
5. Infant ventilator.
6. End-tidal carbon dioxide monitor.
7. Invasive and noninvasive blood pressure monitors.
8. IV infusion pumps.
9. Portable blood gas analyzer (state regulations vary regarding use and quality control checks in mobile intensive care environments).
10. Defibrillator/pacer (minimum capacity, 2 watt-seconds).
11. Portable oxygen cylinders.
12. Portable air cylinders or air compressor.
13. Electrical invertor in vehicle.
14. Use by some teams of nitric oxide, extracorporeal membrane oxygenation, and high-frequency ventilation during neonatal transport.

C. **Equipment for neonatal transport (Table 30–1).**

Neonatal Transport Process

A. **Referral call.** The referral call should be handled by a designated physician who is responsible for obtaining adequate information to make a provisional diagnosis, anticipate potential complications during transport, and provide consultation for care of the infant as needed until the transport team arrives. Management given via phone should be recorded or accurately documented. Transport computer data systems are available (Donn, Gates, and Kiska, 1993). During the initial call, minimum information should be obtained to activate the appropriate team (one-way vs two-way transport, team composition) and dispatch the appropriate vehicle. Then additional information may be obtained. Information to be obtained during the referral call includes the following:
1. Time and date of referral call.
2. Patient name and gender.
3. Parent's name and demographic information.
4. Referring physician.

Table 30–1
NEONATAL EQUIPMENT INVENTORY

This equipment list is designed for critical care interfacility neonatal transport.

RESPIRATORY EQUIPMENT
Laryngoscope handle with blades, sizes Miller 0 and 1
Spare laryngoscope bulbs and batteries
ET tube stylet
Anesthesia bag (not to exceed 750 mL) with manometer or self-inflating bag with manometer
Face mask, sizes 0 and 1 (premature and term)
ET tubes, sizes 2.0, 2.5, 3.0, 3.5, and 4.0
Suction catheter and glove sets, sizes 5F, 6F, 8F, and 10F
Meconium aspirator
Blood gas kit
CPAP prongs
Nasal cannula (infant)
Ventilator circuit
Thoracentesis setups:
 Syringe, 60 mL
 Three-way stopcock
 Angiocatheters, 20- and 22-gauge
 Tubing T-connector
Antiseptic solution
Heimlich valves
Chest tubes, sizes 8F, 10F, and 12F
Oxygen hood

INTRAVENOUS THERAPY EQUIPMENT
Bags of D_5W and $D_{10}W$, 250 mL
IV pump tubing
IV filters
Platelet and blood infusion sets
Umbilical catheters, sizes 3.5F and 5F
IV extension tubing
T-connectors, multiport connectors
Sterile drapes
Syringes, sizes 1-60 mL
Needles, assorted sizes, 18-25 gauge; or needleless system
Three-way stopcock and stopcock plugs
Wipes with povidone-iodine (Betadine) and alcohol
Scalp vein needles, 23 and 25 gauge
Intravenous catheters, 22, 24, and 26 gauge
Disposable razors
Medication additive labels
Paper tape measure
Tongue blades
Armboards, sizes premature and infant

Assorted tape
Umbilical tape
Povidone-iodine (Betadine) and alcohol, one bottle each
Size 4.0 silk suture with curved needle
Umbilical catheter and thoracotomy set, including:
 Two sterile drapes
 Iris forceps
 Needle holders
 Scissors
 Curved forceps
 Tongue tissue forceps
 Sterile gauze pads, 2 by 2 inches
 Scalpel and blade
 Blunt-end adapters, 17, 18, and 20 gauge

THERMOREGULATION AND MONITORING EQUIPMENT
Knit hat
Plastic wrap, bubble wrap
Crushable heat packs and mattress
Space blankets
Thermometer
Chest electrodes; limb leads
Lead wires for heart monitor
Capillary tubes
Glucose monitoring device
Lancets
Arterial transducer tubing

MISCELLANEOUS
Intraosseous needles
Camera, film
Parent information
Blood culture bottles
Scissors and hemostat
Flashlight
Gauze pads, 2 by 2 inches
Limb restraints
Safety pins
Rubber bands
Pacifiers (various sizes)
Cottonballs
Liquid adhesive tape
Christmas tree adapters
Feeding tubes, sizes 5F and 8F
Salem sump tubes, sizes 10F and 12F
Dual flow gastric tubes, sizes 10F and 12F
Sterile glove packs (assorted sizes)

Sphygmomanometer with blood pressure cuffs, sizes premature, neonate, and infant
Neonatal stethoscope
Trash bag; needle disposal system
Bulb syringe
Personal protective equipment (goggles, gowns, masks, gloves)
Visceral pack: normal saline solution, sterile gauze, sterile operating-room drape or sterile plastic bag
Glass filter needles

MEDICATIONS
Epinephrine 1 : 10,000
Sodium bicarbonate ($NaHCO_3$), 4.2%
$NaHCO_3$, 8.4%
Naloxone hydrochloride (Narcan)
Atropine
Calcium gluconate 10%
Dopamine
Dobutamine
Isoproterenol (Isuprel)
Tolazoline (Priscoline)
Prostaglandin E_1
Phenobarbital
Phenytoin (Dilantin)
Diazepam (Valium)
Paralytic agent: pancuronium bromide (Pavulon)
Analgesics
Concentrated sodium chloride and potassium acetate
Lidocaine (Xylocaine), 1%
Heparin (1000 U/mL)
Normal saline diluent, 0.9%
Sterile water diluent
Flush solution
Broad-spectrum antibiotics
Albumin 5% and/or normal saline solution
$D_{50}W$
Hyaluronidase (Wydase)
Adenosine
Digoxin (Lanoxin)
Surfactant
Ophthalmic ointment
Vitamin K
Lorazepam (Ativan)
Sedative(s)

ET, Endotracheal; *CPAP*, continuous positive airway pressure; D_5W and $D_{10}W$, 5% and 10% dextrose in water.

5. Referring institution, including city, state, and phone number.
6. Maternal prenatal, labor, and delivery history.
7. Date and time of birth.
8. Gestational age, birth weight, and current weight.
9. Apgar scores.
10. Details of delivery room stabilization.
11. Subsequent neonatal course, including reason for transfer request.
    a. Significant findings of physical examination.

    b. Laboratory data.

    c. X-ray findings.

    d. Vital signs.

    e. Respiratory support.

    f. Fluid management. To prevent aspiration, the infant should receive nothing by mouth before transport.

    g. Other pertinent patient findings or medical management.

B. Selection and notification of team members.

C. Selection and dispatch of appropriate vehicles.

D. Selection of appropriate equipment and supplies.

E. Procedures while en route to referring hospital.

1. Team members will discuss provisional and differential diagnoses, a proposed plan of care, and division of responsibilities.
2. Referring hospital should be notified of team's dispatch, mode of transport, and estimated time of arrival at referring hospital.
3. Emergency and anticipated medication dosages and IV fluid amounts are calculated on the basis of weight.
4. Potential complications are anticipated.
5. History and diagnostic study results to be obtained at referring hospital are identified.

F. Stabilization at referral hospital (James, 1993; Kissoon, 1992; Kronick et al., 1996; Morton, Pollack, and Wallace, 1997; Paxton, 1990; Sayler, 1991).

1. Introduce transport team members to referring physicians, staff, and family members. Check identification band on infant. All patients should be transported with identification band on. Parents' religious, cultural, and ethnic preferences should be noted.
2. Assess infant to determine need for any immediate interventions.
3. Obtain further details of history and current management.
4. Review x-ray films.
5. Obtain vital signs and glucose screening results. Determine blood gas values if clinical situation warrants.
6. Perform physical assessment.
7. Initiate monitoring systems as appropriate; may include direct arterial blood pressure monitoring, transcutaneous oxygen and carbon dioxide measurements, and pulse oximetry.
8. Consult with designated transport physician regarding management plan and anticipated complications en route.
9. Attempt to achieve normal or optimal blood gas values, blood pressure, temperature, perfusion, serum glucose level, and acid-base balance according to the plan of care.
10. Begin switching to transport equipment, including ventilator and IV pumps, carefully monitoring changes in patient status.
11. Notify receiving nursery of estimated time of arrival, current patient status, and anticipated patient needs on admission.
12. Speak with parents.
    a. Update current patient status; discuss anticipated complications during transport and treatment plans.
    b. Assess the parents' understanding of the infant's condition, plans for traveling to the receiving center, and their needs for physical and emotional support.
    c. Provide information about the receiving center, including location, phone numbers, directions, attending physician, primary/admitting nurse, and visiting policy.

d. Obtain written transport consents.
e. Take a picture of the infant or provide a set of footprints of the infant to leave with the parents.
f. Depending on the team's policy, one parent may be allowed to accompany the infant (Lewis, 1997).
g. Obtain copies of prenatal, maternal, and neonatal records; obtain x-ray films.
h. Place an identification band on the infant.

13. Distribute transport evaluation form to referring hospital staff and/or parents.
14. En route to receiving hospital:
    a. Infant should be secured in incubator with safety strap(s) and blanket rolls. Loose equipment should not be placed inside the incubator.
    b. Continuously monitor temperature, pulse, respirations, blood pressure, and oxygenation/ventilation status, as indicated.
    c. Documentation at regular intervals, as indicated by infant's condition.
       (1) Vital signs, blood pressure, color, tone.
       (2) Readings of oxygenation and ventilation monitors and of respiratory support settings (including altitude if appropriate).
       (3) Serum glucose screening.
       (4) Important documentation times for status of infant, including arrival at referring hospital, departure from referring hospital, and time of transfer of care to receiving hospital staff.
15. On arrival at receiving center, notification of parents and referring staff regarding safe completion of transport. Follow-up may be provided to referring staff and physicians during the infant's hospitalization at the receiving center, maintaining patient confidentiality.

Documentation

A. **Necessity of documentation.** Patient status and the care provided must be documented throughout transport (Whitfield and Buser, 1993).

B. **Logistical documentation.**

1. Time of transport call.
2. Time of departure en route to referring hospital.
3. Time of arrival at referring hospital.
4. Time of departure from referring hospital.
5. Time of arrival at receiving hospital.
6. Transport delays.
7. Transport staff.
8. Mode of transport.

C. **Patient care documentation.**

1. Significant maternal history, including medical history before pregnancy and prenatal, labor, and delivery history.
2. Date and time of birth.
3. Gestational age.
4. Birth weight.
5. Delivery room resuscitation, including Apgar scores.
6. Care provided before the team's arrival, including laboratory and x-ray findings and medication administered.
7. Patient status on arrival of the transport team, including physical assessment, vital signs, and current patient management.
8. Problem list, including current and resolved problems.

9. Ongoing documentation of patient assessment, management, and consultations with designated transport physician.

Transport Environment

A. **Safety.** Make safety the highest priority in any transport program (Miller, 1994; NANN, 1998).

B. **Securing of all equipment and articles in the vehicle or aircraft.**

C. **Restraint of all passengers, including the patient, during transport.**

D. **Regular training in safety and emergency procedures for team members.**

E. **Evaluation for extubation and pulmonary air leaks: possibly difficult during transport, especially in rotor-wing aircraft.** Anticipate problems during transport on the basis of diagnosis and clinical presentation.

F. **Cautious use of lights and sirens.** Follow the transport program's policy.

G. **Altitude.**

1. Anticipate increased oxygen requirement or ventilatory support at higher altitudes.
2. Provide supplemental oxygen for staff above 10,000 feet if in a nonpressurized aircraft.

H. **Dysbarism.**

1. Increased atmospheric pressure results in expansion of gases.
2. Anticipate expansion of "trapped" gases in body spaces (pulmonary air leaks, necrotizing enterocolitis, bowel obstruction).
   a. Gastrointestinal tract. Insert orogastric tube and empty stomach of air.
   b. Pulmonary air leaks. Consider needle thoracentesis or tube thoracostomy for decompression.
   c. Middle ear. Provide pacifier if appropriate.

I. **Effects of motion.**

1. Staff should recognize and understand the stresses of transport and flight.
2. Anticipate patient instability on ascent and descent.

J. **Noise and vibration (Sherwood, Donze, and Giebe, 1994).**

1. Provide ear protection for staff and for the neonate (especially in rotor-wing aircraft).
2. Provide routine hearing screens for staff.
3. Minimize noise levels in patient compartment of vehicle.
4. Anticipate patient instability.
5. Use mattress and padding to minimize vibration in incubator.

K. **Eye protection for the neonate from vehicle lighting.**

Legal and Ethical Considerations

A. **Legal issues (Rice, 1991; NANN, 1998).**

1. Determination of the level of responsibility of the receiving and referring staffs and institutions during the transport process has not been clearly established and is open to legal interpretations (Lazar, 1991; McCloskey and Orr, 1995).
   a. Referring institution's level of responsibility gradually decreases as the receiving physician and transport team assume increasing responsibility for the management and care of the infant.

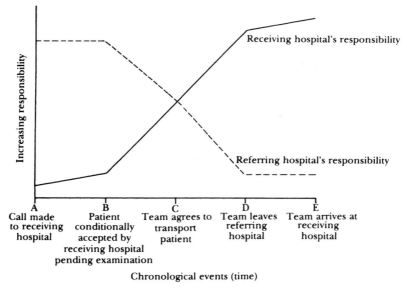

Figure 30–1
Changing levels of responsibility for patient care. (From Brimhall, D.C.: The hospital administrator's perspective. *In* MacDonald, M.G., and Miller, M.K.: Emergency Transport of the Perinatal Patient. Boston, Little, Brown, 1989.)

   b. Transport team should be aware of national and state regulations regarding transport and professional standards: Federal Aviation Administration, local and state departments of transportation, Joint Commission on Accreditation of Healthcare Organizations, the Clinical Laboratories Improvement Act, and the Consolidated Omnibus Budget Reconciliation Act.

   c. Receiving institution acquires increasing responsibility from the time of the transport call and the initial consultation, increasing until the time of admission to the receiving hospital (Fig. 30–1).

2. Transport team should ensure that the parents have adequate information regarding the infant's status and specific transport considerations and risks at the time that informed consent was obtained.

3. Expanded responsibilities of transport team members should be clearly outlined in their job functions and responsibilities and should be compatible with practice acts.

4. The team should be knowledgeable regarding out-of-state and international transport regulations and issues.

B. Ethical issues. Dilemmas regarding the transport of neonates should be addressed by administrative, medical, and transport staff and should include information on the following:

1. Infants with expected poor outcomes, including those with genetic disorders, severely asphyxiated infants, extremely low birth weight infants, and those with lethal anomalies.

2. Cost constraints.

Quality Assurance and Continuous Quality Improvement

A. Quality control issues may include the following:

1. Transport statistics.

2. Equipment malfunction or failure.
3. Transport delays.
4. Equipment issues.
5. Stabilization times.
6. Completion of safety in-service training.

B. **Quality assurance may be attained through a number of mechanisms. A combination of these mechanisms is probably most effective (NANN, 1998).**
1. Case review by the team, medical director, and transport director.
2. Use of peer review.
3. Regular staff meetings.
4. Case review with team members, which can be effectively accomplished by review of selected cases, including the following:
   a. Initial referral call.
   b. Transport logistics.
   c. Stabilization of the infant by the referring hospital as well as the transport team.
   d. Care provided during transport.
   e. Patient outcome.

C. **Peer review may be used to provide input to individuals.**
1. Appropriateness of care provided.
2. Clarity of treatment plan.
3. Treatment plan rationale and outcome.
4. Documentation.

D. **Issues identified through any of these mechanisms should be addressed with recommendations and plans for follow-up.**

REFERENCES

American Academy of Pediatrics: Guidelines for Air and Ground Transport of Neonatal and Pediatric Patients. Elk Grove Village, Ill., Author, 1993.

Association of Air Medical Services: Position paper on the appropriate use of emergency air services. Air Med. J., 11(9):29–33, 1990.

Beyer, A.J., Land, G., and Zaritsky, A.: Nonphysician transport of intubated pediatric patients: A system evaluation. Crit. Care Med., 20:961–966, 1992.

Butterfield, L.J.: Historical perspectives of neonatal transport. Pediatr. Clin. North Am., 40:221–239, 1993.

Chester, G.: Prescheduled neonatal return transports. Neonatal Network, 13(7):23–26, 1994.

Chou, M., and MacDonald, M.G.: Landmarks in the development of patient transport systems. In MacDonald, M.G., and Miller, M.K. (Eds.): Emergency Transport of the Perinatal Patient. Boston, Little, Brown, 1989.

Committee on Perinatal Health: Toward Improving the Outcome of Pregnancy. White Plains, N.Y., National Foundation–March of Dimes, 1976.

Cone, T.E.: History of the Care and Feeding of the Premature Infant. Boston, Little, Brown, 1985, p. 46.

Croop, L.H., and Kenner, C.: Protocol for reverse neonatal transports. Neonatal Network, 9(1):49–53, 1990.

Donn, S.M., Gates, M.R., and Kiska, D.J.: User-friendly computerized quality assurance program for regionalized neonatal care. J. Perinatol., 12(3):190–192, 1993.

Donovan, T.L., and Schmitt, R.: Discharge planning for neonatal back transport. J. Perinatal Neonatal Nurs., 5(1):64–70, 1991.

Harding, J.E., and Morton, S.M.: Adverse effects of neonatal transport between level III centres. J. Paediatr. Child Health, 29(2):146–149, 1993.

James, A.G.: Resuscitation, stabilization, and transport in perinatology. Curr. Opin. Pediatr., 5(2):150–155, 1993.

Kissoon, N.: Triage and transport of the critically ill child. Crit. Care Clin., 8(1):37–57, 1992.

Kollee, L.A., Brand, R., Schreuder, A.M., et al.: Five-year outcome of preterm and very low birth weight infants: A comparison between maternal and neonatal transport. Obstet. Gynecol., 80:635–638, 1992.

Kronick, J.B., Frewen, T.C., Kissoon, N., et al.: Pediatric and neonatal critical care transport: A comparison of therapeutic intervention. Pediatr. Emerg. Care 12(1):23–26, 1996.

Kuhnly, J.E., and Freston, M.S.: Back transport: Exploration of parents' feelings regarding the transition. Neonatal Network, 12(1):49–56, 1993.

Lazar, R.A.: Selecting an air ambulance service: Avoiding negligence in the air. Medic-Air, 10–11, March 1991.

Lee, G. (Ed.): Flight nursing: Principles and practice. St. Louis, Mosby–Year Book, 1991.

Lewis, M.M.: Parents as passengers during pediatric transport. Air Med. J., 16(2):38–43, 1997.

Losty, M.S., Orlofsky, I., and Boles, T.: A transport service for premature babies. Am. J. Nurs., 50:10–12, 1950.

McCloskey, K., and Johnston, C.: Pediatric critical care transport survey: Team composition and training, mobilization time, and mode of transportation. Pediatr. Emerg. Care, 6(1):1–3, 1990.

McCloskey, K., and Johnston, C.: Critical care interhospital transports: Predictability of the need for a pediatrician. Pediatr. Emerg. Care, 6(2):89–92, 1992.

McCloskey, K.A., King, W.D., and Byron, L.: Pediatric critical care transport: Is a physician always needed on the team? Ann. Emerg. Med., 18:247–249, 1989.

McCloskey, K., and Orr, R.: Pediatric transport medicine. St. Louis, Mosby–Year Book, 1995.

McCormick, M.C., and Richardson, D.K.: Access to neonatal intensive care. The Future of Children, 5(1):162–175, 1995.

Miller, C.: The physiologic effects of air transport on the neonate. Neonatal Network, 13(7):7–10, 1994.

Morton, N.S., Pollack, M.M., and Wallace, P.G.M.: Stabilization and Transport of the Critically Ill. New York, Churchill Livingstone, 1997.

National Association of Neonatal Nurses: Neonatal Nursing Transport Guidelines. Petaluma, Calif., Author, 1998.

National Flight Nurses Association: Flight Nursing Core Curriculum. Park Ridge, Ill., Author, 1997.

Paxton, J.M.: Transport of the surgical neonate. J. Perinatal Neonatal Nurs., 3(3):43–49, 1990.

Phibbs, C., and Mortensen, L.: Back transporting infants from neonatal intensive care units to community hospitals for recovery care: Effect on total hospital charges. Pediatrics 90(1 Pt. 1):22–26, 1992.

Rice, M.M.: Medicolegal issues in pediatric and adolescent emergencies. Emerg. Med. Clin. North Am., 9:677–695, 1991.

Sayler, J.W.: Respiratory care in the transport of critically ill and injured infants and children. Respir. Care, 36:720–734, 1991.

Schneider, C., Gomez, M., Lee, R., et al.: Evaluation of ground ambulance, rotor-wing, and fixed-wing aircraft services. Crit. Care Clin., 8:533–564, 1992.

Schwab, S.V., and O'Dowd, S.: Partnerships in neonatal care: A model in reverse neonatal transport. J. Obstet. Gynecol. Neonatal Nurs., 23(3):210–213, 1994.

Scott, S., Smith, C., and O'Connor, T.: A multidisciplinary approach to neonatal ambulance design. Neonatal Network, 13(7):13–17, 1994.

Segal, S.: Transfer of a premature or other high-risk newborn infant to a referral hospital. Pediatr. Clin. North Am., 13:1195–1205, 1966.

Segal, S. (Ed.): Manual for the Transport of High-Risk Newborn Infants. Sherbrooke, Quebec, Canadian Pediatric Society, 1972.

Sherwood, H.B., Donze, A., and Giebe, J.: Mechanical vibration in ambulance transport. J. Obstet. Gynecol. Neonatal Nurs., 23:457–463, 1994.

Thomas, F.T., Wicham, J., Clemmer, T.P., et al.: Outcome, transport times and costs of patients evacuated by helicopter versus fixed-wing aircraft. West. J. Med., 153:40–43, 1990.

Wallace, H.M., Losty, M.A., and Baumgartner, L.: Report of two years' experience in the transportation of premature infants in New York City. Pediatrics, 22:439–447, 1952.

Werman, H.A., and Neely, B.N.: One-way neonatal transport: A new approach to increase effective utilization of air medical resources. Air Med. J., 15(1):13–17, 1996.

Whitfield, J.M., and Buser, M.K.: Transport stabilization times for neonatal and pediatric patients prior to interfacility transfer. Pediatr. Emerg. Care, 9(2):69–71, 1993.

ADDITIONAL READINGS

Buck, M.: Prostaglandin E_1 treatment of congenital heart disease: Use prior to neonatal transport. D.I.C.P.: Ann. Pharmacother., 25:408–409, 1991.

Hulsey, T.C., Pittard, W.B., and Ebeling, M.: Regionalized perinatal transport systems: Association with changes in location of birth, neonatal transport, and survival of very low birth weight deliveries. J. South Carolina Med. Assoc., 87:581–584, 1991.

Jaimovich, D.G., and Vidyasagar, D.: Handbook of Pediatric and Neonatal Transport Medicine. Philadelphia, Hanley & Belfus, 1996.

Jain, L., and Vidyasagar, D.: Cardiopulmonary resuscitation of newborns: Its application to transport medicine. Pediatr. Clin. North Am., 40:287–302, 1993.

Pon, S., and Notterman, D.A.: The organization of a pediatric critical care transport program. Pediatr. Clin. North Am., 40:241–261, 1993.

Reimer, J.M., Schreiber, M.D., and Dimand, R.J.: Portable transcutaneous O_2 and CO_2 monitors and pulse oximeters during transport of critically ill newborn infants. Air Med. J., 11(8):9–13, 1992.

Reynolds, J.W.: The use of surfactant replacement therapy on neonatal transport: A commentary. Air Med. J., 11(9):6–8, 1992.

Squire, S.J., and Kirchhoff, K.T.: Positional oxygenation changes in air-transported neonates. Heart Lung, 21:255–259, 1992.

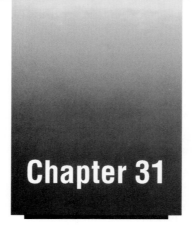

Chapter 31

Common Invasive Procedures

Ann M. Gross

Objectives

1. Explain the indications for intubation, thoracentesis, peripheral IV line placement, umbilical vessel catheterization, capillary blood sampling, radial artery puncture, and bladder catheterization.

2. List the equipment and supplies needed to perform common invasive procedures.

3. Describe care and support necessary for each patient undergoing invasive procedures.

4. Identify anatomic landmarks for determining placement of needles or catheters for various invasive procedures.

5. Describe the precautions to be familiar with for various invasive procedures.

6. Describe common complications of various invasive procedures.

Procedures common to the neonatal intensive care setting were once performed only by physicians. Today, both the bedside nurse and the nurse with an expanded role frequently perform these procedures with proficiency. Hospital protocols determine the qualifications necessary for nurses to perform these procedures.

However vital a procedure might be, the potential for complications must be considered. The patient's ability to tolerate the procedure must be assessed against the necessity of the procedure. The patient must be monitored closely during any procedure, and optimal care and support must not be compromised. Provisions must be made for adequate oxygenation, thermoregulation, and pain control. Documentation of the procedure and the patient's tolerance of the procedure on the patient's chart is also necessary. Informed consent may be necessary for some procedures. The nurse should be familiar with hospital protocol for obtaining informed consent. Discussing procedures with parents and family is important even if consent is not necessary.

For every procedure, standard precautions and aseptic and/or sterile technique must be implemented. These basic procedures should be adapted as necessary to conform to regulatory, institutional, and unit protocols, guidelines, and procedures.

Airway Procedures

ENDOTRACHEAL INTUBATION: ADVANCED PRACTICE PROCEDURE

A. Indications.

1. Bag-and-mask ventilation is ineffective or undesirable.
2. Need for mechanical ventilation is ongoing.
3. Tracheal suctioning is required.
4. Protection of the airway is required.
5. Diaphragmatic hernia is present.

B. Precautions.

1. Patient's heart rate must be monitored continuously during the procedure. Optimally, oxygen saturation is also monitored.
2. Hypoxia during the procedure should be minimized.
   a. Free-flow oxygen should be held near the mouth and nose of any infant with respiratory effort, to maximize oxygenation during the procedure.
   b. Intubation attempts should be limited to 20 seconds, and the infant's condition should be stabilized with bag-and-mask ventilation between attempts.

C. Equipment/supplies.

1. Laryngoscope.
2. Laryngoscope blade.
   a. Size 0 for preterm infant or for infant weighing less than 3.5 kg.
   b. Size 1 for term infant or for infant weighing more than 3.5 kg.
3. Endotracheal tube (American Heart Association, 1994).
   a. Internal diameter (ID) 2.5 mm for infants weighing less than 1.0 kg.
   b. ID 3.0 mm for 1–2 kg infant.
   c. ID 3.5 mm for 2–4 kg infant.
   d. ID 4.0 mm may be necessary for infants weighing more than 4.0 kg.
4. Stylet, if desired.
5. Suction catheter and suction source.
6. Resuscitation bag and mask of appropriate size.
7. Oxygen source.
8. Supplies to secure endotracheal tube according to hospital policy.

D. Procedure.

1. Select endotracheal tube of the appropriate size.
2. Insert stylet, if used, and shape the endotracheal tube as desired. The stylet must be secured so that it does not extend below the tip of the endotracheal tube and cannot advance during the procedure. This should be done while maintaining the tube and stylet as clean as possible.
3. Prepare the resuscitation bag so that the infant may be given bag-and-mask ventilation before and after the procedure.
4. Aspirate the gastric contents and suction the oropharynx.
5. Position the patient on a flat surface, with the head at midline and the neck slightly extended with the use of a flat roll. The person performing intubation must have easy access to the airway and equipment while positioned at the patient's head.
6. Hold the laryngoscope in the left hand between the thumb and first finger, with the blade pointing away.
7. Open the patient's mouth with the fingers of the right hand and gently slide the blade into the right side of the mouth.
8. Stabilize the left hand against the left side of the patient's face, advance the blade tip to the base of the tongue, and move the blade to the midline, pushing the tongue to the left.

9. Expose the pharynx by lifting the entire blade upward in the direction in which the handle is pointing. Do not rock the tip of the blade upward or use the upper gum as a fulcrum.

10. If unable to see the glottis, apply gentle pressure over the trachea with the fifth finger of the left hand and withdraw the blade slowly until the glottis is visible.

11. Any secretions that interfere with visualization should be removed with suctioning. Direct suctioning under laryngoscopy is ideal.

12. Identify anatomic landmarks (Fig. 31–1).
    a. Epiglottis is uppermost.
    b. Glottis is anterior, with vocal cords closing side to side.
    c. Esophagus is posterior.

13. After identifying the vocal cords, and with the cords in clear view, place the endotracheal tube into the right side of the patient's mouth with the right hand. Do not interfere with visualization by threading the tube through the curved laryngoscope blade.

14. Keeping the cords in view, pass the endotracheal tube between the cords to the level of the vocal cord guide mark on the endotracheal tube. This should position the tip of the tube approximately halfway between the vocal cords and the carina.

15. With the right hand, firmly grasp the endotracheal tube at the level of the patient's lip, stabilize the right hand against the patient's face, and carefully remove the laryngoscope with the left hand.

16. Carefully remove the stylet, if used, from the endotracheal tube.

17. Attach the resuscitation bag to the endotracheal tube and deliver manual breaths.

18. Assess tube placement.
    a. Auscultate both sides of the chest for the presence and intensity of breath sounds.
    b. Assess chest movement with manual breaths.
    c. The stomach is auscultated and assessed for distention.

19. If the tube is in too far and placed in a right or left main-stem bronchus, auscultation may reveal unilateral or unequal breath sounds. The tube should be withdrawn 0.5–1 cm and placement reassessed.

20. If the tube is in the esophagus.
    a. Air may be heard entering the stomach with manual breaths.
    b. The stomach may become distended.
    c. No breath sounds will be heard on auscultation of the chest during manual breaths, though air movement may be heard, especially over the lower portion of the chest.
    d. The endotracheal tube should be removed and discarded.
    e. In very small infants, breath sounds may be audible even with an endotracheal tube in the esophagus.

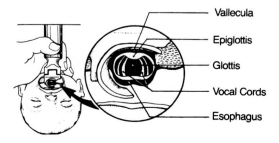

— Vallecula

— Epiglottis

— Glottis

— Vocal Cords

— Esophagus

Figure 31–1
Anatomic landmarks for endotracheal intubation. (Reproduced with permission © *Textbook of Neonatal Resuscitation*, 1987. Copyright American Heart Association.)

21. When the tube is assessed to be in good position, note the markings relative to the upper gum, and secure the tube according to hospital policy.
22. Position of the tube must be confirmed by x-ray film, 1 cm above the carina.
23. After tube placement has been confirmed by x-ray film, any length of tube that extends more than 4 cm beyond the lip should be cut off to limit dead space and prevent kinking.

E. **Complications.**

1. Hypoxia (American Heart Association, 1994).
   a. During the procedure.
   b. Due to misplacement of tube.
2. Bradycardia (American Heart Association, 1994).
   a. Due to hypoxia.
   b. Due to vagal stimulation from the laryngoscope, endotracheal tube, or suction catheter.
3. Infection.
4. Perforation of esophagus or trachea (Page, Giehl, and Luke, 1998).
5. Trauma to oropharyngeal and laryngeal tissues (Holzki, 1997).
6. Pulmonary air leak, especially with tube placement in a main-stem bronchus.
7. Loss of endotracheal tube into the esophagus or stomach if the tube is misplaced into the esophagus and the endotracheal tube adapter is disconnected (Wu et al., 1997).
8. Pain.

THORACENTESIS: ADVANCED PRACTICE PROCEDURE

A. **Indications:** emergency evacuation of pneumothorax.

B. **Precautions.**

1. Infection near the selected site of puncture.
2. Loss of skin integrity at puncture site.

C. **Equipment/supplies.**

1. Skin antiseptics for thoracentesis according to hospital policy.
2. Butterfly needle, 23 gauge, ¾ inch.
3. Three-way stopcock.
4. Syringe, 20 mL.

D. **Technique (Swift, 1996).**

1. Attach butterfly-needle tubing to syringe and stopcock. The stopcock allows for aspiration of free air into the syringe and emptying of the syringe while maintaining a closed system.
2. Position the infant on the back, and restrain if necessary.
3. Identify puncture site.
   a. Identify and avoid breast tissue.
   b. Use second or third intercostal space in mid-clavicular line.
4. Prepare skin with antiseptic.
5. Puncture skin at 45-degree angle, angling over third or fourth rib, and advance needle at 90-degree angle while assistant aspirates gently. Angling over the rib avoids the intercostal vessels, which are located on the inferior surface of the ribs (Swift, 1996).
6. When free air is obtained, stabilize the needle and continue to aspirate until preparation for chest tube insertion is complete, or until the air leak is evacuated.

E. **Complications.**

1. Hemorrhage (Quak, Szatmari, and van den Anker, 1993).

2. Infection.
3. Needle injury to lung or adjacent structures (Arya, Williams, Ponsford, and Bissenden, 1991).
4. Damage to breast tissue.

Circulatory Access Procedures

PERIPHERAL INTRAVENOUS LINE PLACEMENT

A. Indications.

1. Administration of medications.
2. Administration of fluids.
3. Administration of parenteral nutrition.

B. Precautions.

1. Areas of infection near selected puncture site.
2. Coagulation defects.
3. Loss of skin integrity at selected puncture site.
4. Need to preserve venous site for possible central venous cannulation.

C. Equipment/supplies.

1. Padded arm board of appropriate size for gestational age if an extremity is to be used.
2. Tape and/or dressing supplies per hospital policy.
3. Skin antiseptics per hospital policy.
4. Tourniquet or rubber band.
5. Normal saline solution or flush solution in a 1 or 3 mL syringe.
6. Butterfly needle, 23 or 25 gauge (scalp vein set), or catheter-over-the-needle, 24 to 22 gauge.

D. Procedure.

1. Flush needle and tubing with flush solution. Flushing catheter-over-the-needle is optional.
2. Select vein (Fig. 31–2). Distending of the vessel may be accomplished by applying a gentle tourniquet or having an assistant encircle area with hand and apply direct pressure.
3. Position and stabilize puncture site to allow puncture in direction of blood flow.
4. Prepare skin with antiseptics.
5. At a point 0.5 cm distal to the anticipated site of vessel puncture, insert the needle point, bevel up, at a 15- to 45-degree angle.
6. Advance needle until blood appears in the tubing.
   a. If resistance is met or vessel is not punctured, withdraw needle slowly to just below the level of the skin, relocate vessel, and advance the needle again.
   b. If a hematoma develops or bleeding occurs, occlude the vessel with pressure just proximal to the puncture site, withdraw the needle, and apply pressure until hemostasis is ensured.
7. Remove the tourniquet and inject some of the flush solution gently to ensure patency of the needle. If flush solution infiltrates the tissues surrounding the needle or catheter tip, occlude the vessel with pressure just proximal to the puncture site, withdraw the needle or angiocatheter, and apply pressure until hemostasis is ensured.
8. Connect IV tubing and fluid to needle and tape needle in position per hospital policy. Tape, dressing, and restraint must allow for easy inspection of insertion site and circulation of the distal extremity, as well as patency of the IV tubing.

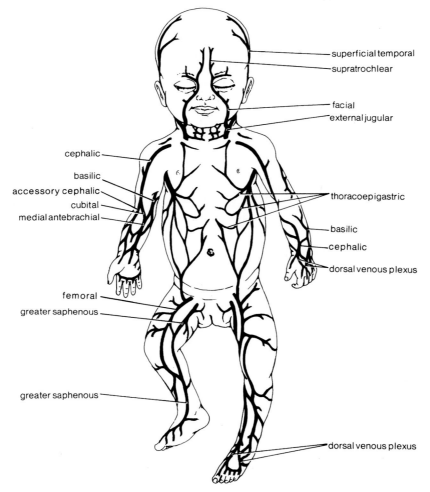

superficial temporal
supratrochlear

facial
external jugular

cephalic

basilic

accessory cephalic

cubital

medial antebrachial

thoracoepigastric

basilic

cephalic

dorsal venous plexus

femoral

greater saphenous

greater saphenous

dorsal venous plexus

Figure 31–2
Peripheral veins. (From Fletcher, M.A., MacDonald, M.G., and Avery, G.B. (Eds.): Atlas of Procedures in
Neonatology. Philadelphia, J.B. Lippincott, 1983.)

E. Complications.

1. Hemorrhage.
2. Infection (Schlager et al., 1997).
3. Hematoma.
4. Air or clot embolus.
5. Tissue injury and possible necrosis after infiltration of infused solutions and/or
   medications.
   a. Hyaluronidase can be injected around the periphery of any extravasation
      site to prevent tissue injury.
   b. Hyaluronidase is indicated for extravasation involving irritants to veins:
      aminophylline, amphotericin B, calcium, diazepam, erythromycin, methi-
      cillin, nafcillin, oxacillin, phenytoin, potassium chloride, sodium bicarbon-
      ate, vancomycin, and total parenteral nutrition.
   c. Hyaluronidase is not indicated for treatment of extravasations of vaso-
      constrictive drugs (e.g., dopamine, epinephrine, norepinephrine); in such
      instances, phentolamine (Regitine) is indicated (Young and Mangum,
      1996).

6. Injury of extremity from restraint.
   a. Compromised distal circulation.
   b. Pressure necrosis over bony areas.
   c. Limb deformity after prolonged immobilization.
   d. Pressure damage to peripheral nerves.
7. Inadvertent arterial line placement.
8. Pain.

UMBILICAL VESSEL CATHETERIZATION: ADVANCED PRACTICE PROCEDURE

A. Indications.

1. Arterial catheterization.
   a. Frequent arterial blood sampling.
   b. Continuous arterial blood pressure monitoring.
   c. Vascular access when other sites are not available or suitable.
   d. Exchange transfusion.
   e. Cardiac catheterization.
2. Venous catheterization.
   a. Emergency administration of drugs.
   b. Emergency measurement of P_{CO_2} and pH.
   c. Fluid administration (hypertonic solutions or inadequate pheripheral access).
   d. Exchange transfusion.
   e. Central venous pressure monitoring.

B. Precautions.

1. Abdominal wall defects.
2. Necrotizing enterocolitis.
3. Vascular compromise below level of umbilicus.
4. Omphalitis.

C. Equipment/supplies.

1. Sterile instrument tray for umbilical catheterization.
   a. Gauze pads.
   b. Drapes.
   c. Umbilical catheter of appropriate size.
      (1) Size 3.5F for infants weighing less than 1250–1500 g.
      (2) Size 5.0F for infants weighing more than 1250–1500 g.
   d. Small container for antiseptic solution.
   e. Blunt needle adapter if catheter is not designed with minimal dead space at hub.
   f. Three-way Luer-Lok stopcock.
   g. Scissors.
   h. Umbilical tape.
   i. Syringe, 10 mL.
   j. Scalpel, No. 11.
   k. Mosquito hemostats (2).
   l. Curved, nontoothed iris forceps.
   m. Needle holder.
   n. Silk suture, size 4–0, with curved needle.
2. Sterile IV flush solution.
3. Sterile antiseptic solution.

D. Umbilical artery catheterization (for alternative side-entry method, see Squire, Harnung, and Kirchhoff, 1990).
 1. Place infant in supine position and restrain limbs.

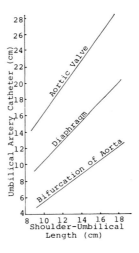

Figure 31–3
Umbilical artery catheter insertion length for shoulder-umbilical length. (Adapted from Dunn, P.M.: Arch. Dis. Child, *41*:69, 1966; *in* Cole, C.H. (Ed.): The Harriet Lane Handbook, 10th ed. Chicago, Year Book Medical Publishers, 1984, p. 278.)

2. Measure shoulder to umbilical distance and determine length of catheter to be inserted (Fig. 31–3).
   a. "Low position," with catheter tip placed between the third and fourth lumbar vertebrae.
   b. "High position," with catheter tip placed between the sixth and tenth thoracic vertebrae.
3. Prepare catheter.
   a. Trim flared end of catheter, if not designed with minimal dead-space hub, and securely insert blunt-end needle adapter.
   b. Attach Luer-Lok stopcock to catheter or blunt-end adapter.
   c. Connect flush-filled syringe to stopcock.
   d. Fill stopcock and catheter with flush solution.
   e. Turn stopcock off to catheter.
4. Prepare umbilical cord and surrounding abdomen, having assistant hold umbilical cord up and out of procedure area. Do not let antiseptic drip down infant's side as this may cause burns, especially in extremely premature infants.
5. Drape procedure area.
6. Tie umbilical tape loosely at base of cord, to be used for hemostasis if bleeding occurs.
7. Using scalpel, cut through umbilical cord 1–1.5 cm from skin.
8. Identify cord vessels.
   a. Arteries: two small, thick-walled constricted vessels.
   b. Vein: single, large, thin-walled vessel, often open.
9. Stabilize cord stump.
   a. Grasp portion of cut edge of cord with hemostat and apply gentle traction.
   b. Apply hemostat to opposite sides of the cord and roll them away from each other, causing the arteries to protrude from the cut surface of the cord.
10. Dilate artery.
    a. Insert one tip of curved iris forceps into selected artery and probe gently to about 0.5 cm.
    b. With tips of forceps together, gently probe artery to about 0.5 cm.
    c. Gently spread forceps apart, and then slowly withdraw forceps from artery, dilating lumen as forceps is withdrawn.
    d. Continue to dilate lumen until forceps can easily be inserted about 1.0 cm.
11. Insert catheter.
    a. Insert catheter into dilated artery while applying gentle traction on the cord stump in the direction of the patient's head.

b. Thread catheter to predetermined distance.
   (1) If resistance is met, *do not force catheter.* Apply gentle, steady pressure to catheter, applying gentle traction on cord.
   (2) If catheter cannot be advanced to the desired distance, discontinue attempts and catheterize second artery.
   (3) Observe for blanching of legs, toes, and/or buttocks.
12. Aspirate blood to ensure placement in vessel. If blood cannot be aspirated, remove catheter and attempt catheterization of second artery.
13. Secure catheter.
    a. Place purse-string suture around cord. Avoid piercing vessels and skin.
    b. Knot suture securely in cord close to catheter, and then loop suture around catheter and secure with additional knots.
    c. Suture around catheter must be tight to prevent catheter from sliding, but not so tight that flow through catheter is obstructed.
14. Loosen umbilical tape.
15. Tape flat loop of catheter to abdomen until x-ray examination confirms position.
16. Confirm position with x-ray examination.
    a. If catheter tip is too high, remove securing suture, pull catheter back to proper position, and resuture.
    b. If catheter tip is too low for "high position," pull back to "low position."
    c. If catheter tip is too low for "low position," it must be removed.
    d. A catheter that is no longer sterile may not be advanced.
17. Remove antiseptic as soon as possible from skin to prevent burns.
18. Tape catheter to abdomen with "bridge" or "goalpost" taping technique (Fig. 31–4).

E. Umbilical venous catheterization.

1. Emergency placement (low).
   a. Encircle cord with umbilical tape and cut the cord.
   b. Identify the thin-walled vein and insert catheter 2–3 cm.
   c. Aspirate blood into the syringe; clear air from the line.
   d. Infuse emergency medications and fluid.
   e. Remove catheter once infant is stabilized.
2. Indwelling venous catheterization.
   a. Measure the infant to estimate depth of insertion (Shukla and Ferrara, 1986).
   b. Prepare cord as for artery catheter and identify the thin-walled vein.
   c. Grasp the edge of the vein and the side of the cord with forceps.
   d. Insert the catheter while maintaining traction on the cord toward the left foot.

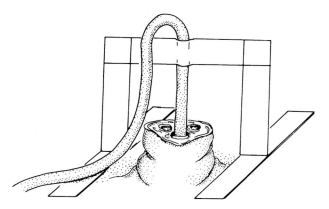

Figure 31–4
"Bridge," or "goalpost," taping technique.

e. If resistance is met, withdraw the catheter 2–3 cm, twist, and reinsert.
f. Connect and secure catheter and confirm (and, if necessary, adjust and re-confirm) position at or just above the diaphragm.

F. **Complications of using umbilical catheters.**

1. Vasospasm, embolism, and/or thrombosis (Kempley et al., 1993; Schneider, Hartl, and Fendel, 1989; Seibert, Northington, Miers, and Taylor, 1991).
   a. Blanching, cyanosis, and mottling of skin.
   b. Sloughing of skin.
   c. Necrosis of extremities (Fullilove and Fixsen, 1997).
   d. Paraplegia (Lemke et al., 1996).
   e. Hypertension.
   f. Necrotizing enterocolitis.
   g. Intestinal necrosis and perforation.
2. Infection.
3. Mechanical complications.
   a. Perforation of vessels.
   b. Perforation of peritoneum.
   c. False aneurysm.
   d. Knot in catheter.
4. Hypoglycemia.
5. Skin burns from antiseptics.
6. Hemorrhage; exsanguination.

Blood Sampling Procedures

CAPILLARY BLOOD SAMPLING

A. **Indications.**

1. Small blood sample is needed.
2. Arterial sample not possible or necessary.
3. Venous sample not possible or necessary.

B. **Precautions.**

1. Infection near selected puncture site.
2. Coagulation defects.
3. Loss of skin integrity at selected puncture site.
4. Impaired or inadequate circulation in selected limb.
5. Inaccurate laboratory values may result from the following:
   a. Contamination of specimen with tissue fluid.
   b. Contamination of specimen with skin-preparation solution(s).
   c. Poor circulation at the puncture site.
   d. Hemolysis of specimen.

C. **Equipment/supplies.**

1. Antiseptic skin preparation supplies for capillary blood sample per hospital policy.
2. Lancet, with tip not longer than 2.5 mm.
3. Container(s) for specimen(s).
4. Sterile gauze pad.
5. Warm (not more than 40° C) compress.

D. **Technique for heel stick.**

1. Select puncture site on lateral or medial aspect of the heel (Fig. 31–5). Avoid other areas because of possibility of nerve damage.

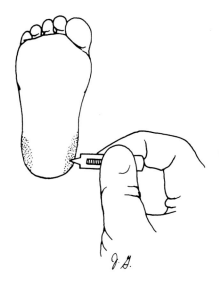

Figure 31–5
Capillary blood sampling from the heel. (From Fletcher, M.A., MacDonald, M.G., and Avery, G.B. (Eds.): Atlas of Procedures in Neonatology. Philadelphia, J.B. Lippincott, 1983.)

2. Warm heel with compress.
3. Prepare area selected for skin puncture per hospital policy.
4. Puncture heel perpendicular to the skin.
5. Wipe away first drop of blood with sterile gauze pad.
6. Collect specimen as drops form at puncture site.
   a. Blood flow is increased if the puncture site is dependent relative to the extremity.
   b. Gentle "milking" of the extremity above the puncture site may encourage blood flow.
   c. Squeezing and pinching at the puncture site may cause hemolysis of specimen, contamination of specimen with tissue fluid, and/or bruising of extremity.
7. After specimen is collected, apply pressure with sterile gauze pad until hemostasis is ensured.

E. **Complications.**

1. Bruising.
2. Loss of skin integrity.
3. Infection.
4. Scarring.
5. Calcified nodules.
6. Hematoma.
7. Difficulty in walking, related to multiple heel sticks in the neonatal period.
8. Pain.

VEINPUNCTURE

A. **Indications.**

1. Arterial sample not possible or necessary.
2. Capillary sample not necessary or possible.

B. **Precautions.**

1. Infection near selected puncture site.
2. Coagulation defects.
3. Loss of skin integrity at selected puncture site.

4. Inadequate or impaired circulation in selected limb.
5. Need to preserve venous site for possible cannulation.

C. Equipment/supplies.

1. Antiseptic skin preparation for venipuncture per hospital policy.
2. Butterfly needle (scalp vein set) or 25- or 23-gauge needle on syringe.
3. Syringe(s) for specimen collection.
4. Sterile gauze pad.
5. Laboratory tubes.

D. Procedure.

1. Choose vein to be used (Fig. 31–2). Distention of the vessel(s) may be accomplished by applying a gentle tourniquet or having an assistant encircle the area with the hand to apply direct pressure.
2. Stabilize and position the selected puncture site to allow puncture in direction of blood flow.
3. Prepare area selected per hospital policy.
4. Puncture skin at 15- to 45-degree angle just distal to planned puncture site, using shallow angle for smaller infants or superficial vessels.
5. Advance needle slowly to puncture vessel.
   a. If resistance is met or vessel is not punctured, withdraw needle slowly to just below level of the skin, relocate vessel, and advance the needle again.
   b. If a hematoma develops or bleeding occurs, occlude the vessel with pressure just proximal to the puncture site, withdraw needle, and apply pressure until hemostasis is ensured.
6. On entrance of blood into tubing, attach syringe and gently aspirate to obtain specimen.
7. After specimen is obtained, occlude vessel with pressure, using gauze pad just proximal to puncture site, and withdraw needle.
8. Apply pressure to site until hemostasis is obtained.

E. Complications.

1. Hemorrhage.
2. Hematoma.
3. Infection.
4. Needle injury to adjacent structures.
5. Pain.

RADIAL ARTERY PUNCTURE: ADVANCED PRACTICE PROCEDURE

A. Indications.

1. Venous and/or capillary sites are not satisfactory.
2. Arterial line is unavailable or nonfunctioning.

B. Precautions.

1. Infection near selected puncture site.
2. Coagulation defects.
3. Loss of skin integrity at selected puncture site.
4. Inadequate or impaired circulation in selected limb.
5. Need to preserve arterial site for possible cannulation.
6. Inadequate collateral circulation distal to the selected puncture site.

C. Equipment/supplies.

1. Antiseptic supplies to prepare for arterial puncture per hospital policy.
2. Butterfly needle set (scalp, vein set) or 25-gauge needle attached to syringe.

3. Syringe(s) to collect specimen(s).
4. Sterile gauze pad.

D. Technique.

1. Determine puncture site.
   a. Extend wrist.
   b. Palpate artery at distal crease of wrist.
2. Perform modified Allen's test to assess collateral circulation.
   a. Elevate hand.
   b. Apply pressure to occlude radial and ulnar arteries.
   c. Milk hand from fingers to wrist to blanch hand.
   d. Release pressure on ulnar artery.
   e. If color returns to hand in less than 10 seconds, adequate collateral circulation is present.
3. Position and stabilize extended wrist to allow puncture against direction of arterial flow.
4. Prepare area with antiseptic for skin puncture (middle of outer third of wrist).
5. Puncture skin with needle (bevel up) at 15- to 45-degree angle, using shallower angle for smaller infants or more superficial arteries.
6. Advance needle slowly to puncture artery.
   a. If resistance is met or blood is not obtained, withdraw needle slowly to just below skin level, palpate artery, and advance needle again in direction of artery.
   b. If hematoma or bleeding develops, occlude artery with gauze and pressure just proximal to the puncture site, withdraw needle, and apply pressure until hemostasis is ensured (may take up to 5 minutes of direct pressure).
7. When blood enters the tubing, attach syringe and aspirate gently to obtain sample.
8. Occlude artery with gauze and pressure just proximal to puncture site and withdraw needle.
9. Apply pressure to site for 5 minutes or until hemostasis is ensured.

E. Complications.

1. Hematoma.
2. Hemorrhage.
3. Infection.
4. Thrombosis, embolism.
5. Arteriospasm, distal ischemia.
6. Needle injury to adjacent structures.
7. Pain.

Miscellaneous Procedures

BLADDER CATHETERIZATION

A. Indications.

1. To obtain urine specimen when clean-catch specimen or suprapubic aspiration cannot be obtained.
2. To monitor urinary output.
3. To relieve urinary retention.
4. To accompany genitourinary testing such as cystogram or voiding cystourethrogram.

B. Equipment and materials.

1. Urethral catheters.
   a. Size 3.5F umbilical artery catheter for infants weighing less than 1000 g.

    b. Size 6F Foley catheter or 5F feeding tube for infants weighing 1000–1800 g.

    c. Size 8F feeding tube or Foley catheter for infants weighing more than 1800 g.

2. Urinary catheter tray.

    a. Sterile gloves.

    b. Cotton balls.

    c. Povidone-iodine (Betadine) solution.

    d. Sterile drapes.

    e. Lubricant.

    f. Sterile specimen container.

PROCEDURES

A. Male catheterization.

1. Place infant on back and restrain legs or have assistant hold legs.
2. Clean penis with povidone-iodine solution, starting at meatus and moving down the penis.
3. Put on sterile gloves and drape area with sterile towels.
4. Apply sterile lubricant to catheter tip.
5. Hold the penis perpendicular to the body. Place the catheter in the urethra and advance until urine appears in the catheter. Slight resistance may be felt as the catheter passes through the external sphincter. Steady, gentle pressure is usually needed to pass beyond this area; however, *never force the catheter.*
6. Collect the urine specimen in the sterile container and send to the laboratory.
7. If a Foley catheter is used, inflate the catheter per manufacturer's recommendation.
8. If catheter is to remain in place, tape securely to the lower abdomen.

B. Female catheterization.

1. Place infant on back and secure legs in frog-leg position. You may secure with restraints or have an assistant hold the legs.
2. Separate the labia and clean the area around the meatus with povidone-iodine solution, using front-to-back strokes.
3. Put on sterile gloves and apply sterile drapes around the labia.
4. Spread the labia and identify the urethra.
5. Apply sterile lubricant to the tip of the catheter.
6. Insert the catheter in the urethra and advance until urine appears.
7. Inflate bulb of Foley catheter if applicable and tape catheter to leg.

C. Complications.

1. Infection.
2. Hematuria.
3. Trauma to urethra.
4. Stricture.
5. Pain.

REFERENCES

American Heart Association: Textbook of Neonatal Resuscitation. Dallas, Author, 1994.

Arya, H., Williams, J., Ponsford, S.N., and Bissenden, J.G.: Neonatal diaphragmatic paralysis caused by chest drains. Arch. Dis. Child., 66:441–442, 1991.

Fullilove, S., and Fixsen, J.: Major limb deformities as complications of vascular access in neonates. Paediatr. Anaesth. 7:247–250, 1997.

Holzki, J.: Laryngeal damage from tracheal intubation. Paediatr. Anaesth., 7:435–437, 1997.

Kempley, J., Bennett, S., Loftus, B.G., et al.: Randomized trial of umbilical artery catheter position: Clinical outcome. Acta Paediatr. 82:173–176, 1993.

Lemke, R.P., Idiong, N., al-Saedi, S., et al.: Spinal cord infarct after arterial switch associated with an umbilical artery catheter. Ann. Thorac. Surg., 62:1532–1534, 1996.

Page, N.E., Giehl, M., and Luke, S.: Intubation complications in the critically ill child. AACN Clinical Issues, 9(1):25–35, 1998.

Quak, J.M., Szatmari, A., and van den Anker, J.N.: Cardiac tamponade in a preterm neonate secondary to a chest tube. Acta Paediatr., 82:490–491, 1993.

Schlager, T.A., Hidde, M., Rodger, P., et al.: Intravascular catheter colonization in critically ill children. Infect. Control Hosp. Epidemiol., 18:347–348, 1997.

Schneider, K., Hartl, M., and Fendel, H.: Umbilical and portal vein calcifications following umbilical vein catheterization. Pediatr. Radiol. 19:468–470, 1989.

Seibert, J.J., Northington, F.J., Miers, J.F., and Taylor, B.J.: Aortic thrombosis after umbilical artery catheterization in neonates: Prevalence of complications on long-term follow-up. A.J.R. Am. J. Roentgenol., 156:567–569, 1991.

Shukla, H., and Ferrara, A.: Rapid estimation of insertional length of umbilical catheters in newborns. Am. J. Dis. Child., 140:786–788, 1986.

Squire, S.S., Harnung, T.L., and Kirchhoff, K.T.: Comparing two methods of umbilical arterial catheter placement. Am. J. Perinatol., 7:8, 1990.

Stavis, R.L., and Krauss, A.N.: Complications of neonatal intensive care. Clin. Perinatol., 7(1):107–124, 1980.

Swift, J.: Thoracentesis and thoracostomy tubes. In Taeusch, H.W., Christiansen, R.O., and Buescher, E.S. (Eds.): Pediatric and neonatal tests and procedures. Philadelphia, W.B. Saunders, 1996, p. 77.

Young, T.E., and Mangum, O.B.: Neofax: A Manual of Drugs Used in Neonatal Care, 11th ed. Raleigh, N.C.: Acorn Publishing, 1998.

Wu, C., Li, C., Wong, C.S., et al.: The lost endotracheal tube: A rare complication of accidental esophageal intubation. Acta Anaesthesiol. Sin., 35(1):55–58, 1997.

SECTION
VI

CURRENT ISSUES AND
TRENDS IN NEONATAL CARE

Chapter 32

Research

Wendy Cornell

Objectives

1. Discuss how neonatal intensive care nurses can become involved with research projects that improve the quality of neonatal care.

2. Demonstrate an understanding and use of research results.

3. Describe how to use research findings in daily practice.

4. Examine issues of patient advocacy in neonatal research participation.

5. Discuss ideas that can become the basis for neonatal nursing research.

Neonatal care environments are ripe for nursing research. The situations that NICU nurses encounter daily can provide the basis for a myriad of nursing studies. Through research, effective care practices can be demonstrated, the impact of nursing care on patient outcomes can be studied, and unnecessary interventions can be identified and eliminated. This chapter is designed to provide the bedside practitioner with basic research information to stimulate creative ideas and critical thinking. Use of research findings requires commitment and awareness of the research process but is within the realm of the practicing nurse. Nursing participation in biomedical and clinical nursing research studies is essential to the promotion and verification of quality patient care.

Basic Principles of Research

A. Purposes of nursing research (Polit and Hungler, 1997, pp 5–10).

1. Contributes to nursing science through:
   a. Generation of new knowledge that improves understanding of human health-related experiences.
   b. Replication of studies contributing to existing knowledge.
   c. Expansion of existing nursing knowledge.
2. Facilitates nursing practice improvement by:
   a. Discovery and/or verification of information that develops the scientific

knowledge base for nursing practice (rather than relying on ritual as the determiner of practice).

   b. Testing models for care delivery that enhance efficient use of available resources while ensuring quality care.

   c. Shaping practice through improving decision-making ability.

   d. Defining specific populations and their unique needs.

3. Determines cost-effectiveness in care delivery to:
   a. Document the efficacy of nursing care.
   b. Demonstrate the cost savings of nursing interventions.
   c. Examine the practices that may lead to more efficient patterns of caregiving.

4. Identifies the impact of nursing care on patient outcomes in:
   a. Assessing alterations in complication rates, length of stay, mortality and morbidity rates, and quality of life related to nursing interventions.
   b. Demonstrating use of interventions that foster restoration of health.
   c. Demonstrating effectiveness of anticipatory guidance and education to support optimal development and promote wellness.

B. **Methods of nursing research.**

1. Study designs provide a variety of ways to answer research questions or test research hypotheses (LoBiondo-Wood and Haber, 1998, pp. 176–189).
   a. Laboratory studies create special environments within which subjects can be analyzed under controlled circumstances (most frequently used with animal models).
   b. Clinical investigations are conducted in real-life surroundings.
   c. Retrospective studies examine phenomena of current interest, using information available from the past. In contrast, prospective studies involve a future-oriented approach to data gathering.
   d. Experimental (quantitative) studies manipulate or control one or more independent variables to allow observation of the intervention effects.
   e. Nonexperimental studies (descriptive and correlational research) do not include manipulation or control of an independent variable. The status of the variables of interest is summarized (or relationships are studied as they naturally occur).
   f. Longitudinal studies involve long-term study of the topic of interest. Cross-sectional studies examine the topic of interest at one point in time.
   g. Qualitative research (e.g., with phenomenologic or grounded-theory methods) involves findings that are not generated through statistical analysis. Data may be gathered from observations, interviews, or a variety of other means, but the process of analysis is nonmathematic.

2. The most appropriate means of answering the research questions or testing the research hypothesis influences decisions regarding study methods, including:
   a. Target population identification.
   b. Reliable and valid measurement of the variables.
   c. Sample size and method of selection.
   d. Data analysis methods.

C. **Research ethics.**

1. Each researcher has a fundamental responsibility to safeguard the individual subject's rights (Polit and Hungler, 1997, p. 127).
   a. Parental consent is required for unemancipated minors.
   b. Informed consent includes provision of sufficient information—with some measure of assurance of individual understanding regarding what is expected, to allow noncoercive participation.
   c. Confidentiality ensures that an individual subject's identity will not be made public or available to others, so that the privacy and dignity of the subjects can be maintained.

    d. Anonymity ensures that a subject's identity cannot be linked with his or her data, even by the researcher.

    e. Subjects have a right to refuse to participate (or drop out of the study at any time) and still receive standard-quality care.

    f. An institutional review board approves the study process to ensure appropriate consent procedures and protection measures (to prevent undue risk or loss of personal rights and dignity).

2. Study benefit.

    a. Benefits of the study must be assessed to ensure that the risks are minimized and are balanced by the magnitude of potential benefit that can be obtained.

    b. Avoidance of harm to subjects addresses the issues of vulnerability of study subjects, including:

      (1) Subjection to additional tests or procedures.

      (2) Temporary discomfort versus permanent damage.

      (3) Loss of privacy or confidentiality.

3. Responsibilities of the researcher include scientific objectivity, truthfulness, and integrity; impeccable care of data gathered; honest disclosure of findings; and clarification and communication of results.

4. Research competency denotes the ability of the researcher to complete the study successfully, through understanding of the complexities of the process and of the potential risks and benefits to the study population.

Identifying Research Questions

A. **Clinical patient care experience** can stimulate curiosity, excite special interests, and promote insights that generate nursing care questions.

1. Nurses may provide ideas and limitless questions regarding why practices and observations are as they are; how trends and patterns emerge and relate; what research has been done; and when enough knowledge is gathered to justify changes in or continuation of current practices.

    a. Issues related to treatment differences can help define and determine whether outcomes related to varied practices can be demonstrated and replicated, to provide generalizability to additional situations or populations.

    b. Creative ideas related to unresolved patient concerns provide hunches and strong beliefs that can be systematically studied, so that solutions to recurrent questions or bothersome problems can be generated.

    c. Through use of research methods, nonpublished experiences can be transformed from multiple individual occurrences into a logical pattern.

2. Problems previously researched often provide suggestions for additional study and may describe findings that are not working as predicted. Discrepancies that need further review, and alternative explanations for findings that need to be tested, may also be described.

    a. A need for further research is indicated when inconclusive or contradictory results are identified. Inconsistent findings, or variations from anticipated results in practical application, also suggest a need for further research.

    b. Generalizability of results to a larger population, or to different populations beyond the study sample, requires continued exploration and study.

B. **Nursing practice questions** can assist in the development of a scientific base for clinical practice to advance nursing knowledge.

1. Systematic inquiry into nursing interventions that influence patient care outcomes will verify the value of those practices in improving patient care and will promote effective use of time and resources.

2. Theory generation involves the development and testing of existing theories to generate knowledge and guide practice.

C. **Study feasibility issues** denote a responsible assurance that the study can be carried out once research questions are identified.
1. Study variables must be measurable.
2. Sample size must be sufficient to show statistical significance.
3. Time, money, equipment, and personnel issues include:
    a. Time needed for development and completion of the study, as well as the involvement of the participants.
    b. Expenses for printing, testing, participating, facilities, and computation of results.
    c. Research support for methodologic review, statistical analysis, and budget and financial administration.
    d. Availability of clinical experts and support staff.
    e. Exploration of possible funding sources, which may involve grant writing.

Steps in the Research Process

A. **Problem identification** specifies the topic of interest to be studied (Nieswiadomy, 1998, pp. 26–35).
1. Narrowing the topic involves the selection of a few high-priority (very specific) variables that are measurable and may have potential for generalizing the findings.
2. Formulating the question provides a statement of what provided the impetus for the study, the scope of the problem, the significance of the research, and the questions to be answered by the study.
3. Study variables comprise independent variables that define the intervention or relationship that is manipulated or observed by the investigator and that have an effect on the dependent or outcome variables.

B. **Definition of the study purpose** and significance to nursing.
1. Justification for study specifies the value of the results to nursing practice and who will benefit from the information (generalizability of the knowledge to others).
2. Expectation for use of results may include:
    a. Validation of existing knowledge.
    b. Exploration of new ideas that will introduce new practices or change current practice.
    c. Documentation of outcomes.

C. **Review of the literature** summarizes and critiques existing research related to the topic of interest (Nieswiadomy, 1998, pp. 74–83).
1. Methods and sources used in organizing and approaching an analysis of existing literature include:
    a. Computer searches involving selection of key words of the research question, which may use headings from literature indices. Reference librarian assistance is most helpful. Online searches can be conducted at most libraries or health care facilities.
    b. Indices and abstracts that have reference listings and overviews of that content in published literature. These resources are available in most medical or nursing libraries.
    c. A variety of literature sources that may provide valuable information on nursing and related topics.
        (1) Nursing and medical research can be shared through the Internet, practice guidelines, journals, abstracts, books, bibliographies, unpublished theses, published reports of presentations at professional conferences, and personal communication with other researchers.
        (2) Theoretical knowledge pursuits involve review of nursing's and other disciplines' frameworks, which may stimulate new practice ideas and

offer recommendations or directions for appropriate methods to answer research questions.

(3) Methodologic reports provide studies of the development, evaluation, and testing of various research methods and instruments.

(4) Research studies from other disciplines may contain applicable content for nursing.

(5) Information available on the Internet, as well as in popular books, articles, and the lay literature, can produce ideas and approaches to conceptualizing research questions.

2. Note taking facilitates a critical analysis of results and an exploration of the effectiveness of previous methods. Use of computer software (e.g., spreadsheets, databases, and statistical programs) can facilitate the management of this process for ease of future use.

a. *Examining knowns versus unknowns* involves contemplating the adequacy of research to the present.

(1) The extent of knowledge currently available supplies parameters of known information to define the direction for additional study.

(2) Support for previous results may be verified with additional research that demonstrates consistent findings or may be rebutted by studies that obtain different results (outcomes).

(3) Identification of conceptual or theoretical frameworks that have guided study of the research question may be provided.

b. *Methods* used in previous studies should indicate the reliability, validity, and effectiveness attained.

(1) Study design includes a definition of participants, observations of variables, setting, time, and the role of the researcher.

(2) Sample size considers calculated adequacy to achieve maximal validity of the results.

(3) Results support or dispute the framework of study, note limitations, and describe significance.

(4) Conclusions incorporate a demonstration of the meaning and worth of the research and can provide data-based generalizations.

c. *Preparing the text* includes summarizing significant earlier work, with interpretations and their relationship to the present study.

3. Compilation of individual reports documents the citations in a consistent, approved format that organizes the information in logical sequences. The content contains an outline of reviews, concepts relating to proposed study, and notations of consistencies and inconsistencies that underscore the importance of further study.

D. **Development of a conceptual or theoretical framework** integrates diverse information to clarify assumptions, define variables, and provide direction for the conduct of the research (Polit and Hungler, 1997, pp. 106–107).

1. Clarification of concepts communicates the focus of the study, to aid understanding of complex ideas related to the topic of interest under investigation.

2. Assumptions relate to statements that are accepted as true for the purposes of the study.

3. Definitions of relationships among concepts provide the blueprint of how the generalizations in the study fit together.

E. **Limitations of the study** influence the generalizability of the findings and may include:

1. Other relevant (uncontrolled) variables that may confuse interpretation of the results.

2. Lack of identification of relationships among concepts, or unclear definition of relationships in the study.

3. Concerns regarding sample size and representativeness, instrument validity and reliability, appropriateness of statistical analysis, and other study design issues that may result in limitations of the findings.

F. **Hypothesis formation** and research questions describe the prediction of relationships between variables.
1. Independent variables are naturally occurring or can be manipulated or controlled to have an effect on the outcome variable.
2. Dependent variables describe the effect (outcome) that is contingent on another variable.

G. **Study terms** and variable definitions specify the terminology to ensure clarity of meaning for readers.
1. Operational definitions convey an explanation of how the variables will be measured or observed.
2. Specification of population defines to whom the study results apply.
    a. Inclusion criteria designate guidelines for characteristics required to participate in the study.
    b. Exclusion criteria eliminate some participants who do not fit sample criteria for the target population.
    c. Study setting considerations include the availability of relevant subjects in a feasible population and location, to ensure a representative sample.

H. **Selection of research design** involves a determination of the most workable plan to answer the research question.
1. Types (approaches to data gathering and analysis).
    a. Descriptive designs are used to identify or describe concepts.
    b. Comparative designs explore the contrasts between two or more groups.
    c. Experimental designs integrate scientific inquiry into the study of cause-and-effect relationships.
2. Data collection possibilities may include observation, recording of available data, and administration of standardized, preexisting, or newly developed instruments.
    a. Interviews facilitate the study process by helping researchers to understand participants' perceptions through verbal questioning.
    b. Participant observation involves researcher interaction with subjects and observations of behaviors that can be covert or overt.
    c. Document analysis includes examination of records for analysis relating to research questions, regardless of whether the data source was developed for that specific purpose.
    d. Correlation surveys examine the strength of the relationship between or among variables.
    e. Comparative surveys involve a retrospective look at relationships between what is existing and something that occurred in the past.
    f. Case studies employ an intensive investigation of people, groups, or situations that usually are naturally occurring.
    g. Prospective studies plan a futuristic approach to the study of the effect that an intervention or event will have on outcome variables.
    h. Retrospective studies provide a historical review of known effects and their potential causes.

I. **Sample selection** incorporates decisions regarding whom to study to ensure systematic and representative selection from the larger population.
1. Following are four types of probability sampling:
    a. Random sampling connotes that every element of the population has an equal chance to be a participant.
    b. Systematic sampling defines a preset strategy of selection from the population (e.g., every third person).

    c. Stratified sampling divides the population into stratified subsets and randomly selects a proportionate number of subjects from the subsets.

    d. Cluster sampling includes successive random sampling that breaks down the population into smaller and smaller units, in stages.

2. Nonprobability sampling is nonrandom selection, which can decrease the chance of attaining a representative sample.

    a. Convenience sampling uses a relevant, available subject group.

    b. Expert sampling employs a choice of samples from experts in the area of the research question.

    c. Quota sampling involves dividing the population into stratified subsets and then selecting the sample in a nonrandom fashion that may be representative.

3. Sample size calculations take into consideration the variance error, anticipated effect size, type of design planned (number of variables being studied), and the power and significance level.

    a. Homogeneity versus heterogeneity of study phenomena influences the sample size, because greater numbers are needed to demonstrate an effect when the sample and population are less alike in as many ways as possible.

    b. Achievement of statistical significance requires adequate sample size to note that a significant relationship exists. Use of a power analysis technique to determine sample size is recommended.

    c. Effect size connotes the expected degree of magnitude of findings in the population studied.

    d. Study participation expectations acknowledge reluctance to participate, usual response rates for different methodologies, and availability of subjects.

J. Data measurement planning outlines a systematic process for gathering information from sources, for ease of analysis.

1. Organization of data is outlined before implementation of the study and provides a logical summarization framework.

    a. Instrument development and evaluation specify data to be measured and how the information will be recorded.

    b. Computer technology for the coding, entry, and analysis of data is determined.

    c. Promotion of legibility and completeness (which influences the usefulness of data) and a standard approach to interpretation and methods of collection are described.

        (1) Plan the method by which incomplete data will be used and analyzed.

        (2) Interim analysis can allow for additional clarification of incomplete or questionably interpretable data.

2. Statistical analysis provides systematic interpretation of findings in relation to the study problem and is influenced by the type of data collected. Use of statistician consultation is recommended.

    a. Descriptive statistics organize and summarize information.

        (1) Frequency distributions arrange number values from lowest to highest.

        (2) Measures of central tendency describe the middle and general trends of the number findings (mean, median, and mode).

        (3) Measures of variability define ways that measure groups together (range, interquartile range, standard deviation, confidence intervals, and standard error).

        (4) Measures of correlation denote the extent to which variables are related to each other (correlation coefficients).

    b. Inferential statistics assist in generalization of the sample characteristics to the larger population but cannot be used with all types of data.

(1) The null hypothesis is a statement that the variable being investigated is without effect.

(2) A defined level of significance denotes the probability that differences between sets of data are due to chance (conventional levels are usually 0.01 or 0.05).

K. **Interpretation of findings** describes the search for the meaning and implication of the results.

1. Substantiation of the research hypothesis or question, and affirmation of the conceptual framework of the study, warrant pursuit of the broader meaning of the results.

2. Analysis of the study design verifies that the validity of the results are considered in light of the methods used and that plausible alternative explanations are examined.

3. Comparison with previous studies explores the relationship of new results to earlier study and theory.

4. The implications for nursing incorporate an assessment of what changes may be needed in practice, education, and research, based on study findings.

L. **Dissemination of research findings** promotes communication of results; provides suggested changes in approaches for practice; and supplies ideas for concentration of research efforts.

1. Submission of articles and/or abstracts to journals, books, and other publications provides opportunities to discuss the study and findings. Research findings also may provide data for development of research-based practice protocols.

2. Poster sessions involve preparation of abstracts and poster presentations regarding the study results for conferences, in hospitals, and in public displays.

3. Oral presentations contain concise, descriptive study reviews that are audience focused and that communicate findings to others.

4. Findings may also be shared while networking with colleagues, during roundtable or practice change discussions, with hospital-based research committees, in journal clubs, during interviews, and through use of online chat rooms and bulletin boards.

Role of Research in Neonatal Nursing

A. **Quality-of-care issues** have heightened concern regarding quality improvement, consumer advocacy, and patient satisfaction, providing a renewed impetus to review practice.

1. Systematic evaluation of care, through use of the research process, can document nursing care interventions in relation to patient outcomes and effective use of nursing time and expertise.

   a. Efforts to promote efficiency in nursing care delivery, as a replacement for routine (historical) methods of care provision, require exploration to determine their effectiveness, cost, and impact on neonates.

      (1) Development of standards of care provides anticipated outcome measures, which need to be defined and tested in the hospital setting. The standardization of practice, through consistent knowledge bases of neonatal nursing care providers, assists in the evaluation of care delivery and in assessment of which variables influence deviations from expected outcomes (Johnson & Maas, 1997, p. 69).

      (2) Exploration of the long-term effects of neonatal practice, practice implications for morbidity and mortality, and mechanisms to promote staff satisfaction through professional practice are needed.

    b. Avoidance of the "cookbook method" of caregiving, with reliance on strict adherence to policies and procedures rather than critical thinking, focuses attention on assessment of the individual infant. The use of new research findings and a willingness to explore new methods of caregiving can be facilitated by nurses who integrate research mindfulness in their daily activities.

      (1) Critiques of research results provide a forum to evaluate the validity of findings and to determine whether sufficient reliability exists to justify acceptance and changes in practice.

      (2) Credibility that findings may be replicated and demonstrated for more than just the study situation promotes incorporation into individual practice patterns.

2. The communication and value of the research to the practitioner has an impact on the use of study findings.

    a. Progressive change involves frequent review of new information that has been introduced in a manner that is perceived as useful and timely.

      (1) Critical analysis of new data, by respected colleagues with neonatal expertise, facilitates changes in nursing practice. New material is better accepted when existing care practices are understood and rationale for change can be readily explained.

      (2) When practice changes involve skill development, sufficient time and teaching must be allotted. Experienced nurses may exhibit skepticism regarding practice changes unless their expertise is supported. Subtle outcomes may be more difficult to see, thereby reducing the visibility of the reinforcement for practice changes.

    b. A balance needs to be maintained between the value of intuitive, sensible nursing caregiving and the development of high-technology tools in neonatal practice.

      (1) Rapid changes in caregiving, with limited supporting evidence, increases the need for studies regarding the impact of recent advances. Research may provide the reassurance that approaches to care have been productive and cost-effective, or it may suggest that further change is needed. Some resistance to change is inherent in rapid technologic development, where there is limited time for testing and gaining of expertise.

      (2) Substantiating clinical observations in day-to-day practice provides fruitful ground for questions that need to be studied and verified. Caregivers have the expertise in observing patterns and suggesting relationships between variables.

B. **Experts in neonatal nursing** need continued opportunities for intellectual stimulation and demonstration of their value to practice to promote their full professional growth. Research provides the foundation of knowledge for development of expertise.

1. Establishment of a specific interest area, through familiarization with a body of specialized knowledge and development of expertise in that area, is useful in professional presentations and for consultation with other, less expert staff.

    a. Creating experts among neonatal nurses involves:

      (1) Development of a particular area of interest, concern, or growth.

      (2) Use of opportunities for exploration and advanced knowledge development, which is then acknowledged and valued by colleagues. The opportunities may include participation in study protocols and/or review and dissemination of research results related to the topic of interest.

b. Acceptance of a lifelong need to continue learning includes:
(1) Acknowledgment of the time limitations of initial knowledge base development and the rapidity of new information transmission.
(2) Taking risks in questioning practice, thus encouraging and facilitating the development and practical use of specialized knowledge.
2. Recognition and rewards for advanced knowledge are personally valuable and marketable.
a. Professional growth, through use of research and critical thinking, promotes expert practice and respect among interdisciplinary team members.
b. Expansion of personal goals, to develop expertise related to the research process, improves marketability and provides additional career opportunities.
3. Peer support and education can be provided through thoughtful, rational explanation of study results and nursing implications. This method can assist in the introduction of change and enhancement of patient care.
a. Appropriate evaluation of the nursing implications by bedside care providers increases the likelihood of improved patient care through use of new knowledge.
b. Encouraging peer involvement in unit-based research increases commitment to the process and interest in the outcomes.
4. Much opportunity exists for developing the unique knowledge base of neonatal nursing through nursing research, and many people will be needed to fill the gaps in what is beneficial practice versus historical routine. Neonatal nurses aspiring to increase their knowledge and expertise related to research can help fill the anticipated needs.

Interdisciplinary Research: Implications for Nursing

A. **Participation in research** is influenced by the level of commitment to research and the extent to which participation is considered to be a priority by institutional leadership (Nieswiadomy, 1998, pp. 11, 12).
1. The study benefit must be considered in regard to the time expenditure (nursing investment) in the study process, because more resources may be required than are available.
a. Proposal development feasibility considerations include the anticipated workload for all participating, ensuring that efficient use of time is promoted.
b. Coordinating research studies that require interventions with infants necessitates consideration of:
(1) Care patterns and unique patient needs (to avoid interference or additional stress).
(2) Needs of staff in determining methods to incorporate study requirements into their care delivery process. Adherence to study procedures while maintaining care standards is important and yet, at times, challenging.
c. Before implementation of studies, obtaining the approval and support of unit nurse managers and clinical specialists is helpful for clinical studies that involve patients and staff.
2. Ethical considerations incorporate patient advocacy as a hallmark of NICU nursing and are a major factor in the acceptance and involvement of staff in research studies. This fundamental concept should be considered, to avoid conflicts for staff between personal values and plans for study. This may be more evident in randomized, placebo-controlled studies when nurses notice care changes during the study process.

a. Recognition of the intensity of nursing involvement with infants and families in the NICU encourages researchers to educate staff adequately regarding the study process. Support of studies is remarkably strong when staff can appreciate the value of the results to their patients or practice, even when the time requirements may seem excessive.

b. Nursing leadership support and encouragement are essential to the progress and promotion of research efforts (Penticuff, 1987).

3. Multiple research protocols may be concurrently conducted in the NICU and can have an impact on the availability of subjects. Interference in the progress of any particular study may also be noted, requiring coordination among study protocols.

a. Awareness of the methods of ongoing research can assist in ensuring that infants are not overwhelmed by study interventions and yet receive the benefit of experimental therapies that promote improved health and development.

b. Data collection issues can be minimized by systematic study coordination. This helps decrease confusion with staff, improves efficiency, and ultimately increases the reliability of the results achieved.

c. Coordination and preparation help to avoid potential delays in treatment related to enrollment and start-up processes (e.g., assembling equipment, completing data collection forms).

4. The dynamic nature and seemingly constant change that are inherent in the NICU environment necessitate an ability of nursing staff to update their knowledge and skills continually.

a. Organizing for efficiency involves establishing communication pathways and education for periodic updates, to maintain awareness of changes and of care practice improvements.

b. Critical analysis of studies, through journal review forums and community meetings with other care providers, can provide opportunities for discussion of new information and generate plans for research.

B. **Nurses can provide research questions** and concerns for others to consider, in addition to participating directly in research efforts.

1. Clinical insights regarding the patterns and potential relationships noted in caregiving can provide fertile topics for practical research.

2. Changes in the care delivery environment may elicit concerns that can be addressed through research.

C. **Promoting acceptance of research** with families and/or staff needs to be incorporated into the repertoire of staff practice, because research is a fundamental component in many NICUs.

1. Acceptance of participation in study protocols is balanced with the caregiving needs and the ethical concerns that research elicits. Staff members need orientation to the studies and research mileu of the unit, with appropriate opportunities to discuss their concerns and suggestions. Education related to the rationale and need of support for various study practices should be incorporated into this orientation process.

2. Nursing leadership's provision of a welcoming environment for expression of feelings and concerns relating to research will enhance the ability of staff to participate in studies and may allow for development of a more efficient research process. Study coordinators can be helpful in working with unit leadership to facilitate this goal (LoBiondo-Wood and Haber, 1998, p. 492).

D. **Mechanisms for ensuring that staff are informed of research outcomes** can provide positive feedback for involvement as well as enhance knowledge.

1. Expert staff analysis and review of new information in discussion with staff nurses are helpful in ensuring that research is evaluated for merit.

2. Integration of findings and suggestions for change require attention to staff acceptance and acknowledgment of the benefit of the changes to their practice. Effective change strategies need to be employed.
3. The extensive amount of neonatal information can be overwhelming to staff, and finding creative methods to promote continued attention to new ideas is imperative.

REFERENCES

Johnson, M., and Maas, M. (Eds.): Nursing Outcomes Classification (NOC). St. Louis, Mosby, 1997.

LoBiondo-Wood, G., and Haber, J.: Nursing Research Methods, Critical Appraisal, and Utilization, 4th ed. St. Louis, Mosby, 1998.

Nieswiadomy, R.M.: Foundations of Nursing Research, 3rd ed. Stamford, Conn., Appleton & Lange, 1998.

Penticuff, J.H.: Neonatal nursing ethics: Toward a consensus. Neonatal Network, 5(6):7–16, 1987.

Polit, D., and Hungler, B.: Essentials of Nursing Research Methods, Appraisal, and Utilization, 4th ed. Philadelphia, J.B. Lippincott, 1997.

ADDITIONAL READINGS

Abdellah, F.G., and Levine, E.: Preparing Nursing Research for the 21st Century: Evolution, Methodologies, Challenges. New York, Springer Publishing, 1994.

Burns, N., and Grove, S.K. (Eds.): Understanding Nursing Research. Philadelphia, W.B. Saunders, 1995.

Donabedian, A.: Criteria and standards for quality assessment and monitoring. Quality Review Bulletin, 12(3): 99–108, 1986.

Meier, P.: Research methodologies in neonatal nursing. Neonatal Network, 2(2):16–22, 1983.

Sexton, D.L.: Presentation of research findings: The poster session. Nurs. Res., 33:374–375, 1984.

Strauss, A., and Corbin, J.: Basics of Qualitative Research. Newbury Park, Calif., Sage Publications, 1990.

Tanner, C.A., and Lindeman, C.A.: Using Nursing Research. Philadelphia, National League for Nursing, 1989.

Ward, M.J., and Fetler, M.E.: What guidelines should be followed in critically evaluating research reports? Nurs. Res., 28:120–125, 1979.

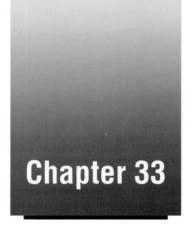

Chapter 33

Ethical Issues in Neonatal Nursing

Bonnie Barndt-Maglio

Neonatal nurses face ethical issues in their practice every day. Advanced technology, extreme measures of care, a new awareness of patient rights, and financial constraints are just a few of the reasons that ethical concerns have become so prevalent. We can expect that concerns about ethical care and treatment will only escalate in the coming years as we continue to examine issues of quality and cost while at the same time science and technology forge ahead in the discovery of new avenues of treatment.

Principles of Ethics

Ethical dilemmas can occur when any member of the health care team, the patient, or the family decision maker disagrees with the type, course, or aggressiveness of treatment. In the NICU, the patient is a minor, and therefore the patient's parents or legal guardian are placed in the position of decision making. This situation is particularly complex because not only do the parents act in the baby's behalf, but, unlike other pediatric situations, the relationship between the parent and child is new and the emotional ties forged in the bonding process are just beginning to form. In contrast, parents of patients of older children may have a greater sense of their children's wishes and desires regarding life and quality of life than a parent of a new and sick baby. Therefore situations regarding neonates are different and at times much more complex than in other pediatric situations.

DECISION SCIENCE

Ethical decision making comprises two fields of study that do not fit comfortably together. The first field of study is that of decision science, or the rational consideration of problems and issues to find a reasonable conclusion (Pierce, 1997, p. 1). As clinicians, we rely heavily on the use of decision science to plan, implement, and evaluate care for patients. We are usually most comfortable when we can assemble facts based on proven scientific data before intervening in a patient issue.

MORAL REASONING

The second field of study used in ethical decisions is that of moral reasoning, which is based on philosophic, religious, and cultural beliefs and perspectives.

Moral reasoning often defies rational explanation but carries with it the power of belief that is inexplicably tied to an individual's family, experiences, relationships, values, and religion. An individual's moral beliefs are unique and cannot be fully explained or understood. It is important to remember that in any ethical dilemma, the parents, family, nurses, physicians, and other participants bring with them a system of moral beliefs that are not always fully identifiable or tangible but will affect their perception of the situation (Pierce, 1997, p. 1).

INTEGRATION OF MORAL REASONING AND DECISION SCIENCE

The integration of decision science with moral reasoning engages nurses and other health care professionals in the most difficult and complex issues in practice, because they move those involved from a state of scientific certainty into a state of uncertainty and instability. When the equilibrium of the normal state of security is upset, an individual feels spiritually, emotionally, physically, and intellectually stressed. The most natural reaction in this state is to take immediate action that will relieve this overwhelming feeling of vulnerability and discomfort. In families of neonates the feelings are intensified by the responsibility of making decisions for the care of a new baby with an uncertain future (Pierce, 1997, p. 2).

Principles of Moral Reasoning

Principles of moral reasoning are useful in examining the components of an ethical dilemma. Understanding commonly used frameworks for moral reasoning enhances the ability of nurses to maintain a therapeutic and respectful relationship with parents even in situations of great disagreement. Although health care professionals and parents alike tend to use a combination of these frameworks, a working knowledge of each is important both to understand and effectively to work through an ethical situation.

UTILITARIANISM

The ethical perspective of utilitarianism strives to achieve the greatest benefit for the most people through the balancing of the interests and priorities of the people involved. There are no right or wrong actions, but each possible course of action is evaluated in comparison with all others (Beauchamp and Childress, 1994, p. 47). Parents use this frame of reference when considering the effect that the neonate's illness and condition will have on the family in both the near and long term. For example, they may express concerns regarding the family's financial stability, time constraints, the alteration of personal and professional goals, and the effect on the other children already present in the family.

Using the principle of utilitarian thinking means to evaluate the situation on the basis of the obligation of the individuals involved. This principle views individuals as thinking, rational beings capable of intellectually reviewing the situation and arriving at a solution. The consequences of the action, not a predetermined moral principle or rule, determine whether it is right or wrong (Beauchamp and Childress, 1994, p. 56). For example, the parental role in our society is to care for and protect the children. When a parent is faced with a critically ill neonate, the performance of parental duties and the meeting of parental obligations are carried out in a context that necessitates a partnership with the health care team. The parents consent, even though the treatment regimens prescribed seem to the parents to violate their roles of protector and caregiver of the newborn infant.

VIRTUE ETHICS

Virtue ethics is based on the belief that behavior is governed by an individual's moral character. Implicit in this framework is the idea that a person's acts are reflective of his or her inner self and that a moral or virtuous person constantly strives to act in a manner that is just and right (Beauchamp and Childress, 1994, p. 66). Principles and rules that govern professional conduct fall under the ethical framework of deontologic behavior, such as autonomy, nonmaleficence, beneficence, justice, veracity, and confidentiality. The principle of autonomy recognizes an individual's right to chose and act freely with regard to the decisions made for his or her care. In the case of a neonate, parents act as surrogate decision makers and are considered autonomous. The purpose of nonmaleficence is to protect a patient from harm, whereas that of beneficence is to promote good and to work only in the patient's best interest. Treating a patient with justice means to be fair in judgments and to treat all patients in a like manner. Professional veracity is to give patients full, complete, and truthful information with regard to all issues of care. Confidentiality is to honor the patient's right to privacy and to refrain from disclosing patient information to any unauthorized person (Beauchamp and Childress, 1994, p. 39). In the NICU these principles are applied holistically to the neonate and to his or her family.

Ethic of Care

Unlike the other ethical framework, the ethic of care has been identified and discussed only in the past 20 years. Care, in this instance, refers to the action of caring for an individual through an emotional commitment and willingness to act in the best interest of the person with whom the relationship is maintained (Beauchamp and Childress, 1994, p. 85). Caring implies emotions such as empathy, compassion, and concern. Implicit in the relationship is the respect for and acknowledgment of human vulnerability, interdependence, and inequity. The ethical framework of care epitomizes the relationship that nurses have traditionally maintained with patients. Respect for patient dignity and quality of life and a comprehensive concern for the patient's overall well-being are the hallmarks of the care ethic.

Special Considerations in the NICU

Neonatal nurses face special challenges when dealing with ethical issues in their practice. The NICU environment is foreign and even frightening to most parents, making them feel as though they have little or no control over the care of their babies. Mingled with the feelings of fear and apprehension over the NICU environment is the perception that modern health care technology and the advanced medical knowledge of health care providers have immense capacity to cure almost any condition regardless of severity. As time in the NICU progresses, parents may become increasingly disillusioned and disappointed with the limitations still present in neonatal care. Unclear information from a variety of health care providers, emotional weariness, and the urgency and gravity of decisions converge together to cause a crisis in the relationship between the parents and the health care team.

Thorne and Robinson (1989) studied the relationship that families of chronically ill children developed with the health care system. Describing the relationship, the researchers identified three stages of development. The first stage is termed "naive trust" and is characterized by a belief that the health care team has great power to treat the family member and will always work in the best interest of the patient, without error. The second stage progresses to "disenchantment," when the family's often unrealistic expectations are not met and the feelings of disappointment and abandonment begin to dominate. The last stage is described as a "guarded alliance" as the family members realize that they must collaborate with the health care team and accept the limitations of modern health care technology and the individuals who practice in it. In the NICU, parental behavior progresses along this continuum and is evidenced by the request for only certain nurses to care for the infant, extreme reactions to any human error in the care of the baby, parental depression, and defensive reactions to a health care team member's suggestions.

Ethical Conflict

As time progresses in the NICU, the neonate is continually assessed and data are gathered with regard to current condition and future prognosis. The very presence of the neonate in the NICU serves as an indicator that the parents desire full treatment for their baby. The seemingly endless string of examinations, tests, diagnostic procedures, and specialists produces massive amounts of information, all intended to contribute to a continuing plan of care and treatment. Communication to the parents comes through the attending physician, neonatal nurse, social worker, and nurse practitioner, as well as other health care team members. Parents take the information given to them and discuss it between themselves and with others whose opinions and counsel they value.

In the ideal situation, there is enough time before a procedure to discuss fully with the parents the purpose, process, benefits, and risks of a procedure. If the parents agree, the procedure takes place as planned. Conflict arises, however, when the parents do not agree and refuse to consent to a procedure, regardless of what the health care team recommend. The health care team may react in a number of different ways to parental refusal of treatment. One reaction may be to abide by the parents' wishes and to accept that the parents are working in the baby's best interest. Immediate acceptance on the part of the health care team is extremely rare, and further discussions with the parents usually ensue.

Initially, the health care team's approach to parents may be based on the assumption that the parents are not sufficiently informed or do not adequately understand the importance of the procedure. Even if the assumption is true, the health care team, and particularly the neonatal nurse, should proceed with extreme caution. The rationale that the parents used to arrive at the decision may be the result of a combination of one or more factors, including inadequate education, family concerns, the need to protect the baby from further pain or prolonged suffering, or a clash of values with the health care team. The neonatal nurse, through ongoing interaction with the family, is in an excellent position to gain insight into the key issues for the parents and may resolve the conflict before it advances further.

At times, parents cannot be convinced to give consent for a treatment or procedure that the health care team believes to be beneficial or lifesaving. These conflicts are common when the baby's expected survival is minimal even with the treatment or when the baby has been ill for an extended period and the treatment will prolong life but will cause great pain or discomfort to the baby. Conflict then exists that must be resolved to treat the infant appropriately while at the same time respecting the legal and cultural duties, rights, and obligations of the parents.

Legal resolution of these situations occurs when the hospital seeks legal custody of the patient or a court order is obtained to proceed with the treatment despite the parents' objections. In most instances a telephone call to a judge, detailing the medical rationale and necessity of the treatment, is all that is needed to secure custody for the purpose of treatment. These remedies work well to alleviate the immediate medical crisis, but a long-term solution needs to be found to resolve the conflict between the family and the health care team.

Parents as Decision Makers

Parents of babies in an NICU are faced with a particularly difficult set of circumstances with regard to decision making for their child. Whether and to what extent they are involved with decision making may be influenced to a great degree by the accepted culture and routines of the unit and the hospital where their baby is a patient. Criteria for decision making are also affected by the attending health care team's values, the ability of the team to communicate, and the level of compassion that the team has for the situation in which the parents find themselves (Kirschbaum, 1996, p. 52). However, the parents must deal with less objective data than the health care team has, must consider global information that affects other individuals besides the baby, and must be able to live with the consequences of the decisions throughout the rest of their lives. The interests of the family and their baby are so closely intertwined that they are not easily separated, and there are no adequate guidelines or protocols at this time to be of real use in the resolution of these difficult situations.

MEDICALIZATION PROCESS OF ETHICS

The general practice in NICUs has long been to initiate aggressive treatment immediately and to evaluate outcome once treatment has taken place. Judgments with regard to the "rightness" of the procedure must be evaluated retrospectively. Therefore, in practice, the role of the parent in decision making in the NICU is limited, at least during the first few critical hours or days. In an ethnographically based study of NICUs, the role of the parents in meaningful decision making was found to be extremely limited from the point of admission. Physicians and nurses did not readily engage in discussion of ethical issues or use words that connote an ethical dilemma. The researcher labeled the persistent use of medical jargon rather that ethical language consistent with a "medicalization" process of ethics. That is, decision making was based on the medical parameters of success, rather than being a part of a more globally comprehensive aspect of the patient's and family's current and future existence (Jennings, 1988, p. 264).

PARENTAL VALUES

When Kirschbaum (1996) conducted a study of parents with critically ill children, several key themes of parental values emerged that provide insight for nurses into the thoughts and ethical processing of parents. The study's implications for the NICU are evident.

1. The first and initially impeachable value was that of preservation of life. Parents stated that they often chose treatment because they wanted more time with their child and because they, in essence, were not ready to let the child die. At this point, they did not always consider the type of life their child would have or the long-lasting implications of the child's condition for the family. What remained for the parents was a single-minded, instinctual devotion to life (Kirschbaum, 1996, p. 56).
2. The next stage for parents in the study was deep concern for the child's suffering and ongoing pain. This realization seemed to occur after a child had been ill for some time and the parents had witnessed considerable suffering, ranging from routine laboratory sticks and intravenous "starts" to suffering

resulting from a major procedure. Once parents began to question the efficacy of a particular treatment and the possible long-term outcome, the question of quality of life became an overriding concern (Kirschbaum, 1996, p. 57).

3. Quality of life was defined by the parents within the context of the child's life, rather than their own or the family's life. The parents in the study could not define "quality of life" but could discuss only what it is not. The quality-of-life yardstick for some parents was normalcy, a concept that was influenced by the long critical care experience. However, for many parents the mental and functional status of their child was a defining parameter. Parents were in agreement that an existence without the capacity to care for himself or herself demonstrated an absence of quality of life (Kirschbaum, 1996, p. 59).

4. Family issues were also important to parents in several ways. Membership in the family was essential to the parents, and they began to fear that the child mattered only to them and would eventually be forgotten by others in both the immediate and the extended family. Involvement of the extended family throughout the hospitalization and in the preparation for death eased some of that burden because these family members also served as witnesses to the child's existence and importance. For first-time parents, the baby may represent their entire family, and the loss of the baby therefore takes away their status as a family. Other parents expressed great fear of having more babies, stating that they could not go through such an ordeal again and survive. Parents with other children worried about the effect the baby would have on the siblings, and these concerns were present whether the baby lived or died. One concern was that the monetary expense and over-riding time commitment might not be fair to the baby's siblings (Kirschbaum, 1996, p. 62).

STAGES OF ADAPTATION

Worries and concerns about the care of the neonate subsequent to the NICU period constituted a prevalent finding in a study of former NICU parents. Interviews of 32 families 4 years after discharge indicated that the memories of the NICU experience remained strong, with parents able to recall the NICU experience in great detail. Three stages of adaptation that emerged from the parent interviews give insight into the parents' moral reasoning.

1. The first stage was processing the story, in which the parents discussed the NICU experience as a segment of both their own and the baby's life. Parents reported emotional stress and feelings of not being connected to their baby during the NICU stay. Memories of treatments remained superficial, but the parents remembered accepting whatever was being done for their infant by the health care team. Significantly, parents reported an inability to evaluate treatment options because of the medical terminology used and the overwhelming NICU environment. Further, they did not associate ethics and moral decision making with the NICU period, believing without question that giving the necessary treatment was the right thing to do (Pinch and Speilman, 1996, p. 77).

2. Next, the parents began to integrate the responsibility of parenting a high-risk infant as the baby grew and developed into childhood. Parents discussed the impact that the baby had on the other members of the household and their anxiety over their inability to predict the future development of the child. Although parents seldom used words such as "disability" or "handicap," they often compared their infant to siblings or to other children born healthy. Money became an issue for the parents, with the initial hospital charges being the first of many expenses. Dealing with the insurance carrier throughout the experience was a huge stressor for parents, as was the subsequent job immobility caused by the employment-based insurance system (Pinch and Speilman, 1996, p. 78).

3. The final stage for parents was concern for the family's future welfare and the desire to assist and support other parents of premature infants. If a possibility existed that the child would be "normal" in the long term, the belief was expressed that the future would be secure. One parent in the study expressed the wish that the child did not exist, because the child had created a great amount of work and stress in their lives. Some parents described feelings of great worry related to their child's lifetime requirement of care, assistance, and intervention (Pinch and Speilman, 1996, p. 79).

The Nurse's Role in Ethical Dilemmas

ETHICAL DILEMMAS IN THE NICU

Ethical dilemmas in the NICU are the products of several different patient scenarios. First, such dilemmas are likely to occur when an infant has received treatment in the NICU for an extended period, the likelihood of an optimal outcome seems remote, and the baby has endured a great deal of pain and discomfort. At this time the parents may want to discontinue treatment when the health care team desires to continue, or the health care team may want to discontinue treatment but the parents are not in agreement. In either case a conflict exists that must be resolved in the baby's best interest.

PREVENTION OF ETHICAL CONFLICT

Another time when ethical issues arise for families is once the baby is at home with the parents and the care responsibilities become a reality. This is unique among NICU patients because the ethical issues become prevalent long after the decisions were made and the care rendered. In an interview a father contrasted his own assessment of his baby's survival in the NICU with that of the health care professional: "It's a great miracle to read about in the paper, but I've got to take the miracle home and, ah, I have to be up with him at 2 or 3 o'clock in the morning, and then I gotta be up at 5:30 and go to work. Because he was screaming and uncomfortable and he . . . we have a lot of, an awful lot of, ah . . . problems. When all the cameras are gone, the parents take home a very sickly child. When the cameras are gone, the burden lies in a very quiet place, you know" (Pinch and Speilman, 1996, p. 82).

The best way to deal with ethical conflict in the NICU is always to work toward prevention. Neonatal nurses are in the best position throughout the NICU stay to partner with the parents to resolve conflicts and prepare families for what lies ahead. The NICU nurse accomplishes this first and foremost through communication with the parents and the other health care team members. Communication among health care team members must also be frequent, clear, and concise. Any ambiguous messages given to parents by health care communicators must be immediately clarified to the parents' satisfaction. Communication to the parents needs to be clear and as free of medical jargon as possible. Parents do not always know the questions to ask, and therefore the nurse should supply a great deal of information and do so repeatedly. Arranging for the parents to meet with former NICU parents will allow them to receive important information in a less threatening manner and will facilitate a rapid growth of their objective knowledge base. Speak to parents early regarding the baby's current status, usual recovery course, and potential problems or complications. Identify decisions or potential decisions that need to be made and the information and support necessary to make them. This enables the parents to take counsel with other family members, the physician, clergy, social worker, or others who can provide insight into the problem. When an ethical conflict appears to be forming, early consultation with the institutional ethics committee can facilitate the open airing of concern, discussion, and counseling that can ward off a full-scale confrontation.

Respect and empathy for the parents is the most important action that the NICU nurse can take in the care of the neonate and the family. Understanding that it is the parent who has the lifelong duty to care for the infant enables the neonatal nurse to work with the parents in an atmosphere of care. The decisions that the parents make will shape the future of their lives and those of their family. Facilitating the parents' ability to make choices that are meaningful for their baby and themselves is neonatal nursing at its best.

Using Institutional Ethics Committees

In some instances, conflicts between and among the health care team members and the parents of the infant cannot be resolved without the intervention of an outside agent. In these instances the institutional ethics committee (IEC) should be contacted to provide consultation for both the family and the caregivers. Early involvement by the IEC can help prevent the uncertainty and differences in treatment positions between the parents and the health care team from becoming emotional conflicts that are difficult or impossible to resolve. The goal of the IEC is to resolve conflict and provide a structure for due process.

CONSULTATION AND GUIDANCE

The work of the IEC begins with the provision of consultation and guidance to the NICU health care team during the time when policies and procedures for care are formulated. Working with the NICU team as the policies are formed enables the IEC to ensure that uniform standards are established and maintained, that they are consistent with the most current ethical thought, and that they meet legal and regulatory requirements. The IEC can ensure that policies are written in broad terms that allow the diversity of each situation to be considered in decision making while at the same time providing consistent guidance to staff members (Nelson and Shapiro, 1995, p. 29).

EDUCATION

Another, equally important role of the IEC is to provide education to staff and parents regarding ethical decision making. Educational programming for the staff can be accomplished easily in a variety of forums, such as in-service training, continuing education programs, or staff meetings. For parents the forums are not as readily available, but information about the IEC should be clearly outlined in the parents' handbook, which they receive at admission to the NICU, and through individual consultation during the stay (Nelson and Shapiro, 1995, p. 29).

ROLE OF THE IEC

The most common use of the IEC is consultation in a situation that already has become conflictual. Any individual on the health care team or the parents of the infant can contact the IEC for consultation. The IEC is required to have established procedures that allows for reasonable accessibility, timely response, documentation of the process, and evaluation of the situation. The role of the IEC is to explore issues, provide a forum for open discussion, delineate options, facilitate communications among all participants, and mediate disagreements. However, it must be remembered that the IEC is not a decision-making body but a group that makes recommendations regarding the process and issues that should be considered by both the health care team and the provider (Leeman, Fletcher, Spencer, and Fry-Revere, 1997, p. 260).

GOAL OF THE IEC

It is the goal of this process to build consensus between those caring for the infant and the parents. Consultation by the IEC may be conducted initially by an individual from the committee who evaluates the situational variables and develops a plan to further explore the issues. Strategies used by the IEC include interviews and counseling on an individual basis, use of two or three other committee members to work with the participants, and group meetings that facilitate the expression of thoughts and feelings while providing a forum for education.

Of last resort is the convening of the full IEC, with parents and health care team members providing testimony to the IEC regarding the status, care, and prognosis of the infant. When this occurs, the IEC makes nonbinding recommendations regarding the process for further care (Nelson and Shapiro, 1995, p. 31).

Advancing technology, federal regulations, and the continuing national debate over the issues of life make the NICU an environment where uncertainty and conflict is commonplace. Dealing effectively with these situations requires nurses to know the components of decision making, understand the issues from the perspective of the patients and their families, and use the resources made available through the IEC.

REFERENCES

Beauchamp, T.L., and Childress, J.F.: Principles of Biomedical Ethics, 4th ed. New York, Oxford University Press, 1994.

Jennings, B.: Ethics and ethnography in neonatal intensive care. In Weisz, G. (Ed): Social Science Perspectives on Medical Ethics. Dordrecht, The Netherlands, Kluwer Academic Publishers, 1988.

Kirschbaum, M.S.: Life support decisions for children: What do parents value? Adv. Nurs. Sci., 19(1):51–71, 1996.

Leeman, C.P., Fletcher, J.C., Spenser, E.M., and Fry-Revere, S.: Quality control for hospitals' clinical ethics services: Proposed standards. Cambridge Quarterly of Healthcare Ethics, 6(3):257–268.

Nelson, R.M., and Shapiro, R.S.: The role of an ethics committee in resolving conflict in the neonatal intensive care unit. Journal of Law, Medicine, and Ethics, 23(1):27–32, 1995.

Pierce, P.F.: What is an ethical decision? Crit. Care Nurs. Clin. North Am., 9(1):1–11, 1997.

Pinch, W.J., and Speilman, M.L.: Ethics in the neonatal intensive care unit: Parental perceptions at four years postdischarge. Adv. Nurs. Sci., 19(1):72–85, 1996.

Thorne, S.E, and Robinson, C.A.: Guarded alliance: Health care relationships in chronic illness. Image Journal of Nursing Scholarship, 21(1):153–157, 1989.

Chapter 34

Legal Issues in the NICU

M. Terese Verklan

Objectives

1. Identify how an attorney may use the nursing process for litigation.

2. Define standards of care and guidelines for establishing the standard of care.

3. Define malpractice and the conditions that constitute malpractice.

4. Define concepts of liability and negligence.

5. Discuss the importance of documentation in the patient's record and guidelines for charting.

6. Discuss the nurse's role in informed consent.

7. Identify scope of practice issues in providing patient care functions.

8. Identify the risks and benefits of possessing professional liability insurance.

In the past, the specialty of obstetrics was considered the "high risk" area for malpractice suits and loss of licensure. Today, litigation is not uncommon in our own area of specialization. Neonates are seen as a "special" population that are afforded extra protections (Verklan, 1996). Thus neonatal nurses must be cognizant of the minimum standards of professional conduct that they, as health care providers, must adhere to. The purpose of this chapter is to familiarize the nurse with the concepts and ramifications of legal concerns as they pertain to the realm of neonatal intensive care nursing. Topics that will be discussed include standards of care, liability, documentation, informed consent, scope of practice and malpractice issues, and professional liability insurance.

Nursing Process

A. **The nursing process has formed the foundation for nursing education, practice, and documentation, regardless of whether the nurse graduated from a diploma, associate degree, or baccalaureate program for many years.** Even though nurses are beginning to leave the description "nursing process" out of their practice standards and teaching strategies, nursing documentation should still reflect the nursing process. Failure to follow the following five steps is the number one cause of all patient injuries:

1. **Assessment:** gathers data related to the neonate's physiologic and psychosocial status.
   a. Vital sign records, flowsheets, and nursing progress records.
   b. Body and organ-system findings (e.g., cardiopulmonary findings).
   c. Laboratory and diagnostic reports.
   d. Medical progress notes.
   e. Intake and output.
   f. Progress notes from other disciplines (e.g., respiratory, social work, pharmacy).
   g. Information from the family.
2. **Diagnosis:** correctly identifies the neonate's condition, using the data obtained from the assessment step; documents on the nursing care plan and in the progress notes.
3. **Planning:** develops a plan of care that incorporates all aspects of the neonate's condition.
   a. Uses multidisciplinary approach.
   b. Documents interventions and anticipated outcomes for the targeted diagnosis on the nursing care plan.
4. **Implementation:** carries out the plan of care.
   a. Follows neonatologist and/or advanced practice nurse orders, provides direct care, supervises the care given by another, teaches and/or counsels the family, provides referrals for care by other disciplines.
   b. Documents all pertinent information on the neonate's medical record.
5. **Evaluation:** evaluates the neonate's response to the plan of care as outlined by the multidisciplinary team, noting any revisions and/or changes to the plan.
   a. Implementation process is not complete without evaluating the effectiveness of the intervention.
   b. Communicates patient response to treatment to members of the multidisciplinary team.
   c. Documents pertinent findings in the patient's medical record.

B. The attorney, as well as all interested parties involved in the legal process, will use the steps of the nursing process to:

1. Interpret the medical record.
2. Identify possible deviations from the standard of care.
3. Speak the same language as the nurse.
4. Pose questions that will be used to depose a nurse defendant.
5. Use the reports of expert witnesses who will outline how the nurse did or did not follow the nursing process.

Standard of Care

In the legal system, the standard of care is established by defining what a reasonable and prudent nurse would have done in the same or similar circumstances (Meissner-Cutler and Gardner, 1997). The issue of excellence in practice or quality of care given does not pertain to the argument—what is being sought is reasonableness and prudence. A reasonable and prudent nurse is a nurse with like education, background, and experience who would behave in a corresponding manner, given a parallel set of events.

In addition, it is expected that the standard of care given to neonates everywhere is the same. *Ewing v. Aubert* (1988) set out that a maternal-child nurse is held to the standard of care of a nurse practicing in the maternal-child specialty.

Nurses today are evaluated by a national standard because advances in communication, technology, transportation, and the law have made obsolete the "locality rule" (Tammelleo, 1994). The locality rule permitted nurses to be judged according to the standard of care evidenced by nurses working in the same geographic area. In addition, accredited schools of nursing across the nation have similar curricula and textbooks, and nurses attend similar continuing education conferences. Thus it is expected that the professional nurse will be and remain competent and continually updated on the standards of care and practice (American Nurses Association, [ANA], 1991).

Five basic types of evidence are used to establish the legal standard of care: (1) state and federal regulations, (2) institutional policies, procedures, and protocols, (3) testimony from expert witnesses, (4) standards of professional organizations, and (5) current professional literature.

STATE AND FEDERAL REGULATIONS

These agencies establish the standards of care and scope of practice. The national standards tend to be written in broad language to permit flexibility without compromising standards to accommodate differences within each state. The standard of practice is also defined by the state nurse practice act as mandated by each state's legislature. Here the scope of practice is delineated for each level of nursing (e.g., licensed vocational nurse, registered nurse, advanced practice nurse). For example, a registered nurse may not delegate the act of assessment and the formulation of a nursing diagnosis to any assistive personnel who are unqualified to perform this task (ANA, 1994). In addition, standards of nursing practice are also regulated by the state board of nursing, the department of health, the Joint Commission for Accreditation of Healthcare Organizations (JCAHO), and the Health Care Financing Administration, in addition to other regulatory agencies (Iyer, 1996a).

INSTITUTIONAL POLICIES, PROCEDURES, AND PROTOCOLS

The hospital's policies, procedures, and protocols also outline the standard of care. The policy establishes the purposes for performing a procedure, whereas the procedure is the guideline for how that procedure should be carried out. These guidelines must reflect the national and state standards of care, should be reviewed at least annually, and should be revised to reflect current acceptable nursing practice (JCAHO, 1996). In addition, these guidelines must also be (1) prepared by a qualified committee of professionals who practice in the specialty, (2) consistent with current research and practice literature, (3) archived for the length of liability, and (4) accessible to staff (Meissner-Cutler & Gardner, 1997). The policy and procedures manual is approved by both the unit and the hospital's nursing and medical administrations.

Being unaware of the policy and procedures for the standard clinical practice at your establishment is not an acceptable excuse for not being held accountable for your realm of practice. Because this is often the best source for specific standards by which to evaluate a specific nurse's care, this is usually one of the first documents requested by the both the plaintiff and the defense attorneys. Because the statutes of limitations endure for 18–21 years and standard care practices change dramatically across the years, keeping the policy and procedures manual will also help to determine what the standard of care was at the time the infant was hospitalized.

TESTIMONY FROM EXPERT WITNESSES

A nurse expert is typically required to articulate what the standard of care is or was in the situation in which the nurse has deviated from the usual and customary standard of care. A nursing expert opinion requires that the person expressing that opinion possess special skill, knowledge, and experience in the neonatal area, and knowledge of the standards applicable at the time the occurrence took place (Iyer and Yudkoff, 1996). The judge and jury have little knowledge related to neonatal physiology, pathophysiology, and the relevant neonatal nursing care. They therefore need assistance in understanding just what a reasonable and prudent nurse would have done in the given circumstances. (For example, did the nurse meet the accepted standard of care?)

As discussed above, both liability and damages have to be proved in nursing malpractice cases. Thus two types of experts are usually necessary: a nurse to address the nursing standard of care, and a physician to determine causation, that is, to link the breach of standard to the injuries suffered by the neonate. Professional nursing philosophies dictate that nurses be the only witnesses permitted to testify as experts outlining what the nursing standard of care is in a nursing malpractice suit. However, it is the quality of the expert's experience and education that determines the competency and credibility of the testimony (Tammelleo, 1994).

STANDARDS OF PROFESSIONAL ORGANIZATIONS

Professional associations represent the interests of nurses. The ANA has developed standards with measurable criteria that define professional nursing practice. Specialty organizations such as the National Association of Neonatal Nurses (NANN), Association of Women's Health, Obstetrics and Neonatal Nurses (AWHONN), American Association of Critical Care Nurses (AACN), and National Association of Pediatric Nurse Associates and Practitioners (NAPNAP) have adapted these standards to define the standards of care and professional practice guidelines applicable to the care of neonates.

CURRENT PROFESSIONAL LITERATURE

Current texts and journal articles, although technically hearsay, aid in establishing the legal standard of care. A number of journals specific to the care of neonates focus on clinical, management, and research articles. Clinical articles are useful in helping to determine the applicable standard of care at the time of the malpractice suit, whereas nursing textbooks provide information related to the standard of care associated with nursing techniques and care (Iyer, 1996a). Research articles are beginning to assume more importance in the legal arena because of the desire to document evidence-based practice. Keeping theory and clinical practice on par with the literature and remaining current with regard to continuing education will assist the nurse in ensuring that his or her professional standards are synonymous with those of his or her peers.

FURTHER ISSUES: PRACTICE GUIDELINES AND ETHICAL STANDARDS

Standards of care are often confused with practice guidelines. Standards of care are the basis for proving that the nurse had a duty to the patient and that there was a breach of that duty. Clinical practice guidelines, with reference to the standards of care, are meant to assist the health care provider in the delivery of care in specific clinical circumstances (Bergman, 1994). For example, *Guidelines for Perinatal Care* outlines recommendations regarding nurse providers, nursing ratios, staffing guidelines, and outreach education for inpatient perinatal care facilities providing basic, specialty, and subspecialty care (American Academy of Pediatrics and American College of Obstetricians and Gynecologists [AAP/ ACOG], 1997). Critical pathways are another example of a practice guideline that is modified to reflect the neonate's clinical progress. Therefore the difference between a standard of care and a practice guideline is that the standard always must be adhered to, whereas the guideline suggests a voluntary approach to achieve a desirable patient outcome (Iyer, 1996a).

The ethical standards of nursing practice may also be the issue in a malpractice suit:

> An obstetrician began the incision for the Cesarean section even though the woman's epidural anesthesia had not taken full effect. The nurses did not believe this to be an emergent delivery as the obstetrician did not communicate a difficulty in delivering the neonate. He did not stop and wait a few minutes to give the anesthesia time to take full effect. Five nurses signed incident reports. They testified that they had never seen a patient express their pain as vocally as this woman. County (MN) District Court, Case No. C7-92-5925. The nurses felt compelled to act under the third item of the ANA's Code for Nurses (1978) which states that the nurse is to "safeguard the client and the public when health care and safety are affected by the incompetent, unethical or illegal practice of any person" (Laska, 1993).

Malpractice

The term "malpractice" means negligence on the part of the nurse, in that she or he has violated the standards of ordinary nursing practiced by nurses of similar background in the same specialty of nursing:

> By undertaking professional services to the patient, a nurse represents that she possesses, and it is her duty to possess only that degree of learning of skill ordinarily possessed by nurses of good standing practicing in the same community under similar circumstances. It is her further duty to use the care ordinarily exercised in like cases by reputable members of her/his profession practicing in the same/similar locality and under similar circumstances. S/he is to use reasonable diligence and her/his best judgment in the exercise of skill and application of learning in an effort to accomplish the purpose for which s/he is employed. A defendant nurse must violate one of these duties before s/he is guilty of malpractice (Davis and Neggers, 1996, p. 974).

It must be emphasized that the nurse need possess only the knowledge and skill possessed by the *average* reasonable, prudent nurse:

> The difficulties and uncertainties in the practice of nursing are such that no nurse can be required to guarantee results. A nurse is not responsible for unexpected occurrences during the course of treatment or care s/he is providing or for an unsuccessful result unless the same can be attributed to negligence on her/his part (Davis and Neggers, 1996, p. 974).

Occasionally an unexpected situation arises so quickly that one's actions on hindsight may not be considered to have been the perfect course of action. These behaviors do not automatically constitute malpractice:

> A nurse who is suddenly and unexpectedly confronted with an emergency situation arising either from actual danger or the appearance of an emergency and imminent danger to the patient, is not expected or required to use the same judgment and prudence that is required of him/her in the exercise of care in a calmer and more deliberate moment. Her/his duty is to exercise only the care that an ordinarily prudent nurse would exercise in the same situation. If at that moment s/he does what appears to him/her to be the best thing to do, and if his/her choice and manner of action are the same as might have been followed by any ordinarily prudent nurse

under the same circumstances, s/he does all that the law requires of him/her even if in the light of after-events it should appear that a different course would have been better and safer (Davis and Neggers, 1996, p. 975).

A mistake in judgment is not considered malpractice:

A mistake in judgment on the part of the nurse is not evidence of negligence. If a nurse possesses reasonable and ordinary learning skill and uses care such as is ordinarily used in like or similar situations by nurses of reasonable and average skill practicing in the community at the time in question, s/he is not guilty of negligence even though the judgment which s/he arrives at may be subsequently proven incorrect (Davis and Neggers, 1996, p. 974).

Liability

Today nurses are recognized as professionals who are responsible and accountable for the care they give to their patients. If the nurse is liable to the patient because of negligent conduct, that nurse can be held legally responsible for the harm caused to that patient (Bernzweig, 1996). Malpractice occurs when a professional nurse is negligent in conducting a professional activity. This is not the same as carelessness, because a nurse's careful conduct may still constitute legal negligence if what she or he does is not what another reasonable and prudent nurse would have done, given the same situation. Harm must result from the act, because without damage, no legal wrong has been committed.

A newborn male was discharged from the defendant XYZ hospital two days after birth with a diagnosis of physiologic jaundice. Four days later, he was admitted to ABC hospital with a diagnosis of *E. coli* sepsis and meningitis. The boy was later diagnosed with galactosemia which had not been diagnosed when he was treated for meningitis. The plaintiffs alleged that the neonate's jaundice was the first sign of infection and should have led the XYZ hospital to conduct further tests. It was also claimed that the XYZ hospital failed to communicate results of a newborn screening that was done while the child was hospitalized for meningitis at the second hospital. The plaintiffs further alleged that ABC hospital failed to recognize symptoms and the results of diagnostic testing which should have led to a diagnosis of galactosemia. Furthermore, this delay resulted in brain damage, mild retardation and right-sided weakness. According to the *Ohio Trial Reporter,* a $1,200,000 settlement was reached. (*Anonymous Minor, et al., v. Anonymous Pediatricians, ABC Hospital and XYZ Hospital,* Cuyahoga County [OH] Court of Common Pleas, Case No. 280713 [Laska, 1997b].)

The plaintiff, the party bringing the suit, must prove the following four elements in a malpractice case:
1. The nurse had a duty to her/his patient.
2. There was a breach of that duty.
3. Harm or damages did occur to the patient.
4. Breach of that duty resulted in harm (proximal cause).

An infant, born in a depressed state, had a one minute Apgar of 3. Although his condition improved, the five minute Apgar was 8, he continued to have raspy breathing, that required suctioning. It was alleged that the defendants failed to provide adequate special care and observation, causing the baby to suffocate on its own secretions. The neonate was discovered in a cyanotic state two hours after birth. Resuscitative techniques restored the heartbeat in eighteen minutes. He was transferred to another hospital, declared to be brain-dead, and was removed from life support four days later. The plaintiff claimed that resuscitation was both delayed and improperly performed. The defendants argued that the baby appeared normal, that the cause of the respiratory arrest is unknown, and that inborn errors of metabolism caused the death. They also countered that failure to respond to resuscitation does not imply negligence. (Du Page County [IL] Circuit Court, Case No. 94L-318 [Laska, 1997a].)

In this case the plaintiff proved that the defendant owed a duty to the neonate, in that the baby and his parents should expect the care received to be at least equal to the standard of care. However, the plaintiff was not able to prove that the defendant breached the duty (failure to respond to resuscitation does not imply negligence) or that there was proximal cause (inborn errors of metabolism may have contributed to or caused the injury). Thus, despite the neonate's death (damages), a malpractice suit cannot be won if all four elements are not present.

A. Although an individual nurse is accountable only for his or her own practice, there are three additional theories of liability that may be pursued against a facility or its management (Speid, 1996):

1. *Respondeat superior,* which, in essence, says that the employer can be held liable for the actions or intentions of the employee. This doctrine:
   a. Holds an employer liable for the negligent acts of employees that arise in the course of the employment (i.e., employers are held responsible for the acts of those whom they have a right to supervise or control).
   b. Holds the institution responsible for ensuring that the policies and procedures meet the standard of care, and that employees follow these policies.
   c. Will not impose liability in most circumstances on a nursing supervisor for negligent acts of the nursing personnel he or she is supervising. This responsibility rests with the person who makes changes in the policies and procedures (Fiesta, 1990b).
   d. Obligates the nursing supervisor to ensure that the licensed and nonlicensed nursing personnel under his or her supervision is able to provide patient care safely (Aiken, 1994). If the supervisor does not document the personnel's deficiencies and use the chain of command, she or he can be held liable for any damages that befall a patient.
   e. Holds that negligent employees are always liable for their own conduct.
2. *Corporate negligence* holds the institution's management and board of trustees liable for any breach of its duties:
   a. The institution must provide a safe physical setting and monitor the quality of care provided, along with the equipment necessary for patient care (Hospital Risk Control, 1995).
   b. An equipment standard must be implemented.
      (1) The institution must have a management plan documenting competency validation for the proper use of medical equipment by the institution's employees (JCAHO, 1996).
      (2) The institution may also name the equipment manufacturer as a third-party defendant in an attempt to shift the blame (Verklan, 1996).

> In a case in which a neonate was burned while being warmed under an infrared lamp, it was the plaintiff's contention that the neonatal intensive care unit negligently monitored the preterm infant. The neonate sustained second- and third-degree burns to her legs, resulting in the amputation of her leg. It was further contended that the neonate will need surgery to her breast area, and further surgeries, including prosthetic devices for her leg, as she continues to grow. The hospital named the company that assembled and distributed the lamp as a third-party defendant, contending that the company did not provide sufficient education with respect to the procedures to follow when using the lamp. The hospital also contended that the intensity of the heat was poorly controlled because of a defective switch. The third party contended that the design was proper and that if the nurse had provided appropriate observation and monitoring of the

neonate, the incident would not have occurred. The third-party defendant argued that the information contained in the accompanying literature was adequate, because this hospital had previous experience with similar equipment. The case was settled before summations for $4,500,000, with the third-party defendant responsible for $500,000 (Zarin, 1995).

    c. The facility may be found liable for advertising a service for which it lacks the proper equipment or personnel or for failure to keep these services at the acceptable standard of care.

    d. The institution must verify the credentials of those who apply for clinical privileges (e.g., advanced practice nurses) and must also query the National Practitioner Data Bank at the time clinical privileges are requested, and subsequently every two years, regarding those who hold practice privileges (NSO Risk Advisor, 1992). The data bank maintains records of disciplinary action taken on licenses, hospital privileges, and payment in conjunction with malpractice suits. In addition to health care organizations, professional societies and attorneys have access to the data bank. Each advanced practice nurse should be familiar with the database and should periodically verify that the information it contains regarding herself or himself is accurate.

    e. Clinical competencies must also be evaluated and documented every year (JCAHO, 1996).

3. *Apparent/ostensible authority* holds an institution liable for the acts of an independent contractor—for example, the advanced practice nurse in private practice with hospital privileges or the agency nurse (Fiesta, 1990a). The hospital should maintain a file for each agency nurse that contains his or her nursing license, required certifications, and a current competency skills checklist.

B. **An area of considerable controversy in the liability arena are the risk management and quality assurance activities.**

1. Risk management deals with errors, and the goal of quality assurance is excellence. The coordination of both areas results in an improvement in patient care and a decrease in malpractice claims (Fiesta, 1991).
2. The task of these departments is to determine the standard of care for their institution.
3. By documenting occurrences and maintaining related records, such as the organization's claims history, quality assurance and utilization review activities, and risk management and analysis, this area may have information valuable for a plaintiff's malpractice case. For that reason, many jurisdictions have provided a protective shield for quality assurance and risk management activities, which renders the materials generated and the thought processes engaged in during those activities "privileged" or otherwise nondiscoverable (defendant cannot be asked to produce the materials) (Ament, 1997).

C. **The costs of liability when a neonate is involved are high for three reasons (Cohn, 1986):**

1. The cost of caring for a damaged infant with a normal life expectancy is high.
2. With the longer statute of limitations for minors, charges may be made years later, applicable to other medical malpractice actions.
3. There is sympathy toward the family, who may not be able to afford the needed care for the child, as opposed to the "cold corporation with ample insurance coverage who will not really miss the money anyway."

Scope of Practice

    Each state has its own nurse practice act, composed of statutes passed by its legislature and defining the boundaries of nursing practice. These laws vary from state to state in their demarcation of nursing practice. In contrast to state medical practice acts, the nurse practice statutes delineate nursing responsibilities in broad, universal nomenclature that generally must be examined with reference to the pertinent local law. The crucial issue regarding the scope of practice is whether or not the procedure performed by the nurse is legally within or beyond the scope of a nursing license to practice (Verklan, 1996).

There are numerous areas of medical and nursing practice that overlap one another, especially in the NICU. Depending on the unit and its written protocols, the same procedure may be considered within the realm of medicine when performed by a physician and within the realm of nursing when performed by a nurse. These "gray areas" have evolved partly in response to the nurse's increased level of educational preparation and advanced practice role and partly in response to the "high tech" environment found in the NICU. Neonatal nursing is considered a specialty area of practice, and the high-risk neonatal nursing in the NICU is considered a subspecialty area of practice. Certification for both the low-risk and the high-risk neonatal nurse is available through several specialty organizations (ANA, AACN, National Certification Corporation [NCC], NAPNAP).

Increasing the scope of practice, autonomy, and authority is likely to result in greater exposure to liability situations. Critical legal-liability and scope-of-practice problems arise whenever the nurse assumes patient care functions of an independent nature that:
1. Have long been held to be solely within the province of physicians.
2. Are not the subject of standing orders.
3. Lack definition in the nurse practice act.
4. Are not generally recognized as legitimate nursing functions by accredited professional organizations.
The standard of care and liability for negligence may be determined by:
1. Nurse's level of training and experience
2. Manuals and textbooks written for the specialty
3. Actions and inactions of the nurse
4. Protocols and instructions referred to by the nurse
5. The accepted professional nursing practice (Samuels, 1993)

The following case of *Dent v. Memorial Hospital of Adel, Inc.*, highlights many of these principles:

> The infant was admitted to the hospital as the result of an apneic event, with orders to place him on an apnea monitor. The nursing supervisor had difficulty in setting up the equipment. Once the monitoring was established, she and a nurse's aide began to assess the boy once an hour on a rotating basis. During the night, the mother found that he was not breathing. The alarm had not sounded, even though the cardiac and respiratory "waves" on the bedside monitor were straight lines. The nurses and physicians responded immediately to the mother's alert; however, the resuscitation was complicated by numerous problems involving missing equipment and supplies on the resuscitation cart. Heart rate returned with intubation, but no spontaneous respirations could be obtained. The boy was transferred to another hospital, where he subsequently died.
>
> The Court found that the hospital was negligent in the care given by the nursing staff. It was also determined that the equipment, facilities, and other personnel at the hospital did not meet the required standard of care in that it took an unnecessarily long period of time to begin proper operation of the monitor. This was seen as an indication of the staff being poorly trained in the use of the equipment. The monitor was also thought to be negligently operated, as the alarm had never sounded. No one was able to definitely establish if the monitor alarm had actually been in the "on" position. There was also evidence that the delayed resuscitation was related to the inadequately equipped resuscitation cart (Tammelleo, 1992b).

The reasonable, prudent nurse besides being responsible to the patient, is also accountable to herself or himself and to the profession (Verklan, 1996). Both the nurse and the employer have the responsibility to determine the level of competence of the nurse who is asked to provide care outside her or his specialty area. The right of a nurse's refusal to "float" has been upheld by the Wisconsin Supreme Court (*Winkelman v. Beloit Memorial Hospital*, 1992):

> A nursery nurse, Nurse Winkelman, was asked to float to a unit that provided postoperative and geriatric care. She discussed the situation with the supervisor, indicating that she had never floated, that she was exclusively a nursery nurse, and that she was not qualified to provide the type of care being requested. It was her opinion that the floating would put the patients and her license at risk, and thus, the hospital in jeopardy. The supervisor gave her three options, (a) float; (b) find another nurse to float; or (c) take an unexcused absence day. Nurse Winkelman left the hospital, and later received a letter informing her that the hospital took her actions to be a voluntary resignation. Although she denied that she had ever resigned, the hospital refused to reinstate her. Nurse Winkelman filed a complaint of wrongful discharge against the hospital. The case was decided in her favor, and the hospital appealed. The Supreme Court affirmed that she had identified the fundamental policy that provides for only qualified nurses to render care, and that nurses who provide care for which they are not qualified are subject to sanctions under the law (Tammelleo, 1992a).

Advanced Practice

Coincident with evolving health care delivery systems, neonatal advanced practice nurses can be found in hospitals, ambulatory care centers, and private practice. The advanced practice nurse (APN) is often the only health care provider in many rural areas. According to the American Nurses Association (ANA) APNs are those who have further knowledge and practice experiences that have prepared them for specialization, expansion, and advancement in the practice role (Barnard et al., 1994):
1. Specialization: focusing on one aspect of the field of nursing.
2. Expansion: acquisition of new practice skills.
3. Advancement: encompassing both specialization and expansion and involving:
   a. New integration of theories and skills.
   b. Graduate education.

The licensing statute in each state controls advanced practice and thereby protects the use of the title of APN. Almost all states have also passed additional legislation defining the scope of practice of the APN. The ANA defined APNs as:

> nurses in advanced clinical practice with a graduate degree in nursing. They conduct comprehensive health assessments, and demonstrate a high level of autonomy and expert skill in the diagnosis and treatment of complex responses of individuals, families and communities to actual or potential health problems. They formulate clinical decisions to manage acute and chronic illness and promote wellness. Nurses in advanced practice integrate education, research, management, leadership, and consultation into their clinical role and function in collegial relationships with nursing peers, physicians, and others who influence the health environment (ANA, 1993, p. 1).

In the neonatal area, the two recognized APNs are the neonatal nurse practitioner (NNP) and the clinical nurse specialist (CNS). As APN roles continue to expand, there will be further debate on what constitutes nursing functions.

A. **Neonatal nurse practitioner.**

1. One of the most common APNs found in the tertiary care setting.

2. Is responsible for managing a caseload of neonatal patients with general supervision, collaboration, and consultation from a physician.
3. Exercises independent judgment in the assessment, diagnosis, and initiation of delegated medical processes and procedures by using extensive knowledge of pathophysiology, pharmacology, and physiology (NANN, 1992).
4. Is involved in education, consultation, and research (NANN, 1992).
5. Received certification through the NCC.
6. Will require a master's degree for certification as of the year 2000.

B. **Clinical nurse specialist.**

1. Focuses on patient care, staff education, research, and consultation.
2. Responsibilities are (Nurses Association of the American College of Obstetricians and Gynecologists [NAACOG], 1990):
   a. Acting as a resource for neonatal nurses, NNPs, and other care providers.
   b. Establishing and evaluating patient care standards.
   c. Assessing and identifying educational needs of the family, nursery, and community.
   d. Designing and implementing appropriate educational programs based on identified needs.
   e. Providing consultation to health care providers.
   f. Initiating research projects, participating in data collection, and instituting changes based on research findings (evidence-based practice).

Each state decides the scope of practice for APNs and who the regulating authority will be. Thus there are no national laws or regulations exercising authority over the APN.

In the majority of the states the board of nursing is the sole authority (Pearson, 1995). Advanced practice continues to lack national standards for the credentialing of APNs. Although certificate programs continue, most APN curriculums today bestow a master's degree on those who successfully complete the requirements. In addition, most states require certification by either the ANA or the APN's specialty organization. By virtue of the necessary education and training required to become an APN, they are held to a higher standard than a general-duty nurse, but *only while performing services in their specialty* (Bernzweig, 1996). Thus the standard of care expected of the APN is the degree of care expected of any reasonable and prudent APN who practices in the same specialty. However, in general, the greater any nurse's background and training, the higher the standard of care expected by the law (Bernzweig, 1996).

Depending on the state, the APN may have his or her own practice in an independent setting, whereas another state may require the APN to practice with a supervising or collaborating physician. The issue of independence continues to be a major problem for both the NNP and the physician (Bernzweig, 1996). When nurses are involved in advanced practice, a question has been raised in those states that have broad statutory regulations: Are APNs legally empowered to perform the functions they render? A nurse who functions as an NNP in a state that does not recognize the NNP role has a high chance of being charged with practicing medicine without a license (Bernzweig, 1996).

An essential component of advanced practice nursing is having the legal authority to prescribe medications. Legislation authorizing prescriptive authority to APNs currently exists in 43 states, with similar legislation pending in several other states (Bernzweig, 1996). Because there is no federal barrier, each APN is allowed to obtain his or her own Drug Enforcement Administration number. Because legislation changes are ongoing in most areas, an annual summary of pending legislation affecting advanced practice can be found each year in the January issue of *Nurse Practitioner: The American Journal of Primary Health Care.*

Documentation

A. It is a professional responsibility of the nurse to document on the medical record. This will:

1. Facilitate care.
2. Enhance continuity and coordination of care.
3. Assist in the evaluation of the patient's response to treatment.
4. Provide a legal and official record of the care provided.

B. Thus the medical record is used by the attorney as a tool to provide evidence in legal proceedings because it also verifies that the nurse (Iyer, 1996b):

1. Provided the standard of care.
2. Did so within the scope of his or her nursing practice act.
3. Provided "routine care." Negligence could be proved if this information is absent or inappropriate. Flowsheets that list these routines, along with times, dates, patient and caregiver identification, and nursing care outcomes are valuable in providing a means of documenting repetitious nursing activities.

C. Although nursing notes need to be as complete as possible, the comment "If it's not documented, then it wasn't done" doesn't always hold true. Patient care is always the number one priority. Once the emergency is past, the nurse should strive to document the events, using as much detail as possible. However, if the needs of other patients were placed on hold during a crisis, those needs must be met immediately once the crisis is past. When the medical record is incomplete, the nurse may testify as to what constitutes her or his usual practice.

D. The most common charting systems in the NICU are (Iyer, 1996b):

1. Flowsheets.
   a. Decrease the need to document repetitive, *routine* nursing functions in the narrative notes.
   b. Have column-and-row format organized according to time and/or shift.
   c. Use abbreviations, symbols, and checkmarks to enter information.
2. Narrative charting.
   a. Patient care is documented by using chronologic format.
   b. Entries describe the neonate's status, interventions, evaluation of care, medical treatments and equipment (e.g., ventilator, bed, phototherapy lights) used, and the neonate's response to care.
3. Problem-oriented charting.
   a. Problem list outlines the patient's priority problems.
   b. Updates should be entered on a regular basis as problems resolve and new ones emerge.
   c. Documentation may be directly on the care plan or in the narrative notes.
   d. Specific format is followed:
      (1) S = subjective information that the patient tells the nurse.
      (2) O = objective information the nurse observes (including laboratory results).
      (3) A = assessment of the above-mentioned data, leading to a nursing diagnosis.
      (4) P = plan that the nurse will implement to address the care issue.
4. *Problem, intervention,* and *evaluation* of problems (PIE) charting: uses flowsheets, progress notes, and nursing diagnoses.
5. Charting by exception.
   a. Narrative notes are completed only when the neonate's progress and/or condition deviates from the expected or when an untoward occurrence arises.

b. Charting system contains nursing care plans, nursing database, flowsheets, and progress notes.

c. Standards of practice, determined by the institution, are incorporated into the charting system to record routine, repetitive nursing interventions (e.g., observation of intravenous site, checking ventilator settings).

E. Table 34–1 outlines the advantages and disadvantages of each charting strategy.

F. Guidelines for documentation (Iyer, 1996b; Iyer and Camp, 1995).

1. Sign at the end of every entry by using full name and credentials or only initials (full name and credentials noted in the appropriate space). Ensure that no vacant lines are left. An empty space may later prompt someone to fill in a "missing" piece of information.

2. Cosigning means that you have observed and/or approved the care given and that you are accepting joint responsibility (and liability) for that care. Nurses who are required by hospital policy routinely to countersign documents or information in the patient's chart should protect themselves in one of two ways:
   a. By personally verifying the information being recorded.
   b. By noting in the record that the signature is included in accordance with hospital policy and is not based on personal knowledge of the information in question (Bernzweig, 1996).

3. Illegible, sloppy handwriting with spelling and/or grammatical errors will convey a negative impression of the nurse. Examples: *fecal* heart tones heard; large, brown BM up walking in halls; vaginal packing out. Dr. in (Iyer and Camp, 1995).

Table 34–1
ADVANTAGES AND DISADVANTAGES OF CHARTING SYSTEMS

Charting Systems	Advantages	Disadvantages
Flowsheets	Easy to use. Decrease time spent.	No note on narrative sheet. Duplication of documentation on narrative sheet.
Narrative charting	Easy to document events as they occur in time.	Information may be disorganized and may not contain all elements of nursing process. Key patient issues may vary from shift to shift and from nurse to nurse; thus it may be difficult, years later, for hospital, nurse, and/or attorney to tease out relevant information related to specific patient complaint.
Problem-oriented charting	Documentation is organized. All disciplines use same progress notes, permitting increased collaboration and continuity of care.	Continuing same format on all patient problems becomes redundant, with same information appearing over and over. Time-consuming because of repetitious nature of note.
PIE charting	Documentation is organized. Evaluation of each problem requires only the information that is specific to that particular problem, intervention, and evaluation.	Novice nurses may have difficulty where there is no traditional care plan but, instead, an ongoing plan of care that is documented daily.
Charting by exception	Complete, detailed patient information is easily accessible to the health care provider. Standard of practice for documentation outlines expected normal findings.	Exceptions to the standards of practice may not be documented because nurses become accustomed to "checking off" the flowsheets.

PIE, Problem, intervention, and evaluation.
Data from Iyer, P. (Ed.): Nursing malpractice. Tucson, Lawyers and Judges Publishing, 1996, pp. 85–143.

4. Late charting is always suspect because it is typically key information that is added. Chart the information as soon as possible, beginning with the words "late entry for [date and time]."

5. To correct a mistaken entry:
   a. Draw one line through the entry.
   b. Write "mistaken entry" above the line. (The term "error" is no longer advised because juries tend to associate it with a clinical error.)
   c. Initial/sign document and add date next to "mistaken entry."
   d. What if a nurse is instructed *not to chart* an error by the attending physician? Nurses who accede to the demands of a physician to cover up the true facts of an unusual clinical episode by deliberately not mentioning it in the patient's chart not only may be subject to possible loss of licensure but, in flagrant circumstances, may even subject themselves to criminal action, leading to a fine or jail sentence (Bernzweig, 1996).

6. Avoid inappropriate comments concerning:
   a. The patient's or family's personality traits or idiosyncrasies (unless such remarks are relevant to the infant's treatment).
   b. Subjective views to the effect that the patient or family is a potential litigant.
   c. Admissions of legal liability with respect to untoward medical or nursing events. Examples are:
      (1) "The IV infiltrated because the night staff forgot to check it" (Solberg, 1986, p. 13).
      (2) "Patient going into shock. Could not get Dr. Jones to come. We never can!!!" (Fox and Imbiorski, 1979, p. 1).

7. Document occurrences accurately and concisely. For example, the neonate's parents (plaintiffs) may have a different view of what actually took place. In a malpractice action the burden of proof rests with the plaintiff. In the case of *Coleman v. Touro Infirmary of New Orleans* (506 So. 2d 571-LA, 1993), the plaintiff alleged that the defendants had been negligent by failing to treat an abruptio placentae before the premature delivery of the infant and that the defendants' actions or inaction had caused the child's death. There were several discrepancies between the patient's recollection of events and the medical record. The court consulted the chart and the physician, determined that the nurses' notes stated another set of events, and concluded that the plaintiff failed to prove any act or omission by the obstetrician or hospital that resulted in the wrongful death of the Coleman infant.

8. Document objectively.
   a. Avoid using "appears to be" and "seems to be." These phrases are not consistent with the judgments/diagnosis made by the critical thinking nurse of today.
   b. Quantify in measurable aliquots when possible. For example, "approximately 30 cc emesis" gives more information than "large emesis."
   c. The patient record is not an appropriate place to refer to an incident report's having been made. What should be documented is a factual account of what transpired and what was done. Incident reports enable the hospital or agency to make necessary investigations of the situation while the patient is still hospitalized, to identify situations of increased risk, and to trend these events to determine whether they are preventable (Ament, 1997).

9. Document promptly:
   a. Any significant changes in the patient's status.
   b. Nursing actions undertaken to intercede in the situation, including notifying the physician of the concern. Note the time of the phone call notifying the physician, the information relayed, any orders received, and what you did next.

The case of *Mark and Debbie Easter, etc. v. Baylor University Medical Center* (Laska, 1993) illustrates the way in which nurses can place themselves in a liability situation by ignoring the above-noted standard of conduct.

> The defendant was a 29-week gestational age neonate delivered by cesarean section at the defendant hospital. His serum potassium was not measured during the first 6 days of his life, and the blood glucose level was measured once on the day of his birth. As a result, hyperkalemia and hypoglycemia were undetected until he had a severe episode of bradycardia and/or cardiac arrest, stopped breathing, and required cardiopulmonary resuscitation. He suffered permanent brain damage. A subsequent laboratory report revealed severe hyperkalemia and hypoglycemia; however, the report was not forwarded to the neonatalogists for approximately 7 hours. The plaintiff brought a complaint of gross negligence for failure to properly diagnose and timely treat the hyperkalemia and hypoglycemia. The jury returned a $4,500,000 verdict.

Medical records are crucial in a court case because they provide the sequence of events, the time frame in which they occurred, and the participants in the care of the patient. If a nurse is named in a suit or is called to testify with regard to what took place, sometimes many years later, the chart serves as a memory aid. Statements contained in the medical record are not, in themselves, admitted into evidence; rather, the testimony of the witness concerning the particular event, as reinforced by the medical record, becomes the direct evidence given under oath (Bernzweig, 1996).

Informed Consent

Legally, for a person to be able to give informed consent, that person must have the capability of "capacity." This usually entails that the person (1) has reached the age of majority and (2) can understand the information that is being given by the health care provider. Neonates therefore do not meet the criteria to give informed consent legally. Thus the parents typically are the surrogate decision makers for the neonate, as long as they appear to be acting in the best interests of their infant. If the parents are married (to each other), either may consent on behalf of the neonate. However, in situations involving divorce, custody battles, and teenaged and foster parenting, issues related to informed consent and patient privacy can become convoluted (Rutherford, 1994). A *guardian ad litum* may be appointed by the court to act in the neonate's best interests, instead of or in addition to the parent(s). To meet the legal standard of informed consent, the surrogate decision maker must receive sufficient information regarding the proposed plan of treatment, including the risks and benefits of treatment, alternative treatment strategies, and the repercussions of not consenting (Ballard, 1994). The only exception to treating before obtaining informed consent is when delay of treatment could place the neonate at risk of further harm, such as in an emergency situation.

It is outside the boundaries of nursing practice to provide the patient and/or family with information regarding medical-surgical risks and benefits of treatment or to suggest alternative medical-surgical therapies. It is appropriate for the nurse to inform the physician that the family members need further clarification to enable them to come to a decision comfortably. Obtaining the informed consent is the responsibility of the physician providing the treatment. Ideally, this physician should also be responsible for obtaining the signatures on the appropriate form once the parent(s) has consented, because she or he is truly the only one who can ensure that the parent(s) has no further questions and fully comprehends all treatment issues.

A. If nurses are required to obtain patient and/or family signatures on consent forms, they should limit their clarification of patient and/or family understanding to two questions:

1. Has your physician discussed your baby's surgery (i.e., treatment approach) with you?
2. Are you ready to sign this consent form? This means that you consent to the procedure.

B. It is recommended that the name of the person able to give informed consent on behalf of the neonate be recorded in the medical record/nursing care plan once identified (Rutherford, 1994).

C. What if the parents or guardian will not give consent?

1. If physicians heed the parents' wishes and do not treat the infant, they may be guilty of child abuse or neglect, because laws stipulate that parents must provide needed medical care. Denial of this care can constitute a form of child neglect or abuse.
2. If physicians proceed to treat the infant, ignoring parental objections, they could be liable for battery, because their touching of the infant was intentional and there was a lack of consent.
3. Physicians may petition the court for an authorization to provide the infant with the necessary treatment (i.e., obtain a court order). The most common example of physicians' seeking court orders to intervene in treatment is that of refused consent for blood transfusions based on religious beliefs. This request is almost always granted—certainly in emergency situations.

D. When parents refuse treatment for other reasons, the court will base its decision on several factors (Rhodes, 1987).

1. The infant's overall health and development.
2. The immediacy of danger to the infant if treatment is withheld.
3. The risks and benefits of the proposed treatment.

Professional Liability Insurance

There is a growing trend to hold nurses personally liable for their acts of negligence, especially when they have assumed additional responsibility as APNs. Some believe that nurses should not carry insurance, because this only provides them with "deep pockets," making them more attractive to the plaintiff. Others insist that being well insured will serve as good protection. How much insurance is enough? Is the insurance coverage provided by the employer enough, or should nurses also invest in a personal policy for additional protection. These questions need to be answered by the individual nurse after examination of her or his practice.

A. Principal benefits afforded by an individual malpractice policy (Bernzweig, 1996).

1. Insurer's agreement to defend *all* malpractice claims filed against the nurse. Also generally included are claims alleging assault, battery, invasion of privacy, and defamation of character and claims that the nurse/APN practiced outside the scope of his or her license.
2. Insurer's agreement to pay the amount that the nurse is legally liable to pay the plaintiff, up to the limits of the policy.
3. Coverage of all costs associated with an appeal of an adverse verdict.
4. Coverage for instructional and supervisory activities, as well as off-duty and non-hospital-related nursing activities, such as volunteer work.

B. **Reasons to obtain malpractice insurance (Bernzweig, 1996).**

1. If you are named as a defendant alleging negligent conduct, your liability is primary in nature. The hospital's insurance policy covers your typical activities as an employee under the doctrine of *respondeat superior,* meaning that the hospital's liability is secondary in nature. If the hospital decides that what you did was not covered under its policy, it will not defend you. In fact, the hospital may actually assume an adversarial position to demonstrate that you are the legally responsible party. You will now have to defend yourself on your own.
2. You will be protected if the hospital is not insured.

> The case of *Wake County Hospital System v. National Causalty Co.* (1992) involved alleged nursing malpractice of a neonatal nurse. The hospital had a self-insured retention, or a deductible, of up to $750,000 per person/event before its commercial insurance coverage became effective. The defendant nurse's policy was deemed to be excess coverage over other valid and collectible insurance. The U.S. District Court ruled that self-insurance by a hospital is not really insurance in the legal sense. It also ruled that the nurse's insurer had to pay the full amount awarded in the case. This case is a good illustration of a nurse's needing her or his own malpractice coverage.

3. When an insurance carrier makes payment to a plaintiff on the basis of malpractice, the insurer is legally entitled to sue the nurse to obtain reimbursement for the amount paid.
4. No institutional policy covers a nurse for any acts or omissions that occur outside the normal work environment.
5. Cost of a policy for staff nurses is low; however, the insurance for the APN may cost several hundred dollars a year.

C. **Most health care providers do carry their own professional liability insurance.** There are two types of insurance policies.
1. Claims-made policy: covers damages only when the damages occurred during the policy period and only if the claim is reported to the insurance company during the policy period or the extending reporting endorsement (tail) (Smith, 1991). This is typical of policies held by institutions.
2. Occurrence-basis policy: covers damages occurring during the period covered by the policy, even if the claim is made after the policy period has ended (Aiken, 1994). This is typical of policies held by *individuals.*

D. **There are differences in coverage between an institutional and an individual liability policy (Hagedorn, Gardner, Laux, and Gardner, 1997).**

1. Institutional liability policy.
   a. Employer purchased and provided as typical "claims made" coverage.
   b. Institution is the primary insured party, holding fullest rights and responsibilities.
   c. Policy covers specific professional activities in the work environment.
   d. Institution may be able to sue the nurse for all or part of the money paid in settlement, judgment, and legal fees.
   e. Insurance company employs the attorney; the individual nurse may not have a right to select counsel.
   f. Individual nurse has no right to refuse or authorize settlement.
2. Individual liability policy.
   a. Commercially purchased insurance that typically has an "occurrence" coverage.
   b. Individual nurse is the primary insured party.
   c. Policy covers specific professional activities of the insured at any time and place.

E. As discussed above, the APN is held to a higher standard of care than a registered nurse because of the APN's advanced education and practice level. Moreover, many APNs practice in nontraditional settings. These are some of the reasons that APNs have difficulty in obtaining appropriate malpractice coverage. Typically, the insurance contains limitations on coverage amounts or requires physician supervision as a condition of coverage (Cronenwett, 1994). Most legal educators advise that the APN carry individual professional liability insurance coverage (Wise and Green, 1996). Although there is the fear of becoming an additional "deep pocket," there is also the fear that the attorney for the employer's insurance company will not have the nurse's best interests at heart because of conflicts of interest (Wise and Green, 1996). Others advocate the use of personal attorneys to monitor the insurance company's attorney's defense and negotiations.

F. All nurses can practice preventive legal maintenance by avoiding eighteen legal pitfalls (Fiesta, 1994):

1. Neglecting to make safety a high priority.
2. Failing to spot and report possible violence. For example, the number of kidnapping occurrences has increased in recent years. Nurses play a role in the security plan by wearing photographic identification badges, enforcing visiting policies, and, along with risk management, developing a preventive program to anticipate neonatal kidnapping.
3. Not following institutional policies and standards of care.
4. Responding unwisely in a short-staffing or floating situation. Courts have generally upheld the validity of the hospital's floating policy; thus a nurse's refusal to accept the assignment may place the nurse in jeopardy. It is suggested that the prudent course is to accept the assignment after clearly informing the nurse manager/charge nurse concerning your limitations and concerns.
5. Neglecting to use due care in physical procedures, such as the dispensing of medications.
6. Not checking equipment.
7. Assuming that others are responsible for your duties.
8. Assuming responsibility for informed consent.
9. Wrongfully disclosing confidential information.
10. Making reckless accusations.
11. Failing to act like a professional.
12. Confusing licensure issues with malpractice.
13. Failing to communicate.
14. Failing to monitor and assess.
15. Failing to listen to information provided by family and friends, and to patient's or parent's requests for assistance.
16. Neglecting to follow principles of risk management.
17. Not following documentation principles.
18. Confusing legal and ethical questions.

REFERENCES

Aiken, T.: Legal, ethical and political issues in nursing. Philadelphia, F.A. Davis, 1994.

Ament, L.A.: Risk management and continuous quality improvement. In: Gardner, S.L., and Hagedorn, M.I.E. (Eds.): Legal Aspects of Maternal-Child Nursing Practice: Concepts and Strategies in Risk Management. Menlo Park, Calif., Addison-Wesley, 1997, pp. 51–66.

American Academy of Pediatrics and the American College of Obstetricians and Gynecologists: Guidelines for Perinatal Care, 4th ed. Elk Grove Village, Ill., American Academy of Pediatrics, 1997.

American Nurses Association: Standards of Clinical Nursing Practice. Washington, D.C., Author, 1991.

American Nurses Association: Nurses in Advanced Practice. Washington, D.C., Author, 1993.

American Nurses Association: Registered Nurses and Unlicensed Assistive Personnel. Washington, D.C., Author, 1994.

Ballard, D.: Permission isn't consent. Am. J. Nurs., 6:48, 1994.

Barnard, K., et al.: Nursing: A Social Policy Statement, 1994 Revision [Draft]. Washington, D.C.: American Nurses Association, 1994.

Bergman, R.: Getting the goods on guidelines. Hosp. Health Netw., 10:70–74, 1994.

Bernzweig, E.P.: The Nurse's Liability for Malpractice: A Programmed Course, 6th ed. St. Louis, Mosby, 1996.

Cohn, S.: Trends in professional liability for OGN nurses (NAACOG Update Services, vol. 4, lesson 11). Princeton, N.J., Continuing Professional Education Center, 1986.

Coleman v. Touro Infirmary of New Orleans, 506 So.2d 571–LA, 1993.

Creighton, J.: Legal significance of charting. Part I. Nursing Management, 18:17, 20, 22, 1987.

Cronenwett, L.: Regulation of nurses in advanced practice (ANA House of Delegates Report CNP-1 A-94). Washington, D.C., American Nurses Association, 1994.

Davis, S.L., and Neggers, W.F.: Trial techniques. In Iyer, P. (Ed.): Nursing Malpractice. Tucson, Lawyers & Judges Publishing, 1996, pp. 895–979.

Ewing v. Aubert, 532 S.2d 876 (Lo. App. 1988).

Fiesta, J.: Agency nurses: Whose liability? Nursing Management, 21(3):16–17, 1990a.

Fiesta, J.: The nursing shortage: Whose liability problem? Nursing Management, 21(2):22–23, 1990b.

Fiesta, J.: QA and risk management: Reducing liability exposure. Nursing Management, 22(2):14–15, 1991.

Fiesta, J.: Twenty legal pitfalls for nurses to avoid. Albany, Delmar Publishers, 1994.

Fox, L., and Imbiorski, W.: The record that defends its friends. Chicago, Care Communications, 1979.

Hagedorn, M.I.E., Gardner, S.L., Laux, M.G., and Gardner, G.L.: A model for professional nursing practice. In Gardner, S.L., and Hagedorn, M.I.E. (Eds.): Legal Aspects of Maternal-Child Nursing Practice: Concepts and Strategies in Risk Management. Menlo Park, Calif., Addison-Wesley, 1997, pp. 67–94.

Hospital Risk Control: Risk analysis: Corporate liability. Tucson, Lawyers & Judges Publishing, 1995.

Iyer, P.: Foundations of nursing practice. In Iyer, P. (Ed.): Nursing Malpractice. Tucson, Lawyers & Judges Publishing, 1996a, pp. 3–36.

Iyer, P.: Nursing documentation. In Iyer, P. (Ed.): Nursing Malpractice. Tucson, Lawyers & Judges Publishing, 1996b, pp. 85–143.

Iyer, P., and Camp N.: Nursing Documentation: A Nursing Process Approach, 2nd ed. St. Louis, Mosby–Year Book, 1995.

Iyer, P., and Yudkoff, M.: Working with nursing expert witnesses. In Iyer, P. (Ed.): Nursing Malpractice. Tucson, Lawyers & Judges Publishing, 1996, pp. 797–865.

Joint Commission for the Accreditation of Healthcare Organizations: Accreditation Manual for Hospitals. Vol. 1: Standards. Oakbrook Terrace, Ill., Author, 1996.

Laska, L. (Ed.): Failure to timely diagnose and treat hyperkalemia and hypoglycemia in premature infant: Brain damage—$4.5 million texas verdict. Medical Malpractice Verdicts, Settlements & Experts, 9:1, 1993.

Laska, L. (Ed.): Newborn suffers cyanosis soon after birth due to lack of suctioning: Brain damage leads to death—defense verdict. Medical Malpractice Verdicts, Settlements & Experts, 1:25–26, 1997a.

Laska, L. (Ed.): Ohio boy's retardation blamed on failure to recognize signs of galactosemia. Medical Malpractice Verdicts, Settlements & Experts, 13:8, 1997b.

Meissner-Cutler, S., and Gardner S.L.: Maternal-child nursing and the law. In Gardner, S.L., and Enzman-Hagedorn, M.I. (Eds.): Legal Aspects of Maternal-Child Nursing Practice: Concepts and Strategies in Risk Management. Menlo Park, Calif., Addison-Wesley, 1997, pp. 25–50.

National Association of Neonatal Nurses: Role definitions for advanced practice. Petaluma, Calif., Author, 1992.

NSO Risk Advisor: How to Stay Out of the Malpractice Data Bank. Trevose, Pa., Author, 1992.

Nurses Association of the American College of Obstetricians and Gynecologists: Nurse Providers of Neonatal Care. Washington, D.C., Author, 1990.

Pearson, L.J.: Annual update of how each state stands on legislative issues affecting advanced nursing practice. Nurs. Pract., 20(1):13–51, 1995.

Rhodes, A.M.: When parents refuse to consent. MCN, Am. J. Matern. Child Nurs., 12:289, 1987.

Rutherford, M.: Small patients, big legal risks. RN, 9:51–57, 1994.

Samuels, A.: The legal liability of the nurse: The lawyer's view. Med. Sci. Law, 33:305–309, 1993.

Smith, J.: Hospital Liability. New York, Law Journal Seminars Press, 1991.

Solberg, P.: Legal Implications of Patient Charting. Fayetteville, N.C.: Nursing Business News, 1986.

Speid, M.H.: An inside look at today's healthcare environment. In: Iyer, P. (Ed.): Nursing Malpractice. Tucson, Lawyers & Judges Publishing, 1996, pp. 37–84.

Tammelleo, A.D.: Court upholds nurse's refusal to float. Regan Report on Nursing Law, 7:4, 1992a.

Tammelleo, A.D.: Was apnea monitor on or off? Expert testimony. Regan Report on Nursing Law, 7:4, 1992b.

Tammelleo, A.D.: Dr. testifies as to national standards of nursing care. Regan Report on Nursing Law, 4:1, 1994.

Verklan, M.T.: Neonatal and pediatric malpractice issues. In Iyer, P. (Ed.): Nursing Malpractice. Tucson, Lawyers & Judges Publishing, 1996, pp. 207–250.

Wake County Hospital System v. National Causalty Co., 804 F. Supp. 768 (N.C. 1992).

Wise D.J., and Green S.: Psychiatric nursing malpractice issues. In Iyer, P. (Ed.): Nursing Malpractice. Tucson, Lawyers & Judges Publishing, 1996, pp. 463–498.

Zarin, I. (Ed.): $4,500,000 recovery. New Jersey Jury Verdict Review and Analysis, 16(2):27, 1995.

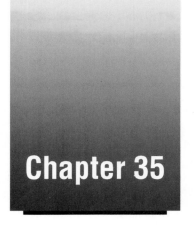

Chapter 35

Transition of the High-Risk Neonate to Home Care

Paula L. Forsythe

Objectives

1. Identify the clinical criteria for the transition to home care.

2. Describe parental participation in the transition process.

3. Define case-managed care.

4. Identify the follow-up needs of high-risk neonates.

Successful transition of the high-risk neonate from hospital to home care requires a thorough understanding of the identified criteria for discharge, coordination and progression of activities that ready the neonate and parent for home, appropriate identification and referral for community-based services, and both the psychologic and the physical preparation required as parents accept their role as independent caregivers. Case-managed care is one method that facilitates this transition from hospital care to home and community-based care.

Basic Principles of Transition Planning

A. Neonates and families admitted to a NICU undergo many transitions during hospitalization. The most anticipated and significant transition is the discharge to home; however, for many of these families, home care supplants hospital care. Effective transitional planning ensures that the processes of care remain coordinated and continuous for families as they transfer from hospital to home.

B. Families partner with health care professionals to identify outcome goals and discharge criteria and to plan and clarify the sequencing of preparatory events.

C. Transition process begins at admission and actively involves parents in a meaningful caregiving and decision-making role throughout the hospital stay.

Discharge teaching is most effectively accomplished in a transitional parent-rooming-in setting, where distractions are minimal and the parents can concentrate on their own infant and the preparation for home care (Damato, 1991; Kenner and Bagwell, 1993).

D. **Case-managed care, using clinical pathways and/or case managers,** is one model of care rapidly gaining credence as a system that effectively promotes consistency in provision of care, is outcome oriented and cost-effective, and provides ongoing communication between parents and members of all health care disciplines (Bell, 1994; Kimberlin and Bregman, 1996; Ladden, 1993; Thompson, 1994).

1. The primary focus of case-managed care is the integration, coordination, and advocacy provided for neonates and their families requiring extensive health care services (Bell, 1994). Case management particularizes the information and support given to families.
2. Case managers coordinate the care, discharge, and access to health care services and resources for a specific patient population. Case management, a role usually undertaken by advanced practice nurses, provides continuous relationships between neonates and parents exposed to numerous health care providers and variables that affect the transition to home care (Bell, 1994; McKim 1993). Case managers must conceptualize a long-term view of care and follow-up, and they determine the feasibility of actual discharge on the basis of the daily medical updates of the neonate's stability (Bell, 1994).
3. Clinical pathways, a key ingredient of the case management model, outline the crucial incidents that normally occur during a hospital stay and the appropriate interventions, time referenced and sequenced, used to achieve the anticipated outcome measures and results (Thompson, 1994). Crucial incidents represent categories of events and interventions required for patient care, such as physical assessments, diet, medications, consultations, tests, and activity and developmental care, as well as the plan for discharge and required parent teaching. Pathways are collaboratively developed; are organized to meet specified patient outcomes; improve cost containment and appropriate resource utilization; and streamline documentation (Kimberlin and Bregman, 1996; Malnight and Wohl, 1997; Terhaar, 1997). Pathways determine the core management of a neonate on the basis of weight or developmental or age milestones (gestational or postconception).
4. The following outcome measures are identified:
   a. Specific behaviors that must be evidenced by the infant before discharge, such as making the transition to an open crib and advancing to oral feedings.
   b. Family education and competency that must be learned and demonstrated for safe care at home.
   c. Health care referrals that are required for families to safely provide care in the home and follow-up care in the community.

E. **The process of case-managing ill neonates is multifaceted,** extends beyond the acute care setting into the long-term follow-up care setting, and requires facile information exchange and collaboration among all parties involved in the neonate's care. This process is particularly important for optimal outcomes for infants at risk of having chronic health problems and/or social, cognitive, language, and interactive disturbances (Bell, 1994).

Goals and Objectives of Discharge Planning

With case-managed care, the clinical goals of care remain unchanged; however, the focus is placed on efficiency and efficacy in reaching those goals. Today's practitioners are being required to demonstrate favorable clinical outcomes concurrently with cost containment and markedly abbreviated hospital stays (Terhaar, 1997). Goals and objectives are:

A. **Defined, and often predetermined, clinical and functional outcome measures, and discharge criteria for neonates and their families** that reflect the neonate's recovery from and stabilization of the birth problems, and competency in the parent's ability to provide care. Neonatal outcome measures are based on the predictable sequencing of infant maturation and development, as demonstrated by an ability to maintain body temperature in an open crib, tolerate adequate nutrition, consistently gain weight, and outgrow apnea and bradycardia episodes (Kimberlin and Bregman, 1996).

B. **Early, active, and meaningful parental involvement in providing physical and developmental care and making care decisions for the infant,** promoting parental competency, confidence, and autonomy, and the enhanced recovery of the neonate.

C. **Coordination of care through case management and the use of "critical pathways"** to promote a smooth transition from hospital to home and community care.

D. **Cost-effective, reimbursed care** through efficient discharge planning and the provision of care in the most appropriate settings, including the use of transitional care hospital settings with rooming-in accommodations for convalescing high-risk neonates and their parents.

E. **Active, interdisciplinary team participation** in the planning, teaching, documentation, and evaluation of the care provided.

F. **Access to decentralized, ongoing community services** to support the provision of quality, comprehensive care for children and families.

G. **Identification of and arrangement for additional financial sources** to support the neonate's required level of health care and technology needs. Federal and state funding sources include Supplemental Security Income (SSI); Women, Infants, and Children (WIC) programs; Medicaid; and waiver programs for neonates requiring assistive technology (Damato, 1991; Parette, 1993).

Health Care Trends That Affect Transitional Planning

A. **Increasing numbers of infants are surviving with complex and often chronic conditions.** An estimated 10.2% of U.S. births are of preterm infants (Simpson, 1997). Prematurity, identified as the number one perinatal and neonatal problem in the United States, is both emotionally and financially costly (Ladden, 1991; Simpson, 1997). Neonatal intensive care is one of the most expensive types of hospitalization, accounting for 5 million neonatal intensive care unit days per year at a cost of more than $5 billion (Bell, 1994; Damato, 1991; Simpson, 1997). The government funds the majority of care in NICUs through Medicaid or other agencies (Bell, 1994).

B. **The potential negative effects of long-term hospitalization, NICU environments, and family separation** are well substantiated in the literature and research studies.

C. **Advances in home care technology programs and resources** support the treatment and management of complex clinical problems at home.

D. **The competitive health care market requires that hospitals develop business strategies that reflect fiscal responsibility for the care provided** (i.e., appropriate lengths and costs of hospital stays in association with measurable patient outcomes) (Bell, 1994).

E. **Reimbursement sources are participating in care delivery decisions, demanding containment of rising health care costs and the identification of cost-effective alternatives to lengthy hospitalizations.** Many insurance companies hire nurses as case managers, and their decisions may affect the length of hospital stay, the choice of home care providers, and the equipment and supplies that will be covered by insurance. Studies have shown that early hospital discharge with proper home care follow-up is a cost-saving measure and is safe and beneficial to the infant and family as well (Damato, 1991).

F. **Legislative initiatives** affect long-term care innovations, access to care, and the efficient use of resources of both state and federal levels (Parette, 1993; Therrien, 1993).

G. **The parent is recognized as the most constant person in the neonate's life and therefore as the best person to care for the infant.** However, parents also require complex support and education during the hospital stay and after discharge (Bell, 1994).

Transition Plan

A. **All patients and families require a transition-to-home plan** developed by an interdisciplinary team; however, the complexity of the plan will vary according to the practitioners' initial and ongoing assessments of the individual neonate's and family's needs. Though most neonates discharged to home are growing premature infants, many continue to have complications that will require extensive home management (Bell, 1994). Oxygen supplementation for infants with chronic lung disease, cardiorespiratory monitoring for infants with episodes of apnea and bradycardia, ventilator and tracheostomy care, and parenteral nutrition are therapies that can be managed at home (Damato, 1991; Parette, 1993).

B. **The family members are active participants in the development, implementation, and ongoing evaluation of the plan.** The family's identified needs for information, education, and psychosocial and financial support, with assigned team member responsibility for meeting those needs, are an integral part of the transition plan. Evaluation of the safety and adequacy of the home environment to support the neonate's level of care occurs early during the hospital course to allow adequate time for interventions when deficiencies are observed. Remedies for identified deficiencies, or an alternative to home placement at the time of discharge, may need to be investigated and integrated into the plan.

C. **Barriers to parental learning and participation in care are assessed, and resources to alleviate the barriers are identified.** Environmental barriers that prevent a parent from interacting with and developing a relationship with the neonate must be removed (Bell, 1994).

D. **The neonate's level of medical stability is assessed, and the physical, developmental, and behavioral needs** requiring planned therapies for management are identified. Criteria for hospital discharge and the sequencing of therapies and events to prepare for discharge are established with parents. Ongoing interdisciplinary discharge planning conferences are scheduled to update the team about the neonate's medical status, level of recovery, and progress toward outcome goals; alternative therapies are discussed when lack of progress is noted.

E. **A well-implemented transition plan provides opportunities for the neonate to achieve the highest level of function before discharge, thereby simplifying**

medical management and minimizing the type and frequency of care that will be required at home. A well-implemented transition plan also provides for the progressive integration of parents into the management of their neonate's care, adequate time for teaching, the coordination of home care services irrespective of the level of need complexity, and the completion of infant discharge testing, by the time discharge criteria are met (Damato, 1991; Kimberlin and Bregman, 1996).

F. **Posthospital services and equipment are identified and arranged with suggested providers.** Community resources, identified to provide ongoing services, support, and financial assistance, are involved in planning and preparing for the transition to home. Home care equipment should be brought to the hospital so that parents can learn their use and maintenance. Vendors will often meet the family at home on the day of discharge to ensure that the equipment is functioning properly and parents are knowledgeable regarding its operation (Damato, 1991).

G. **A realistic, cohesive, and effective discharge plan should simulate care as it will be provided at home,** thereby shortening the length of hospital stay and enhancing the transition to home care and/or other community services.

H. **Neonates with a recognized history or potential for abuse or neglect, or who require county services for transition** to the community, require social work assessment and ongoing management. Evaluating the family's stability and support systems and the need for linking the family to community resources for continuing support is imperative for a successful transition plan (Donohue and Gleason, 1991).

Transition Process

A. **Parents play a crucial role in the transition process.**

1. Prematurity and illness represent a major event in life and motivate families to learn.
2. Parents require anticipatory guidance to alleviate unnecessary concerns and to prepare for the reality of the neonate's effect on home life (Damato, 1991; Dresden, 1997).
3. Parents learn about parenting by observing caregivers and actively participating in and/or demonstrating care on a daily basis. This form of education, identified as modeled interventions, teaches parents what is valued in their neonate's care and patterns of successful interaction with their infant (Cusson and Lee, 1993). Modeled interventions assist parents in their ability to assimilate what is taught in the hospital and to apply those skills to the home environment. Ongoing instruction, encouragement, and participation in care during hospitalization enable parents to practice and successfully demonstrate their caregiving skills and to gain confidence in their ability to make decisions independently and to care competently for their infant at home (Cusson and Lee, 1993; Kenner and Bagwell, 1993).
4. Parents have a taxonomy of learning needs (Kenner and Bagwell, 1993).
   a. Informational needs: how to provide daily care, feedings, medications, and therapies; how to gain access to community services.
   b. Instructional needs: how to recognize problems/illness and what to do when illness occurs; how to promote development and to recognize and respond to infant cues and behaviors, and what to do about child care; how to perform cardiopulmonary resuscitation (CPR) and respond to complications or emergent situations.
   c. Support needs: how to arrange for home visits and follow-up care; how to gain access to reference materials, economic assistance.

5. Parents' learning must be outcome oriented, organized, and particularized to their neonate's need. Written and video information should be used to reinforce verbal and demonstrated teaching.
6. Centralized family learning centers, staffed by nurse educators, have been implemented in hospital settings as cost-effective, quality-based programs to provide parent education.

B. **Nurses play a critical role in the education and modeling of interventions for parents.** The most crucial role in preparing families for discharge is the sequencing of required education, beginning with general infant care, progressing to more complex medical/technologic care, and building on the parents' previously acquired competencies and confidences (Damato, 1991; Forsythe, 1995; Therrien, 1993).

1. Involve and educate parents in the management of their neonate's needs.
   a. Skin care, bathing, and weighing.
   b. Crib and car seat safety.
   c. Nutrition and growth: how to feed the infant and make or gain access to specialized formulas.
   d. Medication scheduling and administration, and the need for immunizations.
   e. Appropriate identification of and response to behavioral cues and sleep needs and patterns.
   f. Provision of developmentally appropriate stimulation and follow-up care; arranging for early intervention services.
   g. Ability to recognize signs of illness and when and how to gain access to medical care.
   h. Ability to perform CPR and gain access to emergency care.
   i. Inclusion of siblings in care and discussion of how siblings will react once the neonate is at home.
   j. Demonstration of how to provide specialized care and treatments. Provision of written material for use at home:
      (1) Oxygen and related equipment; cardiorespiratory monitor.
      (2) Tracheostomy and/or ventilator care; suctioning; humidification.
      (3) Ostomy care and application of appliances.
      (4) Central line care; dressing changes; administration of medication and/or parenteral nutrition.
2. Determine the need for home services, their frequency and duration, and the specific provider, supplies, and equipment required.
   a. Arrange with providers the resources for all postdischarge needs. Investigate credentials and competencies and determine the orientation and training needs of the home care team.
   b. Identify pathways to replenish home supplies.
   c. Order home equipment early so that the family will have time to become familiar with use before discharge.
   d. Teach equipment cleaning, safety, and repair.
3. Negotiate home care benefits and financial coverage with the insurance company and identify additional reimbursement resources needed to cover the required services (Damato, 1991). In collaboration with the social worker, determine family eligibility for state-funded programs such as Medicaid and disabled children's programs.
4. Use a checklist format (component of the "critical pathway") to document outcomes and progress toward and time frames for meeting requirements.
5. Determine a tentative date for discharge in collaboration with the physician, the family, and other members of the health care team.
6. Coordinate team conferences.

7. Develop a response to emergencies occurring at home, identifying specific contact people with telephone numbers. Contact or correspond with the local fire department, rescue squad, and utility companies for emergency situations, including power outages.

8. Complete all written instructions for care at home. In collaboration with parents, develop a schedule for medications, feedings, and treatments that can be realistically implemented at home.

9. Assist the family in scheduling all necessary follow-up appointments.

C. **The neonate undergoes various tests and meets discharge criteria.**

1. All appropriate screening tests are performed before discharge, when possible, because the results will guide treatment and follow-up care (Dresden, 1997).
   a. Metabolic screening test and thyroid function tests.
   b. Complete blood cell count with reticulocyte count; additional blood tests based on concerns related to birth weight and history of interventions.
   c. Ophthalmologic examination for retinopathy of prematurity.
   d. Hearing evaluation and/or screening test.
   e. Blood drug levels measured at discharge: theophylline, caffeine, and phenobarbital.
   f. Chest x-ray film or echocardiogram.
   g. Cranial ultrasonography for interventricular hemorrhage.
   h. Pneumogram or thermistor reading for neonates with clinical symptoms of apnea or bradycardia.

2. Criteria for discharge are met; general guidelines include (Table 35–1):
   a. Stabilization of birth problem(s).
   b. Attainment of a weight parameter or of developmental or gestational maturity.
   c. Ability to maintain body temperature in an open crib.
   d. Ability to take nourishment by mouth and consistently gain weight or tolerate an alternative mode of feeding (e.g., gastrostomy).
   e. Completion of family's discharge education and demonstration of their ability to provide competent care.
   f. Discharge medication prescriptions; immunize if age and weight appropriate.
   g. Postdischarge referrals for follow-up care.
   h. Primary care physician contacted and given medical information (Donohue and Gleason, 1991; Dresden, 1997).

3. Successful transitional management.
   a. Transitions to open crib when medically stable (weighs approximately 1500 g and is >32 weeks, corrected age).
   b. Advancement of feedings to home-going formula or breast milk.
   c. Minimal medication regimen and dosing schedule.
   d. Minimal oxygen settings.
   e. Immunizations if age and weight are appropriate.
   f. Able to sit in car seat for at least 60 minutes without evidencing respiratory distress.

Evaluation of the Transition Plan

A. **Effectiveness of the transitional plan is best evaluated** by correlating how well the processes of care match the patient outcomes.

1. Outcome goals/discharge criteria were met by the predetermined time for discharge.

Table 35–1
EXAMPLE OF DISCHARGE CHECKLIST

Discharge Planning and Outcomes	Met/Initials	Comments
Newborn Metabolic Screen completed		
GA >34 weeks		
Weight 1900 g _____; gain 20-30 g qd _____		
Open crib/stable temperature		
No apneas/bradycardias for 1 week Room air: _____ Wean to room air: _____ Oxygen _____; D/C on oxygen _____ Theophylline: _____	_____ _____ _____	
Medications: discharge scripts filled _____ Discharge meds to division to review concentration and directions _____ Parent education completed _____	_____ _____ _____	
Parent education: well child care complete Feedings: PO _____; NG _____; GT _____ CPR: _____ Equipment: CR monitor _____; POX _____ Oxygen: _____; Fd. Pump _____	_____ _____ _____	
Hearing screen _____; Test (AER) _____ ENT consult: _____; BAER _____	_____	
Eye exam: _____		
HUS: #1 _____#2 _____#3 _____@D/C _____		
Hepatitis B: #1 Consent _____ DTaP: Consent _____ HIB: Consent _____ IPV: #1 Consent _____	_____ _____ _____ _____	Hepatitis B: #2 Consent _____ OPV: Consent _____ IPV: #2 Consent _____
Passed car-seat challenge		
Circumcision arranged		
RSV prophylaxis: insurance approved _____ Enrolled _____Dose #1 _____	_____	
Early intervention referral _____ County custody _____	_____	

Follow-up care:
   PMD/clinic _____
   Eye exam scheduled _____
   Other specialities _____
   _____
   WIC referral _____
   Home care: _____
		Parent information sheets:
		Breast-feeding _____
		Circumcision _____ Home care _____
		Medication administration _____
		Respiratory distress _____
		Early intervention _____

GA, Gestational age; *D/C*, discharged; *PO*, per os (by mouth); *NG*, nasogastric; *GT*, gastrostomy; *CPR*, cardiopulmonary resuscitation; *CR*, cardiorespiratory; *POX*, pulse oximetry; *Fd*, feeding; *AER*, acoustic evoked response; *BAER*, brain-stem evoked response; *ENT*, ear-nose-throat; *HUS*, head ultrasound; *@D/C*, at discharge; *DTaP*, diphtheria, tetanus, acellular pertussis; *HIB*, *Haemophilus influenzae* type B; *IPV*, inactivated poliomyelitis vaccine; *OPV*, oral poliomyelitis vaccine; *RSV*, respiratory syncytial virus; *PMD*, pediatrician; *WIC*, women, infants, and children.

2. Family members and community care providers competently provided care for the infant at home.

3. Arranged resources adequately met the neonate's requirements at home.

B. No care complications or liabilities were incurred.

C. Infant was not readmitted to the hospital within the first month of discharge.

D. Institution's outcome data compare favorably with those of equivalent neonatal centers.

Summary

Nurses who manage high-risk neonates must meet the physical, developmental, and psychosocial needs of the neonate in the hospital while enabling parents to meet those needs at home (Bell, 1994). Effective transitional planning results in a medically safe and resource-supported discharge to home at the earliest opportunity, with a significant reduction in costs, in comparison with the costs of hospitalization.

REFERENCES

Bell, P.: Neonatal case management: A challenge for advanced practice nurses. J. Perinat. Neonat. Nurs., 8(2):48–56, 1994.

Cusson, R., and Lee, A.: Parental interventions and the development of the preterm infant. J. Obstet. Gynecol. Neonatal Nurs., 23(1):60–68, 1993.

Damato, E.: Discharge planning from the neonatal intensive care. J. Perinat. Neonat. Nurs., 5(1):43–53, 1991.

Donohue, P., and Gleason, C.: Discharge planning. In Jones, M., Gleason, C., and Lipstein, S. (Eds.): Hospital Care of the Recovering NICU Infant. Baltimore, Williams & Wilkins, 1991.

Dresden, S.: A family medicine approach to the premature infant. J. Am. Board. Fam. Pract., 10(2):117–124, 1997.

Forsythe, P.: Changing the ecology of the NICU. Designing Child Health, 3(1):7–8, 1995.

Kenner, C., and Bagwell, G.: Assessment and management of the transition to home. In Kenner, C., Brueggemeyer, A., and Gunderson, L. (Eds.): Comprehensive Neonatal Nursing. Philadelphia, W.B. Saunders, 1993.

Kimberlin, L., and Bregman, J.: Postconceptual age as the basis for neonatal case management. Neonatal Network, 15(2):5–13, 1996.

Ladden, M.: On-site perinatal case management: An HMO model. J. Perinat. Neonat. Nurs., 5(1):27–32, 1991.

Malnight, M., and Wahl, J.R.F.: An alternative approach for neonatal clinical pathways. Neonatal Network, 16(4):41–49, 1997.

McKim, E.: The information and support needs of mothers of premature infants. J. Pediatr. Nurs., 8(4): 233–244, 1993.

Parette, H.: High-risk infant case management and assistive technology: Funding and family enabling perspectives. M.C.N. J. Matern. Child Nurs. J., 21(2): 53–64, 1993.

Simpson, K.R.: Preterm birth in the United States: Current issues and future perspectives. J. Perinat. Neonat. Nurs., 10(4):11–15, 1997.

Terhaar, M.: The promise of clinical pathways. J. Perinat. Neonat. Nurs., 10(4):16–20, 1997.

Therrien, L.: Discharge planning for the high-risk neonate. In Beachy, P., and Deacon, J. (Eds.): Core Curriculum for Neonatal Intensive Care Nursing. Philadelphia, W.B. Saunders, 1993.

Thompson, D.: Critical pathways in the intensive care and intermediate care nurseries. M.C.N. Am. J. Matern. Child Nurs., 19(1):29–33, 1994.

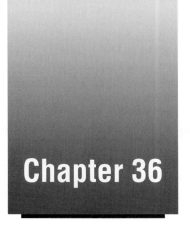

Chapter 36

Follow-up of the Preterm Infant and Outcome of Prematurity

Glenda Louch

Objectives

1. Define and discuss morbidity and mortality in preterm infants.

2. Identify problems that premature infants may encounter after discharge from neonatal intensive care.

3. Discuss management techniques for postdischarge problems.

4. Describe common developmental problems resulting from prematurity.

5. Discuss the importance of follow-up for premature infants.

6. Discuss the impact of a premature infant on the family after discharge from the hospital.

Approximately 450,000 premature infants are born in the United States each year. With increased knowledge and technologic advances, smaller and younger infants are surviving. Although most infants who are born early do well, there is still significant mortality and morbidity associated with prematurity. Many infants have ongoing medical and developmental problems after discharge. Those caring for premature infants and their families need to know which infants are at risk and to help prepare the families to care for the infants. This chapter discusses morbidity and mortality and outlines the follow-up required for outpatient management of premature infants.

Morbidity and Mortality in Premature Infants

Mortality is the incidence of death in a given population, whereas morbidity is the incidence of disease and complications in a given population. It is important to look at the morbidity and mortality rates to determine whether treatment modalities are working and whether the incidence of morbidity and death is decreasing. This is particularly true for premature infants. The advent of surfactant has made it possible for these infants to survive, and with new ventilation modalities, improved equipment, regionalization of care, advances in medical and nursing care such as developmentally supportive care, and multiple other factors, the outcome for premature infants is improving. Other factors influencing outcome for preterm infants include:

A. **Obstetric and prenatal factors (Allen, 1998; Bartram, Clewell, and Kasnic, 1993).**

1. Medical problems such as diabetes mellitus, cardiac disease, thyroid disease, neurologic disorders. Appropriate medical management of these diseases during pregnancy improves outcome, whereas lack of medical care during pregnancy increases morbidity and mortality rates for both mother and infant.
2. Substance use/abuse.
3. Smoking.
4. Complications of pregnancy.
   a. Antepartum bleeding.
   b. Premature rupture of the membranes, uterine infection.
   c. Pregnancy-induced hypertension, gestational diabetes, HELLP syndrome (*h*emolysis, *e*levated *l*iver enzymes, *l*ow *p*latelets), preeclampsia, eclampsia.
   d. Placenta previa or placental abruption.
   e. Multiple gestation.
5. Lack of antenatal steroids with premature labor (<34 weeks' gestation).

B. **Neonatal characteristics (Allen, 1998).**

1. Gestational age, intrauterine growth restriction, gender, congenital anomalies, dysmorphic features.
2. Condition at birth, including Apgar scores, cord pH, presence of meconium, response to resuscitation.
3. Neonatal complications, such as hypoxia, acidosis, hypotension, chronic lung disease, apnea and bradycardia, sepsis, meningitis, seizures, hypoxic-ischemic encephalopathy.
4. Problems with the CNS structure or function, including intraventricular or intraparenchymal hemorrhage, ventricular dilation, cortical atrophy, periventricular leukomalacia.

C. **Low socioeconomic status has been associated with an increased rate of prematurity and poorer neurodevelopmental outcome (Thompson, Gustafson, Oehler, and Catlett, 1997; Watson, Kirby, Kelleher, and Bradley, 1996).**

MORTALITY

A. **The infant mortality rates listed below are the rates for the United States based on weight at the time of birth (Guyer et al., 1997).** Infant mortality is the incidence of death for infants less than 1 year of age. Although a few of these infants could die of causes other than prematurity, the figures also account for late deaths resulting from prematurity that studies which end on discharge from the NICU would not account for. Mortality rates based on weight are:

1. Birth weight (BW) <500 g: 90%.
2. BW 500–750 g: 53%.
3. BW 750–999 g: 18%.
4. BW 1000–1299 g: 9%.
5. BW 1250–1499 g: 5%.

B. **The data based on gestational age (GA) represent the range of survival of the extremely low birth weight (ELBW) infant based on several studies (Allen, Donohue, and Dusman, 1993; Cartlidge and Stewart, 1997; Lefebvre, Glorieux, and St. Laurent–Gagnon, 1996; Synnes et al., 1994).** Mortality rates based on GA are:

1. GA 23 weeks: 15–42%.

2. GA 24 weeks: 25–56%.
3. GA 25–26 weeks: 59–80%.
4. GA 27–28 weeks: 84%.

MORBIDITY

Morbidity in the premature population is difficult to define and establish. The incidence of ongoing medical problems such as chronic lung disease (CLD) and poor growth is well established, although actual incidence is difficult to determine. The neurodevelopmental outcome of premature infants is of great concern to all who are caring for premature infants. Unfortunately, there is no standardization of mild, moderate, or severe disabilities, so each study defines the criteria used in each study. Moreover, the ability to measure the quality of life for a child and the difficulty in measuring the impact on the family make statistical numbers problematic. However, recent studies have looked at the incidence of neurodevelopmental complications in the very low birth weight (VLBW) infant and the ELBW infant. The reader should keep in mind that the morbidity statistics are based on NICU care provided several years before the publication of the data. For instance, for statistics on the school-age child, the child must be more than 5 years of age before follow-up studies can be completed.

A. Survival rates without major neurologic conditions, as defined by a grade 3 or grade 4 intraventricular hemorrhage or periventricular leukomalacia (Kramer et al., 1997).

1. GA 23 weeks: 13%.
2. GA 24 weeks: 40%.
3. GA 25 weeks: 48%.
4. GA 26 weeks: 70%.
5. GA 27 weeks: 71%.

B. Neurodevelopmental outcome.

1. Intelligence quotient (IQ) in infants with BW less than 750 g (Hack, Friedman, and Fanaroff, 1996).
   a. IQ <70: 20%.
   b. IQ 70–84: 14%.
   c. IQ >85: 66%.
2. Neurosensory abnormality (Allen, 1998).
   a. Cerebral palsy.
      (1) BW <1500 g: 5–11%.
      (2) BW <1000 g: 9–11%.
   b. Visual impairment.
      (1) BW <1500 g: 1–5%.
      (2) BW <1000 g: 4–11%.
   c. Hearing impairment.
      (1) BW <1500 g: 1–5%.
      (2) BW <800 g: 5–20%.
   d. Multiple disabilities.
      (1) BW <1500 g: 1.2–4.5%.
      (2) BW <800 g: 14–16%.

C. Problems associated with learning and education.

1. Learning disorders in one area (Whitfield, Grunau, and Holsti, 1997).
   a. Premature infants, BW <800 g: 47%.
   b. Term infants: 18%.
2. Learning disorders in more than one area in infants with BW <800 g: 41%.

3. Children requiring special education services in school (Halsey, Collin, and Anderson, 1996).
   a. BW <1000 g: 50%.
   b. BW 1500–2500 g: 30%.
   c. BW >2500 g: 7%.

D. Both ELBW and VLBW infants who seem to do well initially appear to have more school problems, behavior problems, and difficulties with visual-motor tasks (Goldson, 1996).

Follow-up of the Preterm Infant

Prematurity is defined as the condition of any infant born at less than 37 weeks' gestation. Most infants who are born prematurely are healthy at the time of discharge and have no long-term sequelae. A small percentage, especially of those who were very young, small, or ill, are at risk of having ongoing medical or developmental problems. In general, ELBW infants are at the highest risk of having problems, the VLBW infants are at risk and should be monitored closely, and preterm infants with BW greater than 1500 g are at the lowest risk. The goal for neonatal follow-up care should focus on providing the high-risk neonate and the family with a continuum of high-quality care toward improving outcomes (NANN, 1997). Monitoring at-risk infants and children for both medical and developmental problems is important so that problems can be identified early and treatment initiated. Neonatal follow-up care must be available to all high-risk neonates (NANN, 1997). Many centers have developed clinics to monitor the progress of the preterm infant for early identification of potential deficits. Infants should be referred to these clinics if they have ongoing medical or developmental issues or are at an increased risk of having problems related to their prematurity. Issues that are closely followed in high-risk follow-up clinics include:

A. Growth.

1. Premature infants may be less than 2 standard deviations below the mean or at less than the 5th percentile on premature growth curves at the time of discharge. Ideally, the infant will exhibit "catch-up" growth. However, many preterm infants require more calories than their term counterparts. Growth may be slow. Close monitoring is required to adjust preterm infants' diet to meet their nutritional needs.
2. Some infants who are small for GA exhibit good catch-up growth, but many will be shorter and slimmer than preterm infants who are average in size for GA (Crouse and Cassady, 1994).
3. Corrected age is used for the purpose of assessing growth and development for the first 2 years (Groothuis, Louch, and VanEman, 1996). The child born prematurely thus has time to "catch up" in the areas of growth and development during a time of rapid changes. It also helps prevent a diagnosis of failure to thrive merely because the infant is small or a diagnosis of developmental delay in a child who fails to develop on the same schedule as a term infant. However, the issue of "correcting" age for prematurity is controversial. Some practitioners choose not to do so, and some choose to use corrected age longer that 2 years (Allen, 1998). It is important to know if the corrected age or the true age is used.
   a. Corrected age equals postdelivery age minus the number of weeks the infant was born prematurely. For instance, an infant born on Jan. 1 at 28 weeks' gestation will be 4 weeks' corrected age on April 9 (4 months [16 weeks] postdelivery age – 3 months [12 weeks], which would equal 44 weeks' postconceptional age, or 1 month of corrected age).
   b. An alternative is to use the expected date of delivery as the birth date.

4. Standard growth charts or growth charts for premature infants (not intrauterine growth charts) are used after 36 weeks of (corrected) age. Height, weight, occipitofrontal circumference, and weight/length ratio should be plotted at each visit. The weight/length ratio is a good indicator of whether the child's weight is appropriate for height.
   a. A healthy premature infant who is average in size for GA should grow at the same velocity for all parameters as a term infant of the same corrected age.
   b. Healthy preterm infants, especially ELBW infants, may grow at or below the 5th percentile but should parallel standard curves for weight and length.
   c. Weight/length ratio should be within or slightly below standard percentiles. Weight/length ratios for the growing preterm infant have been developed (Guo et al., 1996).
   d. Occipitofrontal circumference should be within 2 standard deviations of the mean by 8 months (corrected age). Tables of the ratio of head circumference to length may also be useful in monitoring head growth in preterm, low birth weight infants (Roche, Guo, Wholihan, and Casey, 1997).

B. **Nutrition.**

1. Premature infants often have increased caloric needs but may have problems consuming adequate calories for growth. This can be due to feeding difficulties or other problems related to prematurity, such as necrotizing enterocolitis, bowel loss, and malabsorption.
2. Babies who fail to follow the expected growth curve may need increased caloric density in their formula (22–30 calories per ounce). Formulas for the growing, recovering preterm infant, such as Neosure and Enfamil 22, are commercially available. The amount of protein, some of the vitamins, and some of the minerals are higher than in regular infant formula but lower than in premature formulas. If additional caloric supplementation is needed, commercially prepared products such as glucose polymers or microlipids are available to further increase caloric density. Adding oil such as medium-chain triglycerides is not generally recommended because of the risk of aspiration and the possibility of lipid pneumonia.
3. Caloric requirements of 120–180 calories per kilogram per day may be required to sustain catch-up growth if metabolic needs are increased because of chronic illness such as CLD (deGamarra, 1992). These children will have increased work of breathing, as exhibited by an elevated respiratory rate, continual mild to moderate retractions, and an elevated heart rate. In addition, infants with CLD may tire easily when eating or may have oral aversions, making adequate caloric intake impossible (Koops, Abman, and Accurso, 1984). Special feeding techniques or aids, such as a nasogastric tube or a gastrostomy tube or gastrostomy button, may be required to help these children receive adequate calories.
4. Breast-feeding the preterm child can be particularly challenging. Many former NICU patients have nipple confusion from bottle feeding, in addition to the previously mentioned feeding problems. Referral to a lactation specialist can provide assistance to help the infant successfully breast-feed. Some infants will need increased caloric supplementation. Breast-milk fortifier is expensive, is not readily available for use at home, and does not have the right balance of nutrients for the growing preterm infant. Parents may need to be reminded that breast-fed infants may nurse more frequently than formula-fed infants and that waiting 4 hours between feedings may not be appropriate.
5. Solid foods are introduced around 4–6 months of corrected age.
   a. Signs of readiness.
      (1) Good head and neck control.
      (2) Coordinated swallow, no tongue thrust.
      (3) Ability to sit with support.

    b. Children who are not gaining weight well but are taking solid food will benefit from food that is high in calories (Groothuis and Louch, 1992). A nutritionist can help the family determine what foods to add to the child's diet. Caloric content of baby foods is available from baby food manufacturers. An infant nutritional supplement (Pediasure or Kindercal [30 calories per ounce]) is recommended for children older than 1 year of age who need a supplement for weight gain (Dusick, 1997). This can be given orally or via a gastrostomy button or gastrostomy tube.

6. Additional supplements.

    a. Liquid multivitamins are needed if the total caloric intake is less than 300 calories per day on a standard formula.

    b. Fluoride is needed starting at 6 months of age if the infant is breast fed, the water supply used to prepare formula is not fluoridated, or the formula is "ready to feed" commercial formula (American Academy of Pediatrics [AAP] Committee on Nutrition, 1995). Families should be aware that some water filters eliminate fluoride.

    c. Breastfed infants may benefit from iron, multivitamins, including vitamin D, and minerals especially calcium, phosphorus, and zinc.

C. **Anemia.**

1. Defined as a hematocrit of less than 34%.

2. A preterm infant's formula should be changed from a low iron formula to a standard iron-containing formula by 36 weeks' gestation to help prevent anemia. Standard formula, at a normal daily volume of consumption, contains approximately 2 mg/kg per day.

3. Anemic infants should be started on therapeutic doses of iron at 5–6 mg/kg per day for the total daily intake. The dose can be rounded up or down for easy administration by the caregiver. Standard formulation of supplemental iron is 15 mg/0.6 mL.

    a. If the infant does not have anemia at the time of discharge, a complete blood cell count and reticulocyte count should be checked between 2 and 4 months of age. The hematocrit of an infant recently receiving erythropoietin may decrease slightly after the erythropoietin therapy is stopped. These infants are at risk of having late anemia of prematurity. If the infant has anemia at discharge, the hematocrit should be checked sooner, depending on the hematocrit level.

D. **Immunizations.**

1. The preterm infant's immune response is most closely related to postdelivery age, not corrected age.

2. Immunization dosages and contraindications are the same as for term infants. Infants who are in the hospital for a prolonged period should receive their first diphtheria-tetanus-pertussis or diphtheria–tetanus–acellular pertussis (DTaP), *Haemophilus influenzae* B, rotavirus, and poliomyelitis vaccines at 2 months of age and the second dose of each vaccine at 4 months of age (AAP Committee on Infectious Diseases, 1998). Other immunizations should be given according to the current recommended schedule (see schedule in Appendix B, AAP Committee on Infectious Diseases, 1998).

3. The AAP recommends beginning the hepatitis B vaccination series at more than 2000 g of body weight (AAP Committee on Infectious Diseases, 1994). However, Patel et al. (1997) found that neither birth weight nor weight at the first immunization appeared to influence response rate and suggested that hepatitis B vaccine can be given to infants with BW of less than 1500 g when they have reached 1 month of age.

4. Delay all immunizations until there is adequate muscle mass to absorb the immunization.

5. Infants older than 6 months with CLD or other risk factors should also receive influenza vaccine in the fall (Abman and Groothuis, 1994).
6. Varicella immunization should be delayed in children who are receiving immunosuppressive drugs.

E. **Vision (AAP, American Association for Pediatric Ophthalmology, and American Academy of Ophthalmology, 1997).**

1. Premature infants are at risk of having a variety of visual problems. Those in whom retinopathy of prematurity (ROP) develops are at the highest risk, all extremely premature infants are at a higher risk than other infants of having visual impairment. The first eye examination is usually done in the nursery at 4–6 weeks of life, and many children continue to require frequent testing after discharge. The number of examinations required depends on the degree of ROP and the maturity of the retina. Frequent ophthalmologic examinations will continue until the eyes are mature and/or the ROP is resolved. Long-term ophthalmologic follow-up is recommended for all extremely premature infants (Hebbandi et al., 1997). The use of oxygen does not increase the risk of ROP if the vessels in the retina are mature.
2. Visual impairment related to prematurity with or without ROP.
   a. Myopia.
   b. Strabismus.
   c. Amblyopia.
   d. Astigmatism.
   e. Other refractive errors.
3. Sequelae of severe ROP.
   a. All problems listed under item 2, above.
   b. Retinal detachment.
   c. Severe myopia: 80% incidence in infants with severe ROP.
   d. Blindness.
   e. Glaucoma.
4. Cortical blindness occurs when the brain is unable to interpret the visual input. It is usually the result of severe injury to the optic nerve or occipital cortex. The damage can be caused by bleeding, hypoxia, or any other event causing ischemic injury. Cortical blindness can be partial or complete, and parents often state that their child appears to see sometimes but not at other times.
5. Treatment of the diseases listed under items 2 and 3, above.
   a. Patching of the "better" eye for treatment of amblyopia or strabismus.
   b. Corrective lenses for myopia and other refractive errors.
   c. Surgery for severe strabismus, glaucoma, or ROP (surgery for ROP is usually done before discharge).
   d. There is no current medical treatment for cortical blindness.
6. Development of the visually impaired child.
   a. Encourage independent motor skills such as sitting, crawling, and feeding.
   b. Vocal stimulation is important because the visually impaired child cannot rely on visual cues to know what is happening around him or her.
   c. Early intervention.
      (1) Early intervention programs provide extra stimulation to help develop the other senses, such as touch, hearing, and smell, as well as to provide the family with guidance.
      (2) Special preschools are helpful if available.
   d. The diagnosis of blindness is very difficult for the family members. Support groups may help them cope with raising a visually impaired child.

F. **Hearing.** The National Institutes of Health recommends that all infants have hearing screening before discharge from the hospital (National Institutes of Health Consensus Development Conference Statement, 1993).

1. Sensorineural loss may affect 1–5% of NICU population.
   a. Risk factors.
      (1) Positive family history of hearing loss.
      (2) TORCH (*t*oxoplasmosis, *o*ther [congenital syphilis and viruses], *r*ubella, *c*ytomegalovirus, and *h*erpes simplex virus).
      (3) Extremely elevated bilirubin levels.
      (4) Severe birth asphyxia.
      (5) Persistant pulmonary hypertension.
      (6) Aminoglycosides plus diuretics.
      (7) Birth defects.
      (8) Meningitis.
      (9) Extracorporeal membrane oxygenation (ECMO).
   b. Test before discharge from the hospital at near term gestation.
      (1) False-positive results are common with the auditory brain-stem response.
      (2) May need retesting after discharge.
      (3) Follow hearing milestones carefully and refer for further testing if concerns arise.
      (4) Discuss hearing milestones with parents and refer if parental concerns exist.
2. Central auditory dysfunction occurs when the brain is unable to interpret sound and causes a decrease in auditory comprehension.
3. Conductive hearing loss. Preterm infants have a high incidence of recurrent otitis media and persistent fluid behind the tympanic membrane.
   a. Recurrent ear infections can cause scarring or thickening of the tympanic membrane, which can decrease the transmission of sound.
   b. Fluid behind the tympanic membrane causes sounds to be muffled or diminished.
   c. Consider pressure equalization tubes if fluid persists longer than 12 weeks.
4. Children in whom hearing loss is suspected should be referred to an audiologist for testing and to determine whether hearing aids will be beneficial. Hearing aids can help many children with neurosensory hearing loss.

Chronic Medical Problems of Prematurity

A. **Chronic lung disease (see also Chapter 7, Respiratory Distress).**

1. Incidence: 11–40% in infants born at less than 1500 g (Allen, 1998).
2. Readmissions. More than 50% of infants with CLD are rehospitalized in the first 2 years of life, usually for respiratory illness. Viral respiratory infections can cause severe coughing, wheezing, or pneumonia. The viruses most likely to cause severe respiratory disease are respiratory syncytial virus, influenza virus, and adenovirus, although other respiratory viral infections can cause severe disease in children with CLD (Chye and Gray, 1995).
3. Treatment of CLD.
   a. Oxygen requirements are a concern in children with CLD.
      (1) Oxygen saturation (SaO$_2$) should be maintained in the upper normal range. The oxygen level should be such that the heart rate or the work of breathing is not increased to maintain an adequate saturation. A saturation of 95% or greater will allow for maximal reversal of pulmonary vasoconstriction and optimal pulmonary vasodilation (Groothuis et al., 1996).
         (a) Increased pulmonary artery pressure resulting in pulmonary hypertension may affect some children with CLD (Gill and Weindling, 1995).

      (b) Prolonged SaO_2 of less than 92% may result in pulmonary hypertension or cor pulmonale (Abman and Groothuis, 1994).

  (2) Factors contributing to a decrease in oxygen saturation (Groothuis et al., 1996).

      (a) Formula feeding or breast-feeding—usually in infants less than 44–48 weeks of age.

      (b) Sleeping.

      (c) Reactive airways disease.

      (d) Gastroesophageal reflux.

      (e) Upper respiratory tract infection.

      (f) Lower respiratory tract infection.

      (g) Fever or other acute nonrespiratory illness.

      (h) High altitude: PO_2 drops by 5 mm Hg for each 1000 feet of elevation.

  (3) Additional causes of supplemental oxygen requirement.

      (a) Cardiac: atrial or ventricular septal defect, patent ductus arteriosus, hypertension.

      (b) Large-airway abnormalities (tracheomalacia, bronchomalacia).

      (c) Reactive airways disease.

      (d) Gastroesophageal reflux.

  (4) Weaning from oxygen supplementation (Groothuis et al., 1996).

      (a) Decrease the liter flow by small amounts (½ to ¼ to ⅛ L). Young infants should be weaned from ⅛ to 1/16 L before discontinuing oxygen therapy.

      (b) Weaning criteria for decreasing or discontinuing oxygen therapy.

         (i) SaO_2 of 95% or greater after 40 minutes without oxygen supplementation.

        (ii) Good weight gain.

       (iii) No compensatory tachycardia or tachypnea.

       (iv) No signs of hypoxia.
   - Pallor.
   - Poor feeding.
   - Poor weight gain.
   - Irritability, lethargy.
   - Poor sleeping.

        (v) Parental instruction. Parents should be taught to watch for these signs of subtle hypoxia and to call their care provider if the child exhibits any of them.

      (c) Continuous or nighttime supplemental oxygen should be considered in children with bronchopulmonary dysplasia (BPD) who are not gaining adequate weight but are getting adequate calories, even if the saturations are normal (Groothuis and Rosenberg, 1987).

  (5) Discontinuing supplemental oxygen (Groothuis et al., 1996).

      (a) Supplemental oxygen is discontinued for 1–2 hours once or twice a day and extended to all daytime hours after 2–4 weeks if the criteria listed above are met.

      (b) Nighttime weaning can be attempted after a minimum of 1 month if all the criteria are met. Nocturnal hypoxia can lead to poor weight gain (Moyer-Mileur, Nielson, Pferrer, and Witte, 1996). Nighttime oxygen may need to be resumed. A nocturnal sleep study may be needed to document desaturations during sleep.

      (c) Monitor SaO_2 and clinical progress for 3–6 months after oxygen therapy is discontinued, especially during times of acute illness.

 b. Inhaled medication such as bronchodilators may be indicated for children with CLD and bronchospasm.

 c. Diuretics may be helpful in children with severe CLD.

   d. Secondhand smoke and the smoke from wood-burning fireplaces and stoves are an irritant and cause chronic inflammation in the respiratory tract, especially in children with CLD (Dusick, 1997). Smoking in another room does not decrease the infant's smoke exposure (Greenberg et al., 1989). This should be explained to caregivers, and those who smoke should be encouraged to quit smoking. Children with CLD should not be placed in day care situations where they are exposed to secondhand smoke.

4. Prevention of infection with respiratory syncytial virus (RSV) in high-risk children.
   a. Recommendations for the use of palivizumab (Synagis) (AAP Committee on Infectious Diseases and Committee on the Fetus and Newborn, 1998).
      (1) All children less than 2 years of age with BPD/CLD who have required oxygen or other medical management for their CLD within the 6 months before the onset of the RSV season.
      (2) Infants who were born at 28 weeks' gestation or less may benefit from palivizumab until 12 months of age, and infants who were born at 29–32 weeks' gestation may benefit from the prophylaxis for the first 6 months. Management should be individualized.
      (3) Infants who were born at less than 35 weeks' gestation, are less than 6 months of age at the onset of the RSV season, and are at high risk (e.g., day care, secondhand smoking).
      (4) All immunizations can be given according to the regular schedule to children receiving palivizumab
   b. RSV-IVIG may still be indicated in some children at high risk of infection with other viruses in addition to RSV. The AAP (1997) suggests that intravenously administered immune globulin be considered for the first dose for children at extremely high risk who are being discharged from the NICU during RSV season.

5. Decreasing the incidence of respiratory illness after discharge.
   a. Infants and children with BPD and VLBW infants frequently have exacerbations of BPD during respiratory illnesses (Cunningham, McMillan, and Gross, 1991).
   b. Educate the family on how to reduce the risk of infection (Groothuis et al., 1996).
      (1) Avoid crowds during the winter.
      (2) Attend day care with fewer than 2–3 children.
      (3) Do not allow others with colds to interact with the infant.
      (4) Exposure to secondhand smoke increases the incidence of RSV.
      (5) Avoid elective surgery during the winter months whenever possible.

B. **Gastroesophageal reflux.**

1. Symptoms.
   a. Feeding problems, such as food refusal.
   b. Arching of the back during feeding.
   c. Irritability.
   d. Vomiting.
   e. Poor weight gain or weight loss.
2. Treatment options.
   a. Positioning. Elevate the head of the bed 30 degrees and hold the infant in place with special positioning devices such as blankets or commercially available antireflux harnesses. Research indicates that this may be of limited benefit in infants less than 6 months of age (Orenstein, 1990).
   b. Thicken feedings. Use up to 2 tablespoons of rice cereal per ounce of formula.

c. Medication, usually a combination of an antireflux agent and an H$_2$ blocker. Care providers need to be aware of all the contraindications and adverse reactions associated with some of the common antireflux medications.

d. Surgical intervention with a fundoplication (antireflux procedure).

3. Delayed gastric emptying can be a problem in this population and should be evaluated. Children with neurologic abnormalities are most likely to have a delayed emptying time in addition to gastroesophageal reflux (Fonkalsrud et al., 1995).

C. **Reactive airways disease is common in preterm infants, especially the extremely premature or those with CLD.** Severity of disease is dependent on many variables, including initial lung disease, family history, and early severe respiratory viral illness, especially resulting from RSV and adenovirus infection.

1. Symptoms.
   a. Persistent cough.
   b. Decreased breath sounds.
   c. Wheezing.

2. Treat with nebulizer therapy as indicated; however, each treatment regimen should be individualized. Use of bronchodilators such as albuterol and/or ipratropium, mass cell inhibitors such as cromolyn sodium or nedocromil sodium, and/or inhaled steroids is common. Some infants require daily medication, whereas others may require medication only with respiratory illness.

3. Infants with CLD and reactive airways disease who require general anesthesia may benefit from oral steroids given 48 hours before and after surgery, as well as treatment with bronchodilators (Groothuis et al., 1996).

4. Children with a history of reactive airways disease are more likely to have asthma or exercise-induced bronchospasm.

D. **Pulmonary hypertension (Flanagan and Flyer, 1994).**

1. One cause of pulmonary hypertension: chronic alveolar hypoxia, seen in children with CLD due to pulmonary parenchymal disease.

2. Results in right ventricular hypertrophy or cor pulmonale.

3. Generally improves as parenchymal disease resolves.

4. Treatment.
   a. Adequate oxygenation to promote pulmonary vasodilation.
   b. Bronchodilators and/or diuretics to treat the underlying parenchymal disease.

E. **Systemic hypertension:** observed in some patients with severe BPD (Anderson et al., 1993). Untreated hypertension can result in left ventricular hypertrophy (Flanagan and Flyer, 1994). Blood pressure should be monitored in all patients with BPD and treated if indicated. Blood pressure should be in the normal range for the child's age. In general, infants respond well to antihypertensive medication (Dusick, 1997).

F. **Seizures:** possible complication of intraventricular hemorrhage, periventricular leukomalacia, or other neurologic injury. Adequate seizure management is required for optimal outcome (Bernbaum, 1997).

Associated Problems of Prematurity

A. Developmental sequelae.

1. Head circumference less than 2 standard deviations below the mean by 8 months of corrected age may correlate with suboptimal developmental outcome (Goldson, 1996).

2. Early developmental intervention is indicated when "preemie" behavior does not end in the nursery.

3. Motor abnormalities such as cerebral palsy or other static-movement disorders are commonly found in premature infants. These can occur with or without cognitive impairment.
   a. Hypertonic extremities; hypotonic head, neck, and trunk; and other abnormal tone patterns.
   b. Hemiplegia: cerebral palsy affecting one side.
   c. Diplegia: cerebral palsy affecting the lower extremities.
   d. Quadriplegia: cerebral palsy affecting all extremities and sometimes the facial muscles.
   e. Athetosis: cerebral palsy causing abnormal and uncontrollable movement of the extremities.
   f. Persistence of premature reflexes.
   g. Both gross and fine motor delays.

4. Subtle motor problems may result in delayed milestones, clumsiness, or frustration. Tone abnormalities may not be dramatic and are often overlooked. Though these may resolve in some children, they may be predictors of later developmental and cognitive delays. Referral for early evaluation and treatment is indicated. The therapist should be specifically trained in techniques for infants and children.

5. Sensory integration abnormalities are commonly seen.
   a. Infant may be resistant to different textures, temperatures, or kinds of touch.
   b. Infant may have difficulty in knowing where his or her "body is in space."
   c. Infant may have trouble assimilating the input received from the environment.
   d. Early identification and treatment are believed not only to help the child interact but also possibly to improve school performance.

B. Speech and language delays.

1. Expressive language, or what the child can say, is frequently delayed, even for corrected age. Receptive language, or what the child can understand, often is better than expressive language.

2. Monitor infant's babbling by talking to caregivers about what he or she is verbalizing as early as 4 months corrected age.

3. Look for specific causes of delayed vocalization. Infants who do not make consonant sounds by 11 months of age (corrected) (e.g., "dada," "baba," "yaya") should be tested for hearing impairment.

4. Early detection and intervention is important. Speech evaluations such as the Receptive Expressive Emergent Language (REEL) screening tools are often used to evaluate expressive and receptive language.

C. Cognitive delays and learning disorders.

1. It is difficult to measure cognitive ability in young children who have motor delays. Older children are better able to respond even if they have poor motor skills.

2. Patterns of cognitive development in the preterm infant with BW less than 1500 g during the first 6 years of life (Koller, et al., 1997) are:
   a. Average and stable: 13%.
   b. Average but declined to low average: 24%.
   c. Average but declined to below average: 43%.
   d. Very low and increased to low average: 8%.
   e. Very low and stable: 12%.

3. Observe the child for attention deficit disorder (ADD) and other learning disabilities such as dyslexia. Learning disorders become more apparent in early

school years. Children with ADD or learning disabilities can be mislabeled as cognitively delayed.

4. Initiate early intervention, such as infant stimulation programs or special pre-schools, for children at risk of having delays.

5. Encourage extra help before the child begins to fail in school.

D. **Testing.** Most cognitive and psychologic testing corrects results for prematurity for at least the first 2 years of life (Allen, 1998).

1. Testing for children with delays or at high risk of having delays is mandated by law. Availability and services for follow-up vary from state to state and from county to county.

2. VLBW children should have complete developmental testing at 4–5 years of age. This includes gross and fine motor skills, speech, and IQ. A screening test for ADD should be done if there is any concern about attention.

3. Test for visual and hearing defects before the child starts school.

4. Test in school as needed. Schools are required to administer appropriate tests to children who are having problems in school.

5. Common developmental tests are:
   a. Denver Developmental Screening Test, version II: not a useful screening test for preterm infants (Groothuis and Louch, 1992).
   b. Bayley Scales of Infant Development—Second Edition: measures both physical development and mental development and should be administered between 12 and 18 months (corrected age) and again at 3 years of age. The Bayley Scales should be used earlier in children who are not receiving interventions and are not periodically being screened for early delays.
   c. Other cognitive tests: the Clinical Adaptive Test/Clinical Linguistic and Auditory Milestone Scale; Gesell Developmental Schedules; Stanford-Binet Intelligence Scale—Fourth Edition; the Wechsler Preschool and Primary Scale of Intelligence—Revised; and the Wechsler Intelligence Scale for Children—Third Edition (Allen, 1998).

E. **Behavior disorders.**

1. There are multiple causes of behavior disorders, including parenting skills, socioeconomic class, and genetic differences. Thus the effect of prematurity on behavior is difficult to determine.

2. Behavior disorders frequently accompany ADD.

3. Poor impulse control and wide mood swings are common.

4. Child may have limited response to "time out" and other forms of punishment.

5. Management requires caregiver cooperation and follow-through.

6. Encourage early psychiatric or mental health intervention if indicated.

F. **Psychosocial concerns.**

1. Family disruption and financial stress are common, with a high incidence of separation, divorce, abuse, and neglect.

2. Emotional needs.
   a. Parental anger and guilt may be delayed until the infant goes home.
   b. Parents may need additional support when baby is first discharged.
      (1) Infants are often more time-consuming and demanding than parents anticipate.
      (2) Other family members may be afraid to help care for the infant.
      (3) Parents have little time to themselves, with each other, or with the other children.

3. Compensatory parenting. The parent(s) or other family members treat the child differently because of their medical history or ongoing problems.
   a. Infant may be viewed by parents as fragile or chronically ill, and minor illness may be viewed as major (Miles and Holditch-Davis, 1995).

   b. Parents and other relatives may become overprotective and overindulgent, allowing the child to be in charge.

   c. Parents may have trouble allowing the child to progress through normal stages of development.

   d. Child's own fear may prevent him or her from normal exploration and independence.

4. Financial concerns.

   a. Many third-party payers may limit reimbursement for therapies.

   b. Consider Supplemental Security Income, Handicapped Children's Program, and other entitlement programs when applicable.

5. Assessment and intervention.

   a. Assess family interactions and coping mechanisms.

   b. Anticipatory intervention may help.

   c. Provide referral to support groups for parents if family interested.

   d. Parents may benefit from counseling.

   e. Consider other ways to help the family.

     (1) Handicapped parking for families with infants receiving oxygen or with motor disabilities.

     (2) Extension for public service shut-off notice if needed.

     (3) Subsidies for telephone service, gas, electricity, and water may be available through various resources.

REFERENCES

Abman, S.H., and Groothuis, J.R.: Pathophysiology and treatment of bronchopulmonary dysplasia. Pediatr. Clin. North Am. *41*:277–315, 1994.

Allen, M.C.: Outcome and follow-up of high-risk infants. *In* Taeusch, H.W., and Ballard, J.A. (Eds.): Schaffer and Avery's Diseases of the Newborn. Philadelphia, W.B. Saunders, 1998, pp. 413–425.

Allen, M.C., Donohue, P.K., and Dusman, A.E.: The limit of viability: neonatal outcome of infants born at 22 to 25 weeks' gestation. N. Engl. J. Med., *329*:1597–1601, 1993.

American Academy of Pediatrics. Respiratory syncytial virus. *In* Peters, G. (Ed.): 1997 Red Book: Report of the Committee on Infectious Diseases. Elk Grove Village, Ill., Author, 1997, pp. 443–447.

American Academy of Pediatrics, American Association for Pediatric Ophthalmology and Strabismus, and the American Academy of Ophthalmology: Screening examination of premature infants for retinopathy of prematurity. Pediatrics, *100*:273, 1997.

American Academy of Pediatrics Committee on Infectious Diseases: Update on timing of hepatitis B vaccination for premature infants and for children with lapsed immunizations. Pediatrics, *94*:403–404, 1994.

American Academy of Pediatrics Committee on Infectious Diseases: 1998 recommended childhood immunization schedule. Pediatrics, *101*:154–155, 1998.

American Academy of Pediatrics Committee on Infectious Diseases and Committee of Fetus and Newborn: Prevention of respiratory syncytial virus infections: Indications for the use of palivizumab and update on the use of RSV-IGIV. Pediatrics, *102*(5):1211–1216, 1998.

American Academy of Pediatrics Committee on Nutrition: Fluoride supplementation for children: Interim policy recommendations. Pediatrics, *95*:777, 1995.

Anderson, A.H., Warady, B.A., Daily, D.K., et al.: Systemic hypertension in infants with severe bronchopulmonary dysplasia: Associated clinical factors. Am. J. Perinatol., *10*:190–193, 1993.

Bartram, J., Clewell, W.H., and Kasnic, T.: Prenatal environment: Effect on neonatal outcome. *In* Merenstein, G.B., and Gardner, S.L. (Eds.): Handbook of Neonatal Intensive Care. St. Louis, C.V. Mosby, 1993, pp. 21–39.

Bernbaum, J.C.: Follow-up of the high-risk neonate. *In* Spitzer, A.R. (Ed.): Intensive care of the fetus and neonate. St Louis, Mosby–Year Book, 1997, pp. 729–741.

Cartlidge, P.H., and Stewart, J.H.: Survival of the very low birth weight and very preterm infants in a geographically defined population. Acta Pediat., *86*:105–110, 1997.

Chye, J.D., and Gray, P.H.: Rehospitalization and growth of infants with bronchopulmonary dysplasia: A matched control study. J. Paediatr. Child Health, *31*: 105–111, 1995.

Crouse, D.T., and Cassady, G.: The small-for-gestational-age infant. *In* Avery, G.B., Fletcher, M.A., and MacDonald, M.G. (Eds.): Neonatology, pathophysiology, and management of the newborn, 4th ed. Philadelphia, J.B. Lippincott, 1994, pp. 369–398.

Cunningham, C.K., McMillan, J.A., and Gross, S.J.: Rehospitalization for respiratory illness in infants of less than 32 weeks' gestation. Pediatrics, *88*:527–532, 1991.

deGamarra, E.: Energy expenditure in premature newborns with bronchopulmonary disease. Biol. Neonate, *61*:337–344, 1992.

Dusick, M.: Medical outcomes in preterm infants. Semin. Perinatol., *21*:164–177, 1997.

Flanagan, M.F., and Flyer, D.C.: Cardiac disease. *In* Avery, G.B., Fletcher, M.A., and MacDonald, M.G. (Eds.): Neonatology, pathophysiology, and management of the newborn, 4th ed. Philadelphia, J.B. Lippincott, 1994, pp. 516–567.

Fonkalsrud, E.W., Ellis, D.G, Shaw, A., et al.: A combined hospital experience with fundoplication and gastric emptying procedure for gastroesophageal reflux in children. J. Am. Coll. Surgeons *180*:449–455, 1995.

Gill, A.B., and Weindling, A.M.: Raised pulmonary artery pressure in very low birth weight infants requiring supplemental oxygen at 36 weeks after conception. Arch. Dis. Child. *72:*20–22, 1995.

Goldson, E.: The developmental consequences of prematurity. *In* Wolraich, M.L. (Ed.): Disorders of Development and Learning: A Practical Guide to Assessment and Management. St. Louis, Mosby–Year Book, 1996, pp. 483–508.

Greenberg, J.R., Bauman, D.E., Glover, L.H., et al.: Ecology of passive smoking by young infants. J. Pediatr., *114:*774–780, 1989.

Groothuis, J.R., and Louch, G.K.: When the premature infant goes home: Follow-up issues. Journal of the U.S. Army Medical Department, PB 8–92–*5/6:*3–5, 1992.

Groothuis, J.R., Louch, G.K., and VanEman, C.: Outpatient management of the preterm infant. J. Respir. Care, *9:*(June/July) 69–73, 1996.

Groothuis, J.R., and Rosenberg, A.A.: Home oxygen promotes weight gain in infants with bronchopulmonary dysplasia. Am. J. Dis. Child., *141:*992–995, 1987.

Guo, S.S., Wholihan, K., Roche, A., et al.: Weight-for-length reference data for preterm, low-birth-weight infants. Arch. Pediatr. Adolesc. Med., *150:*964–970, 1996.

Guyer, B., Martin, J.A., MacDorman, M.F., et al.: Annual summary of vital statistics—1996. Pediatrics, *100:*905–918, 1997.

Hack, M., Friedman, H., and Fanaroff, A.A.: Outcomes of extremely low birth weight infants. Pediatrics, *98:*931–935, 1996.

Halsey, C.L., Collin, M.F., and Anderson, C.L.: Extremely low-birth-weight children and their peers: A comparison of school-age outcomes. Arch. Pediatr. Adolesc. Med., *150:*790–794, 1996.

Hebbandi, S.B., Bowen, J.R., Hipwell, G.C., et al.: Ocular sequelae in extremely premature infants at 5 years of age. J. Pediatr. Child Health *33:*339–342, 1997.

Koller, H., Lawson, K., Rose, S.A., et al.: Patterns of cognitive development in VLBW children during the first six years of life. Pediatrics, *99:*383–389, 1997.

Koops, B., Abman, S., and Accurso, F.J.: Outpatient management and follow-up of bronchopulmonary dysplasia. Clin. Perinatol., *11:*101–122, 1984.

Kramer, W.B., Saade, G.R., Goodrum, L., et al.: Neonatal outcome after active perinatal management of the very premature infant between 23 and 27 weeks' gestation. J. Perinatol., *17:*439–443, 1997.

Lefebvre, F., Glorieux, J., and St.-Laurent–Gagnon, T.: Neonatal survival and disability rate at age 18 months for infants born between 23 and 28 weeks of gestation. Am. J. Obstet. Gynecol., *174:*833–838, 1996.

Miles, M.S., and Holditch-Davis, D.: Compensatory parenting: How mothers describe parenting their 3-year-old, prematurely born children. J. Pediatr. Nurs. *10:* 243–253, 1995.

Moyer-Mileur, L.F., Nielson, D.W., Pferrer, K.D., and Witte, M.K.: Eliminating sleep-associated hypoxemia improves growth in infants with bronchopulmonary dysplasia. Pediatrics, *98:*779–783, 1996.

National Association of Neonatal Nurses: Position Statement on Neonatal Follow-up Care of the High Risk Neonate. Petaluma, CA, Author, 1997.

National Institutes of Health Consensus Development Conference Statement: Early identification of hearing impairment in infants and young children. Int. J. Pediatr. Otorhinolaryngol., *27:*215–227, 1993.

Orenstein, S.R.: Prone positioning in infant gastroesophageal reflux: Is elevation of the head worth the trouble? J. Pediatr., *117:*184–187, 1990.

Patel, D.M., Butler, J., Feldman, S., et al.: Immunogenicity of hepatitis B vaccine in healthy VLBW infants. J. Pediatr., *131:*641–643, 1997.

Roche, A.F., Guo, S.S., Wholihan, K., and Casey, P.H.: Reference data for head circumference–for–length in preterm low-birth-weight infants. Arch. Pediatr. Adolesc. Med., *151:*50–57, 1997.

Synnes, A.R., Emily, W.Y.L., Whitfield, M.F., et al.: Perinatal outcomes of a large cohort of extremely low gestational age infants (twenty-three to twenty-eight completed weeks of gestation). J. Pediatr., *125:*952–960, 1994.

Thompson, R.J., Gustafson, K.E., Oehler, J.M., and Catlett, A.T.: Developmental outcome of VLBW infants at four years of age as a function of biological risk and psychosocial risk. J. Dev. Behav. Pediatr., *18:*91–96, 1997.

Watson, J.E., Kirby, R.S., Kelleher, K.J., and Bradley, R.H.: Effects of poverty on home environment: An analysis of three-year outcome data for low birth weight premature infants. J. Pediatr. Psychol., *21:*419–431, 1996.

Whitfield, M.F., Grunau, R.V., and Holsti, L.: Extremely premature (< or = 800 g) schoolchildren: Multiple areas of hidden disability. Arch. Dis. Child. Fetal Neonatal Ed., *77:*F85–90, 1997.

A
Appendix

Newborn Metric Conversion Tables

Table A–1
TEMPERATURE

Fahrenheit (F) to Centigrade (C)							
°F	°C	°F	°C	°F	°C	°F	°C
95.0	35.0	98.0	36.7	101.0	38.3	104.0	40.0
95.2	35.1	98.2	36.8	101.2	38.4	104.2	40.1
95.4	35.2	98.4	36.9	101.4	38.6	104.4	40.2
95.6	35.3	**98.6**	**37.0**	101.6	38.7	104.6	40.3
95.8	35.4	98.8	37.1	101.8	38.8	104.8	40.4
96.0	35.6	99.0	37.2	102.0	38.9	105.0	40.6
96.2	35.7	99.2	37.3	102.2	39.0	105.2	40.7
96.4	35.8	99.4	37.4	102.4	39.1	105.4	40.8
96.6	35.9	99.6	37.6	102.6	39.2	105.6	40.9
96.8	36.0	99.8	37.7	102.8	39.3	105.8	41.0
97.0	36.1	100.0	37.8	103.0	39.4	106.0	41.1
97.2	36.2	100.2	37.9	103.2	39.6	106.2	41.2
97.4	36.3	100.4	38.0	103.4	39.7	106.4	41.3
97.6	36.4	100.6	38.1	103.6	39.8	106.6	41.4
97.8	36.6	100.8	38.2	103.8	39.9	106.8	41.6

Note: $°C = (°F - 32) \times 5/9$. Centigrade temperature equivalents rounded to one decimal place by adding 0.1 when second decimal place is 5 or greater.

The metric system replaces the term "Centigrade" with "Celsius" (the inventor of the scale). Reprinted with permission of Ross Laboratories, Columbus, OH, 43216, © Ross Laboratories.

Table A–2
LENGTH

Inches to Centimeters

1 inch increments Example: To obtain centimeters equivalent to 22 inches, read "20" on top scale, "2" on side scale; equivalent is 55.9 centimeters.

Inches	0	10	20	30	40
0	0	25.4	50.8	76.2	101.6
1	2.5	27.9	53.3	78.7	104.1
2	5.1	30.5	55.9	81.3	106.7
3	7.6	33.0	58.4	83.8	109.2
4	10.2	35.6	61.0	86.4	111.8
5	12.7	38.1	63.5	88.9	114.3
6	15.2	40.6	66.0	91.4	116.8
7	17.8	48.2	68.6	94.0	119.4
8	20.3	45.7	71.1	96.5	121.9
9	22.9	48.3	73.7	99.1	124.5

One-Quarter (¼) inch increments Example: To obtain centimeters equivalent to 14¾ inches, read "14" on top scale, "¾" on side scale; equivalent is 37.5 centimeters.

10–15 Inches

	10	11	12	13	14	15
0	25.4	27.9	30.5	33.0	35.6	38.1
¼	26.0	28.6	31.1	33.7	36.2	38.7
½	26.7	29.2	31.8	34.3	36.8	39.4
¾	27.3	29.8	32.4	34.9	37.5	40.0

16–21 Inches

	16	17	18	19	20	21
0	40.6	43.2	45.7	48.3	50.8	53.3
¼	41.3	43.8	46.4	48.9	51.4	54.0
½	41.9	44.5	47.0	49.5	52.1	54.6
¾	42.5	45.1	47.6	50.2	52.7	55.2

Note: 1 inch = 2.540 centimeters. Centimeter equivalents rounded one decimal place by adding 0.1 when second decimal place is 5 or greater; for example, 33.48 becomes 33.5.
Reprinted with permission of Ross Laboratories, Columbus, OH, 43216, © Ross Laboratories.

Table A–3
WEIGHT (MASS)

Pounds and Ounces to Grams

Example: To obtain grams equivalent to 6 pounds, 8 ounces, read "6" on top scale, "8" on side scale; equivalent is 2948 grams.

Ounces \ Pounds	0	1	2	3	4	5	6	7	8	9	10	11	12	13	14
0	0	454	907	1361	1814	2268	2722	3175	3629	4082	4536	4990	5443	5897	6350
1	28	482	936	1389	1843	2296	2750	3203	3657	4111	4564	5018	5471	5925	6379
2	57	510	964	1417	1871	2325	2778	3232	3685	4139	4593	5046	5500	5953	6407
3	85	539	992	1446	1899	2353	2807	3260	3714	4167	4621	5075	5528	5982	6435
4	113	567	1021	1474	1928	2381	2835	3289	3742	4196	4649	5103	5557	6010	6464
5	142	595	1049	1503	1956	2410	2863	3317	3770	4224	4678	5131	5585	6038	6492
6	170	624	1077	1531	1984	2438	2892	3345	3799	4252	4706	5160	5613	6067	6520
7	198	652	1106	1559	2013	2466	2920	3374	3827	4281	4734	5188	5642	6095	6549
8	227	680	1134	1588	2041	2495	2948	3402	3856	4309	4763	5216	5670	6123	6577
9	255	709	1162	1616	2070	2523	2977	3430	3884	4337	4791	5245	5698	6152	6605
10	283	737	1191	1644	2098	2551	3005	3459	3912	4366	4819	5273	5727	6180	6634
11	312	765	1219	1673	2126	2580	3033	3487	3941	4394	4848	5301	5755	6209	6662
12	340	794	1247	1701	2155	2608	3062	3515	3969	4423	4876	5330	5783	6237	6690
13	369	822	1276	1729	2183	2637	3090	3544	3997	4451	4904	5358	5812	6265	6719
14	397	850	1304	1758	2211	2665	3118	3572	4026	4479	4933	5386	5840	6294	6747
15	425	879	1332	1786	2240	2693	3147	3600	4054	4508	4961	5415	5868	6322	6776

Note: 1 pound = 453.59237 grams; 1 ounce = 28.349523 grams; 1000 grams = 1 kilogram. Gram equivalents have been rounded to whole numbers by adding one when the first decimal place is 5 or greater.

Reprinted with permission of Ross Laboratories, Columbus, OH, 43216, © Ross Laboratories.

B
Appendix

Recommended Childhood Immunization Schedule
United States, January–December 1999

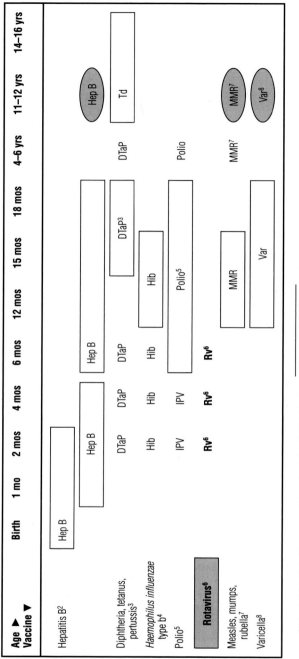

[1]This schedule indicates the recommended ages for routine administration of currently licensed childhood vaccines. Combination vaccines may be used whenever any components of the combination are indicated and its other components are not contraindicated. Providers should consult the manufacturers' package inserts for detailed recommendations.

[2] *Infants born to HBsAg–negative mothers* should receive the 2nd dose of hepatitis B vaccine at least 1 month after the 1st dose. The 3rd dose should be administered at least 4 months after the 1st dose and at least 2 months after the 2nd dose, but not before 6 months of age for infants.

Infants born to HBsAg–positive mothers should receive hepatitis B vaccine and 0.5 mL hepatitis B immune globulin (HBIG) within 12 hours of birth at separate sites. The 2nd dose is recommended at 1–2 months of age and the 3rd dose at 6 months of age.

Infants born to mothers whose HBsAg status is unknown should receive hepatitis B vaccine within 12 hours of birth. Maternal blood should be drawn at the time of delivery to determine the mother's HBsAg status; if the HBsAg test is positive, the infant should receive HBIG as soon as possible (no later than 1 week of age).

All children and adolescents (through 18 years of age) who have not been immunized against hepatitis B may begin the series during any visit. Special efforts should be made to immunize children who were born in or whose parents were born in areas of the world with moderate or high endemicity of HBV infection.

[3] DTaP (diphtheria and tetanus toxoids and acellular pertussis vaccine) is the preferred vaccine for all doses in the immunization series, including completion of the series in children who have received 1 or more doses of whole-cell DTP vaccine. Whole-cell DTP is an acceptable alternative to DTaP. The 4th dose (DTP or DTaP) may be administered as early as 12 months of age, provided 6 months have elapsed since the 3rd dose and if the child is unlikely to return at age 15–18 months. Td (tetanus and diphtheria toxoids) is recommended at 11–12 years of age if at least 5 years have elapsed since the last dose of DTP, DTaP, or DT. Subsequent routine Td boosters are recommended every 10 years.

[4] Three *H. influenzae* type b (Hib) conjugate vaccines are licensed for infant use. If PRP-OMP (PedvaxHIB and COMVAX [Merck]) is administered at 2 and 4 months of age, a dose at 6 months is not required. Because clinical studies in infants have demonstrated that using some combination products may induce a lower immune response to the Hib vaccine component, DTaP/Hib combination products should not be used for primary immunization in infants at 2, 4, or 6 months of age, unless FDA-approved for these ages.

[5] Two poliovirus vaccines currently are licensed in the United States: inactivated poliovirus vaccine (IPV) and oral poliovirus vaccine (OPV). The ACIP, AAP, and AAFP now recommend that the first two doses of poliovirus vaccine should be IPV. The ACIP continues to recommend a sequential schedule of two doses of IPV administered at ages 2 and 4 months, followed by two doses of OPV at 12–18 months and 4–6 years. Use of IPV for all doses also is acceptable and is recommended for immunocompromised persons and their household contacts. OPV is no longer recommended for the first two doses of the schedule and is acceptable only for special circumstances such as children of parents who do not accept the recommended number of injections; late initiation of immunization, which would require an unacceptable number of injections; and imminent travel to polio-endemic areas. OPV remains the vaccine of choice for mass immunization campaigns to control outbreaks due to wild poliovirus.

[6] Rotavirus (Rv) vaccine is printed in boldface to indicate (1) the health care providers may require time and resources to incorporate this new vaccine into practice and (2) the AAFP believes that the decision to use rotavirus vaccine should be made by the parent or guardian in consultation with the physician or other health care provider. The first dose of Rv vaccine should not be administered before 6 weeks of age, and the minimum interval between doses is 3 weeks. The Rv vaccine series should not be initiated at 7 months of age or older, and all doses should be completed by the 1st birthday.

[7] The 2nd dose of measles, mumps, and rubella vaccine (MMR) is recommended routinely at 4–6 years of age, but may be administered during any visit, provided at least 4 weeks have elapsed since receipt of the 1st dose and that both doses are administered beginning at or after 12 months of age. Those who have not previously received the second dose should complete the schedule by the 11– to 12-year-old visit.

[8] Varicella vaccine is recommended at any visit on or after the 1st birthday for susceptible children, i.e., those who lack a reliable history of chickenpox (as judged by a health care provider) and who have not been immunized. Susceptible persons 13 years of age or older should receive 2 doses, given at least 4 weeks apart.

Approved by the Advisory Committee on Immunization Practices (ACIP), the American Academy of Pediatrics (AAP), and the American Academy of Family Physicians (AAFP).

Vaccines[1] are listed under routinely recommended ages. *Bars* indicate range of recommended ages for immunization. Any dose not given at the recommended age should be given as a "catch-up" immunization at any subsequent visit when indicated and feasible. *Ovals* indicate vaccines to be given if previously recommended doses were missed or given earlier than the recommended minimum age.

Neonatal Abstinence Scoring System

System	Signs and Symptoms	Score	Time (Hour of the Day at Which Interval Began Interval Duration [2 Hours or 4 Hours])												
Central Nervous System	Excessive high-pitched or other cry Continuous high-pitched or other cry	2 3													
	Sleeps <1 hour after feeding Sleeps <2 hour after feeding Sleeps <3 hour after feeding	3 2 1													
	Hyperactive Moro reflex Markedly hyperactive Moro reflex	2 3													
	Mild tremors disturbed Moderate–severe tremors disturbed	1 2													
	Mild tremors undisturbed Moderate–severe tremors undisturbed	3 4													
	Increased muscle tone	2													
	Excoriation (specific area)	1													
	Myoclonic jerks	3													
	Generalized convulsions	5													
Metabolic/ Vasomotor/ Respiratory	Sweating Fever <38.4°C (37.2°–38.2°) Fever >38.4°C	1 1													
	Frequent yawning (>3–4 times)	1													
	Mottling	1													
	Nasal stuffiness	1													
	Sneezing (>3–4 times)	1													
	Nasal flaring	2													
	Respiratory rate >60/min Respiratory rate >60/min + retractions	1 2													
Gastrointestinal	Excessive sucking	1													
	Poor feeding	2													
	Regurgitation Projectile vomiting	2 3													
	Loose stools Watery stools	2 3													
	Total score														
	Initials of scorer														

Adapted from Finnegan, L.P.: Neonatal abstinence syndrome. *In* Nelson, N.M. (Ed.): Current Therapy in Neonatal-Perinatal Medicine. Philadelphia, BC Decker Inc, 1990, pp. 314–320. With permission.
  See text on page 627 for scoring technique.

Note: Page numbers in *italics* refer to illustrations; page numbers followed by t refer to tables.